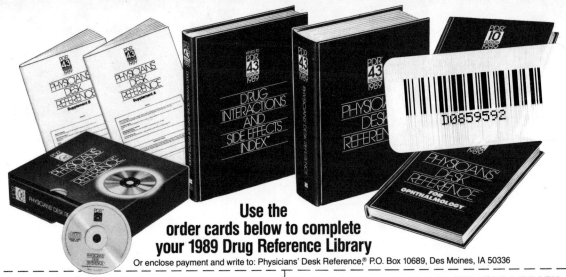

Use the
order cards below to complete
your 1989 Drug Reference Library

Or enclose payment and write to: Physicians' Desk Reference® P.O. Box 10689, Des Moines, IA 50336

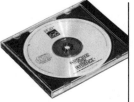

The exact drug information you need... in seconds!

1989 PDR® on CD-ROM

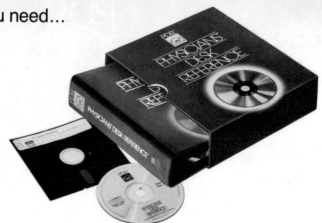

Every vital, must-have fact: Physicians' Desk Reference... PDR For Nonprescription Drugs...PDR Drug Interactions and Side Effects Index...PDR For Ophthalmology—on one CD-ROM disk! Four complete volumes united under a single index for quickest access possible. The text appears instantly, and you can even call up more than one drug at the same time!

It's also easy to use. The screen always tells you exactly what to do next!

Put the power of today's technology—and the vital information contained in all four PDR volumes—to work for you as never before. Order on the other side today! $595.00 for a one year (3 disks) subscription.

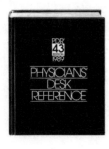

1989 PHYSICIANS' DESK REFERENCE®

The new 43rd Edition of PDR® is the most complete and up-to-date edition yet published of this must-have drug reference. Locate drugs by product name, manufacturer, category, or generic and chemical name. PDR includes complete medical information, usages, and warnings, plus full-color photographs. You also get a key to controlled substances, FDA use-in-pregnancy ratings, clinical pharmacology, and all other FDA-required information. PDR is THE Source for vital drug information.

Use order forms on previous page.

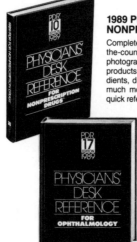

1989 PDR FOR NONPRESCRIPTION DRUGS®

Complete, precise information on over-the-counter drugs, along with full-color photographs of the most widely used products and preparations. Active ingredients, drug interactions, dosages, and much more. Four separate indices for quick reference.

1989 PDR FOR OPHTHALMOLOGY®

This is the reference volume eye-care professionals reach for. Complete information on products and drugs relating to ophthalmology and optometry. Specialized instrumentation, equipment, and lenses.

Use order forms on previous page.

ALL THE INFORMATION FROM ALL FOUR PDR® VOLUMES IN SECONDS...
PDR® ON CD-ROM!

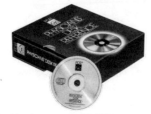

Combine the power of today's technology with the vital information in all four PDR volumes...and get complete, up-to-the-minute information within seconds!

See other side for more complete information and how to order the 1989 PDR on CD-ROM.

The volume medical professionals asked for!
PDR 1989 DRUG INTERACTIONS AND SIDE EFFECTS INDEX™

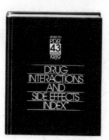

The 1989 PDR Index covers *every* drug found in your 1989 PDR. The Interactions Index alerts you to every combination to watch out for —all the brands and compounds.

The Side Effects Index lets you quickly look up signs, symptoms, and abnormalities and identify the drugs that might be the cause. Save hours of searching for the vital information you need.

Use order forms on previous page.

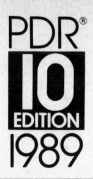

PDR 10 EDITION 1989

PHYSICIANS' DESK REFERENCE

FOR NONPRESCRIPTION DRUGS®

Publisher: Edward R. Barnhart

Director of Production: MARY TRELEWICZ

Production Manager: CARRIE HENWOOD

Manager of Production Services:
ELIZABETH H. CARUSO

Managing Editor: BARBARA B. HUFF

Index Editor: ADELE L. DOWD

Medical Consultant: NATHAN W. NEMIROFF, M.D.

Art Associate: JOAN AKERLIND

Editorial Assistants:
CATHLEEN BUNNELL
JANE T. PASINSKI

Editorial Consultant: DAVID W. SIFTON

Administrative Assistants: SONIA C. RYAN
HELENE WATTMAN

Marketing and Circulation Director:
THOMAS C. MILLER

Assistant Circulation Director:
ANNETTE G. VERNON

Book Fulfillment Manager: ANITA MOORE

Professional Relations Manager:
ANNA E. BARBAGALLO

Circulation Coordinator: MARY J. CADLEY

National Sales Manager: PETER J. MURPHY

Account Managers: JEFFERY J. BONISTALLI
CHARLES MEITNER
JOANNE TERZIDES

Senior Research Analyst: VICKI FAVRE

Design Director: JOHN NEWCOMB

ISBN 0-87489-701-7

Foreword to the Tenth Edition

Responsible self-medication is becoming ever more important in the health care of Americans. Self-medication continues to offer quick and inexpensive relief for minor health discomforts. Consumers of all socioeconomic levels have found the convenient availability and low cost of over-the-counter medicines (OTCs) an invaluable and welcome adjunct to the professional health care system.

Of great interest to health professionals is a trend that began with the OTC Review (the government's exhaustive evaluation of the ingredients and labeling in OTC products), and is now continuing through several regulatory avenues: that of transferring some ingredients and dosages from prescription to OTC (nonprescription) status. This is broadening the range of effective products available to consumers for self-medication, while improved labeling helps ensure appropriate use.

Manufacturers of nonprescription drug products have agreed to voluntarily list inactive ingredients, in addition to active ingredients on their labels. This will be of help to consumers who may have a sensitivity to certain ingredients.

The PHYSICIANS' DESK REFERENCE For NONPRESCRIPTION DRUGS® is published annually by Medical Economics Company Inc., with the cooperation of the manufacturers whose products are described in the Product Information and Diagnostics, Devices and Medical Aids Sections. Its purpose is to make available essential information on nonprescription products.

The function of the Publisher is the compilation, organization, and distribution of this information. Each product description has been prepared by the manufacturer, and edited and approved by the manufacturer's medical department, medical director, and/or medical consultant. In organizing and presenting the material in PHYSICIANS' DESK REFERENCE For NONPRESCRIPTION DRUGS®, the Publisher does not warrant or guarantee any of the products described herein or perform any independent analysis in connection with any of the product information contained herein. PHYSICIANS' DESK REFERENCE For NONPRESCRIPTION DRUGS® does not assume, and expressly disclaims, any obligation to obtain and include information other than that provided to it by the manufacturer. In making this material available it should be understood that the Publisher is not advocating the use of any product described herein. Besides the information given here, additional information on any product may be obtained through the manufacturer.

EDWARD R. BARNHART
Publisher

HOW TO USE THIS EDITION

If you want to find . . .	And you already know . . .	Here's where to look . . .
the brand name of a product	the manufacturer's name	White Section: Manufacturers' Index
	its generic name	Yellow Section: Active Ingredients Index*
the manufacturer's name	the product's brand name	Pink Section: Product Name Index*
	the product's generic name	Yellow Section: Active Ingredients Index*
essential product information, such as: active ingredients indications actions warnings drug interaction precautions symptoms & treatment of oral overdosage dosage & administration how supplied	the product's brand name	Pink Section: Product Name Index*
	the product's generic name	Yellow Section: Active ingredients Index*
a product with a particular chemical action	the chemical action	Yellow Section: Active Ingredients Index*
a product with a particular active ingredient	the active ingredient	Yellow Section: Active Ingredients Index*
a similar acting product	the product classification	Blue Section: Product Category Index*
generic name of a brand name product	the product's brand name	Pink Section: Product Name Index. Generic name will be found under "Active Ingredients" in Product Information Section.

*In the Pink, Blue and Yellow Sections, the page
numbers following the product name refer to the pages
in the Product Identification Section where the product
is pictured and the Product Information Section where
the drug is comprehensively described.*

Contents

SECTION 1
Manufacturers' Index

The manufacturers whose names appear in this index have provided information concerning their products in either the Product Information Section, Product Identification Section, or the Diagnostics, Devices and Medical Aids Section.

Included in this index are the names and addresses of manufacturers, individuals or departments to whom you may address inquiries, a partial list of products as well as emergency telephone numbers wherever available.

The symbol ◆ indicates that the product is shown in the Product Identification Section.

(◆ Shown in Product Identification Section)

Manufacturing and Distribution
Main St. at Perimeter Rd.
Conestee, SC 29605
Toll Free 1-(800) 845-8210
Address inquiries to:
Victor De Oreo, R Ph, V.P., Sales
(803) 277-7282
Richard Stephen Jenkins, Exec. V.P.
(813) 839-6565
OTC Products Available
Beelith Tablets

**BECTON DICKINSON CONSUMER 508
PRODUCTS**
One Becton Drive
Franklin Lakes, NJ 07417-1883
Address inquiries to:
Consumer Service (201) 848-6574
OTC Products Available
B-D Glucose Tablets

BEECHAM PRODUCTS USA 508
P.O. Box 1467
Pittsburgh, PA 15230
Address inquiries to:
Professional Services Dept.
(800) BEECHAM
(412) 928-1050
OTC Products Available
B.F.I. Antiseptic First-Aid Powder
Children's Hold
Deep-Down Pain Relief Rub
Eno Sparkling Antacid
FemIron Tablets
FemIron Multi-Vitamins and Iron
Geritol Complete Tablets
Geritol Liquid - High Potency Iron &
Vitamin Tonic
Hold
Massengill Baby Powder Soft Cloth
Towelette
Massengill Disposable Douche
Massengill Liquid Concentrate
Massengill Medicated Disposable
Douche
Massengill Medicated Liquid
Concentrate
Massengill Powder
Massengill Towelettes
N'ICE Medicated Sugarless Sore Throat
and Cough Lozenges
N'ICE Sore Throat Spray
S.T.37
Scott's Emulsion
Serutan Concentrated Powder - Fruit
Flavored
Serutan Toasted Granules
Sominex
Sominex Liquid
Sominex Pain Relief Formula
Sucrets (Regular and Mentholated)
Sucrets Children's Cherry Flavored
Sore Throat Lozenges
Sucrets Cold Decongestant Formula
Sucrets Cold Relief Formula
Sucrets Cough Control Formula
Sucrets Maximum Strength Sore Throat
Lozenges
Sucrets Maximum Strength Spray
Thermotabs
Vivarin Stimulant Tablets

BIO-TECH PHARMACAL, INC. 515
P.O. Box 1992
Fayetteville, AR 72702
Address inquiries to:
Director, Customer Service
(800) 345-1199
(501) 443-9148
OTC Products Available
Bromase

BLAINE COMPANY, INC. 515
2700 Dixie Highway
Fort Mitchell, KY 41017
Address inquiries to:
Mr. Alex M. Blaine (606) 341-9437
OTC Products Available
Mag-Ox 400
Uro-Mag

BLISTEX INC. 515
1800 Swift Drive
Oak Brook, IL 60521

(312) 571-2870
(800) 323-7343
Address inquiries to:
Vice President, Technical Services
For Medical Emergencies Contact:
Manager, Quality Control
OTC Products Available
Blistex Daily Conditioning Treatment for
Lips
Blistex Medicated Lip Ointment
Blistik Medicated Lip Balm
Foille First Aid Liquid, Ointment &
Spray
Ivarest Medicated Cream & Lotion
Kank•a Medicated Formula
Lip Medex

BLOCK DRUG COMPANY, INC. 516
257 Cornelison Avenue
Jersey City, NJ 07302
Address inquiries to:
Steve Gattanella (201) 434-3000
For Medical Emergencies Contact:
James Gingold (201) 434-3000
OTC Products Available
Arthritis Strength BC Powder
BC Powder
Nytol Tablets
Promise Toothpaste
Original Sensodyne Toothpaste
Mint Sensodyne Toothpaste
Tegrin for Psoriasis Lotion, Cream &
Soap
Tegrin Medicated Shampoo

**BOEHRINGER INGELHEIM 404, 518
PHARMACEUTICALS, INC.**
90 East Ridge
P.O. Box 368
Ridgefield, CT 06877
Address inquiries to:
Medical Services Dept.
(203) 798-9988
OTC Products Available
◆Dulcolax Suppositories
◆Dulcolax Tablets
Nōstril Nasal Decongestant
Nōstrilla Long Acting Nasal
Decongestant

**BOEHRINGER MANNHEIM 760
DIAGNOSTICS**
Division of Boehringer Mannheim Corp.
9115 Hague Road
Indianapolis, IN 46250
Address inquiries to:
Medical Service Department
(800) 858-8072
OTC Products Available
Accu-Chek II Blood Glucose Monitor
Accu-Chek II Diabetes Care Kit
Chemstrip bG Test Strips
Chemstrip K Test Strips
Chemstrip MatchMaker Visual Reader
Chemstrip uG Test Strips
Chemstrip uGK Test Strips
Soft Touch Lancet Device
Soft Touch Lancets
Tracer bG Care Kit
Tracer bG Test Strips
Tracer II Blood Glucose Monitor

BOIRON-BORNEMAN, INC. 404, 520
1208 Amosland Road
Norwood, PA 19074
Address inquiries to:
Robert Matsuk, R.Ph.
National Sales Manager
(215) 532-2035
For Medical Emergencies Contact:
Technical Services Department
(215) 532-2035
OTC Products Available
◆Oscillococcinum

BRISTOL LABORATORIES 520
A Bristol-Myers Company
2400 W. Lloyd Expressway
Evansville, IN 47721
(812) 429-5000
OTC Products Available
Naldecon CX Adult Liquid
Naldecon DX Adult Liquid
Naldecon DX Children's Syrup

Naldecon DX Pediatric Drops
Naldecon EX Children's Syrup
Naldecon EX Pediatric Drops
Naldecon Senior DX
Naldecon Senior EX

BRISTOL-MYERS PRODUCTS 404, 523
(Division of Bristol-Myers Company)
345 Park Avenue
New York, NY 10154
Address Product Inquiries to:
Products Division
Public Affairs Department
345 Park Avenue
New York, NY 10154
*Address Medical Inquiries about
OTC Products to:*
Department of Medical Services
1350 Liberty Avenue
Hillside, NJ 07207
In Emergencies Call:
(212) 546-4616 (9 AM-5 PM)
(212) 546-4700 (Other times)
OTC Products Available
AMMENS Medicated Powder
B.Q. Cold Tablets
BAN Antiperspirant Cream Deodorant
BAN Basic Non-aerosol Antiperspirant
Spray
BAN Roll-on Antiperspirant
BAN Solid Antiperspirant Deodorant
BAN Wide Ball Antiperspirant
BODY ON TAP Beer Enriched Shampoo
◆Tri-Buffered BUFFERIN Analgesic
Tablets and Caplets
◆Arthritis Strength Tri-Buffered
BUFFERIN Analgesic Caplets
◆Extra Strength Tri-Buffered BUFFERIN
Analgesic Tablets
◆COMTREX Multi-Symptom Cold
Reliever-Tablets/Caplets/Liquid
◆COMTREX A/S Multi-Symptom
Allergy/Sinus Formula Tablets &
Caplets
◆CONGESPIRIN For Children Aspirin
Free Chewable Cold Tablets
◆CONGESPIRIN For Children Aspirin
Free Liquid Cold Medicine
◆CONGESPIRIN For Children Cough
Syrup
◆DATRIL Extra Strength Analgesic
Tablets & Caplets
◆EXCEDRIN Extra-Strength Analgesic
Tablets & Caplets
◆EXCEDRIN P.M. Analgesic/Sleeping Aid
Tablets and Caplets
◆Sinus EXCEDRIN Analgesic,
Decongestant Tablets & Caplets
◆4-WAY Cold Tablets
◆4-WAY Fast Acting Nasal Spray
(regular and mentholated)
◆4-WAY Long Acting Nasal Spray &
Metered Spray Pump
MINIT-RUB Analgesic Ointment
MUM Antiperspirant Cream Deodorant
◆NO DOZ Fast Acting Keep Alert Tablets
◆NUPRIN Ibuprofen/Analgesic Tablets
and Caplets
◆PAZO Hemorrhoid Ointment &
Suppositories
TICKLE Antiperspirant
ULTRA BAN Aerosol Antiperspirant
ULTRA BAN Roll-on Antiperspirant
ULTRA BAN Solid
Antiperspirant/Deodorant

**BURROUGHS WELLCOME 405, 530
CO.**
3030 Cornwallis Road
Research Triangle Park, NC 27709
(919) 248-3000
For Medical or Drug Information:
Contact: Drug Information Service
Business hours only
(8:15 AM to 4:15 PM EST)
(800) 443-6763
For 24 hour Medical Emergency
Information, call (800) 443-6763
For Sales Information:
Contact: Sales Distribution
Department

(◆ Shown in Product Identification Section)

Address Other Inquiries to:
Public Affairs Department
Branch Office
Burlingame, CA 94010
1760 Rollins Road   (415) 697-5630
OTC Products Described
◆Actidil Tablets & Syrup
◆Actifed Capsules
◆Actifed 12-Hour Capsules
◆Actifed Syrup
◆Actifed Tablets
◆AllerAct Tablets
◆AllerAct Decongestant Caplets
◆AllerAct Decongestant Tablets
Ammonia Aromatic, Vaporole
Borofax Ointment
◆Empirin Aspirin
Lubafax Surgical Lubricant, Sterile
◆Marezine Tablets
◆Neosporin Cream
◆Neosporin Ointment
◆Polysporin Ointment
◆Polysporin Powder
◆Polysporin Spray
◆Sudafed Children's Liquid
◆Sudafed Cough Syrup
◆Sudafed Plus Liquid
◆Sudafed Plus Tablets
◆Sudafed 12 Hour Capsules
◆Sudafed Tablets, 30 mg
◆Sudafed Tablets, Adult Strength, 60
mg
◆Sudafed Sinus Caplets
◆Sudafed Sinus Tablets
Wellcome Lanoline

CAMPBELL LABORATORIES INC.   536
300 East 51st Street
New York, NY 10022
Address Inquiries to:
Richard C. Zahn, President
P.O. Box 812, FDR Station
New York, NY 10150
(212) 688-7684
OTC Products Available
Herpecin-L Cold Sore Lip Balm

CARTER PRODUCTS   407, 537
Division of Carter-Wallace, Inc.
767 Fifth Avenue
New York, NY 10153   (212)758-4500
OTC Products Available
◆Carter's Little Pills

CHATTEM INC., CONSUMER   537
PRODUCTS DIVISION
Division of Chattem, Inc.
1715 West 38th Street
Chattanooga, TN 37409
Address Inquiries to:
Mike Modzelewski   (615) 821-4571
For Medical Emergencies Contact:
Walt Ludwig   (615) 821-4571
OTC Products Available
Black-Draught Granulated
Black-Draught Lax-Senna Tablets
Black-Draught Syrup
Blis-To-Sol Liquid
Blis-To-Sol Powder
Nullo Deodorant Tablets
Pamprin Extra Strength Multi-Symptom
Pain Relief Formula Tablets
Pamprin Maximum Cramp Relief
Formula Tablets & Caplets
Pamprin-IB
PREMSYN PMS Capsules & Caplets
Soltice Quick-Rub

CHURCH & DWIGHT CO.,   407, 537
INC.
469 North Harrison Street
Princeton, NJ 08540
Address inquiries to:
Mr. Stephen Lajoie   (609) 683-5900
For Medical Emergencies Contact:
Mr. Stephen Lajoie   (609) 683-5900
OTC Products Available
Arm & Hammer Pure Baking Soda
◆Otix Drops Ear Wax Removal Aid

CIBA CONSUMER   407, 538
PHARMACEUTICALS
Division of CIBA-GEIGY Corporation
Raritan Plaza III
Edison, NJ 08837
Address inquiries to:
(201) 225-6000
(201) 906-6000
For Medical Emergencies Contact:
(201) 277-5000
OTC Products Available
◆Acutrim Late Day Appetite Suppressant
◆Acutrim 16 Hour Appetite Suppressant
◆Acutrim II Maximum Strength Appetite
Suppressant
◆Doan's - Original Analgesic
◆Doan's - Extra Strength Analgesic
Fiberall Chewable Tablets
Fiberall Fiber Wafers - Oatmeal Raisin
Fiberall, Natural Flavor
Fiberall, Orange Flavor
◆Nupercainal Hemorrhoidal Ointment
◆Nupercainal Hemorrhoidal
Suppositories
◆Nupercainal Pain Relief Cream
◆Otrivin Nasal Spray & Nasal Drops
◆Otrivin Pediatric Nasal Drops
◆Privine Nasal Solution
◆Privine Nasal Spray
◆Q-vel Muscle Relaxant Pain Reliever
◆Slow Fe Tablets
◆Sunkist Children's Chewable
Multivitamins - Complete
◆Sunkist Children's Chewable
Multivitamins - Plus Extra C
◆Sunkist Children's Chewable
Multivitamins - Plus Iron
◆Sunkist Children's Chewable
Multivitamins - Regular
◆Sunkist Vitamin C

COLGATE-PALMOLIVE   408, 542
COMPANY
A Delaware Corporation
300 Park Avenue
New York, NY 10022
Address inquiries to:
Consumers:
Consumer Affairs
300 Park Avenue
New York, NY 10022
(212) 310-2000
Physicians:
Medical Director
909 River Road
Piscataway, NJ 08854
(201) 878-7500
For Medical Emergencies Contact:
9 AM to 5 PM   (201) 878-7500
5 PM to 9 AM   (201) 547-2500
OTC Products Available
Colgate Dental Cream
◆Colgate Junior Fluoride Gel Toothpaste
◆Colgate MFP Fluoride Gel
◆Colgate MFP Fluoride Toothpaste
◆Colgate Mouthwash Tartar Control
Formula
◆Colgate Tartar Control Formula
◆Colgate Tartar Control Gel
Colgate Toothbrushes
Curad Bandages
Dermassage Dish Liquid
◆Fluorigard Anti-Cavity Fluoride Rinse
Mersene Denture Cleanser
Ultra Brite Toothpaste

CUMBERLAND-SWAN, INC.   408, 543
Corporate Headquarters:
Cumberland-Swan, Inc.
One Swan Drive
Smyrna, TN 37167
(615) 459-8900
Watts: (800) 251-3068
Address inquiries to:
Vice President, Regulatory Affairs
Vice President of Marketing
Regional Sales Office
Cumberland-Swan, Inc., West Coast
9817 7th Street
Rancho, Cucamonga, CA 91730
(714) 980-5522
Watts: (800) 624-9137

OTC Products Available
Swan Acetaminophen Tablets, Caplets
Swan Aspirin Tablets, Coated Tablets,
Caplets
Swan Calamine Lotion
◆Swan Citroma (Citrate of Magnesia)
Swan Epsom Salt
Swan Hydrogen Peroxide Solution (3%)
Swan Ibuprofen Coated Tablets, Caplets
Swan Milk of Magnesia
Swan Mineral Oil

DAYWELL LABORATORIES   544
CORPORATION
78 Unquowa Place
Fairfield, CT 06430
Address inquiries to:
M. E. Norton   (203) 255-3154
OTC Products Available
Vergo Cream

DERMIK LABORATORIES, INC.   544
790 Penllyn Pike
Blue Bell, PA 19422
Distribution Centers
Oak Forest, IL 60452
4325 Frontage Road
(312) 687-7440
Langhorne, PA 19047
P.O. Box 247   (215) 752-1211
Reno, NV 89502
4902 Ampere Dr.
(702) 785-7666
Tucker, GA 30084
4660 Hammermill Road
(404) 934-3091
OTC Products Available
Hytone Cream 1/2%
Loroxide Acne Lotion (Flesh Tinted)
Shepard's Formulations for Dry Skin
Care
Shepard's Cream Lotion
Shepard's Skin Cream
Shepard's Soap
Vanoxide Acne Lotion
Vlemasque Acne Mask
Zetar Shampoo

FISONS   545
CONSUMER HEALTH DIVISION
Fisons Pharmaceuticals
P.O. Box 1212
Rochester, NY 14603
Address inquiries to:
Product Service Department
P.O. Box 1212
Rochester, NY 14603
(716) 475-9000
FAX (716) 383-1637
For Medical Emergencies Contact
(716) 475-9000
OTC Products Available
Allerest Allergy Tablets
Allerest Eye Drops
Allerest Headache Strength Tablets
Allerest No Drowsiness Tablets
Allerest Sinus Pain Formula
Allerest 12 Hour Caplets
Allerest 12 Hour Nasal Spray
Americaine Hemorrhoidal Ointment
Americaine Topical Anesthetic Ointment
Americaine Topical Anesthetic Spray
CaldeCORT Anti-Itch Hydrocortisone
Cream
CaldeCORT Anti-Itch Hydrocortisone
Spray
CaldeCORT Light Creme
Caldesene Medicated Ointment
Caldesene Medicated Powder
Cruex Antifungal Cream
Cruex Antifungal Powder
Cruex Antifungal Spray Powder
Desenex Antifungal Cream
Desenex Antifungal Foam
Desenex Antifungal Liquid
Desenex Antifungal Ointment
Desenex Antifungal Powder
Desenex Antifungal Spray Powder
Desenex Foot & Sneaker Spray
Desenex Soap
Sinarest Nasal Spray

(◆ Shown in Product Identification Section)

Sinarest No Drowsiness Tablets
Sinarest Regular & Extra Strength
Tablets
Ting Antifungal Cream
Ting Antifungal Powder
Ting Antifungal Spray Powder

FLEMING & COMPANY   548
1600 Fenpark Dr.
Fenton, MO 63026
Address inquiries to:
John J. Roth, M.D.   (314) 343-8200
For Medical Emergencies Contact:
John R. Roth, M.D.   (314) 343-8200
OTC Products Available
Chlor-3
Deter Tablets
Impregon Concentrate
Magonate Tablets and Liquid
Marblen Suspension Peach/Apricot
Marblen Suspension Unflavored
Marblen Tablets
Nephrox Suspension
Nicotinex Elixir
Ocean Nasal Mist
Ocean-A/S Mist
Ocean-Plus Mist
Purge Concentrate

GLENBROOK   408, 549
LABORATORIES
Division of Sterling Drug Inc.
90 Park Avenue
New York, NY 10016
Address inquiries to:
Medical Director   (212) 907-2764
OTC Products Available
◆Children's Bayer Chewable Aspirin
◆Bayer Children's Cold Tablets
◆Bayer Children's Cough Syrup
◆Children's Panadol Chewable Tablets,
Liquid, Infants' Drops
◆Diaparene Corn Starch Baby Powder
◆Diaparene Cradol
◆Diaparene Medicated Cream
◆Diaparene Peri-Anal Medicated
Ointment
◆Diaparene Supers Baby Wash Cloths
◆8-Hour Bayer Timed-Release Aspirin
◆Genuine Bayer Aspirin Tablets &
Caplets
◆Haley's M-O
◆Maximum Bayer Aspirin Tablets &
Caplets
◆Maximum Strength Midol
Multi-Symptom Formula
◆Maximum Strength Midol PMS
Premenstrual Syndrome Formula
◆Original Midol Multi-Symptom Formula
◆Midol 200 Advanced Pain Formula
Junior Strength Panadol
◆Maximum Strength Panadol Tablets
and Caplets
◆Phillips' LaxCaps
◆Phillips' Milk of Magnesia
Phillips' Milk of Magnesia Tablets
◆Stri-Dex Maximum Strength Pads
◆Stri-Dex Regular Strength Pads
◆Vanquish Analgesic Caplets

GULF BIO-SYSTEMS, INC.   557
5310 Harvest Hill Road
Dallas, TX 75230
Address inquiries to:
Pat W. Haragan   (214) 386-0442
For Medical Emergencies Contact:
William R. Weaver, MD
(214) 386-2969
OTC Products Available
SuperChar Aqueous - Suspension in
water
Super-Char Liquid with Sorbitol -
Suspension in sorbitol solution &
water
SuperChar Powder - Reconstitute in tap
water as directed

HERALD PHARMACAL, INC.   557
6503 Warwick Road
Richmond, VA 23225
Address inquiries to:
Henry H. Kamps
(804) 745-3400

For Medical Emergencies Contact:
Henry H. Kamps
(804) 745-3400
OTC Products Available
Aqua Glycolic Lotion
Aqua Glycolic Shampoo
Aqua Glyde Cleanser
Cam Lotion

HERBERT LABORATORIES   557
2525 Dupont Drive
Irvine, CA 92715
Address inquiries to:
Product Information Services
(714) 955-6200
For Medical Emergencies Contact:
Product Information Services
(714) 955-6200
OTC Products Available
AquaTar Therapeutic Tar Gel
Bluboro Powder Astringent Soaking
Solution
Danex Dandruff Shampoo
Vanseb Cream and Lotion Dandruff
Shampoos
Vanseb-T Cream and Lotion Tar
Dandruff Shampoos

HOECHST-ROUSSEL   410, 558
PHARMACEUTICALS INC.
Routes 202-206 North
Somerville, NJ 08876
Address medical inquiries to:
Scientific Services Dept.
(201) 231-2611
(8:30 AM-5:00 PM EST)
For medical emergency information
only, after hours and on weekends,
call: (201) 231-2000
OTC Products Available
◆Doxidan
◆Festal II
◆Surfak

HYNSON, WESTCOTT   410, 559
& DUNNING PRODUCTS
Becton Dickinson Microbiology Systems
250 Schilling Circle
Cockeysville, MD 21030
(301) 771-0100
OTC Products Available
◆Lactinex Tablets & Granules

INTER-CAL CORPORATION   559
421 Miller Valley Road
Prescott, AZ 86301
Address inquiries to:
Richard Markham   (602) 445-8063
OTC Products Available
Ester-C Tablets

JACKSON-MITCHELL   560
PHARMACEUTICALS, INC.
1485 East Valley Road
Santa Barbara, CA 93108
Address inquiries to:
Carol Jackson   (805) 565-1538
For Medical Emergencies Contact:
Carol Jackson   (805) 565-1538
Branch Offices
Turlock, CA 95380
P.O. Box 934   (209) 667-2019
OTC Products Available
Meyenberg Evaporated Goat Milk - 12
1/2 fl. oz.
Meyenberg Powdered Goat Milk - 4 oz.
& 14 oz.

JOHNSON & JOHNSON   410, 560
BABY PRODUCTS
COMPANY
Grandview Road
Skillman, NJ 08558
Address inquiries to:
(800) 526-3967
For Medical Emergencies Contact:
(800) 526-3967
OTC Products Available
◆JOHNSON'S Baby Sunblock Cream
(SPF 15)
◆JOHNSON'S Baby Sunblock Lotion
(SPF 15)

Purpose Dry Skin Cream
Purpose Dual Treatment Moisturizer
(SPF 12)
Purpose Soap
◆SUNDOWN Broad Spectrum Cream
Ultra Sunblock (SPF 30)
◆SUNDOWN Broad Spectrum Lotions
Ultra Sunblock (SPF 15)
Ultra Sunblock (SPF 25)
SUNDOWN Sunblock Cream, Ultra
Protection (SPF 24)
◆SUNDOWN Sunblock Stick, Ultra
Protection (SPF 15)
SUNDOWN Sunblock Stick, Ultra
Protection (SPF 20)
SUNDOWN Sunscreen Lotions
Moderate Protection (SPF 4)
Extra Protection (SPF 6)
Maximal Protection (SPF 8)
◆ Ultra Protection Sunblock (SPF 15)
Ultra Protection Sunblock (SPF 20)
SUNDOWN Sunscreen Stick, Maximal
Protection (SPF 8)

JOHNSON & JOHNSON   410, 561
CONSUMER PRODUCTS,
INC.
501 George Street
New Brunswick, NJ 08903
Address inquiries to:
Room J526
(800) 526-3967
For Medical Emergencies Contact:
(800) 526-3967
OTC Products Available
Johnson & Johnson First Aid Cream
◆K-Y Brand Lubricating Jelly

KREMERS URBAN COMPANY   692
See SCHWARZ PHARMA

LACLEDE RESEARCH   562
LABORATORIES
15011 Staff Court
Gardena, CA 90248
Address inquiries to:
Laclede Research Center
(213) 770-0463
For Medical Emergencies Contact:
Medical Director   (213) 770-0497
OTC Products Available
Biotene Dental Chewing Gum
Biotene Dry Mouth Relief Toothpaste
Biotene Gentle Antibacterial Mouthwash
Biotene SuperSoft Toothbrush
Oral Balance Long Lasting Moisturizing
Gel

LAKESIDE   410, 562
PHARMACEUTICALS
Division of Merrell Dow
Pharmaceuticals Inc.
Cincinnati, OH 45242-9553
(513) 948-9111
Address inquiries to:
Professional Information Department
Business hours only
(8:15 AM to 5:00 PM EST)
(513) 948-6040
For Medical Emergency Information
Only after hours or on weekends
(513) 948-9111
OTC Products Available
◆Cēpacol Anesthetic Lozenges (Troches)
◆Cēpacol/Cēpacol Mint
Mouthwash/Gargle
◆Cēpacol Throat Lozenges
◆CEPASTAT Cherry Flavor Sore Throat
Lozenges
◆CEPASTAT Sore Throat Lozenges
◆CITRUCEL
◆CITRUCEL Orange Flavor
◆Novahistine DMX
◆Novahistine Elixir
Simron Capsules
Simron Plus Capsules
Singlet

LAVOPTIK COMPANY, INC.   566, 760
661 Western Avenue North
St. Paul, MN 55103
Address inquiries to:
661 Western Avenue North
St. Paul, MN 55103 (612) 489-1351

(◆ Shown in Product Identification Section)

For Medical Emergencies Contact:
B. C. Brainard   (612) 489-1351
OTC Products Available
Lavoptik Eye Cup
Lavoptik Eye Wash

LEDERLE LABORATORIES   411, 566
Division of American Cyanamid Co.
One Cyanamid Plaza
Wayne, NJ 07470
*Address inquiries on
medical matters to:*
Professional Services Dept.
Lederle Laboratories
Pearl River, NY 10965
8 AM to 4:30 PM EST
    (914) 735-2815
All other inquiries and
after hours emergencies
    (914) 732-5000
Distribution Centers
ATLANTA
Contact EASTERN (Philadelphia)
Distribution Center
CHICAGO
Bulk Address
Mt. Prospect, IL 60056
1100 East Business Center Drive
Mail Address
Mt. Prospect, IL 60056-7614
P.O. Box 7614   (800) 533-3753
    (312) 827-8871
DALLAS
Bulk Address
Dallas, TX 75247
7611 Carpenter Freeway
Mail Address
Dallas, TX 75265
P.O. Box 655731   (800) 533-3753
    (214) 631-2130
LOS ANGELES
Bulk Address
Los Angeles, CA 90040
2300 S. Eastern Ave.
Mail Address
Los Angeles, CA 90051
T.A. Box 2202   (800) 533-3753
    (213) 726-1016
EASTERN (Philadelphia)
Bulk Address
Horsham, PA 19044
202 Precision Drive
Mail Address
Horsham, PA 19044
P.O. Box 993   (800) 533-3753
    (215) 672-5400
OTC Products Available
Acetaminophen Capsules, Tablets, Elixir
Ascorbic Acid Tablets
Aureomycin Ointment 3%
◆Caltrate 600
◆Caltrate 600 + Iron and Vitamin D
◆Caltrate 600 + Vitamin D
◆Caltrate, Jr.
◆Centrum
◆Centrum, Jr. + Extra C
◆Centrum, Jr. + Extra Calcium
◆Centrum, Jr. + Iron
Docusate Sodium (DSS) Capsules &
  Syrup
Docusate Sodium w/Casanthranol
  Capsules & Syrup
◆Ferro-Sequels
Ferrous Gluconate Iron Supplement
Ferrous Sulfate
◆FiberCon Bulk Laxative
Filibon Prenatal Vitamin Tablets
Gevrabon Liquid
Gevral Protein Powder
Gevral Tablets
Gevral T Tablets
Guaifenesin Syrup
Guaifenesin w/D-Methorphan
  Hydrobromide Syrup
Incremin w/Iron Syrup
Lederplex Capsules and Liquid
Neoloid Emulsified Castor Oil
Peritinic Tablets
Pseudoephedrine Syrup & Tablets
Pyridoxine HCl (Vitamin B₆) Tablets
Quinine Capsules
Stresscaps Capsules
◆Stresstabs 600 Tablets

◆Stresstabs 600 + Iron
◆Stresstabs 600 + Zinc
Thiamine HCl (Vitamin B-1) Tablets
Triprolidine with Pseudoephedrine
  Syrup & Tablets
Vitamin A, Natural
Vitamin C Chewable
Vitamin E, Natural, USP
Vitamin E, USP
◆Zincon Dandruff Shampoo

LEEMING DIVISION   412, 572
Pfizer Inc.
100 Jefferson Rd.
Parsippany, NJ 07054
Address inquiries to:
Research and Development Dept.
    (201) 887-2100
OTC Products Available
Ben-Gay External Analgesic Products
Bonine
◆Desitin Ointment
Rheaban Maximum Strength Tablets
RID Lice Control Spray
RID Lice Treatment Kit
Unisom Dual Relief Nighttime Sleep
  Aid/Analgesic
Unisom Nighttime Sleep Aid
◆Visine a.c. Eye Drops
◆Visine Eye Drops
◆Visine Extra Eye Drops
Wart-Off

**LEVER BROTHERS   412, 577
COMPANY**
390 Park Avenue
New York, NY 10022
    (212) 688-6000
OTC Products Available
◆Dove Bar

LOMA LINDA FOODS INC.   577
Address inquiries to:
Marketing Office
11503 Pierce Street
Riverside, CA 92515 (714) 687-7800
    (800) 932-5525
CA only (800) 442-4917
OTC Products Available
Soyalac: Liquid Concentrate,
  Ready-to-Serve and Powder
I-Soyalac: Liquid Concentrate and
  Ready-to-Serve

LUYTIES PHARMACAL COMPANY   578
P. O. Box 8080
St. Louis, MO 63156
Address Inquiries to:
Customer Service   (800) 325-8080
OTC Products Available
Yellolax

3M COMPANY   578
Personal Care Products
Consumer Specialties Division/3M
3M Center
St. Paul, MN 55144-1000
Address Inquiries to:
Sandy Holman
3M Center   (612) 736-0894
For Medical Emergencies Contact:
3M Center   (612) 733-1110
OTC Products Available
Titralac Antacid Tablets
Titralac Plus Antacid/Anti-Gas Liquid
Titralac Plus Antacid/Anti-Gas Tablets

MACSIL, INC.   579
1326 Frankford Avenue
Philadelphia, PA 19125
    (215) 739-7300
OTC Products Available
Balmex Baby Powder
Balmex Emollient Lotion
Balmex Ointment

**MARION LABORATORIES,   412, 579
INC.**
Pharmaceutical Products Division
Marion Industrial Park
Marion Park Drive
Kansas City, MO 64137

Address inquiries to:
Product Surveillance Dept.
P.O. Box 9627
Kansas City, MO 64134
    (816) 966-5000
OTC Products Available
◆Debrox Drops
◆Gaviscon Antacid Tablets
◆Gaviscon Extra Strength Relief Formula
  Antacid Tablets
◆Gaviscon Liquid Antacid
◆Gaviscon-2 Antacid Tablets
◆Gly-Oxide Liquid
◆Os-Cal 250+D Tablets
◆Os-Cal 500 Chewable Tablets
◆Os-Cal 500 Tablets
◆Os-Cal 500+D Tablets
◆Os-Cal Forte Tablets
◆Os-Cal Plus Tablets
◆Throat Discs Throat Lozenges

MARLYN HEALTH CARE   582
6324 Ferris Square
San Diego, CA 92121
    (619) 453-5600
OTC Products Available
C Speridin Tablets, Sustained Release
Daily Nutritional Packs
  Care-4
  MARLYN PMS
  Pro-Formance
  Soft Stress
4 Hair
4 Nails
Hep-Forte Capsules
Marbec Tablets
Marlyn Formula 50 Capsules
Marlyn Prolonged Release Vitamins
  Clock E, 400 I.U.
  Iron-L
  Niacin, 400 mg.
  Super One Daily
  Super Citro Cee
  Ultimate One
  Vitamin B Complex 50
  Vitamin C, 1000 mg.
Pro Skin-E (Face Capsule)
Pro-Skin Nutribloxx

**McNEIL CONSUMER   413, 582
PRODUCTS CO.**
Camp Hill Road
Fort Washington, PA 19034
    (215) 233-7000
Address inquiries to:
Consumer Affairs Department
Fort Washington, PA 19034
Manufacturing Divisions
Fort Washington, PA 19034
Southwest Manufacturing Plant
4001 N. I-35
Round Rock, TX 78664
OTC Products Available
◆Children's CoTYLENOL Chewable Cold
  Tablets & Liquid Cold Formula
◆Children's TYLENOL acetaminophen
  Chewable Tablets & Elixir
◆DELSYM Cough Suppressant Syrup
Extra-Strength TYLENOL
  acetaminophen Adult Liquid Pain
  Reliever
◆Extra-Strength TYLENOL
  acetaminophen Caplets, Gelcaps and
  Tablets
◆IMODIUM A-D Liquid
◆Infants' TYLENOL Drops (see Children's
  TYLENOL Acetaminophen)
◆Junior Strength TYLENOL
  acetaminophen Coated Caplets
◆Maximum Strength TYLENOL Sinus
  Medication Tablets and Caplets
◆MEDIPREN ibuprofen Caplets and
  Tablets
◆PEDIACARE Cold Formula Liquid
◆PEDIACARE Cough-Cold Formula Liquid
  and Chewable Tablets
◆PEDIACARE Infants' Oral Decongestant
  Drops
◆Regular Strength TYLENOL
  acetaminophen Tablets & Caplets

(◆ Shown in Product Identification Section)

◆SINE-AID Sinus Headache Tablets
◆Maximum Strength SINE-AID Sinus Headache Caplets
◆TYLENOL Cold Medication Caplets & Tablets
◆TYLENOL Cold Medication Liquid
◆TYLENOL Cold Medication No Drowsiness Formula Caplets

MEAD JOHNSON   **414, 594**
NUTRITIONALS
A Bristol-Myers Company
2400 W. Lloyd Expressway
Evansville, IN 47721
            (812) 429-5000
Address inquiries to:
Scientific Information Section
   Medical Department
OTC Products Available
Casec
Ce-Vi-Sol
Criticare HN
◆Enfamil Concentrated Liquid, Powder, and Ready-To-Use
Enfamil Nursette
◆Enfamil w/Iron Concentrated Liquid, Powder and Ready-To-Use
Fer-In-Sol
Isocal Complete Liquid Diet
Isocal HCN
Isocal Tube Feeding Set
Lofenalac
Lonalac
Lytren
MCT Oil
Nutramigen
◆Poly-Vi-Sol Vitamins, Chewable Tablets & Drops
◆Poly-Vi-Sol Vitamins, Circus Shapes, Chewable with & without Iron
◆Poly-Vi-Sol Vitamins with Iron, Chewable Tablets
◆Poly-Vi-Sol Vitamins w/Iron, Drops
Portagen
Pregestimil
ProSobee
Smurf Chewable Vitamins
Smurf Chewable Vitamins with Iron and Zinc
Sustacal Liquid
Sustacal Powder & Pudding
Sustacal HC
Sustagen
◆Tempra
TraumaCal
Trind
Trind-DM
◆Tri-Vi-Sol Vitamin Drops
◆Tri-Vi-Sol Vitamin Drops w/Iron

MEAD JOHNSON   **414, 606**
PHARMACEUTICALS
A Bristol-Myers Comapny
2400 W. Lloyd Expressway
Evansville, IN 47721
            (812) 429-5000
Address Inquiries to:
Scientific Information Section
   Medical Department
OTC Products Available
◆Colace
Natalins
◆Peri-Colace

MEDICONE COMPANY   **414, 607**
225 Varick St.
New York, NY 10014
Address inquiries to:
Medical Director   (212) 924-5166
OTC Products Available
◆Medicone Derma Ointment
◆Medicone Dressing Cream
◆Medicone Rectal Ointment
◆Medicone Rectal Suppositories
◆Mediconet Cleansing Cloths

MERICON INDUSTRIES, INC.   **608**
8819 North Pioneer Rd.
Peoria, IL 61615
Address inquiries to:
Thomas P. Morrissey (800) 242-6464
   In IL Collect (309) 693-2150

OTC Products Available
Delacort
Orazinc Capsules
Orazinc Lozenges

MILES INC.   **415, 608**
1127 Myrtle Street
Elkhart, IN 46514
Address inquiries to:
Manager, Consumer Affairs Dept.
            (219) 264-8955
For Medical Emergencies Contact:
Medical Department   (219) 262-7886
OTC Products Available
◆Alka-Mints Chewable Antacid
◆Alka-Seltzer Effervescent Antacid
◆Alka-Seltzer Effervescent Antacid & Pain Reliever
◆Alka-Seltzer (Flavored) Effervescent Antacid & Pain Reliever
◆Alka-Seltzer Extra Strength Effervescent Antacid & Pain Reliever
◆Alka-Seltzer Plus Cold Medicine
◆Alka-Seltzer Plus Night-Time Cold Medicine
◆Bactine Antiseptic/Anesthetic First Aid Spray
◆Bactine First Aid Antibiotic Ointment
◆Bactine Hydrocortisone Skin Care Cream
◆Biocal 500 mg Tablet Calcium Supplement
◆Bugs Bunny Children's Chewable Vitamins (Sugar Free)
◆Bugs Bunny Children's Chewable Vitamins + Minerals with Iron & Calcium (Sugar Free)
◆Bugs Bunny Plus Iron Children's Chewable Vitamins (Sugar Free)
◆Bugs Bunny With Extra C Children's Chewable Vitamins (Sugar Free)
◆Flintstones Children's Chewable Vitamins
◆Flintstones Children's Chewable Vitamins Plus Iron
◆Flintstones Children's Chewable Vitamins With Extra C
◆Flintstones Complete With Iron, Calcium & Minerals Children's Chewable Vitamins
◆Miles Nervine Nighttime Sleep-Aid
◆One-A-Day Essential Vitamins
◆One-A-Day Maximum Formula Vitamins and Minerals
◆One-A-Day Plus Extra C Vitamins
◆Stressgard Stress Formula Vitamins
◆Within Multivitamin for Women with Calcium, Extra Iron and Zinc

MORE DIRECT RESPONSE, INC.   **615**
6351-E Yarrow Drive
Carlsbad, CA 92009
Address inquiries to:
            (619) 438-1935
For Medical Emergencies Contact:
            (619) 438-1935
OTC Products Available
CigArrest Tablets

MURO PHARMACEUTICAL, INC.   **615**
890 East Street
Tewksbury, MA 01876-9987
Address inquiries to:
Professional Service Dept.
            (800) 225-0974
            (508) 851-5981
OTC Products Available
Bromfed Syrup
Salinex Nasal Mist & Drops

NATREN INC.   **615**
10935 Camarillo Street
North Hollywood, CA 91602
Address inquiries to:
   Toll-Free (800) 992-3323
   CA Only (800) 992-9393
OTC Products Available
Bifido Factor (Bifidobacterium bifidum)
Bulgaricum I.B. (Lactobacillus bulgaricus)
Life Start (Bifidobacterium infantis)
M.F.A.-Milk Free Acidophilus (Dairy Free Lactobacillus acidophilus)
Superdophilus (Lactobacillus acidophilus)

NATURE'S BOUNTY, INC.   **616**
90 Orville Drive
Bohemia, NY 11716
Address inquiries to:
Professional Service Dept.
            (516) 567-9500
            (800) 645-5412
OTC Products Available
B-12 & B-12 Sublingual Tablets
B-50 Tablets
B-100 Tablets-Ultra B Complex
B-Complex +C (Long Acting) Tablets
Beta-Carotene Capsules
Calciday-667
Calmtabs Tablets
Ener-B Vitamin B_{12} Nasal Gel Dietary Supplement
KLB6 Capsules
KLB6 Complete Tablets
KLB6 Grapefruit Diet
l-Lysine 500 mg Tablets
M-KYA
Nature's Bounty 1 Tablets
Oyster Calcium Tablets
Oystercal-D 250
Oystercal-500
Slim with Fiber Tablets
Stress "1000" Tablets
l-Tryptophan (200 mg, 500 mg, & 667 mg)
Ultra Vita-Time Tablets
Vitamin C with Rose Hips
Vitamin E (d-alpha tocopheryl)
Water Pill (Natural Diuretic)
Water Pill with Potassium (Natural Diuretic)
Zacne Tablets

NORCLIFF THAYER INC.   **416, 616**
303 South Broadway
Tarrytown, NY 10591
            (914) 631-0033
OTC Products Available
◆A-200 Pediculicide Shampoo and Gel Concentrates
AsthmaHaler Mist Epinephrine Bitartrate Bronchodilator
AsthmaNefrin Solution "A" Bronchodilator
◆Avail
Esotérica Medicated Fade Cream
◆Liquiprin Children's Elixir
◆Liquiprin Infants'Drops
◆Nature's Remedy Natural Vegetable Laxative
◆NoSalt Salt Alternative, Regular
◆NoSalt Salt Alternative, Seasoned
◆Oxy Clean Lathering Facial Scrub
◆Oxy Clean Medicated Cleanser
◆Oxy Clean Medicated Pads - Regular and Maximum Strength
◆Oxy Clean Medicated Soap
◆Oxy-5 Tinted Formula with Sorboxyl
◆Oxy-10 Tinted Formula with Sorboxyl
◆Oxy-5 & Oxy-10 Vanishing Formula with Sorboxyl
◆Oxy-10 Wash Antibacterial Skin Wash
◆Tums Antacid Tablets
◆Tums E-X Antacid Tablets
◆Tums Liquid Extra-Strength Antacid
◆Tums Liquid Extra-Strength Antacid with Simethicone

NOXELL CORPORATION   **417, 621**
11050 York Road
Hunt Valley MD 21030-2098
For Medical Emergencies Contact:
Edward M. Jackson, Ph.D.
            (301) 785-4397
OTC Products Available
◆Noxzema Antiseptic Skin Cleanser-Extra Strength Formula
◆Noxzema Antiseptic Skin Cleanser-Regular Formula
◆Noxzema Antiseptic Skin Cleanser-Sensitive Skin Formula
◆Noxzema Clear-Ups Anti-Acne Gel

(◆ Shown in Product Identification Section)

◆Noxzema Clear-Ups Maximum Strength
Lotion, Vanishing
◆Noxzema Clear-Ups Medicated
Pads-Maximum Strength 2.0%
Salicylic Acid
◆Noxzema Clear-Ups Medicated
Pads-Regular Strength 0.5%
Salicyclic Acid
◆Noxzema Clear-Ups On-the-Spot
Treatment, Tinted & Vanishing
Noxzema Clear-Ups Peel-Off Mask
Noxzema Medicated Shave Cream
◆Noxzema Medicated Skin Cream

NUAGE LABORATORIES, LTD.   622
4200 Laclede Avenue
St. Louis, MO 63108
   Address inquiries to:
Customer Service   (314) 533-9600
   OTC Products Available
Biochemic Tissue Salts
Bioplasma
Calcium Fluoride
Calcium Phosphate
Calcium Sulfate
Ferrous Phosphate
Magnesium Phosphate
Potassium Chloride
Potassium Phosphate
Potassium Sulfate
Silica
Sodium Chloride
Sodium Phosphate
Sodium Sulfate
Tissue A
Tissue B
Tissue C
Tissue D
Tissue E
Tissue G
Tissue H
Tissue I
Tissue J
Tissue K
Tissue M
Tissue N
Tissue O
Tissue P

NUMARK LABORATORIES, INC.   622
P. O. Box 6321
Edison, NJ 08818
   Address inquiries to:
Susan Wilson   (201) 417-1871
              (800) 338-8079
   OTC Products Available
Certan-dri Antiperspirant

ORAL-B LABORATORIES   417, 623
One Lagoon Drive
Redwood City, CA 94065
   Address inquiries to:
P. J. Brochier
Product Manager
              (800) 874-5772
              (415) 598-5000
   OTC Products Available
◆Amosan

ORTHO   417, 623, 760
PHARMACEUTICAL
CORPORATION
Advanced Care Products Division
Route #202
Raritan, NJ 08869   (201) 524-0400
   For Medical Emergencies Contact:
Dr. B. Malyk   (201) 524-5211
   OTC Products Available
◆Advance Pregnancy Test
◆Conceptrol Single Use Contraceptives
◆Daisy 2 Pregnancy Test
◆Delfen Contraceptive Foam
◆Fact Plus Pregnancy Test
◆Gynol II Contraceptive Jelly
◆Intercept Contraceptive Inserts
◆Masse Breast Cream
◆Micatin Antifungal Cream
◆Micatin Antifungal Powder
◆Micatin Antifungal Spray Liquid
Micatin Antifungal Deodorant Spray
Powder
◆Micatin Antifungal Spray Powder
Micatin Jock Itch Cream
Micatin Jock Itch Spray Powder

◆Ortho Personal Lubricant
◆Ortho-Creme Contraceptive Cream
◆Ortho-Gynol Contraceptive Jelly

ORTHO PHARMACEUTICAL
CORPORATION
See JOHNSON & JOHNSON BABY
PRODUCTS COMPANY

PADDOCK LABORATORIES, INC.   626
3101 Louisiana Ave. North
Minneapolis, MN 55427
   Address inquiries to:
Robert E. Freye   (612) 546-4676
Roscoe D. Heim   (800) 328-5113
   For Medical Emergencies Contact:
Bruce G. Paddock   (800) 328-5113
   OTC Products Available
Actidose-Aqua
Actidose with Sorbitol
Emulsoil
Glutose
Ipecac Syrup

PARKE-DAVIS   418, 627, 761
Consumer Health Products Group
Division of Warner-Lambert Company
201 Tabor Road
Morris Plains, New Jersey 07950
See also Warner-Lambert Company
              (201) 540-2000
   For product information call:
         1-(800) 223-0432
   For medical information call:
         (201) 540-3950
   Regional Sales Offices
Atlanta, GA 30328
  1140 Hammond Drive
             (404) 396-4080
Baltimore (Hunt Valley), MD 21031
  11350 McCormick Road
             (301) 666-7810
Chicago (Schaumburg), IL 60195
  1111 Plaza Drive   (312) 884-6990
Dallas (Grand Prairie), TX 75234
  12200 Ford Road   (214) 484-5566
Detroit (Troy), MI 48084
  500 Stephenson Highway
             (313) 589-3292
Los Angeles (Tustin), CA 92680
  17822 East 17th Street
             (714) 731-3441
Memphis, TN 38119
  1355 Lynnfield Road
             (901) 767-1921
New York (Paramus, NJ) 07652
  12 Route 17 North
             (201) 368-0733
Pittsburgh, PA 15220
  1910 Cochran Road
             (412) 343-9855
Seattle (Bellevue), WA 98004
  301 116th Avenue, SE
             (206) 451-1119
   OTC Products Available
Agoral
Agoral, Marshmallow Flavor
Agoral, Raspberry Flavor
Alcohol, Rubbing (Lavacol)
Alophen Pills
◆Anusol Hemorrhoidal Suppositories
◆Anusol Ointment
◆Benadryl Anti-Itch Cream
◆Benadryl Decongestant Elixir
◆Benadryl Decongestant Kapseals
◆Benadryl Decongestant Tablets
◆Benadryl Elixir
◆Benadryl 25 Kapseals
◆Benadryl 25 Tablets
◆Benadryl Plus Tablets
◆Benadryl Spray
◆Benylin Cough Syrup
◆Benylin DM
◆Benylin Decongestant
◆Benylin Expectorant
◆Caladryl Cream, Lotion
◆e.p.t. plus In-Home Early Pregnancy
Test
◆e.p.t Stick Test
◆Gelusil Liquid & Tablets
Gelusil-M Liquid & Tablets
Gelusil-II Liquid & Tablets
Geriplex-FS Kapseals

Geriplex-FS Liquid
Hydrogen Peroxide Solution
Lavacol
◆Mediquell Chewy Cough Squares
◆Mediquell Decongestant Formula
◆Myadec
Natabec Kapseals
Peroxide, Hydrogen
◆Promega
◆Promega Pearls
Rubbing Alcohol (Lavacol)
Siblin Granules
◆Sinutab Maximum Strength Caplets
◆Sinutab Maximum Strength Tablets
◆Sinutab Tablets
◆Sinutab Maximum Strength Without
Drowsiness Tablets & Caplets
Thera-Combex H-P Kapseals
Tucks Cream
Tucks Ointment
◆Tucks Premoistened Pads
Tucks Take-Alongs
◆Ziradryl Lotion

PHARMAFAIR, INC.   636
205-C Kelsey Lane
Silo Bend
Tampa, FL 33619
   Address inquiries to:
Saul Schwartz, National Field Manager
              (800) 227-1427
              (813) 972-7705
   OTC Products Available
Benzoyl Peroxide Gel 5% and 10%
Boric Acid Ointment 5%
Cortifair Cream 0.5% and Lotion 0.5%
Delicate Eyes Cleaning Solution
Delicate Eyes Lubricating & Rewetting
Solution
Delicate Eyes Rinsing & Storage
Solution
Delicate Eyes Saline Solution
(non-preserved)
Delicate Eyes Saline Solution
(preserved)
Ear Drops
Eye Drops 15ml
Eye Wash
Lubrifair Ointment
Lubrifair Solution
Meclizine HCl Chewable Tablets 25mg
Ocugestrin Solution
Petrolatum Ointment
Pseudoephedrine HCl Tablets 30mg
Senna Tabs 217mg
Tearfair Dry Eyes Solution
Tearfair Ointment
Tolnaftate 1% Cream and 1% Solution
Topisporin Ointment
Wetting Solution for Hard Contact
Lenses

PLOUGH, INC.   419, 636
3030 Jackson Avenue
Memphis, TN 38151
   Address inquiries to:
Consumer Relations Dept.
              (901) 320-2386
   For Medical Emergencies Contact:
Clinical Affairs Dept.
              (901) 320-2011
   OTC Products Available
◆Aftate for Athlete's Foot
◆Aftate for Jock Itch
Aspergum
◆Coppertone Sunscreen Lotion SPF 6
◆Coppertone Sunscreen Lotion SPF 8
◆Coppertone Sunblock Lotion SPF 15
◆Coppertone Sunblock Lotion SPF 25
◆Coppertone Sunblock Lotion SPF 30
Coppertone Sunblock Lotion SPF 44
Coppertone Sun Spray Mist SPF 10
◆Correctol Laxative Tablets
Cushion Grip Denture Adhesive
◆Di-Gel Antacid/Anti-Gas
◆Duration Long Acting Nasal
Decongestant Tablets
◆Duration 12 Hour Mentholated Nasal
Spray
◆Duration 12 Hour Nasal Spray
◆Duration 12 Hour Nasal Spray Pump
◆Feen-A-Mint Gum
◆Feen-A-Mint Pills

(◆ Shown in Product Identification Section)

Muskol Insect Repellent Aerosol Liquid
Muskol Insect Repellent Lotion
Muskol Insect Repellent Pump Spray
Muskol Insect Repellent Roll-on
◆Regutol Stool Softener
St. Joseph Adult Aspirin (325 mg.)
St. Joseph Adult Chewable Aspirin (81 mg.)
◆St. Joseph Anti-Diarrheal for Children
◆St. Joseph Aspirin-Free Fever Reducer for Children Chewable Tablets, Liquid & Infant Drops
St. Joseph Cold Tablets for Children
◆St. Joseph Cough Suppressant for Children
◆St. Joseph Measured Dose Nasal Decongestant
◆St. Joseph Nighttime Cold Medicine
◆Solarcaine
◆Stay Trim Diet Gum
◆Stay Trim Diet Mints
Super Shade Clear Gel SPF 15
◆Super Shade Sunblock Lotion SPF 15
◆Super Shade Sunblock Lotion SPF 25
◆Super Shade Sunblock Lotion SPF 30
Super Shade Sunblock Lotion SPF 44
Super Shade Sunblock Stick SPF 25
◆Water Babies Sunblock Cream
◆Water Babies Sunblock Lotion

PROCTER & GAMBLE   420, 640
P.O. Box 171
Cincinnati, OH 45201
Also see Richardson-Vicks
Health Care Products
Address inquiries to:
Lawrence W. Farrell   (513) 983-7469
For Medical Emergencies Contact:
J.B. Lucas, M.D.   (513) 530-3350
After hours, call Collect
           (513) 751-5525
OTC Products Available
Denquel Sensitive Teeth Toothpaste
◆Head & Shoulders
◆Metamucil, Effervescent, Sugar Free, Lemon-Lime Flavor
◆Metamucil, Effervescent, Sugar Free, Orange Flavor
◆Metamucil Powder, Orange Flavor
◆Metamucil Powder, Regular Flavor
◆Metamucil Powder, Strawberry Flavor
◆Metamucil Powder, Sugar Free, Orange Flavor
◆Metamucil Powder, Sugar Free, Regular Flavor
◆Pepto-Bismol Liquid & Tablets
◆Maximum Strength Pepto-Bismol Liquid

REED & CARNRICK   421, 643
1 New England Avenue
Piscataway, NJ 08855
Address Inquiries to:
Professional Service Dept.
           (201) 981-0070
For Medical Emergencies Contact:
Medical Director   (201) 981-0070
OTC Products Available
Alphosyl Lotion
Phazyme Tablets
◆Phazyme-95 Tablets
◆Phazyme-125 Capsules Maximum Strength
◆proctoFoam/non-steroid
◆R&C Lice Treatment Kit
◆R&C Shampoo
◆R&C Spray III
Trichotine Liquid, Vaginal Douche
Trichotine Powder, Vaginal Douche

REID-ROWELL   421, 645
901 Sawyer Road
Marietta, GA 30062
and
210 Main Street W.
Baudette, MN 56623
Address Inquiries to:
Director, Medical Services
           (404) 578-9000
For Medical Emergencies Contact:
Director, Medical Services
           (404) 578-9000

OTC Products Available
◆Balneol
Colrex Capsules
Colrex Expectorant
Colrex Syrup
Colrex Troches
◆Hydrocil Instant

REQUA, INC.   645
Box 4008
1 Seneca Place
Greenwich, CT 06830
Address inquiries to:
Geoffrey Geils   (203) 869-2445
OTC Products Available
Charcoaid
Charcoal Tablets
Charcocaps

**RICHARDSON-VICKS USA,   421, 646
HEALTH CARE PRODUCTS
DIVISION**
Richardson-Vicks Inc.
10 Westport Road
Wilton, CT 06897
Address inquiries to:
Director of Scientific & Regulatory Affairs
Vicks Research Center
           (203) 929-2500
For Medical Emergencies Contact
Medical Director
Vicks Research Center
           (203) 929-2500
OTC Products Available
◆Chloraseptic Children's Lozenges
◆Chloraseptic Liquid and Spray
◆Chloraseptic Liquid - Nitrogen Propelled Spray
◆Chloraseptic Lozenges
Cremacoat 1
Cremacoat 2
Cremacoat 3
Cremacoat 4
◆Dramamine Liquid
◆Dramamine Tablets and Chewable Tablets
Head & Chest Cold Medicine
◆Icy Hot Balm
◆Icy Hot Cream
◆Icy Hot Stick
◆Norwich Aspirin
Norwich Extra Strength Aspirin
◆Percogesic Analgesic Tablets
Vicks Children's Cough Syrup
◆Vicks Children's NyQuil
Vicks Cough Silencers Cough Drops
◆Vicks Daycare Colds Caplets
◆Vicks Daycare Colds Liquid
Vicks Formula 44 Cough Control Discs
◆Vicks Formula 44 Cough Mixture
◆Vicks Formula 44D Decongestant Cough Mixture
◆Vicks Formula 44M Multisymptom Cough Mixture
Vicks Inhaler
◆Vicks NyQuil Nighttime Colds Medicine-Regular & Cherry Flavor
Vicks Oracin Cherry Flavor Cooling Throat Lozenges
Vicks Oracin Cooling Throat Lozenges
◆Vicks Sinex Decongestant Nasal Spray
◆Vicks Sinex Decongestant Nasal Ultra Fine Mist
◆Vicks Sinex Long-Acting Decongestant Nasal Spray
◆Vicks Sinex Long-Acting Decongestant Nasal Ultra Fine Mist
Vicks Throat Drops
     Cherry Flavor
     Ice Blue
     Lemon Flavor
     Regular Flavor
Vicks Throat Lozenges
◆Vicks Vaporub
Vicks Vaporsteam
Vicks Vatronol Nose Drops
Victors Menthol-Eucalyptus Vapor Cough Drops
     Cherry Flavor
     Regular

**RICHARDSON-VICKS USA,   422, 653
PERSONAL CARE
PRODUCTS DIVISION**
10 Westport Road
Wilton, CT 06897
Address inquiries to:
Vicks Research Center
           (203) 929-2500
For Medical Emergencies Contact
Medical Director
Vicks Research Center
           (203) 929-2500
OTC Products Available
◆Clearasil Adult Care Medicated Blemish Cream
Clearasil Adult Care Medicated Blemish Stick
Clearasil Antibacterial Soap
Clearasil 10% Benzoyl Peroxide Medicated Anti-Acne Lotion
◆Clearasil Maximum Strength Medicated Anti-Acne Cream, Tinted
◆Clearasil Maximum Strength Medicated Anti-Acne Cream, Vanishing
◆Clearasil Medicated Astringent

ORAL HEALTH PRODUCTS
Benzodent Analgesic Denture Ointment
Complete Denture Cleanser and Toothpaste in One
Extra Hold Fasteeth for Lowers Denture Adhesive Powder
Fasteeth Denture Adhesive Powder
Fixodent Denture Adhesive Cream
Kleenite Denture Cleanser

**A. H. ROBINS COMPANY,   422, 654
INC.
CONSUMER PRODUCTS
DIVISION**
3800 Cutshaw Avenue
Richmond, VA 23230
Address inquiries to:
The Medical Department
           (804) 257-2000
For Medical Emergencies Contact:
Medical Department   (804) 257-2000
(day or night)
If no answer, call answering service
           (804) 257-7788
OTC Products Available
◆Allbee C-800 Plus Iron Tablets
◆Allbee C-800 Tablets
◆Allbee with C Caplets
◆Chap Stick Lip Balm
◆Chap Stick Petroleum Jelly Plus
◆Chap Stick Petroleum Jelly Plus with Sunblock 15
◆Chap Stick SUNBLOCK 15 Lip Balm
Cough Calmers Lozenges
◆Dimacol Caplets
◆Dimetane Decongestant Caplets
◆Dimetane Decongestant, Elixir
◆Dimetane Elixir
◆Dimetane Extentabs 8 mg
◆Dimetane Extentabs 12 mg
◆Dimetane Tablets
◆Dimetapp Elixir
◆Dimetapp Extentabs
◆Dimetapp Plus Caplets
◆Dimetapp Tablets
◆Donnagel
◆Robitussin
◆Robitussin-CF
◆Robitussin-DM
◆Robitussin-PE
◆Robitussin Night Relief
◆Z-Bec Tablets

**RORER CONSUMER   424, 661
PHARMACEUTICALS**
a division of
Rorer Pharmaceutical Corporation
500 Virginia Drive
Fort Washington, PA 19034
*For Medical Emergencies/
Product Information Contact:*
Medical Services
           (215) 628-6627
           (215) 628-6065

(◆ Shown in Product Identification Section)

For Reports of Adverse Drug Experiences Contact:
Product Surveillance (215) 956-5136
For Quality Assurance Questions Contact:
John Chiles
Complaint Coordinator
(215) 628-6416
For Regulatory Affairs Questions Contact:
Ron Panner
Director, Regulatory Affairs
(215) 956-5119
For Product Information Contact:
Medical Services
(215) 628-6627
(215) 628-6065
OTC Products Available
◆Regular Strength Ascriptin Tablets
◆Ascriptin A/D Caplets
◆Extra Strength Ascriptin Caplets
◆Camalox Suspension
Camalox Tablets
Fermalox Tablets
◆Maalox Suspension
◆Maalox Tablets
◆Extra Strength Maalox Tablets
◆Extra Strength Maalox Whip
◆Extra Strength Maalox Plus Suspension
(reformulated Maalox Plus)
◆Maalox Plus Tablets
◆Maalox TC Suspension
◆Maalox TC Tablets
◆Myoflex Creme
◆Perdiem Granules
◆Perdiem Fiber Granules

ROSS LABORATORIES   425, 667
Division of Abbott Laboratories USA
P.O. Box 1317
Columbus, OH 43216-1317
Address Inquiries to:
Medical Director   (614) 227-3333
OTC Products Available
Advance Nutritional Beverage With Iron
◆Clear Eyes Lubricating Eye Redness
Reliever
◆Ear Drops by Murine
(See Murine Ear Wax Removal
System/Murine Ear Drops)
Isomil Soy Protein Formula With Iron
Isomil SF Sucrose-Free Soy Protein
Formula With Iron
◆Murine Ear Wax Removal
System/Murine Ear Drops
◆Murine Eye Lubricant
◆Murine Plus Lubricating Eye Redness
Reliever
Pedialyte Oral Electrolyte Maintenance
Solution
RCF Ross Carbohydrate Free Low-Iron
Soy Protein Formula Base
Rehydralyte Oral Electrolyte
Rehydration Solution
◆Selsun Blue Dandruff Shampoo
(selenium sulfide lotion 1%)
◆Selsun Blue Extra Conditioning
Dandruff Shampoo
◆Selsun Blue Extra Medicated Dandruff
Shampoo
Similac Low-Iron Infant Formula
Similac PM 60/40 Low-Iron Infant
Formula
Similac With Iron Infant Formula
◆Tronolane Anesthetic Cream for
Hemorrhoids
◆Tronolane Anesthetic Suppositories for
Hemorrhoids

**RYDELLE LABORATORIES,   425, 674
INC.**
Subsidiary of S.C. Johnson & Son, Inc.
1525 Howe Street
Racine, WI 53403
Address inquiries to:
Carol Hansen
Consumer Affairs Director
(414) 631-4000
For Medical Emergencies Contact:
Richard D. Stewart M.D., M.P.H.,
F.A.C.P.
(414) 631-2111

OTC Products Available
◆Aveeno Bath Oilated
◆Aveeno Bath Regular
◆Aveeno Cleansing Bar for Acne
◆Aveeno Cleansing Bar for Dry Skin
◆Aveeno Cleansing Bar for Normal to
Oily Skin
◆Aveeno Lotion
◆Aveeno Shower and Bath Oil
◆Rhuligel
◆Rhulispray

SANDOZ CONSUMER   425, 675
59 Route 10
East Hanover NJ 07936
Address Medical Inquiries To:
Medical Department
Sandoz Pharmaceuticals Corporation
East Hanover, NJ 07936
(201) 503-7500
Address Other Inquiries To:
Drug Regulation and Regulatory
Affairs Department
Sandoz Pharmaceuticals Corporation
East Hanover, NJ 07936
(201) 503-6462
OTC Products Available
Acid Mantle Creme
◆BiCozene Creme
Cama Arthritis Pain Reliever
Chexit Tablets
Denclenz Denture Cleanser
Derma-Soft Medicated Softening Cream
◆Dorcol Children's Cough Syrup
◆Dorcol Children's Decongestant Liquid
◆Dorcol Children's Fever & Pain Reducer
◆Dorcol Children's Liquid Cold Formula
◆Ex-Lax Chocolated Laxative
◆Ex-Lax Pills, Unflavored
◆Extra Gentle Ex-Lax
◆Extra Strength Gas-X Tablets
◆Gas-X Tablets
◆Gentle Nature Natural Vegetable
Laxative
Kanulase Tablets
Triaminic Allergy Tablets
Triaminic Chewables
◆Triaminic Cold Syrup
◆Triaminic Cold Tablets
◆Triaminic Expectorant
◆Triaminic Nite Light
◆Triaminic-DM Cough Formula
◆Triaminic-12 Tablets
◆Triaminicin Tablets
◆Triaminicol Multi-Symptom Cold Syrup
◆Triaminicol Multi-Symptom Cold Tablets
Tussagesic Tablets
Ursinus Inlay-Tabs

SCHERING CORPORATION   426, 682
Galloping Hill Road
Kenilworth, NJ 07033
Address inquiries to:
Professional Services Department
9:00 AM to 5:00 PM EST
(800) 526-4099
After regular hours and on weekends:
(201) 298-4000
OTC Products Available
A and D Cream
◆A and D Ointment
◆Afrin Menthol Nasal Spray 0.05%
◆Afrin Nasal Spray 0.05%, Nasal Spray
Pump, Nose Drops 0.05%, Chilren's
Strength Nose Drops 0.025%
◆Afrinol Repetabs Tablets
◆Chlor-Trimeton Allergy Syrup, Tablets &
Long-Acting Repetabs Tablets
◆Chlor-Trimeton Decongestant Tablets
◆Chlor-Trimeton Long Acting
Decongestant Repetabs Tablets
◆Chlor-Trimeton Maximum Strength
Timed Release Allergy Tablets
◆Chlor-Trimeton Sinus Caplets
◆Cod Liver Oil Concentrate Tablets,
Capsules
◆Cod Liver Oil Concentrate Tablets
w/Vitamin C
Complex 15 Hand & Body Moisturizing
Cream
Complex 15 Hand & Body Moisturizing
Lotion
Complex 15 Moisturizing Face Cream

◆Coricidin 'D' Decongestant Tablets
Coricidin Decongestant Tablets
◆Coricidin Demilets Tablets for Children
◆Coricidin Maximum Strength Sinus
Headache Caplets
◆Coricidin Tablets
◆Demazin Nasal Decongestant/
Antihistamine Repetabs Tablets &
Syrup
Dermolate Anti-Itch Cream
Diasorb
Disophrol Chronotab Sustained-Action
Tablets
Disophrol Tablets
◆Drixoral Antihistamine/Nasal
Decongestant Syrup
◆Drixoral Sustained-Action Tablets
◆Drixoral Plus Extended Release Tablets
◆Emko Because Contraceptor Vaginal
Contraceptive Foam
◆Emko Vaginal Contraceptive Foam
◆Mol-Iron Tablets
◆Mol-Iron Tablets w/Vitamin C
◆OcuClear Eye Drops
◆Tinactin Aerosol Liquid 1%
◆Tinactin Aerosol Powder 1%
◆Tinactin Antifungal 1%, Cream,
Solution & Powder
◆Tinactin Jock Itch Cream 1%
◆Tinactin Jock Itch Spray Powder 1%

SCHWARZ PHARMA   428, 692
Kremers Urban Company
P.O. Box 2038
Milwaukee, WI 53201
Address inquiries to:
Technical Services Department
(414) 354-4300
(800) 558-5114
For Medical Emergencies Contact:
(414) 354-4300
(800) 558-5114
OTC Products Available
◆Fedahist Decongestant Syrup
◆Fedahist Expectorant Pediatric Drops
◆Fedahist Expectorant Syrup
◆Fedahist Tablets
Gemnisyn Tablets
Kudrox Suspension
◆Lactrase Capsules

**SCOT-TUSSIN PHARMACAL   693
COMPANY, INC.**
50 Clemence Street
Cranston, RI 02920-0217
Address inquiries to:
Professional Service Department
(800) 638-SCOT
(401) 942-8555
OTC Products Available
Febrol Liquid Sugar-Free, Dye-Free &
Alcohol-Free
Ferro-Bob Tablets
Hayfebrol Liquid Sugar-Free, Dye-Free,
Alcohol-Free & Sodium-Free
Scot-Tussin Sugar-Free DM (No Sugar,
Alcohol or Decongestant) Cough &
Cold Medicine
Scot-Tussin DM 2 Syrup (with sugar)
Scot-Tussin Sugar-Free Expectorant (No
Sugar, Sodium, Dye)
Scot-Tussin Sugar-Free Original
5-Action Cold Formula
Scot-Tussin Syrup (with sugar) Original
5-Action Cold Formula
Vita-Bob Softgels
Vita-Plus E Softgels Natural 400 I.U.
Vita-Plus G (geriatric) Softgels
Vita-Plus H (hematinic) Softgels
Vitalize (hematinic) Sugar-Free,
Alcohol-Free, Dye-Free, Sodium-Free
Liquid

**SMITHKLINE CONSUMER   428, 694
PRODUCTS**
a SmithKline Beckman Company
One Franklin Plaza
P.O. Box 8082
Philadelphia, PA 19101
Address inquiries to:
Medical Department   (215) 751-5000
OTC Products Available
◆A.R.M. Allergy Relief Medicine Caplets
◆Acnomel Cream

(◆ Shown in Product Identification Section)

◆Aqua Care Cream
◆Aqua Care Lotion
◆Benzedrex Inhaler
◆Clear by Design Gel
◆Congestac Caplets
◆Contac Caplets
◆Contac Capsules
◆Contac Cough Formula
◆Contac Cough & Sore Throat Formula
◆Contac Jr. Children's Cold Medicine
◆Contac Nighttime Cold Medicine
◆Contac Severe Cold Formula Caplets
◆Ecotrin Regular Strength Tablets and Caplets
◆Ecotrin Maximum Strength Tablets and Caplets
◆Feosol Capsules
◆Feosol Elixir
◆Feosol Tablets
◆Ornex Caplets
◆Sine-Off Maximum Strength Allergy/Sinus Formula Caplets
◆Sine-Off Maximum Strength No Drowsiness Formula Caplets
◆Sine-Off Sinus Medicine Tablets-Aspirin Formula
◆Teldrin Allergy Tablets, 4 mg.
◆Teldrin Timed-Release Capsules, 12 mg.
◆Troph-Iron Liquid
◆Trophite Liquid & Tablets

E. R. SQUIBB & SONS, INC.　430, 704
General Offices
P.O. Box 4000
Princeton, NJ 08540 (609) 921-4000
Address Inquiries to:
Squibb Professional Services Dept.
P.O. Box 4000
Princeton, NJ 08540 (609) 921-4006
Distribution Centers
ATLANTA, GEORGIA
P.O. Box 16503
Atlanta, GA 30321
All Customers Call　(800) 241-5364
CHICAGO, ILLINOIS
P.O. Box 788
Arlington Heights, IL 60006
State of IL Customers Call
(800) 942-0674
All Others Call　(800) 323-0665
DALLAS, TEXAS
Mail or telephone orders and customer service inquiries should be directed to Atlanta, GA (see above)
State of MS Customers Call
(800) 241-1744
All others call　(800) 241-5364
LOS ANGELES, CALIFORNIA
P.O. Box 428
La Mirada, CA 90638
State of CA Customers Call
(800) 422-4254
State of HI Customers Call
(714) 521-7050
All Others Call　(800) 854-3050
SEATTLE, WASHINGTON
Mail or telephone orders and customer service inquiries should be directed to Los Angeles, CA (see above)
States of AK and MT Customers Call
(714) 521-7050
State of CA Customers Call
(800) 422-4254
All Others Call　(800) 854-3050
NEW YORK AREA
P.O. Box 2013
New Brunswick, NJ 08903
State of NJ Customers Call
(800) 352-4865
State of ME Customers Call
(201) 469-5400
All Others Call　(800) 631-5244
OTC Products Available
Engran-HP Tablets
◆Proto-Chol Natural Fish Oil Gelcaps
◆Proto-Chol Mini-caps Natural Fish Oil Gelcaps
Spec-T Sore Throat Anesthetic Lozenges

Spec-T Sore Throat/Cough Suppressant Lozenges
Spec-T Sore Throat/Decongestant Lozenges
Spectrocin Plus Ointment
◆Theragran Jr. Chewable Tablets
◆Theragran Jr. Chewable Tablets with Extra Vitamin C
◆Theragran Jr. Chewable Tablets with Iron
◆Theragran Liquid
◆Theragran Stress Formula
◆Theragran Tablets
◆Theragran-M Tablets
Trigesic Tablets
Valadol Liquid
Valadol Tablets
Vigran Tablets
Vigran Plus Iron Tablets

STELLAR PHARMACAL　431, 706 CORP.
1990 N.W. 44th Street
Pompano Beach, FL 33064-1278
Address inquiries to:
Scott L. Davidson　(305) 972-6060
Customer Service & Order Department
(800) 845-7827
OTC Products Available
◆Star-Otic Ear Solution

STUART　431, 706 PHARMACEUTICALS
Div. of ICI Americas, Inc.
Wilmington, DE 19897
Address inquiries to:
Yvonne A. Graham, Manager
Professional Services
(302) 575-2231
For Medical Emergencies:
After hours & on weekends
(302) 575-3000
OTC Products Available
◆ALternaGEL Liquid
◆Dialose Capsules
◆Dialose Plus Capsules
◆Effer-Syllium Natural Fiber Bulking Agent
Ferancee Chewable Tablets
◆Ferancee-HP Tablets
◆Hibiclens
Hibistat Germicidal Hand Rinse
Hibistat Towelette
◆Kasof Capsules
◆Mylanta Liquid
◆Mylanta Tablets
◆Mylanta-II Liquid
◆Mylanta-II Tablets
◆Mylicon (Tablets & Drops)
◆Mylicon-80 Tablets
◆Mylicon-125 Tablets
◆Orexin Softab Tablets
◆Probec-T Tablets
◆The Stuart Formula Tablets
◆Stuart Prenatal Tablets
◆Stuartinic Tablets

SYNTEX LABORATORIES, INC.　713
3401 Hillview Avenue
P.O. Box 10850
Palo Alto, CA 94304
Direct General/Sales/Order inquiries for U.S. Marketed products to:
Marketing Information Department
Specify product　(415) 855-5050
Direct Medical inquiries on U.S. marketed products to:
Medical Services Department
General Medical Inquiries
(415) 855-5545
Adverse Reactions Inquiries
(415) 852-1386
OTC Products Available
Carmol 10, 10% Urea Lotion
Carmol 20, 20% Urea Cream

TAMBRANDS INC.　432, 763
Lake Success, NY 11042
OTC Products Available
◆First Response Ovulation Predictor Test
◆First Response Pregnancy Test

THOMPSON MEDICAL　432, 713 COMPANY, INC.
919 Third Avenue
New York, NY 10022
Address inquiries to:
Medical Services　(212) 688-4420
OTC Products Available
Appedrine, Maximum Strength Tablets
Aqua-Ban Tablets
Aqua-Ban, Maximum Strength Plus Tablets
◆Aspercreme Creme & Lotion
Cardi-Omega 3
Control Capsules
◆Cortizone-5 Creme & Ointment
Dexatrim Capsules
◆Dexatrim Maximum Strength Caffeine-Free Caplets
Dexatrim Maximum Strength Caffeine-Free Capsules
◆Dexatrim Maximum Strength Plus Vitamin C/Caffeine-free Caplets
◆Dexatrim Maximum Strength Plus Vitamin C/Caffeine-free Capsules
Dexatrim Maximum Strength Pre-Meal Caplets
Diar Aid Tablets and Liquid
Encare
End Lice
Ibuprin
◆NP-27 Cream, Solution, Spray Powder & Powder
Prolamine Maximum Strength Capsules
◆Sleepinal Night-time Sleep Aid Capsules
Slim-Fast
Sportscreme
Tempo Antacid with Antigas Action
◆Ultra Slim Fast

TRITON CONSUMER PRODUCTS,　716 INC.
5105 Tollview Drive, Suite 190
Rolling Meadows, IL 60008
Address inquiries to:
Karen Shrader　(312) 577-5900
For Medical Emergencies Contact
(312) 577-5900
OTC Products Available
MG 217 Psoriasis Ointment
MG 217 Psoriasis Shampoo
MG 400 Severe Dandruff Shampoo
ProTech First-Aid Stik
Skeeter Stik Insect Bite Medication
Skeeter Stop 100 Insect Repellent

UAS LABORATORIES　717
9201 Penn Avenue South #10
Minneapolis, MN 55431
Address inquiries to:
Dr. S. K. Dash　(612) 881-1915
(800) 422-3371
OTC Products Available
DDS-Acidophilus

ULTRABALANCE PRODUCTS　717
3215 56th Street NW
Gig Harbor, WA 98335
Address inquiries to:
(800) 843-9660
(206) 851-3943
For Medical Emergencies Contact:
Dr. Pattabi Raman　(800) 843-9660
(206) 851-3943
OTC Products Available
UltraBalance Weight Management Products - Herbulk
UltraBalance Weight Management Products - Protein Formula

UNITED MEDICAL　717
Division of Pfizer Hospital Products Group, Inc.
11775 Starkey Road
Largo, FL 34643-4799
Address inquiries to:
(813) 392-1261
OTC Products Available
Soft Guard Sheer Plus One-Piece System
Soft Guard XL One-Piece System
Soft Guard XL Skin Barrier
Soft Guard XL Two-Piece System
UniFlex Transparent Dressings and Drapes

(◆ Shown in Product Identification Section)

THE UPJOHN COMPANY 432, 718
7000 Portage Road
Kalamazoo, MI 49001
Direct inquiries to:
Medical Information (616) 323-6615
*Pharmaceutical Sales Areas
and Distribution Centers*
Atlanta (Chamblee)
GA 30341-2626 (404) 451-4822
Boston (Wellesley)
MA 02181 (617) 431-7970
Buffalo (Cheektowaga)
NY 14225 (716) 681-7160
Chicago (Oak Brook Terrace)
IL 60181 (312) 574-3300
Cincinnati, OH 45237
(513) 242-4574
Dallas, TX 75205 (214) 520-7855
Denver, CO 80216 (303) 399-3113
Hartford (Enfield)
CT 06082 (203) 741-3421
Honolulu, HI 96818 (808) 422-2777
Kalamazoo, MI 49001
(616) 323-4000
Kansas City, MO 64131
(816) 361-2286
Los Angeles, CA 90038
(213) 463-8101
Memphis, TN 38138 (901) 756-1476
Minneapolis (Bloomington), MN 55437
(612) 921-8484
New York (Uniondale)
NY 11553 (516) 745-6100
Orlando, FL 32809 (407) 859-4591
Philadelphia (Wayne)
PA 19087 (215) 265-2100
Pittsburgh (Bridgeville)
PA 15017 (412) 257-0200
Portland, OR 97232 (503) 232-2133
St. Louis, MO 63146 (314) 872-8626
San Francisco (Palo Alto)
CA 94306-2117 (415) 493-8080
Shreveport, LA 71129
(318) 688-3700
Washington, DC 20011
(202) 882-6163
OTC Products Available
Alkets Tablets
Baciguent Antibiotic Ointment
Calcium Gluconate Tablets, USP
Calcium Lactate Tablets, USP
Cheracol Cough Syrup
◆Cheracol D Cough Formula
◆Cheracol Plus Head Cold/Cough
Formula
Citrocarbonate Antacid
Clocream Skin Cream
◆Cortaid Cream with Aloe
◆Cortaid Lotion
◆Cortaid Ointment with Aloe
◆Cortaid Spray
Cortef Feminine Itch Cream
Diostate D Tablets
◆Haltran Tablets
◆Kaopectate Concentrated Anti-Diarrheal,
Peppermint Flavor
◆Kaopectate Concentrated Anti-Diarrheal,
Regular Flavor
◆Maximum Strength Kaopectate Tablets
Anti-Diarrhea Medicine
Lipomul Oral Liquid
Myciguent Antibiotic Cream
Myciguent Antibiotic Ointment
◆Mycitracin Triple Antibiotic Ointment
Orthoxicol Cough Syrup
P-A-C Revised Formula Analgesic
Tablets
Phenolax Wafers
◆Pyrroxate Capsules ·
Sigtab Tablets
Super D Perles
Unicap Capsules & Tablets
Unicap Jr Chewable Tablets
◆Unicap M Tablets
Unicap Plus Iron Tablets
◆Unicap Senior Tablets
◆Unicap T Tablets
Zymacap Capsules

WAKUNAGA OF AMERICA 433, 722
CO., LTD.
Subsidiary of Wakunaga Pharmaceutical
Co., Ltd.

23501 Madero
Mission Viejo, CA 92691
Address inquires to:
(714) 855-2776
OTC Products Available
◆Kyolic
◆ Kyolic-Aged Garlic Extract Flavor &
Odor Modified Enriched with
Vitamins B_1 & B_{12}
Kyolic-Aged Garlic Extract Flavor &
Odor Modified Plain
Kyolic-Aged Garlic Extract Liquid
Enriched with Vitamins B_1 & B_{12}
Kyolic-Aged Garlic Extract Liquid
Plain
◆ Kyolic-Formula 101 Capsules:
Aged Garlic Extract (270 mg)
Kyolic-Formula 101 Tablets: Aged
Garlic Extract (270 mg)
Kyolic-Formula 103 Capsules:
Aged Garlic Extract Powder
(220 mg)
Kyolic Formula 106 Capsules:
Aged Garlic Extract Powder
(300 mg) & Vitamin E
Kyolic Super Formula 100
Capsules & Tablets: Aged Garlic
Extract Powder (300 mg)
Kyolic Super Formula 100 Tablets:
Aged Garlic Extract Powder
(270 mg)
Kyolic-Super Formula 101, Tablets
& Capsules: Aged Garlic
Extract Powder (270 mg)
with Brewer's Yeast, Kelp & Algin
Kyolic-Super Formula 102, Tablets
& Capsules: Aged
Garlic Extract Powder
(350 mg) with Enzyme Complex
Kyolic-Super Formula 103,
Capsules: Aged Garlic Extract
Powder (220 mg) with Vitamin C,
Astragalus, Calcium
Kyolic Super Formula 104
Capsules: Aged Garlic Extract
Powder (300 mg)
Kyolic-Super Formula 104,
Capsules: Aged Garlic Extract
Powder (300 mg) with
Lecithin
Kyolic Super Formula 105
Capsules: Aged Garlic Extract
Powder (200 mg)
Kyolic-Super Formula 105,
Capsules: Aged Garlic Extract
Powder (250 mg) with
Selenium, Vitamins A & E
Kyolic-Super Formula 106,
Capsules: Aged Garlic Extract
Powder (300 mg) with Vitamin
E, Cayenne Pepper, Hawthorn
Berry
Kyo-Dophilus, Capsules: Acido-
philus, Bifidus, S. Faecalis
Kyo-Green, Powder: Barley &
Wheat Grass, Chlorella,
Brown Rice, Kelp

WALKER, CORP & CO., INC. 433, 722
203 E. Hampton Place
Syracuse, NY 13206
Address inquiries to:
P.O. Box 1320
Syracuse, NY 13201 (315) 463-4511
For Medical Emergencies Contact:
Robert G. Long (315) 638-4763
OTC Products Available
◆Evac-U-Gen Mild Laxative

WALKER PHARMACAL CO. 723
4200 Laclede
St. Louis, MO 63108
Address Inquiries to:
Customer Service (314) 533-9600
OTC Products Available
HIKE Antiseptic Ointment
PRID Salve

WALLACE LABORATORIES 433, 723
Half Acre Road
Cranbury, NJ 08512
Address inquiries to:
Wallace Laboratories
Div. of Carter-Wallace, Inc.
P.O. Drawer #5
Cranbury, NJ 08512 (609) 655-6000
For Medical Emergencies:
(609) 799-1167
OTC Products Available
◆Maltsupex
◆Ryna
◆Ryna-C
◆Ryna-CX
◆Syllact

WARNER-LAMBERT 433, 725, 764
COMPANY
Consumer Health Products Group
201 Tabor Road
Morris Plains, NJ 07950
See also Parke-Davis
Address Inquiries to:
Robert Kirpitch (201) 540-3204
For Medical Emergencies Call:
(201) 540-2000
OTC Products Available
Bromo-Seltzer
Corn Husker's Lotion
◆Early Detector
Efferdent Extra Strength Denture
Cleanser
◆Professional Strength Efferdent
Halls Cough Formula
◆Halls Mentho-Lyptus Cough
Suppressant Tablets
Halls Vitamin C Drops
Listerex Lotion
◆Listerine Antiseptic
◆Listerine Lozenges Regular Strength
◆Listerine Maximum Strength Lozenges
◆Listermint with Fluoride
◆Lubriderm Cream
◆Lubriderm Lotion
◆Lubriderm Lubath Bath-Shower Oil
◆Remegel
◆Rolaids
◆Rolaids (Calcium Rich)
◆Rolaids (Sodium Free)
Sloan's Linament
Super Anahist Tablets

WESTWOOD 434, 727
PHARMACEUTICALS INC.
100 Forest Avenue
Buffalo, NY 14213
(716) 887-3400
Address inquiries to:
Consumer Affairs Department
(716) 887-3773
OTC Products Available
◆Alpha Keri Moisture Rich Body Oil
◆Alpha Keri Moisture Rich Cleansing Bar
Balnetar
Estar Gel
Fostex 5% Benzoyl Peroxide Gel
◆Fostex 10% Benzoyl Peroxide
Cleansing Bar
◆Fostex 10% Benzoyl Peroxide Gel
Fostex 10% Benzoyl Peroxide Tinted
Cream
Fostex 10% Benzoyl Peroxide Wash
◆Fostex Medicated Cleansing Bar
Fostex Medicated Cleansing Cream
Fostril Lotion
Keri Creme
Keri Facial Soap
◆Keri Lotion-Herbal Scent
◆Keri Lotion-Original Formula
◆Keri Lotion-Silky Smooth Formula
Lowila Cake
◆Moisturel Cream
◆Moisturel Lotion
◆Moisturel Sensitive Skin Cleanser
Pernox Lotion
Pernox Medicated Scrub
Pernox Shampoo
PreSun for Kids
◆PreSun 8, 15 and 39 Creamy
Sunscreens
PreSun 15 Facial Stick/Lip Protector
Sunscreen

(◆ Shown in Product Identification Section)

PreSun 15 Facial Sunscreen
PreSun 15 and 29 Sensitive Skin Sunscreen
Sebucare Lotion
Sebulex
◆Sebulex Shampoo with Conditioners
Sebulon Dandruff Shampoo
◆Sebutone and Sebutone Cream

WHITEHALL LABORATORIES 434, 734, 766

Division of American Home Products Corporation
685 Third Avenue
New York, NY 10017

Address inquiries to:
Medical Department (212) 878-5188

OTC Products Available
◆Advil Ibuprofen Caplets & Tablets
◆Anacin Analgesic Coated Caplets
◆Anacin Analgesic Coated Tablets
Anacin Maximum Strength Coated Analgesic Tablets
Anacin-3 Children's Acetaminophen Chewable Tablets, Alcohol-Free Liquid and Infants' Drops
◆Anacin-3 Maximum Strength Acetaminophen Film Coated Caplets
◆Anacin-3 Maximum Strength Acetaminophen Film Coated Tablets
◆Anacin-3 Regular Strength Acetaminophen Film Coated Tablets
◆Anbesol Baby Teething Gel Anesthetic
◆Anbesol Gel Antiseptic-Anesthetic
◆Anbesol Gel Antiseptic-Anesthetic - Maximum Strength
◆Anbesol Liquid Antiseptic-Anesthetic
◆Anbesol Liquid Antiseptic-Anesthetic - Maximum Strength
◆Arthritis Pain Formula by the Makers of Anacin Analgesic Tablets and Caplets
Arthritis Pain Formula Aspirin-Free by the Makers of Anacin Analgesic Tablets
Beminal 500 Tablets
Beminal Forte
Beminal Stress Plus with Iron
Beminal Stress Plus with Zinc
Bisodol Antacid Powder & Tablets
Bronitin Asthma Tablets
Bronitin Mist
◆Clearblue Easy
◆Clearplan Ovulation Predictor
Clusivol Capsules and Syrup
Compound W Gel & Solution
Denalan Denture Cleanser
◆Denorex Medicated Shampoo & Conditioner
◆Denorex Medicated Shampoo, Extra Strength
◆Denorex Medicated Shampoo, Mountain Fresh Herbal
◆Denorex Medicated Shampoo, Regular
◆Dermoplast Lotion & Spray
◆Dristan Decongestant/Antihistamine Analgesic Coated Caplets & Tablets
◆Maximum Strength Dristan Decongestant/Analgesic Coated Caplets
Dristan Inhaler
◆Dristan Long Lasting Nasal Spray
◆Dristan Long Lasting Menthol Nasal Spray
◆Dristan Nasal Spray
◆Dristan Menthol Nasal Spray
Dristan Room Vaporizer
Dristan-AF Decongestant/ Antihistamine/Analgesic Tablets
Dry and Clear Acne Medicated Lotion & Double Strength Cream
Enzactin Cream
Fiber Guard
Freezone Solution
Heather Feminine Deodorant Spray
Heet Analgesic Liniment & Spray
InfraRub Analgesic Cream
Kerodex Cream 51(for dry or oily work)
Kerodex Cream 71 (for wet work)
Larylgan Throat Spray
Medicated Cleansing Pads by the Makers of Preparation H Hemorrhoidal Remedies
Momentum Muscular Backache Formula

Neet Bikini Line Hair Remover
Neet Depilatory Cream & Lotion
Outgro Solution
Oxipor VHC Lotion for Psoriasis
Posture 300 mg
◆Posture 600 mg
Posture-D 300 mg
◆Posture-D 600 mg
◆Preparation H Hemorrhoidal Cream, Ointment & Suppositories
◆Primatene Mist & Mist Suspension
◆Primatene Tablets - M Formula
◆Primatene Tablets - Regular Formula
◆Primatene Tablets - P Formula
Quiet World Nighttime Pain Formula
◆Riopan Antacid Chew Tablets
◆Riopan Antacid Suspension
Riopan Antacid Swallow Tablets
Riopan Rollpacks
◆Riopan Plus Chew Tablets
Riopan Plus Rollpacks
◆Riopan Plus Suspension
◆Riopan Plus 2 Chew Tablets
◆Riopan Plus 2 Suspension
◆Semicid Vaginal Contraceptive Inserts
Sleep-eze 3 Tablets
Sudden Action Breath Freshener
Sudden Beauty Country Air Mask
Sudden Beauty Hair Spray
Today Personal Lubricant
◆Today Vaginal Contraceptive Sponge
Trendar Ibuprofen Tablets
Viro-Med Tablets
Youth Garde Moisturizer Plus PABA

WINTHROP CONSUMER PRODUCTS 436, 745

Division of Sterling Drug Inc.
90 Park Avenue
New York, NY 10016

Address inquiries to:
Winthrop Consumer Products

For Medical Emergencies Contact:
Medical Department (212) 907-3027
(212) 907-3029

OTC Products Available
◆Bronkaid Mist
Bronkaid Mist Suspension
◆Bronkaid Tablets
◆Campho-Phenique Cold Sore Gel
◆Campho-Phenique Liquid
Campho-Phenique Sting Relief Formula
Campho-Phenique Triple Antibiotic Ointment Plus Pain Reliever
◆Fergon Capsules & Tablets
Fergon Elixir
Fergon Iron Plus Calcium Caplets
NTZ Long Acting Spray & Drops
◆NāSal Saline Nasal Spray
◆NāSal Saline Nose Drops
Neo-Synephrine Jelly
◆Neo-Synephrine Nasal Sprays
◆Neo-Synephrine Nasal Spray (Mentholated)
Neo-Synephrine Nose Drops
◆Neo-Synephrine 12 Hour Nasal Spray
◆Neo-Synephrine 12 Hour Nasal Spray Pump
Neo-Synephrine 12 Hour Nose Drops (Adult Strength)
Neo-Synephrine 12 Hour Vapor Nasal Spray
◆pHisoDerm for Baby
◆pHisoDerm Oily Skin Formula
◆pHisoDerm Regular Skin Formula - Unscented
◆pHisoPUFF
◆pHisoPUFF Disposa-PUFFS
WinGel Liquid & Tablets

WINTHROP PHARMACEUTICALS 750

90 Park Avenue
New York, NY 10016

Address inquiries to:
Professional Services Department
(800) 446-6267

Main Office
90 Park Avenue
New York, NY 10016 (212) 907-2000

OTC Products Available
Anti-Rust Tablets
Breonesin Capsules
Bronkolixir

Bronkotabs
Drisdol
Measurin Caplets
pHisoDerm (see Winthrop Consumer)
Pontocaine Cream & Ointment
Zephiran Chloride Aqueous Solution
Zephiran Chloride Concentrate Solution
Zephiran Chloride Spray
Zephiran Chloride Tinted Tincture
Zephiran Towellettes

WYETH-AYERST LABORATORIES 436, 753

Division of American Home Products Corporation
P.O. Box 8299
Philadelphia, PA 19101

Address inquiries to:
Professional Service (215) 688-4400

For EMERGENCY Medical Information
Day or night call (215) 688-4400

Wyeth-Ayerst Distribution Centers
Andover, MA 01810
P.O. Box 1776 (617) 475-9075
Atlanta, GA 30302
P.O. Box 4365 (404) 873-1681
Boston Distribution Center
see under Andover, MA
Buena Park, CA 90622-5000
P.O. Box 5000 (714) 523-5500
(Los Angeles) (213) 627-5374
Chamblee, GA 30341
3600 American Dr. (404) 457-2510
Chicago Distribution Center
see under Wheaton, IL
Cleveland, OH 44101
P.O. Box 91549 (216) 238-9450
Dallas, TX 75265-0231
P.O. Box 650231 (214) 341-2299
Foster City, CA 94404
1147 Chess Drive (415) 574-6065
Kansas City Distribution Center,
see under North Kansas City, MO
Kent, WA 98064-5609
P.O. Box 5609 (206) 872-8790
Los Angeles Distribution Center,
see under Buena Park, CA
Memphis, TN 38101
P.O. Box 1698 (901) 353-4680
North Kansas City, MO 64116
P.O. Box 7588 (816) 842-0680
Pearl City, HI 96782
96-1185 Waihona Street, Unit C-1
(808) 456-4567
Philadelphia Distribution Center
Paoli, PA 19301 (215) 644-8000
P.O. Box 61 (Phila.) (215) 878-9500
Seattle Distribution Center, see under Kent, WA
South Plainfield, NJ 07080
4000 Hadley Road
(201) 754-6220 (NJ)
(212) 964-3903 (NY)
Wheaton, IL 60189-0140
P.O. Box 140 (312) 462-7200

OTC Products Available
◆Aludrox Oral Suspension
◆Amphojel Suspension & Suspension without Flavor
◆Amphojel Tablets
◆Basaljel Capsules & Tablets
◆Basaljel Suspension
◆Cerose-DM
◆Collyrium Fresh
◆Collyrium for Fresh Eyes
◆Nursoy Soy Protein Infant Formula
◆Resol
◆SMA Iron Fortified Infant Formula
◆SMA lo-iron
◆Wyanoids Relief Factor Hemorrhoidal Suppositories

ZILA PHARMACEUTICALS, INC. 437, 757

777 East Thomas Road
Phoenix, AZ 85014
Address inquiries to:
Ed Pomerantz,
Vice President, Marketing
(602) 957-7887

OTC Products Available
◆Zilactin Medicated Gel

(◆ Shown in Product Identification Section)

SECTION 2

Product Name Index

In this section only described products are listed in alphabetical sequence by brand name or generic name. They have page numbers to assist you in locating the descriptions. For additional information on other products, you may wish to contact the manufacturer directly. The symbol ◆ indicates the product is shown in the Product Identification Section.

(◆ Shown in Product Identification Section)

(◆ Shown in Product Identification Section)

(◆ Shown in Product Identification Section)

(◆ Shown in Product Identification Section)

(◆ **Shown in Product Identification Section**)

(◆ Shown in Product Identification Section)

(◆ Shown in Product Identification Section)

◆Visine a.c. Eye Drops (Leeming) p 412, 576
◆Visine Eye Drops (Leeming) p 412, 575
◆Visine Extra Eye Drops (Leeming) p 412, 576
  Vivarin Stimulant Tablets (Beecham Products) p 514
  Vlemasque Acne Mask (Dermik) p 545

W

  Wart-Off (Leeming) p 576
◆Water Babies Sunblock Cream (Plough) p 420
◆Water Babies Sunblock Lotion (Plough) p 420

  Wellcome Lanoline (Burroughs Wellcome) p 536
  WinGel Liquid & Tablets (Winthrop Consumer Products) p 750
◆Within Multivitamin for Women with Calcium, Extra Iron and Zinc (Miles Inc.) p 416, 614
◆Wyanoids Relief Factor Hemorrhoidal Suppositories (Wyeth-Ayerst) p 437, 757

X

◆Xylocaine 2.5% Ointment (Astra) p 403, 507

Y

  Yellolax (Luyties) p 578

Z

◆Z-Bec Tablets (Robins) p 424, 661
  Zephiran Chloride Aqueous Solution (Winthrop Pharmaceuticals) p 751
  Zephiran Chloride Spray (Winthrop Pharmaceuticals) p 751
  Zephiran Chloride Tinted Tincture (Winthrop Pharmaceuticals) p 751
  Zetar Shampoo (Dermik) p 545
◆Zilactin Medicated Gel (Zila Pharmaceuticals) p 437, 757
◆Zincon Dandruff Shampoo (Lederle) p 411, 572
◆Ziradryl Lotion (Parke-Davis) p 419, 635

(◆ Shown in Product Identification Section)

SECTION 3
Product Category Index

Products described in the Product Information (White) Section are listed according to their classifications. The headings and subheadings have been determined by the OTC Review process of the U.S. Food and Drug Administration. Classification of products have been determined by the Publisher with the cooperation of individual manufacturers. In cases where there were differences of opinion or where the manufacturer had no opinion, the Publisher made the final decision.

A

ACNE PRODUCTS
(see under DERMATOLOGICALS, Acne Preparations)

AEROSOLS
Americaine Topical Anesthetic Spray (Fisons) p 545
CaldeCORT Anti-Itch Hydrocortisone Spray (Fisons) p 546
Cruex Antifungal Spray Powder (Fisons) p 546
Desenex Antifungal Foam (Fisons) p 547
Desenex Antifungal Spray Powder (Fisons) p 547
Desenex Foot & Sneaker Spray (Fisons) p 547
Micatin Antifungal Spray Liquid (Ortho Pharmaceutical) p 418, 624
Micatin Antifungal Spray Powder (Ortho Pharmaceutical) p 418, 624
Primatene Mist (Whitehall) p 435, 741
Primatene Mist Suspension (Whitehall) p 435, 741
R&C Spray III (Reed & Carnrick) p 421, 644
Rhulispray (Rydelle) p 425, 675
Tinactin Aerosol Liquid 1% (Schering) p 428, 691
Tinactin Aerosol Powder 1% (Schering) p 428, 691
Tinactin Jock Itch Spray Powder 1% (Schering) p 428, 691

ALLERGY RELIEF PRODUCTS
A.R.M. Allergy Relief Medicine Caplets (SmithKline Consumer Products) p 428, 694
Actidil Tablets & Syrup (Burroughs Wellcome) p 405, 530
Actifed Capsules (Burroughs Wellcome) p 405, 530
Actifed 12-Hour Capsules (Burroughs Wellcome) p 406, 531
Actifed Syrup (Burroughs Wellcome) p 406, 531

Actifed Tablets (Burroughs Wellcome) p 406, 531
Afrin Menthol Nasal Spray (Schering) p 426, 682
Afrin Nasal Spray, Nasal Spray Pump, Nose Drops, Children's Strength Nose Drops (Schering) p 426, 682
Afrinol Repetabs Tablets (Schering) p 426, 683
AllerAct Tablets (Burroughs Wellcome) p 406, 532
AllerAct Decongestant Caplets (Burroughs Wellcome) p 406, 532
AllerAct Decongestant Tablets (Burroughs Wellcome) p 406, 532
Allerest Allergy Tablets (Fisons) p 545
Allerest Headache Strength Tablets (Fisons) p 545
Allerest No Drowsiness Tablets (Fisons) p 545
Allerest Sinus Pain Formula (Fisons) p 545
Allerest 12 Hour Caplets (Fisons) p 545
Ayr Saline Nasal Drops (Ascher) p 403, 506
Ayr Saline Nasal Mist (Ascher) p 403, 506
Benadryl Decongestant Elixir (Parke-Davis) p 418, 628
Benadryl Decongestant Kapseals (Parke-Davis) p 418, 628
Benadryl Decongestant Tablets (Parke-Davis) p 418, 628
Benadryl Elixir (Parke-Davis) p 418, 628
Benadryl 25 Kapseals (Parke-Davis) p 418, 629
Benadryl 25 Tablets (Parke-Davis) p 418, 629
Benadryl Plus Tablets (Parke-Davis) p 418, 629
Bromfed Syrup (Muro) p 615
Caladryl Cream & Lotion (Parke-Davis) p 418, 631
Chlor-Trimeton Allergy Syrup, Tablets & Long-Acting Repetabs Tablets (Schering) p 427, 683

Chlor-Trimeton Decongestant Tablets (Schering) p 427, 684
Chlor-Trimeton Long Acting Decongestant Repetabs Tablets (Schering) p 427, 684
Comtrex A/S Multi-Symptom Allergy/Sinus Formula Tablets and Caplets (Bristol-Myers) p 404, 525
Congespirin For Children Aspirin Free Chewable Cold Tablets (Bristol-Myers) p 404, 526
Congespirin For Children Aspirin Free Liquid Cold Medicine (Bristol-Myers) p 404, 526
Contac Caplets (SmithKline Consumer Products) p 429, 695
Contac Capsules (SmithKline Consumer Products) p 429, 696
Coricidin Decongestant Nasal Mist (Schering) p 685
Coricidin Demilets Tablets for Children (Schering) p 427, 686
Delacort (Mericon) p 608
Demazin Nasal Decongestant/ Antihistamine Repetabs Tablets & Syrup (Schering) p 427, 687
Dimetane Decongestant Caplets (Robins) p 423, 657
Dimetane Decongestant Elixir (Robins) p 423, 657
Dimetane Elixir (Robins) p 423, 656
Dimetane Extentabs 8 mg (Robins) p 423, 656
Dimetane Extentabs 12 mg (Robins) p 423, 656
Dimetane Tablets (Robins) p 423, 656
Dimetapp Elixir (Robins) p 423, 657
Dimetapp Extentabs (Robins) p 423, 658
Dimetapp Plus Caplets (Robins) p 423, 658
Dimetapp Tablets (Robins) p 423, 658
Disophrol Chronotab Sustained-Action Tablets (Schering) p 688
Dorcol Children's Liquid Cold Formula (Sandoz Consumer) p 425, 677
Dristan Decongestant/Antihistamine (Whitehall) p 435, 738

Vicks Formula 44M Multisymptom Cough Mixture (Richardson-Vicks Health Care) p 422, 650
Vicks NyQuil Nighttime Colds Medicine-Regular & Cherry Flavor (Richardson-Vicks Health Care) p 422, 651

Aspirin
Children's Bayer Chewable Aspirin (Glenbrook) p 409, 549
8-Hour Bayer Timed-Release Aspirin (Glenbrook) p 408, 551
Empirin Aspirin (Burroughs Wellcome) p 406, 532
Genuine Bayer Aspirin Tablets & Caplets (Glenbrook) p 408, 549
Maximum Bayer Aspirin Tablets & Caplets (Glenbrook) p 408, 551

Aspirin & Combinations
Alka-Seltzer Effervescent Antacid & Pain Reliever (Miles Inc.) p 415, 608
Alka-Seltzer (Flavored) Effervescent Antacid & Pain Reliever (Miles Inc.) p 415, 609
Alka-Seltzer Extra Strength Effervescent Antacid & Pain Reliever (Miles Inc.) p 415, 611
Alka-Seltzer Plus Night-Time Cold Medicine (Miles Inc.) p 415, 611
Anacin Analgesic Coated Caplets (Whitehall) p 434, 734
Anacin Analgesic Coated Tablets (Whitehall) p 434, 734
Anacin Maximum Strength Coated Analgesic Tablets (Whitehall) p 734
Arthritis Pain Formula by the Makers of Anacin Analgesic Tablets and Caplets (Whitehall) p 435, 736
Arthritis Strength BC Powder (Block) p 516
Regular Strength Ascriptin Tablets (Rorer Consumer) p 424, 661
Ascriptin A/D Caplets (Rorer Consumer) p 424, 662
Extra Strength Ascriptin Caplets (Rorer Consumer) p 424, 662
BC Powder (Block) p 516
Bayer Children's Cold Tablets (Glenbrook) p 409, 549
Tri-Buffered Bufferin Analgesic Tablets and Caplets (Bristol-Myers) p 404, 523
Arthritis Strength Tri-Buffered Bufferin Analgesic Caplets (Bristol-Myers) p 404, 524
Extra Strength Tri-Buffered Bufferin Analgesic Tablets (Bristol-Myers) p 404, 524
Cama Arthritis Pain Reliever (Sandoz Consumer) p 675
Ecotrin Regular Strength Tablets and Caplets (SmithKline Consumer Products) p 429, 699
Ecotrin Maximum Strength Tablets and Caplets (SmithKline Consumer Products) p 429, 699
Excedrin Extra-Strength Analgesic Tablets & Caplets (Bristol-Myers) p 405, 527
4-Way Cold Tablets (Bristol-Myers) p 405, 528
Measurin Caplets (Winthrop Pharmaceuticals) p 751
Momentum Muscular Backache Formula (Whitehall) p 739
Ursinus Inlay-Tabs (Sandoz Consumer) p 681
Vanquish Analgesic Caplets (Glenbrook) p 410, 556

Cold Gels
Rhuligel (Rydelle) p 425, 674

Ibuprofen
Advil Ibuprofen Caplets (Whitehall) p 434, 734
Advil Ibuprofen Tablets (Whitehall) p 434, 734
Haltran Tablets (Upjohn) p 432, 719
Medipren ibuprofen Caplets and Tablets (McNeil Consumer Products) p 413, 584
Midol 200 Advanced Pain Formula (Glenbrook) p 409, 553

Nuprin Ibuprofen/Analgesic Tablets and Caplets (Bristol-Myers) p 405, 529
Trendar Ibuprofen Tablets (Whitehall) p 745

Topical-Analgesic
Americaine Topical Anesthetic Ointment (Fisons) p 545
Americaine Topical Anesthetic Spray (Fisons) p 545
Anbesol Baby Teething Gel Anesthetic (Whitehall) p 435, 736
Anbesol Gel Antiseptic-Anesthetic (Whitehall) p 435, 736
Anbesol Gel Antiseptic-Anesthetic - Maximum Strength (Whitehall) p 435, 736
Anbesol Liquid Antiseptic-Anesthetic (Whitehall) p 435, 736
Anbesol Liquid Antiseptic-Anesthetic - Maximum Strength (Whitehall) p 435, 736
Bactine Antiseptic/Anesthetic First Aid Spray (Miles Inc.) p 415, 612
BiCozene Creme (Sandoz Consumer) p 425, 675
Blistex Medicated Lip Ointment (Blistex) p 515
Campho-Phenique Cold Sore Gel (Winthrop Consumer Products) p 436, 746
Campho-Phenique Liquid (Winthrop Consumer Products) p 436, 746
Cēpacol Anesthetic Lozenges (Troches) (Lakeside Pharmaceuticals) p 410, 563
Cēpastat Cherry Flavor Sore Throat Lozenges (Lakeside Pharmaceuticals) p 410, 563
Cēpastat Sore Throat Lozenges (Lakeside Pharmaceuticals) p 410, 563
Chloraseptic Children's Lozenges (Richardson-Vicks Health Care) p 421, 646
Chloraseptic Liquid and Spray (Richardson-Vicks Health Care) p 421, 646
Chloraseptic Liquid - Nitrogen Propelled Spray (Richardson-Vicks Health Care) p 421, 646
Chloraseptic Lozenges (Richardson-Vicks Health Care) p 421, 646
Dermoplast Lotion (Whitehall) p 435, 737
Dermoplast Spray (Whitehall) p 435, 737
Ivarest Medicated Cream & Lotion (Blistex) p 515
Kank•a Medicated Formula (Blistex) p 516
Medicone Dressing Cream (Medicone) p 414, 607
Medicone Rectal Ointment (Medicone) p 415, 607
Medicone Rectal Suppositories (Medicone) p 415, 607
Nupercainal Hemorrhoidal Ointment (CIBA Consumer) p 407, 539
Nupercainal Pain Relief Cream (CIBA Consumer) p 407, 539
proctoFoam/non-steroid (Reed & Carnrick) p 421, 644
Rhuligel (Rydelle) p 425, 674
Rhulispray (Rydelle) p 425, 675
Solarcaine (Plough) p 420, 639
Sucrets Maximum Strength Spray (Beecham Products) p 514
Tronolane Anesthetic Cream for Hemorrhoids (Ross) p 425, 673
Tronolane Anesthetic Suppositories for Hemorrhoids (Ross) p 425, 673
Vicks Cough Silencers Cough Drops (Richardson-Vicks Health Care) p 648
Vicks Formula 44 Cough Control Discs (Richardson-Vicks Health Care) p 649
Vicks Throat Lozenges (Richardson-Vicks Health Care) p 652
Xylocaine 2.5% Ointment (Astra) p 403, 507

Zilactin Medicated Gel (Zila Pharmaceuticals) p 437, 757

Topical-Counterirritant
Ben-Gay External Analgesic Products (Leeming) p 572
Deep-Down Pain Relief Rub (Beecham Products) p 508
Icy Hot Balm (Richardson-Vicks Health Care) p 422, 647
Icy Hot Cream (Richardson-Vicks Health Care) p 422, 647
Icy Hot Stick (Richardson-Vicks Health Care) p 422, 647
Vicks Vaporub (Richardson-Vicks Health Care) p 422, 652
Zilactin Medicated Gel (Zila Pharmaceuticals) p 437, 757

Topical-Salicylates & Combinations
Aspercreme Creme & Lotion (Thompson Medical) p 432, 713
Ben-Gay External Analgesic Products (Leeming) p 572
Deep-Down Pain Relief Rub (Beecham Products) p 508
Icy Hot Balm (Richardson-Vicks Health Care) p 422, 647
Icy Hot Cream (Richardson-Vicks Health Care) p 422, 647
Icy Hot Stick (Richardson-Vicks Health Care) p 422, 647
Mobisyl Analgesic Creme (Ascher) p 403, 506
Myoflex Creme (Rorer Consumer) p 425, 666

Other
Biochemic Tissue Salts (NuAGE Laboratories) p 622
Doan's - Original Analgesic (CIBA Consumer) p 407, 539
Doan's - Extra Strength Analgesic (CIBA Consumer) p 407, 539
Magonate Tablets and Liquid (Fleming) p 548
Mobigesic Analgesic Tablets (Ascher) p 403, 506
Momentum Muscular Backache Formula (Whitehall) p 739

ANEMIA PREPARATIONS
(see under HEMATINICS)

ANESTHETICS, TOPICAL
(see under ANALGESICS)

ANORECTAL PRODUCTS

Creams, Foams, Lotions, Ointments
Americaine Hemorrhoidal Ointment (Fisons) p 545
Anusol Ointment (Parke-Davis) p 418, 627
Balneol (Reid-Rowell) p 421, 645
BiCozene Creme (Sandoz Consumer) p 425, 675
Cortaid Cream with Aloe (Upjohn) p 432, 719
Cortaid Lotion (Upjohn) p 432, 719
Cortaid Ointment with Aloe (Upjohn) p 432, 719
Hytone Cream 1/2% (Dermik) p 544
Medicone Rectal Ointment (Medicone) p 415, 607
Nupercainal Hemorrhoidal Ointment (CIBA Consumer) p 407, 539
Nupercainal Pain Relief Cream (CIBA Consumer) p 407, 539
Pazo Hemorrhoid Ointment & Suppositories (Bristol-Myers) p 405, 530
Preparation H Hemorrhoidal Cream (Whitehall) p 435, 741
Preparation H Hemorrhoidal Ointment (Whitehall) p 435, 741
proctoFoam/non-steroid (Reed & Carnrick) p 421, 644
Tronolane Anesthetic Cream for Hemorrhoids (Ross) p 425, 673
Tucks Cream (Parke-Davis) p 635
Tucks Ointment (Parke-Davis) p 635

Suppositories
Anusol Suppositories (Parke-Davis) p 418, 627

Other

Anbesol Gel Antiseptic-Anesthetic (Whitehall) p 435, 736
Anbesol Gel Antiseptic-Anesthetic - Maximum Strength (Whitehall) p 435, 736
Anbesol Liquid Antiseptic-Anesthetic (Whitehall) p 435, 736
Anbesol Liquid Antiseptic-Anesthetic - Maximum Strength (Whitehall) p 435, 736
Biotene Dental Chewing Gum (Laclede Research) p 562
Chloraseptic Lozenges (Richardson-Vicks Health Care) p 421, 646
Gly-Oxide Liquid (Marion) p 412, 580
Kank•a Medicated Formula (Blistex) p 516
Oral Balance Long Lasting Moisturizing Gel (Laclede Research) p 562
Zilactin Medicated Gel (Zila Pharmaceuticals) p 437, 757

DENTURE PREPARATIONS

Anbesol Gel Antiseptic-Anesthetic (Whitehall) p 435, 736
Anbesol Gel Antiseptic-Anesthetic - Maximum Strength (Whitehall) p 435, 736
Anbesol Liquid Antiseptic-Anesthetic (Whitehall) p 435, 736
Anbesol Liquid Antiseptic-Anesthetic - Maximum Strength (Whitehall) p 435, 736
Denclenz Denture Cleanser (Sandoz Consumer) p 676
Professional Strength Efferdent (Warner-Lambert) p 433, 725
Medicone Derma Ointment (Medicone) p 414, 607

DEODORANTS

Certan-dri Antiperspirant (Numark) p 622
Nullo Deodorant Tablets (Chattem) p 537

DERMATOLOGICALS

Abradant

Oxy Clean Lathering Facial Scrub (Norcliff Thayer) p 416, 618
pHisoPUFF (Winthrop Consumer Products) p 436, 749
pHisoPUFF Disposa-PUFFS (Winthrop Consumer Products) p 436, 750

Acne Preparations

Acnomel Cream (SmithKline Consumer Products) p 428, 694
Aqua Glyde Cleanser (Herald Pharmacal) p 557
Aveeno Cleansing Bar for Acne (Rydelle) p 425, 674
Biochemic Tissue Salts (NuAGE Laboratories) p 622
Clear by Design (SmithKline Consumer Products) p 429, 695
Clearasil Adult Care Medicated Blemish Cream (Richardson-Vicks Personal Care) p 422, 653
Clearasil 10% Benzoyl Peroxide Medicated Anti-Acne Lotion (Richardson-Vicks Personal Care) p 653
Clearasil Maximum Strength Medicated Anti-Acne Cream, Tinted (Richardson-Vicks Personal Care) p 422, 653
Clearasil Maximum Strength Medicated Anti-Acne Cream, Vanishing (Richardson-Vicks Personal Care) p 422, 653
Clearasil Medicated Astringent (Richardson-Vicks Personal Care) p 422, 654
DDS-Acidophilus (UAS Laboratories) p 717
Fostex 5% Benzoyl Peroxide Gel (Westwood) p 728
Fostex 10% Benzoyl Peroxide Cleansing Bar (Westwood) p 434, 729

Fostex 10% Benzoyl Peroxide Gel (Westwood) p 434, 729
Fostex 10% Benzoyl Peroxide Tinted Cream (Westwood) p 729
Fostex 10% Benzoyl Peroxide Wash (Westwood) p 729
Fostex Medicated Cleansing Bar (Westwood) p 434, 728
Fostex Medicated Cleansing Cream (Westwood) p 728
Fostril Lotion (Westwood) p 730
Loroxide Acne Lotion (Flesh Tinted) (Dermik) p 544
Noxzema Antiseptic Skin Cleanser-Extra Strength Formula (Noxell) p 417, 621
Noxzema Antiseptic Skin Cleanser-Regular Formula (Noxell) p 417, 621
Noxzema Clear-Ups Anti-Acne Gel (Noxell) p 417, 621
Noxzema Clear-Ups Maximum Strength Lotion, Vanishing (Noxell) p 417, 621
Noxzema Clear-Ups Medicated Pads-Maximum Strength 2.0% Salicylic Acid (Noxell) p 417, 622
Noxzema Clear-Ups Medicated Pads-Regular Strength 0.5% Salicyclic Acid (Noxell) p 417, 621
Noxzema Clear-Ups On-the-Spot Treatment, Tinted & Vanishing (Noxell) p 417, 622
Oxy Clean Medicated Cleanser (Norcliff Thayer) p 416, 619
Oxy Clean Medicated Pads - Regular and Maximum Strength (Norcliff Thayer) p 416, 619
Oxy Clean Medicated Soap (Norcliff Thayer) p 416, 619
Oxy-5 Tinted Formula with Sorboxyl (Norcliff Thayer) p 416, 619
Oxy-10 Tinted Formula with Sorboxyl (Norcliff Thayer) p 416, 619
Oxy-5 & Oxy-10 Vanishing Formula with Sorboxyl (Norcliff Thayer) p 416, 619
Oxy-10 Wash Antibacterial Skin Wash (Norcliff Thayer) p 416, 619
Pernox Lotion (Westwood) p 731
Pernox Medicated Scrub (Westwood) p 731
Pernox Shampoo (Westwood) p 731
Stri-Dex Maximum Strength Pads (Glenbrook) p 410, 556
Stri-Dex Regular Strength Pads (Glenbrook) p 410, 556
Vanoxide Acne Lotion (Dermik) p 544
Vlemasque Acne Mask (Dermik) p 545

Analgesic

Americaine Topical Anesthetic Ointment (Fisons) p 545
Americaine Topical Anesthetic Spray (Fisons) p 545
Aspercreme Creme & Lotion (Thompson Medical) p 432, 713
Benadryl Anti-Itch Cream (Parke-Davis) p 418, 628
Benadryl Spray (Parke-Davis) p 418, 629
Campho-Phenique Sting Relief Formula (Winthrop Consumer Products) p 747
Campho-Phenique Triple Antibiotic Ointment Plus Pain Reliever (Winthrop Consumer Products) p 747
Icy Hot Balm (Richardson-Vicks Health Care) p 422, 647
Icy Hot Cream (Richardson-Vicks Health Care) p 422, 647
Icy Hot Stick (Richardson-Vicks Health Care) p 422, 647
Vicks Vaporub (Richardson-Vicks Health Care) p 422, 652

Anesthetics, Topical

Americaine Topical Anesthetic Ointment (Fisons) p 545
Americaine Topical Anesthetic Spray (Fisons) p 545
Bactine Antiseptic/Anesthetic First Aid Spray (Miles Inc.) p 415, 612

Campho-Phenique Sting Relief Formula (Winthrop Consumer Products) p 747
Campho-Phenique Triple Antibiotic Ointment Plus Pain Reliever (Winthrop Consumer Products) p 747
Dermoplast Lotion (Whitehall) p 435, 737
Dermoplast Spray (Whitehall) p 435, 737
Medicone Derma Ointment (Medicone) p 414, 607
Solarcaine (Plough) p 420, 639

Antibacterial

B.F.I. (Beecham Products) p 508
Bactine Antiseptic/Anesthetic First Aid Spray (Miles Inc.) p 415, 612
Bactine First Aid Antibiotic Ointment (Miles Inc.) p 415, 612
Campho-Phenique Cold Sore Gel (Winthrop Consumer Products) p 436, 746
Campho-Phenique Liquid (Winthrop Consumer Products) p 436, 746
Campho-Phenique Triple Antibiotic Ointment Plus Pain Reliever (Winthrop Consumer Products) p 747
Diaparene Cradol (Glenbrook) p 409, 552
Diaparene Medicated Cream (Glenbrook) p 409
Diaparene Peri-Anal Medicated Ointment (Glenbrook) p 409
Fostex 5% Benzoyl Peroxide Gel (Westwood) p 728
Fostex 10% Benzoyl Peroxide Cleansing Bar (Westwood) p 434, 729
Fostex 10% Benzoyl Peroxide Gel (Westwood) p 434, 729
Fostex 10% Benzoyl Peroxide Tinted Cream (Westwood) p 729
Fostex 10% Benzoyl Peroxide Wash (Westwood) p 729
Hibiclens Antimicrobial Skin Cleanser (Stuart) p 431, 708
Hibistat Germicidal Hand Rinse (Stuart) p 709
Hibistat Towelette (Stuart) p 709
Listerine Antiseptic (Warner-Lambert) p 433, 725
Loroxide Acne Lotion (Flesh Tinted) (Dermik) p 544
Neosporin Cream (Burroughs Wellcome) p 406, 533
Neosporin Ointment (Burroughs Wellcome) p 406, 533
Noxzema Clear-Ups Maximum Strength Lotion, Vanishing (Noxell) p 417, 621
Noxzema Clear-Ups Medicated Pads-Maximum Strength 2.0% Salicylic Acid (Noxell) p 417, 622
Noxzema Clear-Ups Medicated Pads-Regular Strength 0.5% Salicyclic Acid (Noxell) p 417, 621
Noxzema Clear-Ups On-the-Spot Treatment, Tinted & Vanishing (Noxell) p 417, 622
Oxy Clean Medicated Cleanser (Norcliff Thayer) p 416, 619
Oxy Clean Medicated Pads - Regular and Maximum Strength (Norcliff Thayer) p 416, 619
Oxy Clean Medicated Soap (Norcliff Thayer) p 416, 619
Oxy-5 Tinted Formula with Sorboxyl (Norcliff Thayer) p 416, 619
Oxy-10 Tinted Formula with Sorboxyl (Norcliff Thayer) p 416, 619
Oxy-5 & Oxy-10 Vanishing Formula with Sorboxyl (Norcliff Thayer) p 416, 619
Oxy-10 Wash Antibacterial Skin Wash (Norcliff Thayer) p 416, 619
Polysporin Ointment (Burroughs Wellcome) p 406, 533
Polysporin Powder (Burroughs Wellcome) p 406, 533
Polysporin Spray (Burroughs Wellcome) p 406, 534

Bugs Bunny Children's Chewable Vitamins + Minerals with Iron & Calcium (Sugar Free) (Miles Inc.) p 415, 613

Bugs Bunny With Extra C Children's Chewable Vitamins (Sugar Free) (Miles Inc.) p 415, 613

Centrum, Jr. + Extra C (Lederle) p 411, 567

Centrum, Jr. + Extra Calcium (Lederle) p 411, 568

Centrum, Jr. + Iron (Lederle) p 411, 568

Ce-Vi-Sol (Mead Johnson Nutritionals) p 594

Flintstones Children's Chewable Vitamins (Miles Inc.) p 416, 613

Flintstones Children's Chewable Vitamins With Extra C (Miles Inc.) p 416, 613

Flintstones Complete With Iron, Calcium & Minerals Children's Chewable Vitamins (Miles Inc.) p 415, 613

Poly-Vi-Sol (Mead Johnson Nutritionals) p 414, 599

Poly-Vi-Sol Vitamins w/Iron, Drops (Mead Johnson Nutritionals) p 414, 600

Smurf Chewable Vitamins (Mead Johnson Nutritionals) p 602

Sunkist Children's Chewable Multivitamins - Complete (CIBA Consumer) p 408, 541

Sunkist Children's Chewable Multivitamins - Plus Extra C (CIBA Consumer) p 408, 541

Sunkist Children's Chewable Multivitamins - Plus Iron (CIBA Consumer) p 408, 541

Sunkist Children's Chewable Multivitamins - Regular (CIBA Consumer) p 408, 541

Tri-Vi-Sol Vitamin Drops (Mead Johnson Nutritionals) p 414, 605

Tri-Vi-Sol Vitamin Drops w/Iron (Mead Johnson Nutritionals) p 414, 606

Unicap Jr Chewable Tablets (Upjohn) p 721

Prenatal

Filibon Prenatal Vitamin Tablets (Lederle) p 569

Natabec Kapseals (Parke-Davis) p 633

Stuart Prenatal Tablets (Stuart) p 432, 712

Therapeutic

Beminal 500 Tablets (Whitehall) p 736

Centrum, Jr. + Extra C (Lederle) p 411, 567

Centrum, Jr. + Extra Calcium (Lederle) p 411, 568

Centrum, Jr. + Iron (Lederle) p 411, 568

Gevral T Tablets (Lederle) p 570

Orexin Softab Tablets (Stuart) p 431, 712

Sigtab Tablets (Upjohn) p 720

Stresstabs 600 (Lederle) p 411, 571

Stresstabs 600 + Iron (Lederle) p 411, 572

Stresstabs 600 + Zinc (Lederle) p 411, 572

Vitamins

Drisdol (Winthrop Pharmaceuticals) p 751

Ester-C Tablets (Inter-Cal) p 559

Fergon Iron Plus Calcium Caplets (Winthrop Consumer Products) p 747

Other

Beelith Tablets (Beach) p 507

Cod Liver Oil Concentrate Tablets, Capsules (Schering) p 427, 684

Halls Vitamin C Drops (Warner-Lambert) p 725

Mol-Iron Tablets w/Vitamin C (Schering) p 428, 691

Nicotinex Elixir (Fleming) p 548

Orexin Softab Tablets (Stuart) p 431, 712

Sunkist Vitamin C (CIBA Consumer) p 407, 542

W

WART REMOVERS (see under DERMATOLOGICALS, Wart Removers)

WEIGHT CONTROL PREPARATIONS (see under APPETITE SUPPRESSANTS or FOODS)

WET DRESSINGS (see under DERMATOLOGICALS, Wet Dressings)

WOUND MANAGEMENT DEVICE

Soft Guard Sheer Plus One-Piece System (United Medical) p 717

Soft Guard XL One-Piece System (United Medical) p 717

Soft Guard XL Skin Barrier (United Medical) p 717

Soft Guard XL Two-Piece System (United Medical) p 718

UniFlex Transparent Dressings and Drapes (United Medical) p 718

SECTION 4

Active Ingredients Index

In this section the products described in the Product Information (White) Section are listed under their chemical (generic) name according to their principal ingredient(s). Products have been included under specific headings by the Publisher with the cooperation of individual manufacturers.

Vicks Formula 44M Multisymptom Cough Mixture (Richardson-Vicks Health Care) p 422, 650

Vicks NyQuil Nighttime Colds Medicine-Regular & Cherry Flavor (Richardson-Vicks Health Care) p 422, 651

Pseudoephedrine Sulfate

Afrinol Repetabs Tablets (Schering) p 426, 683

Chlor-Trimeton Decongestant Tablets (Schering) p 427, 684

Chlor-Trimeton Long Acting Decongestant Repetabs Tablets (Schering) p 427, 684

Disophrol Chronotab Sustained-Action Tablets (Schering) p 688

Drixoral Antihistamine/Nasal Decongestant Syrup (Schering) p 427, 688

Drixoral Sustained-Action Tablets (Schering) p 427, 688

Drixoral Plus Extended Release Tablets (Schering) p 427, 689

Duration Long Acting Nasal Decongestant Tablets (Plough) p 419, 637

Psyllium Preparations

Effer-Syllium Natural Fiber Bulking Agent (Stuart) p 431, 707

Hydrocil Instant (Reid-Rowell) p 421, 645

Metamucil, Effervescent, Sugar Free, Lemon-Lime Flavor (Procter & Gamble) p 420, 642

Metamucil, Effervescent, Sugar Free, Orange Flavor (Procter & Gamble) p 420, 642

Metamucil Powder, Orange Flavor (Procter & Gamble) p 420, 641

Metamucil Powder, Regular Flavor (Procter & Gamble) p 420, 640

Metamucil Powder, Strawberry Flavor (Procter & Gamble) p 420, 641

Metamucil Powder, Sugar Free, Orange Flavor (Procter & Gamble) p 420, 642

Metamucil Powder, Sugar Free, Regular Flavor (Procter & Gamble) p 420, 641

Perdiem Granules (Rorer Consumer) p 425, 666

Perdiem Fiber Granules (Rorer Consumer) p 425, 667

Serutan Concentrated Powder - Fruit Flavored (Beecham Products) p 511

Serutan Toasted Granules (Beecham Products) p 511

Syllact (Wallace) p 433, 724

UltraBalance Weight Management Products - Herbulk (UltraBalance Products) p 717

Pyrethrins

A-200 Pediculicide Shampoo and Gel Concentrates (Norcliff Thayer) p 416, 616

R&C Shampoo (Reed & Carnrick) p 421, 644

RID Lice Treatment Kit (Leeming) p 574

Pyrethroids

R&C Spray III (Reed & Carnrick) p 421, 644

Pyridoxine

Beelith Tablets (Beach) p 507

Bugs Bunny Children's Chewable Vitamins (Sugar Free) (Miles Inc.) p 415, 613

Bugs Bunny Plus Iron Children's Chewable Vitamins (Sugar Free) (Miles Inc.) p 415, 613

Bugs Bunny With Extra C Children's Chewable Vitamins (Sugar Free) (Miles Inc.) p 415, 613

Flintstones Children's Chewable Vitamins (Miles Inc.) p 416, 613

Flintstones Children's Chewable Vitamins Plus Iron (Miles Inc.) p 416, 613

Flintstones Children's Chewable Vitamins With Extra C (Miles Inc.) p 416, 613

Geritol Liquid - High Potency Iron & Vitamin Tonic (Beecham Products) p 509

One-A-Day Essential Vitamins (Miles Inc.) p 416, 614

One-A-Day Maximum Formula Vitamins and Minerals (Miles Inc.) p 416, 614

One-A-Day Plus Extra C Vitamins (Miles Inc.) p 416, 614

Pyridoxine Hydrochloride (see under Vitamin B₆)

Pyrilamine Maleate

Chexit Tablets (Sandoz Consumer) p 675

4-Way Fast Acting Nasal Spray (regular & mentholated) (Bristol-Myers) p 405, 529

Maximum Strength Midol Multi-Symptom Formula (Glenbrook) p 409, 554

Maximum Strength Midol PMS Premenstrual Syndrome Formula (Glenbrook) p 409, 553

Original Midol Multi-Symptom Formula (Glenbrook) p 409, 552

Premsyn PMS (Chattem) p 537

Primatene Tablets - M Formula (Whitehall) p 435, 742

Robitussin Night Relief (Robins) p 424, 660

Tussagesic Tablets (Sandoz Consumer) p 681

Pyrithione Zinc

Danex Dandruff Shampoo (Herbert) p 557

Head & Shoulders (Procter & Gamble) p 420, 640

Q

Quinine Sulfate

Q-vel Muscle Relaxant Pain Reliever (CIBA Consumer) p 407, 541

R

Racepinephrine Hydrochloride

AsthmaNefrin Solution "A" Bronchodilator (Norcliff Thayer) p 617

Resorcinol

Acnomel Cream (SmithKline Consumer Products) p 428, 694

BiCozene Creme (Sandoz Consumer) p 425, 675

Clearasil Adult Care Medicated Blemish Cream (Richardson-Vicks Personal Care) p 422, 653

Riboflavin

Allbee C-800 Plus Iron Tablets (Robins) p 422, 654

Allbee C-800 Tablets (Robins) p 422, 654

Allbee with C Caplets (Robins) p 423, 654

Bugs Bunny Children's Chewable Vitamins (Sugar Free) (Miles Inc.) p 415, 613

Bugs Bunny Plus Iron Children's Chewable Vitamins (Sugar Free) (Miles Inc.) p 415, 613

Bugs Bunny With Extra C Children's Chewable Vitamins (Sugar Free) (Miles Inc.) p 415, 613

Flintstones Children's Chewable Vitamins (Miles Inc.) p 416, 613

Flintstones Children's Chewable Vitamins Plus Iron (Miles Inc.) p 416, 613

Flintstones Children's Chewable Vitamins With Extra C (Miles Inc.) p 416, 613

Geritol Liquid - High Potency Iron & Vitamin Tonic (Beecham Products) p 509

One-A-Day Essential Vitamins (Miles Inc.) p 416, 614

One-A-Day Maximum Formula Vitamins and Minerals (Miles Inc.) p 416, 614

One-A-Day Plus Extra C Vitamins (Miles Inc.) p 416, 614

Probec-T Tablets (Stuart) p 431, 712

The Stuart Formula Tablets (Stuart) p 431, 712

Stuart Prenatal Tablets (Stuart) p 432, 712

Stuartinic Tablets (Stuart) p 432, 713

Z-Bec Tablets (Robins) p 424, 661

Rosin

PRID Salve (Walker Pharmacal) p 723

S

Salicylic Acid

Aqua Glyde Cleanser (Herald Pharmacal) p 557

Aveeno Cleansing Bar for Acne (Rydelle) p 425, 674

Clearasil Medicated Astringent (Richardson-Vicks Personal Care) p 422, 654

Compound W Gel (Whitehall) p 736

Compound W Solution (Whitehall) p 736

Fostex Medicated Cleansing Bar (Westwood) p 434, 728

Fostex Medicated Cleansing Cream (Westwood) p 728

Freezone Solution (Whitehall) p 739

MG 217 Psoriasis Ointment (Triton Consumer Products) p 716

MG 217 Psoriasis Shampoo (Triton Consumer Products) p 716

Noxzema Clear-Ups Anti-Acne Gel (Noxell) p 417, 621

Noxzema Clear-Ups Medicated Pads-Maximum Strength 2.0% Salicylic Acid (Noxell) p 417, 622

Noxzema Clear-Ups Medicated Pads-Regular Strength 0.5% Salicyclic Acid (Noxell) p 417, 621

Oxipor VHC Lotion for Psoriasis (Whitehall) p 740

Oxy Clean Medicated Cleanser (Norcliff Thayer) p 416, 619

Oxy Clean Medicated Pads - Regular and Maximum Strength (Norcliff Thayer) p 416, 619

Oxy Clean Medicated Soap (Norcliff Thayer) p 416, 619

Pernox Lotion (Westwood) p 731

Pernox Medicated Scrub (Westwood) p 731

Sebucare Lotion (Westwood) p 732

Sebulex (Westwood) p 733

Sebulex Shampoo with Conditioners (Westwood) p 434, 733

Sebutone and Sebutone Cream (Westwood) p 434, 733

Stri-Dex Maximum Strength Pads (Glenbrook) p 410, 556

Stri-Dex Regular Strength Pads (Glenbrook) p 410, 556

Vanseb Cream and Lotion Dandruff Shampoo (Herbert) p 558

Vanseb-T Cream and Lotion Tar Dandruff Shampoo (Herbert) p 558

Wart-Off (Leeming) p 576

Saline Solution

Delicate Eyes Saline Solution (non-preserved) (Pharmafair) p 636

Delicate Eyes Saline Solution (preserved) (Pharmafair) p 636

Salt Substitutes

NoSalt Salt Alternative, Regular (Norcliff Thayer) p 416, 618

NoSalt Salt Alternative, Seasoned (Norcliff Thayer) p 416, 618

Scopolamine Hydrobromide

Donnagel (Robins) p 423, 659

Selenium Sulfide

Selsun Blue Dandruff Shampoo (selenium sulfide lotion 1%) (Ross) p 425, 671

Selsun Blue Extra Conditioning Dandruff Shampoo (Ross) p 425, 671

Selsun Blue Extra Medicated Dandruff Shampoo (Ross) p 425, 671

Senna

Perdiem Granules (Rorer Consumer) p 425, 666

Senna Concentrate

Senna Tabs 217mg (Pharmafair) p 636

Sennosides (A & B)

Gentle Nature Natural Vegetable Laxative (Sandoz Consumer) p 426, 678

Sesame Oil

Shepard's Cream Lotion (Dermik) p 544

Shark Liver Oil

Preparation H Hemorrhoidal Cream (Whitehall) p 435, 741

Preparation H Hemorrhoidal Ointment (Whitehall) p 435, 741

Preparation H Hemorrhoidal Suppositories (Whitehall) p 435, 741

Wyanoids Relief Factor Hemorrhoidal Suppositories (Wyeth-Ayerst) p 437, 757

Silica

Biochemic Tissue Salts (NuAGE Laboratories) p 622

Simethicone

Di-Gel Antacid/Anti-Gas (Plough) p 419, 637

Extra Strength Gas-X Tablets (Sandoz Consumer) p 426, 678

Gas-X Tablets (Sandoz Consumer) p 426, 678

Gelusil Liquid & Tablets (Parke-Davis) p 419, 631

Gelusil-II Liquid & Tablets (Parke-Davis) p 631

Extra Strength Maalox Plus Suspension (reformulated Maalox Plus) (Rorer Consumer) p 424, 664

Maalox Plus Tablets (Rorer Consumer) p 424, 664

Mylanta Liquid (Stuart) p 431, 710

Mylanta Tablets (Stuart) p 431, 710

Mylanta-II Liquid (Stuart) p 431, 710

Mylanta-II Tablets (Stuart) p 431, 710

Mylicon (Tablets & Drops) (Stuart) p 431, 711

Mylicon-80 Tablets (Stuart) p 431, 711

Mylicon-125 Tablets (Stuart) p 431, 711

Phazyme Tablets (Reed & Carnrick) p 643

Phazyme-95 Tablets (Reed & Carnrick) p 421, 643

Phazyme-125 Capsules Maximum Strength (Reed & Carnrick) p 421, 644

Riopan Plus Chew Tablets (Whitehall) p 743

Riopan Plus Suspension (Whitehall) p 435, 743

Riopan Plus 2 Chew Tablets (Whitehall) p 436, 743

Riopan Plus 2 Suspension (Whitehall) p 436, 743

Titralac Plus Antacid/Anti-Gas Liquid (3M Company) p 578

Titralac Plus Antacid/Anti-Gas Tablets (3M Company) p 578

Tums Liquid Extra-Strength Antacid with Simethicone (Norcliff Thayer) p 417, 620

Sodium Benzoate

Donnagel (Robins) p 423, 659

Sodium Bicarbonate

Alka-Seltzer Effervescent Antacid (Miles Inc.) p 415, 610

Alka-Seltzer Effervescent Antacid & Pain Reliever (Miles Inc.) p 415, 608

Alka-Seltzer (Flavored) Effervescent Antacid & Pain Reliever (Miles Inc.) p 415, 609

Alka-Seltzer Extra Strength Effervescent Antacid & Pain Reliever (Miles Inc.) p 415, 611

Arm & Hammer Pure Baking Soda (Church & Dwight) p 537

Citrocarbonate Antacid (Upjohn) p 718

Massengill Liquid Concentrate (Beecham Products) p 510

Sodium Borate

Collyrium Fresh with Tetrahydrozoline HCl plus Glycerin Sterile Eye Drops (Wyeth-Ayerst) p 437, 755

Collyrium for Fresh Eyes (Wyeth-Ayerst) p 437, 755

Sodium Carboxymethylcellulose

Soft Guard XL Skin Barrier (United Medical) p 717

Sodium Chloride

Ayr Saline Nasal Drops (Ascher) p 403, 506

Ayr Saline Nasal Mist (Ascher) p 403, 506

Chlor-3 (Fleming) p 548

NāSal Saline Nasal Spray (Winthrop Consumer Products) p 436, 748

NāSal Saline Nose Drops (Winthrop Consumer Products) p 436, 748

Ocean Mist (Fleming) p 548

Resol (Wyeth-Ayerst) p 437, 756

Salinex Nasal Mist & Drops (Muro) p 615

Thermotabs (Beecham Products) p 514

Sodium Citrate

Citrocarbonate Antacid (Upjohn) p 718

Eno (Beecham Products) p 508

Resol (Wyeth-Ayerst) p 437, 756

Sodium Fluoride

Colgate Mouthwash Tartar Control Formula (Colgate-Palmolive) p 408, 542

Colgate Tartar Control Formula (Colgate-Palmolive) p 408, 543

Colgate Tartar Control Gel (Colgate-Palmolive) p 408, 543

Fluorigard Anti-Cavity Fluoride Rinse (Colgate-Palmolive) p 408, 543

Listermint with Fluoride (Warner-Lambert) p 433, 725

Sodium Lactate

Massengill Baby Powder Soft Cloth Towelette (Beecham Products) p 510

Sodium Monofluorophosphate

Biotene Dry Mouth Relief Toothpaste (Laclede Research) p 562

Colgate Junior Fluoride Gel Toothpaste (Colgate-Palmolive) p 408, 542

Colgate MFP Fluoride Gel (Colgate-Palmolive) p 408, 542

Colgate MFP Fluoride Toothpaste (Colgate-Palmolive) p 408, 542

Sodium Perborate

Professional Strength Efferdent (Warner-Lambert) p 433, 725

Sodium Peroxyborate Monohydrate

Amosan (Oral-B Laboratories) p 417, 623

Sodium Tallowate

Shepard's Soap (Dermik) p 544

Sodium Tartrate

Eno (Beecham Products) p 508

Sorbitol

Actidose with Sorbitol (Paddock) p 626

Super Char Liquid with Sorbitol (Gulf Bio-Systems) p 557

Soybean Preparations

Isomil Soy Protein Formula With Iron (Ross) p 668

Isomil SF Sucrose-Free Soy Protein Formula With Iron (Ross) p 669

ProSobee (Mead Johnson Nutritionals) p 601

RCF Ross Carbohydrate Free Low-Iron Soy Protein Formula Base (Ross) p 670

Soyalac: Liquid Concentrate, Ready-to-Serve and Powder (Loma Linda) p 577

I-Soyalac (Loma Linda) p 577

Starch

Balmex Baby Powder (Macsil) p 579

Strontium Chloride Hexahydrate

Sensodyne Toothpaste (Block) p 517

Sulfur

Acnomel Cream (SmithKline Consumer Products) p 428, 694

Aveeno Cleansing Bar for Acne (Rydelle) p 425, 674

Clearasil Adult Care Medicated Blemish Cream (Richardson-Vicks Personal Care) p 422, 653

Fostex Medicated Cleansing Bar (Westwood) p 434, 728

Fostex Medicated Cleansing Cream (Westwood) p 728

Fostril Lotion (Westwood) p 730

Pernox Lotion (Westwood) p 731

Pernox Medicated Scrub (Westwood) p 731

Sebulex (Westwood) p 733

Sebulex Shampoo with Conditioners (Westwood) p 434, 733

Sebutone and Sebutone Cream (Westwood) p 434, 733

Vanseb Cream and Lotion Dandruff Shampoo (Herbert) p 558

Vanseb-T Cream and Lotion Tar Dandruff Shampoo (Herbert) p 558

Sulfur (Colloidal)

MG 217 Psoriasis Ointment (Triton Consumer Products) p 716

MG 217 Psoriasis Shampoo (Triton Consumer Products) p 716

Sulfurated Lime Solution

Vlemasque Acne Mask (Dermik) p 545

T

Tannic Acid

Outgro Solution (Whitehall) p 740

Zilactin Medicated Gel (Zila Pharmaceuticals) p 437, 757

Tar Preparations

Zetar Shampoo (Dermik) p 545

Tartaric Acid

Eno (Beecham Products) p 508

Terpin Hydrate

Chexit Tablets (Sandoz Consumer) p 675

Tussagesic Tablets (Sandoz Consumer) p 681

Tetrachlorosalicylanilide

Impregon Concentrate (Fleming) p 548

Tetrahydrozoline Hydrochloride

Collyrium Fresh with Tetrahydrozoline HCl plus Glycerin Sterile Eye Drops (Wyeth-Ayerst) p 437, 755

Eye Drops 15ml (Pharmafair) p 636

Murine Plus Lubricating Eye Redness Reliever (Ross) p 425, 670

Visine a.c. Eye Drops (Leeming) p 412, 576

Visine Eye Drops (Leeming) p 412, 575

Visine Extra Eye Drops (Leeming)
p 412, 576

Theophylline
Bronkaid Tablets (Winthrop Consumer
Products) p 436, 746
Bronkolixir (Winthrop Pharmaceuticals)
p 750
Bronkotabs (Winthrop Pharmaceuticals)
p 751

Theophylline Anhydrous
Primatene Tablets - M Formula
(Whitehall) p 435, 742
Primatene Tablets - Regular Formula
(Whitehall) p 435, 742

Theophylline Hydrous
Primatene Tablets - P Formula
(Whitehall) p 435, 742

Thiamine
Bugs Bunny Children's Chewable
Vitamins (Sugar Free) (Miles Inc.)
p 415, 613
Bugs Bunny Plus Iron Children's
Chewable Vitamins (Sugar Free)
(Miles Inc.) p 415, 613
Bugs Bunny With Extra C Children's
Chewable Vitamins (Sugar Free)
(Miles Inc.) p 415, 613
Flintstones Children's Chewable
Vitamins (Miles Inc.) p 416, 613
Flintstones Children's Chewable
Vitamins Plus Iron (Miles Inc.) p 416,
613
Flintstones Children's Chewable
Vitamins With Extra C (Miles Inc.)
p 416, 613
Geritol Liquid - High Potency Iron &
Vitamin Tonic (Beecham Products)
p 509
One-A-Day Essential Vitamins (Miles
Inc.) p 416, 614
One-A-Day Maximum Formula Vitamins
and Minerals (Miles Inc.) p 416, 614
One-A-Day Plus Extra C Vitamins (Miles
Inc.) p 416, 614
Probec-T Tablets (Stuart) p 431, 712
The Stuart Formula Tablets (Stuart)
p 431, 712
Stuartinic Tablets (Stuart) p 432, 713

Thiamine Mononitrate
Allbee C-800 Plus Iron Tablets
(Robins) p 422, 654
Allbee C-800 Tablets (Robins) p 422,
654
Allbee with C Caplets (Robins) p 423,
654
Orexin Softab Tablets (Stuart) p 431,
712
Stuart Prenatal Tablets (Stuart) p 432,
712
Z-Bec Tablets (Robins) p 424, 661

Thymol
Listerine Antiseptic (Warner-Lambert)
p 433, 725

Tincture of Benzoin Compound
Kank•a Medicated Formula (Blistex)
p 516

Titanium Dioxide
Johnson's Baby Sunblock Cream (SPF
15) (Johnson & Johnson Baby
Products) p 410, 560
Johnson's Baby Sunblock Lotion (SPF
15) (Johnson & Johnson Baby
Products) p 410, 560
Sundown Broad Spectrum Cream, Ultra
Sunblock (SPF 30) (Johnson &
Johnson Baby Products) p 410, 561
Sundown Broad Spectrum Lotion, Ultra
Sunblock (SPF 15) (Johnson &
Johnson Baby Products) p 410, 561
Sundown Broad Spectrum Lotion, Ultra
Sunblock (SPF 25) (Johnson &
Johnson Baby Products) p 561
Sundown Sunblock Lotion, Ultra
Protection (SPF 20) (Johnson &
Johnson Baby Products) p 561

Sundown Sunblock Stick, Ultra
Protection (SPF 20) (Johnson &
Johnson Baby Products) p 561

Tolnaftate
Aftate for Athlete's Foot (Plough)
p 419, 636
Aftate for Jock Itch (Plough) p 419,
636
NP-27 (Thompson Medical) p 432,
715
Tinactin Aerosol Liquid 1% (Schering)
p 428, 691
Tinactin Aerosol Powder 1% (Schering)
p 428, 691
Tinactin 1% Cream, Solution & Powder
(Schering) p 428, 691
Tinactin Jock Itch Cream 1%
(Schering) p 428, 691
Tinactin Jock Itch Spray Powder 1%
(Schering) p 428, 691
Tolnaftate 1% Cream and 1% Solution
(Pharmafair) p 636

Triclosan
Solarcaine (Plough) p 420, 639

Triprolidine Hydrochloride
Actidil Tablets & Syrup (Burroughs
Wellcome) p 405, 530
Actifed Capsules (Burroughs Wellcome)
p 405, 530
Actifed 12-Hour Capsules (Burroughs
Wellcome) p 406, 531
Actifed Syrup (Burroughs Wellcome)
p 406, 531
Actifed Tablets (Burroughs Wellcome)
p 406, 531
AllerAct Tablets (Burroughs Wellcome)
p 406, 532
AllerAct Decongestant Caplets
(Burroughs Wellcome) p 406, 532
AllerAct Decongestant Tablets
(Burroughs Wellcome) p 406, 532

Trolamine Salicylate
Aspercreme Creme & Lotion
(Thompson Medical) p 432, 713
Mobisyl Analgesic Creme (Ascher)
p 403, 506
Myoflex Creme (Rorer Consumer)
p 425, 666

U

Undecylenic Acid
Cruex Antifungal Cream (Fisons) p 546
Cruex Antifungal Spray Powder (Fisons)
p 546
Desenex Antifungal Cream (Fisons)
p 547
Desenex Antifungal Foam (Fisons)
p 547
Desenex Antifungal Liquid (Fisons)
p 547
Desenex Antifungal Ointment (Fisons)
p 547
Desenex Antifungal Powder (Fisons)
p 547
Desenex Antifungal Spray Powder
(Fisons) p 547

Urea
Aqua Care Cream (SmithKline
Consumer Products) p 428, 694
Aqua Care Lotion (SmithKline
Consumer Products) p 428, 694
Carmol 10 Lotion (Syntex) p 713
Carmol 20 Cream (Syntex) p 713
Pen•Kera Creme (Ascher) p 403, 507

Urea Preparations
Debrox Drops (Marion) p 412, 579
Gly-Oxide Liquid (Marion) p 412, 580

V

Vinegar
Massengill Disposable Douche
(Beecham Products) p 510

Vinyl Film with Oxygen Barrier
Soft Guard Sheer Plus One-Piece
System (United Medical) p 717
Soft Guard XL One-Piece System
(United Medical) p 717
Soft Guard XL Two-Piece System
(United Medical) p 718

Vitamin A
Bugs Bunny Children's Chewable
Vitamins (Sugar Free) (Miles Inc.)
p 415, 613
Bugs Bunny Plus Iron Children's
Chewable Vitamins (Sugar Free)
(Miles Inc.) p 415, 613
Bugs Bunny With Extra C Children's
Chewable Vitamins (Sugar Free)
(Miles Inc.) p 415, 613
Flintstones Children's Chewable
Vitamins (Miles Inc.) p 416, 613
Flintstones Children's Chewable
Vitamins Plus Iron (Miles Inc.) p 416,
613
Flintstones Children's Chewable
Vitamins With Extra C (Miles Inc.)
p 416, 613
Myadec (Parke-Davis) p 419, 632
One-A-Day Essential Vitamins (Miles
Inc.) p 416, 614
One-A-Day Maximum Formula Vitamins
and Minerals (Miles Inc.) p 416, 614
One-A-Day Plus Extra C Vitamins (Miles
Inc.) p 416, 614
Pro Skin-E (Face Capsule) (Marlyn)
p 582
Stressgard Stress Formula Vitamins
(Miles Inc.) p 416, 614
Tri-Vi-Sol Vitamin Drops (Mead Johnson
Nutritionals) p 414, 605
Tri-Vi-Sol Vitamin Drops w/Iron (Mead
Johnson Nutritionals) p 414, 606
Within Multivitamin for Women with
Calcium, Extra Iron and Zinc (Miles
Inc.) p 416, 614

Vitamins A & D
Cod Liver Oil Concentrate Tablets,
Capsules (Schering) p 427, 684
Cod Liver Oil Concentrate Tablets
w/Vitamin C (Schering) p 427, 684
Scott's Emulsion (Beecham Products)
p 511
Sigtab Tablets (Upjohn) p 720
The Stuart Formula Tablets (Stuart)
p 431, 712
Stuart Prenatal Tablets (Stuart) p 432,
712

Vitamin B₁
Allbee C-800 Plus Iron Tablets
(Robins) p 422, 654
Allbee C-800 Tablets (Robins) p 422,
654
Allbee with C Caplets (Robins) p 423,
654
Beminal 500 Tablets (Whitehall) p 736
Bugs Bunny Children's Chewable
Vitamins (Sugar Free) (Miles Inc.)
p 415, 613
Bugs Bunny Plus Iron Children's
Chewable Vitamins (Sugar Free)
(Miles Inc.) p 415, 613
Bugs Bunny With Extra C Children's
Chewable Vitamins (Sugar Free)
(Miles Inc.) p 415, 613
Flintstones Children's Chewable
Vitamins (Miles Inc.) p 416, 613
Flintstones Children's Chewable
Vitamins Plus Iron (Miles Inc.) p 416,
613
Flintstones Children's Chewable
Vitamins With Extra C (Miles Inc.)
p 416, 613
One-A-Day Essential Vitamins (Miles
Inc.) p 416, 614
One-A-Day Maximum Formula Vitamins
and Minerals (Miles Inc.) p 416, 614
One-A-Day Plus Extra C Vitamins (Miles
Inc.) p 416, 614
Orexin Softab Tablets (Stuart) p 431,
712
Stressgard Stress Formula Vitamins
(Miles Inc.) p 416, 614

HEALTH ASSOCIATIONS AND ORGANIZATIONS

AARP Pharmacy Service
1 Prince Street
Alexandria, VA 22314
(703) 684-0244

**Alcohol and Drug Problems
Association of North America**
444 North Capitol St., N.W.
Washington, DC 20001
(202) 737-4340

**Alcoholics Anonymous World
Services, Inc.**
P.O. Box 459
Grand Central Station
New York, NY 10163
(212) 686-1100

**Alzheimer's Disease and
Related Disorders Association, Inc.**
70 E. Lake St., Suite 600
Chicago, IL 60601
(800) 621-0379
Illinois only: (800) 572-6037

**American Anorexia Bulimia
Association, Inc.**
133 Cedar Lane
Teaneck, NJ 07666
(201) 836-1800

**American Association of
Poison Control Centers**
c/o Arizona Poison Center
Rm. 3240K
1501 N. Campbell Avenue
Tucson, AZ 85724
(602) 626-7899

American Cancer Society
3340 Peachtree Road
Atlanta, GA 30326
(404) 320-3333

**American Council on
Alcohol Problems**
3426 Bridgeland Drive
Bridgeton, MO 63044
(314) 739-5944

American Dental Association
211 E. Chicago Avenue
Chicago, IL 60611
(312) 440-2500

American Diabetes Association, Inc.
National Service Center
1660 Duke St.
Alexandria, VA 22314
(703) 549-1500

American Dietetic Association
216 W. Jackson Blvd. Suite 800
Chicago, IL 60606-6995
(312) 899-0040

American Foundation for the Blind
15 W. 16th Street
New York, NY 10011
(212) 620-2000
(800) 232-5463

American Heart Association
7320 Greenville Avenue
Dallas, TX 75231
(214) 373-6300

HEALTH ASSOCIATIONS AND ORGANIZATIONS

American Liver Foundation
998 Pompton Avenue
Cedar Grove, NJ 07009
(201) 857-2626

American Lung Association
1740 Broadway
New York, NY 10019
(212) 315-8700

American Medical Association
535 N. Dearborn Street
Chicago, IL 60610-4377
(312) 645-4818

**American Nutritional
Medical Association, Inc.**
1326 Dearborn St.
Gary, IN 46403
(219) 938-6548

American Osteopathic Association
142 E. Ohio Street
Chicago, IL 60611
(312) 280-5800

**American Osteopathic
Hospital Association**
1454 Duke Street
Alexandria, VA 22314
(703) 684-7700

**American Physical Therapy
Association**
1111 North Fairfax Street
Alexandria, VA 22314
(703) 684-2782

**American Red Cross
Medical Operations**
National Headquarters
1730 E. St., NW
Washington, DC 20006
(202) 639-3011

American Society of Internal Medicine
1101 Vermont Ave., NW
Suite 500
Washington, DC 20005
(202) 298-1700

Arthritis Foundation
1314 Spring Street, NW
Atlanta, GA 30309
(404) 872-7100

**Asthma and Allergy Foundation
of America**
1717 Massachusetts Ave. NW
Suite 305
Washington, DC 20036
(202) 265-0265

Autism Society of America
1234 Massachusetts Ave., NW
Suite C1017
Washington, DC 20005
(202) 783-0125

Center for Sickle Cell Disease
2121 Georgia Ave., NW
Washington, DC 20059
(202) 636-7930

Citizens Alliance for VD Awareness
222 W. Adams Street
Chicago, IL 60606
(312) 236-6339

Cystic Fibrosis Foundation
6931 Arlington Rd.
Bethesda, MD 20814
(301) 951-4422

**Division of Sexually Transmitted
Diseases
Centers for Disease Control**
Atlanta, GA 30333
(404) 639-2580

HEALTH ASSOCIATIONS AND ORGANIZATIONS

**The Epilepsy Foundation
of America**
4351 Garden City Drive
Landover, MD 20785
(301) 459-3700

**Food and Drug Administration
Press Office**
15-05
5600 Fishers Lane
Rockville, MD 20857
(301) 443-4177; (301) 443-3285

**Food and Nutrition Board
Institute of Medicine
National Academy of Sciences**
2101 Constitution Ave., NW
Washington, DC 20418
(202) 334-2238

**Huntington's Disease Society
of America**
140 W. 22nd Street
6th Floor
New York, NY 10011-2420
(212) 242-1968
(800) 345-HDSA

Joslin Diabetes Center
1 Joslin Place
Boston, MA 02215
(617) 732-2400

**Juvenile Diabetes Foundation
International**
432 Park Ave. South
New York, NY 10016-8013
(800) 223-1138

Leukemia Society of America
733 Third Avenue
New York, NY 10017
(212) 573-8484

**March of Dimes
Birth Defects Foundation**
1275 Mamaroneck Avenue
White Plains, NY 10605
(914) 428-7100

**Medic Alert Foundation
International**
2323 Colorado Ave.
Turlock, CA 95381-1009
(800) IDALERT

Muscular Dystrophy Association
810 7th Avenue
New York, NY 10019
(212) 586-0808

**National Association of Anorexia
Nervosa & Associated Disorders**
Box 7
Highland Park, IL 60035
(312) 831-3438

National Association of the Deaf
814 Thayer Avenue
Silver Spring, MD 20910
(301) 587-1788

National Association of the Deaf
Branch Office
445 N. Pennsylvania Street
Suite 804
Indianapolis, IN 46204

**National Association of
Rehabilitation Facilities**
Box 17675
Washington, DC 20041
(703) 648-9300

**National Association for
Sickle Cell Disease, Inc.**
4221 Wilshire Blvd.
Suite 360
Los Angeles, CA 90010-3503
(213) 936-7205 1 (800)-421-8453

National Council on Alcoholism
12 West 21st St.
New York, NY 10010
(212) 206-6770

HEALTH ASSOCIATIONS AND ORGANIZATIONS

National Federation of the Blind
1800 Johnson Street
Baltimore, MD 21230
(301) 659-9314

**National Foundation for
Ileitis and Colitis**
444 Park Avenue South
New York, NY, 10016
(212) 685-3440

National Health Council, Inc.
622 Third Ave., 34th Floor
New York, NY 10017-6765
(212) 972-2700

National Hemophilia Foundation
The Soho Bldg
110 Greene St., Rm 406
New York, NY 10012
(212) 219-8180

**National Clearinghouse for
Alcohol and Drug Information**
P.O. Box 2345
Rockville, MD 20852
(301) 468-2600

National Institutes of Health
9000 Rockville Pike
Bethesda, MD 20892
(301) 496-4000

National Kidney Foundation
30 East 33rd Street
New York, NY 10016
(212) 889-2210

National Mental Health Association
1021 Prince Street
Alexandria, VA 22314-2971
(703) 684-7722

National Multiple Sclerosis Society
205 E. 42nd Street
New York, NY 10017
(212) 986-3240

National Parkinson Foundation
1501 NW 9th Avenue
Bob Hope Road
Miami, FL 33136-9990
(305) 547-6666
(800) 327-4545

National Rehabilitation Association
633 S. Washington Street
Alexandria, VA 22314
(703) 836-0850

National Society to Prevent Blindness
500 East Remington Road
Schaumberg, IL 60173
(312) 843-2020

**National Spinal Cord Injury
Association**
600 West Cummings Park, Suite 2000
Woburn, MA 01801
(617) 935-2222
(800) 962-9629

**Office on Smoking and Health
Technical Information Center**
5600 Fishers Lane
Park Building Room 1-16
Rockville, MD 20857
(301)443-1690

**Planned Parenthood Federation
of America, Inc.**
810 Seventh Avenue
New York, NY 10019
(212) 603-4695

Psoriasis Research Institute
(formerly the International Psoriasis
Research Foundation)
Post Office Box V
Stanford, CA 94305
(415) 326-1848

HEALTH ASSOCIATIONS AND ORGANIZATIONS

**Rusk Institute of
Rehabilitation Medicine
NYU Medical Center**
400 East 34th Street
New York, NY 10016
(212) 340-6105

**United Cerebral Palsy Associations,
Inc.**
66 E. 34th Street
New York, NY 10016
(212) 481-6300

United Ostomy Association
36 Executive Park
Suite 120
Irvine, CA 92714
(714) 660-8624

**Wellness and Health Activation
Networks**
P.O. Box 923
Vienna, VA 22180
(703) 281-3830

Product Identification Section

This section is designed to help you identify products and their packaging.

Participating manufacturers have included selected products in full color. Where capsules and tablets are included they are shown in actual size. Packages generally are reduced in size.

For more information on products included, refer to the description in the PRODUCT INFORMATION SECTION or check directly with the manufacturer.

While every effort has been made to reproduce products faithfully, this section should be considered only as a quick-reference identification aid.

INDEX BY MANUFACTURER

ADRIA

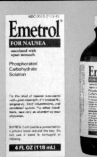

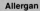

EMETROL®
(phosphorated carbohydrate solution)

Adria

MODANE®
(phenolphthalein)

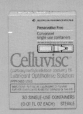

MODANE® PLUS
(phenolphthalein and docusate sodium)

ALLERGAN

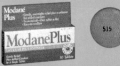

30 single-use containers
(0.01 fl oz each)

CELLUVISC™
Lubricant Ophthalmic Solution

Allergan

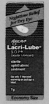

7 g   3.5 g

Also available: 0.7 g unit dose (24 pack)

LACRI-LUBE® S.O.P.®
Sterile Ophthalmic Ointment

Allergan

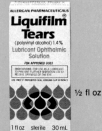

½ fl oz

1 fl oz   sterile   30 mL

Also available: 1 fl oz

LIQUIFILM TEARS®
Lubricant Ophthalmic Solution

Allergan

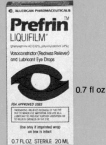

0.7 fl oz

0.7 OZ STERILE 20 ML

PREFRIN™ LIQUIFILM®
Vasoconstrictor (Redness Reliever)
and Lubricant Eye Drops
(phenylephrine HCl 0.12%,
polyvinyl alcohol 1.4%)

Allergan

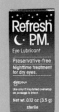

0.12 oz (3.5 g)

Preservative-free
Nighttime treatment for
dry eyes.

REFRESH® P.M.
Eye Lubricant

Allergan

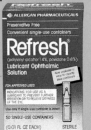

50 single-use containers
(0.01 fl oz each)

Also available:
30 single-use containers

REFRESH®
Lubricant Ophthalmic Solution

Allergan

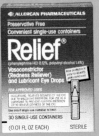

30 single-use containers
(0.01 fl oz each)

RELIEF®
Vasoconstrictor (Redness Reliever)
and Lubricant Eye Drops

Allergan

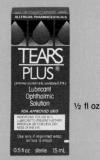

½ fl oz

0.5 fl oz   sterile   15 mL

Also available: 1 fl oz

TEARS PLUS®
Lubricant Ophthalmic Solution

ASCHER

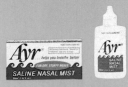

AYR® SALINE NASAL MIST

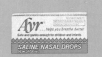

AYR® SALINE NASAL DROPS

B. F. Ascher & Co., Inc.

Available: 18's, 50's & 100's

MOBIGESIC®
ANALGESIC TABLETS

B. F. Ascher & Co., Inc.

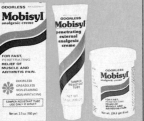

Also Available: 1.25 oz

MOBISYL®
ANALGESIC CREME

B. F. Ascher & Co., Inc.

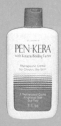

Available in 8 oz bottle

PEN•KERA®

Therapeutic Creme
for Chronic Dry Skin

B. F. Ascher & Co., Inc.

Available in 15's
& 60's

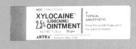

UNILAX®
Softgel
Capsules

ASTRA

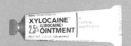

Available in 35g Tube

XYLOCAINE® 2.5% OINTMENT
(lidocaine)

Boehringer Ingelheim

15 minutes to 1 hour
Fast Predictable Relief
Dulcolax
The original brand (bisacodyl USP)
L A X A T I V E
4 SUPPOSITORIES

Available in boxes of 4's, 8's, 16's and 50's

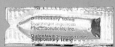

10 mg.
Dulcolax® Suppositories
(bisacodyl USP)

Boehringer Ingelheim

Overnight Relief
Gentle and Predictable
Dulcolax
The original brand (bisacodyl USP)
L A X A T I V E
SODIUM FREE
25 TABLETS

Available in boxes of 10's, 25's, 50's and 100's

12 **BI** 5 mg.

Dulcolax® Tablets
(bisacodyl USP)

BOIRON-BORNEMAN

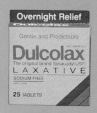

oscillococcinum
NATURAL RELIEF
FROM SYMPTOMS OF FLU
HOMEOPATHIC REMEDY

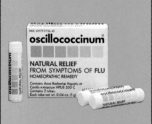

OSCILLOCOCCINUM®

Homeopathic remedy for relief of flu-like symptoms

Bristol-Myers Products

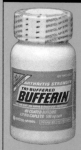

Bottles of 40 and 100 coated caplets

**ARTHRITIS STRENGTH
TRI-BUFFERED BUFFERIN®
CAPLET**
(buffered aspirin)

Bristol-Myers Products

Bottles of 12's, 36's, 60's, 100's, 200's and 1000's

Hospital/Institutional packs of 150 x 2 tablet in foil packets

**TRI-BUFFERED BUFFERIN®
TABLET**
(buffered aspirin)

Bristol-Myers Products

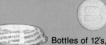

Bottles of 36, 60 and 100 coated caplets

**TRI-BUFFERED BUFFERIN®
CAPLET**
(buffered aspirin)

Bristol-Myers Products

Bottles of 30, 60 and 100 coated tablets

**EXTRA STRENGTH TRI-BUFFERED
BUFFERIN® TABLET**
(buffered aspirin)

Bristol-Myers Products

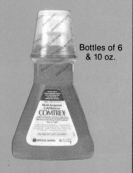

Bottles of 6 & 10 oz.

COMTREX® LIQUID

Bristol-Myers Products

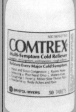

Blister packs of 24's, bottles of 50's

COMTREX® TABLETS

Bristol-Myers Products

Carded 16's and bottles of 36's

COMTREX® CAPLETS

Bristol-Myers Products

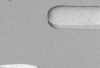

COMTREX
Multi-Symptom
**ALLERGY-SINUS
FORMULA AS**

Available in blister packs of 24 and bottles of 50 tablets

**COMTREX® A/S TABLETS
MULTI-SYMPTOM
ALLERGY-SINUS FORMULA**
(acetaminophen, pseudoephedrine, chlorpheniramine)

Bristol-Myers Products

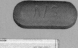

COMTREX
Multi-Symptom
**ALLERGY-SINUS
FORMULA AS**

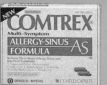

Available in blister packs of 24 and bottles of 36 caplets

**COMTREX® A/S CAPLETS
MULTI-SYMPTOM
ALLERGY-SINUS FORMULA**
(acetaminophen, pseudoephedrine, chlorpheniramine)

Bristol-Myers Products

Congespirin

Bottles of 24

ASPIRIN FREE CONGESPIRIN®
(acetaminophen 81 mg., phenylephrine 1.25 mg.)

Bristol-Myers Products

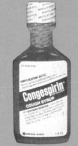

Congespirin
COUGH SYRUP

3 oz. bottles
5 mg. per 5 ml teaspoon

**CONGESPIRIN® COUGH
SYRUP**
(dextromethorphan, hydrobromide)

Bristol-Myers Products

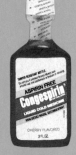

**ASPIRIN FREE
Congespirin**

3 oz. bottles

**CONGESPIRIN® LIQUID COLD
MEDICINE**

Bristol-Myers Products

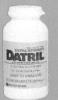

DATRIL   **DATRIL**

Bottles of 24's & 36's

Bottles of 30, 60 & 100 Tablets

**EXTRA STRENGTH DATRIL®
CAPLETS AND TABLETS**
(acetaminophen)

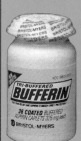
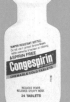

Bristol-Myers Products

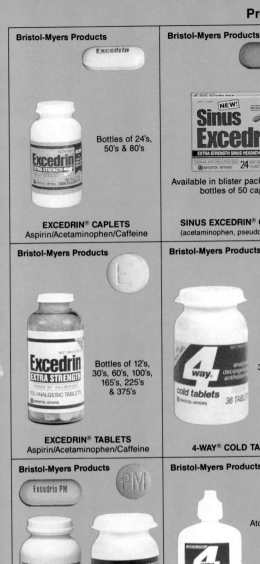

Bottles of 24's, 50's & 80's

EXCEDRIN® CAPLETS
Aspirin/Acetaminophen/Caffeine

Bristol-Myers Products

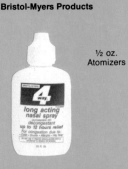

Available in blister packs of 24 and bottles of 50 caplets

SINUS EXCEDRIN® CAPLETS
(acetaminophen, pseudoephedrine)

Bristol-Myers Products

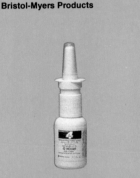

½ oz. Atomizers

4-WAY® LONG ACTING NASAL SPRAY
(oxymetazoline hydrochloride 0.05%)

Bristol-Myers Products

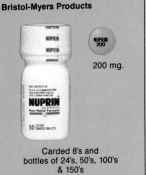

200 mg.

Carded 8's and bottles of 24's, 50's, 100's & 150's

NUPRIN®
(ibuprofen)

Bristol-Myers Products

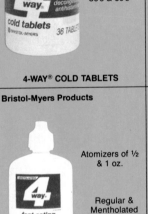

Bottles of 12's, 30's, 60's, 100's, 165's, 225's & 375's

EXCEDRIN® TABLETS
Aspirin/Acetaminophen/Caffeine

Bristol-Myers Products

Bottles of 36's & 60's

4-WAY® COLD TABLETS

Bristol-Myers Products

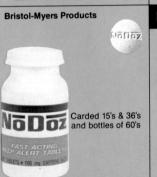

Available in ½ oz. metered spray pump
4-WAY®
LONG ACTING NASAL SPRAY

Bristol-Myers Products

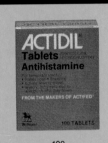

Boxes of 12 & 24 suppositories

PAZO
Hemorrhoid Ointment

Tubes of 1 & 2 oz.

PAZO®
Hemorrhoid Ointment and Suppositories

Bristol-Myers Products

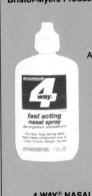

Bottles of 10's, 30's, 50's & 80's

EXCEDRIN P.M.®

Bristol-Myers Products

Atomizers of ½ & 1 oz.

Regular & Mentholated

4-WAY® NASAL SPRAY

Bristol-Myers Products

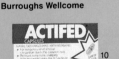

Carded 15's & 36's and bottles of 60's

NO-DOZ® TABLETS
(caffeine)

BURROUGHS WELLCOME

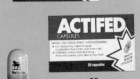

100
Syrup available in pints

ACTIDIL®
TABLETS & SYRUP

Bristol-Myers Products

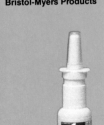

Available in blister packs of 24 and bottles of 50 tablets

SINUS EXCEDRIN® TABLETS
(acetaminophen, pseudoephedrine)

Bristol-Myers Products

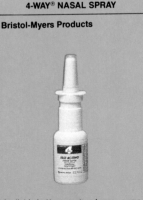

Available in ½ oz. metered spray pump
4-WAY®
FAST ACTING NASAL SPRAY

Bristol-Myers Products

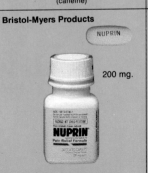

200 mg.

Available in bottles of 24, 50 and 100 caplets

NUPRIN® CAPLET
(ibuprofen)

Burroughs Wellcome

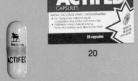

10

20

ACTIFED® CAPSULES

Continued on next page

Burroughs Wellcome

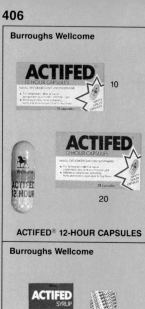

10

20

ACTIFED® 12-HOUR CAPSULES

Burroughs Wellcome

24

24

48

ALLERACT™
DECONGESTANT CAPLETS & TABLETS

Burroughs Wellcome

NEOSPORIN®

Available in ½ and 1 oz. tubes

NEOSPORIN®
ANTIBIOTIC
FIRST AID OINTMENT

Burroughs Wellcome

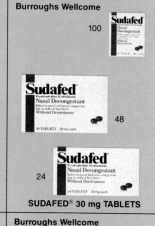

100

48

24

SUDAFED® 30 mg TABLETS

Burroughs Wellcome

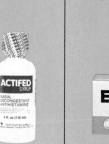

4 fl. oz.

Also available in pints

ACTIFED® SYRUP

Burroughs Wellcome

EMPIRIN ASPIRIN

250

Also available in 50s and 100s

EMPIRIN® ASPIRIN TABLETS

Burroughs Wellcome

Polysporin

Powder, 0.35 oz. (10g)

Spray, 3 oz. (85g)

Ointment Polysporin

½ oz.

1 oz.

POLYSPORIN®
FIRST AID ANTIBIOTIC
SPRAY, POWDER & OINTMENT

Burroughs Wellcome

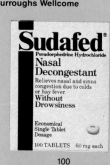

100

SUDAFED®
60 mg TABLETS

Burroughs Wellcome

12

24

Also available in 48s and in
bottles of 100

ACTIFED®
TABLETS

Burroughs Wellcome

marezine

12

Also available in 100s

MAREZINE® TABLETS

Burroughs Wellcome

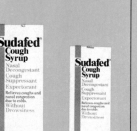

8 fl. oz.

4 fl. oz.

SUDAFED® COUGH SYRUP

Burroughs Wellcome

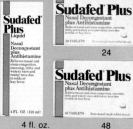

24

48

4 fl. oz.

SUDAFED® PLUS
LIQUID & TABLETS

Burroughs Wellcome

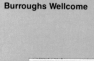

24

ALLERACT™
TABLETS

Burroughs Wellcome

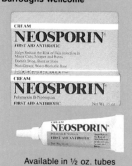

Available in ½ oz. tubes

NEOSPORIN® CREAM
ANTIBIOTIC
FIRST AID CREAM

Burroughs Wellcome

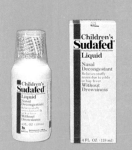

4 fl. oz.

CHILDREN'S SUDAFED® LIQUID

Burroughs Wellcome

Sudafed Sinus

24

Sudafed Sinus

24

Also available in 48s

SUDAFED® SINUS
CAPLETS & TABLETS

Burroughs Wellcome

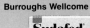
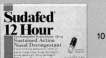
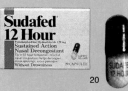

10

20

Also available in 40s

SUDAFED® 12 HOUR CAPSULES

CARTER PRODUCTS

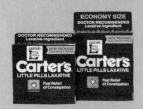

2 sizes: 75 pills
and 25 pills

CARTER'S LITTLE PILLS®
Laxative

(5 mg. bisacodyl)

CHURCH & DWIGHT

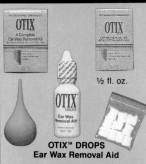

½ fl. oz.

OTIX™ DROPS
Ear Wax Removal Aid

Available: OTIX™ Drops with Cotton
Ear Plugs & Complete Wax Removal
Kit Including Bulb Irrigator

CIBA CONSUMER

ACUTRIM
16 Hour

MAXIMUM
STRENGTH

ACUTRIM II
Maximum

ACUTRIM
Late Day

ACUTRIM®
Appetite Suppressants

Caffeine Free/Precision Release™

CIBA Consumer

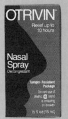
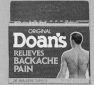

ORIGINAL DOAN'S®

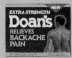

EXTRA STRENGTH DOAN'S®

Available in packages of 24 and
48 caplets

CIBA Consumer

Available in 2 oz and 1 oz tubes

Nupercainal
HEMORRHOIDAL & ANESTHETIC OINTMENT

Prompt, temporary relief of pain,
itching, and burning
due to painful hemorrhoids.

NUPERCAINAL®
Hemorrhoidal & Anesthetic
Ointment

CIBA Consumer

Available in boxes of
12 and 24 suppositories

Nupercainal
HEMORRHOIDAL SUPPOSITORIES

Temporary relief of itching, burning,
and discomfort of hemorrhoids.

NUPERCAINAL®
Hemorrhoidal Suppositories

CIBA Consumer

1½ oz

Nupercainal
PAIN-RELIEF CREAM

Prompt, temporary relief of painful
sunburn, minor burns, scrapes,
scratches, and nonpoisonous
insect bites.

NUPERCAINAL®
Pain-Relief Cream

CIBA Consumer

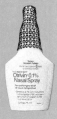

½ fl oz

OTRIVIN®
Nasal Decongestant Spray

CIBA Consumer

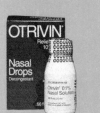

.66 fl oz

OTRIVIN®
Nasal Decongestant Drops

CIBA Consumer

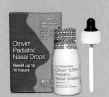
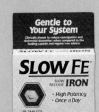

.66 fl oz

OTRIVIN®
Pediatric
Nasal Decongestant Drops

CIBA Consumer

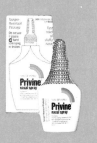

½ fl oz

PRIVINE®
Nasal Decongestant Spray

CIBA Consumer

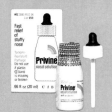

.66 fl oz

PRIVINE®
Nasal Decongestant Solution

CIBA Consumer

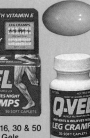

Bottles of 16, 30 & 50
Soft Gels
Q-vel®
Muscle Relaxant
Pain Reliever

CIBA Consumer

SLOW FE
SLOW RELEASE IRON
- High Potency
- Once a Day

Available in packages of
30, 60 & 100 tablets
SLOW FE®
Slow Release Iron

CIBA Consumer

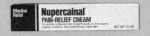
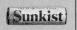

SUNKIST®
Vitamin C Citrus Complex

250 & 500 mg chewable tablets;
500 mg easy to swallow caplets;
60 mg chewable tablets
(11-tablet roll)

Continued on next page

CIBA Consumer

Regular

+Extra C

+Iron

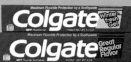

Complete

SUNKIST®
Children's Multivitamins

COLGATE-PALMOLIVE

Available in flip-cap tubes
or in pump dispensers

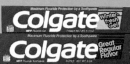

Flip-top Gel Tubes available in 1.4,
2.6, 4.6, 6.4 and 8.2 oz.
Flip-top Toothpaste Tubes available
in 1.5 3.0, 5.0, 7.0 and 9.0 oz.

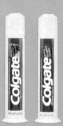

Gel Pumps available in 4.5
and 6.4 oz.
Toothpaste Pumps available in 4.9
and 6.4 oz.

COLGATE® MFP®
FLUORIDE
TOOTHPASTE & GEL

Colgate-Palmolive

Available in flip-cap tubes
or in pump dispensers

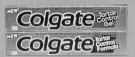

Flip-top Gel and Toothpaste
Tubes available in 1.3, 2.6, 4.6,
6.4 and 8.2 oz.

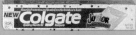

Gel and Toothpaste Pumps
available in 4.5 oz.

COLGATE®
TARTAR CONTROL
FORMULA & GEL

Colgate-Palmolive

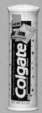

Available in
flip-cap tubes
or in pump
dispensers

Flip-top tube
available in 2.7,
4.5, 6.4 and 8.2 oz.
Pump available
in 4.5 oz.

COLGATE® JUNIOR
Fluoride Gel Toothpaste

Colgate-Palmolive

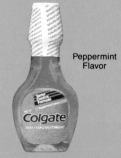

Peppermint
Flavor

COLGATE® MOUTHWASH
Tartar Control Formula

Colgate-Palmolive

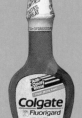

FLUORIGARD™
Anti-Cavity Fluoride Rinse

CUMBERLAND-SWAN

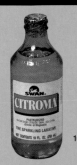

10 fl. oz.

CITROMA®
(citrate of magnesia)
The Sparkling Laxative

For more detailed in-
formation on products
illustrated in this sec-
tion, consult the Prod-
uct Information Sec-
tion or manufacturers
may be contacted di-
rectly.

While every effort has
been made to reproduce
products faithfully, this
section is to be consid-
ered a Quick-Reference
identification aid.

GLENBROOK

Division of Sterling Drug Inc.

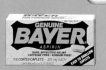

Available in
bottles of
50's and 100's

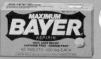

Available in packs of 12 tablets
and bottles of 24's, 50's,
100's, 200's and 300's

GENUINE BAYER® ASPIRIN
Toleraid® Micro-Thin Coating
Sodium Free • Caffeine Free

Glenbrook

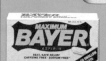

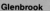

Available in bottles of 60's

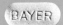

500 mg.

MAXIMUM BAYER® ASPIRIN
Toleraid® Micro-Thin Coating
Sodium Free • Caffeine Free

Glenbrook

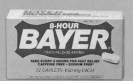

Available in bottles of
30, 72, and 125 caplets

8-HOUR BAYER®
TIMED-RELEASE ASPIRIN
Sodium Free • Caffeine Free

Glenbrook

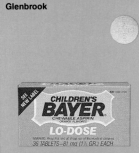

Available in bottle
of 36 tablets

**BAYER® CHILDREN'S
CHEWABLE ASPIRIN
LO-DOSE**

Glenbrook

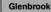
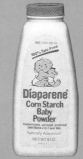

Available in 4 oz., 9 oz., and
14 oz. containers

DIAPARENE® BABY POWDER

Glenbrook

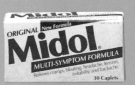

Available in packages of 12, 30
and 60 caplets®

MIDOL®

Glenbrook

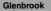
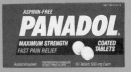
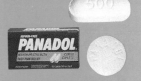

MAXIMUM STRENGTH PANADOL®
Coated Caplets and Tablets
Acetaminophen

Glenbrook

Available in bottle
of 36 tablets

**BAYER® CHILDREN'S
COLD TABLETS**

Glenbrook

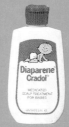

3 oz.

DIAPARENE® CRADOL®

Medicated Scalp Treatment
for Babies

Glenbrook

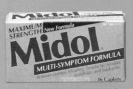

Available in packages of
8, 16 and 32 caplets®

**MIDOL®
MAXIMUM STRENGTH**

Glenbrook

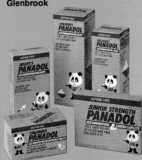

CHILDREN'S PANADOL®
Chewable Tablets, Caplets, Liquid
and Drops
Acetaminophen

Glenbrook

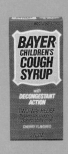

Available in 3 oz. cherry flavor

**BAYER® CHILDREN'S
COUGH SYRUP**

Glenbrook

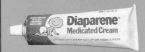
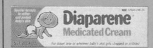

Available in tubes of
1 oz., 2 oz., 4 oz.

**DIAPARENE®
MEDICATED CREAM**

Glenbrook

Available in packages of 16 and 32
coated tablets

MIDOL® 200

Glenbrook

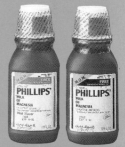

Available in regular and mint flavor
4 oz., 12 oz., 26 oz. plastic bottles

PHILLIPS® MILK OF MAGNESIA

Glenbrook

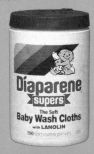

Available in canisters of
70 and 150 wash cloths

**DIAPARENE® SUPERS
BABY WASH CLOTHS**

Glenbrook

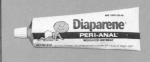
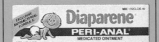

Available in tubes of
1 oz., 2 oz., 4 oz.

**DIAPARENE®
PERI-ANAL OINTMENT**

Glenbrook

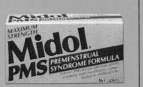

Available in bottles of
16 and 32 caplets

**MIDOL® PMS
MAXIMUM STRENGTH**

Glenbrook

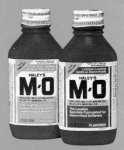

Available in regular and flavored
4 oz., 12 oz. and 26 oz. plastic bottles

HALEY'S M-O®

Continued on next page

410   **Product Identification**

Glenbrook

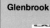

24 capsules

48 capsules

LAXCAPS®
Laxative Plus Softener
Combined Action Formula

Glenbrook

Regular
Strength
Pads

In containers of
42 and 75 pads

Maximum
Strength
Pads

In containers of
12, 42 and 75 pads

STRIDEX®

Glenbrook

VANQUISH
*The Extra-Strength
Pain Formula with
Two Buffers*

Available in packages
of 30, 60 and 100 caplets

VANQUISH®
Extra-Strength Pain Formula
with Two Buffers

HOECHST-ROUSSEL

Doxidan®

DOXIDAN®

Packages
of 10 and 30,
Bottles of 100

Stimulant/Stool Softener Laxative

DOXIDAN®
(docusate calcium USP,
phenolphthalein USP)

Hoechst-Roussel

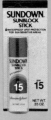

Festal® II
DIGESTIVE AID
100 TABLETS

Bottles
of 100
Tablets

Digestive Aid

FESTAL® II
(digestive enzymes)

Hoechst-Roussel

50 mg
Packages of
30 and 100

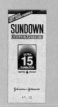

Surfak
docusate calcium USP
Stool Softener
30 CAPSULES
240 MG EACH

240 mg
Packages of
7 and 30,
Bottles of 100

Surfak®

Stool Softener

SURFAK®
(docusate calcium USP)

Hynson, Westcott & Dunning

Product must be refrigerated

Lactinex™ Granules

Lactinex

Granules: 1 gram packet

Tablets: bottles of 50

LACTINEX®
Tablets & Granules
(Lactobacillus acidophilus and
Lactobacillus bulgaricus)

JOHNSON & JOHNSON
Baby Products Company

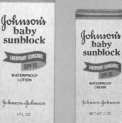

**Johnson's
baby
sunblock**
EVERYDAY SUNCARE
SPF 15
WATERPROOF
LOTION

**Johnson's
baby
sunblock**
EVERYDAY SUNCARE
WATERPROOF
CREAM

Waterproof
Lotion

Waterproof
Cream

**JOHNSON'S BABY SUNBLOCK
SPF 15 Everyday Suncare**

Baby Products Company

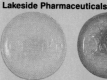

SUNDOWN
SUNBLOCK
STICK
15

SUNDOWN
SUNBLOCK
15

Also available:
SPF 8 and 20

Also available:
SPF 4, 6, 8,
20 and 24

SUNDOWN® SUNBLOCK
Lotion and Stick

Baby Products Company

SUNDOWN
15

SUNDOWN
30

Lotion
Also available:
SPF 25

Cream

**SUNDOWN®
BROAD SPECTRUM**

Sunblock Lotions and Cream

JOHNSON & JOHNSON

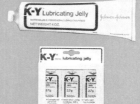

K-Y Lubricating Jelly

K-Y
lubricating jelly

K-Y

Available in 2 oz. and 4 oz. tubes
and single-use packs

K-Y® BRAND LUBRICATING JELLY
Water Soluble, for General
Lubricating Needs

For more detailed information on products illustrated in this section, consult the Product Information Section or manufacturers may be contacted directly.

Lakeside Pharmaceuticals

Cepacol Gold

Available in 4, 12, 18, 24
and 32 fl. oz. bottles

Cepacol Mint

Cepacol

CEPACOL®
Mouthwash/Gargle

Lakeside Pharmaceuticals

**Cepacol
Throat Lozenges**

**Cepacol Anesthetic
Lozenges (Troches)**

18 lozenges per package

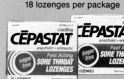

Cepacol
THROAT LOZENGES

Cepacol
ANESTHETIC LOZENGES (TROCHES)

CEPACOL®
Throat Lozenges

Lakeside Pharmaceuticals

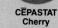

**CEPASTAT
Regular**

**CEPASTAT
Cherry**

18 lozenges per package

CEPASTAT
SORE THROAT
LOZENGES

CEPASTAT
cherry
SORE THROAT
LOZENGES

CEPASTAT®
Sore Throat Lozenges

Lakeside Pharmaceuticals

**CITRUCEL
Orange**
Available in 16 oz.
and 30 oz.
containers

**CITRUCEL
Regular**
Available in 7 oz.
and 10 oz.
containers

CITRUCEL®
Therapeutic Fiber
for Regularity

Lakeside Pharmaceuticals

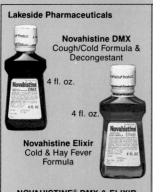

Novahistine DMX
Cough/Cold Formula & Decongestant

4 fl. oz.

4 fl. oz.

Novahistine Elixir
Cold & Hay Fever Formula

NOVAHISTINE® DMX & ELIXIR
Cough/Cold
Products

Lederle

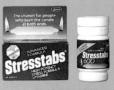

C45

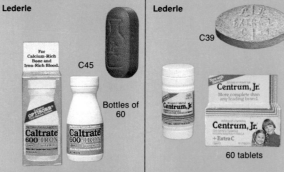

Bottles of 60

CALTRATE® 600+IRON+
VITAMIN D
High Potency Calcium
Supplement

Lederle

C39

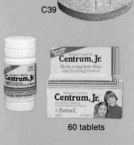

60 tablets

CENTRUM, JR.®
Children's Chewable
Vitamin/Mineral Formula + Extra C

Lederle

S1

Bottles of 30 and 60

Advanced Formula
STRESSTABS® 600

High Potency Stress Formula
Vitamins

LEDERLE

LEDERMARK®
Product Identification
Code

Many Lederle tablets and capsules bear an identification code, and these codes are listed with each product pictured. A current listing appears in the Product Information Section of the 1989 Physicians' Desk Reference.

Lederle

C360

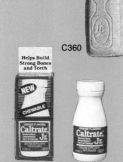

CALTRATE® JR.
Chewable Calcium Supplement
For Children

Lederle

C60

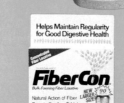

60 tablets

CENTRUM, JR.® +Extra Calcium
Children's Chewable
Vitamin/Mineral Formula

Lederle

S2

Bottles of 30 and 60

Advanced Formula
STRESSTABS® 600
with IRON

High Potency Stress Formula
Vitamins

Lederle
Now available in smaller size tablet

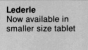

C600

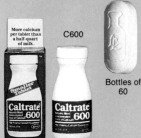

Bottles of 60

CALTRATE® 600
High Potency Calcium
Supplement

Lederle

Bottles of 100 + 30
Bottles of 60

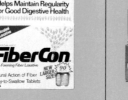

C1

Advanced Formula CENTRUM®
High Potency Multivitamin/
Multimineral Formula

Lederle

F66

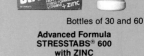

FiberCon

Available in boxes of 36, 60 and 90

FIBERCON®
Calcium Polycarbophil
Bulk-Forming Fiber Laxative

Lederle

S3

Bottles of 30 and 60

Advanced Formula
STRESSTABS® 600
with ZINC

High Potency Stress Formula
Vitamins

Lederle
Now available in smaller size tablet

C45

Bottles of 60

CALTRATE® 600+D
High Potency Calcium
Supplement

Lederle

C2

60 tablets

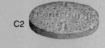
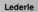
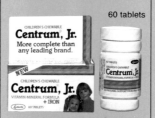

CENTRUM, JR.®
Children's Chewable
Vitamin/Mineral Formula + Iron
More Essential Nutrients

Lederle

F2

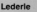
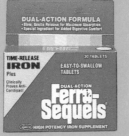

Dual-Action
FERRO-SEQUELS®
High Potency Iron Supplement

Lederle

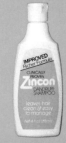

Bottles of 4 fl. oz. and 8 fl. oz.

ZINCON®
Pyrithione Zinc 1%
Dandruff Shampoo

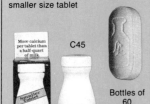
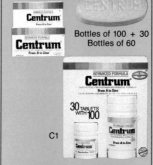
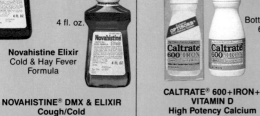
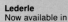

LEEMING

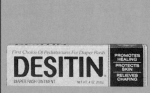

DESITIN®
Diaper Rash Ointment

LEVER BROTHERS

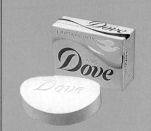

Dove® Bar
Original and New Unscented

Marion

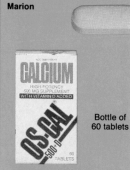

12 fl. oz.   6 fl. oz.

GAVISCON®
Liquid Antacid

Marion

Bottle of
60 tablets

OS-CAL® 500+D
Tablets
(calcium with vitamin D)

Leeming   ½ fl. oz.

VISINE®
Redness
Reliever
Eye Drops

VISINE a.c.®
Astringent/
Redness
Reliever
Eye Drops

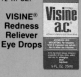

VISINE® EXTRA Redness Reliever/
Lubricant Eye Drops

MARION

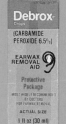

1 fl. oz.   ½ fl. oz.

DEBROX®
Drops

Marion

Box of 48
foil-wrapped
tablets

GAVISCON®-2
Antacid Tablets

Marion

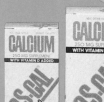

Bottles of 60 and 120 tablets

OS-CAL® 500
Tablets

For more detailed information on products illustrated in this section, consult the Product Information Section or manufacturers may be contacted directly.

Marion

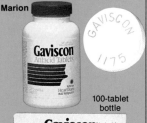

100-tablet
bottle

30-tablet box (foil-wrapped 2s)
GAVISCON®
Antacid Tablets

Marion

2 fl. oz.   ½ fl. oz.

GLY-OXIDE® Liquid

Marion

Bottles of 100 and 240 tablets

OS-CAL® 250+D
Tablets
(calcium with vitamin D)

While every effort has been made to reproduce products faithfully, this section is to be considered a Quick-Reference identification aid.

Marion

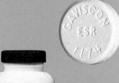

100-tablet
bottle

GAVISCON®
Extra Strength
Relief Formula Antacid Tablets

Marion

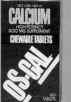

Bottle of
60 tablets

OS-CAL® 500
Chewable Tablets

Marion

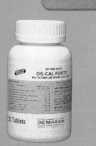

Bottle of 100 tablets

OS-CAL FORTE®
Multivitamin and Mineral
Supplement

Marion

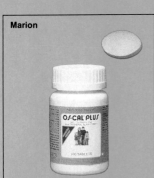

Bottle of 100 tablets

OS-CAL® PLUS
Multivitamin and Multimineral
Supplement

McNeil Consumer

500 mg.

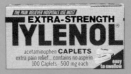

Caplets available in
tamper-resistant bottles
of 10, 24, 50 and 100.

EXTRA-STRENGTH TYLENOL®
acetaminophen
Caplets

McNeil Consumer

SINE-AID®

Available in blister
packs of 24 and bottles
of 50 and 100 tablets. No Drowsiness
Formula

Available in blister packs of 24
and bottles of 50 caplets.

EXTRA-STRENGTH SINE-AID®
For sinus headache pain and pressure

McNeil Consumer

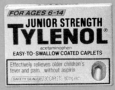

Available in
child-resistant blister-pack of 30.

JUNIOR STRENGTH TYLENOL®
acetaminophen
Swallowable Tablets

Marion

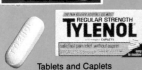

Box of 60 lozenges

THROAT DISCS®
Throat Lozenges

McNeil Consumer

500 mg.

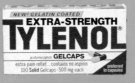

Gelcaps available in
tamper-resistant bottles
of 24, 50 and 100.

EXTRA-STRENGTH TYLENOL®
acetaminophen
GELCAPS®

McNeil Consumer

Available in ½ fl. oz. bottle with
child-resistant safety cap and
calibrated dropper.

INFANTS' TYLENOL®
acetaminophen
Alcohol Free Drops

McNeil Consumer

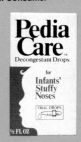

Available in ½ fl. oz. bottle with
child-resistant safety cap and
calibrated dropper.

PEDIACARE®
Oral Decongestant Drops

McNEIL CONSUMER

325 mg.

Tablets and Caplets
Available in 24's, 50's and 100's.

REGULAR STRENGTH TYLENOL®
acetaminophen   Tablets and Caplets

McNeil Consumer

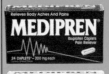

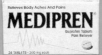

Caplets and Tablets available in
bottles of 24, 50 and 100.

MEDIPREN®
ibuprofen

McNeil Consumer

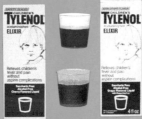
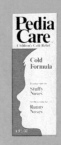

Available in cherry and grape
flavors in 2 and 4 fl. oz. bottles
with child-resistant safety cap and
convenient dosage cup.

CHILDREN'S TYLENOL®
acetaminophen
Alcohol Free Elixir

McNeil Consumer

Available in 4 fl. oz. bottle with
child-resistant safety cap and
convenient dosage cup.

PEDIACARE®
Cold Formula

McNeil Consumer

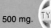

500 mg.

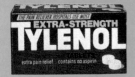

Tablets available in tamper-resistant
vials of 10 and bottles of 30, 60, 100
and 200. Liquid: 8 fl. oz.

EXTRA-STRENGTH TYLENOL®
acetaminophen
Tablets & Liquid

McNeil Consumer

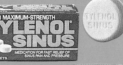

MAXIMUM-STRENGTH
TYLENOL®
SINUS MEDICATION
Caplets: Bottles of 24's and 50's.
Tablets: Bottles of 24's and 50's

McNeil Consumer

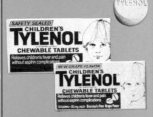
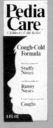

Fruit flavor: available in bottles
of 30 with child-resistant safety
cap and blister-packs of 48.
Grape flavor: available in bottles of
30 with child-resistant safety cap.

CHILDREN'S TYLENOL®
acetaminophen
Chewable Tablets

McNeil Consumer

Available in 4 fl. oz. bottle with
convenient dosage cup and in bottles
of 24 chewable tablets, both with
child-resistant safety cap.

PEDIACARE®
Cough-Cold Formula

McNeil Consumer

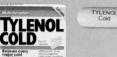

Available in blister-packs of 24 and bottles of 50.

TYLENOL®
COLD MEDICATION
Tablets and Caplets

McNeil Consumer

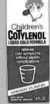

Available in 4 fl. oz. bottle with child-resistant safety cap and convenient dosage cup.

CHILDREN'S COTYLENOL®
Liquid Cold Formula

Mead Johnson Nutritionals

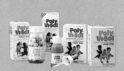

POLY-VI-SOL®
CHEWABLE VITAMINS
with and without iron

POLY-VI-SOL®
VITAMIN DROPS
with and without iron

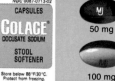

Bottles of 30, 60, 250 and 1000
Stool Softener

†COLACE®
(docusate sodium)

McNeil Consumer

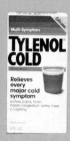

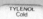

Available in 5 fl. oz. bottle with child-resistant safety cap and convenient dosage cup enclosed.

TYLENOL®
COLD MEDICATION LIQUID

McNeil Consumer

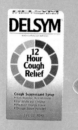
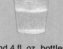

Available in 3 fl. oz. bottle with child-resistant safety cap and convenient dosage spoon enclosed.

DELSYM®
dextromethorphan polistirex
12-HOUR COUGH RELIEF

Mead Johnson Nutritionals

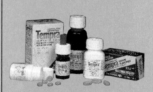

Available in bottles of 60 and 100 tablets

POLY-VI-SOL® CIRCUS SHAPES
CHEWABLE VITAMINS
with and without iron

Mead Johnson Pharmaceuticals

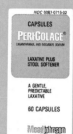

Bottles of 30, 60, 250 and 1000
Laxative and Stool Softener

†PERI-COLACE®
(casanthranol and docusate sodium)

McNeil Consumer

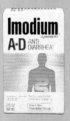

Available in blister-packs of 24 and bottles of 50.

TYLENOL®
COLD MEDICATION
No Drowsiness
Formula Caplets

McNeil Consumer

Available in 2, 3 and 4 fl. oz. bottles with a convenient dosage cup.

IMODIUM® A-D
loperamide HCl
ANTI-DIARRHEAL

Mead Johnson Nutritionals

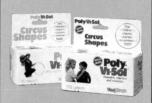

Alcohol-free
Aspirin-free
TEMPRA®
Acetaminophen for children

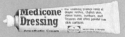

1½ oz.

MEDICONE® DERMA
Anesthetic/Astringent Ointment

McNeil Consumer

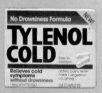

Available in bottles of 24 chewable tablets with child-resistant safety cap.

CHILDREN'S COTYLENOL®
Chewable Cold Tablets

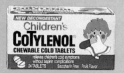

13 fl. oz.

ENFAMIL®   **ENFAMIL®**
               With Iron

Infant Formula for
Baby's First Twelve Months

Mead Johnson Nutritionals

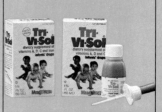

TRI-VI-SOL®
VITAMIN DROPS
with and without iron

Medicone

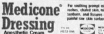

1½ oz.

MEDICONE® DRESSING
Anesthetic Cream

Medicone

MEDICONE® RECTAL OINTMENT

1½ oz.

**MEDICONE®
RECTAL SUPPOSITORIES**

Medicone

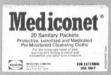

20 Packets

Moist Cleansing
Cloths

**MEDICONET®
CLEANSING CLOTHS**

MILES INC.

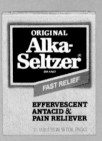

**ALKA-SELTZER® BRAND
EFFERVESCENT
ANTACID & PAIN RELIEVER**

Miles Inc.
Consumer Healthcare Division

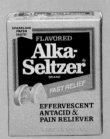

**ALKA-SELTZER® BRAND
FLAVORED EFFERVESCENT
ANTACID & PAIN RELIEVER**

Miles Inc.
Consumer Healthcare Division

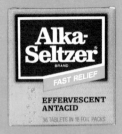

**ALKA-SELTZER® BRAND
EFFERVESCENT ANTACID**

Miles Inc.
Consumer Healthcare Division

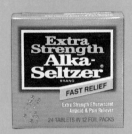

**ALKA-SELTZER® BRAND
EXTRA STRENGTH
EFFERVESCENT ANTACID &
PAIN RELIEVER**

Miles Inc.
Consumer Healthcare Division

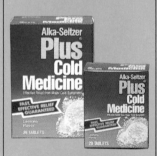

**ALKA-SELTZER PLUS®
COLD MEDICINE**

Miles Inc.
Consumer Healthcare Division

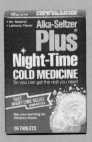

**ALKA-SELTZER PLUS®
NIGHT-TIME
COLD MEDICINE**

Miles Inc.
Consumer Healthcare Division

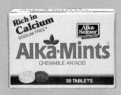

**ALKA-MINTS® CHEWABLE
ANTACID**
(Calcium Carbonate 850 mg)

Miles Inc.
Consumer Healthcare Division

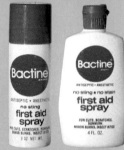

**BACTINE® BRAND
ANTISEPTIC • ANESTHETIC
FIRST AID SPRAY**
Aerosol and Liquid

Miles Inc.
Consumer Healthcare Division

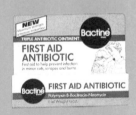

**BACTINE®
FIRST AID
ANTIBIOTIC OINTMENT**

Miles Inc.
Consumer Healthcare Division

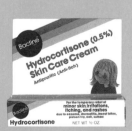

**BACTINE® BRAND
HYDROCORTISONE (0.5%)
SKIN CARE CREAM**

Miles Inc.
Consumer Healthcare Division

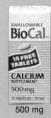

500 mg

**BIOCAL™
CALCIUM SUPPLEMENT**
(Calcium Carbonate)

Miles Inc.
Consumer Healthcare Division

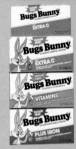

**BUGS BUNNY® BRAND SUGAR FREE
CHILDREN'S CHEWABLE VITAMINS
WITH EXTRA C, REGULAR,
AND PLUS IRON**

Miles Inc.
Consumer Healthcare Division

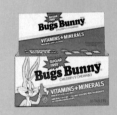

**BUGS BUNNY® BRAND SUGAR FREE
CHILDREN'S CHEWABLE
VITAMINS + MINERALS**

Miles Inc.
Consumer Healthcare Division

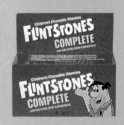

**FLINTSTONES® BRAND COMPLETE
CHILDREN'S CHEWABLE VITAMINS
WITH IRON, CALCIUM & MINERALS**

Continued on next page

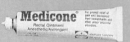

Miles Inc.
Consumer Healthcare Division

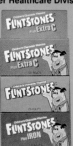

**FLINTSTONES® BRAND
CHILDREN'S CHEWABLE VITAMINS
WITH EXTRA C, REGULAR,
AND PLUS IRON**

Miles Inc.
Consumer Healthcare Division

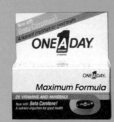

**ONE A DAY® BRAND
MAXIMUM FORMULA
THE MOST COMPLETE
ONE A DAY® BRAND**

Norcliff Thayer

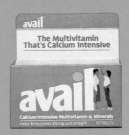

60 tablets

AVAIL™

Norcliff Thayer

OXY® 5
Vanishing   OXY® 5
Tinted

OXY® 10
Vanishing   OXY® 10
Tinted

Miles Inc.
Consumer Healthcare Division

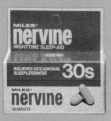

**MILES® NERVINE
NIGHTTIME SLEEP-AID**

(Diphenhydramine HCl 25 mg)

Miles Inc.
Consumer Healthcare Division

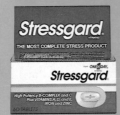

**STRESSGARD®
STRESS FORMULA VITAMINS**

Norcliff Thayer

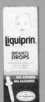

1.16 fl. oz.   4 fl. oz.

Fruit Flavored Drops and
Cherry Elixir
Alcohol Free
Child Resistant Safety Cap

LIQUIPRIN®
Acetaminophen

Norcliff Thayer

Regular   Maximum
Strength   Strength
50 pads
Also available: 90 pads

**OXY CLEAN®
MEDICATED PADS**

Miles Inc.
Consumer Healthcare Division

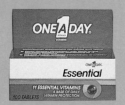

ONE A DAY® BRAND VITAMINS

Miles Inc.
Consumer Healthcare Division

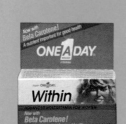

ONE-A-DAY® WITHIN®
Advanced Multivitamin
For Women With Calcium &
Extra Iron

Norcliff Thayer

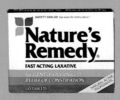

60 tablets

NATURE'S REMEDY®

Also available:
Box 12s and 30s

Norcliff Thayer

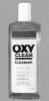

Medicated   Lathering
Cleanser   Facial
4 fl. oz.   Scrub
             2.65 oz.

 Medicated Soap
3.25 oz.

OXY CLEAN®

Miles Inc.
Consumer Healthcare Division

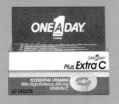

**ONE A DAY® BRAND PLUS EXTRA C
VITAMINS**

11 essential vitamins
with high potency
300 mg Vitamin C

NORCLIFF THAYER

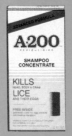

4 fl. oz.

A-200® PEDICULICIDE SHAMPOO

Also available:
A-200® Pediculicide Shampoo, 2 fl. oz.
A-200® Pediculicide Gel, 1 oz.

Norcliff Thayer

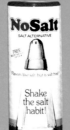

11 oz.   8 oz.

NOSALT®
Salt Alternative

**SEASONED
NOSALT®**
Salt Alternative

Norcliff Thayer

TUMS®
Peppermint   **TUMS®**
Assorted Flavors

TUMS E-X®
Wintergreen   **TUMS E-X®**
Assorted Flavors

Norcliff Thayer

Available in Extra Strength and Extra Strength with Simethicone

12 fl. oz.

TUMS® LIQUID
Extra Strength Antacid
(calcium carbonate)

Noxell

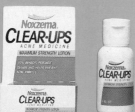

CLEAR-UPS®
Maximum Strength Lotion
Acne Medicine

ORTHO

Ortho—Advanced Care Prods.

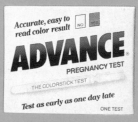

Test as early as one day late
ADVANCE®
Pregnancy Test

Ortho—Advanced Care Prods.

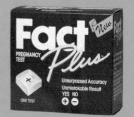

Unmistakable Result
FACT PLUS™
Pregnancy Test

NOXELL

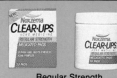

Regular Strength

Maximum Strength

CLEAR-UPS®
Medicated Cleansing Pads

Noxell

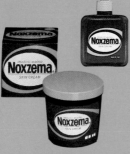

NOXZEMA®
Greaseless   Medicated
Skin Cream

Ortho—Advanced Care Prods.

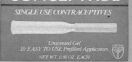

6's (6 easy-to-use prefilled applicators)
10's (10 easy-to-use prefilled applicators)

CONCEPTROL™
Single Use Contraceptives
(nonoxynol 9, 4%)

Ortho—Advanced Care Prods.

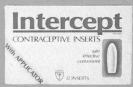

Gynol II is intended for
use with a diaphragm

Starter (2.5 oz. tube with
applicator package)
Refill (2.5 oz. and 3.8 oz.
tube only packages)

GYNOL II®
Contraceptive Jelly
(nonoxynol 9, 2%)

Noxell

Vanishing
(invisible)

Concealing
(tinted)

CLEAR-UPS®
On-The-Spot
Acne Medicine

Noxell

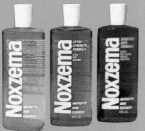

Regular
Formula

Extra
Strength
Formula

Sensitive
Skin
Formula

NOXZEMA®
Antiseptic Skin Cleanser

Ortho—Advanced Care Prods.

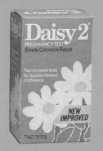

Two complete tests in each kit.

DAISY 2®
Pregnancy Test

Ortho—Advanced Care Prods.

Starter (12 inserts w/applicator
package)
Refill (12 inserts)

INTERCEPT®
Contraceptive Inserts
(nonoxynol 9, 5.56%)

Noxell

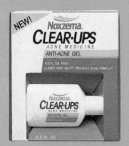

CLEAR-UPS®
Anti-Acne Gel
Acne Medicine

ORAL-B

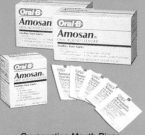

Oxygenating Mouth Rinse

AMOSAN®

For Gum Inflammation and Oral
Discomfort

Ortho—Advanced Care Prods.

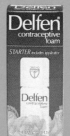

Starter (0.70 oz. vial w/applicator
package)
Refill (0.70 oz. and 1.75 oz. vial
only packages)
DELFEN® Contraceptive Foam
(nonoxynol 9, 12.5%)

Ortho—Advanced Care Prods.

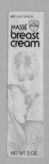

2 oz. tube

MASSÉ® Breast Cream

Ortho—Advanced Care Prods.

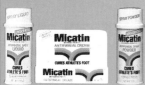

Spray Liquid (3.5 oz.)

Cream (½ oz. and 1 oz.)

Spray Powder and Spray Deodorant (3.0 oz.)

MICATIN® Antifungal
For Athlete's Foot
(miconazole nitrate, 2%)

PARKE-DAVIS

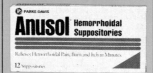

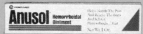

Available in boxes of 12, 24 and 48

Available in 1 Oz. and 2 Oz. Tubes

ANUSOL®
Suppositories and Ointment

Parke-Davis

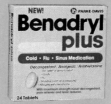

Available in boxes of 24

BENADRYL® PLUS
Decongestant/Analgesic/
Antihistamine

Parke-Davis

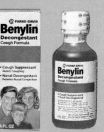

Available in 4 Oz. Bottles

BENYLIN®
Decongestant Cough Formula

Ortho—Advanced Care Prods.

ORTHO-CREME
CONTRACEPTIVE CREAM FOR USE WITH DIAPHRAGM
NET WT. 3.45 OZ.

Ortho-Creme is intended for use with a diaphragm

2.15 oz. and 3.45 oz. tube only packages.

ORTHO-CREME®
Contraceptive Cream
(nonoxynol 9, 2.00%)

Parke-Davis

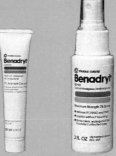

Available in Cream and Spray

BENADRYL®
Topical Antihistamine

Parke-Davis

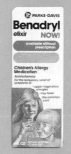

Available in 4 Oz. and 8 Oz. Bottles

BENADRYL®
Elixir

Parke-Davis

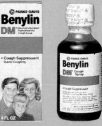

Available in 4 Oz. Bottles

BENYLIN DM®
Cough Syrup

Ortho—Advanced Care Prods.

ORTHO-GYNOL
CONTRACEPTIVE JELLY FOR USE WITH DIAPHRAGM
NET WT. 3.51 OZ.

Ortho-Gynol is intended for use with a diaphragm

ORTHO-GYNOL®
Contraceptive Jelly
(diisobutylphenoxypolyethoxyethanol, 1.00%)

Parke-Davis

Available in boxes of 24

BENADRYL®
Decongestant

Parke-Davis

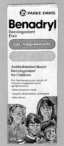

Available in 4 Oz. Bottles

BENADRYL®
Decongestant Elixir

Parke-Davis

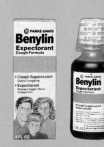

Available in 4 Oz. and 8 Oz. Bottles

BENYLIN® EXPECTORANT

Ortho—Advanced Care Prods.

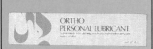

2 oz. and 4 oz. tubes

ORTHO® PERSONAL LUBRICANT

Parke-Davis

Kapseals available in boxes of 24 and 48

Tablets available in boxes of 24 and bottles of 100

BENADRYL® 25

Parke-Davis

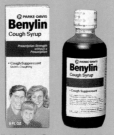

Available in 4 Oz. and 8 Oz. Bottles

BENYLIN®
Cough Syrup

Parke-Davis

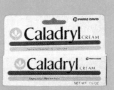

Available in Lotion and Cream
For relief from itching due to:
Poison Ivy, Insect Bites, Poison Oak,
Mild Sunburn, Minor Skin Irritation

CALADRYL®
Topical Antihistamine/Skin Protectant

Parke-Davis

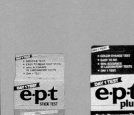

e·p·t®
STICK TEST

e·p·t®
PLUS

Early Pregnancy Test

Parke-Davis

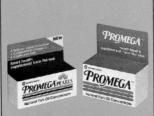

PROMEGA™
PEARLS
600 mg.
Soft Gels

PROMEGA™
1000 mg.
Soft Gels

Parke-Davis

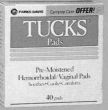

40 pads

Also available in 100 pad packages

**TUCKS®
Pre-Moistened Pads**

Plough, Inc.

Available in
15, 30, 60
and 90 tablet sizes.

CORRECTOL® LAXATIVE
(Tablet contains 100 mg. docusate sodium
and 65 mg. phenolphthalein.)

Parke-Davis

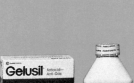

Also available:
50 tablets

**GELUSIL®
Antacid-Anti-gas
Sodium Free**

12 Fl. Oz.

Parke-Davis

Easy-to-open package
(Non-child resistant)

Child-resistant package
REGULAR SINUTAB®

Parke-Davis

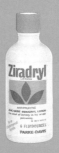

6 Fl. Oz.

ZIRADRYL® LOTION

Plough, Inc.

Liquid   Tablets

Mint and Lemon/Orange flavors,
6 fl. oz. and 12 fl. oz. liquid plus 30
and 90 tablet sizes.
Now also available in 3-roll pack
and 60 tablet bottle (Mint only).

DI-GEL®

Parke-Davis

12 or 24
squares

For 8 hour cough control

12 squares

For nasal congestion and cough relief

**MEDIQUELL®
Chewy Cough Squares**

Parke-Davis

Caplets

Tablets

**MAXIMUM STRENGTH
SINUTAB®**

PLOUGH, INC.

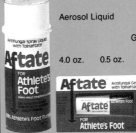

Aerosol Liquid

Gel

4.0 oz.   0.5 oz.

Also available in 3.5 oz. spray powder
and 2.25 oz. shaker powder.

AFTATE® FOR ATHLETE'S FOOT
(tolnaftate)

Plough, Inc.

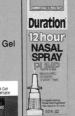

Available in ½ oz., 1 oz.; ½ oz.
measured dosage pump spray;
and ½ oz. mentholated.
(oxymetazoline HCl)

**DURATION®
NASAL SPRAY**

Parke-Davis

Available in bottles of 130 Tablets

**MYADEC®
Multivitamin-Multimineral Supplement**

Parke-Davis

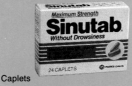

Caplets

Tablets

**MAXIMUM STRENGTH
SINUTAB®
Without Drowsiness**

Plough, Inc.

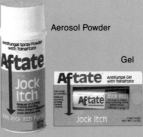

Aerosol Powder

Gel

3.5 oz.   0.5 oz.
Also available in 1.5 oz. shaker powder.

AFTATE® FOR JOCK ITCH
(tolnaftate)

Plough, Inc.

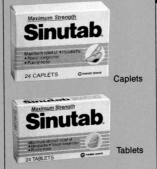

Available in 10's or 20's

**DURATION®
DECONGESTANT TABLETS**
(pseudoephedrine sulfate)

Continued on next page

Plough, Inc.

Pill
Available in 15,
30 and 60's

Gum
Available in 5,
16 and 40's

FEEN-A-MINT® LAXATIVE

Gum contains:
97.2 mg. phenolphthalein.
Pills contain: 100 mg. docusate
sodium and 65 mg. phenolphthalein.

Plough, Inc.

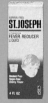

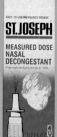

ST. JOSEPH® ASPIRIN-FREE
Fever Reducers
Alcohol-Free, Sugar-Free
Infant Drops — Liquid and Tablets

Plough, Inc.

Gum & Mints
Available in Spear-
mint, Peppermint
& Cinnamint

STAY TRIM®
Appetite Suppressant Products
(phenylpropanolamine HCl)

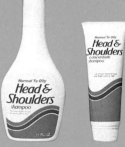

HEAD & SHOULDERS®
Dandruff Care Shampoo

Plough, Inc.

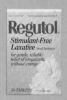

Available in 30, 60 and 90
tablet sizes.

REGUTOL®
STOOL SOFTENER
(100 mg. docusate sodium per tablet)

Plough, Inc.

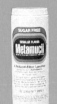

½ fl. oz.
bottle

ST. JOSEPH® MEASURED DOSE
NASAL DECONGESTANT
(phenylephrine HCl 0.125%)

Plough, Inc.

SPF 6   SPF 8

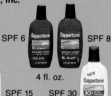

4 fl. oz.

SPF 15   SPF 30

SPF 6–15: padimate O, oxbenzone
SPF 30: also includes ethylhexyl
p-methoxycinnamate, 2-ethylhexyl
salicylate, Padimate O, oxybenzone

Also available in SPF 4, SPF 25 and
SPF 44 Lotion

COPPERTONE® WATERPROOF
SUNSCREENS

Procter & Gamble

METAMUCIL®

Natural Therapeutic Fiber
for Regularity

Plough, Inc.

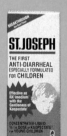

2 fl. oz.
bottle

ST. JOSEPH®
CHILDREN'S ANTI-DIARRHEAL
Each teaspoon contains 750 mg.
of non-fibrous attapulgite

Plough, Inc.

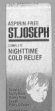

4 fl. oz.
bottle

Each 5 cc (average teaspoon) contains:
Chlorpheniramine maleate 1 mg.,
pseudoephedrine hydrochloride 15 mg.,
acetaminophen 160 mg., dextromethorphan
hydrobromide 5 mg.

ST. JOSEPH®
NIGHTTIME COLD RELIEF

Plough, Inc.

SPF 15   SPF 25   SPF 30
4 fl. oz.

SPF 15: ethylhexyl p-methoxycinnamate,
oxybenzone
SPF 25: ethylhexyl p-methoxycinnamate,
2-ethylhexyl salicylate, homosalate,
oxybenzone
SPF 30: ethylhexyl p-methoxycinnamate,
2-ethylhexyl salicylate, homosalate,
oxybenzone

Also available in SPF 44 Lotion and
.48 oz. SPF 25 Sunblock Stick

SUPER SHADE®
WATERPROOF SUNSCREENS

Procter & Gamble

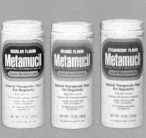

METAMUCIL®

Natural Therapeutic Fiber
for Regularity

Plough, Inc.

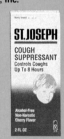

Available in 2 fl. oz. and 4 fl. oz.
sizes.

ST. JOSEPH®
COUGH SUPPRESSANT
FOR CHILDREN
(dextromethorphan hydrobromide)

Plough, Inc.

3 oz.
Spray

3 oz.
Lotion

(benzocaine and triclosan)
SOLARCAINE® FIRST-AID
PRODUCTS
For sunburns, minor burns,
cuts and scrapes

Plough, Inc.

4 fl. oz.   3 fl. oz.   4 fl. oz.

SPF 15: ethylhexyl p-methoxycinnamate,
oxybenzone
SPF 25: ethylhexyl p-methoxycinnamate, oxybenzone, 2-ethylhexyl salicylate, homosalate
SPF 30: ethylhexyl p-methoxycinnamate,
2-ethylhexyl salicylate, homosalate,
oxybenzone

WATER BABIES®
SUNBLOCK LOTION
CHILDREN'S SUNSCREENS

Procter & Gamble

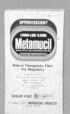

EFFERVESCENT METAMUCIL®
Natural Therapeutic Fiber
for Regularity

Procter & Gamble

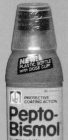
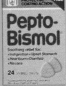

Liquid available in 4 oz., 8 oz., 12 oz. and 16 oz. plastic bottles

Tablets available in cartons of 24 and 42

PEPTO-BISMOL® LIQUID AND TABLETS

Reed & Carnrick

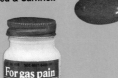

Available in 50s

MAXIMUM STRENGTH PHAZYME® 125
An antiflatulent to alleviate or relieve symptoms of gas. Softgel capsule for ease of swallowing.

Reed & Carnrick

Available in 5 and 10 oz. sizes

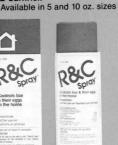

R&C SPRAY®
Controls lice and their eggs in the home. Insecticide: not for use on humans or animals.

RICHARDSON-VICKS

Health Care Products Div.

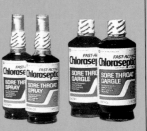

Available: Menthol and Cherry in 6 oz. spray, 12 oz. gargle/refill and 1.5 oz. aerosol spray.
CHLORASEPTIC® LIQUID

Procter & Gamble

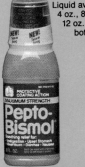

Liquid available in 4 oz., 8 oz. and 12 oz. plastic bottles

MAXIMUM STRENGTH PEPTO BISMOL®

Reed & Carnrick

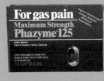

MAXIMUM STRENGTH PHAZYME® 125 Consumer 10 Packs
An antiflatulent to alleviate or relieve symptoms of gas.

Reed & Carnrick

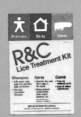

R&C LICE TREATMENT KIT
Contains 4 oz. R&C SHAMPOO, 5 oz. R&C SPRAY and nit comb.

Richardson-Vicks
Health Care Products Div.

Cherry

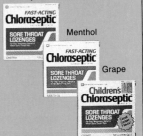

Menthol

Grape

Available: Menthol and Cherry in cartons of 18 and 36; Grape in cartons of 18.
CHLORASEPTIC® LOZENGES

REED & CARNRICK

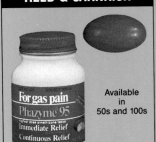

Available in 50s and 100s

PHAZYME® 95
An antiflatulent to alleviate or relieve symptoms of gas.

Reed & Carnrick

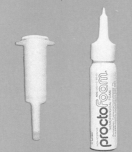

Non-steroid PROCTOFOAM® Hemorrhoidal Foam

REID-ROWELL

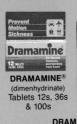

3 fl oz (89 mL)

89 mL

BALNEOL®
Perianal Cleansing Lotion

Richardson-Vicks
Health Care Products Div.

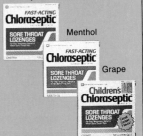

DRAMAMINE®
(dimenhydrinate)
Tablets 12s, 36s & 100s

DRAMAMINE® LIQUID
(dimenhydrinate syrup USP)
Liquid 3 fl. oz.

DRAMAMINE® CHEWABLE
(dimenhydrinate)
Tablets 8s & 24s

Reed & Carnrick

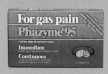

PHAZYME® 95 Consumer 10 Packs
An antiflatulent to alleviate or relieve symptoms of gas.

Reed & Carnrick

Available in 2 and 4 fl. oz. sizes

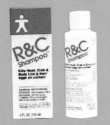

R&C SHAMPOO®
Kills head, crab and body lice and their eggs. Effective nit comb included.

Reid-Rowell

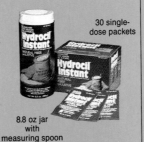

30 single-dose packets

8.8 oz jar with measuring spoon

HYDROCIL® INSTANT
Bulk Forming Agent for Constipation

Richardson-Vicks
Health Care Products Div.

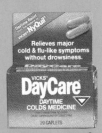
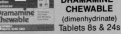

Relieves major cold & flu-like symptoms without drowsiness.

VICKS® DAYCARE®
Daytime Colds Medicine
(acetaminophen, pseudoephedrine hydrochloride, dextromethorphan hydrobromide, guaifenesin)

Continued on next page

Richardson-Vicks
Health Care Products Div.
Bottles of 6 oz. and 10 oz.

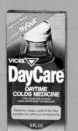
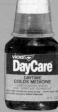

VICKS® DAYCARE®
Daytime Colds Medicine

(acetaminophen, pseudoephedrine
hydrochloride, dextromethorphan
hydrobromide, guaifenesin)

Richardson-Vicks
Health Care Products Div.

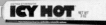

Rub, greaseless,
1¼-oz and 3-oz tubes

Balm, 3½-oz and
7-oz jars

Stick, 1¾ oz

ICY HOT®
Analgesic Balm, Rub, and Stick
for Arthritis and Muscle Aches

Richardson-Vicks
Health Care Products Div.

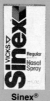
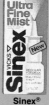

Sinex®

Sinex®
Ultra Fine Mist

Available in ½ oz., 1 oz. squeeze bottles
and new ½ oz. measured dose atomizer.
VICKS® SINEX® ULTRA FINE MIST
Decongestant Nasal Spray

(phenylephrine hydrochloride,
cetylpyridinium chloride)

Richardson-Vicks
Personal Care Products Div.

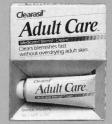

.6 oz. size

CLEARASIL® ADULT CARE™

(sulfur, resorcinol)

Richardson-Vicks
Health Care Products Div.

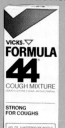
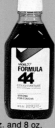

Available in 4 oz. and 8 oz.

VICKS® FORMULA 44®
Cough Mixture

(dextromethorphan hydrobromide,
chlorpheniramine maleate)

Richardson-Vicks
Health Care Products Div.

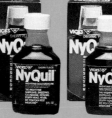

Original Flavor: 6 oz., 10 oz., 14 oz.
Cherry Flavor: 6 oz., 10 oz.
VICKS® NYQUIL®
NIGHTTIME COLDS MEDICINE

(acetaminophen, doxylamine succinate,
pseudoephedrine hydrochloride, dextromethorphan hydrobromide)

Richardson-Vicks
Health Care Products Div.

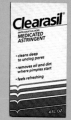

Sinex®
Long-Acting

Sinex® Ultra Fine
Mist 12 Hour

Available in ½ oz., 1 oz. squeeze bottles and
new ½ oz. measured dose atomizer.
VICKS® SINEX® LONG-ACTING
Decongestant Nasal Spray

(oxymetazoline hydrochloride)

Richardson-Vicks
Personal Care Products Div.

4 oz. size
CLEARASIL®
Medicated Astringent

For Oily Skin
(0.5% salicylic acid)

Richardson-Vicks
Health Care Products Div.

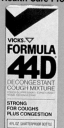
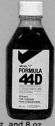

Available in 4 oz. and 8 oz.

VICKS® FORMULA 44D®
Decongestant Cough Mixture

(dextromethorphan hydrobromide,
pseudoephedrine hydrochloride,
guaifenesin)

Richardson-Vicks
Health Care Products Div.

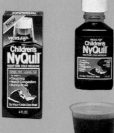

VICKS® CHILDREN'S NYQUIL®

(chlorpheniramine maleate,
pseudoephedrine HCl, dextromethorphan
hydrobromide)

Richardson-Vicks
Health Care Products Div.

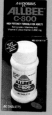

1.5 oz., 3.0 oz., 6 oz. jar
and 2 oz. tube

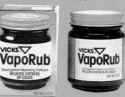

VICKS® VAPORUB®
Decongestant Cough Suppressant

(menthol, camphor, eucalyptus oil)

A. H. ROBINS

Consumer
Products
Division

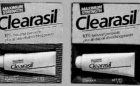

Available in bottles of 60
ALLBEE® C-800 TABLETS

Richardson-Vicks
Health Care Products Div.

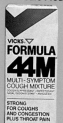
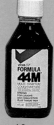

Available in 4 oz. and 8 oz.

VICKS® FORMULA 44M®
MULTI-SYMPTOM
COUGH MIXTURE

(dextromethorphan hydrobromide,
pseudoephedrine hydrochloride,
guaifenesin, acetaminophen)

Richardson-Vicks
Health Care Products Div.

Percogesic
for enhanced relief of pain
aspirin-free analgesic
50 tablets

Available in bottles of
24, 50 and 90
PERCOGESIC®
analgesic

(acetaminophen and
phenyltoloxamine citrate)

RICHARDSON-VICKS

Personal Care Products Div.

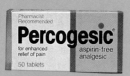

Vanishing   Tinted
Both available in .65 and 1.0 oz.
sizes

CLEARASIL®
Acne Treatment Cream

(10% benzoyl peroxide)

A. H. Robins

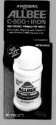

Available in bottles of 60

ALLBEE® C-800 PLUS IRON TABLETS

A. H. Robins

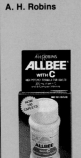

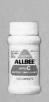

Available in bottles of 130 and 1000

ALLBEE® WITH C CAPLETS

A. H. Robins

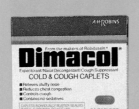

Available in consumer cartons of 12 and 24 and bottles of 100 and 500

DIMACOL® CAPLETS

A. H. Robins

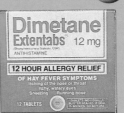

Available in consumer cartons of 12 and bottles of 100

DIMETANE EXTENTABS® 12 mg
(Brompheniramine Maleate, USP)

A. H. Robins

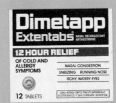

Available in consumer cartons of 12, 24 and 48 and bottles of 100 and 500

DIMETAPP EXTENTABS®

A. H. Robins

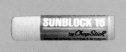

Ultra sunscreen protection (SPF-15)

Helps prevention and healing of dry, chapped, sun- and windburned lips.

CHAP STICK®
SUNBLOCK 15 Lip Balm

A. H. Robins

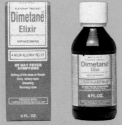

Available in bottles of 4 Fl. Oz. and 16 Fl. Oz.

DIMETANE® ELIXIR
(Brompheniramine Maleate Elixir, USP)

A. H. Robins

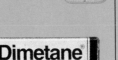

4 Fl. Oz.

DIMETANE®
DECONGESTANT ELIXIR

A. H. Robins

Available in consumer cartons of 24

DIMETAPP® TABLETS

A. H. Robins

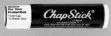
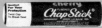

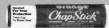
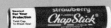
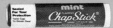

CHAP STICK®
Lip Balm

A. H. Robins

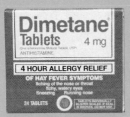

Available in consumer cartons of 24 and bottles of 100 and 500

DIMETANE® TABLETS
(Brompheniramine Maleate Tablets, USP)

A. H. Robins

Available in consumer cartons of 24 and 48

DIMETANE® DECONGESTANT CAPLETS

A. H. Robins

Available in consumer cartons of 24 and bottles of 48

DIMETAPP® PLUS CAPLETS

A. H. Robins

Cherry
Flavored

for Dry, Chapped Lips | for Dry, Chapped Lips with SUNBLOCK 15

CHAP STICK® Petroleum Jelly Plus

A. H. Robins

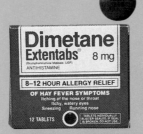

Available in consumer cartons of 12 and bottles of 100

DIMETANE EXTENTABS® 8 mg
(Brompheniramine Maleate, USP)

A. H. Robins

Available in bottles of 4 Fl. Oz., 8 Fl. Oz., 16 Fl. Oz. and 128 Fl. Oz.

DIMETAPP® ELIXIR

A. H. Robins

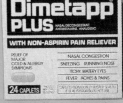

Available in bottles of 4 Fl. Oz., 8 Fl. Oz. and 16 Fl. Oz.

DONNAGEL®

Continued on next page

A. H. Robins

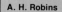
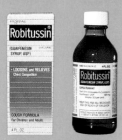

Available in bottles of 4 Fl. Oz.,
8 Fl. Oz., 16 Fl. Oz. and 128 Fl. Oz.

ROBITUSSIN® SYRUP
(Guaifenesin Syrup, USP)

A. H. Robins

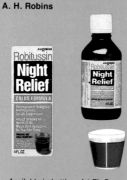

Available in bottles of 4 Fl. Oz. and
8 Fl. Oz. with convenient dosage cup.

ROBITUSSIN NIGHT RELIEF®

Rorer Consumer

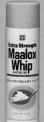

bottles of 36 & 75
caplets

**EXTRA STRENGTH
ASCRIPTIN®**
(Aspirin [500 mg] and Maalox
[magnesium hydroxide 80 mg, dried
aluminum hydroxide gel 80 mg],
buffered with calcium carbonate)

Rorer Consumer

8 oz.
Aerosol
Can

**EXTRA STRENGTH
MAALOX® WHIP™**
Magnesium and Aluminum
Hydroxides Oral Suspension, Rorer
(525 mg dried aluminum hydroxide gel
and 480 mg magnesium hydroxide)

A. H. Robins

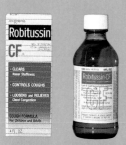

Available in bottles of 4 Fl. Oz.,
8 Fl. Oz. and 16 Fl. Oz.

ROBITUSSIN-CF® SYRUP

A. H. Robins

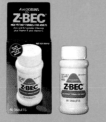

Available in bottles of 60 and 500

Z-BEC® TABLETS

Rorer Consumer

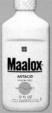

Suspension
12 fl. oz.

Bottles
of 50
Tablets

CAMALOX®

Magnesium and Aluminum
Hydroxides with Calcium Carbonate
Oral Suspension, Rorer

Rorer Consumer

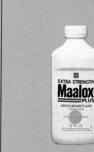

Tablets
12's, 50's, 100's

Single Roll
Triple Roll

MAALOX® PLUS
Alumina, Magnesia and Simethicone
Tablets, Rorer

A. H. Robins

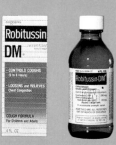

Available in bottles of 4 Fl. Oz.,
8 Fl. Oz., 16 Fl. Oz. and 128 Fl. Oz.

ROBITUSSIN-DM® SYRUP

RORER CONSUMER

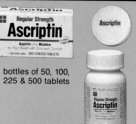

bottles of 50, 100,
225 & 500 tablets

**REGULAR STRENGTH
ASCRIPTIN®**
(Aspirin [325 mg] and Maalox
[magnesium hydroxide 50 mg, dried
aluminum hydroxide gel 50 mg],
buffered with calcium carbonate)

Rorer Consumer

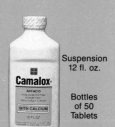

Bottles of
100 tablets

Bottles of
5 fl. oz., 12 fl. oz.
& 26 fl. oz.

MAALOX®
Magnesia and Alumina Oral
Suspension and Tablets, Rorer
(225 mg of aluminum hydroxide [200 mg
tablets] and 200 mg of
magnesium hydroxide)

Rorer Consumer

Suspension
bottles of 12
& 26 fl. oz.

**EXTRA STRENGTH
MAALOX® PLUS**
Alumina, Magnesia and Simethicone
Oral Suspension, Rorer

A. H. Robins

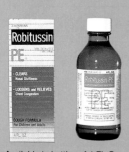

Available in bottles of 4 Fl. Oz.,
8 Fl. Oz. and 16 Fl. Oz.

ROBITUSSIN-PE® SYRUP

Rorer Consumer

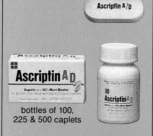

bottles of 100,
225 & 500 caplets

ASCRIPTIN® A/D
(Aspirin [325 mg] and Maalox
[magnesium hydroxide 75 mg, dried
aluminum hydroxide gel 75 mg],
buffered with calcium carbonate)

Rorer Consumer

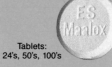

Tablets:
24's, 50's, 100's

**EXTRA STRENGTH
MAALOX®**
Magnesia and Alumina
Tablets, Rorer

Rorer Consumer

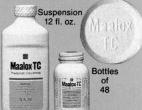

Suspension
12 fl. oz.

Bottles
of
48

**MAALOX® TC
(Therapeutic Concentrate)**
Magnesium and Aluminum
Hydroxides Oral Suspension
and Tablets, Rorer

(300 mg of magnesium hydroxide and
600 mg of aluminum hydroxide
per 5 ml/tablet)

Rorer Consumer

- Odorless
- Stainless
- Non-Burning
- Wrappable

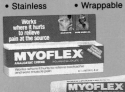

2 oz. and 4 oz.
Tube, 3 oz. Pump,
8 oz. and 16 oz. Jar

MYOFLEX®
Analgesic Creme
(trolamine salicylate)

Rorer Consumer

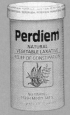

250 grams   100 grams

Granules

PERDIEM®
Natural Vegetable Laxative
82 percent psyllium (Plantago Hydrocolloid)
18 percent senna (Cassia Pod Concentrate)

Rorer Consumer

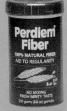

250 grams   100 grams

Granules

PERDIEM® FIBER
100% Natural Fiber
(Plantago Hydrocolloid)

ROSS

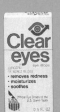

0.5 Fl. Oz.

CLEAR EYES®
Lubricating Eye Redness
Reliever

Also available in 1.0 Fl. Oz.

Ross

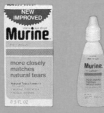

0.5 Fl. Oz.

MURINE® EYE LUBRICANT
More Closely Matches Natural Tears

Also available in 1.0 Fl. Oz.

Ross

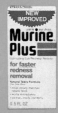

0.5 Fl. Oz.

MURINE® PLUS
Lubricating Eye Redness
Reliever

Also available in 1.0 Fl. Oz.

Ross

 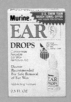

0.5 Fl. Oz.   0.5 Fl. Oz.

MURINE® EAR   **MURINE®**
WAX REMOVAL   EAR DROPS
SYSTEM

Ross   4 Fl. Oz.

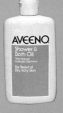

For Oily   For Dry   For Normal   For All
Hair   Hair   Hair   Hair Types

SELSUN BLUE®
Dandruff Shampoo

Also available in 7
and 11 Fl. Oz.

Extra Medicated
For All Hair Types

Ross

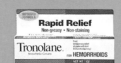

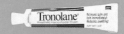 FOR HEMORRHOIDS

1 Oz. Tube With Applicator

TRONOLANE®
Anesthetic Cream for Hemorrhoids

Also available in a 2 oz. tube.

Ross

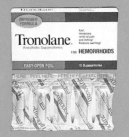

10 Suppositories

TRONOLANE®
Anesthetic Suppositories for
Hemorrhoids

Also available in size 20's.

RYDELLE

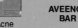

Regular   For Dry Skin
AVEENO® BATH

Normal to Oily Skin   Dry Skin

AVEENO®
BAR

For Acne

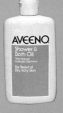

Shower and   Lotion
Bath Oil

AVEENO®
With Natural Colloidal Oatmeal
For the Relief of Dry, Itchy Skin

Rydelle

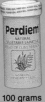

4 oz.   2 oz.

RHULI® SPRAY & RHULI® GEL

SANDOZ

Consumer

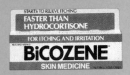

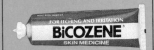

1 oz. (28.4 g.)

BICOZENE® CREME

Sandoz Consumer

4 oz., 8 oz.

DORCOL®
Children's Cough
Syrup

4 oz.

DORCOL®
Children's Liquid
Cold Formula

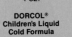

4 oz.

DORCOL®
Children's
Decongestant
Liquid

4 oz.

DORCOL®
Children's
Fever & Pain
Reducer

DORCOL®
PEDIATRIC FORMULAS

Continued on next page

Sandoz Consumer

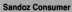
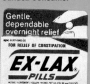

Gentle, dependable overnight relief
FOR RELIEF OF CONSTIPATION

EX-LAX PILLS

30 PILLS – UNFLAVORED

Pill

8's, 30's, 60's

EX-LAX
THE CHOCOLATED LAXATIVE

6's, 18's, 48's and 72's
EX-LAX®

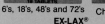

Chocolated Tablet

Sandoz Consumer

16's

(Sennosides)

GENTLE NATURE
from EX-LAX

for natural-feeling relief overnight
Natural Vegetable Laxative

16 tablets

GENTLE NATURE®
(20 mg. sennosides)

Sandoz Consumer

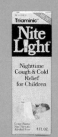

Triaminic Nite Light

Nighttime Cough & Cold Relief for Children

TRIAMINIC® NITE LIGHT™
Nighttime Cough & Cold Relief for Children

Schering

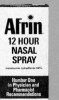

Afrin 12 HOUR NASAL SPRAY

Number One in Physician and Pharmacist Recommendations

Afrin 12 HOUR NASAL SPRAY COOLING MENTHOL ACTION

Afrin–Number One in Physician and Pharmacist Recommendations

Safety Sealed

AFRIN® NASAL SPRAY 0.05%   **AFRIN® MENTHOL NASAL SPRAY 0.05%**

(oxymetazoline hydrochloride, USP)

Sandoz Consumer

Triaminic-12
TWELVE HOUR RELIEF

Oral Nasal Decongestant/Antihistamine

TRIAMINIC-12® Tablets
(Sustained Release)

10's, 20's

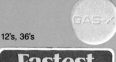

24's

EXTRA GENTLE EX-LAX

Laxative with stool softener

For gentle more comfortable relief

24's

EXTRA GENTLE EX-LAX®

24's
TRIAMINIC® Cold Tablets

Triaminic
COLD TABLETS

4 oz., 8 oz.
TRIAMINIC® Cold Syrup   **TRIAMINIC®**

Sandoz Consumer

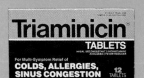

Triaminicin TABLETS

For Multi-Symptom Relief of
COLDS, ALLERGIES, SINUS CONGESTION 12 TABLETS

12's, 24's, 48's, 100's

TRIAMINICIN® TABLETS

Schering

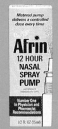

Metered pump delivers a controlled dose every time

Afrin 12 HOUR NASAL SPRAY PUMP

Number One in Physician and Pharmacist Recommendations

Safety Sealed

AFRIN® NASAL SPRAY PUMP
(oxymetazoline hydrochloride 0.05%)

Sandoz Consumer

12's, 36's

Fastest

Gas-X
SIMETHICONE-ANTIFLATULENT
for relieving symptoms of
gas pains and pressure

GAS-X®
(80 mg. simethicone)

Sandoz Consumer

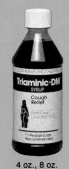

Triaminic-DM SYRUP
Cough Relief

#1 Pediatrician Recommended

4 oz., 8 oz.

TRIAMINIC-DM® COUGH FORMULA

Sandoz Consumer

4 oz., 8 oz.
TRIAMINICOL® MULTI-SYMPTOM COLD SYRUP

Triaminicol
MULTI-SYMPTOM COLD TABLETS

24 Tablets

24's

TRIAMINICOL® MULTI-SYMPTOM COLD TABLETS

Schering

Afrin 12 HOUR NOSE DROPS

Afrin–Number One in Physician and Pharmacist Recommendations

Afrin CHILDREN'S STRENGTH 2 THRU 5 YEARS **12 HOUR NOSE DROPS**

Safety Sealed

Nose Drops 0.05%   Children's Strength Nose Drops 0.025%

AFRIN® NOSE DROPS
(oxymetazoline hydrochloride, USP)

Sandoz Consumer

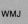

18 tablets

EXTRA STRENGTH Gas-X
SIMETHICONE-ANTIFLATULENT
STRONGEST, FASTEST
doctor prescribed ingredient for relieving symptoms of
gas pains and pressure

125 mg EACH

EXTRA-STRENGTH GAS-X®
(125 mg. simethicone)

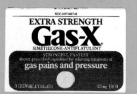

Sandoz Consumer

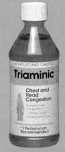

Triaminic
Chest and Head Congestion

#1 Pediatrician Recommended

4 oz., 8 oz.

TRIAMINIC® EXPECTORANT

SCHERING

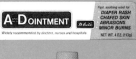

A-D OINTMENT White
Widely recommended by doctors, nurses and hospitals.
NET WT. 4 OZ. (113g)

Fast, soothing relief for
DIAPER RASH
CHAFED SKIN
ABRASIONS
MINOR BURNS

WMJ

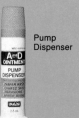

A AND D OINTMENT PUMP DISPENSER

Pump Dispenser

A and D Reg. ™ Ointment

Schering

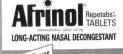
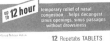

Afrinol Repetabs® TABLETS
pseudoephedrine sulfate 120 mg
LONG-ACTING NASAL DECONGESTANT

up to 12 hour temporary relief of nasal congestion...helps decongest sinus openings, sinus passages without drowsiness

12 Repetabs TABLETS

AFRINOL® REPETABS® TABLETS
(pseudoephedrine sulfate)

Schering

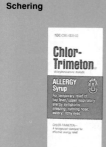

CHLOR-TRIMETON®
ALLERGY SYRUP
(2 mg chlorpheniramine maleate, USP)

Schering

901

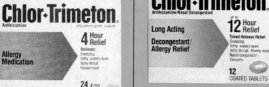

CHLOR-TRIMETON®
DECONGESTANT TABLETS
(4 mg chlorpheniramine maleate, USP and 60 mg pseudoephedrine sulfate)

Schering

PKD or SN or 171 or 522

CORICIDIN® TABLETS
(2 mg chlorpheniramine maleate and 325 mg acetaminophen)

Schering

751

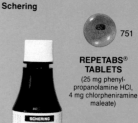

REPETABS®
TABLETS
(25 mg phenyl-propanolamine HCl, 4 mg chlorpheniramine maleate)

SYRUP
(12.5 mg phenyl-propanolamine HCl, 2 mg chlorpheniramine maleate)

DEMAZIN®
DECONGESTANT-ANTIHISTAMINE

Schering

TW

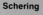

CHLOR-TRIMETON®
ALLERGY TABLETS
(4 mg chlorpheniramine maleate, USP)

Schering

LONG ACTING
CHLOR-TRIMETON®
DECONGESTANT REPETABS®
(8 mg chlorpheniramine maleate, USP and 120 mg pseudoephedrine sulfate)

Schering

871 or 307

CORICIDIN 'D'®
DECONGESTANT TABLETS
(2 mg chlorpheniramine maleate, 12.5 mg phenylpropanolamine HCl, and 325 mg acetaminophen)

Schering

DRIXORAL®
SUSTAINED-ACTION TABLETS
(6 mg dexbrompheniramine maleate and 120 mg pseudoephedrine sulfate)

Schering

374

CHLOR-TRIMETON®
LONG ACTING ALLERGY
REPETABS® TABLETS
(8 mg chlorpheniramine maleate, USP)

Schering

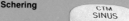

CHLOR-TRIMETON®
SINUS CAPLETS
(2 mg chlorpheniramine maleate, 12.5 mg phenylpropanolamine HCl, and 500 mg acetaminophen)

Schering

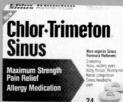

CORICIDIN® DEMILETS®
TABLETS

Schering

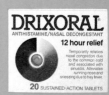

DRIXORAL® PLUS
(60 mg pseudoephedrine sulfate, 3 mg dexbrompheniramine maleate and 500 mg acetaminophen)

Schering

009

CHLOR-TRIMETON®
MAXIMUM STRENGTH
TIMED RELEASE
ALLERGY TABLETS
(12 mg chlorpheniramine maleate, USP)

Schering/White Product Line

COD LIVER OIL CONCENTRATE
CAPSULES

COD LIVER OIL CONCENTRATE
TABLETS

COD LIVER OIL CONCENTRATE
TABLETS W/VITAMIN C

Schering

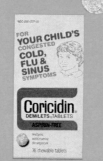

CORICIDIN® SINUS
HEADACHE CAPLETS

(500 mg acetaminophen, 2 mg chlor-pheniramine maleate, and 12.5 mg phenylpropanolamine HCl)

Schering

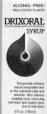

Safety Sealed

DRIXORAL® SYRUP
(2 mg brompheniramine maleate and 30 mg pseudoephedrine sulfate)

Continued on next page

Schering/Emko Product Line

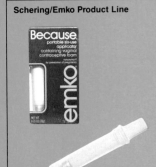
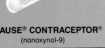

BECAUSE® CONTRACEPTOR®
(nonoxynol-9)

Schering

**TINACTIN®
CREAM AND SOLUTION**
(tolnaftate 1%)

SCHWARZ PHARMA

24 tablets   4 fl oz

Tablets also available in
bottles of 100

Available in Rx timed-release
dosage form

**FEDAHIST®
Tablets and Decongestant
Syrup**

SMITHKLINE

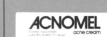

1 oz. tube

ACNOMEL® ACNE CREAM
(resorcinol, sulfate, alcohol)

Schering/Emko Product Line

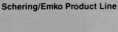

**EMKO®
CONTRACEPTIVE
FOAM**

(nonoxynol-9)

Schering

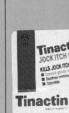

**TINACTIN® JOCK ITCH
CREAM AND SPRAY POWDER**
(tolnaftate 1%)

Schwarz Pharma

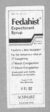

4 fl oz   1 fl oz

**FEDAHIST®
Expectorant Syrup
and Expectorant Pediatric Drops**

SmithKline Consumer Products

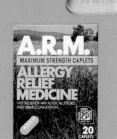

Packages of 20 and 40 caplets
**A.R.M.® ALLERGY RELIEF
MEDICINE**
(chlorpheniramine maleate,
phenylpropanolamine HCl)

Schering/White Product Line

Tablets

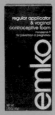

with Vitamin C
Tablets

MOL-IRON®

Schering

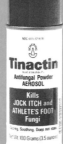

**TINACTIN® POWDER AEROSOL
AND POWDER**
(tolnaftate 1%)

Schwarz Pharma

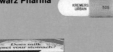

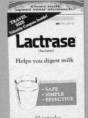

Available in
cartons of
10 and 30 and
bottles of 100

LACTRASE® Capsules
(lactase) 250 mg

SmithKline Consumer Products

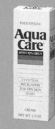

2.5 oz. tube
**AQUA CARE® CREAM
with 10% Urea**

Schering

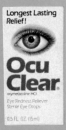

**OCUCLEAR®
EYE DROPS**

(oxymetazoline HCl 0.025%)

Schering

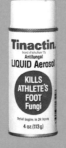

**TINACTIN®
LIQUID AEROSOL**
(tolnaftate 1%)

For more detailed in-
formation on products
illustrated in this sec-
tion, consult the Prod-
uct Information Sec-
tion or manufacturers
may be contacted di-
rectly.

SmithKline Consumer Products

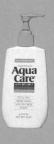

8 oz. bottle
**AQUA CARE® LOTION
with 10% Urea**

SmithKline Consumer Products	**SmithKline Consumer Products**	**SmithKline Consumer Products**	**SmithKline Consumer Products**

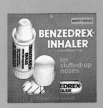

1 inhaler per package

BENZEDREX® INHALER
(propylhexedrine)

Packages of 10, 20 and 40 caplets

**CONTAC®
CONTINUOUS ACTION
NASAL DECONGESTANT
ANTIHISTAMINE CAPLETS**

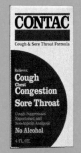

Measured
dose
cup

**CONTAC®
COUGH & SORE THROAT FORMULA**

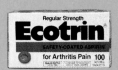

In 100, 250 and 1000
tablet bottles

ECOTRIN® TABLETS
Duentric® coated 5 gr. aspirin

SmithKline Consumer Products	**SmithKline Consumer Products**	**SmithKline Consumer Products**	**SmithKline Consumer Products**

**CLEAR
BY DESIGN®**

For Sensitive Skin

1.5 oz. tube
CLEAR BY DESIGN®
(benzoyl peroxide 2.5%)

**CONTAC®
CAPLETS
Severe Cold Formula**

Packages of 10 and 20 caplets

**CONTAC®
SEVERE COLD FORMULA**

**CONTAC
Nighttime
Cold Medicine**

Measured
dose
cup

**CONTAC®
NIGHTTIME
COLD MEDICINE**

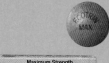

Ecotrin

In 60 and 150
tablet bottles

**MAXIMUM STRENGTH
ECOTRIN® TABLETS**
Duentric® coated 7.7 gr. aspirin

SmithKline Consumer Products	**SmithKline Consumer Products**	**SmithKline Consumer Products**	**SmithKline Consumer Products**

Congestac
CONGESTION
RELIEF MEDICINE

Packages of 12 and 24 caplets

CONGESTAC™
Congestion Relief Medicine
Decongestant/Expectorant

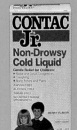

**CONTAC
Jr.
Non-Drowsy
Cold Liquid**

Includes dose-
by-weight cup

**CONTAC JR.®
COLD MEDICINE FOR CHILDREN**

Ecotrin
Regular Strength
SAFETY-COATED ASPIRIN
for Arthritis Pain 75

75 caplet bottle

ECOTRIN® CAPLETS
Duentric® coated 5 gr. aspirin

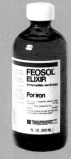

**FEOSOL
ELIXIR**
For Iron

16 oz. bottle
FEOSOL® ELIXIR
(ferrous sulfate USP)

SmithKline Consumer Products	**SmithKline Consumer Products**	**SmithKline Consumer Products**	**SmithKline Consumer Products**

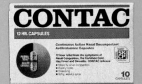

Packages of 10, 20 and 40 capsules

CONTAC
12 HR. CAPSULES

**CONTAC®
CONTINUOUS ACTION
NASAL DECONGESTANT
ANTIHISTAMINE CAPSULES**

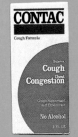

CONTAC
Cough Formula

Cough
Chest
Congestion

Measured
dose
cup

**CONTAC®
COUGH FORMULA**

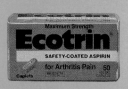

Ecotrin
Maximum Strength
SAFETY-COATED ASPIRIN
for Arthritis Pain 50
Caplets

50 caplet bottle

**MAXIMUM STRENGTH
ECOTRIN® CAPLETS**
Duentric® coated 7.7 gr. aspirin

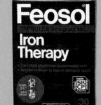

**Feosol
Iron
Therapy**

Packages of 30 and
60 capsules

FEOSOL® CAPSULES
(ferrous sulfate USP)

Continued on next page

SmithKline Consumer Products

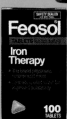

In 100 and 1000 tablet bottles
FEOSOL® TABLETS
(ferrous sulfate USP)

SmithKline Consumer Products

24 caplet package

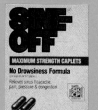

**SINE-OFF®
MAXIMUM STRENGTH
NO DROWSINESS FORMULA CAPLETS**

SmithKline Consumer Products

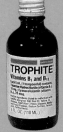

4 oz. liquid and 50 tablet bottle
TROPHITE® LIQUID AND TABLETS
Vitamins B1, B12

E. R. Squibb & Sons

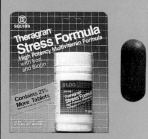

THERAGRAN® STRESS FORMULA
High Potency Multivitamin Formula
with Iron and Biotin

SmithKline Consumer Products

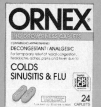

Packages of 24 and 48 caplets
ORNEX® CAPLETS
Decongestant/Analgesic

SmithKline Consumer Products

Packages of 24 and 48 tablets

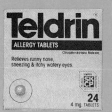

TELDRIN® TABLETS
(chlorpheniramine maleate)

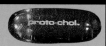

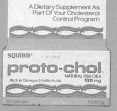

PROTO-CHOL®
Natural Fish Oils, 1000 mg.

E. R. Squibb & Sons

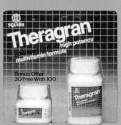

**ADVANCED FORMULA
THERAGRAN®**
High Potency Multivitamin
Formula

SmithKline Consumer Products

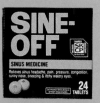

Packages of 24, 48, and 100 tablets
**SINE-OFF® REGULAR STRENGTH
ASPIRIN FORMULA**

SmithKline Consumer Products

Packages of 12, 24 and 48 capsules   12 mg.

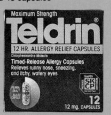

**TELDRIN®
TIMED-RELEASE CAPSULES**
(chlorpheniramine maleate)

E. R. Squibb & Sons

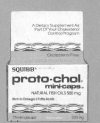

PROTO-CHOL® MINI-CAPS™
Natural Fish Oils, 500 mg.

E. R. Squibb & Sons

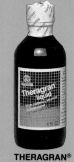

**THERAGRAN®
LIQUID**
High Potency Liquid
Vitamin Supplement

SmithKline Consumer Products

24 caplet package

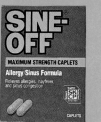

**SINE-OFF®
MAXIMUM STRENGTH ALLERGY/
SINUS FORMULA CAPLETS**

SmithKline Consumer Products

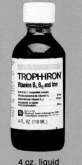

4 oz. liquid
TROPH-IRON®
Vitamins B1, B12 and Iron

E. R. Squibb & Sons

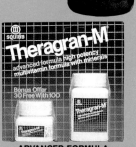

**ADVANCED FORMULA
THERAGRAN-M®**
High Potency Multivitamin
Formula with Minerals

E. R. Squibb & Sons

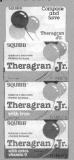

THERAGRAN, JR.®
Children's Chewable Vitamin Formula
Regular, With Iron, and
With Extra Vitamin C

STELLAR

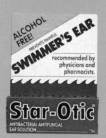

Prevent Swimmer's Ear

STAR-OTIC®
Antibacterial • Antifungal

Stuart

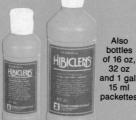

Bottles
of
60 tablets

FERANCEE®-HP
High Potency Hematinic

Stuart

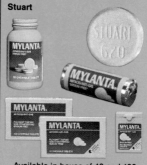

Available in boxes of 40 and 100,
bottles of 180, flip-top Convenience
Packs of 48 and 12 tablet rolls
MYLANTA® TABLETS
Antacid/Anti-Gas

Stuart

Boxes of
12s and 60s

125 mg
simethicone

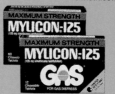

**MAXIMUM STRENGTH
MYLICON®-125**
Antiflatulent

STUART

12 oz

All Stuart products
are packaged with
tamper-resistant fea-
tures as required by
applicable Federal
Regulations.

5 oz

ALternaGEL®
High Potency Aluminum Hydroxide
Antacid

Stuart

Also
bottles
of 16 oz,
32 oz
and 1 gal;
15 ml
packettes

4 oz   8 oz

HIBICLENS®
(chlorhexidine gluconate)
Antiseptic Antimicrobial
Skin Cleanser

Stuart

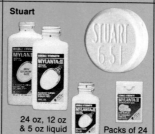

24 oz, 12 oz
& 5 oz liquid

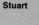

Packs of 24

Boxes of
60 tablets

MYLANTA®-II LIQUID and TABLETS
Double Strength Antacid/Anti-Gas

Stuart

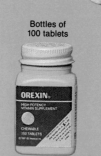

Bottles of
100 tablets

OREXIN®
Therapeutic Vitamin Supplement

Stuart

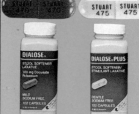

Bottles of 36
and 100 capsules
DIALOSE®
(docusate potassium,
100 mg)

Bottles of 36, 100
and 500 capsules
DIALOSE® PLUS
(docusate potassium,
100 mg and casan-
thranol, 30 mg)
Stool Softeners

Stuart

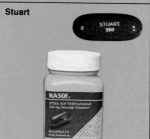

Bottles of 30 and 60 capsules

KASOF®
(docusate potassium, 240 mg)
High Strength Stool Softener

Stuart

40 mg
simethicone

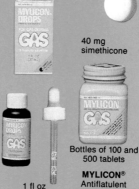

Bottles of 100 and
500 tablets

MYLICON®
Antiflatulent

1 fl oz

Stuart

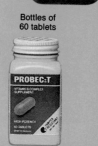

Bottles of
60 tablets

PROBEC®-T
High potency B complex supplement
with 600 mg of vitamin C

Stuart

Available in
9 oz and 16 oz
bottles

24 packet
carton

EFFER-SYLLIUM®
Natural Fiber Bulking Agent

Stuart

Sodium Free

24 oz   12 oz

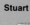

5 oz

MYLANTA® LIQUID
Antacid/Anti-Gas

(magnesium and alumi-
num hydroxides with
simethicone)

Stuart

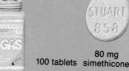

100 tablets

80 mg
simethicone

Convenience
Package
of 48s

Convenience
Package of 12s
MYLICON®-80
Antiflatulent

Stuart

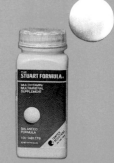

Bottles of 100 and 250 tablets

STUART FORMULA® TABLETS
Multivitamin/Multimineral Supplement

Continued on next page

Stuart

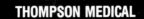
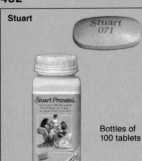

Bottles of
100 tablets

STUART PRENATAL® TABLETS
Multivitamin/Multimineral Supplement
for pregnant or lactating women

THOMPSON MEDICAL

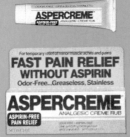

**FAST PAIN RELIEF
WITHOUT ASPIRIN**
Odor-Free...Greaseless, Stainless

ASPERCREME

Available in 1.25, 3, 5 oz. Creme;
6 oz. Lotion

ASPERCREME®

Thompson Medical Company, Inc.

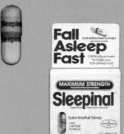

Available in 16, 32 capsule sizes

SLEEPINAL™
(diphenhydramine HCl 50 mg.)

Upjohn

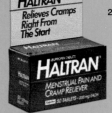

200 mg

Available in Blister Packages of 12;
Bottles of 30 & 50 tablets

HALTRAN® Tablets
(ibuprofen tablets, USP)

Stuart

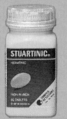

Bottles of 60 tablets

STUARTINIC®
Hematinic

Thompson Medical Company, Inc.

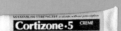

**RASH, ECZEMA,
PSORIASIS?**
Doctor Recommended
Itch & Rash Relief

Cortizone·5

Available in ½, 1, 2 oz. creme;
1 oz. ointment

CORTIZONE-5
(hydrocortisone 0.5%)

Thompson Medical Company, Inc.

Available in Chocolate Royale,
French Vanilla and Strawberry
Supreme; 14 oz. can

ULTRA SLIM-FAST®

Upjohn

KAOPECTATE®
Tablets

Blister packs
of 12 & 20

Regular
8, 12 & 16 oz

Peppermint
8 & 12 oz

KAOPECTATE®
Concentrated Anti-Diarrheal

TAMBRANDS

Ovulation Predictor Test

**Pregnancy
Test**

FIRST RESPONSE®

Thompson Medical Company, Inc.

Available in
10, 20 and 40
capsule sizes

Available in
10, 20 and 40
caplet sizes

**MAXIMUM STRENGTH DEXATRIM®
Capsules & Caplets
Plus Vitamin C**

UPJOHN

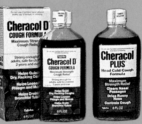

2 oz, 4 oz,
6 oz

4 oz, 6 oz

CHERACOL D®
Cough Formula

CHERACOL PLUS®
Head Cold/Cough
Formula

Upjohn

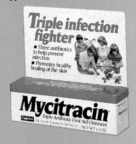

**Triple infection
fighter**
■ Three antibiotics
to help prevent
infection
■ Promotes healthy
healing of the skin

Mycitracin

½ oz & 1 oz tubes
MYCITRACIN®
Triple Antibiotic Ointment

(bacitracin-polymyxin-neomycin
topical ointment)

For more detailed in-
formation on products
illustrated in this sec-
tion, consult the Prod-
uct Information Sec-
tion or manufacturers
may be contacted di-
rectly.

Thompson Medical Company, Inc.

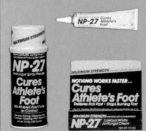

Available in ½, 1 oz. cream; ½ oz.
solution; 3.5 oz. spray powder

NP-27®
(tolnaftate 1%)

Upjohn

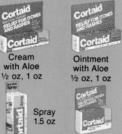

Cream
with Aloe
½ oz, 1 oz

Ointment
with Aloe
½ oz, 1 oz

Spray
1.5 oz

Lotion 1 oz

CORTAID®
Cream & Ointment with Aloe; Lotion
(hydrocortisone acetate)
Spray (hydrocortisone)

Upjohn

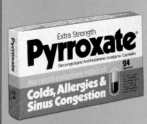

Extra Strength
Pyrroxate
Decongestant/Antihistamine/Analgesic Capsules
24 Capsules

**Colds, Allergies &
Sinus Congestion**

Available in blister packs
of 24 and bottles of 500

Nasal Decongestant/Antihistamine/
Analgesic

PYRROXATE® Capsules

Upjohn

UNICAP M® Tablets
Advanced formula
dietary supplement
Bottle of 120

UNICAP® Senior
Tablets
Multivitamin
supplement
Bottle of 120

UNICAP T® Tablets
Stress Formula
Bottle of 60

WALLACE

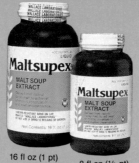

16 fl oz (1 pt)   8 fl oz (½ pt)

MALTSUPEX® LIQUID
(malt soup extract)

Wallace

1 pint
(473 ml)

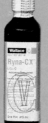

Also available: 4 fl oz (118 ml)

RYNA-CX® LIQUID
(antitussive-decongestant-expectorant)

Warner-Lambert Co.

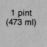

HALLS® Mentho-Lyptus®
Cough Tablets

WAKUNAGA

KYOLIC®
Aged Garlic Extract
with B₁, B₁₂

KYOLIC®
Aged Garlic Extract
Super Formula
101-Capsules

Wallace

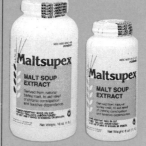

16 oz (1 lb)   8 oz (½ lb)

MALTSUPEX® POWDER
(malt soup extract)

Wallace

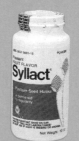

SYLLACT™
(powdered psyllium seed husks)

Warner-Lambert Co.

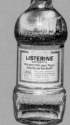

12 oz.

LISTERINE® ANTISEPTIC

WALKER, CORP

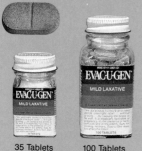

35 Tablets   100 Tablets

EVAC-U-GEN®
Mild Laxative

Wallace

1 pint
(473 ml)

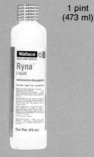

Also available: 4 fl oz (118 ml)

RYNA™ LIQUID
(antihistamine-decongestant)

WARNER-LAMBERT CO.

EARLY DETECTOR®
In-Home Test
for Fecal Occult Blood

Warner-Lambert Co.

24
Lozenges

LISTERINE®
Antiseptic Throat Lozenges

24
Lozenges

**MAXIMUM STRENGTH
LISTERINE®**
Antiseptic Throat Lozenges

For more detailed in-
formation on products
illustrated in this sec-
tion, consult the Prod-
uct Information Sec-
tion or manufacturers
may be contacted di-
rectly.

Wallace

1 pint
(473 ml)

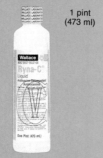

Also available: 4 fl oz (118 ml)

RYNA-C® LIQUID
(antitussive-antihistamine-decongestant)

Warner-Lambert Co.

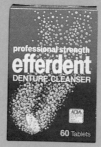

**PROFESSIONAL STRENGTH
EFFERDENT®**

Denture Cleanser

Warner-Lambert Co.

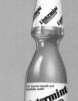

LISTERMINT™ with FLUORIDE
Anticavity Dental Rinse &
Mouthwash

Continued on next page

Warner-Lambert Co.

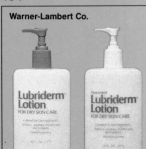

Scented   Unscented

**LUBRIDERM®
LOTION**

For Dry Skin Care

Warner-Lambert Co.

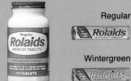

Regular

Wintergreen

Spearmint

ROLAIDS®

Fast, Safe, Lasting Relief from
Heartburn, Sour Stomach or Acid
Indigestion and Upset Stomach
Associated with these Symptoms

**FOSTEX®
10% Benzoyl Peroxide Gel**

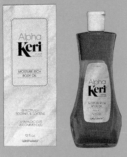

10% Benzoyl
Peroxide   Medicated

**FOSTEX®
Cleansing Bars**

Westwood

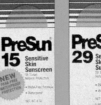

Sensitive Skin   Sensitive Skin
Sunscreen 15   Sunscreen 29

**PRESUN®
Creamy, Lotion, Facial, Sensitive
Skin and Stick Formulas**

Warner-Lambert Co.

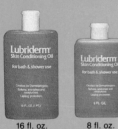

16 fl. oz.   8 fl. oz.

**LUBRIDERM®
SKIN CONDITIONING OIL**

For Dry Skin Care

Warner-Lambert Co.

**SODIUM FREE*
ROLAIDS®**

Sodium Free Relief from Heartburn,
Sour Stomach or Acid Indigestion
and Upset Stomach Associated with
these Symptoms

Westwood
Moisture Rich Body Oil

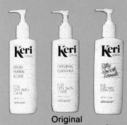

**ALPHA KERI®
Shower and Bath Products**

Westwood

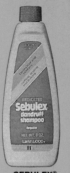

SEBULEX®   **SEBUTONE®**
Medicated Dandruff Shampoos

Warner-Lambert Co.

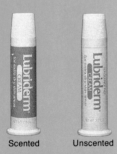

Scented   Unscented

LUBRIDERM® CREAM

For Extra Dry
Skin Areas

Warner-Lambert Co.

Cherry

Assorted Fruit

**CALCIUM RICH
ROLAIDS®**

Calcium Rich, Sodium Free Relief
from Heartburn, Sour Stomach or
Acid Indigestion and Upset Stomach
Associated with these Symptoms

Westwood

Fresh   Original   Silky
Herbal   Formula   Smooth
Scent   Formula

**KERI® LOTION
For Dry Skin Care**

Coated Tablets in Bottles of 8, 24,
50, 100, 165 and 250. Coated Caplets in Bottles of 24, 50, 100 and 165.

ADVIL®
Ibuprofen Tablets and Caplets, USP

Warner-Lambert Co.

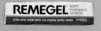
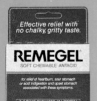

REMEGEL®

Soft, Chewable Antacid
Effective Relief with No Chalky,
Gritty Taste

For more detailed in-
formation on products
illustrated in this sec-
tion, consult the Prod-
uct Information Sec-
tion or manufacturers
may be contacted di-
rectly.

Westwood

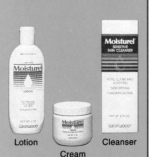

Lotion   Cleanser

Cream

**Fragrance-Free
MOISTUREL®**

Whitehall

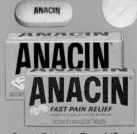

Coated Tablets in Tins of 12 and
Bottles of 30, 50, 100, 200 and 300.
Coated Caplets in Bottles of
30, 50 and 100.

ANACIN®
Analgesic Tablets and Caplets

Whitehall — REGULAR STRENGTH ANACIN-3®

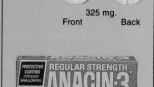

325 mg.
Front — Back

Coated Tablets: Bottles
of 24, 50 and 100.

REGULAR STRENGTH ANACIN-3®
Acetaminophen Tablets

Whitehall — ARTHRITIS PAIN FORMULA

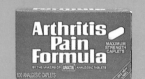

Available in Bottles of 40, 100 and
175 Caplets.

ARTHRITIS PAIN FORMULA
by the makers of ANACIN®
Analgesic Tablets

Whitehall — DRISTAN Nasal Spray

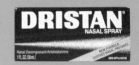
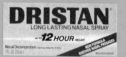

Both Available in Bottles of
15 ml. and 30 ml.
and Metered Dose Pumps of 15 ml.

DRISTAN®
Nasal Spray

Whitehall — PREPARATION H

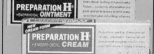

Ointment
1 oz. and 2 oz. Tubes

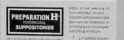

Cream
0.9 oz. and 1.8 oz. Tubes

Suppositories
12s, 24s, 36s and 48s

PREPARATION H®
Hemorrhoidal Ointment, Cream
and Suppositories

Whitehall — MAXIMUM STRENGTH ANACIN-3®

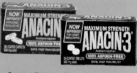

Front — Back
500 mg.

Coated Tablets: Tins of 12, Bottles
of 30, 60 and 100. Coated Caplets:
Bottles of 30, 60 and 100.

MAXIMUM STRENGTH ANACIN-3®
Acetaminophen Tablets and Caplets

Whitehall — CLEARPLAN / CLEARBLUE EASY

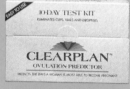

CLEARPLAN™
OVULATION PREDICTOR
10-Day Test Kit

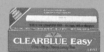

CLEARBLUE EASY™
One-Step Pregnancy Test

Whitehall — DRISTAN Coated Tablets and Caplets

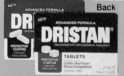

Front — Back

Coated Tablets: Tins of 12, Packages
of 24, 48 and Bottles of 100. Coated
Caplets: Packages of 20 and 40.

DRISTAN®
COATED TABLETS AND CAPLETS
Decongestant/Antihistamine/
Analgesic

Whitehall — PRIMATENE MIST

Available in 15 cc.
Inhaler Unit and
15 cc. and 22.5 cc.
Refills.

PRIMATENE® MIST

Asthma Remedy

Whitehall — ANBESOL

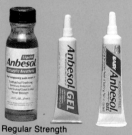

Regular Strength
Liquid
.31 oz.
and
.74 oz.

Gel
.25 oz.

Baby Teething
Gel
.25 oz.

ANBESOL®

Whitehall — DENOREX

Regular — Mountain Fresh Herbal — Shampoo & Conditioner

4 oz., 8 oz.
& 12 oz.
Bottles

Extra Strength

DENOREX®
Medicated Shampoo

Whitehall — MAXIMUM STRENGTH DRISTAN

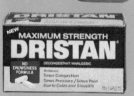

Coated Caplets: Packages of
24, 48 and Bottles of 100.

MAXIMUM STRENGTH DRISTAN®
(acetaminophen 500 mg., pseudoephedrine
HCl 30 mg.)

Whitehall — PRIMATENE TABLETS

Regular — Front Back

P Formula — Front Back

M Formula — Front Back

PRIMATENE® TABLETS
Asthma Remedy

Whitehall — MAXIMUM STRENGTH ANBESOL

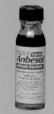

Liquid
.31 oz.

Gel
.25 oz.

**MAXIMUM STRENGTH
ANBESOL®**
Anesthetic for Oral Topical
Pain Relief

Whitehall — DERMOPLAST

DERMOPLAST®
Anesthetic Pain Relief Spray
and Lotion

Available in 2¾ oz. Spray and
3 oz. Lotion

Whitehall — POSTURE and POSTURE-D

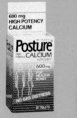

600 mg
HIGH POTENCY
CALCIUM

600 mg
CALCIUM with
VITAMIN D

High Potency Calcium Supplement
and High Potency Calcium
Supplement with Vitamin D

Both available in Bottles of 60
POSTURE® and POSTURE®-D
(elemental calcium/Vitamin D)

Whitehall — RIOPAN and RIOPAN PLUS

RIOPAN®
Antacid
(magaldrate)

RIOPAN PLUS®
Antacid plus
Anti-Gas
(magaldrate and
simethicone)

Both products available in 12 fl. oz.
Suspension, Chew Tablets, 60's and 100's,
and Rollpacks. RIOPAN also available
in Swallow Tablets, 60's and 100's.

Continued on next page

Whitehall Available in 12 fl. oz. Suspension and Chew Tablets (60s) 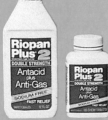 **RIOPAN PLUS® 2** High-Potency Antacid plus Anti-Gas (magaldrate and simethicone)	**Winthrop Consumer Products** 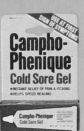 **CAMPHO-PHENIQUE®** **Cold Sore Gel** .23 oz and .5 oz	**Winthrop Consumer Products** 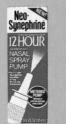 **NEO-SYNEPHRINE®** **Nasal Decongestant** Spray, Spray Pump or Drops	**Wyeth-Ayerst** 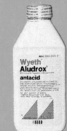 12 Fl. Oz. **ALUDROX® SUSPENSION** Antacid
Whitehall 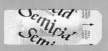 Available in Packages of 10 and 20. **SEMICID®** Vaginal Contraceptive Inserts	**Winthrop Consumer Products** 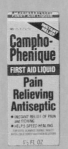 **CAMPHO-PHENIQUE®** **First Aid Liquid** .75 oz, 1.5 oz, 4 oz	**Winthrop Consumer Products** 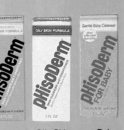 Unscented Regular / Oily Skin Formula / Baby Cleanser Available in 5 oz, 9 oz (regular), 16 oz / 5 oz **pHisoDerm®**	**Wyeth-Ayerst** 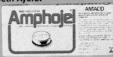 100 tablets 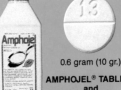 0.6 gram (10 gr.) **AMPHOJEL® TABLETS and SUSPENSION** Antacid 12 Fl. Oz. Also available in 0.3 gram (5 gr.) tablets
Whitehall 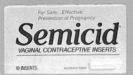 Available in Packages of 3, 6 and 12. **TODAY®** Vaginal Contraceptive Sponge	**Winthrop Consumer Products** 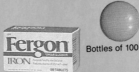 Bottles of 100 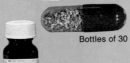 Bottles of 30 **FERGON® (IRON)** Tablets and Capsules	**Winthrop Consumer Products** **pHisoPUFF®** and **pHisoPUFF® Disposa-PUFFS®** Exfoliating Sponges	**Wyeth-Ayerst** 472 Bottles of 100, 500 Bottles of 100 473 **BASALJEL®** TABLETS and CAPSULES Antacid
WINTHROP **Consumer Products** 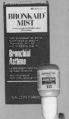 Available in 15 cc Inhaler Units and 15 cc and 22.5 cc Refills. Available in packages of 24 and 60 tablets. **BRONKAID®** Mist and Tablets Asthma Remedy	**Winthrop Consumer Products** 15 ml / 15 ml **NāSal™** Saline Nasal Moisturizing Solution Spray and Drops	**WYETH-AYERST** **Tamper-Resistant/Evident Packaging** Statements alerting consumers to the specific type of Tamper-Resistant/Evident Packaging appear on the bottle labels and cartons of all over-the-counter products of Wyeth-Ayerst. This includes plastic cap seals on bottles, individually wrapped tablets or suppositories, and sealed cartons. This packaging has been developed to better protect the consumer.	**Wyeth-Ayerst** 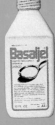 12 Fl. Oz. **BASALJEL® SUSPENSION** Antacid

Wyeth-Ayerst

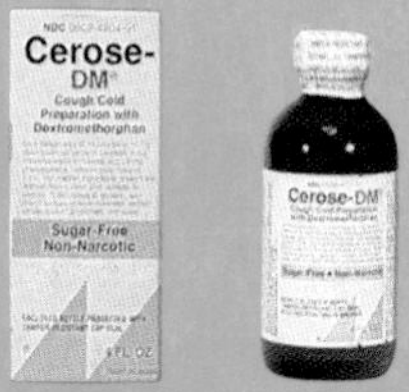

4 Fl. Oz.

CEROSE-DM®

**Cough/Cold Preparation
with Dextromethorphan**

Also available in 1-pint bottles

Wyeth-Ayerst

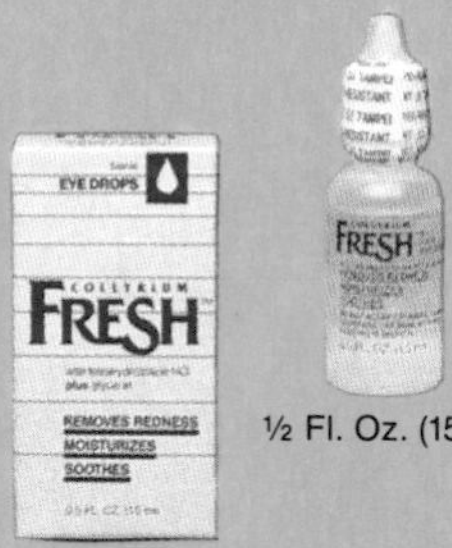

½ Fl. Oz. (15 ml)

COLLYRIUM FRESH™

**Eye drops with tetrahydrozoline
HCl plus glycerin**

Wyeth-Ayerst

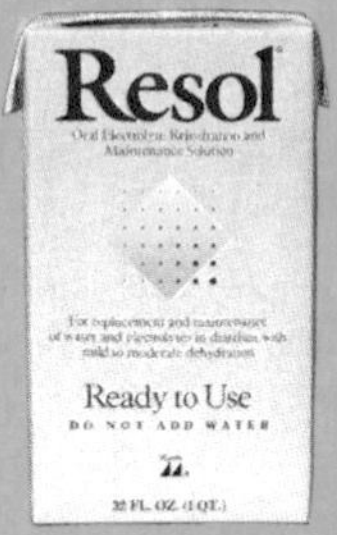

32
Fl. Oz.

**RESOL®
ORAL ELECTROLYTE REHYDRATION
AND MAINTENANCE SOLUTION**
Ready to Use

Wyeth-Ayerst

12 Suppositories

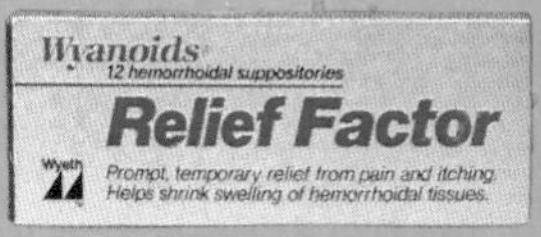

Also available in boxes of 24

**WYANOIDS®
RELIEF FACTOR
Hemorrhoidal Suppositories**

Wyeth-Ayerst

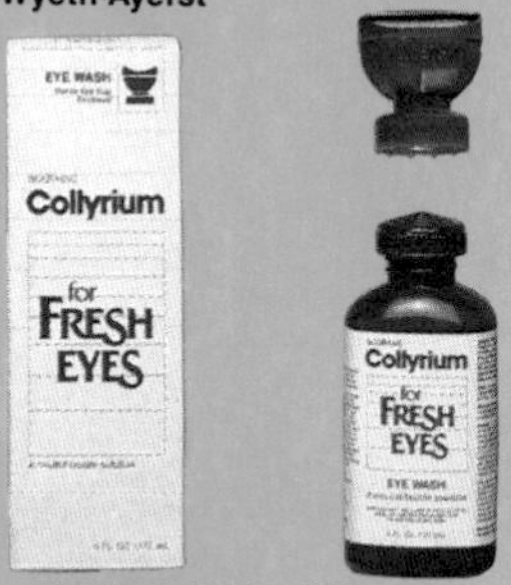

Lotion 6 Fl. Oz. (177 ml) with
separate eyecup bottle cap

**COLLYRIUM For FRESH EYES
Eye Wash**

Wyeth-Ayerst

Also available in
Ready-to-Feed
Liquid and Powder

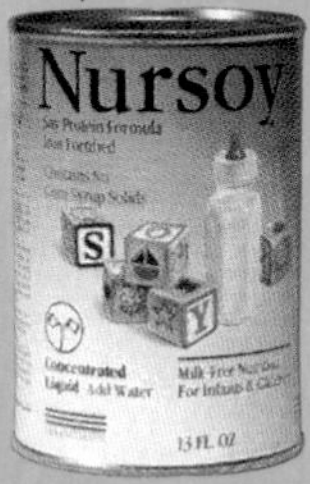

13 Fl. Oz.

Iron Fortified

**NURSOY®
SOY PROTEIN FORMULA
Concentrated Liquid**

Wyeth-Ayerst

Also available in Ready-to-Feed
Liquid and Powder

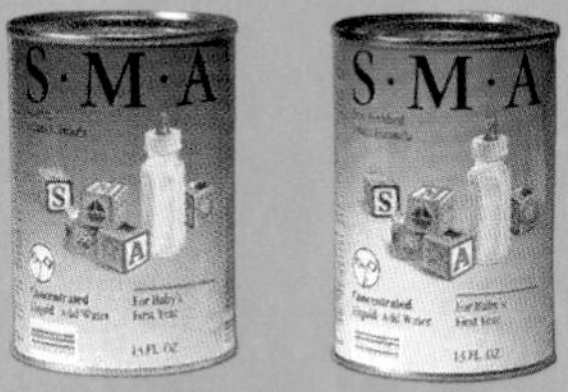

Lo-Iron

Iron
Fortified

13 Fl. Oz.

**S • M • A® INFANT FORMULA
Concentrated Liquid**

ZILA

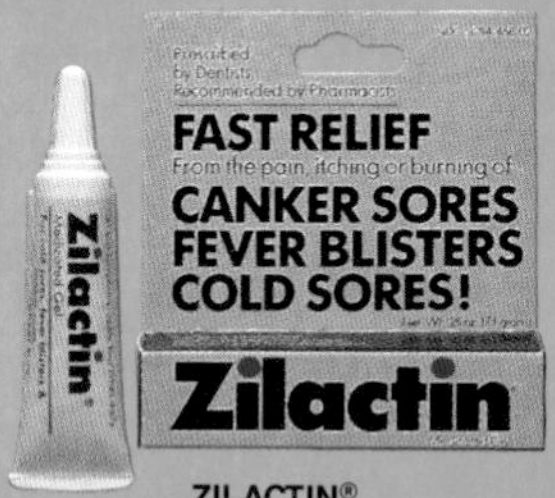

FAST RELIEF
From the pain, itching or burning of
**CANKER SORES
FEVER BLISTERS
COLD SORES!**

Zilactin

**ZILACTIN®
Medicated Gel**

Fast relief from the pain, itching or
burning of canker sores, fever blisters
and cold sores.

Conversion Tables

Metric Doses With Approximate Apothecary Equivalents

The approximate dose equivalents represent the quantities usually prescribed by physicians using, respectively, the metric and apothecary system of weights and measures. When prepared dosage forms such as tablets, capsules, etc. are prescribed in the metric system, the pharmacist may dispense the corresponding approximate equivalent in the apothecary system and vice versa. (Note: A milliliter [mL] is the approximate equivalent of a cubic centimeter [cc]). Exact equivalents, which appear in the United States Pharmacopeia and the National Formulary, must be used to calculate quantities in pharmaceutical formulas and prescription compounding:

| LIQUID MEASURE | | LIQUID MEASURE | | LIQUID MEASURE | | LIQUID MEASURE | |
Metric	Approximate Apothecary Equivalents	Metric	Approximate Apothecary Equivalents	Metric	Approximate Apothecary Equivalents	Metric	Approximate Apothecary Equivalents
1000 mL	1 quart	3 mL	45 minims	30 mL	1 fluid ounce	0.25 mL	4 minims
750 mL	1½ pints	2 mL	30 minims	15 mL	4 fluid drams	0.2 mL	3 minims
500 mL	1 pint	1 mL	15 minims	10 mL	2½ fluid drams	0.1 mL	1½ minims
250 mL	8 fluid ounces	0.75 mL	12 minims	8 mL	2 fluid drams	0.06 mL	1 minim
200 mL	7 fluid ounces	0.6 mL	10 minims	5 mL	1¼ fluid drams	0.05 mL	¾ minim
100 mL	3½ fluid ounces	0.5 mL	8 minims	4 mL	1 fluid dram	0.03 mL	½ minim
50 mL	1¾ fluid ounces	0.3 mL	5 minims				

| WEIGHT | | WEIGHT | | WEIGHT | | WEIGHT | |
Metric	Approximate Apothecary Equivalents	Metric	Approximate Apothecary Equivalents	Metric	Approximate Apothecary Equivalents	Metric	Approximate Apothecary Equivalents
30g	1 ounce	30mg	1/2 grain	500mg	7½ grains	1.2 mg	1/50 grain
15g	4 drams	25mg	3/8 grain	400mg	6 grains	1 mg	1/60 grain
10g	2½ drams	20mg	1/3 grain	300mg	5 grains	800 µg	1/80 grain
7.5g	2 drams	15mg	1/4 grain	250mg	4 grains	600 µg	1/100 grain
6g	90 grains	12mg	1/5 grain	200mg	3 grains	500 µg	1/120 grain
5g	75 grains	10mg	1/6 grain	150mg	2½ grains	400 µg	1/150 grain
4g	60 grains (1 dram)	8mg	1/8 grain	125mg	2 grains	300 µg	1/200 grain
3g	45 grains	6mg	1/10 grain	100mg	1½ grains	250 µg	1/250 grain
2g	30 grains (½ dram)	5mg	1/12 grain	75mg	1¼ grains	200 µg	1/300 grain
1.5g	22 grains	4mg	1/15 grain	60mg	1 grain	150 µg	1/400 grain
1g	15 grains	3mg	1/20 grain	50mg	¾ grain	120 µg	1/500 grain
750mg	12 grains	2mg	1/30 grain	40mg	⅔ grain	100 µg	1/600 grain
600mg	10 grains	1.5mg	1/40 grain				

Approximate Household Equivalents

For household purposes, an American Standard Teaspoon is defined by the American National Standards Institute as containing 4.93 ± 0.24 mL. The USP states that in view of the almost universal practice of employing teaspoons ordinarily available in the household for administration of medicine, the teaspoon may be regarded as representing 5 mL. Household units of measure often are used to inform patients of the size of a liquid dose. Because of difficulties involved in measuring liquids under normal conditions of use, household spoons are not appropriate when accurate measurement of a liquid dose is required. When accurate measurement of a liquid dose is required, the USP recommends that a calibrated oral syringe or dropper be used.

1 fluid dram = 1 teaspoonful = 5 mL
2 fluid drams = 1 dessertspoonful = 10 mL
4 fluid drams = 1 tablespoonful = 15 mL
2 fluid ounces = 1 wineglassful = 60 mL
4 fluid ounces = 1 teacupful = 120 mL
8 fluid ounces = 1 tumblerful = 240 mL

Temperature Conversion Table:

$9 \times °C = (5 \times °F) - 160$
Centigrade to Fahrenheit = $(°C \times 9/5) + 32 = °F$
Fahrenheit to Centigrade = $(°F - 32) \times 5/9 = °C$

Milliequivalents per Liter (mEq/L)

$$mEq/L = \frac{\text{weight of salt (g)} \times \text{valence of ion} \times 1000}{\text{molecular weight of salt}}$$

$$\text{weight of salt (g)} = \frac{mEq/L \times \text{molecular weight of salt}}{\text{valence of ion} \times 1000}$$

Pounds—Kilograms (kg) Conversion

1 pound = 0.453592 kg
1 kg = 2.2 pounds

SECTION 6
Product Information Section

This section is made possible through the courtesy of the manufacturers whose products appear on the following pages. The information concerning each product has been prepared, edited and approved by the manufacturer.

Products described in this edition comply with labeling regulations. Copy may include all the essential information necessary for informed usage such as active ingredients, indications, actions, warnings, drug interactions, precautions, symptoms and treatment of oral overdosage, dosage and administration, professional labeling, and how supplied. In some cases additional information has been supplied to complement the foregoing. The Publisher has emphasized to manufacturers the necessity of describing products comprehensively so that all information essential for intelligent and informed use is available. In organizing and presenting the material in this edition the Publisher is providing all the information made available by manufacturers.

In presenting the following material to the medical profession, the Publisher is not necessarily advocating the use of any product.

Abbott Laboratories
Pharmaceutical Products Division
NORTH CHICAGO, IL 60064

DAYALETS® Filmtab®
[dāy'a-lets]
Multivitamin Supplement for adults and children 4 or more years of age

DAYALETS® PLUS IRON Filmtab®
Multivitamin Supplement with Iron for adults and children 4 or more years of age

Description: Dayalets provide 100% of the recommended daily allowances of essential vitamins. Dayalets Plus Iron provides 100% of the recommended daily allowances of essential vitamins plus the mineral iron.
Daily dosage (one Dayalets tablet) provides:

VITAMINS			% U.S. RDA
Vitamin A.. (1.5 mg)..	5000	IU	100%
Vitamin D.. (10 mcg).	400	IU	100%
Vitamin E	30	IU	100%
Vitamin C	60	mg	100%
Folic Acid	0.4	mg	100%
Thiamine (Vitamin B_1)	1.5	mg	100%
Riboflavin (Vitamin B_2)	1.7	mg	100%
Niacin	20	mg	100%
Vitamin B_6	2	mg	100%
Vitamin B_{12}	6	mcg	100%

Ingredients: Ascorbic acid, cellulose, dl-alpha tocopheryl acetate, niacinamide, povidone, pyridoxine hydrochloride, riboflavin, thiamine hydrochloride, vitamin A acetate, vitamin A palmitate, folic acid, FD&C Yellow No. 6, cholecalciferol, and cyanocobalamin in a filmcoated tablet with vanillin flavoring and artificial coloring added.
Each Dayalets Plus Iron Filmtab® represents all the vitamins in the Dayalets formula in the same concentrations, plus the mineral iron 18 mg (100% U.S. R.D.A.), as ferrous sulfate. Dayalets Plus Iron contain the same ingredients as Dayalets.
These products contain no sugar and essentially no calories.

Indications: Dietary supplement and supplement with iron for adults and children 4 or more years of age.

Administration and Dosage: One Filmtab tablet daily.

How Supplied: Dayalets® Filmtab® in bottles of 100 tablets (NDC 0074-3925-01).
Dayalets® Plus Iron Filmtab in bottles of 100 tablets (NDC 0074-6667-01).
® Filmtab—Film-sealed tablets, Abbott.
Abbott Laboratories
North Chicago, IL 60064
Ref. 02-6903-8/R9, Ref. 02-6906-7/R7

OPTILETS®–500
[op'te-lets]
High potency multivitamin for use in treatment of multivitamin deficiency.

OPTILETS–M–500®
High potency multivitamin for use in treatment of multivitamin deficiency.
Mineral supplementation added.

Description: A therapeutic formula of ten important vitamins, with and without minerals, in a small tablet with the Abbott Filmtab® coating. Each Optilets-500 tablet provides:

Vitamin C (as sodium ascorbate)	500 mg
Niacinamide	100 mg
Calcium Pantothenate	20 mg
Vitamin B_1 (thiamine mononitrate)	15 mg
Vitamin B_2 (riboflavin)	10 mg
Vitamin B_6 (pyridoxine hydrochloride)	5 mg
Vitamin A (as palmitate 1.5 mg, as acetate 1.5 mg— total 3 mg)	10,000 IU
Vitamin B_{12} (cyanocobalamin)	12 mcg
Vitamin D (cholecalciferol)	(10 mcg) 400 IU
Vitamin E (as dl-alpha tocopheryl acetate)	30 IU

Inactive Ingredients: Cellulosic polymers, corn starch, D&C Yellow No. 10, FD&C Yellow No. 6, iron oxide, polyethylene glycol, povidone, stearic acid, talc, titanium dioxide and vanillin.
Each Optilets-M-500 Filmtab contains all the vitamins (vitamin C—ascorbic acid) in the same quantities provided in Optilets-500, plus the following minerals and inactive ingredients:

Magnesium (as oxide)	80 mg
Iron (as dried ferrous sulfate)	20 mg
Copper (as sulfate)	2 mg
Zinc (as sulfate)	1.5 mg
Manganese (as sulfate)	1 mg
Iodine (as calcium iodate)	0.15 mg

Inactive Ingredients: Cellulosic polymers, colloidal silicon dioxide, corn starch, D&C Red No. 7, FD&C Blue No. 1, iron oxide, magnesium stearate, microcrystalline cellulose, polyethylene glycol, povidone, propylene glycol, sorbic acid and titanium dioxide.

Dosage and Administration: Usual adult dosage is one Filmtab tablet daily, or as directed by physician.

How Supplied: Optilets-500 tablets are supplied in bottles of 100 (**NDC 0074-4287-13**). Optilets-M-500 tablets are supplied in bottles of 30 (**NDC 0074-4286-30**) and 100 (**NDC 0074-4286-13**).
®Filmtab—Film-sealed Tablets, Abbott.
Abbott Laboratories
North Chicago, IL 60064
Ref. 07-5628-7/R18, Ref. 07-5627-7/R17

SURBEX®
[sir'bex]
Vitamin B-complex

SURBEX® with C
Vitamin B-complex with vitamin C

Description: Each Surbex Filmtab tablet provides:

Niacinamide	30 mg
Calcium Pantothenate	10 mg
Vitamin B_1 (thiamine mononitrate)	6 mg
Vitamin B_2 (riboflavin)	6 mg
Vitamin B_6 (pyridoxine hydrochloride)	2.5 mg
Vitamin B_{12} (cyanocobalamin)	5 mcg

Each Surbex with C Filmtab tablet provides the same ingredients as Surbex, plus 250 mg Vitamin C (as sodium ascorbate).

Inactive Ingredients
Surbex tablets: Castor oil, cellulosic polymers, corn starch, D&C Yellow No. 10, dibasic calcium phosphate, FD&C Yellow No. 6, magnesium stearate, povidone, propylene glycol, stearic acid, titanium dioxide, and vanillin.
Surbex with C Tablets: Castor oil, cellulosic polymers, corn starch, D&C Yellow No. 10, FD&C Yellow No. 6, lactose, magnesium stearate, microcrystalline cellulose, povidone, propylene glycol, titanium dioxide, and vanillin.

Indications: Surbex is indicated for treatment of Vitamin B-Complex deficiency.
Surbex with C is indicated for use in treatment of Vitamin B-Complex with Vitamin C deficiency.

Dosage and Administration: Usual adult dosage is one tablet twice daily or as directed by physician.

How Supplied: Surbex is supplied as bright orange-colored tablets in bottles of 100 (NDC 0074-4876-13).
Surbex with C is supplied as yellow-colored tablets in bottles of 100 (NDC 0074-4877-13).
Abbott Pharmaceuticals, Inc.
North Chicago, IL 60064
Ref. 03-1306-4/R10, 03-1482-4/R11

SURBEX–T®
High-potency vitamin B-complex with 500 mg of vitamin C

Description: Each Filmtab® tablet provides:

Vitamin C (ascorbic acid)	500 mg
Niacinamide	100 mg
Calcium Pantothenate	20 mg
Vitamin B_1 (thiamine mononitrate)	15 mg
Vitamin B_2 (riboflavin)	10 mg
Vitamin B_6 (pyridoxine hydrochloride)	5 mg
Vitamin B_{12} (cyanocobalamin)	10 mcg

Inactive Ingredients: Cellulosic polymers, colloidal silicon dioxide, corn starch, D&C Yellow No. 10, FD&C Yellow No. 6, magnesium stearate, microcrystalline cellulose, polyethylene glycol, povidone, propylene glycol, titanium dioxide, and vanillin.

Indications: For use in treatment of Vitamin B-Complex with Vitamin C deficiency.

Dosage and Administration: Usual adult dosage is one Filmtab tablet daily, or as directed by physician.

How Supplied: Orange-colored tablets in bottle of 100 (**NDC** 0074-4878-13). Also supplied in Abbo-Pac® unit dose packages of 100 tablets in strips of 10 tablets per strip (**NDC** 0074-4878-11). ®Filmtab—Film-sealed Tablets, Abbott. Abbott Pharmaceuticals, Inc.
North Chicago, IL 60064
Ref. 03-1483-7/R12

SURBEX®-750 with IRON
High-potency B-complex with iron, vitamin E and 750 mg vitamin C

Description: Each Filmtab® tablet provides:
VITAMINS
Vitamin C (as sodium ascorbate) 750 mg
Niacinamide .... 100 mg
Vitamin B$_6$ (pyridoxine
  hydrochloride) .... 25 mg
Calcium Pantothenate .... 20 mg
Vitamin B$_1$ (thiamine
  mononitrate) .... 15 mg
Vitamin B$_2$ (riboflavin) .... 15 mg
Vitamin B$_{12}$ (cyanocobalamin) 12 mcg
Folic Acid .... 400 mcg
Vitamin E (as dl-alpha tocopheryl
  acetate) .... 30 IU
MINERAL
Elemental Iron (as dried
  ferrous sulfate) .... 27 mg
  equivalent to 135 mg ferrous sulfate

Inactive Ingredients: Cellulosic polymers, colloidal silicon dioxide, FD&C Red No. 3, corn starch, iron oxide, magnesium stearate, microcrystalline cellulose, polyethylene glycol, povidone, and vanillin.

Indications: For the treatment of vitamin C and B-complex deficiencies and to supplement the daily intake of iron and vitamin E.

Dosage and Administration: Usual adult dosage is one tablet daily or as directed by physician.

How Supplied: Bottles of 50 tablets (**NDC** 0074-8029-50)
Abbott Pharmaceuticals, Inc.
North Chicago, IL 60064
Ref. 03-1489-4/R8

SURBEX®-750 with ZINC
High-potency B-complex with zinc, vitamin E and 750 mg of vitamin C. For persons 12 years of age or older

Description: Daily dose (one Filmtab® tablet) provides:

VITAMINS		%U.S. R.D.A.*
Vitamin E	30 IU	100%
Vitamin C	750 mg	1250%
Folic Acid	0.4 mg	100%
Thiamine (B$_1$)	15 mg	1000%
Riboflavin (B$_2$)	15 mg	882%
Niacin	100 mg	500%
Vitamin B$_6$	20 mg	1000%
Vitamin B$_{12}$	12 mcg	200%
Pantothenic Acid	20 mg	200%
MINERAL		
Zinc**	22.5 mg	150%

* % U.S. Recommended Daily Allowance for Adults.
** Equivalent to 100 mg of zinc sulfate.

Ingredients: Ascorbic acid, niacinamide, cellulose, dl-alpha tocopheryl acetate, zinc sulfate, povidone, pyridoxine hydrochloride, calcium pantothenate, riboflavin, thiamine mononitrate, cyanocobalamin, magnesium stearate, colloidal silicon dioxide, folic acid, in a film-coated tablet with vanillin flavoring and artificial coloring added.

Usual Adult Dose: One tablet daily.

How Supplied: Bottles of 50 tablets (**NDC** 0074-8152-50).
Abbott Pharmaceuticals, Inc.
North Chicago, IL 60064
Ref. 03-1490-4/R9

If desired, additional information on any Abbott Product will be provided upon request to Abbott Laboratories.

Adria Laboratories
Division of Erbamont Inc.
7001 POST ROAD
DUBLIN, OH 43017

Professional Labeling
EMETROL®
[ĕm ʹĕ-trŏl]
(Phosphorated Carbohydrate Solution)
For the relief of nausea associated with upset stomach.

Description: EMETROL is an oral solution containing balanced amounts of levulose (fructose) and dextrose (glucose) and phosphoric acid with controlled hydrogen ion concentration. Pleasantly lemon-mint flavored.

Ingredients: Each 5 mL teaspoonful contains dextrose (glucose), 1.87 g; levulose (fructose), 1.87 g; and phosphoric acid, 21.5 mg and the following inactive ingredients: D&C yellow No. 10, flavors, glycerin, methylparaben and purified water.

Action: EMETROL quickly relieves nausea by local action on the wall of the hyperactive G.I. tract. It reduces smooth-muscle contractions in proportion to the amount used. Unlike systemic antiemetics, EMETROL works almost immediately to control nausea.

Indications: For the relief of nausea associated with upset stomach. For other conditions, take only as directed by your physician.

Advantages:
1. **Fast Action**—works almost immediately by local action on contact with the hyperactive G.I. tract.
2. **Effectiveness**—reduces smooth-muscle contractions in proportion to the amount used—stops nausea.
3. **Safety**—non-toxic—won't mask symptoms of organic pathology.
4. **Convenience**—can be recommended over the phone for any member of the family, even the children—no ℞ required.
5. **Patient Acceptance**—a low cost that patients appreciate—a pleasant lemon-mint flavor that both children and adults like.

Usual Adult Dose: One or two tablespoonful. Repeat every 15 minutes until distress subsides.
For nausea and upset stomach associated with morning sickness: Take one or two tablespoonful immediately on arising repeated every three hours or when symptoms threaten.

Usual Children's Dose: One or two teaspoonful. Repeat dose every 15 minutes until distress subsides.

Important: Never dilute EMETROL or drink fluids of any kind immediately before or after taking a dose.

Caution: If upset stomach continues or recurs frequently, consult a physician promptly as it may be a sign of a serious condition.

Warning: KEEP THIS AND ALL MEDICATIONS OUT OF THE REACH OF CHILDREN. As with any drug, if you are pregnant or nursing a baby, seek the advice of a health professional before using this product.
This product contains fructose and should not be taken by persons with hereditary fructose intolerance (HFI).

This product contains sugar and should not be taken by diabetics except under the advice and supervision of a physician.

In case of accidental overdose, contact a poison control center, emergency medical facility, or physician immediately for advice.

How Supplied: Each 5 mL teaspoonful of EMETROL contains dextrose (glucose), 1.87 g; levulose (fructose), 1.87 g; and phosphoric acid, 21.5 mg in a yellow, lemon-mint-flavored syrup.
NDC 0013-2113-45 Bottle of 4 fluid ounces (118 mL)
NDC 0013-2113-65 Bottle of 8 fluid ounces (236 mL)
NDC 0013-2113-51 Bottle of 1 pint (473 mL)
Store at room temperature

Notice: Each bottle is protected by a printed band around the cap. Do not use if band is damaged or missing.
ADRIA LABORATORIES
Division of Erbamont Inc.
COLUMBUS, OH 43215
Shown in Product Identification Section, page 403

Continued on next page

Adria—Cont.

Professional Labeling

MODANE
[mō 'dāne]
(phenolphthalein)

Description: MODANE TABLETS (rust red)—Each tablet contains white phenolphthalein 130 mg. Inactive ingredients include acacia, calcium carbonate, calcium sulfate, corn starch, dibasic calcium phosphate, FD&C Red No. 40 aluminum lake, lactose, magnesium stearate, povidone, shellac, sodium benzoate, sucrose, talc, titanium dioxide, water and carnauba wax. MODANE MILD Tablets (pink)—Each tablet contains white phenolphthalein 60 mg. Inactive ingredients include acacia, calcium carbonate, calcium sulfate, corn starch, dibasic calcium phosphate, FD&C Red No. 40 aluminum lake, lactose, magnesium stearate, methylparaben, povidone, propylparaben, shellac, sodium benzoate, sucrose, talc, titanium dioxide, water and carnauba wax.

Clinical Pharmacology: Phenolphthalein, a stimulant laxative, acts primarily on the large intestine to produce a semifluid stool usually in 4–8 hours. It is dissolved by bile salts and alkaline intestinal secretions and may impart a red color to alkaline feces and urine.

Indications: For temporary relief of constipation.

Contraindications: Sensitivity to phenolphthalein.

Warnings: Do not use any laxative preparations when abdominal pain, nausea, or vomiting are present. Frequent and continued use may cause dependence upon laxatives.
KEEP THIS PRODUCT OUT OF REACH OF CHILDREN.
As with any drug, if the patient is pregnant or nursing a baby, she should consult a health professional before using.

Precautions: Phenolphthalein may color alkaline feces and urine red. If skin rash appears, do not use this product or any other preparation containing phenolphthalein.

Adverse Reactions: Excessive bowel activity, usually diarrhea or abdominal discomfort, nausea, vomiting, cramps, weakness, dizziness, palpitations, sweating and fainting may follow the administration of a laxative. Diarrhea may lead to fluid and electrolyte deficits. Allergic reactions, skin rashes attributed to phenolphthalein, have been reported.

Overdosage: Phenolphthalein is relatively nontoxic. Overdosage may be expected to result in excessive bowel activity. Treatment is symptomatic if the duration of effects is prolonged. Fluid and electrolyte deficits might result from prolonged catharsis.

Dosage and Administration:
MODANE Tablet (rust red)—Adults: One tablet daily, or as directed by a doctor. This strength is not recommended for children.

MODANE MILD Tablets (pink)—Adults: One to two tablets daily, or as directed by a doctor. Children (6–12 years): One tablet daily, or as directed by a doctor. Not recommended for children under 6 years of age.

How Supplied: Each MODANE tablet contains white phenolphthalein 130 mg in a rust red, round, sugar coated tablet printed with A on one side and 513 on the other. Store at room temperature.
Packages of 10 tablets.
NDC 0013-5131-07
Package of 30 tablets.
NDC 0013-5131-13
Bottle of 100 tablets.
NDC 0013-5131-17

How Supplied: Each MODANE MILD tablet contains white phenolphthalein 60 mg in a pink, round, sugar coated tablet printed with A on one side and 512 on the other. Store at room temperature.
Package of 10 tablets.
NDC 0013-5121-07
Package of 30 tablets.
NDC 0013-5121-13
Bottle of 100 tablets
NDC 0013-5121-17
Shown in Product Identification Section, page 403

Professional Labeling
MODANE PLUS
[mō 'dāne plŭs]
(phenolphthalein and docusate sodium)

Description: Each tablet contains white phenolphthalein 65mg and docusate sodium 100mg. Inactive ingredients include acacia, calcium carbonate, calcium sulfate, croscarmellose sodium, FD&C yellow #6 aluminum lake, magnesium stearate, microcrystalline cellulose, povidone, shellac, silica gel, sodium benzoate, sucrose, talc, titanium dioxide, water and carnauba wax.
Phenolphthalein is classified as a stimulant laxative. Chemically phenolphthalein is 3, 3-bis (p-hydroxyphenyl) phthalide.
Chemically, docusate sodium is butanedioic acid, sulfo-1, 4-bis (2-ethylhexyl) ester, sodium salt. It is an anionic surfactant.

Clinical Pharmacology: Phenolphthalein, a stimulant laxative, acts primarily on the large intestine to produce a semifluid stool usually in 4–8 hours. It is dissolved by bile salts and alkaline intestinal secretions and may impart a red color to alkaline feces and urine.
Docusate sodium is classified as a stool softener. It is used in conditions in which it is desirable that the feces be kept soft and straining at the stool be avoided.

Indications: For temporary relief of constipation in adults.

Contraindications: Sensitivity to phenolphthalein. Mineral oil administration.

Warnings: Do not use any laxative preparations when abdominal pain, nausea, or vomiting are present. Frequent and continued use may cause dependence upon laxatives.
KEEP THIS PRODUCT OUT OF REACH OF CHILDREN.
As with any drug, if the patient is pregnant or nursing a baby, she should consult a health professional before using.

Precautions: Phenolphthalein may color alkaline feces and urine red. If skin rash appears, do not use this product or any other preparation containing phenolphthalein.
Docusate sodium may increase the intestinal absorption of mineral oil and/or hepatic uptake of other drugs administered concurrently.

Adverse Reactions: Excessive bowel activity, usually diarrhea or abdominal discomfort, nausea, vomiting, cramps, weakness, dizziness, palpitations, sweating and fainting may follow the administration of a laxative. Diarrhea may lead to fluid and electrolyte deficits. Allergic reactions, skin rashes attributed to phenolphthalein, have been reported.

Overdosage: Phenolphthalein is relatively nontoxic. Overdosage may be expected to result in excessive bowel activity. Treatment is symptomatic if the duration of effects is prolonged. Fluid and electrolyte deficits might result from prolonged catharsis.

Dosage and Administration:
Adults: One tablet daily, or as directed by a doctor. This strength is not recommended for children.

How Supplied: Each MODANE PLUS tablet contains white phenolphthalein 65 mg and docusate sodium 100 mg in an orange, round, sugar coated tablet printed with A on one side and 514 on the other.
Package of 10 tablets
NDC 0013-5151-07
Package of 30 tablets.
NDC 0013-5151-13
Bottle of 100 tablets.
NDC 0013-5151-17
Store at room temperature.
Shown in Product Identification Section, page 403

Allergan
Pharmaceuticals
A Division of Allergan, Inc.
2525 DUPONT DRIVE
IRVINE, CA 92715

CELLUVISC™
(carboxymethylcellulose sodium) 1%
Lubricant Ophthalmic Solution

Contains: Carboxymethylcellulose sodium 1% with: calcium chloride, potassium chloride, purified water, sodium chloride, and sodium lactate.

FDA APPROVED USES

Indications: FOR USE AS A LUBRICANT TO PREVENT FURTHER IRRITATION OR TO RELIEVE DRYNESS OF THE EYE.

Warnings: Do not reuse. Once opened, discard. To avoid contamination, do not touch tip of container to any surface. If you experience eye pain, changes in vision, continued redness or irritation of the eye, or if the condition worsens or persists for more than 72 hours, discontinue use and consult a doctor. If solution changes color or becomes cloudy, do not use. Keep out of the reach of children.

Directions: Instill 1 or 2 drops in the affected eye(s) as needed.

How Supplied: Celluvisc™ (carboxymethylcellulose sodium) 1% Lubricant Ophthalmic Solution is supplied in sterile, preservative free, disposable, single-use containers of 0.01 fluid ounces each, in the following size:
30 SINGLE-USE CONTAINERS—
NDC 0023-4554-30
*Shown in Product Identification
Section, page 403*

LACRI–LUBE® S.O.P.®
Sterile Ophthalmic Ointment

Contains: White petrolatum 55%, mineral oil 42.5%, petrolatum (and) lanolin alcohol 2% with chlorobutanol (chloral derivative) 0.5%.

Indications: Dry eye conditions.

Actions: Ocular lubricant.

Note: Do not touch tube tip to any surface since this may contaminate the ointment. Keep out of the reach of children. Store away from heat.

Dosage: Pull lower lid down and apply a small amount of ointment to affected areas as needed or as directed by physician.

Professional Labeling: Same as outlined under Indications.

How Supplied: 3.5 g and 7 g tubes and packs of 24-0.7 g unit-dose containers.
*Shown in Product Identification
Section, page 403*

LIQUIFILM FORTE®
(polyvinyl alcohol) 3.0%
Lubricant Ophthalmic Solution

Contains: Polyvinyl alcohol 3.0% with: edetate disodium, mono- and dibasic sodium phosphates, purified water, sodium chloride, and thimerosal 0.002%. May also contain hydrochloric acid or sodium hydroxide to adjust pH.

FDA APPROVED USES

Indications: FOR USE AS A LUBRICANT TO PREVENT FURTHER IRRITATION OR TO RELIEVE DRYNESS OF THE EYE.

Warnings: To avoid contamination, do not touch tip of container to any surface. Replace cap after using. If you experience eye pain, changes in vision, continued redness or irritation of the eye, or if the condition worsens or persists for more than 72 hours, discontinue use and consult a doctor. This product contains thimerosal 0.002% as a preservative. Do not use this product if you are sensitive to thimerosal or any other ingredient containing mercury. If solution changes color or becomes cloudy, do not use. Keep out of the reach of children.

Directions: Instill 1 or 2 drops in the affected eye(s) as needed.

How Supplied: Liquifilm Forte® (polyvinyl alcohol) 3.0% Lubricant Ophthalmic Solution is supplied in sterile plastic dropper bottles in the following sizes:
½ fl oz—NDC 11980-187-15
1 fl oz—NDC 11980-187-30

LIQUIFILM TEARS®
(polyvinyl alcohol) 1.4%
Lubricant Ophthalmic Solution

Contains: Polyvinyl alcohol 1.4% with: chlorobutanol (chloral deriv.) 0.5%, purified water, and sodium chloride. May also contain hydrochloric acid or sodium hydroxide to adjust pH.

FDA APPROVED USES

Indications: FOR USE AS A LUBRICANT TO PREVENT FURTHER IRRITATION OR TO RELIEVE DRYNESS OF THE EYE.

Warnings: To avoid contamination, do not touch tip of container to any surface. Replace cap after using. If you experience eye pain, changes in vision, continued redness or irritation of the eye, or if the condition worsens or persists for more than 72 hours, discontinue use and consult a doctor. If solution changes color or becomes cloudy, do not use. Keep out of the reach of children.

Directions: Instill 1 or 2 drops in the affected eye(s) as needed.

How Supplied: Liquifilm Tears® (polyvinyl alcohol) 1.4% Lubricant Ophthalmic Solution is supplied in sterile plastic dropper bottles in the following sizes:
½ fl oz—NDC 11980-025-15
1 fl oz—NDC 11980-025-30
*Shown in Product Identification
Section, page 403*

PREFRIN™ Liquifilm®
(phenylephrine HCl 0.12%, polyvinyl alcohol 1.4%)
Vasoconstrictor (Redness Reliever) and Lubricant Eye Drops

Contains: Phenylephrine HCl 0.12% and polyvinyl alcohol 1.4% with: benzalkonium chloride 0.004%, edetate disodium, purified water, sodium acetate, mono- and dibasic sodium phosphates and sodium thiosulfate. May also contain hydrochloric acid or sodium hydroxide to adjust pH.

FDA APPROVED USES

Indications: RELIEVES REDNESS OF THE EYE DUE TO MINOR EYE IRRITATIONS. FOR USE AS A LUBRICANT TO PREVENT FURTHER IRRITATION OR TO RELIEVE DRYNESS OF THE EYE.

Warnings: To avoid contamination, do not touch tip of container to any surface. Replace cap after using. If you experience eye pain, changes in vision, contin-

ued redness or irritation of the eye, or if the condition worsens or persists for more than 72 hours, discontinue use and consult a doctor. If you have glaucoma, do not use this product except under the advice and supervision of a doctor. Overuse of this product may produce increased redness of the eye. If solution changes color or becomes cloudy, do not use. Keep out of the reach of children.

Directions: Instill 1 or 2 drops in the affected eye(s) up to four times daily.

How Supplied: Prefrin™ Liquifilm® (phenylephrine HCl 0.12%, polyvinyl alcohol 1.4%) Vasoconstrictor (Redness Reliever) and Lubricant Eye Drops is supplied in sterile plastic dropper bottles in the following size:
0.7 fl oz—NDC 11980-036-07
*Shown in Product Identification
Section, page 403*

REFRESH®
(polyvinyl alcohol 1.4%, povidone 0.6%)
Lubricant Ophthalmic Solution

Contains: Polyvinyl alcohol 1.4% and povidone 0.6% with: purified water and sodium chloride. May also contain hydrochloric acid or sodium hydroxide to adjust pH.

FDA APPROVED USES

Indications: FOR USE AS A LUBRICANT TO PREVENT FURTHER IRRITATION OR TO RELIEVE DRYNESS OF THE EYE.

Warnings: Do not reuse. Once opened, discard. To avoid contamination, do not touch tip of container to any surface. If you experience eye pain, changes in vision, continued redness or irritation of the eye, or if the condition worsens or persists for more than 72 hours, discontinue use and consult a doctor. If solution changes color or becomes cloudy, do not use. Keep out of the reach of children.

Directions: Instill 1 or 2 drops in the affected eye(s) as needed.

How Supplied: Refresh® (polyvinyl alcohol 1.4%, povidone 0.6%) Lubricant Ophthalmic Solution is supplied in sterile, preservative free, disposable, single-use containers of 0.01 fluid ounces each, in the following sizes:
30 SINGLE-USE CONTAINERS—NDC 0023-0506-01
50 SINGLE-USE CONTAINERS—NDC 0023-0506-50
*Shown in Product Identification
Section, page 403*

REFRESH® P.M.
Eye Lubricant

Contains: White petrolatum 55.0%, mineral oil 41.5%, petrolatum (and) lanolin alcohol 2.0% with purified water and sodium chloride.

Continued on next page

Allergan—Cont.

Indications: Dry eye conditions.

Actions: Ocular lubricant.

Warnings: To avoid contamination of this product, do not touch tip of tube to any surface. Replace cap after use. Keep container tightly closed. If symptoms do not improve, discontinue use and consult your doctor. Keep out of the reach of children.
Note: Store away from heat. Protect from freezing.

Dosage: Pull down lower lid and apply a small strip ($\frac{1}{4}$″–$\frac{1}{2}$″) of the ointment. Use as needed or as directed by your doctor.

Professional Labeling: Same as outlined under Indications.

How Supplied: 3.5 g tubes.
Shown in Product Identification Section, page 403

RELIEF®
(phenylephrine HCl 0.12%, polyvinyl alcohol 1.4%)
Vasoconstrictor (Redness Reliever) and Lubricant Eye Drops

Contains: Phenylephrine HCl 0.12% and polyvinyl alcohol 1.4%, with: edetate disodium, purified water, sodium acetate, mono- and dibasic sodium phosphates and sodium thiosulfate. May also contain hydrochloric acid or sodium hydroxide to adjust pH.

FDA APPROVED USES

Indications: RELIEVES REDNESS OF THE EYE DUE TO MINOR EYE IRRITATIONS. FOR USE AS A LUBRICANT TO PREVENT FURTHER IRRITATION OR TO RELIEVE DRYNESS OF THE EYE.

Warnings: Do not reuse. Once opened, discard. To avoid contamination, do not touch tip of container to any surface. If you experience eye pain, changes in vision, continued redness or irritation of the eye, or if the condition worsens or persists for more than 72 hours, discontinue use and consult a doctor. If you have glaucoma, do not use this product except under the advice and supervision of a doctor. Overuse of this product may produce increased redness of the eye. If solution changes color or becomes cloudy, do not use. Keep out of the reach of children.

Directions: Instill 1 or 2 drops in the affected eyes(s) up to four times daily.

How Supplied: Relief® (phenylephrine HCl 0.12%, polyvinyl alcohol 1.4%) Vasoconstrictor (Redness Reliever) and Lubricant Eye Drops is supplied in sterile, preservative free, disposable, single-use containers of 0.01 fluid ounces each, in the following sizes:
30 SINGLE-USE CONTAINERS—
NDC 0023-0507-01
Shown in Product Identification Section, page 403

TEARS PLUS®
(polyvinyl alcohol 1.4%, povidone 0.6%)
Lubricant Ophthalmic Solution

Contains: Polyvinyl alcohol 1.4% and povidone 0.6% with: chlorobutanol (chloral deriv.) 0.5%, purified water and sodium chloride. May also contain hydrochloric acid or sodium hydroxide to adjust pH.

FDA APPROVED USES

Indications: FOR USE AS A LUBRICANT TO PREVENT FURTHER IRRITATION OR TO RELIEVE DRYNESS OF THE EYE.

Warnings: To avoid contamination, do not touch tip of container to any surface. Replace cap after using. If you experience eye pain, changes in vision, continued redness or irritation of the eye, or if the condition worsens or persists for more than 72 hours, discontinue use and consult a doctor. If solution changes color or becomes cloudy, do not use. Keep out of the reach of children.

Directions: Instill 1 or 2 drops in the affected eye(s) as needed.

How Supplied: Tears Plus® (polyvinyl alcohol 1.4%, povidone 0.6%) Lubricant Ophthalmic Solution is supplied in sterile, plastic dropper bottles in the following sizes:
½ fl oz—NDC 0023-0165-15
1 fl oz—NDC 0023-0165-30
Shown in Product Identification Section, page 403

B. F. Ascher & Company, Inc.
15501 WEST 109th STREET
LENEXA, KS 66219
Mailing address:
P.O. BOX 410827
KANSAS CITY, MO 64141-0827

AYR® Saline Nasal Mist and Drops
[ār]

AYR Mist or Drops restores vital moisture to provide prompt relief for dry, crusted and inflamed nasal membranes due to chronic sinusitis, colds, low humidity, overuse of nasal decongestant drops and sprays, allergies, minor nose bleeds and other minor nasal irritations. AYR provides a soothing way to thin thick secretions and aid their removal from the nose and sinuses. AYR can be used as often as needed without the side effects associated with overuse of decongestant nose drops and sprays.
SAFE & GENTLE ENOUGH FOR CHILDREN AND INFANTS
AYR Drops are particularly convenient for easy application with infants and children. AYR is formulated to prevent stinging, burning and irritation of delicate nasal tissue, even that of babies.

Directions For Use: SPRAY—Squeeze twice in each nostril as often as needed. DROPS—Two to four drops in each nos-

tril every two hours as needed, or as directed by your physician.
AYR is a specially formulated, buffered, isotonic saline solution containing sodium chloride 0.65% adjusted to the proper tonicity and pH with monobasic potassium phosphate/sodium hydroxide buffer to prevent nasal irritation. AYR also contains the non-irritating antibacterial and antifungal preservatives thimerosal and benzalkonium chloride and is formulated with deionized water.

How Supplied: AYR Mist in 50 ml spray bottles, AYR Drops in 50 ml dropper bottles.
Shown in Product Identification Section, page 403

MOBIGESIC® Analgesic Tablets
[mō′bĭ-jē′zĭk]

Active Ingredients: Each tablet contains 325 mg of magnesium salicylate with 30 mg of phenyltoloxamine citrate.

Also Contains: Microcrystalline cellulose, magnesium stearate and colloidal silicon dioxide which aid in the formulation of the tablet and its dissolution in the gastrointestinal tract.

Indications: MOBIGESIC acts fast to provide relief from the pain and discomfort of simple headaches and colds; for temporary relief of the pain and tension accompanying muscle soreness and fatigue, neuralgia, minor menstrual cramps, T.M.J. and pain of tooth extraction. The unique formula provides relief of pain due to sinusitis and in the fever and inflammation of colds.

Caution: When used for the temporary symptomatic relief of colds, if relief does not occur within 7 days (3 days for fever), discontinue use and consult physician. This preparation may cause drowsiness. Do not drive or operate machinery while taking this medication. Do not administer to children under 6 years of age or exceed recommended dosage unless directed by physician.

Warnings: Keep this and all drugs out of the reach of children. In case of accidental overdose, call your doctor or poison control center immediately. As with any drug, if you are pregnant or nursing a baby, seek the advice of a health professional before using this product.

Usual Dosage: Adults—1 or 2 tablets every four hours, up to 10 tablets daily. Children (6 to 12 years)—1 tablet every 4 hours, up to 5 tablets daily. Do not use more than 10 days unless directed by physician.
Store at room temperature (59°–86°F).

How Supplied: Packages of 18's, 50's and 100's.
Shown in Product Identification Section, page 403

MOBISYL® Analgesic Creme
[mō′bĭ-sĭl]

Active Ingredient: Trolamine salicylate 10%. Also Contains: Glycerin, methylparaben, mineral oil, polysorbate 60,

propylparaben, sorbitan stearate, sorbitol, stearic acid, and water.

Description: MOBISYL is a greaseless, odorless, penetrating, non-burning, non-irritating analgesic creme.

Indications: For adults and children, 12 years of age and older, MOBISYL is indicated for the temporary relief of minor aches and pains of muscles and joints, such as simple backache, lumbago, arthritis, neuralgia, strains, bruises and sprains.

Actions: MOBISYL penetrates fast into sore, tender joints and muscles where pain originates. It works to reduce inflammation. Helps soothe stiff joints and muscles and gets you going again.

Warnings: For external use only. Avoid contact with the eyes. Discontinue use if condition worsens or if symptoms persist for more than 7 days, and consult a physician. Do not use on children under 12 years of age except under the advice and supervision of a physician. In case of accidental ingestion, seek professional assistance or contact a Poison Control Center immediately. Close cap tightly. Keep this and all drugs out of the reach of children. Store at room temperature.

Dosage and Administration: Place a liberal amount of MOBISYL Creme in your palm and massage into the area of pain and soreness three or four times a day, especially before retiring. MOBISYL may be worn under clothing or bandages.

How Supplied: MOBISYL is available in 1.25 oz tubes, 3.5 oz tubes, 8 oz jars.
Shown in Product Identification Section, page 403

PEN●KERA® Creme with Keratin Binding Factor
A Therapeutic Creme for Chronic Dry Skin

Ingredients: Water, octyl palmitate, glycerin, mineral oil, polysorbate 60, sorbitan stearate, carbomer 940, triethanolamine, wheat germ glycerides, diazolidinyl urea, polyamino sugar condensate (and) urea, and dehydroacetic acid.

Indications: PEN●KERA Therapeutic Creme for Chronic Dry Skin contains Keratin Binding Factor, a polyamino sugar condensate and urea, which is synthesized to match the same biological components as those found in skin. The Keratin Binding Factor in PEN●KERA Creme replaces the missing elements of dehydrated skin which absorb and retain moisture. The Keratin Binding Factor actually simulates the natural moisturizing mechanism of the skin, relieving itching, flaking, sensitive, dry skin symptoms.
PEN●KERA is fragrance-free, dye-free, paraben-free, lanolin-free and nongreasy for smooth, fast absorption.

Dosage and Administration: Apply in a thin layer. Because it penetrates quickly and is non-greasy, PEN●KERA

may be used under make-up or sun screens. Regular use will reduce the frequency of application and quantity required to achieve moisturized skin.

Precautions: FOR EXTERNAL USE ONLY

How Supplied: PEN●KERA Therapeutic Creme is available in 8 oz. bottles (0225-0440-35).
Shown in Product Identification Section, page 403

UNILAX® Softgel Capsules

Active Ingredients: Docusate sodium, USP 230 mg and yellow phenolphthalein, USP 130 mg.

Inactive Ingredients: D&C Yellow No. 10, FD&C Blue No. 1, FD&C Yellow No. 6, gelatin, glycerin, polyethylene glycol 400, sorbitol and titanium dioxide.

Indications: Constipation (irregularity).

Actions: UNILAX® is a dual-acting stool softener and stimulant laxative.

Warnings: Do not use laxative products when abdominal pain, nausea, or vomiting are present. As with all laxatives, frequent or prolonged use may result in dependence. If skin rash appears, do not use this or any other preparation containing phenolphthalein. As with any drug, if you are pregnant or nursing a baby, seek the advice of a health professional before using this product. Keep this and all drugs out of the reach of children. In case of accidental overdose, seek professional assistance or contact a poison control center immediately.

Dosage and Administration: Adults and children 12 years of age and over: Oral dosage is 1 softgel capsule daily (preferably at bedtime) or as directed by a physician. Do not use in children under 12 years of age.

How Supplied: Bottles of 15 and 60 softgel capsules.
Shown in Product Identification Section, page 403

Astra Pharmaceutical Products, Inc.
50 OTIS ST.
WESTBORO, MA 01581-4428

XYLOCAINE® (lidocaine) 2.5%
[$z\bar{\imath}$ 'lo-caine]
OINTMENT

For temporary relief of pain and itching due to minor burns, sunburn, minor cuts, abrasions, insect bites and minor skin irritations.

Composition: Diethylaminoacet-2, 6-xylidide 2.5% in a water miscible ointment vehicle consisting of polyethylene glycols and propylene glycol.

Action and Uses: A topical anesthetic ointment for fast, temporary relief of pain and itching due to minor burns, sunburn, minor cuts, abrasions, insect bites

and minor skin irritations. The ointment can be easily removed with water. It is ineffective when applied to intact skin.

Administration and Dosage: Apply topically in liberal amounts for adequate control of symptoms. When the anesthetic effect wears off additional ointment may be applied as needed.

Important Warning: *In persistent, severe or extensive skin disorders, advise patient to use only as directed. In case of accidental ingestion advise patient to seek professional assistance or to contact a poison control center immediately. Keep out of the reach of children.*

Caution: *Do not use in the eyes. Not for prolonged use. If the condition for which this preparation is used persists or if a rash or irritation develops, advise patient to discontinue use and consult a physician.*

How Supplied: Available in tube of 35 grams (approximately 1.25 ounces).
Shown in Product Identification Section, page 403

Ayerst Laboratories
Division of American Home Products Corporation
685 THIRD AVE.
NEW YORK, NY 10017-4071

For information for Ayerst's consumer products, see product listings under Whitehall Laboratories.
Please turn to Whitehall Laboratories, page 734.

Beach Pharmaceuticals
Division of BEACH PRODUCTS, INC.
5220 SOUTH MANHATTAN AVE.
TAMPA, FL 33611

BEELITH Tablets
[*bē-lith*]
Magnesium Oxide with Vitamin B$_6$

Description: Each tablet contains magnesium oxide 600 mg and pyridoxine hydrochloride (Vitamin B$_6$) 25 mg equivalent to B$_6$ 20 mg.

Inactive Ingredients: Castor oil, hydroxypropyl methylcellulose, magnesium stearate, microcrystalline cellulose, pharmaceutical glaze, povidone and sodium starch glycolate. May contain hydroxypropyl cellulose, polyethylene glycol and propylene glycol. Also contains: FD&C Blue #2, D&C Yellow #10, FD&C Yellow #6 (Sunset Yellow), and titanium dioxide.

Warning: Keep this and all drugs out of the reach of children. In case of accidental overdose seek professional assistance or contact a Poison Control Center immediately. As with any drug, if you are pregnant or nursing a baby, seek the

Continued on next page

Beach—Cont.

advice of a health professional before using this product.

Actions and Uses: BEELITH is a dietary supplement for patients deficient in magnesium and/or pyridoxine. Each tablet yields approximately 362 mg of elemental magnesium & supplies 1000% of the Adult U.S. Recommended Daily Allowance (RDA) for Vitamin B_6 and 90% of the Adult RDA for magnesium.

Dosage: The usual adult dose is one or two tablets daily.

Precaution: Excessive dosage might cause laxation.

Caution: Use only under the supervision of a physician. Use with caution in renal insufficiency.

Drug Interaction Precautions: Do not take this product if you are presently taking a prescription antibiotic drug containing any form of tetracycline.

Storage: Keep tightly closed. Store at controlled room temperature 15°C–30°C (59°F–86°F).

How Supplied: Golden yellow film coated tablet with the name BEACH and the number 1132 printed on each tablet. Bottles of 100 (NDC 0486-1132-01) tablets.

Shown on page 404 in the 1989 PHYSICIANS' DESK REFERENCE

Becton Dickinson Consumer Products
ONE BECTON DRIVE
FRANKLIN LAKES, NJ
07417-1883

B–D Glucose Tablets

Indications and Usage: For fast relief from hypoglycemia. B-D Glucose tablets contain D-Glucose (Dextrose), the most readily absorbed sugar, and are recommended for treatment of hypoglycemia. The tablets are chewable and dissolve quickly in the mouth to facilitate ingestion.

Adverse Reactions: No adverse reactions have been reported with appropriate use of glucose. Occasional reports of nausea may be due to the hypoglycemia itself.

Dosage and Administration: The recommended dosage is three (3) to (4) tablets (15.0 to 20.0 grams of dextrose) at the first sign of hypoglycemia. Repeat dosage as needed to counter additional hypoglycemic episodes caused by longer acting insulins. Dosage may be regulated by taking fewer or more tablets, depending on severity of the episode. Notify your physician of hypoglycemic episodes. Do not administer to anyone who is unconscious.

How Supplied: Box containing six chewable 5.0 gram tablets. Tablets are packaged in durable three tablet blister packs.

Ingredients: Each tablet contains 5.0 grams dextrose. Other ingredients are flavors and tabletting aids: Microcrystalline cellulose and stearic acid. Contains no preservatives.

EDUCATIONAL MATERIAL

Know Your Diabetes, Know Yourself
A one hour videotape program in which medical experts and persons with diabetes discuss the essential elements of diabetes management. (Paid)

Beecham Products USA
DIVISION OF BEECHAM INC.
POST OFFICE BOX 1467
PITTSBURGH, PA 15230

B.F.I.®
Antiseptic First-Aid Powder

Active Ingredient: Bismuth-Formic-Iodide 16.0%. Other ingredients—Boric Acid, Bismuth Subgallate, Zinc Phenolsulfonate, Potassium Alum, Thymol, Menthol, Eucalyptol, and inert diluents.

Indications: For cuts, abrasions, minor burns, skin irritations, athlete's foot and dermatitis due to poison ivy and poison oak.

Actions: B.F.I. First-Aid Powder promotes healing of cuts, scratches, abrasions and minor burns. Relieves itching, chafing and irritations from prickly heat, sunburn, mosquito bites, athlete's foot and poison ivy and oak.

Warnings: Keep out of reach of children. If redness, irritation, swelling or pain persists or increases or if infection occurs, discontinue use and consult physician. For deep or puncture wounds or serious burns, consult physician. For external use only.

Dosage and Administration: Freely sprinkle B.F.I. on the injured area to completely cover the area. Avoid use on extensive denuded (raw) areas particularly on infants and children.

How Supplied: ¼ oz., 1¼ oz. and 8 oz. shaker top container.

DEEP–DOWN® Pain Relief Rub

Active Ingredients: Methyl salicylate 15%; menthol 5%; camphor 0.5%.

Inactive Ingredients: SD Alcohol, 5%, Cetareth 20, Cetearyl Alcohol, Dimethicone, Glyceryl stearate, Methyl paraben, Mineral oil, Sorbitan stearate, Stearyl alcohol, water, Xanthan gum.

Indications: To relieve the pain of minor arthritis, sore joints, muscle aches and sprains, backache, lumbago.

Actions: Counterirritation: cutaneous stimulation for relief of pain in underlying structures.

Warnings: For external use only. Avoid getting in eyes or on mucous membranes, broken or irritated skin. Discontinue use if excessive skin irritation develops. If pain lasts more than 7 days, or redness is present, or in conditions affecting children under 12 years of age, consult a physician. Keep product out of children's reach. In case of accidental swallowing, call a physician or contact a poison control center immediately.

Dosage and Administration: Rub generously into painful area, then massage gently until ointment is absorbed and disappears. Reapply every 3 to 4 hours or as needed. Do not bandage.

How Supplied: Available in 1.25 and 3 oz. collapsible tubes.

ENO®
[e 'no]
Sparkling Antacid

Active Ingredient: When mixed with water, one level teaspoon of Eno produces 1620 mg. of sodium tartrate and 1172 mg. of sodium citrate. Contains 819 mg. of sodium per teaspoonful.

Indications: For relief from the symptoms of sour stomach, acid indigestion, and heartburn.

Actions: Eno is a good tasting, fast acting and effective antacid. It is free of aspirin or sugar and is 100% antacid.

Warnings: If under 60 years of age, don't take more than 6 teaspoonfuls in a 24 hour period. If over 60, don't take over 3 teaspoonfuls. Don't use maximum dosage for over 2 weeks, or use the product if on a sodium restricted diet, except under the advice of a physician. May have a laxative effect. Keep out of reach of children.

Symptoms and Treatment of Oral Overdosage: In case of a large overdose, consult your physician, your local poison control center, or the Rocky Mt. Poison Control Center at 303-592-1710 (Collect), 24 hours a day.

Dosage and Administration: Adults —1 level teaspoonful in 6 ozs. of water. May be repeated every 4 hours. Children 4–6—¼ level teaspoonful; children 7–15—½ level teaspoonful.

How Supplied: 3½ and 7 oz. bottles.

FEMIRON® Tablets
[fem 'i 'ern]

Active Ingredient: (Per Tablet) Iron (from ferrous fumarate) 20 mg.

Inactive Ingredients: Alginic acid, Carnauba wax, Corn starch, Dibasic calcium phosphate, Hydroxypropyl methylcellulose, Magnesium stearate, Polyethylene glycol, Shellac, Silicon dioxide, White wax, FD&C Blue #2, FD&C Red #3, FD&C Yellow #6, Titanium dioxide.

Indications: For use as an iron supplement.

Actions: Supplements dietary iron intake; helps maintain iron stores.

Warnings: Keep out of reach of children.

Precaution: Alcoholics and individuals with chronic liver or pancreatic disease may have enhanced iron absorption with the potential for iron overload. NOTE: Unabsorbed iron may cause some darkening of the stool.

Drug Interaction Precaution: Taking with antacid or tetracycline may interfere with absorption.

Symptoms and Treatment of Oral Overdose: Toxicity and symptoms are primarily due to iron overdose. Abdominal pain, nausea, vomiting and diarrhea may occur, with possible subsequent acidosis and cardiovasular collapse with severe poisoning. **Treatment:** Induce vomiting immediately. Administer milk, eggs to reduce gastric irritation. Contact a physician immediately.

Dosage and Administration: Women: One tablet daily.

How Supplied: Bottles of 40 and 120 tablets.

FEMIRON® Multi-Vitamins and Iron
[fem 'i 'ern]

Active Ingredients: Iron (from ferrous fumarate) 20 mg; Vitamin A 5,000 I.U.; Vitamin D 400 I.U.; Thiamine (Vitamin B_1) 1.5 mg; Riboflavin (Vitamin B_2) 1.7 mg; Niacinamide 20 mg; Ascorbic Acid (Vitamin C) 60 mg; Pyridoxine (Vitamin B_6) 2 mg; Cyanocobalamin (Vitamin B_{12}) 6 mcg; Calcium Pantothenate 10 mg; Folic Acid .4 mg; and Tocopherol Acetate (Vitamin E) 15 I.U.

Indications: For use as an iron and vitamin supplement.

Actions: Helps insure adequate intake of iron and vitamins.

Warnings: Keep out of reach of children.

Precaution: Alcoholics and individuals with chronic liver or pancreatic disease may have enhanced iron absorption with the potential for iron overload. NOTE: Unabsorbed iron may cause some darkening of the stool.

Symptoms and Treatment of Oral Overdosage: Toxicity and symptoms are primarily due to iron overdose. Abdominal pain, nausea, vomiting and diarrhea may occur, with possible subsequent acidosis and cardiovascular collapse with severe poisoning. **Treatment:** Induce vomiting immediately. Administer milk, eggs to reduce gastric irritation. Contact a physician immediately.

Dosage and Administration: Women: One tablet daily.

How Supplied: Bottles of 35, 60, and 90 tablets.

GERITOL® Liquid
[jer 'e-tol]
High Potency Iron & Vitamin Tonic

Active Ingredients Per Dose (½ fluid ounce): Iron (as ferric ammonium citrate) 50 mg; Thiamine (B_1) 2.5 mg; Riboflavin (B_2) 2.5 mg; Niacinamide 50 mg; Panthenol 2 mg; Pyridoxine (B_6) 0.5 mg; Cyanocobalamin (B_{12}) 0.75 mcg; Methionine 25 mg; Choline Bitartrate 50 mg.

Inactive Ingredients: Alcohol, Benzoic acid, Caramel color, Citric acid, Invert sugar, Sucrose, Water, Flavors.

Indications: For use as a dietary supplement.

Actions: Help treat and prevent iron deficiency.

Warnings: Keep out of reach of children.

Precaution: Alcohol accelerates absorption of ferric iron. Alcoholics and individuals with chronic liver or pancreatic disease may have enhanced iron absorption with the potential for iron overload.
NOTE: Unabsorbed iron may cause some darkening of the stool.

Symptoms and Treatment of Oral Overdose: Toxicity and symptoms are primarily due to iron overdose. Abdominal pain, nausea, vomiting and diarrhea may occur, with possible subsequent acidosis and cardiovascular collapse with severe poisoning. If an overdose is suspected, immediately seek professional assistance by contacting your physician, the local poison control center, or the Rocky Mt. Poison Control Center at 303-592-1710 (Collect), 24 hours a day.

Dosage and Administration (Adults): As an iron supplement and for normal menstrual needs: One (1) tablespoonful (0.5 fl. oz.) daily at mealtime. For iron deficiency: One (1) tablespoonful (0.5 fl. oz.) three times daily at mealtime or as directed by a physician.

How Supplied: Bottles of 4 oz., and 12 oz.

7001M
11/14/83

GERITOL COMPLETE™ Tablets
[jer 'e-tol]
The High Iron Multi-Vitamin/Mineral

Active Ingredients (Per Tablet): Vitamin A (5000 IU, including 1,250 IU from Beta Carotene); Vitamin E (30 IU); Vitamin C (60 mg.); Folic Acid (400 mcg.); Vitamin B_1 (1.5 mg.); Vitamin B_2 (1.7 mg.); Niacin (20 mg.); Vitamin B_6 (2 mg.); Vitamin B_{12} (6 mcg.); Vitamin D (400 IU); Biotin (300 mcg.); Pantothenic Acid (10 mg.); Vitamin K (50 mcg.); Calcium (162 mg.); Phosphorus (125 mg.); Iodine (150 mcg.); Iron (50 mg.); Magnesium (100 mg.); Copper (2 mg.); Manganese (7.5 mg.); Potassium (37.5 mg.); Chloride (34.1 mg.); Chromium (15 mcg.); Molybdenum (15 mcg.); Selenium (15 mcg.); Zinc (15 mcg.); Nickel (5 mcg.); Silicon (80 mcg.).

Inactive Ingredients: Carnauba wax, Crospovidone, Flavors, Gelatin, Glycerides of Stearic and Palmitic acids, Hydroxypropyl cellulose, Hydroxypropyl methylcellulose, Magnesium stearate, Microcrystalline cellulose, Polyethylene glycol, Silicon dioxide, Stearic acid, White wax, FD&C Red #40, FD&C Blue #2, FD&C Yellow #6, Titanium dioxide.

Indications: For use as a dietary supplement.

Actions: Help treat and prevent iron deficiency.

Warnings: Keep out of reach of children.

Precaution: Alcoholics and individuals with chronic liver or pancreatic disease may have enhanced iron absorption with the potential for iron overload. NOTE: Unabsorbed iron may cause some darkening of the stool.

Symptoms and Treatment of Oral Overdose: Toxicity and symptoms are primarily due to iron overdose. Abdominal pain, nausea, vomiting and diarrhea may occur, with possible subsequent acidosis and cardiovascular collapse with severe poisoning. If an overdose is suspected, immediately seek professional assistance by contacting your physician, the local poison control center, or the Rocky Mt. Poison Control Center at 303-592-1710 (Collect), 24 hours a day.

Dosage and Administration (Adults): One (1) tablet daily after mealtime.

How Supplied: Bottles of 14, 40, 100, and 180 tablets.

HOLD®
4 Hour Cough Suppressant Lozenge

Active Ingredient: 5.0 mg. dextromethorphan HBr per lozenge.

Inactive Ingredients: Corn syrup, magnesium trisilicate, sucrose, vegetable oil, flavors, FD&C Yellow #10.

Indications: Suppresses coughs for up to 4 hours.

Actions: Dextromethorphan is the most widely used, non-narcotic/non-habit forming antitussive. A 10-20 mg. dose has been recognized as being effective in relieving the discomfort of coughs up to 4 hours by reducing cough intensity and frequency.

Warnings: If cough persists or is accompanied by high fever, consult a physician promptly. Do not administer to children under 6. Do not exceed recommended dose. Keep this and all other medications out of reach of children.

Drug Interaction: No known drug interaction. As with any drug, if you are pregnant or nursing a baby, seek the advice of a health professional before using this product.

Symptoms and Treatment of Oral Overdosage: The principal symptom of overdose with dextromethorphan HBr is

Continued on next page

Beecham Products—Cont.

slowing of respiration. Should a large overdose be suspected seek professional assistance by contacting your physician, the local poison control center, or The Rocky Mt. Poison Control Center at 303-592-1710 (Collect), 24 hrs. a day.

Dosage and Administration: Adults (12 years and older): Take 2 suppressants one after the other, every 4 hours as needed. Children (6-12 years): One suppressant every 4 hours as needed. Let dissolve fully.

How Supplied: 10 individually wrapped suppressants come packaged in a plastic tube container. Children's Hold also available.

MASSENGILL®
Baby Powder Soft Cloth Towelette

Inactive Ingredients: Water, Lactic Acid, Sodium Lactate, Potassium Sorbate, Octoxynol-9, Disodium EDTA, Cetylpyridinium Chloride, and Fragrance.

Indications: For cleansing and refreshing the external vaginal area.

Actions: Massengill Baby Powder Soft Cloth Towelettes safely cleanse the external vaginal area. The towelette delivery system makes the application soft and gentle.

Warnings: For external use only. Avoid contact with eyes.

Directions: Remove towelette from foil packet, unfold, and gently wipe. Throw away towelette after it has been used once.

How Supplied: Sixteen individually wrapped, disposable towelettes per carton.

MASSENGILL®
Disposable Douches
MASSENGILL®
Liquid Concentrate
MASSENGILL® Powder

Ingredients:
DISPOSABLES: Vinegar & Water-Extra Mild—Water and Vinegar.
Vinegar & Water-Extra Cleansing—Water, Vinegar, Cetylpyridinium Chloride, Diazolidinyl Urea, Disodium EDTA.
Belle-Mai—Water, SD Alcohol 40, Lactic Acid, Sodium Lactate, Octoxynol-9, Cetylpyridinium Chloride, Propylene Glycol (and) Diazolidinyl Urea (and) Methyl Paraben (and) Propyl Paraben, Disodium EDTA, Fragrance, FD&C Blue #1.
Country Flowers—Water, SD Alcohol 40, Lactic Acid, Sodium Lactate, Octoxynol-9, Cetylpyridinium Chloride, Propylene Glycol (and) Diazolidinyl Urea (and) Methyl Paraben (and) Propyl Paraben, Disodium EDTA, Fragrance, D&C Red #28, FD&C Blue #1.
Mountain Herbs—Water, SD Alcohol 40, Lactic Acid, Sodium Lactate, Octoxynol-9, Cetylpyridinium Chloride, Propylene Glycol (and) Diazolidinyl Urea (and) Methyl Paraben (and) Propyl Paraben,

Disodium EDTA, Fragrance, D&C Yellow #10, FD&C Blue #1.
LIQUID CONCENTRATE: Water, SD Alcohol 40, Lactic Acid, Sodium Lactate, Octoxynol-9, Methyl Salicylate, Eucalyptol, Menthol, Thymol, D&C Yellow #10, FD&C Yellow #6.
POWDER: Sodium Chloride, Ammonium alum, PEG-8, Phenol, Methyl Salicylate, Eucalyptus Oil, Menthol, Thymol, D&C Yellow #10, FD&C Yellow #6.
FLORAL POWDER: Sodium Chloride, Ammonium alum, SD Alcohol 23-A, Octoxynol-9, Fragrance, FD&C Yellow #6.

Indications: Recommended for routine cleansing at the end of menstruation, after use of contraceptive creams or jellies (check the contraceptive package instructions first) or to rinse out the residue of prescribed vaginal medication (as directed by physician).

Actions: The buffered acid solutions of Massengill Douches are valuable adjuncts to specific vaginal therapy following the prescribed use of vaginal medication or contraceptives and in feminine hygiene.

Directions:
DISPOSABLES: Twist off flat, wing-shaped tab from bottle containing premixed solution, attach nozzle supplied and use. After douching, simply throw away bottle and nozzle.
LIQUID CONCENTRATE: Fill cap ¾ full and pour contents into douche bag containing 1 quart of warm water. Mix thoroughly.
POWDER: Dissolve two rounded teaspoonfuls in a douche bag containing 1 quart of warm water. Mix thoroughly.

Warning: Vaginal cleansing douches should not be used more than twice weekly except on the advice of a physician. If irritation occurs, discontinue use. Do not douche during pregnancy except under the advice and supervision of your physician. Douching does not prevent pregnancy.
Keep out of reach of children. In case of accidental ingestion, seek professional assistance by contacting your physician, the local poison control center, or the Rocky Mt. Poison Control Center at 303-592-1710 (Collect), 24 hours a day.

How Supplied: Disposable—6 oz. disposable plastic bottle.
Liquid Concentrate—4 oz., 8 oz., plastic bottles.
Powder—4 oz., 8 oz., 16 oz., 22 oz. Packettes—10's, 12's.

MASSENGILL® Medicated
Disposable Douche
MASSENGILL® Medicated Liquid
Concentrate

Active Ingredient: Cepticin™ (0.30% povidone-iodine).

Indications: For symptomatic relief of minor irritation and itching associated with vaginitis due to Candida albicans, Trichomonas vaginalis and Gardnerella vaginalis.

Action: Povidone-iodine is widely recognized as an effective broad spectrum microbicide against both gram negative and gram positive bacteria, fungi, yeasts and protozoa. While remaining active in the presence of blood, serum or bodily secretions, it possesses virtually none of the irritating properties of iodine.

Warnings: If symptoms persist after seven days of use, or if redness, swelling or pain develop during treatment, consult a physician. Women with iodine-sensitivity should not use this product. Women may douche during menstruation if they douche gently. Do not douche during pregnancy, or while nursing, unless directed by a physician. Douching does not prevent pregnancy. Keep out of reach of children. In case of accidental ingestion, seek professional assistance by contacting your physician, the local poison control center, or the Rocky Mt. Poison Control Center at 303-592-1710 (Collect), 24 hours a day.

Dosage and Administration: Disposables: Dosage is provided as a single unit concentrate to be added to 6 oz. of sanitized water supplied in a disposable bottle. A specially designed nozzle is provided. After use, the unit is discarded. Use one bottle daily for seven days. Even if symptoms are relieved earlier, treatment should be continued for the full seven days. Liquid Concentrate: The product is provided in concentrate form, to be mixed with water and administered using a douche bag or bulb syringe.
Fill cap and pour contents into 1 quart of warm water. Mix thoroughly. Use once daily for five days, even though symptoms may be relieved earlier. For maximum relief, use for seven days.

How Supplied: Disposables: 6 oz. bottle of sanitized water with 0.17 oz. vial of povidone-iodine and nozzle. Liquid Concentrate: 4 oz., 8 oz., plastic bottles.

N'ICE® Medicated Sugarless Sore Throat and Cough Lozenges
[ni'ce]

Active Ingredient: Cherry—Each lozenge contains 5.0 mg. menthol in a sorbitol base. Citrus—Each lozenge contains 5.0 mg. menthol in a sorbitol base. Menthol Eucalyptus—Each lozenge contains 5.0 mg. menthol in a sorbitol base. Menthol Mint—Each lozenge contains 5.0 mg. menthol in a sorbitol base. Children's Berry—Each lozenge contains 3.0 mg. menthol in a sorbitol base.

Inactive Ingredients: Cherry—Blue 1, Flavors, Red 40, Sorbitol, Tartaric Acid. Citrus—Citric Acid, Flavors, Saccharin Sodium, Sodium Citrate, Sorbitol, Yellow 10. Menthol Eucalyptus—Citric Acid, Flavors, Sorbitol. Menthol Mint—Blue 1, Flavor, Hydrogenated Glucose Syrup, Sorbitol, Yellow 10. Children's Berry—Citric Acid, Flavor, Red 33, Sodium Citrate, Sorbitol.

Indications: Temporarily suppresses coughs due to minor throat and bronchial irritation associated with a cold or

inhaled ingredients. Temporarily relieves occasional minor sore throat pain.

Actions: Menthol in a sorbitol base soothes irritated throat tissue and leaves the throat feeling cool.

Warnings: Do not administer to children under six years of age unless directed by a physician. Severe or persistent sore throat or sore throat accompanied by high fever, headache, nausea, and vomiting may be serious. Consult a physician in such case, or if sore throat persists more than two days. A persistent cough may be a sign of a serious condition. If cough persists for more than one week, tends to recur, or is accompanied by fever, rash or persistent headache, consult a physician. Do not take this product for persistent or chronic cough such as occurs with smoking, asthma, emphysema, or if cough is accompanied by excessive phlegm, unless directed by a physician. In case of accidental overdose, seek professional assistance or contact a poison control center immediately. Keep this and all medications out of the reach of children.

Drug Interaction: No known drug interaction.

Symptoms and Treatment of Oral Overdosage: Should a large overdose of N'ICE (Cherry, Citrus, Menthol Eucalyptus, Menthol Mint, or Children's Berry) be suspected, with symptoms of nausea, vomiting and diarrhea, seek professional assistance. Contact your physician, the local poison control center, or the Rocky Mountain Poison Control Center at 303-592-1710 (Collect); 24 hours a day.

Dosage and Administration: Cherry, Citrus, Menthol Eucalyptus, Menthol Mint—Let lozenge dissolve slowly in the mouth. Repeat as needed, up to 10 lozenges per day. Children's Berry—Take two lozenges. Let lozenges dissolve slowly in the mouth. Repeat as needed, up to 10 lozenges per day.

Professional Labeling: For the temporary relief of pain associated with tonsilitis, pharyngitis, throat infections or stomatitis.

How Supplied: Available in packages of 4, 8 and 16 lozenges.

N'ICE® Sore Throat Spray
[ni'ce]

Active Ingredient: Menthol 0.13%

Inactive Ingredients: Alcohol, Blue 1, Flavor, Saccharin Sodium, Sorbitol, Water, Xanthan Gum, Yellow 10. Alcohol Content: 26% by volume.

Indications: For temporary relief of occasional minor sore throat pain.

Actions: Menthol in a sugarless spray/gargle soothes irritated throat tissue and leaves the throat feeling cool.

Warnings: Persistent cough or sore throat accompanied by high fever, headache, nausea or vomiting may be serious. Consult a physician promptly in such case. Do not use more than 2 days or give to children under 6 years of age unless directed by a physician. Stop use and consult a physician if irritation persists or increases or a skin rash appears. Keep this and all medications out of the reach of children.

Drug Interaction: No known drug interaction.

Symptoms and Treatment of Oral Overdosage: Should a large overdose of N'ICE Sore Throat Spray be suspected, with symptoms of nausea, vomiting and diarrhea, seek professional assistance. Contact your physician, the local poison control center, or the Rocky Mountain Poison Control Center at 303-592-1710 (Collect), 24 hours a day.

Dosage and Administration: Spray —spray four times and swallow (3 ml). Gargle—rinse affected area for 15 seconds, then spit out. Use as needed, up to ten times daily.

Professional Labeling: For the temporary relief of pain associated with tonsilitis, pharyngitis, throat infections or stomatitis.

How Supplied: In 0.9 fl. oz. and 6 fl. oz. plastic bottles with sprayer, and 12 fl. oz. plastic bottles.

SCOTT'S EMULSION®
Vitamin A and D and Omega-3 Fish Oil Food Supplement

Active Ingredient: Cod Liver Oil which provides 5,000 International Units of Vitamin A (100% of RDA). 400 International Units of Vitamin D and .9 grams of Omega-3 fish oil per 4 teaspoons of Scott's Emulsion (100% of RDA).

Indications: Provides daily requirements of Vitamin A and D.

Actions: Scott's Emulsion supplies natural Vitamins A and D and Omega-3 fish oil from cod liver oil. The product is in a highly emulsified form for more rapid absorption by the body. Flavoring agents are included to help mask the flavor of cod liver oil.

Dosage and Administration: 4 teaspoons per day provides 100% of the adult RDA for Vitamins A and D.

How Supplied: $6\frac{1}{4}$ and $12\frac{1}{2}$ fl. oz. bottles.

SERUTAN®
[sēr'u-tan]
Natural-Fiber Laxative

Active Ingredient: Psyllium (3.4 gm. per dose).

Inactive Ingredients: Dextrose, Oat flour, Silicon dioxide, Wheat germ, Flavors.

Indications: For aiding bowel regularity.

Actions: Softens stools, increases bulk volume and water content.

Warnings: Keep out of the reach of children.

Precaution: Patients with suspected intestinal disorders should consult a physician.

Dosage and Administration: Adults: Stir one heaping teaspoonful into an 8 oz. glass of water or fruit juice. Drink immediately. Take one to three times daily, preferably at mealtime.

How Supplied: Concentrated powder—7 oz., 14 oz., and 21 oz. bottles. Also Fruit flavored powder—6 oz., 12 oz., and 18 oz. bottles.

SERUTAN®
[sēr'u-tan]
Natural-Fiber Laxative
Toasted Granules

Active Ingredient: Psyllium (2.5 gm. per dose).

Indications: For aiding bowel regularity.

Actions: Softens stools, increases bulk volume and water content.

Warnings: Keep out of the reach of children.

Precaution: Patients with suspected intestinal disorders should consult a physician. Not to be taken directly by spoon.

Dosage and Administration: Adults: Sprinkle one heaping teaspoonful on cereal or other food, one to three times daily.

How Supplied: Available in 6 oz., and 18 oz. plastic bottles.

SOMINEX®
[som'in-ex]

Active Ingredients: Each tablet contains Diphenhydramine HCl, 25 mg.

Inactive Ingredients: Corn starch, dibasic calcium phosphate, magnesium stearate, microcrystalline cellulose, silicon dioxide, FD&C Blue #1.

Indications: To induce drowsiness and assist in falling asleep.

Action: An antihistamine with anticholinergic and sedative effects.

Warnings: Do not give to children under 12 years of age. If sleeplessness persists continuously for more than 2 weeks, consult your physician. Insomnia may be a symptom of serious underlying medical illness. Take this product with caution if alcohol is being consumed. Keep this and all drugs out of the reach of children. In case of accidental overdose, seek professional assistance by contacting your physician, the local poison control center, or the Rocky Mountain Poison Control Center at 303-592-1710 (Collect); 24 hours a day. As with any drug, if you are pregnant or nursing a baby, seek the advice of a health professional before using this product. DO NOT TAKE THIS PRODUCT IF YOU HAVE ASTHMA, GLAUCOMA OR ENLARGEMENT OF THE PROS-

Continued on next page

Beecham Products—Cont.

TATE GLAND, EXCEPT UNDER THE ADVICE AND SUPERVISION OF A PHYSICIAN.

Drug Interaction: Monoamine oxidase (MAO) inhibitors prolong and intensify the anticholinergic effects of antihistamines. The CNS depressant effect is heightened by alcohol and other CNS depressant drugs.

Symptoms and Treatment of Oral Overdosage: Antihistamine overdosage reactions may vary from central nervous system depression to stimulation. Stimulation is particularly likely in children. Atropine-like signs and symptoms, such as dry mouth, fixed and dilated pupils, flushing, and gastrointestinal symptoms, may also occur.

Dosage and Administration: Take 2 tablets thirty minutes before bedtime, or as directed by a physician.

How Supplied: Available in blister packs of 16, 32, and 72 tablets.

SOMINEX® Liquid
[som 'in-ex]

Active Ingredients: Each fluid ounce (30 ml.) contains 50 mg. Diphenhydramine HCl. Also contains Alcohol, 10% by volume.

Inactive Ingredients: Citric Acid, Dibasic Sodium Phosphate, Flavors, FD&C Blue No. 1, Glycerin, Polyethylene Glycol, Sodium Saccharin, Sorbitol, Water, Xanthan Gum.

Indications: To help you fall asleep.

Actions: An antihistamine with anticholinergic and sedative effects.

Warnings: Do not give to children under 12 year of age. If sleeplessness persists continuously for more than two weeks, contact your physician. Insomnia may be a symptom of serious underlying medical illness. Take this product with caution if alcohol is being consumed. As with any drug, if you are pregnant or nursing a baby, seek the advice of a health professional before using this product. Keep this and all drugs out of the reach of children. Do not exceed recommended dosage. In case of an accidental overdose, seek professional assistance by contacting your physician, the local poison control center, or the Rocky Mountain Poison Control Center at (303) 592-1710 (Collect), 24 hours a day. DO NOT TAKE THIS PRODUCT IF YOU HAVE ASTHMA, GLAUCOMA OR ENLARGEMENT OF THE PROSTATE GLAND, EXCEPT UNDER THE ADVICE AND SUPERVISION OF A PHYSICIAN.

Drug Interaction: Monoamine oxidase (MAO) inhibitors prolong and intensify the anticholinergic effects of antihistamines. The CNS depressant effect is heightened by alcohol and other CNS depressant drugs.

Symptoms and Treatment of Oral Overdosage: Antihistamine overdosage reactions may vary from central nervous system depression to stimulation. Stimulation is particularly likely in children. Atropine-like signs and symptoms, such as dry mouth, fixed and dilated pupils, flushing, and gastrointestinal symptoms, may also occur.

Dosage and Administration: Dosage is one fluid ounce (30 ml.) thirty minutes before bedtime, or as directed by a physician. Use dosage cup provided, or two (2) measured tablespoons.

How Supplied: Available in 6 oz. bottles.

SOMINEX® Pain Relief Formula
[som 'in-ex]

Active Ingredients: Each tablet contains 25 mg. diphenhydramine HCl and 500 mg. acetaminophen.

Inactive Ingredients: Corn starch, crospovidone, povidone, silicon dioxide, stearic acid, FD&C Blue #1.

Indications: For sleeplessness with accompanying occasional minor aches, pains, or headache.

Action: An antihistamine with sedative effects combined with an internal analgesic.

Warnings: Do not give to children under 12 years of age. If symptoms persist continuously for more than 10 days, or if new ones occur, consult your physician. Do not exceed recommended dosage because severe liver damage may occur. Insomnia may be a symptom of serious underlying medical illness. Take this product with caution if alcohol is being consumed. Do not take this product for the treatment of arthritis, except under the advice and supervision of a physician. As with any drug, if you are pregnant or nursing a baby, seek the advice of a health professional before using this product. Keep this and all drugs out of the reach of children. In case of accidental overdose, seek professional assistance by contacting your physician, the local poison control center, or the Rocky Mountain Poison Control Center at 303-592-1710 (Collect), 24 hours a day. DO NOT TAKE THIS PRODUCT IF YOU HAVE ASTHMA, GLAUCOMA OR ENLARGEMENT OF THE PROSTATE GLAND, EXCEPT UNDER THE ADVICE AND SUPERVISION OF A PHYSICIAN.

Drug Interaction: Monoamine oxidase (MAO) inhibitors prolong and intensify the anticholinergic effects of antihistamines. The CNS depressant effect is heightened by alcohol and other CNS depressant drugs.

Symptoms and Treatment of Oral Overdosage: Antihistamine overdosage reactions may vary from central nervous system depression to stimulation. Stimulation is particularly likely in children. Atropine-like signs and symptoms, such as dry mouth, fixed and dilated pupils, flushing, and gastrointestinal symptoms, may also occur.

Dosage and Administration: Take two tablets thirty minutes before bedtime, or as directed by a physician.

How Supplied: Available in blister packs of 16 tablets and bottles of 32 tablets.

S.T.37®
Antiseptic Solution

Active Ingredients: Hexylresorcinol (0.1%), Glycerin (28.2%).

Inactive Ingredients: Sodium bisulfite; Water.

Indications: For use on cuts, abrasions, burns, scalds, sunburn and the hygienic care of the mouth.

Actions: S.T.37 is a non-stinging, non-staining antiseptic solution that provides soothing protection and helps relieve pain of burns, cuts, abrasions and mouth irritations.

Warnings: If redness, irritation, swelling or pain persists or increases or if infection occurs, discontinue use and consult physician. In case of deep or puncture wounds or serious burns, consult physician. Keep out of reach of children.

Dosage and Administration: For cuts, burns, scalds and abrasions apply undiluted, bandage lightly keeping bandage wet with S.T.37 antiseptic solution. For hygienic care of the mouth, dilute with 1 or 2 parts of warm water. To be used as a rinse and gargle.

How Supplied: 5.5 and 12 fl. oz. bottles.

SUCRETS® (Regular and Mentholated)
Sore Throat Lozenges
[su 'krets]

Active Ingredient: Hexylresorcinol, 2.4 mg. per lozenge.

Inactive Ingredients: Citric acid (Mentholated only), Blue 1, Corn Syrup, Flavors, Sucrose, Yellow 10.

Indications: For temporary relief of occasional minor sore throat pain and mouth irritations.

Actions: Hexylresorcinol's soothing anesthetic action quickly relieves minor throat irritations.

Warnings: If sore throat is severe, persists more than 2 days, is accompanied or followed by fever, rash, nausea or vomiting, see a doctor promptly. If sore mouth symptoms do not improve in 7 days, see a doctor or dentist promptly. KEEP THIS AND ALL MEDICATIONS OUT OF THE REACH OF CHILDREN.

Drug Interaction: No known drug interaction

Symptoms and Treatment of Oral Overdosage: Should a large overdose of Sucrets (Regular or Mentholated) be suspected, with symptoms of profuse sweating, nausea, vomiting and diarrhea, seek professional assistance. Call your physi-

cian, local poison control center or the Rocky Mountain Poison Control Center at 303-592-1710 (Collect), 24 hrs. a day.

Dosage and Administration: Adults and children 2 years of age and older: Dissolve slowly in the mouth. Repeat as needed.

Professional Labeling: For the temporary relief of pain associated with tonsilitis, pharyngitis, throat infections or stomatitis.

How Supplied: Sucrets-Regular: Available in tins of 24 and 48 individually wrapped lozenges. Sucrets-Mentholated: Available in tins of 24 lozenges.

SUCRETS®–Cold Decongestant Formula
[su 'krets]
Decongestant Lozenges

Active Ingredient: Phenylpropanolamine hydrochloride, 25 mg. per lozenge.

Inactive Ingredients: Citric acid, corn syrup, sucrose, titanium dioxide, flavors, D&C Yellow #10, FD&C Red #40.

Indications: For fast temporary relief of nasal congestion.

Warnings: Do not exceed recommended dosage because at higher dosages nervousness, dizziness or sleeplessness may occur. Do not take this product for more than 7 days. If symptoms do not improve or are accompanied by fever, consult a doctor. Do not take this product if you have high blood pressure, heart disease, diabetes, thyroid disease or difficulty in urination due to enlargement of the prostate gland unless directed by a doctor. As with any drug, if you are pregnant or nursing a baby, seek the advice of a health professional before using this product. KEEP THIS AND ALL MEDICATIONS OUT OF THE REACH OF CHILDREN.

Drug Interaction: Do not take this product if you are presently taking a prescription drug for high blood pressure or depression, without first consulting your doctor.

Symptoms and Treatment of Oral Overdosage: The principal symptoms of an overdose are restlessness, dizziness, anxiety. Should these symptoms appear or a large overdose be suspected, seek professional assistance. Call your physician, the local poison control center or the Rocky Mt. Poison Control Center at 303-592-1710 (Collect), 24 hours a day.

Dosage and Administration: Adults (12 years and over): Slowly dissolve one lozenge in the mouth. One additional lozenge every 4 hours, but do not exceed 6 lozenges in 24 hours. Do not exceed recommended dosage. Do not administer to children under 12 years of age unless directed by a doctor.

Professional Labeling: None.

How Supplied: Available in tins of 24 lozenges.

SUCRETS® Cold Relief Formula
[su 'krets]
Lozenges

Active Ingredients: Each lozenge contains Hexylresorcinol 2.4 mg., Menthol 10 mg.

Inactive Ingredients: Blue 1, Corn Syrup, Flavors, Silicon Dioxide, Sucrose.

Indications: For temporary relief of occasional minor sore throat pain, cough, and nasal congestion associated with a cold.

Warnings: A persistent cough may be a sign of a serious condition. If sore throat, cough or congestion is severe, lasts more than 2 days, is accompanied or followed by fever, rash, nausea, vomiting or persistent headache, see a doctor promptly. Do not take this product for chronic cough such as occurs with smoking, asthma, emphysema, or if cough is accompanied by excessive phlegm, unless directed by a doctor. KEEP THIS AND ALL MEDICATIONS OUT OF THE REACH OF CHILDREN.

Drug Interaction: No known drug interaction.

Symptoms and Treatment of Oral Overdosage: Should a large overdose of Sucrets Cold Relief Formula be suspected, with symptoms of profuse sweating, nausea, vomiting and diarrhea, seek professional assistance. Call your doctor, local poison control center, or the Rocky Mountain Poison Control Center at 303/592-1710 (collect) 24 hrs. a day.

Dosage and Administration: Adults and children 2 years of age and older: Dissolve slowly in the mouth. Repeat every two hours as needed. Do not administer to children under 2 years of age, unless directed by a doctor.

Professional Labeling: For the temporary relief of pain associated with tonsilitis, pharyngitis, throat infections or stomatitis.

How Supplied: Available in tins of 24 individually wrapped lozenges.

SUCRETS® Cough Control Formula
[su 'krets]
Cough Control Lozenges

Active Ingredient: Dextromethorphan hydrobromide, 5.0 mg. per lozenge.

Inactive Ingredients: Blue 1, Corn Syrup, Flavors, Red 40, Sucrose, Vegetable Oil, Yellow 10, and other ingredients.

Indications: For temporary suppression of cough due to minor throat and bronchial irritation associated with a cold or inhaled irritants.

Actions: Dextromethorphan is the most widely used non-narcotic/non-habit forming antitussive. A 10-20 mg. dose in adults (5–10 mg. in children over 6, and 2.5–5 mg. in children 2–5) has been recognized as being effective in relieving the frequency and intensity of cough for up to 4 hours.

Warnings: A persistent cough may be a sign of a serious condition. If cough persists for more than 1 week, tends to recur, or is accompanied by fever, rash or persistent headache, consult a doctor. Do not take this product for persistent or chronic cough such as occurs with smoking, asthma, emphysema or if cough is accompanied by excessive phlegm unless directed by a doctor. As with any drug, if you are pregnant or nursing a baby, seek the advice of a health professional before using this product. KEEP THIS AND ALL MEDICATIONS OUT OF THE REACH OF CHILDREN.

Drug Interaction: No known drug interaction.

Symptoms and Treatment of Oral Overdosage: Slowing of respiration is the principal symptom of dextromethorphan HBr overdose. Should a large overdose be suspected, seek professional assistance. Call your physician, the local poison control center, or the Rocky Mt. Poison Control Center at 303-592-1710 (Collect), 24 hours a day.

Dosage and Administration: Adults and children 12 years and older: Take 2 lozenges. Children 2 to under 12 years: Take 1 lozenge. Repeat every 4 hours as needed. Do not administer to children under 2 years of age unless directed by a doctor.

Professional Labeling: Same as those outlined under Indications.

How Supplied: Available in tins of 24 lozenges.

SUCRETS® Maximum Strength
SUCRETS® Children's Cherry
Flavored
Sore Throat Lozenges
[su 'krets]

Active Ingredient: Maximum Strength: Dyclonine Hydrochloride 3.0 mg. per lozenge. Children's Cherry: Dyclonine Hydrochloride 1.2 mg. per lozenge.

Inactive Ingredients: Maximum Strength: Citric Acid, Corn Syrup, Silicon Dioxide, Sucrose, Yellow 10. Children's Cherry: Blue 1, Citric Acid, Corn Syrup, Red 40, Silicon Dioxide, Sucrose.

Indications: For temporary relief of occasional minor sore throat pain and mouth irritations.

Actions: Dyclonine Hydrochloride's soothing anesthetic action relieves minor throat irritations.

Warnings: If sore throat is severe, persists more than 2 days, is accompanied or followed by fever, headache, rash, nausea, or vomiting, consult a doctor promptly. If sore mouth symptoms do not improve in 7 days, see your dentist or doctor promptly. KEEP THIS AND ALL MEDICATIONS OUT OF THE REACH OF CHILDREN.

Drug Interaction: No known drug interaction.

Continued on next page

Beecham Products—Cont.

Symptoms and Treatment of Oral Overdosage: Reactions due to large overdosage are systemic and involve the central nervous system and cardiovascular system. Central nervous system reactions are characterized by excitation and/or depression. Nervousness, dizziness, blurred vision or tremors may occur. Reactions involving the cardiovascular system include depression of the myocardium, hypotension or bradycardia. Should a large overdose be suspected seek professional assistance. Call your physician, local poison control center or the Rocky Mountain Poison Control Center at 303/592-1710 (Collect), 24 hours a day.

Dosage and Administration: Adults and children 2 years of age or older: Allow to dissolve slowly in the mouth. Repeat every two hours as needed. Do not administer to children under 2 years of age unless directed by a doctor.

Professional Labeling: For the temporary relief of pain associated with tonsilitis, pharyngitis, throat infections or stomatitis.

How Supplied: Available in tins of 24 lozenges.

SUCRETS MAXIMUM STRENGTH SPRAY
[su'krets]

Active Ingredients: Dyclonine Hydrochloride 0.1%.

Inactive Ingredients: Alcohol, Blue 1 (Mint Only), Chlorobutanol (Mint Only), Dibasic Sodium Phosphate, Flavors, Glycerin, Monobasic Sodium Phosphate, Phosphoric Acid, Potassium Sorbate, Red 33 (Cherry Only), Sorbitol, Water, Yellow 6 (Cherry Only), Yellow 10 (Mint Only).

Indications: Temporary relief of occasional minor sore throat pain due to colds, throat irritations, and mouth and gum irritations.

Actions: Dyclonine Hydrochloride's soothing anesthetic action quickly relieves minor throat irritations.

Warnings: If sore throat is severe, persists for more than 2 days, is accompanied or followed by fever, headache, rash, nausea or vomiting, consult a doctor promptly. If sore mouth symptoms do not improve in 7 days, see your dentist or doctor promptly.

Drug Interaction: No known drug interaction.

Symptoms and Treatment of Oral Overdosage: Reactions due to large overdosage are systemic and involve the central nervous system and cardiovascular system. Central nervous system reactions are characterized by excitation and/or depression. Nervousness, dizziness, blurred vision or tremors may occur. Reactions involving the cardiovascular system include depression of the myo-

cardium, hypotension or bradycardia. Should a large overdose be suspected seek professional assistance. Call your physician, local poison control center or the Rocky Mountain Poison Control Center at 303-592-1710 (Collect), 24 hours a day.

Dosage and Administration: Spray: Adults and Children 2 years of age or older use full strength: Spray 4 times and swallow.
Gargle/rinse: Gargle or rinse affected area for 15 seconds and then spit out. Use up to 6 times daily or as directed by a dentist or doctor. Do not administer to children under 2 years of age, unless directed by a dentist or doctor.

Professional Labeling: For the temporary relief of pain associated with tonsilitis, pharyngitis, throat infections and stomatitis.

How Supplied: Available in 6 oz. Spray, and 12 oz. Rinse bottles.

THERMOTABS®
[ther'mo-tabs]
Buffered Salt Tablets

Active Ingredients: Per tablet—sodium chloride—450 mg.; potassium chloride—30 mg.

Inactive Ingredients: Acacia, Calcium carbonate, Calcium stearate, Dextrose.

Indications: To minimize fatigue and prevent muscle cramps and heat prostration due to excessive perspiration.

Actions: Thermotabs are designed for tennis players, joggers, golfers and other athletes who experience excessive perspiration. Also for use in steel mills, industrial plants, kitchens, stores, or other locations where high temperatures cause heat fatigue, cramps or heat prostration.

Warnings: Keep out of reach of children.

Precaution: Individuals on a salt-restricted diet should use THERMOTABS only under the advice and supervision of a physician.

Symptoms and Treatment of Oral Overdosage: Signs of salt overdose include diarrhea and muscular twitching. If an overdose is suspected, contact a physician, the local poison control center, or call the Rocky Mt. Poison Control Center at 303-592-1710 (Collect), 24 hours a day.

Dosage and Administration: One tablet with a full glass of water, 5 to 10 times a day depending on temperature and conditions.

How Supplied: 100 tablet bottles.

VIVARIN® Stimulant Tablets
[vi'va-rin]

Active Ingredient: Each tablet contains 200 mg. caffeine alkaloid.

Inactive Ingredients: Dextrose, magnesium stearate, microcrystalline cellulose, silicon dioxide, Starch, Yellow #6, Yellow #10.

Indications: Helps restore mental alertness or wakefulness when experiencing fatigue or drowsiness.

Actions: Stimulates cerebrocortical areas involved with active mental processes.

Warnings: The recommended dose of this product contains about as much caffeine as two cups of coffee. Limit the use of caffeine containing medications, foods, or beverages while taking this product because too much caffeine may cause nervousness, irritability, sleeplessness, and, occasionally, rapid heart beat. For occasional use only. Not intended for use as a substitute for sleep. If fatigue or drowsiness persists or continues to recur, consult a doctor. Do not give to children under 12 years of age. As with any drug, if you are pregnant or nursing a baby, seek the advice of a health professional before using this product. In case of accidental overdose, seek professional assistance or contact a poison control center immediately. Keep this and all drugs out of the reach of children.

Drug Interaction: Use of caffeine should be lowered or avoided if drugs are being used to treat cardiovascular ailments, psychological problems, or kidney trouble.

Precaution: Higher blood glucose levels may result from caffeine use.

Symptoms and Treatment of Oral Overdosage: Convulsions may occur if caffeine is consumed in doses larger than 10 g. Emesis should be induced to empty the stomach. In case of accidental overdose, seek professional assistance by contacting your physician, the local poison control center, or the Rocky Mt. Poison Control Center at 303-592-1710 (Collect), 24 hours a day.

Dosage and Administration: Adults and children 12 years of age and over: Oral dosage is 1 tablet (200 mg.) not more than every 3 to 4 hours.

How Supplied: Available in packages of 16, 40 and 80 tablets.

EDUCATIONAL MATERIAL

Feminine Hygiene and You (Film, Video)
This 14-minute color film begins with a simple explanation of how a woman's body works (reproductive system, menstrual cycle, and vaginal secretions), then explains douching. Free loan to physicians, pharmacists and clinics. Available in 16mm and VHS.
A Personal Guide to Feminine Freshness
A 16-page illustrated booklet on vaginal infections, feminine hygiene and douching. Free to physicians, pharmacists and patients in limited quantities. These items are available by writing Beecham or by calling 800-245-1040. PA residents call 800-242-1718.

Bio-Tech Pharmacal, Inc.
P.O. BOX 1992
FAYETTEVILLE, AR 72702

BROMASE (Proteolytic Enzyme from *Ananus comosus*)
(bromelain)

Active Ingredients: Each **BROMASE** capsule contains 500 mg of Bromelain (2400 mcu/gm), a concentrated complex of sulfhydryl proteolytic (protein digesting) enzymes extracted from the green stem of the pineapple plant (*Ananus comosus*), and 15 mg Ascorbic Acid (Vitamin C) to stabilize the enzymatic activity.

Inactive Ingredients: Contains no yeast, sugar, lactose, starch, wheat, soy, rye, filler, binder, dyes, or preservatives. Microcrystalline cellulose employed as excipient (flow agent).

Indications: Due to its anti-inflammatory, antithrombotic, and fibrinolytic action as a prostaglandin modulator, **BROMASE** is useful as a supplement to augment standard therapy for inflammatory conditions resulting from prostaglandin metabolism, surgical procedures, sports activities, infections, and other trauma.

Actions: Pharmacological actions reported in over 200 scientific papers include: anti-inflammatory action; prevention of induced pulmonary edema; smooth muscle relaxation; antibiotic absorption and wound/surgical healing enhancement; and inhibition of blood platelet aggregation. Up to 40% of orally administered Bromelain reportedly can be absorbed intact.

Warnings: Virtually non-toxic; no LD50 up to 10 g/Kg. Chronic use welltolerated. Can induce IgE mediated response, and cross-react with papain, wheat, rye flour, grass, and birch pollen.

Precaution and Drug Interaction: Concomitant use with Coumadin, or in hemophiliacs and others with bleeding tendencies inadvisable. Safe use during pregnancy not established. Use with caution in severe renal or hepatic patients, and those with sensitivity to pineapple and/or pineapple products.

Dosage and Administration: One to two (1–2) capsules BID or TID (between meals, preferrably), or as prescribed by physician.

Professional Labeling: BROMASE capsules AS A NUTRITIONAL AID FOR PROSTAGLANDIN MODULATION.

How Supplied: BROMASE two-piece clear gelatin capsules, each containing 500 mg 2400 mcu/gm Bromelain and 15 mg Ascorbic Acid, in bottles of 60 (NDC #53191-151-06).

Literature: Available free upon request of health professional.

Blaine Company, Inc.
2700 DIXIE HIGHWAY
FT. MITCHELL, KY 41017

MAG–OX 400

Description: Each tablet contains Magnesium Oxide 400 mg. U.S.P. (Heavy), or 241.3 mg. Elemental Magnesium (19.86 mEq.)

Indications and Usage: Hypomagnesemia, magnesium deficiencies and/or magnesium depletion resulting from malnutrition, restricted diet, alcoholism or magnesium depleting drugs. An antacid. For increasing urinary magnesium excretion.

Warnings: Do not use this product except under the advice and supervision of a physician if you have a kidney disease. May have laxative effect.

Dosage: Adult dose 1 or 2 tablets daily or as directed by a physician.

Professional Labeling: Mag-Ox 400 Tablets for recurring calcium oxalate urinary calculi.
MAGNESIUM OXIDE U.S.P. is indicated in the reduction of crystalluria and calcium oxalate excretion in patients with recurring calcium oxalate lithiasis and to reduce the incidence of calculus formation in idiopathic, recurrent stone formers.

How Supplied: Bottles of 100 and 1000.

URO–MAG

Description: Each capsule contains Magnesium Oxide 140 mg. U.S.P. (Heavy), or 84.5 mg. Elemental Magnesium (6.93 mEq.)

Indications and Usage: Hypomagnesemia, magnesium deficiencies and/or magnesium depletion resulting from malnutrition, restricted diet, alcoholism or magnesium depleting drugs. An antacid. For increasing urinary magnesium excretion.

Warnings: Do not use this product except under the advice and supervision of a physician if you have a kidney disease. May have laxative effect.

Dosage: Adult dose 3–4 capsules daily or as directed by a physician.

Professional Labeling: URO-MAG Capsules for recurring calcium oxalate urinary calculi.
MAGNESIUM OXIDE U.S.P. is indicated in the reduction of crystalluria and calcium oxalate excretion in patients with recurring calcium oxalate lithiasis and to reduce the incidence of calculus formation in idiopathic, recurrent stone formers.

How Supplied: Bottles of 100 and 1000.

EDUCATIONAL MATERIAL

Samples and literature available to physicians upon request.

Blistex Inc.
1800 SWIFT DRIVE
OAK BROOK, IL 60521

BLISTEX®
Medicated Lip Ointment

Indications: Blistex is a medicated ointment in a tube. The product is recommended for symptomatic relief of cold sores and sunburned lips, and for the prevention and relief of severely dry, cracked lips, including angular cheilitis (cracking at the corners of the mouth).

Ingredients:
Actives:
  Allantoin 1.0% (skin protectant)
  Camphor 0.5% (counter-irritant)
  Phenol 0.5% (antiseptic)
Excipients:
  An emollient base with Cetyl Alcohol, Flavor, Glycerin, Lanolin, Mineral Oil, Mixed Waxes, Petrolatum, Polyglyceryl-3 Diisostearate, SD Alcohol 36, Stearyl Alcohol, Water and other ingredients.

Mode of Action: Allantoin affords protection of the lips against external irritants, since it forms complexes with a variety of sensitizing agents rendering them non-sensitizing. Camphor is used to furnish slight local anesthetic and counter-irritant action to sore and chapped lips. Phenol will provide mild antiseptic action. The tissue cleansing properties for this product are contributed by the cationic soap produced in the preparation of finished product. The emollient and lubricant properties are produced by the lipid phase.

Directions: Severely Dry, Cracked Lips and Sunburned Lips: At first symptoms, apply and massage thoroughly. Repeat every half hour until condition is relieved.
Cold Sores: At the first sign of a cold sore, gently apply and massage Blistex into the immediate (sensitive) area.

Cautions: Do not use in the eyes. If the condition persists, or if inflammation develops, the patient should discontinue use and consult a physician. As with all products, a few individuals may prove to be allergic to ingredients contained in this ointment.

Literature Available: Patient and professional pamphlets available on request.

How Supplied: Blistex ointment is available in .21 oz. (NDC 10157-9920-2) and .35 oz. (NDC 10157-9920-3) tubes.

IVAREST®
Medicated Cream & Lotion

Indications: Ivarest is a medicated product for relief of inflammation from

Continued on next page

Blistex—Cont.

poison ivy, poison oak, and minor skin irritations.

Ingredients:
Actives:
  Calamine 14.0% (skin protectant)
  Benzocaine 5.0% (external analgesic)
Excipients:
  A water-washable base with FD&C Yellow #5, FD&C Yellow #6, FD&C Red #33, Fragrance, Hydroxyethylcellulose, Lanolin Oil, Petrolatum, Polysorbate 60, Propylene Glycol, Purified Water, Pyrilamine Maleate, Sorbitan Stearate and other ingredients.

Mode of Action: Benzocaine is used to relieve minor pain and itching caused by irritation from poison ivy, oak or sumac. The analgesic action of Benzocaine is almost entirely on nerve terminals. Calamine is used for its protective, antiseptic and antibacterial action against a wide variety of skin diseases.

Directions: Gently cleanse the affected area and apply a liberal amount of Ivarest. Repeat application 3 or 4 times daily until condition is relieved.

Cautions: Do not use in the eyes. If the condition persists, or if inflammation develops, the patient should discontinue use and consult a physician. The product is not designed for prolonged use.

How Supplied: Ivarest is available in a 2 oz. cream tube (NDC 10157-9004-3) and a 4 oz. lotion bottle (NDC 10157-9104-1).

KANK-A®
Mouth Sore Medication

Indications: Kank-a is a liquid medication for relief of sores inside the mouth; aphthous ulcers, abrasions and cuts. In addition to relieving pain associated with these oral disturbances, Kank-a forms a protective film to protect against further irritation. Kank-a is accepted by the Council on Dental Therapeutics, American Dental Association.

Ingredients:
Actives:
  Compound Benzoin Tincture (oral mucosal protectant)
  Benzocaine 5.0% (oral mucosal analgesic)
  Cetylpyridinium Chloride 0.5% (antiseptic)
Excipients:
  A buffered vehicle with Castor Oil, Flavors, Propylene Glycol and other ingredients.

Mode of Action: Compound Benzoin Tincture forms a protective film when applied to painful vesiculobullous lesions of the oral mucosa, aphthous stomatitis and Vincent's infection.
Benzocaine, a local anesthetic virtually devoid of systemic toxicities, provides prompt, temporary relief of pain, itching, and soreness of mucous membrane. Cetylpyridinium Chloride reduces bacterial flora and helps prevent infection.

Directions: Dry the irritated area. Apply Kank·a (using the sponge applicator) directly to the mouth or canker sore and let dry. Repeat up to four times a day if necessary.

Cautions: Patients with a known sensitivity to Benzocaine or to other para-amino compounds should avoid use of this product. Do not apply to the area of recently extracted teeth. If irritation or inflammation persists, or if a fever develops, the patient should discontinue use of the product and consult a dentist or physician. Kank·a should not be used for a period exceeding seven days.

Literature Available: Patient and professional pamphlets available on request.

How Supplied: Kank·a is available in a ⅙ fl. oz. plastic bottle with a built-in applicator (NDC 10157-0011-2).

EDUCATIONAL MATERIAL

Canker and Mouth Sores: What You Should Know
Canker sores and other oral conditions are discussed in easy-to-understand terms; causes of mouth sores and possible approaches to reducing their incidence are listed.
Smooth, Moist Lips are Healthy Lips
Two separate sections, Lip Health and Lip Beauty, are presented in detail; the health section discusses various lip disorders and their treatment; the beauty section provides tips on cosmetic uses of lip care products.
Products for Lips Care and Oral Care
Brief discussion for professionals of lip care and oral care problems along with technical descriptions of Blistex products.
Products for Topical First Aid
Brief discussion for professionals of burns and other skin disorders; includes information of Blistex topical first aid products.
A Doctor's Guide to Poison Ivy
Prevention, symptoms and treatment of contact dermatitis are discussed to educate the lay person regarding this itchy rash.
Use of Blistex Products in Dental Practice
A guide to the use of Blistex products for lip and oral care in the dental profession.

IDENTIFICATION PROBLEM?
Consult the
Product Identification Section
where you'll find
products pictured
in full color.

Block Drug Company, Inc.
257 CORNELISON AVENUE
JERSEY CITY, NJ 07302

ARTHRITIS STRENGTH BC®
POWDER

Active Ingredients: Aspirin 742 mg in combination with 222 mg Salicylamide and 36 mg Caffeine per powder.

Indications: Arthritis Strength BC Powder is specially formulated with more of the pain relieving ingredients to provide fast temporary relief of minor arthritis pain and inflammation, neuralgia, neuritis and sciatica; relief of muscular aches, discomfort and fever of colds; and pain of tooth extraction.

Warning: Children and teenagers should not use this medicine for chicken pox or flu symptoms before a doctor is consulted about Reye Syndrome, a rare but serious illness reported to be associated with aspirin. Do not exceed recommended dosage or administer to children, including teenagers, with chicken pox or flu, unless directed by a physician. Do not take this product if you are allergic to aspirin, have asthma, gastric ulcer, or are taking a medication that affects the clotting of blood, except under the advice and supervision of a physician. If pain persists for more than 10 days or redness is present, discontinue use of this product and consult a physician immediately. Keep this and all medication out of children's reach. As with any drug, if you are pregnant or nursing a baby, consult your physician before using this product. Discontinue use if ringing in the ears occurs.
In case of accidental overdosage, contact a physician or poison control center immediately.

Dosage and Administration: Place one powder on tongue and follow with liquid. If you prefer, stir powder into glass of water or other liquid. May be used every three to four hours, up to 4 powders each 24 hours. For children under 12, consult a physician.

How Supplied: Available in tamper resistant cellophane wrapped envelopes of 6 powders, and tamper resistant cellophane wrapped boxes of 24 and 50 powders.

BC® POWDER

Active Ingredients: Aspirin 650 mg per powder, Salicylamide 195 mg per powder and Caffeine 32 mg per powder.

Indications: BC Powder is for relief of simple headache; for temporary relief of minor arthritic pain, neuralgia, neuritis and sciatica; for relief of muscular aches, discomfort and fever of colds; and for relief of normal menstrual pain and pain of tooth extraction.

Warning: Children and teenagers should not use this medicine for chicken pox or flu symptoms before a doctor is

consulted about Reye Syndrome, a rare but serious illness reported to be associated with aspirin. Do not exceed recommended dosage or administer to children, including teenagers, with chicken pox or flu, unless directed by a physician. Do not take this product if you are allergic to aspirin, have asthma, gastric ulcer, or are taking a medication that affects the clotting of blood, except under the advice and supervision of a physician. If pain persists for more than 10 days or redness is present, discontinue use of this product and consult a physician immediately. Keep this and all medication out of children's reach. As with any drug, if you are pregnant or nursing a baby, consult your physician before using this product. Discontinue use if ringing in the ears occurs.

In case of accidental overdosage, contact a physician or poison control center immediately.

Dosage and Administration: Stir one powder into a glass of water or other liquid, or, place powder on tongue and follow with liquid. May be used every 3 or 4 hours up to 4 times a day. For children under 12 consult a physician.

How Supplied: Available in tamper resistant cellophane wrapped envelopes of 2 or 6 powders, as well as tamper resistant boxes of 24 and 50 powders.

NYTOL® TABLETS

Active Ingredient: Diphenhydramine Hydrochloride, 25 mg per tablet.

Indications: Diphenhydramine Hydrochloride is an antihistamine with anticholinergic and sedative effects which induces drowsiness and helps in falling asleep.

Warnings: Do not give children under 12 years of age. If sleeplessness persists continuously for more than 2 weeks, consult your physician. Insomnia may be a symptom of serious underlying medical illness. If pregnant or nursing, consult your physician before taking this or any medicine. Do not take this product if you have asthma, glaucoma, or enlargement of the prostate gland except under the advice and supervision of a physician. Take this product with caution if alcohol is being consumed. Keep this and all drugs out of the reach of children. In case of accidental overdose, contact a physician immediately.

Drug Interaction: Alcohol and other drugs which cause CNS depression will heighten the depressant effect of this product. Monoamine oxidase (MAO) inhibitors will prolong and intensify the anticholinergic effects of antihistamines.

Symptoms and Treatment of Oral Overdosage: In adults overdose may cause CNS depression resulting in hypnosis and coma. In children CNS hyperexcitability may follow sedation; the stimulant phase may bring tremor, delirium and convulsions. Gastrointestinal reactions may include dry mouth, appetite loss, nausea and vomiting. Respira-

tory distress and cardiovascular complications (hypotension) may be evident. Treatment includes inducing emesis, and controlling symptoms.

Dosage and Administration: Take 2 tablets 20 minutes before bed or as directed by a physician.

How Supplied: Available in tamper resistant packages of 16, 32, 48, and 72 tablets.

PROMISE® TOOTHPASTE
Desensitizing Dentifrice

Active Ingredients: 5% Potassium Nitrate in a pleasantly mint-flavored dentifrice.

Promise contains Potassium Nitrate for relief of dentinal hypersensitivity resulting from the exposure of tooth dentin due to periodontal surgery, cervical (gumline) erosion, abrasion or recession which causes pain on contact with hot, cold, or tactile stimuli.

Actions: Promise significantly reduces tooth hypersensitivity, with response to therapy evident after two weeks of use. Controlled double-blind clinical studies provide substantial evidence of the safety and effectiveness of Promise. The mechanism of action of potassium nitrate in Promise is not well-defined at this time: it may function by blocking the dentinal tubules to obtund pain transmission or have a direct or indirect effect on neural transmission.

Warning: When used as directed, it is important to remember that you have to brush for at least two weeks before relief begins to occur. If no improvement is seen after three months of use, consult your dentist.

Dosage and Administration: Use twice a day in place of regular toothpaste or as directed by a dental professional.

How Supplied: Promise Toothpaste is supplied in 1.6 oz. and 3.0 oz. tubes.

ORIGINAL SENSODYNE®
TOOTHPASTE
Desensitizing Dentifrice

Description: Each tube contains strontium chloride hexahydrate (10%) in a pleasantly flavored cleansing/polishing dentifrice.

Actions/Indications: Tooth hypersensitivity is a condition in which individuals experience pain from exposure to hot, cold stimuli, from chewing fibrous foods, or from tactile stimuli (e.g. toothbrushing.) Hypersensitivity usually occurs when the protective enamel covering on teeth wears away (which happens most often at the gum line) or if gum tissue recedes and exposes the dentin underneath.

Running through the dentin are microscopic small "tubules" which, according to many authorities, carry the pain impulses to the nerve of the tooth. Sensodyne provides a unique ingredient—strontium chloride which is

believed to be deposited in the tubules where it blocks the pain. The longer Sensodyne is used, the more of a barrier it helps build against pain.

The effect of Sensodyne may not be manifested immediately and may require a few weeks or longer of use for relief to be obtained. A number of clinical studies in the U.S. and other countries have provided substantial evidence of Sensodyne's performance attributes. Complete relief of hypersensitivity has been reported in approximately 65% of users and measurable relief or reduction in hypersensitivity in approximately 90%. Sensodyne has been commercially available for over 25 years and has received wide dental endorsement.

Contraindications: Subjects with severe dental erosion should brush properly and lightly with any dentifrice to avoid further removal of tooth structure.

Dosage: Use regularly in place of ordinary toothpaste or as recommended by dental professional.
NOTE: Individuals should be instructed to use SENSODYNE frequently since relief from pain tends to be cumulative. If relief does not occur after 3 months, a dentist should be consulted.

How Supplied: SENSODYNE Toothpaste is supplied as a paste in tubes of 4 oz. and 2.1 oz.
(U.S. Patent No. 3,122,483)

MINT SENSODYNE®
TOOTHPASTE
Desensitizing Dentifrice

Active Ingredients: 5% Potassium Nitrate in a pleasantly mint-flavored dentifrice.
Mint Sensodyne contains Potassium Nitrate for relief of dentinal hypersensitivity resulting from the exposure of tooth dentin due to periodontal surgery, cervical (gum line) erosion, abrasion or recession which causes pain on contact with hot, cold, or tactile stimuli.

Actions: Mint Sensodyne significantly reduces tooth hypersensitivity, with response to therapy evident after two weeks of use. Controlled double-blind clinical studies provide substantial evidence of the safety and effectiveness of Mint Sensodyne. The mechanism of action of potassium nitrate in Mint Senodyne is not well-defined at this time: it may function by blocking the dentinal tubules to obtund pain transmission or have a direct or indirect effect on neural transmission.

Warning: When used as directed, it is important to remember that you have to brush for at least two weeks before relief begins to occur. If no improvement is seen after three months of use, consult your dentist.

Dosage and Administration: Use twice a day in place of regular toothpaste or as directed by a dental professional.

Continued on next page

Block—Cont.

How Supplied: Mint Sensodyne Toothpaste is supplied in 2.4 and 4.6 oz. tubes.

TEGRIN® MEDICATED SHAMPOO

Highly effective shampoo for moderate-to-severe dandruff and the relief of flaking, itching, and scaling associated with eczema, seborrhea, and psoriasis. Two commercial product versions are available: a lotion shampoo, in three formulas; herbal, original, and extra conditioning, and a gel concentrate, available in herbal scent.

Description: Each tube of gel shampoo or bottle of lotion shampoo contains 5% special alcohol extract of coal tar in a pleasantly scented, high-foaming, cleansing shampoo base with emollients, conditioners and other formula components.

Actions/Indications: Coal Tar is obtained in the destructive distillation of bituminous coal and is a highly effective agent for the local therapy of a number of dermatological disorders. The action of coal tar extract is believed to be keratolytic, antiseptic, antipruritic and astringent. The special extract of coal tar used in the Tegrin products is prepared in such a way as to reduce the pitch and other irritant components found in crude coal tar without reduction in therapeutic potency.

Coal tar extract has been used clinically for many years as a remedy for dandruff and for scaling associated with scalp disorders such as eczema, seborrhea, and psoriasis. Its mechanism of action has not been fully established, but it is believed to retard the rate of turnover of epidermal cells with regular use. A number of clinical studies have demonstrated the performance attributes of Tegrin Shampoo against dandruff and seborrheic dermatitis. In addition to relieving the above symptoms, Tegrin shampoo used regularly, maintains scalp and hair cleanliness and leaves the hair lustrous and manageable.

Contraindications: For External Use Only—Should irritation develop, discontinue use. Avoid contact with eyes. Keep out of reach of children.

Dosage: Use regularly as a shampoo. Wet hair thoroughly. Rub Tegrin liberally into hair and scalp. Rinse thoroughly. Briskly massage a second application of the shampoo into a rich lather. Rinse thoroughly.

How Supplied: Tegrin Concentrated Gel Shampoo is supplied in 2.5 oz. collapsible tubes.
Tegrin Lotion Shampoo is supplied in 3.75 and 6.6 oz. plastic bottles.

TEGRIN® for Psoriasis Lotion, Cream and Soap

Description: Each tube of cream or bottle of lotion contains special crude coal tar extract (5%) and allantoin (1.7%) in a greaseless, stainless vehicle. Tegrin Medicated Soap contains 2.0% crude coal tar extract.

Actions/Indications: Crude coal tar is obtained in the destructive distillation of bituminous coal and is a highly effective agent for the local therapy of a number of dermatological disorders. The action of coal tar extract is believed to be keratolytic, antiseptic, antipruritic and astringent. The special coal tar extract used in the Tegrin products is prepared in such a way as to reduce the pitch and other irritant components found in crude coal tar. Allantoin (5-Ureidohydantoin) is a debriding and dispersing agent for psoriatic scales and is believed to accelerate proliferation of normal skin cells. The combination of coal tar extract and allantoin used in Tegrin has been demonstrated in a number of controlled clinical studies to have a high level of efficacy in controlling the itching and scaling of psoriasis.

Contraindications: Discontinue medication should irritation or allergic reactions occur. Avoid contact with eyes and mucous membranes. Keep out of reach of children.

Dosage and Administration: Apply lotion or cream 2 to 4 times daily as needed, massaging thoroughly into affected areas. Lather with Tegrin Soap in a hot bath before application to help soften heavy scales. Once condition is under control, maintenance therapy should be individually adjusted. Occlusive dressings are not required.

How Supplied: Tegrin Lotion 6 fl. oz., Tegrin Cream 2 oz. and 4.4 oz. tubes, Tegrin Soap 4.5 oz. bars.

Boehringer Ingelheim Pharmaceuticals, Inc.
**90 EAST RIDGE
POST OFFICE BOX 368
RIDGEFIELD, CT 06877**

DULCOLAX®
[dul 'co-lax]
**brand of bisacodyl USP
Tablets of 5 mg.................BI-CODE 12
Suppositories of 10 mg...BI-CODE 52
Laxative**

Description: Dulcolax is a contact laxative acting directly on the colonic mucosa to produce normal peristalsis throughout the large intestine. Its unique mode of action permits either oral or rectal administration, according to the requirements of the patient. Because of its gentleness and reliability of action, Dulcolax may be used whenever constipation is a problem. In preparation for surgery, proctoscopy, or radiologic examination, Dulcolax provides satisfactory cleansing of the bowel, obviating the need for an enema.

The active ingredient in Dulcolax, bisacodyl, is a colorless, tasteless compound that is practically insoluble in water and alkaline solution. It is designated chemically bis(p-acetoxyphenyl)-2-pyridylmethane.

Each tablet contains bisacodyl USP 5 mg. Also contains acacia, acetylated monoglyceride, carnauba wax, cellulose acetate phthalate, corn starch, D&C Red No. 30 aluminum lake, D&C Yellow No. 10 aluminum lake, dibutyl phthalate, docusate sodium, gelatin, glycerin, iron oxides, kaolin, lactose, magnesium stearate, methylparaben, pharmaceutical glaze, polyethylene glycol, povidone, propylparaben, sodium benzoate, sorbitan monooleate, sucrose, talc, titanium dioxide, white wax.

Each suppository contains bisacodyl USP 10 mg. Also contains hydrogenated vegetable oil.

Dulcolax tablets and suppositories are sodium free.

Actions: Dulcolax differs markedly from other laxatives in its mode of action: it is virtually nontoxic, and its laxative effect occurs on contact with the colonic mucosa, where it stimulates sensory nerve endings to produce parasympathetic reflexes resulting in increased peristaltic contractions of the colon. Administered orally, Dulcolax is absorbed to a variable degree from the small bowel but such absorption is not related to the mode of action of the compound. Dulcolax administered rectally in the form of suppositories is negligibly absorbed. The contact action of the drug is restricted to the colon, and motility of the small intestine is not appreciably influenced. Local axon reflexes, as well as segmental reflexes, are initiated in the region of contact and contribute to the widespread peristaltic activity producing evacuation. For this reason, Dulcolax may often be employed satisfactorily in patients with ganglionic blockage or spinal cord damage (paraplegia, poliomyelitis, etc.).

Indications: *Acute Constipation:* Taken at bedtime, Dulcolax tablets are almost invariably effective the following morning. When taken before breakfast, they usually produce an effect within six hours. For a prompter response and to replace enemas, the suppositories, which are usually effective in 15 minutes to one hour, can be used.

Chronic Constipation and Bowel Retraining: Dulcolax is extremely effective in the management of chronic constipation, particularly in older patients. By gradually lengthening the interval between doses as colonic tone improves, the drug has been found to be effective in redeveloping proper bowel hygiene. There is no tendency to "rebound".

Preparation for Radiography: Dulcolax tablets are excellent in eliminating fecal and gas shadows from x-rays taken of the abdominal area. For barium enemas, no food should be given following the administration of the tablets, to prevent reaccumulation of material in the cecum, and a suppository should be given one to two hours prior to examination.

Preoperative Preparation: Dulcolax tablets have been shown to be an ideal laxative in emptying the G.I. tract prior to abdominal surgery or to other surgery under general anesthesia. They may be supplemented by suppositories to replace

the usual enema preparation. Dulcolax will not replace the colonic irrigations usually given patients before intracolonic surgery, but is useful in the preliminary emptying of the colon prior to these procedures.

Postoperative Care: Suppositories can be used to replace enemas, or tablets given as an oral laxative, to restore normal bowel hygiene after surgery.

Antepartum Care: Either tablets or suppositories can be used for constipation in pregnancy without danger of stimulating the uterus.

Preparation for Delivery: Suppositories can be used to replace enemas in the first stage of labor provided that they are given at least two hours before the onset of the second stage.

Postpartum Care: The same indications apply as in postoperative care, with no contraindication in nursing mothers.

Preparation for Sigmoidoscopy or Proctoscopy: For unscheduled office examinations, adequate preparation is usually obtained with a single suppository. For sigmoidoscopy scheduled in advance, however, administration of tablets the night before in addition will result in adequate preparation almost invariably.

Colostomies: Tablets the night before or a suppository inserted into the colostomy opening in the morning will frequently make irrigations unnecessary, and in other cases will expedite the procedure.

Contraindication: There is no contraindication to the use of Dulcolax, other than an acute surgical abdomen.

Caution for Patients: Do not use laxative products when abdominal pain, nausea or vomiting are present unless directed by a doctor. As with all medicines, keep these tablets/suppositories out of reach of children. Frequent or continued use of this preparation may result in dependence on laxatives.

Adverse Reactions: As with any laxative, abdominal cramps are occasionally noted, particularly in severely constipated individuals.

Dosage:
Tablets
Tablets must be swallowed whole, not chewed or crushed, and should not be taken within one hour of antacids or milk.
Adults: Two or three (usually two) tablets suffice when an ordinary laxative effect is desired. This usually results in one or two soft, formed stools. Tablets when taken before breakfast usually produce an effect within 6 hours, when taken at bedtime usually in 8–12 hours.
Up to six tablets may be safely given in preparation for special procedures when greater assurance of complete evacuation of the colon is desired. In producing such thorough emptying, these higher doses may result in several loose, unformed stools.
Children: One or two tablets, depending on age and severity of constipation, administered as above. Tablets should not be given to a child too young to swallow them whole.

Suppositories
Adults: One suppository at the time a bowel movement is required. Usually effective in 15 minutes to one hour.
Children: Half a suppository is generally effective for infants and children under two years of age. Above this age, a whole suppository is usually advisable.
Combined
In preparation for surgery, radiography and sigmoidoscopy, a combination of tablets the night before and a suppository in the morning is recommended (see Indications).

How Supplied: Dulcolax, brand of bisacodyl: Yellow, enteric-coated tablets of 5 mg in boxes of 10, 25, 50 and 100; suppositories of 10 mg in boxes of 4, 8, 16 and 50.

Note: Store Dulcolax suppositories and tablets at temperatures below 77°F (25°C). Avoid excessive humidity.

Also Available: Dulcolax® Bowel Prep Kit. Each kit contains:
1 Dulcolax suppository of 10 mg bisacodyl;
4 Dulcolax tablets of 5 mg bisacodyl;
Complete patient instructions.

Clinical Applications: Dulcolax can be used in virtually any patient in whom a laxative or enema is indicated. It has no effect on the blood picture, erythrocyte sedimentation rate, urinary findings, or hepatic or renal function. It may be safely given to infants and the aged, pregnant or nursing women, debilitated patients, and may be prescribed in the presence of such conditions as cardiovascular, renal, or hepatic diseases.

Shown in Product Identification Section, page 404

NŌSTRIL® Nasal Decongestant
[nō 'stril]
phenylephrine HCl, USP

Active Ingredient: Contains phenylephrine HCl, USP, 0.25% (¼% Mild strength) or phenylephrine HCl, USP, 0.5% (½% Regular strength). Also contains benzalkonium chloride 0.004% as a preservative, boric acid, sodium borate, water.

Indications: For temporary relief of nasal congestion due to the common cold, sinusitis, hay fever or other upper respiratory allergies.

Actions: NŌSTRIL, the first metered one-way pump spray for nasal decongestion delivers measured, uniform doses. The medication constricts the smaller arterioles of the nasal passages, producing a gentle, predictable, decongestant effect. Nōstril penetrates and shrinks swollen membranes, restoring freer breathing and unclogs sinus passages, bringing the effective medication in contact with inflamed, swollen tissues. It will not hurt tender membranes since it is formulated to match the pH of normal nasal secretions. The first one-way pump spray helps prevent draw-back contamination of the medication.

Warnings: Do not exceed recommended dosage because symptoms such as burning, stinging, sneezing, or increased nasal discharge may occur. Do not use for more than 3 days. If symptoms persist, consult a physician. Do not give Nōstril 0.25% to children under 6 or Nōstril 0.5% to children under 12 except under the advice and supervision of a physician. Nōstril 0.5% for adult use only. Use of the dispenser by more than one person may spread infection. Keep this and all drugs out of reach of children.

Symptoms and Treatment of Oral Overdosage: In case of accidental ingestion, seek professional assistance or consult a poison control center immediately.

Dosage and Administration:
0.25% for adults and children 6 years and over: 1 to 2 sprays in each nostril not more frequently than every four hours.
0.5% for adults: 1 to 2 sprays in each nostril not more frequently than every four hours.
Remove protective cap. With head upright, insert metered pump spray nozzle in nostril. Hold bottle with thumb at base, nozzle between first and second fingers. Depress pump once or twice, all the way down with a firm even stroke and sniff deeply.
Note: Before using for the first time, remove the protective cap from the tip and depress the round tab firmly several times to prime the metering pump.

How Supplied: Metered one-way nasal pump spray in white plastic bottles of ½ fl. oz. (15 ml) packaged in tamper-resistant outer cartons.
0.25% (¼% Mild strength): for children 6 years and over and adults who prefer a milder decongestant. (NDC 0597-0083-85)
0.5% (½% Regular strength): for adults and children 12 years or older (NDC 0597-0084-85)

NŌSTRILLA™ Long Acting Nasal
[nō-stril 'a]
Decongestant
oxymetazoline HCl, USP

Active Ingredient: Contains oxymetazoline HCl, USP, 0.05%. Also contains benzalkonium chloride 0.02% as a preservative, glycine, sorbitol solution, water. (Mercury preservatives are not used in this product.)

Indications: For up to 12 hour relief of nasal congestion due to the common cold, sinusitis, hay fever or other upper respiratory allergies.

Actions: NŌSTRILLA, the first metered one-way pump spray for nasal decongestion delivers measured, uniform doses. The medication constricts the smaller arterioles of the nasal passages, producing a prolonged (up to 12 hours), gentle, predictable, decongestant effect. Nōstrilla penetrates and shrinks swollen membranes, restoring freer breathing and unclogs sinus passages, bringing the

Continued on next page

Boehringer Ingelheim—Cont.

effective medication in contact with inflamed, swollen tissues. It will not hurt tender membranes since it is formulated to match the pH of normal nasal secretions. Use at bedtime restores freer nasal breathing through the night. The first one-way pump spray helps prevent drawback contamination of the medication.

Warnings: Do not exceed recommended dosage because symptoms such as burning, stinging, sneezing or increased nasal discharge may occur. Do not use for more than 3 days. If symptoms persist, consult a physician. Do not give this product to children under 6 except under advice and supervision of a physician. Use of the dispenser by more than one person may spread infection. Keep this and all drugs out of reach of children.

Symptoms and Treatment of Oral Overdosage: In case of accidental ingestion, seek professional assistance or contact a poison control center immediately.

Dosage and Administration: Adults and children 6 and over: 1 to 2 sprays in each nostril 2 times daily (in the morning and evening).

Remove protective cap. With head upright, insert metered pump spray nozzle in nostril. Hold bottle with thumb at base, nozzle between first and second fingers. Depress pump once or twice, all the way down with a firm even stroke and sniff deeply.
Note: Before using for the first time, remove the protective cap from the tip and depress the round tab firmly several times to prime the metering pump.

How Supplied: Metered one-way nasal pump spray in white plastic bottles of ½ fl. oz. (15 ml) packaged in tamper-resistant outer cartons. (NDC 0597-0085-85).

EDUCATIONAL MATERIAL

Bowel Evacuation: An Illustrated Teaching Manual
A nurse's guide to bowel care and retraining.

Products are cross-indexed by generic and chemical names
in the
YELLOW SECTION

Boiron-Borneman, Inc.
**1208 AMOSLAND ROAD
NORWOOD, PA 19074**

OSCILLOCOCCINUM®
[ŏ-sĭl′ō-kŏk-sē′nŭm]

Active Ingredient: Anas Barbariae Hepatis et Cordis Extractum HPUS 200C

Indications: For the relief of flu-like symptoms such as fever, chills, body aches and pains.

Actions: Like most Homeopathic remedies, Oscillococcinum® acts gently by stimulating the patient's natural defense mechanisms.

Warnings: If symptoms persist for more than three days or worsen, consult your physician. Keep all medication out of reach of children. As with any drug if you are pregnant or nursing a baby, seek professional advice before using this product.

Dosage and Administration: (Adults and Children over 2 years)
At the onset of symptoms, place the entire contents of one tube in your mouth and allow to dissolve under your tongue. Repeat every 6 hours as necessary. For maximum results, Oscillococcinum® should be taken early, at the onset of symptoms, and at least 15 minutes before or 1 hour after meals.

How Supplied: boxes of 3 unit-doses of 0.04 oz. (1 Gram) each. (NDC 51979-9756-43) Tamper resistant package.
Manufactured by Boiron, France.
Distributor: Boiron-Borneman, Inc.
Shown in Product Identification Section, page 404

EDUCATIONAL MATERIAL

Boiron-Borneman, Inc. Product Catalogue
General description of the most popular Boiron-Borneman, Inc. remedies and lines.
Oscillococcinum ® Brochure
Brochure on Oscillococcinum® describing clinical research on the product and its general use.

IDENTIFICATION PROBLEM?
Consult the
Product Identification Section
where you'll find
products pictured
in full color.

Bristol Laboratories
A Bristol-Myers Company
**2400 W. LLOYD EXPRESSWAY
EVANSVILLE, IN 47721**

NALDECON CX® ADULT LIQUID℃
[nal′dĕ-côn]

Description: Each teaspoonful (5 mL) of Naldecon CX Adult Liquid contains:
Phenylpropanolamine
  hydrochloride .... 18 mg
Guaifenesin (glyceryl
  guaiacolate) .... 200 mg
Codeine Phosphate .... 10 mg
  (Warning: May be Habit Forming)
This combination product is antihistamine-free and alcohol-free.

Indications: Temporarily relieves cough due to minor throat and bronchial irritation as may occur with a cold or inhaled irritants. Helps loosen phlegm (sputum) and bronchial secretions and rid the bronchial passageways of bothersome mucus. For the temporary relief of nasal congestion due to the common cold (cold), hay fever or other respiratory allergies (allergic rhinitis), or associated with sinusitis.

Contraindications: Hypersensitivity to guaifenesin, codeine or sympathomimetic amines.

Warnings: As with any drug, if you are pregnant or nursing a baby, seek the advice of a health professional before using this product. Nervousness, dizziness or sleeplessness may occur if recommended dosage is exceeded. Do not exceed recommended dose or give to children under 12 years of age except as directed by a physician. Do not give this product to a person with high blood pressure, heart disease, diabetes, thyroid disease, high fever, or persistent cough except under the advice and supervision of a physician. Do not give this product to a person presently taking a prescription drug containing a monoamine oxidase inhibitor except under the advice and supervision of a physician. Do not administer this product for persistent or chronic cough such as occurs with asthma or emphysema or when cough is accompanied by excessive secretions, except under the care and advice of a physician. A persistent cough may be a sign of a serious condition. If cough persists for more than 1 week, tends to recur, or is accompanied by high fever, rash or persistent headaches, consult a physician. This product is not intended for use by children. Keep this and all drugs out of the reach of children. In case of accidental overdose, seek professional assistance or contact a Poison Control Center immediately. .

Inactive Ingredients: Citric acid, cool cherry flavor (natural and artificial), FD&C Blue No. 1, FD&C Red No. 40, hydrogenated glucose syrup (lycasin), polyethylene glycol, purified water, saccharin sodium, sodium benzoate, sodium citrate.

Dosage and Administration: Adults: 2 teaspoonsful every 4 to 6 hours, not to

exceed 4 doses every 24 hours, or as directed by a physician.

How Supplied: Naldecon CX Adult Liquid—4 oz. and pint bottles.

NALDECON DX® ADULT LIQUID
[nal 'dĕ-côn]

Description: Each teaspoonful (5 mL) of Naldecon DX Adult Liquid contains:
Phenylpropanolamine
   hydrochloride...............................18 mg
Guaifenesin (glyceryl
   guaiacolate)................................200 mg
Dextromethorphan
   hydrobromide..............................15 mg
This combination product is antihistamine-free, sugar-free and alcohol-free.

Indications: Provides prompt relief of cough and nasal congestion due to the common cold, bronchitis, nasopharyngitis, and flu. Dextromethorphan temporarily quiets nonproductive coughing by its antitussive action while guaifenesin's expectorant action helps loosen phlegm and bronchial secretions. Phenylpropanolamine reduces swelling of nasal passages and shrinks swollen membranes.

Contraindications: Hypersensitivity to guaifenesin, dextromethorphan, or sympathomimetic amines.

Warnings: As with any drug, if you are pregnant or nursing a baby, seek the advice of a health professional before using this product. Nervousness, dizziness or sleeplessness may occur if recommended dosage is exceeded. Do not exceed recommended dose or give to children under 12 years of age except as directed by a physician. Do not give this product to a person with high blood pressure, heart disease, diabetes, thyroid disease, high fever, or persistent cough except under the advice and supervision of a physician. Do not give this product to a person presently taking a prescription drug containing a monamine oxidase inhibitor except under the advice and supervision of a physician. Do not administer this product for persistent or chronic cough such as occurs with asthma or emphysema or when cough is accompanied by excessive secretions except under the care and advice of a physician. A persistent cough may be a sign of a serious condition. If cough persists for more than 1 week, tends to recur, or is accompanied by high fever, rash or persistent headaches, consult a physician. This product is not intended for use by children. Keep this and all drugs out of the reach of children. In case of accidental overdose, seek professional assistance or contact a Poison Control Center immediately.

Inactive Ingredients: Citric acid, FD&C Yellow No. 6, peppermint flavor (natural and artificial), polyethylene glycol, purified water, saccharin sodium, sodium benzoate, sodium citrate, sorbitol solution.

Dosage and Administration: 12 years and older: 2 teaspoonsful 4 times daily.

How Supplied: Naldecon DX Adult Liquid—4 oz. and pint bottles.

NALDECON DX®
[nal 'dĕ-côn]
CHILDREN'S SYRUP

Description: Each teaspoonful (5 mL.) of Naldecon DX Children's Syrup contains:
Phenylpropanolamine
   hydrochloride ....9 mg
Guaifenesin (glyceryl
   guaiacolate)................................100 mg
Dextromethorphan
   hydrobromide ....7.5 mg
Alcohol 0.5%
This combination product is antihistamine-free.

Indications: Provides prompt relief of cough and nasal congestion due to the common cold, bronchitis, nasopharyngitis, flu, and croup. Dextromethorphan temporarily quiets nonproductive coughing by its antitussive action while guaifenesin's expectorant action helps loosen phlegm and bronchial secretions. Phenylpropanolamine reduces swelling of nasal passages and shrinks swollen membranes.

Contraindications: Hypersensitivity to guaifenesin, dextromethorphan or sympathomimetic amines.

Warnings: Nervousness, dizziness or sleeplessness may occur if recommended dosage is exceeded. Do not exceed recommended dose or give to children under 2 years of age except as directed by a physician. Do not give this product to a child with high blood pressure, heart disease, diabetes, thyroid disease, high fever, or persistent cough except under the advice and supervision of a physician. Do not give this product to a child presently taking a prescription drug containing a monamine oxidase inhibitor except under the advice and supervision of a physician. Do not administer this product for persistent or chronic cough such as occurs with asthma or emphysema or when cough is accompanied by excessive secretions except under the care and advice of a physician. A persistent cough may be a sign of a serious condition. If cough persists for more than 1 week, tends to recur, or is accompanied by high fever, rash or persistent headaches, consult a physician. Keep this and all drugs out of the reach of children. In case of accidental overdose, seek professional assistance or contact a Poison Control Center immediately.

Inactive Ingredients: FD&C Yellow No. 6, fructose, glycerin, natural and artificial flavorings, purified water, sodium benzoate, sucrose and tartaric acid.

Dosage and Administration: Children 2–6 years of age (under 50 lbs.): 1 teaspoonful every 4 hours. Children 6–12 years of age (under 100 lbs.): 2 teaspoonsful every 4 hours. Do not exceed 4 doses every 24 hours. Under 2 years: use only as directed by a physician.

How Supplied: Naldecon DX Children's Syrup—4 oz. and pint bottles.

NALDECON DX®
[nal 'dĕ-côn]
PEDIATRIC DROPS

Description: Each 1 mL dropperful of Naldecon DX Pediatric Drops contains:
Phenylpropanolamine
   hydrochloride............................... 9 mg
Guaifenesin (glyceryl
   guaiacolate)................................ 30 mg
Dextromethorphan
   hydrobromide........................... 7.5 mg
Alcohol.. 0.6%
This combination product is antihistamine-free and sugar-free.

Indications: Provides prompt relief of cough and nasal congestion due to the common cold, bronchitis, nasopharyngitis, flu and croup. Dextromethorphan temporarily quiets nonproductive coughing by its antitussive action while guaifenesin's expectorant action helps loosen phlegm and bronchial secretions. Phenylpropanolamine reduces swelling of nasal passages and shrinks swollen membranes.

Contraindications: Hypersensitivity to guaifenesin, dextromethorphan, or sympathomimetic amines.

Warnings: Take by mouth only. Nervousness, dizziness or sleeplessness may occur if recommended dosage is exceeded. Do not exceed recommended dose. Do not give this product to a child with high blood pressure, heart disease, diabetes, thyroid disease, high fever, or persistent cough except under the advice and supervision of a physician. Do not give this product to a child presently taking a prescription drug containing a monamine oxidase inhibitor except under the advice and supervision of a physician. Do not administer this product for persistent or chronic cough such as occurs with asthma or emphysema or when cough is accompanied by excessive secretions except under the care and advice of a physician. A persistent cough may be a sign of a serious condition. If cough persists for more than 1 week, tends to recur, or is accompanied by high fever, rash or persistent headaches, consult a physician. Keep this and all drugs out of the reach of children. In case of accidental overdose, seek professional assistance or contact a Poison Control Center immediately.

Inactive Ingredients: Citric acid, FD&C Yellow No. 6, natural and artificial flavorings, propylene glycol, purified water, sodium benzoate, sodium saccharin and sorbitol.

Dosage and Administration: Dose should be adjusted to age or weight and be given 4 times a day (see calibrations on dropper). Do not exceed 4 doses in 24 hours. Administer by mouth only.

Continued on next page

Bristol—Cont.

1–3 Months:	¼ mL every
(8–12 lbs.)	4–6 hours
4–6 Months:	½ mL every
(13–17 lbs.)	4–6 hours
7–9 Months:	¾ mL every
(18–20 lbs.)	4–6 hours
10 Months or over:	1 mL every
(21 lbs. or more)	4–6 hours

Bottle label dosage reads as follows: Children under 2 years of age: use only as directed by a physician.

How Supplied: Naldecon DX Pediatric Drops—30 mL bottle with calibrated dropper.

NALDECON EX®
[nal 'dĕ-côn]
CHILDREN'S SYRUP

Description: Each teaspoonful (5 mL) of Naldecon EX Children's Syrup contains:

Phenylpropanolamine
hydrochloride..................................9 mg
Guaifenesin (glyceryl
guaiacolate)..................................100 mg
Alcohol..0.5%
This combination product is antihistamine-free and sugar-free.

Indications: Combined decongestant/expectorant designed specifically to promptly reduce the swelling of nasal membranes and to help loosen phlegm and bronchial secretions through productive coughing. This dual action is of particular value in children with common cold, acute bronchitis, nasopharyngitis, flu and croup.

Contraindications: Hypersensitivity to guaifenesin or sympathomimetic amines.

Warnings: Nervousness, dizziness or sleeplessness may occur if recommended dosage is exceeded. Do not exceed recommended dose or give to children under 2 years of age except as directed by a physician. Do not give this product to a child with high blood pressure, heart disease, diabetes, thyroid disease, high fever, or persistent cough except under the advice and supervision of a physician. Do not give this product to a child presently taking a prescription drug containing a monamine oxidase inhibitor except under the advice and supervision of a physician. Do not administer this product for persistent or chronic cough such as occurs with asthma or emphysema or when cough is accompanied by excessive secretions except under the care and advice of a physician. A persistent cough may be a sign of a serious condition. If cough persists for more than 1 week, tends to recur, or is accompanied by high fever, rash or persistent headaches, consult a physician. Keep this and all drugs out of the reach of children. In case of accidental overdose, seek professional assistance or contact a Poison Control Center immediately.

Inactive Ingredients: D&C Yellow No. 10, glycerin, natural and artificial flavorings, propylene glycol, purified water, sodium benzoate, sodium saccharin, sorbitol and tartaric acid.

Dosage and Administration: Children 2–6 years of age (under 50 lbs.): 1 teaspoonful every 4 hours. Children 6–12 years of age (under 100 lbs.): 2 teaspoonsful every 4 hours. Do not exceed 4 doses every 24 hours. Under 2 years: use only as directed by a physician.

How Supplied: Naldecon EX Children's Syrup—4 oz and pint bottles.

NALDECON EX®
[nal 'dĕ-côn]
PEDIATRIC DROPS

Description: Each 1 mL. of Naldecon EX Pediatric Drops contains:
Phenylpropanolamine
hydrochloride ....9 mg
Guaifenesin (glyceryl
guaiacolate) ....30 mg
Alcohol 0.6%
This combination product is antihistamine-free.

Indications: Combined decongestant/expectorant designed specifically to promptly reduce the swelling of nasal membranes and to help loosen phlegm and bronchial secretions through productive coughing. This dual action is of particular value in infants with common cold, acute bronchitis, nasopharyngitis, flu and croup.

Contraindications: Hypersensitivity to guaifenesin or sympathomimetic amines.

Warnings: Take by mouth only. Nervousness, dizziness or sleeplessness may occur if recommended dosage is exceeded. Do not exceed recommended dose. Do not give this product to a child with high blood pressure, heart disease, diabetes, thyroid disease, high fever, or persistent cough except under the advice and supervision of a physician. Do not give this product to a child presently taking a prescription drug containing a monamine oxidase inhibitor except under the advice and supervision of a physician. Do not administer this product for persistent or chronic cough such as occurs with asthma or emphysema or when cough is accompanied by excessive secretions except under the care and advice of a physician. A persistent cough may be a sign of a serious condition. If cough persists for more than 1 week, tends to recur, or is accompanied by high fever, rash or persistent headaches, consult a physician. Keep this and all drugs out of the reach of children. In case of accidental overdose, seek professional assistance or contact a Poison Control Center immediately.

Inactive Ingredients: Citric acid, D&C Yellow No. 10, natural and artificial flavorings, propylene glycol, purified water, sodium benzoate and sucrose.

Dosage and Administration: Dose should be adjusted to age or weight and be given 4 times a day (see calibrations on dropper). Do not exceed 4 doses in 24 hours. Administer by mouth only.

1–3 Months:	¼ mL every
(8–12 lbs.)	4–6 hours
4–6 Months:	½ mL every
(13–17 lbs.)	4–6 hours
7–9 Months:	¾ mL every
(18–20 lbs.)	4–6 hours
10 Months or over	1 mL every
(21 lbs. or more)	4–6 hours

Bottle label dosage reads as follows: children under 2 years of age: use only as directed by a physician.

How Supplied: Naldecon EX Pediatric Drops in 30 mL bottles with calibrated dropper.

NALDECON® SENIOR DX™
Expectorant/Cough Suppressant
Cough/Cold Liquid
for Adults 50 and Over

Description: Each teaspoonful (5 mL) of Naldecon Senior DX Cough/Cold Liquid contains:
Guaifenesin ....200 mg
Dextromethorphan
hydrobromide ....15 mg

Indications: Non-narcotic cough suppressant for the temporary relief of coughing. Helps loosen phlegm (sputum) and bronchial secretions and rid the bronchial passageways of bothersome mucus.

Contraindications: Do not take if hypersensitive to guaifenesin or dextromethorphan.

Warnings: A persistent cough may be a sign of a serious condition. If cough persists for more than 1 week, tends to recur, or is accompanied by fever, rash, or persistent headache, consult a physician. Do not take this product for persistent or chronic cough such as occurs with smoking, asthma, emphysema, or if cough is accompanied by excessive phlegm (mucus) unless directed by a physician. Do not exceed recommended dose or give this product to children under 12 years of age unless directed by a physician. As with any drug, if you are pregnant or nursing a baby, seek the advice of a health professional before using this product. Keep this and all drugs out of the reach of children. In case of accidental overdose, seek professional assistance or contact a Poison Control Center immediately.

Inactive Ingredients: Citric acid, FD&C Blue No. 1, FD&C Red No. 40, natural & artificial flavorings, polyethylene glycol, purified water, sodium benzoate, sodium citrate, sodium saccharin, sorbitol.

Dosage and Administration: Adults: Oral dosage is 2 teaspoonsful every 6 to 8 hours, not to exceed 4 doses in 24 hours, or as directed by a physician. Children under 12 years of age: consult a physician.

How Supplied: Naldecon Senior DX Cough/Cold Liquid—4 oz and pint bottles.

NALDECON® SENIOR EX™
(guaifenesin)
Expectorant
Cough/Cold Liquid
for Adults 50 and Over

Description: Each teaspoonful (5 mL) of Naldecon Senior-EX Cough/Cold Liquid contains:
Guaifenesin.......................................200 mg

Indications: Helps loosen phlegm (sputum) and bronchial secretions and rid the bronchial passageways of bothersome mucus.

Contraindications: Do not take if hypersensitive to guaifenesin.

Warnings: A persistent cough may be a sign of a serious condition. If cough persists for more than 1 week, tends to recur, or is accompanied by fever, rash, or persistent headache, consult a physician. Do not take this product for persistent or chronic cough such as occurs with smoking, asthma, emphysema, or if cough is accompanied by excessive phlegm (mucus) unless directed by a physician. Do not exceed recommended dose or give this product to children under 12 years of age unless directed by a physician. As with any drug, if you are pregnant or nursing a baby, seek the advice of a health professional before using this product. Keep this and all drugs out of the reach of children. In case of accidental overdose, seek professional assistance or contact a Poison Control Center immediately.

Inactive Ingredients: Citric acid, FD&C Blue No. 1, FD&C Red No. 40, natural & artificial flavorings, polyethylene glycol, purified water, sodium benzoate, sodium citrate, sodium saccharin, sorbitol.

Dosage and Administration: Adults: Oral dosage is 2 teaspoonsful every 4 hours, not to exceed 6 doses in 24 hours, or as directed by a physician. Children under 12 years of age: consult a physician.

How Supplied: Naldecon Senior EX Cough/Cold Liquid—4 oz and pint bottles.

Bristol-Myers Products
(Div. of Bristol-Myers Co.)
345 PARK AVENUE
NEW YORK, NY 10154

Tri-Buffered BUFFERIN®
[bŭf'fer-ĭn]
Analgesic

Composition:

Active Ingredient: Each coated tablet or caplet contains Aspirin 325 mg in a formulation buffered with Calcium Carbonate, Magnesium Oxide and Magnesium Carboante.
Other Ingredients: Citric Acid, Corn Starch, FD&C Blue No. 1, Hydroxypropyl Methylcellulose, Mineral Oil, Polysorbate 20, Povidone, Propylene Glycol, Simethicone Emulsion, Sodium

Phosphate, Sorbitan Monolaurate, Titanium Dioxide. May also contain: Benzoic Acid, Carnauba Wax, Magnesium Stearate, Sodium Lauryl Sulfate.

Action and Uses: For effective relief from headaches, pain and fever of colds and flu, muscle aches, temporary relief of minor arthritis pain and inflammation, menstrual pain and toothaches. Buffered formulation helps prevent the stomach upset that plain aspirin can cause. Coated tablets for easy swallowing.

Contraindications: Hypersensitivity to any ingredient in the product.

Caution: If pain persists for more than 10 days or redness is present or, in arthritic or rheumatic conditions affecting children under 12, consult physician immediately. Do not take without consulting physician if under medical care. Consult a dentist promptly for toothache.

Warning: Children and teenagers should not use this medicine for chicken pox or flu symptoms before a doctor is consulted about Reye syndrome, a rare but serious illness reported to be associated with aspirin. KEEP THIS AND ALL MEDICINES OUT OF CHILDREN'S REACH. IN CASE OF ACCIDENTAL OVERDOSE, CONTACT A PHYSICIAN OR POISON CONTROL CENTER IMMEDIATELY. If dizziness, impaired hearing or ringing in the ears occurs, discontinue use. As with any drug, if you are pregnant or nursing a baby, seek the advice of a health professional before using this product.

Administration and Dosage: Adults: 2 tablets or caplets with water every 4 hours as needed. Do not exceed 12 tablets or caplets in 24 hours, unless directed by physician. For children 6 to under 12, one-half dose. Under 6, consult physician.

Overdose: (Symptoms and treatment) Typical of aspirin.

How Supplied: Coated tablets in bottles of 12, 36, 60, 100, and 200. Coated Caplets in bottles of 36, 60, and 100. All sizes have child resistant closures except 100's for tablets and 60's for caplets which sizes are not recommended for households with young children. For hospital and clinical use: bottle—1,000; boxed 200 × 2 tablet foil packets. Professional samples available on request.

Product Identification: Coated circular white tablet with letter "B" debossed on one surface. Coated scored white caplet with the letter "B" debossed on each side of the scoring.

Professional Labeling
1. Tri-Buffered BUFFERIN® FOR RECURRENT TRANSIENT ISCHEMIC ATTACKS

Indication: There is evidence that aspirin is safe and effective for reducing the risk of recurrent transient ischemic attacks or stroke in men who have had transient ischemia of the brain due to fibrin platelet emboli.

There is no evidence that aspirin is effective in reducing TIA's in women, or is of benefit in the treatment of completed strokes in men or women.
Patients presenting with signs and symptoms of TIA's should have a complete medical and neurologic evaluation. Consideration should be given to other disorders which resemble TIA's.
It is important to evaluate and treat, if appropriate, other diseases associated with TIA's and stroke such as hypertension and diabetes.

Clinical Trials: The indication is supported by the results of a Canadian study in which 585 patients with threatened stroke were followed in a randomized clinical trial for an average of 26 months to determine whether aspirin or sulfinpyrazone, singly or in combination, influenced subsequent occurrence of transient ischemic attacks, stroke, or death. The study showed that although sulfinpyrazone had no statistically significant effect, aspirin reduced the risk of continuing transient ischemic attacks by 19 percent and reduced the risk of stroke or death by 31 percent. Both these effects were noted in men only, and aspirin appeared to be more effective in those men who were nondiabetic and who had no history of myocardial infarction.[1]
Another aspirin study, carried out in the U.S. with a smaller number of patients, showed a statistically significant number of "favorable outcomes", including reduced transient ischemic attacks, stroke, and death.[2]
Current data suggest that aspirin acts as an antithrombotic agent by inhibiting platelet adhesion and aggregation by blocking prostaglandin synthesis.[3]
Data on effectiveness are available only for the prevention of transient ischemic attacks or stroke in men who have already experienced at least one TIA. The prophylactic use of aspirin in persons with no history of TIA, or for treatment of completed strokes, is not advocated.

References: 1. Barnett HJ, and the Canadian Cooperative Study Group: A randomized trial of aspirin and sulfinpyrazone in threatened stroke, N Eng J Med, 299 (2): 53–9, 1978. 2. Fields WS, Lemak NA, Frankowski RF: Controlled trial of aspirin in cerebral ischemia, Part I. Stroke, 9(3): 301–16, 1977. 3. Moncada S, and Vane JR: Arachidonic acid metabolites and the interactions between platelets and blood-vessel walls. New Eng. J Med, 300(20): 1142–7, 1979.

Dosage and Administration: The recommended dosage for this indication is 1,300 mg a day (650 mg. twice a day or 325 mg. four times a day).

2. Tri-Buffered BUFFERIN® FOR MYOCARDIAL INFARCTION

Indication: Aspirin is indicated to reduce the risk of death and/or nonfatal myocardial infarction in patients with a previous infarction or unstable angina pectoris.

Continued on next page

Bristol-Myers—Cont.

Clinical Trials: The indication is supported by the results of six, large, randomized multicenter placebo-controlled studies[1-7] involving 10,816, predominantly male, post-myocardial infarction (MI) patients and one randomized placebo-controlled study of 1,266 men with unstable angina. Therapy with aspirin was begun at intervals after the onset of acute MI varying from less than 3 days to more than 5 years and continued for periods of from less than one year to four years. In the unstable angina study, treatment was started within 1 month after the onset of unstable angina and continued for 12 weeks and complicating conditions such as congestive heart failure were not included in the study.

Aspirin therapy in MI patients was associated with about a 20 percent reduction in the risk of subsequent death and/or nonfatal reinfarction, a median absolute decrease of 3 percent from the 12 to 22 percent event rates in the placebo groups. In the aspirin-treated unstable angina patients the reduction in risk was about 50 percent, a reduction in the event rate of 5% from the 10% rate in the placebo group over the 12 weeks of the study.

Daily dosage of aspirin in the post-myocardial infarction studies was 300 mg. in one study and 900 and 1500 mg. in five studies. A dose of 325 mg. was used in the study of unstable angina.

Adverse Reactions: Gastrointestinal Reactions: Doses of 1000 mg. per day of aspirin caused gastrointestinal symptoms and bleeding that in some cases were clinically significant. In the largest postinfarction study (The Aspirin Myocardial Infarction Study (AMIS) with 4,500 people), the percentage incidences of gastrointestinal symptoms for the aspirin (1000 mg. of a standard, solid-tablet formulation) and placebo-treated subjects, respectively, were: stomach pain (14.5%; 4.4%); heartburn (11.9%; 4.8%); nausea and/or vomiting (7.6%; 2.1%); hospitalization for gastrointestinal disorder (4.9%; 3.5%). In the AMIS and other trials, aspirin treated patients had increased rates of gross gastrointestinal bleeding. Symptoms and signs of gastrointestinal irritation were not significantly increased in subjects treated for unstable angina with buffered aspirin in solution.

Cardiovascular and Biochemical: In the AMIS trial, the dosage of 1000 mg. per day of aspirin was associated with small increases in systolic blood pressure (BP) (average 1.5 to 2.1 mm) and diastolic BP (0.5 to 0.6 mm), depending upon whether maximal or last available readings were used. Blood urea nitrogen and uric acid levels were also increased, but by less than 1.0 mg%. Subjects with marked hypertension or renal insufficiency had been excluded from the trial so that the clinical importance of these observations for such subjects or for any subjects treated over more prolonged periods is not known. It is recommended that patients placed on long-term aspirin treatment, even at doses of 300 mg. per day, be seen at regular intervals to assess changes in these measurements.

References: 1. Elwood P.C., et al., "A Randomized Controlled Trial of Acetylsalicylic Acid in the Secondary Prevention of Mortality from Myocardial Infarction," British Medical Journal, 1:436–440, 1974. 2. The Coronary Drug Project Research Group, "Aspirin in Coronary Heart Disease," Journal of Chronic Disease, 29:625–642, 1976. 3. Breddin K, et al., "Secondary Prevention of Myocardial Infarction; Comparison of Acetylsalicylic Acid Phenprocoumon and Placebo," Thromb. Haemost., 41:225–236, 1979. 4. Aspirin Myocardial Infarction Study Research Group, "A Randomized, Controlled Trial of Aspirin in Persons Recovered from Myocardial Infarction," Journal American Medical Association, 243:661–669, 1980. 5. Elwood P.C., and Sweetnam, P.M., "Aspirin and Secondary Mortality after Myocardial Infarction," Lancet, pp. 1313–1315, December 22–29, 1979. 6. The Persantine-Aspirin Reinfarction Study Research Group. "Persantine and Aspirin in Coronary Heart Disease," Circulation 62:449–461, 1980. 7. Lewis H.D., et al., "Protective Effects of Aspirin Against Acute Myocardial Infarction and Death in Men with Unstable Angina, Results of a Veterans Administration Cooperative Study," New England Journal of Medicine, 309:396–403, 1983.

Administration and Dosage: Although most of the studies used dosages exceeding 300 mg., two trials used only 300 mg. and pharmacologic data indicate that this dose inhibits platelet function fully. Therefore, 300 mg. or a conventional 325 mg. aspirin dose is a reasonable, routine dose that would minimize gastrointestinal adverse reactions.

*Shown in Product Identification
Section, page 404*

**Arthritis Strength Tri–Buffered
BUFFERIN®**
[bŭf'fĕr-ĭn]
Analgesic

Composition:
Active Ingredients: Each coated caplet contains Aspirin 500 mg in a formulation buffered with Calcium Carbonate, Magnesium Oxide and Magnesium Carbonate.
Other Ingredients: Citric Acid, Corn Starch, FD&C Blue No. 1, Hydroxypropyl Methylcellulose, Mineral Oil, Polysorbate 20, Povidone, Propylene Glycol, Simethicone Emulsion, Sodium Phosphate, Sorbitan Monolaurate, Titanium Dioxide. May also contain: Benzoic Acid, Carnauba Wax, Magnesium Stearate, Sodium Lauryl Sulfate.

Action and Uses: For temporary relief from the minor aches and pains, stiffness, swelling and inflammation of arthritis. Buffered formulation helps prevent the stomach upset that plain aspirin can cause. Coated caplets for easy swallowing.

Contraindications: Hypersensitivity to any ingredient in the product.

Caution: If pain persists for more than 10 days or redness is present or in arthritic or rheumatic conditions affecting children under 12 consult physician immediately. Do not take without consulting physician if under medical care.

Warning: Children and teenagers should not use this medicine for chicken pox or flu symptoms before a doctor is consulted about Reye syndrome, a rare but serious illness reported to be associated with aspirin. KEEP THIS AND ALL MEDICINES OUT OF CHILDREN'S REACH. IN CASE OF ACCIDENTAL OVERDOSE, CONTACT A PHYSICIAN OR POISON CONTROL CENTER IMMEDIATELY. If dizziness, impaired hearing or ringing in the ears occurs, discontinue use. As with any drug, if you are pregnant or nursing a baby, seek the advice of a health professional before using this product.

Administration and Dosage: Adults: Two caplets with water every 4 hours as needed. Do not exceed 8 caplets in 24 hours, or give to children 12 or under unless directed by a physician. If dizziness, impaired hearing or ringing in the ear occurs, discontinue use.

Overdose: (Symptoms and treatment) Typical of aspirin.

How Supplied: Coated caplets in bottles of 40 and 100. The 40 caplet size does not have a child resistant closure, which is the size not recommended for households with young children. Professional samples available upon request.

Product Identification: Plain white coated caplet with "ASB" debossed on one side.

*Shown in Product Identification
Section, page 404*

**Extra Strength Tri–Buffered
BUFFERIN®**
[bŭf'fĕr-ĭn]
Analgesic

Composition:
Active Ingredients: Each coated tablet contains Aspirin 500 mg in a formulation buffered with Calcium Carbonate, Magnesium Oxide and Magnesium Carbonate.
Other Ingredients: Citric Acid, Corn Starch, FD&C Blue No.1, Hydroxypropyl Methylcellulose, Mineral Oil, Polysorbate 20, Povidone, Propylene Glycol, Simethicone Emulsion, Sodium Phosphate, Sorbitan Monolaurate, Titanium Dioxide. May also contain: Benzoic Acid, Carnauba Wax, Magnesium Stearate, Sodium Lauryl Sulfate.

Action and Uses: For relief from headaches, pain and fever of colds and flu, muscle aches, temporary relief of minor arthritis pain and inflammation, menstrual pain and toothaches. Buffered for-

	COMTREX Per Tablet or Caplet	COMTREX Liquid Per Fl. Ounce
Acetaminophen:	325 mg.	650 mg.
Pseudoephedrine HCl:	30 mg.	60 mg.
Chlorpheniramine Maleate:	2 mg.	4 mg.
Dextromethorphan Hbr:	10 mg.	20 mg.

Also Contains:	Tablet	Coated Caplets	Alcohol (20% by volume)
	Corn Starch	Carnauba Wax	Citric Acid
	D&C Yellow No. 10 Lake	Corn Starch	D&C Yellow No. 10
	Erythorbic Acid	D&C Yellow No. 10 Lake	FD&C Red No. 40
	FD&C Yellow No. 6 Lake	Erythorbic Acid	Flavors
	Magnesium Stearate	FD&C Red No. 40 Lake	Povidone
	Methylparaben	FD&C Yellow No. 6 Lake	Sodium Citrate
	Microcrystaline cellulose	Hydroxypropylmethylcellulose	Sucrose
	Povidone	Magnesium Stearate	Water
	Propylparaben	Methylparaben	
		Microcrystalline Celluose	
		Mineral Oil	
		Polysorbate 20	
		Povidone	
		Propylene Glycol	
		Propylparaben	
		Simethicone Emulsion	
		Sorbitan Monolaurate	
		Titanium Dioxide	
May Also Contain:	Polysorbate 80	Polysorbate 80	
	Silicon Dioxide	Silicon Dioxide	
	Wood Celluose	Wood Cellulose	

mulation helps prevent the stomach upset that plain aspirin can cause. Coated tablets for easy swallowing.

Contraindications: Hypersensitivity to any ingredient in the product.

Caution: If pain persists for more than 10 days, or redness is present, or in arthritic or rheumatic conditions affecting children under 12, consult a physician immediately. Do not take without consulting a physician if under medical care. Consult a dentist for toothache promptly.

Warning: Children and teenagers should not use this medicine for chicken pox or flu symptoms before a doctor is consulted about Reye syndrome, a rare but serious illness reported to be associated with aspirin. KEEP THIS AND ALL MEDICINES OUT OF CHILDREN'S REACH. IN CASE OF ACCIDENTAL OVERDOSE, CONTACT A PHYSICIAN OR POISON CONTROL CENTER IMMEDIATELY. If dizziness, impaired hearing or ringing in the ears occurs, discontinue use. As with any drug, if you are pregnant or nursing a baby, seek the advice of a health professional before using this product.

Administration and Dosage: Adults: Two tablets with water every 4 hours as needed. Do not exceed 8 tablets in 24 hours, or give to children under 12 unless directed by a physician.

Overdose: (Symptoms and treatment) Typical of aspirin.

How Supplied: Coated tablets in bottles of 30, 60 and 100. All sizes have child resistant closures except 60's (for tablets): which are sizes not recommended for households with young children. Professional samples available upon request.

Product Identification: White elongated coated tablet with "ESB" debossed on one side.
Shown in Product Identification Section, page 404

COMTREX®
[cŏm 'trĕx]
Multi-Symptom Cold Reliever

Composition: Each tablet, fluid ounce (30 ml.), and caplet contains:
[See table above].

Actions and Uses: COMTREX® contains a combination of ingredients including a non-aspirin analgesic, a decongestant, an antihistamine and a non-narcotic antitussive. COMTREX is of value in relieving the following cold symptoms when they occur together: nasal and sinus congestion, post nasal drip, coughing due to minor throat and bronchial irritation, fever, minor sore throat pain (systemically), headache, body aches and pain.

Contraindications: Hypersensitivity to any ingredient in the product.

Caution: Do not take without consulting a physician if under medical care. Do not drive a car or operate machinery while taking this cold remedy as it may cause drowsiness.

Warning: Keep this and all medicine out of children's reach. In case of accidental overdose, consult a physician or poison control center immediately. Persistent cough may indicate the presence of a serious condition. Persons with a high fever or persistent cough, or with high blood pressure, diabetes, heart or thyroid disease, asthma, glaucoma or difficulty in urination due to enlargement of the prostate gland should not use this preparation unless directed by a physician. Do not use for more than 10 days unless directed by a physician. As with any drug, if you are pregnant or nursing a baby, seek the advice of a health professional before using this product.

Administration and Dosage:
Tablets or Caplets—Adults: 2 tablets or caplets every 4 hours as needed not to exceed 12 tablets or caplets in 24 hours. Children 6–12 years: ½ the adult dose. Under 6, consult a physician.
Liquid—Adults: 1 fluid ounce (30 ml.) every 4 hours as needed, not to exceed 6 fluid ounces (180 ml.) in 24 hours. Children 6–12 years: ½ the adult dose. Under 6, consult a physician.

Overdose: For overdose treatment information, consult a regional poison control center. (Also see COMTREX A/S, Cough Formula COMTREX.

How Supplied: Tablets in blister packages of 24's and in bottles of 50's. Caplets in 16's and 36's. Liquid in 6 oz. and 10 oz. plastic bottles. All sizes packaged in child resistant closures except 24's (for tablets), 16's (for caplets) and 6 oz. (for liquid). Professional samples available on request.

Product Identification Mark: Yellow tablet with letter "C" debossed on one surface. Yellow caplet with "Comtrex" debossed on one side. Liquid is clear orange in color.
Shown in Product Identification Section, page 404

COMTREX A/S®
[cŏm 'trĕx]
Multi-Symptom Allergy/Sinus Formula

Composition: Active Ingredients: Each coated tablet or caplet contains 500 mg

Continued on next page

Bristol-Myers—Cont.

acetaminophen, 30 mg pseudoephedrine HCl, 2 mg chlorpheniramine maleate. OTHER INGREDIENTS: carnauba wax, corn starch, crospovidone, D&C yellow No. 10 lake, erythorbic acid, FD&C blue No. 1 lake, FD&C Red No. 40 lake, hydroxypropyl methylcellulose, microcrystalline cellulose, mineral oil, polysorbate 20, povidone, propylene glycol, simethicone emulsion, sodium citrate, sorbitan monolaurate, stearic acid, titanium dioxide. May also contain: polysorbate 80, silicon dioxide, wood cellulose.

Action and Uses: COMTREX A/S tablets contains a combination of three ingredients. A maximum dose of non-aspirin analgesic acetaminophen to relieve headache. A decongestant pseudoephedrine HCl to clear nasal and sinus passages and to reduce swollen nasal and sinus tissues. An antihistamine chlorpheniramine maleate to relieve itchy, watery eyes, sneezing, runny nose.

Contraindications: Hypersensitivity to any ingredient in the product.

Warnings: KEEP THIS AND ALL MEDICINE OUT OF CHILDREN'S REACH. In case of accidental overdose, consult a physician or Poison Control Center immediately. Do not give to children under 12 or exceed recommended dosage. Reduce dosage if nervousness, restlessness or sleeplessness occurs. Do not use for more than 10 days unless directed by a physician. Do not take without consulting a physician if under medical care. Individuals with high blood pressure, diabetes, heart or thyroid disease, asthma, glaucoma, or difficulty in urination due to enlargement of the prostate gland should not take this preparation unless directed by a physician. As with any drug, if you are pregnant or nursing a baby, seek the advice of a health professional before using this product. Do not drive or operate machinery while taking this medicine as it may cause drowsiness.

Administration and Dosage: Adults, two tablets or caplets every 6 hours, as needed, not to exceed 8 tablets or caplets in 24 hours.

Overdose: For overdose treatment information, consult a regional poison control center. (See COMTREX Tablets, Caplets and Liquid Cough Formula COMTREX).

How Supplied: Tablets in blister packages of 24's and in bottles of 50's. Caplets in blister packages of 16's and in bottles of 36's. Tablets 24's and caplets 16's do not have child resistant closures.

Product Identification: Tablets green imprinted "Comtrex A/S."
Caplets green with "A/S" debossed on one surface.
Shown in Product Identification Section, page 404

CONGESPIRIN® for Children COUGH SYRUP
[con "gĕs 'pir-in]

Composition: Each 5 ml teaspoon contains Dextromethorphan hydrobromide —5 mg. Also Contains: Benzoic Acid, Citric Acid, D&C Yellow #10, FD&C Red #40, Flavor, Sodium Citrate, Sorbitol, Sucrose, Water.

Actions and Uses: Contains a non-narcotic antitussive comparable in potency to codeine, in an orange flavored syrup. Reduces coughs due to colds and to minor throat irritations.

Warning: Do not administer without consulting a physician if child is under medical care. Persistent cough may indicate the presence of a serious condition. Children with a cough persisting for more than 10 days, with high fever, or with fever lasting more than 3 days should not be given this preparation unless directed by a physician. Do not administer to children under two years of age, except as directed by physician. KEEP THIS AND ALL MEDICINES OUT OF THE REACH OF CHILDREN.

Administration and Dosage: Children 2–5, one teaspoon every 4 hours as needed. Do not exceed 6 teaspoons in 24 hours. Children 6–12, two teaspoons every 4 hours as needed. Do not exceed 12 teaspoons in 24 hours.

Overdose: For overdose treatment information, consult a regional poison control center. See also: Congespirin for Children Aspirin Free Chewable Cold Tablets and Congespirin for Children Aspirin Free Liquid Cold Medicine.

How Supplied: Available in 3 oz plastic bottles.

Product Identification: Clear Orange Liquid.
Shown in Product Identification Section, page 404

CONGESPIRIN® for Children Aspirin Free Chewable Cold Tablets
[cŏn "gĕs 'pir-in]

Composition: Each tablet contains acetaminophen 81 mg. (1¼ grains), phenylephrine hydrochloride 1¼ mg. Also Contains: Calcium Stearate, Ethyl Cellulose, FD&C Yellow No. 6 Aluminum Lake, Flavor, Mannitol, Microcrystalline Cellulose, Polyethylene, Saccharin Calcium, Sucrose.

Action and Uses: A non-aspirin analgesic/nasal decongestant to temporarily reduce fever and relieve aches, pains and nasal congestion associated with colds and flu.

Warnings: KEEP THIS AND ALL MEDICINES OUT OF CHILDREN'S REACH. IN CASE OF ACCIDENTAL OVERDOSE, CONTACT A PHYSICIAN IMMEDIATELY.

Caution: If child is under medical care, do not administer without consulting physician. Do not exceed recommended dosage. Consult your physician if symp-

toms persist or if high fever, high blood pressure, heart disease, diabetes or thyroid disease is present. Do not administer for more than 10 days unless directed by physician.

Dosage and Administration: Under 2, consult your physician.
2–3 years	2 tablets
4–5 years	3 tablets
6–8 years	4 tablets
9–10 years	5 tablets
11–12 years	6 tablets
Over 12 years	8 tablets

Repeat dose in four hours if necessary. Do not give more than four doses per day unless prescribed by your physician.

Overdose: For overdose treatment information consult a regional poison control center. See also: Congespirin for Children Aspirin Free Liquid Cold Medicine and Congespirin for Children Cough Syrup.

Product Identification: Scored orange tablet with "C" on one side.

How Supplied: Tablets, in bottles of 24.
Shown in Product Identification Section, page 404

CONGESPIRIN® for Children Aspirin Free Liquid Cold Medicine
[con "gĕs 'pir-in]

Composition: Each 5 ml. teaspoon contains Acetaminophen 130 mg., Phenylpropanolamine Hydrochloride 6 ¼ mg. Also Contains: Alcohol (10% by volume), Citric Acid, FD&C Red No. 40, Flavor, Methylparaben, Polyethylene Glycol, Povidone, Sodium Citrate, Sucrose, Water.

Action and Uses: An effective aspirin free analgesic and nasal decongestant that temporarily reduces fever and relieves aches, pains and nasal congestion associated with colds and "flu."

Dosage and Administration:
Children 3–5, 1 teaspoon every 3–4 hours.
Children 6–12, 2 teaspoons every 3–4 hours.
Children under 3 years use only as directed by your physician.
Do not give more than 4 doses a day unless directed by your physician.

Caution: If child is under medical care, do not administer without consulting physician. Do not exceed recommended dosage. Consult your physician if symptoms persist or if high fever, high blood pressure, heart disease, diabetes or thyroid disease is present. Do not administer for more than 10 days unless directed by your physician.

Warning: KEEP THIS AND ALL MEDICINES OUT OF CHILDREN'S REACH. IN CASE OF ACCIDENTAL OVERDOSAGE, CONTACT A PHYSICIAN IMMEDIATELY.

Overdose: For overdose treatment information, consult a regional poison control center. See also: Congespirin for Children Aspirin Free Chewable Cold

Tablets and Congespirin for Children Cough Syrup.

How Supplied: In 3 oz. plastic, unbreakable bottles.

Product Identification: Clear red liquid.

Shown in Product Identification Section, page 404

Extra–Strength DATRIL®
[dā′trĭl]
Analgesic

Composition: Each tablet or caplet contains acetaminophen, 500 mg. Tablets Also Contain: Corn Starch, Stearic Acid.
May Also Contain: Croscamellose Sodium, Povidone, Silicon Dioxide, Sodium Lauryl Sulfate, Wood Cellulose.
Caplets Also Contain: Carnauba Wax, Corn Starch, FD&C Blue No. 1, Hydroxypropyl Methylcellulose, Mineral Oil, Polysorbate 20, Povidone, Propylene Glycol, Simethicone Emulsion, Sorbitan Monolaurate, Stearic Acid, Titanium Dioxide. May also contain: Croscarmellose Sodium, Crospovidone, Erythorbic Acid, Methylparaben, Propylparaben, Silicon Dioxide, Sodium Lauryl Sulfate, Wood Cellulose.

Actions and Uses: Extra-Strength DATRIL contains non-aspirin acetaminophen which is less likely to irritate the stomach than plain aspirin. Extra-Strength DATRIL is intended for the temporary relief of minor aches, pains, headaches and fever. For most persons with peptic ulcer Extra-Strength DATRIL may be used when taken as directed for recommended conditions.

Contraindications: There have been rare reports of skin rash or glossitis attributed to acetaminophen. Discontinue use if a sensitivity reaction occurs. However, acetaminophen is usually well tolerated by aspirin-sensitive patients.

Caution: Severe or recurrent pain or high or continued fever may be indicative of serious illness. Under these conditions consult a physician. Do not take without consulting a physician if under medical care.

Warning: Do not give to children 12 and under or use for more than 10 days unless directed by a physician. KEEP THIS AND ALL MEDICINES OUT OF REACH OF CHILDREN. IN CASE OF ACCIDENTAL OVERDOSE CONTACT A PHYSICIAN IMMEDIATELY. As with any drug, if you are pregnant or nursing a baby, seek the advice of a health professional before using this product.

Dosage: Adults: Two tablets or caplets. May be repeated in 4 hours if needed. Do not exceed 8 tablets or caplets in any 24 hour period.

Overdose:
MUCOMYST (acetylcysteine) As An Antidote For Acetaminophen Overdose)

Actions: Acetaminophen is rapidly absorbed from the upper gastrointestinal tract with peak plasma levels occurring between 30 and 60 minutes after therapeutic doses and usually within 4 hours following an overdose. The parent compound, which is nontoxic, is extensively metabolized in the liver to form principally the sulfate and glucuronide conjugates which are also nontoxic and are rapidly excreted in the urine. A small fraction of an ingested dose is metabolized in the liver by the cytochrome P-450 mixed function oxidase enzyme system to form a reactive, potentially toxic, intermediate metabolite which preferentially conjugates with hepatic glutathione to form the nontoxic cysteine and mercapturic acid derivatives which are then excreted by the kidney. Therapeutic doses of acetaminophen do not saturate the glucuronide and sulfate conjugation pathways and do not result in the formation of sufficient reactive metabolite to deplete glutathione stores. However, following ingestion of a large overdose (150 mg/kg or greater) the glucuronide and sulfate conjugation pathways are saturated resulting in a larger fraction of the drug being metabolized via the P-450 pathway. The increased formation of reactive metabolite may deplete the hepatic stores of glutathione with subsequent binding of the metabolite to protein molecules within the hepatocyte resulting in cellular necrosis. Acetylcysteine has been shown to reduce the extent of liver injury following acetaminophen overdose.
Early symptoms following a potentially hepatotoxic overdose may include: nausea, vomiting, diaphoresis and general malaise. Clinical and laboratory evidence of hepatic toxicity may not be apparent until 48 to 72 hours postingestion. In adults and adolescents, regardless of the quantity of acetaminophen reported to have been ingested, administer MUCOMYST® acetylcysteine immediately. MUCOMYST acetylcysteine therapy should be initiated and continued for a full course of therapy. Its effectiveness depends on early administration, with benefit seen principally in patients treated within 16 hours of the overdose.
If acetaminophen plasma assay capability is not available, and the estimated acetaminophen ingestion exceeds 150 mg/kg, MUCOMYST acetylcysteine therapy should be initiated and continued for a full course of therapy.
For full prescribing information, refer to the MUCOMYST package insert. Do not await the results of assays for acetaminophen level before initiating treatment with MUCOMYST acetylcysteine. The following additional procedures are recommended: The stomach should be emptied promptly by lavage or by induction of emesis with syrup of ipecac. A serum acetaminophen assay should be obtained as early as possible, but no sooner than four hours following ingestion. Liver function studies should be obtained initially and repeated at 24-hour intervals.

For additional emergency information call your regional poison center or toll-free (1-800-525-6115) to the Rocky Mountain Poison Center for assistance in diagnosis and for directions in the use of MUCOMYST acetylcysteine as an antidote.

How Supplied: Tablets in bottles of 30's, 60's and 100's. Caplets in bottles of 24's and 50's. All sizes packaged in child resistant closures except 50 caplet size and 60 tablet size.

Product Identification Mark: White tablet with "DATRIL" debossed on one surface. White caplet with "DATRIL" debossed on one side.

Shown in Product Identification Section, page 404

EXCEDRIN® Extra-Strength
Analgesic
[ĕx″cĕd′rĭn]

Composition: Each tablet or caplet contains Acetaminophen 250 mg.; Aspirin 250 mg.; and Caffeine 65 mg. Tablets Also Contain: Microcrystalline Cellulose, Stearic Acid. Caplets Also Contain: Carnauba Wax, FD&C Blue No. 1, Hydoxypropyl Methylcellulose, Microcrystalline Cellulose, Mineral Oil, Polysorbate 20, Povidone, Propylene Glycol, Simethicone Emulsion, Sorbitan Monolaurate, Stearic Acid, Titanium Dioxide, Hydroxypropylcellulose.

Action and Uses: Extra-Strength EXCEDRIN is intended for the relief of pain from: headache, sinusitis, colds or 'flu', muscular aches and menstrual discomfort. Also recommended for temporary relief of toothaches and minor arthritic pains.

Contraindications: Hypersensitivity to any ingredient in the product.

Caution: If pain persists for more than 10 days, or if redness is present, or in arthritic conditions affecting children under 12, consult physician immediately. Consult dentist for toothache promptly. Do not take without consulting physician if under medical care. Store at room temperature.

Warning: Children and teenagers should not use this medicine for chicken pox or flu symptoms before a doctor is consulted about Reye syndrome, a rare but serious illness reported to be associated with aspirin. Do not exceed 8 tablets or caplets in 24 hours or use for more than 10 days unless directed by physician, or give to children under 12. KEEP THIS AND ALL MEDICINES OUT OF CHILDREN'S REACH. IN CASE OF ACCIDENTAL OVERDOSE, CONTACT A PHYSICIAN IMMEDIATELY. As with any drug, if you are pregnant or nursing a baby, seek the advice of a health professional before using this product.

Administration and Dosage: Tablets or Caplets—Individuals 12 and over,

Continued on next page

Bristol-Myers—Cont.

take 2 tablets or caplets every 4 hours as needed. Do not exceed 8 tablets or caplets in any 24 hour period.

Overdose: For overdose treatment information, consult a regional poison control center.

How Supplied: Bottles of 12, 30, 60, 100, 165 and 225 tablets. Caplets in bottles of 24's, 50's and 80's. A metal tin of 12 tablets. All sizes packaged in child resistant closures except 100's (for tablets); 80's (for caplets).

Product Identification Mark: White, circular tablet with letter "E" debossed on one side. White caplets with "Excedrin" printed in red on one side.
Shown in Product Identification Section, page 405

EXCEDRIN P.M.®
[ĕx ″cĕd ′rĭn]
Analgesic/Sleeping Aid

Composition: Each tablet or caplet contains Acetaminophen 500 mg. and Diphenhydramine citrate 38 mg. Tablets also Contain: Corn Starch Pregelatinized, D&C Yellow No. 10, D&C Yellow No. 10 Aluminum Lake, FD&C Blue No. 1, FD&C Blue No. 1 Aluminum Lake, Magnesium Stearate, Methylparaben, Microcrystalline Cellulose, Povidone, Propylparaben, Stearic Acid.
Caplets also Contain: Benzoic Acid; Carauba Wax; Corn Starch; D&C Yellow No. 10; D&C Yellow No. 10 Aluminum Lake; FD&C Blue No. 1; FD&C Blue No. 1 Aluminum Lake; Hydroxypropyl Methylcellulose; Methylparaben; Magnesium Stearate; Propylene Glycol; Propylparaben; Simethicone Emulsion; Stearic Acid; Titanium Dioxide.

Action and Uses: For the temporary relief of occasional headaches and minor aches and pains with accompanying sleeplessness. Also for fever with accompanying sleeplessness.

Contraindications: Hypersensitivity to any ingredient in the product.

Caution: Do not drive a car or operate machinery while taking this medication. Do not take without consulting physician if under medical care.

Warning: KEEP THIS AND ALL MEDICINES OUT OF CHILDREN'S REACH. IN CASE OF ACCIDENTAL OVERDOSE, CONTACT A PHYSICIAN IMMEDIATELY. Do not give to children under 12 years of age or use for more than 10 days unless directed by a physician. Consult your physician if symptoms persist or new ones occur or if fever persists more than 3 days (72 hours) or recurs or if sleeplessness persists continuously for more than two weeks. Insomnia may be a symptom of serious underlying medical illness. Take this product with caution if alcohol is being consumed. DO NOT TAKE THIS PRODUCT IF YOU HAVE ASTHMA, GLAUCOMA OR ENLARGEMENT OF THE PROSTATE GLAND EXCEPT UNDER THE ADVICE AND SUPERVISION OF A PHYSICIAN. As with any drug, if you are pregnant or nursing a baby, seek the advice of a health professional before using this product.

Administration and Dosage: Adults take two tablets at bedtime or as directed by a physician. Do not exceed recommended dosage.

Overdose: For overdose treatment information, consult a regional poison control center.

How Supplied: Bottles of 10, 30, 50, and 80 tablets. Caplets in bottles of 30's and 50's. All sizes packaged in child resistant closures except 50's, which is a size not recommended for households with young children.

Product Identification Mark: Blue/green circular tablet with letters "PM" debossed on one side. Light blue caplet with "Excedrin PM" imprinted on one side.
Shown in Product Identification Section, page 405

Sinus EXCEDRIN®
[ex ″cĕd ′rĭn]
Analgesic, Decongestant

Composition: Each coated tablet or caplet contains 500 mg Acetaminophen and 30 mg Pseudoephedrine HCl.

Other Ingredients: Corn Starch, D&C Yellow No. 10, FD&C Red No. 40 Lake, Hydroxypropylcellulose, Hydroxpropyl Methylcellulose, Mineral Oil, Polysorbate 20, Povidone, Propylene Glycol, Simethicone Emulsion, Sorbitan Monolaurate, Stearic Acid, Titanium Dioxide. May also contain: Carnauba Wax.

Action and Uses: Sinus EXCEDRIN is intended for the temporary relief of headache and sinus pain and for the relief of sinus pressure due to sinusitis or the common cold.

Contraindications: Hypersensitivity to any ingredient in the product.

Warnings: KEEP THIS AND ALL MEDICINES OUT OF CHILDREN'S REACH. In case of accidental overdose, consult a physician or Poison Control Center immediately. Do not exceed recommended dosage. Reduce dosage if nervousness, dizziness or sleeplessness occurs. Do not take this product for more than 7 days. If symptoms do not improve or are accompanied by a fever, consult a doctor. If you have heart disease, diabetes, high blood pressure, thyroid disease or difficulty in urination due to enlargement of the prostate gland, or are presently taking a prescription drug for high blood pressure or depression, do not take this medicine unless directed by a physician. As with any drug, if you are pregnant or nursing a baby, seek the advice of a health professional before using this product.

Administration and Dosage: Adults and Children over 12: two tablets or caplets every 6 hours as needed, not to exceed 8 tablets or caplets in 24 hours. Children 12 and under should use only as directed by a doctor.

How Supplied: Bottles of 50's and Blister Pack 24's. Bottles have a child resistant closure.

Product Identification Mark: Orange caplets and circular orange tablets have "Sinus Excedrin" imprinted in green on one side.
Shown in Product Identification Section, page 405

4-WAY® Cold Tablets

Composition: Each tablet contains aspirin 324 mg., phenylpropanolamine HCl 12½ mg., and chlorpheniramine maleate 2 mg. Also Contains: Corn Starch, Corn Starch Pregelatinized, D&C Red No. 30 Lake, Lactose.

Action and Uses: For temporary relief of minor aches and pains, fever, nasal congestion and runny nose as may occur in the common cold.

Dosage and Administration:
Adults—2 tablets every 4 hours, if needed. Do not exceed 8 tablets in 24 hours. Children 6–12 years—1 tablet every 4 hours. Do not exceed 4 tablets in 24 hours. Under age 6, consult a physician.

Caution: This preparation may cause drowsiness. Do not drive or operate machinery while taking this medication.

Warning: Children and teenagers should not use this medicine for chicken pox or flu symptoms before a doctor is consulted about Reye syndrome, a rare but serious illness reported to be associated with aspirin. KEEP THIS AND ALL MEDICINES OUT OF CHILDREN'S REACH. IN CASE OF ACCIDENTAL OVERDOSE, CONTACT A PHYSICIAN IMMEDIATELY. Do not exceed recommended dosage or use for more than 10 days unless directed by a physician. Individuals with high blood pressure, diabetes, heart or thyroid disease, asthma, glaucoma or difficulty in urination due to enlargement of the prostate gland should not use this preparation unless directed by a physician. Do not take without consulting a physician if under medical care. As with any drug, if you are pregnant or nursing a baby, seek the advice of a health professional before using this product.

Overdose: For overdose treatment information, consult a regional poison control center.

How Supplied: Bottles of 36's and 60's.

Product Identification Mark: Pink and White tablet with number "4" debossed on pink surface.
Shown in Product Identification Section, page 405

4–WAY® Fast Acting Nasal Spray

Composition: Phenylephrine hydrochloride 0.5%, naphazoline hydrochloride 0.05%, pyrilamine maleate 0.2%, in a buffered isotonic aqueous solution with thimerosal, 0.005% added as a preservative. Also contains: Benzalkonium Chloride, Poloxamer 188, Potassium Phosphate, Sodium Chloride, Sodium Phosphate, Water. Also available in a **mentholated formula** containing Phenylephrine hydrochloride 0.5%, naphazoline hydrochloride 0.05%, pyrilamine maleate 0.2%, in a buffered isotonic aqueous solution with thimerosal 0.005% added as a preservative. Also Contains: Benzalkonium Chloride, Camphor, Eucalyptol, Menthol, Poloxamer 188, Polysorbate 80, Potassium Phosphate, Sodium Chloride, Sodium Phosphate, Water.

Action and Uses: For prompt, temporary relief of nasal congestion due to the common cold, sinusitis, hay fever or other upper respiratory allergies.

Dosage and Administration: With head in a normal upright position, put atomizer tip into nostril. Squeeze atomizer with firm, quick pressure while inhaling. Adults spray twice into each nostril. Repeat in six hours, if needed. Do not give to children under 12 years of age unless directed by a doctor.

Warning: KEEP OUT OF CHILDREN'S REACH. Overdosage in young children may cause marked sedation. Do not exceed recommended dosage because symptoms may occur such as burning, stinging, sneezing or increase of nasal discharge. Follow directions carefully. Do not use this product for more than 3 days. If symptoms persist, consult physician. The use of this dispenser by more than one person may spread infection.

Overdosage: For overdose treatment information, consult a regional poison control center.

How Supplied: Atomizers of ½ fluid ounce and 1 fluid ounce.
Metered pump of ½ fluid ounce.
Shown in Product Identification Section, page 405

4–WAY® Long Acting Nasal Spray

Composition: Oxymetazoline Hydrochloride 0.05% in a buffered isotonic aqueous solution. Phenylmercuric Acetate 0.002% added as a preservative. Also Contains: Benzalkonium Chloride, Glycine, Sorbitol Water.

Action and Uses: Provides temporary relief of nasal congestion due to the common cold, sinusitis, hayfever or other upper respiratory allergies.

Dosage and Administration: With head in a normal upright position, put atomizer tip into nostril. Squeeze atomizer with firm, quick pressure while inhaling. Adults: Spray 2 or 3 times in each nostril twice daily—once in the morning and once in the evening. Not recommended for children under 6.

Warning: KEEP OUT OF CHILDREN'S REACH. For adult use only. Do not give this product to children under 6 years of age except under the advice and supervision of a physician. Do not exceed recommended dosage because symptoms may occur such as burning, stinging, sneezing, or an increase of nasal discharge. Do not use this product for more than 3 days. If symptoms persist, consult a physician. The use of this dispenser by more than one person may spread infection.

Overdosage: For overdose treatment information, consult a regional poison control center.

How Supplied: Metered pump and Atomizers of ½ fluid ounce.
Shown in Product Identification Section, page 405

NO DOZ® Fast Acting Keep Alert Tablets

[nō´dōz]

Composition: Each tablet contains 100 mg. Caffeine. Also Contains: Flavors, Mannitol, Microcrystalline Cellulose, Stearic Acid, Sucrose.

Action and Uses: Helps restore mental alertness.

Dosage and Administration:
For Adults: 2 tablets initially, thereafter, 1 tablet every three hours should be sufficient.

Caution: Do not take without consulting physician if under medical care. No stimulant should be substituted for normal sleep in activities requiring physical alertness.

Warning: For occasional use only. Not intended for use as a substitute for sleep. If fatigue or drowsiness persists or continues to recur, consult a doctor. The recommended dose of this product contains about as much caffeine as a cup of coffee. Limit the use of caffeine-containing medications, foods, or beverages while taking this product because too much caffeine may cause nervousness, irritability, sleeplessness and, occasionally, rapid heart beat. Do not give to children under 12 years of age. KEEP THIS AND ALL MEDICINES OUT OF THE REACH OF CHILDREN. As with any drug, if you are pregnant or nursing a baby, seek the advice of a health professional before using this product.

Overdose: Typical of caffeine.

How Supplied: Carded 15's and 36's and bottles of 60's.

Product Identification Mark: Circular white tablet with "No Doz" debossed on one side.
Shown in Product Identification Section, page 405

NUPRIN®
(ibuprofen)
Analgesic

Warning: ASPIRIN SENSITIVE PATIENTS should not take this product if they have had a severe allergic reaction to aspirin, e.g.—asthma, swelling, shock or hives, because even though this product contains no aspirin or salicylates, cross-reactions may occur in patients allergic to aspirin.

Composition: Each coated tablet or caplet contains ibuprofen USP, 200 mg.
Other Ingredients: Carnauba wax, cornstarch, D&C Yellow No. 10, FD&C Yellow No. 6, hydroxypropyl methylcellulose, propyleneglycol, silicon dioxide, stearic acid, titanium dioxide.

Action and Uses: For the temporary relief of minor aches and pains associated with the common cold, headache, toothache, muscular aches, backache, for the minor pain of arthritis, for the pain of menstrual cramps and for reduction of fever.

Warnings: The following warnings are stated on the Nuprin label: Do not take for pain for more than 10 days or for fever for more than 3 days unless directed by a doctor. If pain or fever persists or gets worse, if new symptoms occur, or if the painful area is red or swollen, consult a doctor. These could be signs of serious illness. If you are under a doctor's care for any serious condition, consult a doctor before taking this product. As with aspirin and acetaminophen, if you have any condition which requires you to take prescription drugs or if you have had any problems or serious side effects from taking any non-prescription pain reliever, do not take NUPRIN without first discussing it with your doctor. If you experience any symptoms which are unusual or seem unrelated to the condition for which you took ibuprofen, consult a doctor before taking any more of it. Although ibuprofen is indicated for the same conditions as aspirin and acetaminophen, it should not be taken with them except under a doctor's direction. Do not combine this product with any other ibuprofen—containing product. As with any drug, if you are pregnant or nursing a baby, seek the advice of a health professional before using this product. IT IS ESPECIALLY IMPORTANT NOT TO USE IBUPROFEN DURING THE LAST 3 MONTHS OF PREGNANCY UNLESS SPECIFICALLY DIRECTED TO DO SO BY A DOCTOR BECAUSE IT MAY CAUSE PROBLEMS IN THE UNBORN CHILD OR COMPLICATIONS DURING DELIVERY. Keep this and all drugs out of the reach of children. In case of accidental overdose, seek professional assistance or contact a poison control center immediately.

Caution: Store at room temperature. Avoid excessive heat 40°C (104°F).

Continued on next page

Bristol-Myers—Cont.

Administration and Dosage:
Directions. Adults: Take 1 tablet or caplet every 4 to 6 hours while symptoms persist. If pain or fever does not respond to 1 tablet or caplet, 2 tablets or caplets may be used but do not exceed 6 tablets or caplets in 24 hours, unless directed by a doctor. The smallest effective dose should be used. Take with food or milk if occasional and mild heartburn, upset stomach, or stomach pain occurs with use. Consult a doctor if these symptoms are more than mild or if they persist. Children: Do not give this product to children under 12 except under the advice and supervision of a doctor.

Overdosage: For overdose treatment information, consult a regional poison control center.
How Supplied: Tablets in bottles of: Trial size 8, 24's, 50's, 100's and 150's. Caplets in bottles of: 24's, and 100's.

Product Identification: Golden yellow round tablet with "NUPRIN" 200 printed in black on one side. Golden yellow caplet with "Nuprin" printed in black on one side.
Distributed by Bristol-Myers Company
Shown in Product Identification Section, page 405

PAZO® Hemorrhoid Ointment/Suppositories

Composition:
Ointment: Triolyte®, [Bristol-Myers brand of the combination of benzocaine (0.8%) and ephedrine sulphate (0.2%)]; zinc oxide (4.0%); camphor (2.18%). Also Contains: Lanolin, Petrolatum.

Suppositories (per suppository): Triolyte® [Bristol-Myers brand of the combination of benzocaine (15.44 mg) and ephedrine sulfate (3.86 mg)]; zinc oxide (77.2 mg); camphor (42.07 mg). Also Contains: Hydrogenated Vegetable Oil.

Action and Uses: Pazo helps shrink swelling of inflamed hemorrhoid tissue. Provides prompt, temporary relief of burning itch and pain in many cases.

Administration:
Ointment—Apply Pazo well up in rectum night and morning, and after each bowel movement. Repeat as often during the day as may be necessary to maintain comfort. Continue for one week after symptoms subside. When applicator is used, lubricate applicator first with Pazo. Insert slowly, then simply press tube.
Suppositories—Remove foil and insert one Pazo suppository night and morning, and after each bowel movement. Repeat as often during the day as may be necessary to maintain comfort. Continue for one week after symptoms subside.

Warning: If the underlying condition persists or recurs frequently, despite treatment, or if any bleeding or hard irreducible swelling is present, consult your physician.

Keep out of children's reach. Keep in a cool place.

How Supplied:
Ointment—1-ounce and 2-ounce tubes with plastic applicator.
Suppositories—Boxes of 12 and 24 wrapped in silver foil.
Shown in Product Identification Section, page 405

Burroughs Wellcome Co.
**3030 CORNWALLIS ROAD
RESEARCH TRIANGLE PARK,
NC 27709**

**ACTIDIL® Syrup
ACTIDIL® Tablets**
[ăk 'tuh-dĭl]

Syrup
Active Ingredients: Each 5 ml (1 teaspoonful) contains triprolidine hydrochloride 1.25 mg.

Inactive Ingredients: alcohol 4%; methylparaben 0.1% and sodium benzoate 0.1% (added as preservatives), FD&C Yellow No. 6, flavor, glycerin, purified water, and sorbitol.
Store at 15°–30°C (59°–86°F) and protect from light.

Tablets
Active Ingredients: Each scored tablet contains triprolidine hydrochloride 2.5 mg.

Inactive Ingredients: Corn and potato starch, lactose, magnesium stearate.
Store at 15°–30°C (59°–86°F) in a dry place and protect from light.

Indications: For the temporary relief of running nose, sneezing, itching of the nose or throat and itchy and watery eyes as may occur in allergic rhinitis (such as hay fever).

Directions: Tablets: Adults and children 12 years of age and over, 1 tablet every 4 to 6 hours. Children 6 to under 12 years of age, ½ tablet every 4 to 6 hours. Children under 6 years of age, consult a physician. Do not exceed 4 doses in 24 hours.
Syrup: Adults and children 12 years of age and over, 2 teaspoonfuls every 4 to 6 hours. Children 6 to under 12 years of age, 1 teaspoonful every 4 to 6 hours. Children under 6 years of age, consult a physician. Do not exceed 4 doses in 24 hours.

Warnings: May cause excitability especially in children. May cause drowsiness. Do not take this product if you have asthma, glaucoma or difficulty in urination due to enlargement of the prostate gland except under the advice and supervision of a physician. Do not give this product to children under 6 years except under the advice and supervision of a physician. As with any drug, if you are pregnant or nursing a baby, seek the advice of a health professional before using this product.

Caution: Avoid driving a motor vehicle or operating heavy machinery. Avoid

alcoholic beverages while taking this product.
KEEP THIS AND ALL DRUGS OUT OF THE REACH OF CHILDREN. In case of accidental overdose, seek professional assistance or contact a Poison Control Center immediately.

How Supplied: Tablets, bottle of 100; Syrup, 1 pint.
Shown in Product Identification Section, page 405

ACTIFED® Capsules
[ăk 'tuh-fĕd]

Indications: For temporary relief of nasal congestion due to the common cold, hay fever or other upper respiratory allergies. Helps decongest sinus openings, sinus passages. For temporary relief of running nose, sneezing, itching of the nose or throat and itchy and watery eyes as may occur in allergic rhinitis (such as hay fever).

Directions: Adults and children 12 years of age and over, 1 capsule every 4 to 6 hours. Do not exceed 4 capsules in a 24 hour period. Children under 12 years of age, consult a physician.

Warnings: May cause excitability especially in children. Do not give this product to children under 12 years except under the advice and supervision of a physician. May cause drowsiness. Do not exceed recommended dosage because at higher doses nervousness, dizziness or sleeplessness may occur. If symptoms do not improve within 7 days or are accompanied by high fever, consult a physician before continuing use. Do not take this product if you have high blood pressure, heart disease, diabetes, thyroid disease, asthma, glaucoma or difficulty in urination due to enlargement of the prostate gland except under the advice and supervision of a physician. As with any drug, if you are pregnant or nursing a baby, seek the advice of a health professional before using this product.

Drug Interaction Precaution: Do not take this product if you are presently taking a prescription antihypertensive or antidepressant drug containing a monoamine oxidase inhibitor except under the advice and supervision of a physician.

Caution: Avoid driving a motor vehicle or operating heavy machinery. Avoid alcoholic beverages while taking this product.
KEEP THIS AND ALL DRUGS OUT OF THE REACH OF CHILDREN. In case of accidental overdose, seek professional assistance or contact a Poison Control Center immediately.

Active Ingredients: Each capsule contains pseudoephedrine hydrochloride 60 mg and triprolidine hydrochloride 2.5 mg.

Inactive Ingredients: Corn starch and magnesium stearate. The capsule shell consists of gelatin, D&C Yellow No. 10, FD&C Yellow No. 6 and titanium dioxide. May contain one or more parab-

ens. Printed with edible black ink. Store at 15°–30°C (59°–86°F) in a dry place and protect from light.

How Supplied: Boxes of 10, 20.
Shown in Product Identification Section, page 405

ACTIFED® 12–Hour Capsules
[ăk 'tuh-fĕd]

Indications: For temporary relief of nasal congestion due to the common cold, hay fever or other upper respiratory allergies. Helps decongest sinus openings, sinus passages. For temporary relief of running nose, sneezing, itching of the nose or throat and itchy and watery eyes as may occur in allergic rhinitis (such as hay fever).

Directions: Adults and children 12 years of age and over—One capsule every 12 hours. Do not exceed two capsules in a 24 hour period. Children under 12 years of age, consult a physician.

Warnings: May cause excitability especially in children. Do not give this product to children under 12 years except under the advice and supervision of a physician. May cause drowsiness. Do not exceed recommended dosage because at higher doses nervousness, dizziness or sleeplessness may occur. If symptoms do not improve within 7 days or are accompanied by high fever, consult a physician before continuing use. Do not take this product if you have high blood pressure, heart disease, diabetes, thyroid disease, asthma, glaucoma or difficulty in urination due to enlargement of the prostate gland except under the advice and supervision of a physician. As with any drug, if you are pregnant or nursing a baby, seek the advice of a health professional before using this product.

Drug Interaction Precaution: Do not take this product if you are presently taking a prescription antihypertensive or antidepressant drug containing a monoamine oxidase inhibitor except under the advice and supervision of a physician.

Caution: Avoid driving a motor vehicle or operating heavy machinery. Avoid alcoholic beverages while taking this product.
KEEP THIS AND ALL DRUGS OUT OF THE REACH OF CHILDREN. In case of accidental overdose, seek professional assistance or contact a Poison Control Center immediately.

Active Ingredients: Each capsule contains pseudoephedrine hydrochloride 120 mg and triprolidine hydrochloride 5 mg.

Inactive Ingredients: Corn starch, D&C Yellow No. 10, sucrose, and other ingredients. The capsule shell consists of gelatin, D&C Yellow No. 10, FD&C Yellow No. 6, and titanium dioxide. May contain one or more parabens. Printed with edible black ink.
Store at 15°–25°C (59°–77°F) in a dry place and protect from light.

How Supplied: Boxes of 10, 20.
Shown in Product Identification Section, page 406

ACTIFED® Syrup
[ăk 'tuh-fĕd]

Indications: For temporary relief of nasal congestion due to the common cold, hay fever or other upper respiratory allergies. Helps decongest sinus openings, sinus passages. For temporary relief of running nose, sneezing, itching of the nose or throat and itchy and watery eyes as may occur in allergic rhinitis (such as hay fever).

Directions: Adults and children 12 years of age and over, 2 teaspoonfuls every 4 to 6 hours. Children 6 to under 12 years of age, 1 teaspoonful every 4 to 6 hours. Children under 6 years of age, consult a physician. Do not exceed 4 doses in 24 hours.

Warnings: May cause excitability especially in children. Do not give this product to children under 6 years except under the advice and supervision of a physician. May cause drowsiness. Do not exceed recommended dosage because at higher doses nervousness, dizziness or sleeplessness may occur. If symptoms do not improve within 7 days or are accompanied by high fever, consult a physician before continuing use. Do not take this product if you have high blood pressure, heart disease, diabetes, thyroid disease, asthma, glaucoma or difficulty in urination due to enlargement of the prostate gland except under the advice and supervision of a physician. As with any drug, if you are pregnant or nursing a baby, seek the advice of a health professional before using this product.

Drug Interaction Precaution: Do not take this product if you are presently taking a prescription antihypertensive or antidepressant drug containing a monoamine oxidase inhibitor except under the advice and supervision of a physician.

Caution: Avoid driving a motor vehicle or operating heavy machinery. Avoid alcoholic beverages while taking this product.
KEEP THIS AND ALL DRUGS OUT OF THE REACH OF CHILDREN. In case of accidental overdose, seek professional assistance or contact a Poison Control Center immediately.

Active Ingredients: Each 5 ml (1 teaspoonful) contains pseudoephedrine hydrochloride 30 mg and triprolidine hydrochloride 1.25 mg.

Inactive Ingredients: sodium benzoate 0.1% and methylparaben 0.1% (added as preservatives), D&C Yellow No. 10, glycerin, purified water, and sorbitol.
Store at 15°–30°C (59°–86°F) and protect from light.

How Supplied: Bottles of 4 fl oz and 1 pint.
Shown in Product Identification Section, page 406

ACTIFED® Tablets
[ăk 'tuh-fĕd]

Indications: For temporary relief of nasal congestion due to the common cold, hay fever or other upper respiratory allergies. Helps decongest sinus openings, sinus passages. For temporary relief of running nose, sneezing, itching of the nose or throat and itchy and watery eyes as may occur in allergic rhinitis (such as hay fever).

Directions: Adults and children 12 years of age and over, 1 tablet every 4 to 6 hours. Children 6 to under 12 years of age, ½ tablet every 4 to 6 hours. Children under 6 years of age, consult a physician. Do not exceed 4 doses in 24 hours.

Warnings: May cause excitability especially in children. Do not give this product to children under 6 years except under the advice and supervision of a physician. May cause drowsiness. Do not exceed recommended dosage because at higher doses nervousness, dizziness or sleeplessness may occur. If symptoms do not improve within 7 days or are accompanied by high fever, consult a physician before continuing use. Do not take this product if you have high blood pressure, heart disease, diabetes, thyroid disease, asthma, glaucoma or difficulty in urination due to enlargement of the prostate gland except under the advice and supervision of a physician. As with any drug, if you are pregnant or nursing a baby, seek the advice of a health professional before using this product.

Drug Interaction Precaution: Do not take this product if you are presently taking a prescription antihypertensive or antidepressant drug containing a monoamine oxidase inhibitor except under the advice and supervision of a physician.

Caution: Avoid driving a motor vehicle or operating heavy machinery. Avoid alcoholic beverages while taking this product.
KEEP THIS AND ALL DRUGS OUT OF THE REACH OF CHILDREN. In case of accidental overdose, seek professional assistance or contact a Poison Control Center immediately.

Active Ingredients: Each scored tablet contains pseudoephedrine hydrochloride 60 mg and triprolidine hydrochloride 2.5 mg.

Inactive Ingredients: Flavor, hydroxypropyl methylcellulose, lactose, magnesium stearate, polyethylene glycol, potato starch, povidone, sucrose, and titanium dioxide. Store at 15°–25°C (59°–77°F) in a dry place and protect from light.

How Supplied: Boxes of 12, 24, 48 and bottles of 100 and 1000; unit dose pack box of 100.
Shown in Product Identification Section, page 406

Continued on next page

Burroughs Wellcome—Cont.

ALLERACT™ Tablets
[ˈal-ər-ˈakt]

Indications: For the temporary relief of running nose, sneezing, itching of the nose or throat and itchy and watery eyes as may occur in allergic rhinitis (such as hay fever).

Directions: Adults and children 12 years of age and over, 1 tablet every 4 to 6 hours. Children 6 to under 12 years of age, ½ tablet every 4 to 6 hours. Children under 6 years of age, consult a physician. Do not exceed 4 doses in 24 hours.

Warnings: May cause excitability especially in children. May cause drowsiness. Do not take this product if you have asthma, glaucoma or difficulty in urination due to enlargement of the prostate gland except under the advice and supervision of a physician. Do not give this product to children under 6 years except under the advice and supervision of a physician. As with any drug, if you are pregnant or nursing a baby, seek the advice of a health professional before using this product.

Caution: Avoid driving a motor vehicle or operating heavy machinery. Avoid alcoholic beverages while taking this product. **KEEP THIS AND ALL DRUGS OUT OF THE REACH OF CHILDREN.** In case of accidental overdose, seek professional assistance or contact a Poison Control Center immediately.

Active Ingredients: Each scored tablet contains triprolidine hydrochloride 2.5 mg.
Also Contains: Corn and potato starch, hydroxypropyl methylcellulose, lactose, magnesium stearate, polyethylene glycol, and titanium dioxide.
Store at 15°–25°C (59°–77°F) in a dry place and protect from light.

How Supplied: Boxes of 24.
Shown in Product Identification Section, page 406

ALLERACT™ DECONGESTANT Caplets
[ˈal-ər-ˈakt]

Indications: For temporary relief of running nose, sneezing, itching of the nose or throat and itchy and watery eyes as may occur in allergic rhinitis (such as hay fever). For temporary relief of nasal congestion due to hay fever or other upper respiratory allergies.

Directions: Adults and children 12 years of age and over, 1 caplet every 4 to 6 hours. Children 6 to under 12 years of age, ½ caplet every 4 to 6 hours. Children under 6 years of age, consult a physician. Do not exceed 4 doses in 24 hours.

Warnings: May cause excitability especially in children. Do not give this product to children under 6 years except under the advice and supervision of a physician. May cause drowsiness. Do not

exceed recommended dosage because at higher doses nervousness, dizziness or sleeplessness may occur. If symptoms do not improve within 7 days or are accompanied by high fever, consult a physician before continuing use. Do not take this product if you have high blood pressure, heart disease, diabetes, thyroid disease, asthma, glaucoma or difficulty in urination due to enlargement of the prostate gland except under the advice and supervision of a physician. As with any drug, if you are pregnant or nursing a baby, seek the advice of a health professional before using this product.
Drug Interaction Precaution: Do not take this product if you are presently taking a prescription antihypertensive or antidepressant drug containing a monoamine oxidase inhibitor except under the advice and supervision of a physician.

Caution: Avoid driving a motor vehicle or operating heavy machinery. Avoid alcoholic beverages while taking this product. **KEEP THIS AND ALL DRUGS OUT OF THE REACH OF CHILDREN.** In case of accidental overdose, seek professional assistance or contact a Poison Control Center immediately.

Active Ingredients: Each scored caplet contains pseudoephedrine hydrochloride 60 mg and triprolidine hydrochloride 2.5 mg. **Also Contains:** Carnauba wax, hydroxypropyl methylcellulose, lactose, magnesium stearate, polyethylene glycol, potato starch, povidone, and titanium dioxide.
Store at 15°–25°C (59°–77°F) in a dry place and protect from light.

How Supplied: Boxes of 24.
Shown in Product Identification Section, page 406

ALLERACT™ DECONGESTANT Tablets
[ˈal-ər-ˈakt]

Indications: For temporary relief of running nose, sneezing, itching of the nose or throat and itchy and watery eyes as may occur in allergic rhinitis (such as hay fever). For temporary relief of nasal congestion due to hay fever or other upper respiratory allergies.

Directions: Adults and children 12 years of age and over, 1 tablet every 4 to 6 hours. Children 6 to under 12 years of age, ½ tablet every 4 to 6 hours. Children under 6 years of age, consult a physician. Do not exceed 4 doses in 24 hours.

Warnings: May cause excitability especially in children. Do not give this product to children under 6 years except under the advice and supervision of a physician. May cause drowsiness. Do not exceed recommended dosage because at higher doses nervousness, dizziness or sleeplessness may occur. If symptoms do not improve within 7 days or are accompanied by high fever, consult a physician before continuing use. Do not take this product if you have high blood pressure, heart disease, diabetes, thyroid disease,

asthma, glaucoma or difficulty in urination due to enlargement of the prostate gland except under the advice and supervision of a physician. As with any drug, if you are pregnant or nursing a baby, seek the advice of a health professional before using this product.
Drug Interaction Precaution: Do not take this product if you are presently taking a prescription antihypertensive or antidepressant drug containing a monoamine oxidase inhibitor except under the advice and supervision of a physician.

Caution: Avoid driving a motor vehicle or operating heavy machinery. Avoid alcoholic beverages while taking this product. **KEEP THIS AND ALL DRUGS OUT OF THE REACH OF CHILDREN.** In case of accidental overdose, seek professional assistance or contact a Poison Control Center immediately.

Active Ingredients: Each scored tablet contains pseudoephedrine hydrochloride 60 mg and triprolidine hydrochloride 2.5 mg.
Also Contains: Hydroxypropyl methylcellulose, lactose, magnesium stearate, polyethylene glycol, potato starch, povidone, and titanium dioxide.
Store at 15°–25°C (59°–77°F) in a dry place and protect from light.

How Supplied: Boxes of 24 and 48.
Shown in Product Identification Section, page 406

BOROFAX® Ointment
[bôr ˈuh-fǎks]

Description: Contains boric acid 5% and lanolin.
Inactive Ingredients: fragrances, glycerin, mineral oil, purified water and sodium borate.

Indications: A soothing application for burns, abrasions, chafing, and for infants' tender skin.

Directions: Apply topically as required.
Keep this and all medicines out of children's reach.
Store at 15°–25°C (59°–77°F).

How Supplied: Tube, 1¾ oz.

EMPIRIN® ASPIRIN
[ěm ˈpuh-rŭn]

For relief of headache, minor muscular aches and pains, toothache, discomfort and fever of colds and flu, pain of the premenstrual and menstrual periods, and temporary relief of minor arthritis pain (see CAUTION below).

Directions: **Adults:** 1 or 2 tablets with a full glass of water. Repeat every 4 hours as needed, up to 12 tablets a day.
Children: Consult a physician (see WARNINGS).

Caution: In arthritic conditions, if pain persists for more than 10 days or redness is present, consult a physician immediately.

Warnings: Children and teenagers should not use this medicine for chicken pox or flu symptoms before a doctor is consulted about Reye syndrome, a rare but serious illness reported to be associated with aspirin. Keep this and all medicines out of children's reach. In case of accidental overdose, contact a physician immediately.

High or continued fever, severe or persistent sore throat especially when accompanied by high fever, headache, nausea or vomiting, may be serious. Consult your physician. Do not exceed dose unless directed by a physician. Do not take this product if you are allergic to aspirin, have asthma, a gastric ulcer or its symptoms, or are taking a medication that affects the clotting of blood, except under the advice of a physician. As with any drug, if you are pregnant or nursing a baby, seek the advice of a health professional before using this product.

Active Ingredients: Each tablet contains aspirin 325 mg (5 gr).

Inactive Ingredients: microcrystalline cellulose and potato starch.
Store at 15°–30°C (59°–86°F) in a dry place.

How Supplied: Bottles of 50, 100, 250.
Shown in Product Identification Section, page 406

MAREZINE® Tablets
[mâr 'uh-zēn]

FDA APPROVED USES

Indications: For the prevention and treatment of the nausea, vomiting or dizziness associated with motion sickness.

Directions: Adults and children 12 years of age and older: 1 tablet every 4 to 6 hours, not to exceed 4 tablets in 24 hours or as directed by a doctor. Children 6 to under 12 years of age: ½ tablet every 6 to 8 hours, not to exceed 1½ tablets in 24 hours or as directed by a doctor. For prevention, take the first dose one-half hour before departure.

Warnings: Do not take this product if you have asthma, glaucoma, emphysema, chronic pulmonary disease, shortness of breath, difficulty in breathing or difficulty in urination due to enlargement of the prostate gland unless directed by a doctor. Do not give to children under 6 years of age unless directed by a doctor. May cause drowsiness; alcohol, sedatives and tranquilizers may increase the drowsiness effect. Avoid alcoholic beverages while taking this product. Do not take this product if you are taking sedatives or tranquilizers without first consulting your doctor. Use caution when driving a motor vehicle or operating machinery. As with any drug, if you are pregnant or nursing a baby, seek the advice of a health professional before using this product. Keep this and all drugs out of the reach of children. In case of accidental overdose, seek professional as-

sistance or contact a Poison Control Center immediately.

Active Ingredients: Each scored tablet contains cyclizine hydrochloride 50 mg.

Inactive Ingredients: corn and potato starch, dextrin, lactose, and magnesium stearate.
Store at 15°–25°C (59°–77°F) in a dry place and protect from light.

How Supplied: Box of 12, bottle of 100.
Shown in Product Identification Section, page 406

NEOSPORIN® Cream
[nē 'uh-spō 'rŭn]

Indications: First aid to help prevent infection in minor cuts, scrapes, and burns.

Directions: Clean the affected area. Apply a small amount of this product (an amount equal to the surface area of the tip of a finger) on an area 1 to 3 times daily. May be covered with sterile bandage.

Warnings: For external use only. Do not use in the eyes or apply over large areas of the body. In case of deep or puncture wounds, animal bites, or serious burns, consult a physician. Stop use and consult a physician if the condition persists or gets worse. Do not use longer than 1 week unless directed by a physician. Keep this and all drugs out of the reach of children. In case of accidental ingestion, seek professional assistance or contact a Poison Control Center immediately.

Each gram contains: Aerosporin® (polymyxin B sulfate) 10,000 units and neomycin 3.5 mg. Also contains: methylparaben 0.25% (added as a preservative), emulsifying wax, mineral oil, polyoxyethylene polyoxypropylene compound, propylene glycol, purified water and white petrolatum.
Store at 15° to 25°C (59° to 77°F).

How Supplied: ½ oz tube; $\frac{1}{32}$ oz (approx.) foil packets packed 144 per carton.

Professional Labeling: Consult 1989 Physicians' Desk Reference.
Shown in Product Identification Section, page 406

NEOSPORIN® Ointment
[nē 'uh-spō 'rŭn]

Indications: First aid to help prevent infection in minor cuts, scrapes and burns.

Directions: Clean the affected area. Apply a small amount of this product (an amount equal to the surface area of the tip of a finger) on the area 1 to 3 times daily. May be covered with sterile bandage.

Warnings: For external use only. Do not use in the eyes or apply over large areas of the body. In case of deep or puncture wounds, animal bites, or serious burns, consult a physician. Stop use and

consult a physician if the condition persists or gets worse. Do not use longer than 1 week unless directed by a physician. Keep this and all drugs out of the reach of children. In case of accidental ingestion, seek professional assistance or contact a Poison Control Center immediately.

Each gram contains: Aerosporin® (polymyxin B sulfate) 5,000 units, bacitracin zinc 400 units and neomycin 3.5 mg in a special white petrolatum base.
Store at 15° to 25°C (59° to 77°F).

How Supplied: Tubes, ½ oz (with applicator tip), 1 oz; $\frac{1}{32}$ oz (approx.) foil packets packed 144 per carton.

Professional Labeling: Consult 1989 Physicians' Desk Reference.
Shown in Product Identification Section, page 406

POLYSPORIN® Ointment
[pŏl 'ē-spō 'rŭn]

Indications: First aid to help prevent infection in minor cuts, scrapes and burns.

Directions: Clean the affected area. Apply a small amount of this product (an amount equal to the surface area of the tip of a finger) on the area 1 to 3 times daily. May be covered with a sterile bandage.

Warnings: For external use only. Do not use in the eyes or apply over large areas of the body. In case of deep or puncture wounds, animal bites, or serious burns, consult a physician. Stop use and consult a physician if the condition persists or gets worse. Do not use longer than 1 week unless directed by a physician. Keep this and all drugs out of the reach of children. In case of accidental ingestion, seek professional assistance or contact a Poison Control Center immediately.

Each Gram Contains: Aerosporin® (Polymyxin B Sulfate) 10,000 units and bacitracin zinc 500 units in a special white petrolatum base.
Store at 15° to 25°C (59° to 77°F).

How Supplied: Tubes, ½ oz with applicator tip, 1 oz; $\frac{1}{32}$ oz (approx.) foil packets packed in cartons of 144.
Shown in Product Identification Section, page 406

POLYSPORIN® Powder
[pŏl 'ē-spō 'rŭn]

Indications: First aid to help prevent infection in minor cuts, scrapes and burns.

Directions: Clean the affected area. Apply a light dusting of the powder on the area 1 to 3 times daily. May be covered with a sterile bandage.

Warnings: For external use only. Do not use in the eyes or apply over large areas of the body. In case of deep or puncture wounds, animal bites, or serious burns, consult a physician. Stop use and

Continued on next page

Burroughs Wellcome—Cont.

consult a physician if the condition persists or gets worse.

Do not use longer than 1 week unless directed by a physician. Keep this and all drugs out of the reach of children. In case of accidental ingestion, seek professional assistance or contact a Poison Control Center immediately.

Each Gram Contains: Aerosporin® (polymyxin B sulfate) 10,000 units and bacitracin zinc 500 units in a lactose base.

Store at 15° to 30°C (59° to 86°F). Do not store under refrigeration.

How Supplied: 0.35 oz (10 g) shaker-vial.

Shown in Product Identification Section, page 406

POLYSPORIN® Spray
[pŏl 'ē-spō 'rŭn]

Description: Each 85 gram can contains: Aerosporin® (polymyxin B sulfate) 200,000 units and bacitracin zinc 10,000 units. Propellant—dichlorodifluoromethane and trichloromonofluoromethane.

Each 1 second spray delivers approximately 2300 units of polymyxin B sulfate and 115 units of bacitracin zinc.

Indications: First aid to help prevent infection in minor cuts, scrapes and burns. Decreases the number of bacteria on the treated area.

Directions: Clean the affected area. SHAKE WELL before each spraying. Remove cap and press button to spray affected area. Hold container upright when spraying. Use one-second intermittent sprays from a distance of about eight inches. Prolonged spraying is unnecessary and wastes medication. Apply a small amount of this product one to three times daily. May be covered with a sterile bandage.

Warnings: Avoid spraying in eyes. Contents under pressure. Do not puncture or incinerate. Do not store at temperatures above 120°F. For external use only. Do not use in the eyes or apply over large areas of the body. In case of deep or puncture wounds, animal bites, or serious burns, consult a doctor. Stop use and consult a doctor if the condition persists or gets worse. Do not use longer than 1 week unless directed by a doctor. Keep this and all drugs out of the reach of children. In case of accidental ingestion, seek professional assistance or contact a Poison Control Center immediately.

Store at 15°–30°C (59°–86°F).

How Supplied: 3 oz (85 g) spray can.

Shown in Product Identification Section, page 406

Children's
SUDAFED® Liquid
[sū 'duh-fĕd]

Each 5 ml (1 teaspoonful) contains pseudoephedrine hydrochloride 30 mg. Also

contains: methylparaben 0.1% and sodium benzoate 0.1% (added as preservatives), citric acid, FD&C Red No. 40, flavor, glycerin, purified water, sorbitol and sucrose.

Indications: For temporary relief of nasal congestion due to the common cold, hay fever or other upper respiratory allergies, and nasal congestion associated with sinusitis; promotes nasal and/or sinus drainage.

Directions: To be given every 4 to 6 hours. Do not exceed 4 doses in 24 hours. Children 6 to under 12 years of age, 1 teaspoonful. Children 2 to under 6 years of age, ½ teaspoonful. For children under 2 years of age, consult a physician.

Warnings: Do not exceed recommended dosage because at higher doses nervousness, dizziness or sleeplessness may occur. Do not give this product to children for more than 7 days. If symptoms do not improve or are accompanied by high fever, consult a physician. Do not give this product to children who have heart disease, high blood pressure, thyroid disease or diabetes unless directed by a physician.

Drug Interaction Precaution: Do not give this product to a child who is taking a prescription drug for high blood pressure or depression, without first consulting the child's physician.
KEEP THIS AND ALL MEDICINES OUT OF CHILDREN'S REACH. In case of accidental overdose, seek professional assistance or contact a Poison Control Center immediately.

Store at 15°–25°C (59°–77°F) and protect from light.

How Supplied: Bottles of 4 fl oz.
Shown in Product Identification Section, page 406

SUDAFED® Cough Syrup
[sū 'duh-fĕd]

Each 5 ml (1 teaspoonful) contains pseudoephedrine hydrochloride 15 mg, dextromethorphan hydrobromide 5 mg and guaifenesin 100 mg. Also contains: alcohol 2.4%, sodium benzoate 0.1% and methylparaben 0.1% (added as preservatives), citric acid, D&C Yellow No. 10, FD&C Blue No. 1, flavor, glycerin, purified water, saccharin sodium, sodium chloride and sucrose.

Indications: For temporary relief of cough due to minor throat and bronchial irritation as may occur with the common cold or inhaled irritants. For temporary relief of nasal congestion due to the common cold. Helps loosen phlegm and bronchial secretions and rid the bronchial passageways of bothersome mucus.

Directions: To be given every 4 to 6 hours. Do not exceed 4 doses in 24 hours. Adults and children 12 years of age and over, 4 teaspoonfuls. Children 6 to under 12 years of age, 2 teaspoonfuls. Children 2 to under 6 years of age, 1 teaspoonful. For children under 2 years of age, consult a physician.

Warnings: Do not give this product to children under 2 years of age unless directed by a physician. Do not exceed recommended dosage because at higher doses, nervousness, dizziness or sleeplessness may occur. Do not take this product for persistent or chronic cough such as occurs with smoking, asthma or emphysema, or where cough is accompanied by excessive secretions unless directed by a physician. A persistent cough may be a sign of a serious condition. If cough persists for more than 1 week, tends to recur, or is accompanied by fever, rash or persistent headache, consult a physician. Do not take this preparation if you have high blood pressure, heart disease, diabetes, thyroid disease, or difficulty in urination due to enlargement of the prostate gland, except under the advice and supervision of a physician. As with any drug, if you are pregnant or nursing a baby, seek the advice of a health professional before using this product.

Drug Interaction Precaution: Do not take this product if you are presently taking a prescription antihypertensive or antidepressant drug containing a monoamine oxidase inhibitor except under the advice and supervision of a physician.
KEEP THIS AND ALL DRUGS OUT OF THE REACH OF CHILDREN. In case of accidental overdose, seek professional assistance or contact a Poison Control Center immediately.
Store at 15°–30°C (59°–86°F).
DO NOT REFRIGERATE.

How Supplied: Bottles of 4 fl oz and 8 fl oz.
Shown in Product Identification Section, page 406

SUDAFED® Tablets 30 mg
[sū 'duh-fĕd]

Each tablet contains pseudoephedrine hydrochloride 30 mg. Also contains: acacia, carnauba wax, dibasic calcium phosphate, FD&C Red No. 3 Lake and Yellow No. 6 Lake, magnesium stearate, polysorbate 60, potato starch, povidone, sodium benzoate, stearic acid, sucrose and titanium dioxide.

Indications: For temporary relief of nasal congestion due to the common cold, hay fever or other upper respiratory allergies, and nasal congestion associated with sinusitis; promotes nasal and/or sinus drainage.

Directions: To be given every 4 to 6 hours. Do not exceed 4 doses in 24 hours. Adults and children 12 years of age and over, 2 tablets. Children 6 to under 12 years of age, 1 tablet. Children 2 to under 6 years of age, use Children's Sudafed Liquid. For children under 2 years of age, consult a physician.

Warnings: Do not exceed recommended dosage because at higher doses nervousness, dizziness or sleeplessness may occur. If symptoms do not improve within 7 days, or are accompanied by a high fever, consult a physician before continuing use. Do not take this prepara-

tion if you have high blood pressure, heart disease, diabetes, thyroid disease, or difficulty in urination due to enlargement of the prostate gland, except under the advice and supervision of a physician. As with any drug, if you are pregnant or nursing a baby, seek the advice of a health professional before using this product.

Drug Interaction Precaution: Do not take this product if you are presently taking a prescription antihypertensive or antidepressant drug containing a monoamine oxidase inhibitor, except under the advice and supervision of a physician.

KEEP THIS AND ALL MEDICINES OUT OF CHILDREN'S REACH. In case of accidental overdose, seek professional assistance or contact a Poison Control Center immediately.
Store at 15°–30°C (59°–86°F) in a dry place and protect from light.

How Supplied: Boxes of 24, 48. Bottles of 100, 1000.
Shown in Product Identification Section, page 406

SUDAFED® Tablets 60 mg (Adult Strength)
[sū 'duh-fĕd]

Each tablet contains pseudoephedrine hydrochloride 60 mg. Also contains: acacia, carnauba wax, corn starch, dibasic calcium phosphate, hydroxypropyl methylcellulose, magnesium stearate, polysorbate 60, sodium starch glycolate, stearic acid, sucrose, titanium dioxide, and white shellac. Printed with edible red ink.

Indications: For temporary relief of nasal congestion due to the common cold, hay fever or other upper respiratory allergies, and nasal congestion associated with sinusitis; promotes nasal and/or sinus drainage.

Directions: To be given every 4 to 6 hours. Do not exceed 4 doses in 24 hours. Adults and children 12 years of age and over, 1 tablet. Children 6 to under 12 years of age, use Sudafed 30 mg Tablets. Children 2 to under 6 years of age, use Children's Sudafed Liquid. For children under 2 years of age, consult a physician.

Warnings: Do not exceed recommended dosage because at higher doses nervousness, dizziness or sleeplessness may occur. If symptoms do not improve within 7 days, or are accompanied by a high fever, consult a physician before continuing use. Do not take this preparation if you have high blood pressure, heart disease, diabetes, thyroid disease, or difficulty in urination due to enlargement of the prostate gland, except under the advice and supervision of a physician. As with any drug, if you are pregnant or nursing a baby, seek the advice of a health professional before using this product.

Drug Interaction Precaution: Do not take this product if you are presently taking a prescription antihypertensive or antidepressant drug containing a

monoamine oxidase inhibitor, except under the advice and supervision of a physician.

KEEP THIS AND ALL MEDICINES OUT OF CHILDREN'S REACH. In case of accidental overdose, seek professional assistance or contact a Poison Control Center immediately.
Store at 15°–30°C (59°–86°F) in a dry place and protect from light.

How Supplied: Bottles of 100.
Shown in Product Identification Section, page 406

SUDAFED® PLUS Liquid
[sū 'duh-fĕd]

Each 5 ml (1 teaspoonful) contains pseudoephedrine hydrochloride 30 mg and chlorpheniramine maleate 2 mg. Also contains: methylparaben 0.1% and sodium benzoate 0.1% (added as preservatives), citric acid, D&C Yellow No. 10, FD&C Yellow No. 6, flavor, glycerin, purified water and sucrose.

Indications: For the temporary relief of nasal/sinus congestion associated with the common cold; also sneezing; watery, itchy eyes; runny nose and other hay fever/upper respiratory allergy symptoms.

Directions: To be given every 4 to 6 hours. Do not exceed 4 doses in 24 hours. Adults and children 12 years of age and over, 2 teaspoonfuls. Children 6 to under 12 years of age, 1 teaspoonful. Children under 6 years of age, consult a physician.

Warnings: May cause excitability, especially in children. Do not give to children under 6 years except as directed by a physician. May cause drowsiness. Do not exceed recommended dosage because at higher doses nervousness, dizziness or sleeplessness may occur. If symptoms do not improve within 7 days, or are accompanied by a high fever, consult a physician before continuing use. Do not take this product if you have high blood pressure, heart disease, diabetes, thyroid disease, asthma, glaucoma or difficulty in urination due to enlargement of the prostate gland except under the advice and supervision of a physician. As with any drug, if you are pregnant or nursing a baby, seek the advice of a health professional before using this product.

Drug Interaction Precaution: Do not take this product if you are presently taking a prescription antihypertensive or antidepressant drug containing a monoamine oxidase inhibitor except under the advice and supervision of a physician.

Caution: Avoid driving a motor vehicle or operating heavy machinery. Avoid alcoholic beverages while taking this product.
KEEP THIS AND ALL MEDICINES OUT OF CHILDREN'S REACH. In case of accidental overdose, seek professional assistance or contact a Poison Control Center immediately.
Store at 15°–30°C (59°–86°F) and protect from light.

How Supplied: Bottles of 4 fl oz.
Shown in Product Identification Section, page 406

SUDAFED® PLUS Tablets
[sū 'duh-fĕd]

Each scored tablet contains pseudoephedrine hydrochloride 60 mg and chlorpheniramine maleate 4 mg. Also contains: lactose, magnesium stearate, potato starch and povidone.

Indications: For the temporary relief of nasal/sinus congestion associated with the common cold; also sneezing; watery, itchy eyes; runny nose and other hay fever/upper respiratory allergy symptoms.

Directions: To be given every 4 to 6 hours. Do not exceed 4 doses in 24 hours. Adults and children 12 years of age and over, 1 tablet. Children 6 to under 12 years of age, ½ tablet. Children under 6 years of age, consult a physician.

Warnings: May cause excitability, especially in children. Do not give to children under 6 years except as directed by a physician. May cause drowsiness. Do not exceed recommended dosage because at higher doses nervousness, dizziness or sleeplessness may occur. If symptoms do not improve within 7 days, or are accompanied by a high fever, consult a physician before continuing use. Do not take this product if you have high blood pressure, heart disease, diabetes, thyroid disease, asthma, glaucoma or difficulty in urination due to enlargement of the prostate gland except under the advice and supervision of a physician. As with any drug, if you are pregnant or nursing a baby, seek the advice of a health professional before using this product.

Drug Interaction Precaution: Do not take this product if you are presently taking a prescription antihypertensive or antidepressant drug containing a monoamine oxidase inhibitor except under the advice and supervision of a physician.

Caution: Avoid driving a motor vehicle or operating heavy machinery. Avoid alcoholic beverages while taking this product.
KEEP THIS AND ALL MEDICINES OUT OF CHILDREN'S REACH. In case of accidental overdose, seek professional assistance or contact a Poison Control Center immediately.
Store at 15°–30°C (59°–86°F) in a dry place and protect from light.

How Supplied: Boxes of 24, 48.
Shown in Product Identification Section, page 406

SUDAFED® SINUS Caplets
[sū 'dah-fĕd " 'sī-nəs]

Product Benefits:
● Maximum allowable levels of non-aspirin pain reliever and nasal decongestant provide temporary relief of sinus headache pain, pressure and nasal con-

Continued on next page

Burroughs Wellcome—Cont.

gestion due to colds or hay fever and other allergies.
- Contains no ingredients which may cause drowsiness.

Directions: Adults and children 12 years and over, 2 caplets every 6 hours, not to exceed 8 caplets in a 24-hour period. Not recommended for children under 12 years of age.

Each Caplet Contains: acetaminophen 500 mg and pseudoephedrine hydrochloride 30 mg. Also contains FD&C Yellow No. 6 Lake, magnesium stearate, microcrystalline cellulose, povidone and sodium starch glycolate.

Warnings: Do not exceed recommended dosage because at higher doses nervousness, dizziness, or sleeplessness may occur. If symptoms do not improve within 7 days or are accompanied by high fever, consult a physician before continuing use. Do not take this product for more than 10 days. Do not take this product if you have high blood pressure, heart disease, diabetes, thyroid disease, or difficulty in urination due to enlargement of the prostate gland except under the advice and supervision of a physician. As with any drug, if you are pregnant or nursing a baby, seek the advice of a health professional before using this product.

Drug Interaction Precaution: Do not take this product if you are presently taking a prescription antihypertensive or antidepressant drug containing a monoamine oxidase inhibitor except under the advice and supervision of a physician.
KEEP THIS AND ALL DRUGS OUT OF THE REACH OF CHILDREN. In case of accidental overdose, seek professional assistance or contact a Poison Control Center immediately.
Store at 15°–25°C (59°–77°F) in a dry place and protect from light.

How Supplied: Boxes of 24 and 48.
Shown in Product Identification Section, page 406

SUDAFED® SINUS Tablets
[sū 'dah-fĕd " 'sī-nəs]

Product Benefits:
- Maximum allowable levels of non-aspirin pain reliever and nasal decongestant provide temporary relief of sinus headache pain, pressure and nasal congestion due to colds or hay fever and other allergies.
- Contains no ingredients which may cause drowsiness.

Directions: Adults and children 12 years and over, 2 tablets every 6 hours, not to exceed 8 tablets in a 24-hour period. Not recommended for children under 12 years of age.

Each Tablet Contains: acetaminophen 500 mg and pseudoephedrine hydrochloride 30 mg. Also contains FD&C Yellow No. 6 Lake, magnesium stearate,

microcrystalline cellulose, povidone and sodium starch glycolate.

Warnings: Do not exceed recommended dosage because at higher doses nervousness, dizziness, or sleeplessness may occur. If symptoms do not improve within 7 days or are accompanied by high fever, consult a physician before continuing use. Do not take this product for more than 10 days. Do not take this product if you have high blood pressure, heart disease, diabetes, thyroid disease, or difficulty in urination due to enlargement of the prostate gland except under the advice and supervision of a physician. As with any drug, if you are pregnant or nursing a baby, seek the advice of a health professional before using this product.

Drug Interaction Precaution: Do not take this product if you are presently taking a prescription antihypertensive or antidepressant drug containing a monoamine oxidase inhibitor except under the advice and supervision of a physician.
KEEP THIS AND ALL DRUGS OUT OF THE REACH OF CHILDREN. In case of accidental overdose, seek professional assistance or contact a Poison Control Center immediately.
Store at 15°–25°C (59°–77°F) in a dry place and protect from light.

How Supplied: Boxes of 24 and 48.
Shown in Product Identification Section, page 406

SUDAFED® 12 Hour Capsules
[sū 'duh-fĕd]

Each capsule contains pseudoephedrine hydrochloride 120 mg. Also contains: corn starch, sucrose and other ingredients. The capsule shell consists of gelatin, FD&C Blues No. 1 and 2, and Red No. 3. May contain one or more parabens. Printed with edible black ink.

Indications: For temporary relief of nasal congestion due to the common cold, hay fever, or other upper respiratory allergies, and nasal congestion associated with sinusitis; promotes nasal and/or sinus drainage.

Directions: Adults and children 12 years and over—One capsule every 12 hours, not to exceed two capsules in 24 hours. Sudafed 12 Hour is not recommended for children under 12 years of age.

Warnings: Do not exceed recommended dosage because at higher doses nervousness, dizziness, or sleeplessness may occur. If symptoms do not improve within 7 days, or are accompanied by a high fever, consult a physician before continuing use. Do not take this preparation if you have high blood pressure, heart disease, diabetes, thyroid disease, or difficulty in urination due to enlargement of the prostate gland, except under the advice and supervision of a physician. As with any drug, if you are pregnant or nursing a baby, seek the advice of a health professional before using this product.

Drug Interaction Precaution: Do not take this product if you are presently taking a prescription antihypertensive or antidepressant drug containing a monoamine oxidase inhibitor, except under the advice and supervision of a physician.
KEEP THIS AND ALL DRUGS OUT OF THE REACH OF CHILDREN. In case of accidental overdose, seek professional assistance or contact a Poison Control Center immediately.
Store at 15°–30°C (59°–86°F) in a dry place and protect from light.

How Supplied: Boxes of 10, 20, 40.
Shown in Product Identification Section, page 407

WELLCOME® LANOLINE
[lăn 'ō-lŭn]

Description: Lanolin with solid and liquid petrolatum, fragrances, and glycerin.

Indications: A soothing and softening application for dry, rough skin and a protective application against the effects of harsh weather.

Directions: Apply topically to the hands and face as required.
Keep this and all medicines out of children's reach.
Store at 15°–25°C (59°–77°F).

How Supplied: Tubes, 1¾ oz.

Campbell Laboratories Inc.
300 EAST 51st STREET
P.O. BOX 812, F.D.R. STATION
NEW YORK, NY 10150

HERPECIN–L® Cold Sore Lip Balm
[her "puh-sin-el "]

Composition: A soothing, emollient, cosmetically pleasant lip balm incorporating pyridoxine HCl; allantoin; the sunscreen, octyl p-(dimethylamino)-benzoate (Padimate O); and titanium dioxide in a balanced, acidic lipid system. (All ingredients appear on the package. Has no "caines", antibiotics, phenol or camphor.) (NDC 38083-777-31)

Actions and Uses: HERPECIN-L® relieves dryness and chapping by providing a lipid barrier to help restore normal moisture balance to labial tissues. The sunscreen is effective in 2900-3200 AU range while titanium dioxide helps to block, scatter and reflect the sun's rays.

Administration: (1) *Recurrent "cold sores, sun and fever blisters":* Simply put, users report the sooner and more often applied, the better the results. Frequent sufferers report that with *prophylactic* use (B.I.D./P.R.N.), their attacks are fewer and less severe. Most recurrent herpes labialis patients are aware of the *prodromal* symptoms: tingling, itching, burning. At this stage, or if the lesion has already developed, HERPECIN-L should

be applied liberally as often as convenient—at least *every hour* (qq. hor.). The prodrome will often persist and remind the patient to continue to reapply HERPECIN-L. (2) *Outdoor sun/winter protection:* Apply during and after exposure (and after swimming) and again at bedtime (h.s.). (3) *Dry, chapped lips:* Apply as needed.

Note: HERPECIN-L is for peri-oral use only; not for "canker sores" (aphthous stomatitis). Primary attacks, usually in children and young adults, are normally intra-oral and accompanied by foul breath, pain and fever. Lasting up to six weeks, they are resistant to most treatments. Adjunctive therapy for pain, fever and secondary infection may be indicated. Excessive chapping may be from mouth breathing.

Adverse Reactions: A few, rare instances of topical sensitivity to pyridoxine HCl (Vitamin B_6) and/or the sunscreen have been reported. Discontinue use if allergic reaction develops.

Contraindications: HERPECIN-L does not contain any steroids. (Corticosteroids are normally contraindicated in *herpes* infections.)

How Supplied: 2.8 gm. swivel tubes.

Samples Available: Yes. (Request on your Professional letterhead.)

Carter Products
Division of Carter-Wallace, Inc.
767 FIFTH AVENUE
NEW YORK, NY 10153

CARTER'S LITTLE PILLS®
A Stimulant Laxative

Active Ingredient: 5 mg bisacodyl, U.S.P. in each enteric coated pill.

Indications: For effective short-term relief of simple constipation (infrequent or difficult bowel movement).

Actions: Bisacodyl is a stimulant laxative that promotes bowel movement by one or more direct actions on the intestine.

Directions for Use: Adult oral dosage is 1 to 3 pills (usually 2) in a single daily dose. Children 6 to under 12 years of age, 1 pill a day. For children under 6 years of age, consult a doctor.

Warnings: Do not chew. Do not give to children under 6 years of age without consulting a doctor or to persons who cannot swallow without chewing. Do not use this product when abdominal pain, nausea, or vomiting are present. Do not take this product within one hour before or after taking an antacid and/or milk. This product may cause abdominal discomfort, faintness or mild cramps. Store in a cool place at temperatures not above 86°F (30°C). Prolonged or continued use of this product can lead to laxative dependence and loss of normal bowel function. Serious

side effects from prolonged use or overdose can occur.

If you have noticed a sudden change in bowel habits that persists over a period of two weeks, consult a physician before using a laxative. This product should be used only occasionally, but in any event, no longer than daily for one week, except on the advice of a physician.

As with any drug, if you are pregnant or nursing a baby, seek the advice of a health professional before using this product.

Drug Interaction Precaution: No known drug interaction.

Treatment of Overdosage: In case of accidental overdose seek professional assistance or contact a Poison Control Center immediately.

Professional Labeling: For effective short-term relief of simple constipation. For use in preparation of the patient for surgery or for preparation of the colon for x-ray and endoscopic examination.

How Supplied: Available in packages of 25 pills and 75 pills.

Shown in Product Identification Section, page 407

Chattem Consumer Products
Division of Chattem, Inc.
1715 WEST 38TH STREET
CHATTANOOGA, TN 37409

NULLO Deodorant Tablets

Active Ingredient: Each tablet contains 33.3 mg. Chlorophyllin Copper Complex.

Indications: Taken orally to control body odors due to fecal and urinary incontinence and odor due to colostomy and ileostomy.

Warning: Keep this and all drugs out of the reach of children. In case of accidental overdose, seek professional assistance or contact a poison control center immediately.

Drug Interaction: None has ever been reported.

Toxicity: None has ever been reported.

Dosage and Administration: Adult twelve years and older: swallow one or two tablets three times a day, before meals, until odor is eliminated, (from two to seven days). Then take one tablet three times a day or as needed to control odor. For children under 12 years of age, consult a physician.

Ostomates may also place one or two tablets in empty pouch each time it is reused or changed.

Side Effects: Few side effects have been reported following the administration of chlorophyllin copper complex in oral doses of up to 800 mg. (in divided doses) daily for varying durations, each exceeding one week. Temporary mild diarrhea has occurred with a few humans along with the expected green col-

oration of the stool. One case of abdominal cramps and one case of excessive gas was reported.

How Supplied: Tamper resistant bottles containing 30, 60 and 135 tablets.

PRĒMSYN PMS™
[preem 'sin pms]
Premenstrual Syndrome
Capsules/Caplets

Active Ingredients: Each capsule and caplet contains Acetaminophen 500 mg., Pamabrom 25 mg., and Pyrilamine Maleate 15 mg.

Indications: PRĒMSYN PMS™ has been clinically proven to safely and effectively relieve premenstrual tension, irritability, nervousness, edema, backaches, legaches, and headaches that often accompany premenstrual syndrome. The formula in PRĒMSYN PMS™ has been approved by an FDA-appointed panel.

Warning: KEEP THIS AND ALL DRUGS OUT OF THE REACH OF CHILDREN. In case of accidental overdose, seek professional assistance or contact a poison control center immediately.

Precautions: If drowsiness occurs, do not drive or operate machinery. As with any drug, if pregnant or nursing a baby, seek the advice of a health professional before using this product.

Dosage and Administration: Two capsules or caplets at first sign of premenstrual discomfort and repeat every three or four hours as needed not to exceed 8 capsules/caplets in a 24 hour period.

How Supplied: Tamper-resistant bottles of 20 and 40 capsules and caplets.

Church & Dwight Co., Inc.
469 N. HARRISON STREET
PRINCETON, NJ 08540

ARM & HAMMER®
Pure Baking Soda

Active Ingredient: Sodium Bicarbonate U.S.P.

Indications: For alleviation of acid indigestion, also known as heartburn or sour stomach. Not a remedy for other types of stomach complaints such as nausea, stomachache, abdominal cramps, gas pains, or stomach distention caused by overeating and/or overdrinking. In the latter case, one should not ingest solids, liquids or antacid but rather refrain from all physical activity and—if uncomfortable—call a physician.

Actions: ARM & HAMMER® Pure Baking Soda provides fast-acting, effective neutralization of stomach acids. Each level ½ teaspoon dose will neutralize 20.9 mEq of acid.

Continued on next page

Church & Dwight—Cont.

Warnings: Except under the advice and supervision of a physician: (1) do not take more than eight level ½ teaspoons per person up to 60 years old or four level ½ teaspoons per person 60 years or older in a 24-hour period, (2) do not use this product if you are on a sodium restricted diet, (3) do not use the maximum dose for more than two weeks, (4) do not ingest food, liquid or any antacid when stomach is overly full to avoid possible injury to the stomach.

Dosage and Administration: Level ½ teaspoon in ½ glass (4 fl. oz.) of water every two hours up to maximum dosage or as directed by a physician. Accurately measure level ½ teaspoon. Each level ½ teaspoon contains 20.9 mEq (.476 gm) sodium.

How Supplied: Available in 8 oz., 16 oz., 32 oz., and 64 oz. boxes.

OTIX™ DROPS
EAR WAX REMOVAL AID

Description: OTIX™ DROPS with Cotton Ear Plugs is an external ear wax removal aid that contains the active ingredient carbamide peroxide, 6.5%. OTIX™ DROPS Complete Ear Wax Removal Kit includes cotton ear plugs and a soft rubber bulb ear irrigator. Application of carbamide peroxide drops followed by warm water irrigation is an effective, medically recommended way to loosen excessive ear wax. OTIX™ DROPS is the only ear wax removal brand that supplies cotton ear plugs, which are recommended for use as a means to keep each product application in the ear for several minutes.

Indication: For occasional use as an aid to gently soften, loosen and remove excessive ear wax.

Ingredients: Carbamide Peroxide 6.5% in a base of Anhydrous Glycerin and Glyceryl Succinate.

Actions: OTIX™ DROPS patent pending formulation provides the foaming action of hydrogen peroxide with the solvent action of glycerin. In the bottle the carbamide peroxide is stabilized with the unique stabilizer glyceryl succinate. When contact is made with natural enzymes in the ear, oxygen is released. This oxygen release results in a foaming action which together with the solvent action of glycerin helps loosen and remove impacted ear wax. It is usually necessary to remove the loosened wax by gently flushing the ear with warm water using a soft rubber bulb ear irrigator.

Directions: FOR USE IN THE EAR ONLY. Adults and children over 12 years of age: Tilt head sideways and place 5 to 10 drops into ear. Tip of applicator should not enter ear canal. Keep drops in ear for several minutes by keeping head tilted or placing cotton in the ear. Use twice daily for up to 4 days if needed, or as directed by a physician.

Any wax remaining after treatment may be removed by gently flushing the ear with warm water, using a soft rubber bulb ear irrigator. Children under 12 years of age: Consult a physician.

Warnings: Do not use if you have ear drainage or discharge, ear pain, irritation, or rash in the ear or are dizzy; consult a physician. Do not use if you have an injury or perforation (hole) of the eardrum or after ear surgery, unless directed by a physician.
Do not use for more than 4 days; if excessive ear wax remains after use of this product, consult a physician. Avoid contact with the eyes. Keep this and all drugs out of the reach of children. In case of accidental ingestion, consult a physician.

Caution: Avoid exposing bottle to excessive heat and direct sunlight.

How Supplied:
For Patients
OTIX™ DROPS with Cotton Ear Plugs and OTIX™ DROPS Complete Ear Wax Removal Kit with Cotton Ear Plugs and Rubber Bulb Irrigator each contain a ½ fl. oz. bottle which will provide 30 to 60 applications. Both are available in the eye/ear sections of leading food and drug stores.
For Physicians
OTIX™ DROPS is also available in a 0.03 fl. oz. unit dose application for professional use only.
Shown in Product Identification Section, page 407

CIBA Consumer Pharmaceuticals
Division of CIBA-GEIGY Corporation
RARITAN PLAZA III
EDISON, NJ 08837

ACUTRIM® 16 HOUR* PRECISION RELEASE™ APPETITE SUPPRESSANT TABLETS
Caffeine Free

ACUTRIM® II—MAXIMUM STRENGTH PRECISION RELEASE™ APPETITE SUPPRESSANT TABLETS
Caffeine Free

ACUTRIM LATE DAY® PRECISION RELEASE™ APPETITE SUPPRESSANT TABLETS
Caffeine Free

Description:
ACUTRIM® Precision Release™ tablets deliver their maximum strength dosage of appetite suppressant at a precisely controlled, even rate.
This steady release is scientifically targeted to effectively distribute the appetite suppressant all day.
ACUTRIM makes it easier to follow the kind of reduced calorie diet needed for best weight control results.

A diet plan developed by an expert dietitian is included in the package for your personal use as a further aid.

ACUTRIM 16 Hour* *Breakfast to Bedtime* ™* Appetite Suppressant Contains no caffeine.

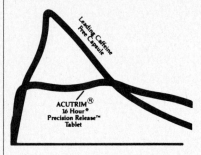

Hours 4   8   12   16

Formula: Each Precision Release™ tablet contains: Active Ingredient—phenylpropanolamine HCl 75 mg. (appetite suppressant).

Inactive Ingredients—ACUTRIM® 16 HOUR*: Cellulose Acetate, Hydroxypropyl Methylcellulose, Stearic Acid—ACUTRIM® II MAXIMUM STRENGTH: Cellulose Acetate, D&C Yellow #10, FD&C Blue #1, FD&C Yellow #6, Hydroxypropyl Methylcellulose, Povidone, Propylene Glycol, Stearic Acid, Titanium Dioxide—ACUTRIM LATE DAY®: Cellulose Acetate, FD&C Yellow #6, Hydroxypropyl Methylcellulose, Isopropyl Alcohol, Propylene Glycol, Riboflavin, Stearic Acid, Titanium Dioxide.
*Extent of duration relates solely to blood levels.

Dosage: For best results, take one tablet daily directly after breakfast. Do not take more than one tablet every 24 hours. Recommended dosage may be used up to three months.

Caution: Do not give this product to children under 12. Do not exceed recommended dosage. If nervousness, dizziness, or sleeplessness occurs, stop taking this medication and consult your physician. If you are being treated for high blood pressure or depression, or have heart disease, diabetes, or thyroid disease, do not take this product, except under the supervision of a physician. If you are taking a cough/cold allergy medication containing any form of phenylpropanolamine, do not take this product.

Warning: As with any drug, if you are pregnant or nursing a baby, seek the advice of a health professional before using this product.

KEEP THIS AND ALL MEDICATION OUT OF THE REACH OF CHILDREN. In case of accidental overdose, seek professional assistance or contact a poison control center immediately.

Drug Interaction Precaution: If you are taking any prescription drugs, or any type of nasal decongestant, antihypertensive or antidepressant drug, do not take this product, except under the supervision of a physician.

How Supplied: Tamper-evident blister packages of 20 and 40 tablets. Do not use if individual seals are broken.
DO NOT STORE ABOVE 86°F
PROTECT FROM MOISTURE

12/86

Shown in Product Identification
Section, page 407

ORIGINAL DOAN'S®
Analgesic Caplets

Indications: For temporary relief of occasional minor backache pain.

Directions: Adults—Two caplets every 4 hours as needed, not to exceed 12 caplets during a 24 hour period or as directed by a physician. Not intended for use by children or teenagers except under the advice of a physician. If pain persists for more than 10 days, discontinue use and consult your physician.

Warning: Children and teenagers should not use this medicine for chicken pox or flu symptoms before a doctor is consulted about Reye Syndrome, a rare but serious illness. As with any drug, if you are pregnant or nursing a baby, seek the advice of a health professional before using this product. Do not use this product if you are under medical care or are allergic to aspirin or salicylates, except under the advice and supervision of your physician. **Keep this and all medicines out of the reach of children.** In case of accidental overdose, seek professional assistance or consult a Poison Control Center immediately.

Active Ingredient: Each caplet contains Magnesium Salicylate 325 mg.
Also Contains: Magnesium Stearate, Microcrystalline Cellulose, Opadry Olive Green, Polyethylene Glycol, Purified Water, Stearic Acid.

How Supplied: Tamper-evident blister packages of 24 and 48 caplets. Do not use if individual seals are broken.
Shown in Product Identification
Section, page 407

EXTRA STRENGTH DOAN'S®
Analgesic Caplets

Indications: For temporary relief of occasional minor backache pain.

Directions: Adults—Two caplets 3 or 4 times daily, not to exceed 8 caplets during a 24 hour period or as directed by a physician. Not intended for use by children or teenagers except under the advice of a physician. If pain persists for more than 10 days, discontinue use and consult your physician.

Warning: Children and teenagers should not use this medicine for chicken pox or flu symptoms before a doctor is consulted about Reye Syndrome, a rare but serious illness. As with any drug, if you are pregnant or nursing a baby, seek the advice of a health professional before using this product. Do not use this product if you are under medical care or are allergic to aspirin or salicylates, except under the advice and supervision of your physician. **Keep this and all medicines out of the reach of children.** In case of accidental overdose, seek professional assistance or consult a Poison Control Center immediately.

Active Ingredient: Each caplet contains Magnesium Salicylate 500 mg.
Also Contains: calcium stearate, gelatin, lactose and purified water.

How Supplied: Tamper-evident blister packages of 24 and 48 caplets. Do not use if individual seals are broken.
Shown in Product Identification
Section, page 407

NUPERCAINAL®
Hemorrhoidal and Anesthetic Ointment
Pain-Relief Cream

Caution:
Nupercainal products are not for prolonged or extensive use and should never be applied in or near the eyes. If the symptom being treated does not subside, or rash, irritation, swelling, pain, bleeding or other symptoms develop or increase, discontinue use and consult a physician.
Consult labels before using.
Keep this and all medications out of reach of children.
NUPERCAINAL SHOULD NOT BE SWALLOWED. IN CASE OF ACCIDENTAL INGESTION CONSULT A PHYSICIAN OR POISON CONTROL CENTER IMMEDIATELY.

Indications: Nupercainal Ointment and Cream are fast-acting, long-lasting pain relievers that you can use for a number of painful skin conditions. **Nupercainal Hemorrhoidal and Anesthetic Ointment** is for hemorrhoids as well as for general use. **Nupercainal Pain-Relief Cream** is for general use only. The **Cream** is half as strong as the **Ointment**.
How to use Nupercainal Anesthetic Ointment (for general use). This soothing Ointment helps lubricate dry, inflamed skin and gives fast, temporary relief of pain, itching and burning. It is recommended for sunburn, nonpoisonous insect bites, minor burns, cuts and scratches. **DO NOT USE THIS PRODUCT IN OR NEAR YOUR EYES.**
Apply to affected areas gently. If necessary, cover with a light dressing for protection. Do not use more than 1 ounce of Ointment in a 24-hour period for an adult. Do not use more than one-quarter of an ounce in a 24-hour period for a child. If irritation develops, discontinue use and consult your doctor.

How to use Nupercainal Hemorrhoidal and Anesthetic Ointment for fast, temporary relief of pain and itching due to hemorrhoids (also known as piles).
Remove cap from tube and set it aside. Attach the white plastic applicator to the tube. Squeeze the tube until you see the Ointment begin to come through the little holes in the applicator. Using your finger, lubricate the applicator with the Ointment. Now insert the entire applicator gently into the rectum. Give the tube a good squeeze to get enough Ointment into the rectum for comfort and lubrication. Remove applicator from rectum and wipe it clean. Apply additional Ointment to anal tissues to help relieve pain, burning, and itching. For best results use Ointment morning and night and after each bowel movement. After each use detach applicator, and wash it off with soap and water. Put cap back on tube before storing. In case of rectal bleeding, discontinue use and consult your doctor.
Pain-Relief Cream for general use. This Cream is particularly effective for fast, temporary relief of pain and itching associated with sunburn, cuts, scrapes, scratches, minor burns and nonpoisonous insect bites. **DO NOT USE THIS PRODUCT IN OR NEAR YOUR EYES.** Apply liberally to affected area and rub in gently. This Cream is water-washable, so be sure to reapply after bathing, swimming or sweating. If irritation develops, discontinue use and consult your doctor.
Nupercainal Hemorrhoidal and Anesthetic Ointment contains 1% dibucaine USP. Also contains acetone sodium bisulfite, lanolin, light mineral oil, purified water, and white petrolatum. Available in tubes of 1 and 2 ounces. Store between 59°–86°F.
Nupercainal Pain-Relief Cream contains 0.5% dibucaine USP. Also contains acetone sodium bisulfite, fragrance, glycerin, potassium hydroxide, purified water, stearic acid, and trolamine. Available in 1½ ounce tubes.
Dibucaine USP is officially classified as a "topical anesthetic" and is one of the strongest and longest lasting of all topical pain relievers. It is not a narcotic.

C86-62 (Rev. 11/86)

Shown in Product Identification
Section, page 407

NUPERCAINAL®
Suppositories

Caution: Nupercainal suppositories are not for prolonged or extensive use. Contact with the eyes should be avoided.

Continued on next page

The full prescribing information for each CIBA Consumer Pharmaceuticals product is contained herein and is that in effect as of December 1, 1988.

CIBA Consumer—Cont.

Consult labels before using.
Keep this and all medications out of reach of children.
NUPERCAINAL SUPPOSITORIES SHOULD NOT BE SWALLOWED. SWALLOWING CAN BE HAZARDOUS, PARTICULARLY TO CHILDREN. IN THE EVENT OF ACCIDENTAL SWALLOWING CONSULT A PHYSICIAN OR POISON CONTROL CENTER IMMEDIATELY.

Indications: Nupercainal Rectal Suppositories are for the temporary relief from itching, burning, and discomfort due to hemorrhoids or other anorectal disorders.

Hov. to use Nupercainal Suppositories for hemorrhoids (also known as piles) or other anorectal disorders.
Tear off one suppository along the perforated line. Remove foil wrapper. Insert the suppository, rounded end first, well into the anus until you can feel it moving into your rectum. For best results, use one suppository after each bowel movement as needed, but not to exceed 6 in a 24-hour period. Each suppository is sealed in its own foil packet to reduce danger of leakage when carried in pocket or purse. **To prevent melting, do not store above 86°F (30°C).**
Each Nupercainal Suppository contains 2.4 gram cocoa butter, and .25 gram zinc oxide. Also contains acetone sodium bisulfite and bismuth subgallate.

C86-42 (Rev. 9/86)
*Shown in Product Identification
Section, page 407*

OTRIVIN®
**xylometazoline hydrochloride USP
Decongestant
Nasal Spray and Nasal Drops 0.1%
Pediatric Nasal Drops 0.05%**

One application provides rapid and long-lasting relief of nasal congestion for up to 10 hours.
Quickly clears stuffy noses due to common cold, sinusitis, hay fever.
Nasal congestion can make life miserable—you can't breathe, smell, taste, or sleep comfortably. That is why Otrivin is so helpful. It clears away that stuffy feeling, usually within 5 to 10 minutes, and your head feels clear for hours.
Otrivin has been prescribed by doctors for many years. Here is how you use it:
Nasal Spray 0.1%—for adults and children 12 years and older. Spray 2 or 3 times into each nostril every 8–10 hours. With head upright, squeeze sharply and firmly while inhaling (sniffing) through the nose.
Nasal Drops 0.1%—for adults and children 12 years and older. Put 2 or 3 drops into each nostril every 8 to 10 hours. Tilt head as far back as possible. Immediately bend head forward toward knees, hold for a few seconds, then return to upright position.

Do not give Nasal Spray 0.1% or Nasal Drops 0.1% to children under 12 years except under the advice and supervision of a physician.
Pediatric Nasal Drops 0.05%—for children 2 to 12 years of age. Put 2 or 3 drops into each nostril every 8 to 10 hours. Tilt head as far back as possible. Immediately bend head forward toward knees, hold a few seconds, then return to upright position.
Do not give this product to children under 2 years except under the advice and supervision of a physician.
Otrivin Nasal Spray/Nasal Drops contain 0.1% xylometazoline hydrochloride, USP. Also contains benzalkonium chloride, potassium chloride, potassium phosphate monobasic, purified water, sodium chloride and sodium phosphate dibasic. They are available in an unbreakable plastic spray package of ½ fl oz (15 ml) and in a plastic dropper bottle of .66 fl oz (20 ml).
Otrivin Pediatric Nasal Drops contain 0.05% xylometazoline hydrochloride, USP. Also contains benzalkonium chloride, potassium chloride, potassium phosphate monobasic, purified water, sodium chloride and sodium phosphate dibasic. It is available in a plastic dropper bottle of .66 fl oz (20 ml).

Warnings: Do not exceed recommended dosage, because symptoms such as burning, stinging, sneezing, or increase of nasal discharge may occur. Do not use this product for more than 3 days. If symptoms persist, consult a physician. The use of this dispenser by more than one person may cause infection.
Keep this and all medicines out of the reach of children. Overdosage in young children may cause marked sedation. In case of accidental ingestion, seek professional assistance or contact a Poison Control Center immediately.
Store between 33°–86°F

C86-44 (9/86)
*Shown in Product Identification
Section, page 407*

PRIVINE®
**naphazoline hydrochloride, USP
0.05% Nasal Solution
0.05% Nasal Spray**

Caution: Do not use Privine if you have glaucoma. Privine is an effective nasal decongestant **when you use it in the recommended dosage.** If you use too much, too long, or too often, Privine may be harmful to your nasal mucous membranes and cause burning, stinging, sneezing or an increased runny nose.
Do not use Privine by mouth.
Keep this and all medications out of the reach of children. Do not use Privine with children under 12 years of age, except with the advice and supervision of a doctor.
OVERDOSAGE IN YOUNG CHILDREN MAY CAUSE MARKED SEDATION AND IF SEVERE, EMERGENCY TREATMENT MAY BE NECESSARY. IF NASAL STUFFINESS PERSISTS AFTER 3 DAYS OF TREATMENT,

DISCONTINUE USE AND CONSULT A DOCTOR.
Privine is a nasal decongestant that comes in two forms: Nasal Solution (in a bottle with a dropper) and Nasal Spray (in a plastic squeeze bottle). Both are for prompt, and prolonged relief of nasal congestion due to common colds, sinusitis, hay fever, etc.
How to use Nasal Solution. Squeeze rubber bulb to fill dropper with proper amount of medication. For best results, tilt head as far back as possible and put two drops of solution into your right nostril. Then lean head forward, inhaling and turning your head to the left. Refill dropper by squeezing bulb. Now tilt head as far back as possible and put two drops of solution into your left nostril. Then lean head forward, inhaling, and turning your head to the right.
Use only 2 drops in each nostril. Do not repeat this dosage more than every 3 hours.
The Privine dropper bottle is designed to make administration of the proper dosage easy and to prevent accidental overdosage. Privine will not cause sleeplessness, so you may use it before going to bed.

Important: After use, be sure to rinse the dropper with very hot water. This helps prevent contamination of the bottle with bacteria from nasal secretions. Use of the dispenser by more than one person may spread infection.

Note: Privine Nasal Solution may be used on contact with glass, plastic, stainless steel and specially treated metals used in atomizers. Do not let the solution come in contact with reactive metals, especially aluminum. If solution becomes discolored, it should be discarded.
How to use Nasal Spray. For best results do **not** shake the plastic squeeze bottle.
Remove cap. With head held upright, spray twice into each nostril. Squeeze the bottle sharply and firmly while sniffing through the nose.
For best results use every 4 to 6 hours. Do not use more often than every 3 hours. Avoid overdosage. Follow directions for use carefully.
Privine Nasal Solution contains 0.05% naphazoline hydrochloride USP. It also contains benzalkonium chloride, disodium edetate dihydrate, hydrochloric acid, purified water, sodium chloride, and trolamine. It is available in bottles of .66 fl. oz. (20 ml) with dropper, and bottles of 16 fl. oz. (473 ml).
Privine Nasal Spray contains 0.05% naphazoline hydrochloride USP. It also contains benzalkonium chloride, disodium edetate dihydrate, hydrochloric acid, purified water, sodium chloride, and trolamine. It is available in plastic squeeze bottles of ½ fl. oz. (15 ml).
Store the nasal solution and nasal spray between 59°–86°F.

C86-43 (Rev. 9/86)
*Shown in Product Identification
Section, page 407*

Q–VEL®
Muscle Relaxant Pain Reliever

Active Ingredient: Quinine Sulfate 1 gr. (64.8 mg).

Contains: Vitamin E (400 I.U. *dl*-alpha tocopheryl acetate) in a lecithin base.

Indications: For prevention and temporary relief of night leg cramps.

Warnings: Do not take if pregnant, nursing a baby or of childbearing potential, if sensitive to quinine, or under 12 years of age. Discontinue use and consult your physician if ringing in the ears, deafness, diarrhea, nausea, skin rash, bruising or visual disturbances occur. In case of accidental overdose, seek medical assistance or contact Poison Control Center at once. Keep this and all medicine out of reach of children.

Dosage: To prevent night leg cramps take 2 soft caplets after the evening meal plus 2 at bedtime. For relief in case of sudden attack, take 2 soft caplets at once plus 2 after ½ hour if needed. Do not exceed 4 soft caplets daily.

How Supplied: Bottles of 16, 30 and 50 softgels.

Shown in Product Identification Section, page 407

SLOW FE®
Slow Release Iron Tablets

Description: SLOW FE supplies ferrous sulfate for the treatment of iron deficiency and iron deficiency anemia with a significant reduction in the incidence of common iron side effects. The wax matrix delivery system of SLOW FE is designed to maximize the release of ferrous sulfate in the duodenum and the jejunum where it is best tolerated and absorbed. SLOW FE has been clinically shown to significantly reduce constipation, diarrhea and abdominal discomfort when compared to regular iron tablets and a leading capsule.

Formula: Each tablet contains 160 mg. dried ferrous sulfate USP, equivalent to 50 mg. elemental iron. Also contains cetostearyl alcohol, colloidal silicon dioxide, hydroxypropyl methylcellulose, shellac, lactose, magnesium stearate, polyethylene glycol.

Dosage: ADULTS—one or two tablets daily or as recommended by a physician. A maximum of four tablets daily may be taken. CHILDREN—one tablet daily. Tablets must be swallowed whole.

Warning: The treatment of any anemic condition should be under the advice and supervision of a physician. As oral iron products interfere with absorption of oral tetracycline antibiotics, these products should not be taken within two hours of each other. As with any drug, if you are pregnant or nursing a baby, seek the advice of a health professional before using this product.
Keep this and all medicines out of reach of children. In case of accidental

VITAMINS	QUANTITY PER TABLET	PERCENT U.S. RDA	
		FOR CHILD. 2 TO 4 YRS OF AGE (1 TABLET)	FOR ADULTS & CHILD. OVER 4 YRS OF AGE (1 TABLET)
Vitamin A (as Palmitate + Beta Carotene)	2500 IU	100	50
Vitamin D-3	400 IU	100	100
Vitamin E	15 IU	150	50
Vitamin C	60 mg	150	100
Folic Acid	0.3 mg	150	75
Niacinamide	13.5 mg	150	68
Vitamin B-6	1.05 mg	150	53
Vitamin B-12	4.5 mcg	150	75
Vitamin B-1	1.05 mg	150	70
Vitamin B-2	1.20 mg	150	71
Vitamin K-1	5 mcg	*	*

*Recognized as essential in human nutrition, but no U.S. RDA established.

overdose, contact your physician or poison control center immediately.
Tamper Resistant Packaging.

How Supplied: Packages of 30, 60 and 100.

Shown in Product Identification Section, page 407

SUNKIST CHILDREN'S CHEWABLE MULTIVITAMINS—REGULAR

Vitamin Ingredients: Each tablet contains:
[See table above].

Indication: Dietary supplementation.

Dosage and Administration: One chewable tablet daily for children two years and older.

Warning: Phenylketonurics: Contains Phenylalanine

How Supplied: SUNKIST Children's Multivitamins-Regular are supplied in bottles of 60 chewable tablets with child resistant caps.

Shown in Product Identification Section, page 408

SUNKIST CHILDREN'S CHEWABLE MULTIVITAMINS—PLUS EXTRA C

Vitamin Ingredients: Each tablet contains the ingredients of the Regular vitamin product plus extra Vitamin C (a total of 250 mg).

Indication: Dietary supplementation.

Dosage and Administration: One chewable tablet daily for adults and children two years and older.

Warning: Phenylketonurics: Contains Phenylalanine.

How Supplied: SUNKIST Children's Multivitamins Plus Extra C are supplied in bottles of 60 chewable tablets with child resistant caps.

Shown in Product Identification Section, page 408

SUNKIST CHILDREN'S CHEWABLE MULTIVITAMINS—PLUS IRON

Vitamin Ingredients: Each tablet contains the vitamins of the Regular product plus 15 mg of Iron.

Indication: Dietary supplementation.

Dosage and Administration: One chewable tablet daily for children two years and older.

Warning: Phenylketonurics: Contains Phenylalanine.

Precaution: Contains iron, which can be harmful in large doses. Close tightly and keep out of reach of children. In case of overdose, contact a physician or poison control center immediately.

How Supplied: SUNKIST Children's Multivitamins Plus Iron are supplied in bottles of 60 chewable tablets with child resistant caps.

Shown in Product Identification Section, page 408

SUNKIST CHILDREN'S CHEWABLE MULTIVITAMINS—COMPLETE

Vitamin Ingredients: Each tablet contains the following ingredients:
[See table on next page].

Indication: Dietary supplementation.

Dosage and Administration: Children ages 2 to 4 one-half chewable tablet daily; One chewable tablet daily for children four years and older.

Warning: Phenylketonurics: Contains Phenylalanine.

Precautions: Contains iron, which can be harmful in large doses. Close tightly and keep out of reach of children. In case of overdose, contact a physician or poison control center immediately.

How Supplied: SUNKIST Children's Multivitamins Complete are supplied in bottles of 60 chewable tablets with child resistant caps.

Shown in Product Identification Section, page 408

Continued on next page

The full prescribing information for each CIBA Consumer Pharmaceuticals product is contained herein and is that in effect as of December 1, 1988.

CIBA Consumer—Cont.

SUNKIST® VITAMIN C
Citrus Complex
Chewable Tablets
Easy to Swallow Caplets

Description: All Sunkist Vitamin C chewable tablets have a delicious orange flavor unlike any other Vitamin C tablet. Each 60 mg chewable tablet contains 100% of the U.S. RDA* of Vitamin C. Each 250 mg chewable tablet contains 417% of the U.S. RDA* of Vitamin C. Each 500 mg chewable tablet contains 833% of the U.S. RDA* of Vitamin C.

Each 500 mg easy to swallow caplet contains 833% of the U.S. RDA* of Vitamin C.

Sunkist Vitamin C chewable tablets and easy to swallow caplets do not contain artificial flavors, colors or preservatives.

*U.S. Recommended Daily Allowance for adults and children over 4 years of age.

Indication: Dietary supplement.

How Supplied: 60 mg Chewable Tablets—Rolls of 11.
250 mg and 500 mg Chewable Tablets—Bottles of 60.
500 mg Easy to Swallow Caplets—Bottles of 60.

Store in a cool dry place.

Sunkist® is a registered trademark of Sunkist Growers, Inc., Sherman Oaks, CA 91423.©

(12/86)
Shown in Product Identification Section, page 407

Colgate-Palmolive Company
A Delaware Corporation
300 PARK AVENUE
NEW YORK, NY 10022

COLGATE® JUNIOR FLUORIDE GEL TOOTHPASTE

Active Ingredient: Sodium Monofluorophosphate (MFP®) 0.76% in a fruit-flavored toothpaste base.

Other Ingredients: Sorbitol, Glycerin, Hydrated Silica, Water, PEG-12, Sodium Lauryl Sulfate, Sodium Benzoate, Flavor, Cellulose Gum, Sodium Saccharin, Titanium Dioxide, FD&C Blue No. 1, D&C Yellow No. 10.

Indications: This toothpaste, with its anti-cavity ingredient MFP® Fluoride, provides clinically proven fluoride protection. It has been specially formulated to appeal to children 12 and under.

Actions: Clinical tests have shown Colgate® with MFP® Fluoride to be an effective aid in the reduction of the incidence of cavities. It is approved as a decay-preventive agent by the American Dental Association.

Contraindications: Sensitivity to any ingredient in the product.

Directions: Brush regularly as part of a dental health program.

How Supplied: 2.7 oz., 4.5 oz., 6.4 oz., and 8.2 oz. tubes. Also available in 4.5 oz. pump.
Shown in Product Identification Section, page 408

COLGATE MFP® FLUORIDE GEL

Active Ingredient: Sodium Monofluorophosphate (MFP®) 0.76% in a spearmint flavored gel toothpaste base.

Other Ingredients: Sorbitol, Glycerin, Hydrated Silica, Water, PEG-12, Sodium Lauryl Sulfate, Flavor, Sodium Benzoate, Cellulose Gum, Sodium Saccharin, Titanium Dioxide, FD&C Blue No. 1.

Indications: The gel toothpaste with the anti-cavity ingredient MFP® Fluoride providing maximum fluoride protection by a toothpaste and a fresh clean taste for the whole family.

Actions: Clinical tests have shown COLGATE® with MFP® Fluoride to be an effective aid in the reduction of the incidence of cavities. It is approved as a decay-preventive dentifrice by the American Dental Association.

Contraindications: Sensitivity to any ingredient in this product.

Directions: Brush regularly as part of a dental health program.

How Supplied: 1.4 oz., 2.6 oz., 4.6 oz., 6.4 oz., 8.2 oz. tubes. Also available in 4.5 and 6.4 oz. pumps.
Shown in Product Identification Section, page 408

COLGATE MFP® FLUORIDE TOOTHPASTE

Active Ingredient: Sodium Monofluorophosphate (MFP®) 0.76% in a doublemint flavored toothpaste base.

Other Ingredients: Dicalcium Phosphate Dihydrate, Water, Glycerin, Sodium Lauryl Sulfate, Cellulose Gum, Flavor, Sodium Benzoate, Tetrasodium Pyrophosphate, Sodium Saccharin.

Indications: The toothpaste with the anti-cavity ingredient MFP® Fluoride providing maximum fluoride protection by a toothpaste.

Actions: Clinical tests have shown COLGATE® with MFP® Fluoride to be an effective aid in the reduction of the incidence of cavities. It is approved as a decay-preventive dentifrice by the American Dental Association.

Contraindications: Sensitivity to any ingredient in this product.

Directions: Brush regularly as part of a dental health program.

How Supplied: 1.50 oz., 3.0 oz., 5.0 oz., 7.0 oz., 9.0 oz. tubes. Also available in 4.9 and 6.4 oz. pumps.
Shown in Product Identification Section, page 408

COLGATE® MOUTHWASH TARTAR CONTROL FORMULA

Ingredients: Water, SD Alcohol 38-B (15.3%), Glycerin, Tetrapotassium Pyrophosphate, Poloxamer 336, Poloxamer 407, Tetrasodium Pyrophosphate, Benzoic Acid, PVM/MA Copolymer, Flavor, Sodium Saccharin, Sodium Fluoride, FD&C Blue #1, FD&C Yellow #5.

VITAMINS	QUANTITY PER TABLET	PERCENT U.S. RDA FOR CHILD. 2 TO 4 YRS OF AGE (½ TABLET)	PERCENT U.S. RDA FOR ADULTS & CHILD. OVER 4 YRS OF AGE (1 TABLET)
Vitamin A (as Palmitate + Beta Carotene)	5000 IU	100	100
Vitamin D-3	400 IU	50	100
Vitamin E	30 IU	150	100
Vitamin C	60 mg	75	100
Folic Acid	0.4 mg	100	100
Biotin	40 mcg	13	13
Pantothenic Acid	10 mg	100	100
Niacinamide	20 mg	111	100
Vitamin B-6	2 mg	143	100
Vitamin B-12	6 mcg	100	100
Vitamin B-1	1.5 mg	107	100
Vitamin B-2	1.7 mg	106	100
Vitamin K-1	110 mcg	*	*
MINERALS			
Iron	18 mg	90	100
Magnesium	20 mg	5	5
Iodine	150 mcg	107	100
Zinc	10 mg	63	67
Manganese	1 mg	*	*
Calcium	100 mg	6	10
Phosphorus	78 mg	5	8
Copper	2 mg	100	100

*Recognized as essential in human nutrition, but no U.S. RDA established.

Indications: Highly effective in the inhibition of supragingival calculus, Colgate Mouthrinse Tartar Control Formula also provides effective breath odor control.

Actions: Clinical studies have shown that Colgate's exclusive combination of pyrophosphate and PVM/MA copolymer reduces calculus build-up by up to 37.7%.

Contraindications: Sensitivity to any ingredient in the product.

Directions: Adults and children 6 years of age and older. Use twice daily after brushing teeth with a toothpaste. Vigorously swish 10 ml. (2 teaspoons; or up to mark on cap) of rinse between teeth for 1 minute and then expectorate. Do not swallow rinse. Do not eat or drink for 30 minutes after rinsing. Children under 6 years of age: Consult a dentist or physician. Children under 12 years of age should be supervised in the use of this product.

How Supplied: 2 oz., 6 oz., 24 oz. and 32 oz. plastic bottles with dose-measure cap.

Shown in Product Identification Section, page 408

COLGATE® TARTAR CONTROL FORMULA

Active Ingredient: Sodium Fluoride 0.24% in a mint flavored toothpaste base.

Other Ingredients: Water, Hydrated Silica, Sorbitol, Glycerine, PEG-12, Tetrapotassium Pyrophosphate, Tetrasodium Pyrophosphate, Sodium Lauryl Sulfate, Flavor, PVM/MA Copolymer, Titanium Dioxide, Carrageenan, Sodium Saccharin, CONTAINS NO SUGAR.

Indications: This toothpaste with the anti-cavity ingredient sodium fluoride provides maximum fluoride protection by a toothpaste and is highly effective in inhibiting the formation of calculus. Repeated clinical studies have demonstrated an average 46% inhibition of calculus buildup.

Actions: Clinical tests have shown Colgate Tartar Control Formula to be effective in the reduction of calculus accumulation. It is also approved as a decay preventive dentifrice by the American Dental Association.

Contraindications: Sensitivity to any ingredient in the product.

Directions: Brush regularly as part of a dental health program.

How Supplied: 1.3 oz., 2.6 oz., 4.6 oz., 6.4 oz., and 8.2 oz. tubes. Also available in 4.5 oz. Pump.

Shown in Product Identification Section, page 408

COLGATE® TARTAR CONTROL GEL

Active Ingredient: Sodium Fluoride 0.24% in a mint flavored gel toothpaste base.

Other Ingredients: Water, Hydrated Silica, Sorbitol, Glycerine, PEG-12, Tetrapotassium Pyrophosphate, Tetrasodium Pyrophosphate, Sodium Lauryl Sulfate, PVM/MA Copolymer, Carrageenan, Sodium Saccharin, FD&C Blue No. 1. CONTAINS NO SUGAR.

Indications: This gel toothpaste with the anti-cavity ingredient sodium fluoride provides maximum fluoride protection by a toothpaste and is highly effective in inhibiting the formation of calculus. Repeated clinical studies have demonstrated an average 46% inhibition of calculus buildup.

Actions: Clinical tests have shown Colgate Tartar Control Gel to be effective in the reduction of calculus accumulation. It is also approved as a decay preventive dentifrice by the American Dental Association.

Contraindications: Sensitivity to any ingredient in the product.

Directions: Brush regularly as part of a dental health program.

How Supplied: 1.3 oz., 2.6 oz., 4.6 oz., 6.4 oz., and 8.2 oz. tubes. Also available in 4.5 oz. Pump.

Shown in Product Identification Section, page 408

FLUORIGARD ANTI–CAVITY FLUORIDE RINSE

Fluorigard is accepted by the American Dental Association.

Active Ingredient: Sodium Fluoride (0.05%) in a neutral solution.

Other Ingredients: Water, Glycerin, SD Alcohol 38-B (6%), Poloxamer 338, Poloxamer 407, Sodium Benzoate, Sodium Saccharin, Benzoic Acid, Flavor, FD & C Blue No. 1, FD & C Yellow No. 5.

Indications: Good tasting Fluorigard Anti-Cavity Fluoride Rinse is fluoride in liquid form. It helps get cavity-fighting fluoride to back teeth, as well as front teeth; even floods those dangerous spaces between teeth where brushing might miss. 70% of all cavities happen in back teeth and between teeth.

Actions: Fluorigard Anti-Cavity Fluoride Rinse is a 0.05% Sodium Fluoride solution which has been proven effective in reducing cavities.

Contraindications: Sensitivity to any ingredient in this product.

Warnings: Do not swallow. For rinsing only. Not to be used by children under 6 years of age unless recommended by a dentist. Keep out of reach of young children. If an amount considerably larger than recommended for rinsing is swallowed, give as much milk as possible and contact a physician immediately.

Directions: Use once daily after thoroughly brushing teeth. For persons 6 years of age and over, fill measuring cap to 10 ml. level (2 teaspoons), rinse around and between teeth for one minute, then spit out. For maximum benefit, use every day and do not eat or drink for at least 30 minutes afterward. Rinsing may be most convenient at bedtime. This product may be used in addition to a fluoride toothpaste.

How Supplied: 6 oz., 12 oz., 18 oz. in shatterproof plastic bottles.
1 Gallon Professional Size for use in dentists offices only.

Shown in Product Identification Section, page 408

Cumberland-Swan, Inc.
ONE SWAN DRIVE
SMYRNA, TN 37167

SWAN CITROMA®, Laxative
Magnesium Citrate Oral Solution
Saline Laxative

Available in 3 Formulas:
1. REGULAR LEMON
2. LOW SODIUM SUGAR FREE LEMON
3. LOW SODIUM SUGAR FREE CHERRY

LOW SODIUM SUGAR FREE FORMULAS CONTAIN ONLY 2 mg. (0.085 mEq) OF SODIUM PER FL. OZ. AND ARE SUGAR FREE.

Description: Pleasant tasting, effervescent pasteurized liquid laxative. Also referred to as Citrate of Magnesia.

Active Ingredient: 1.745g Magnesium Citrate per fl. oz.

Indications: For the relief of constipation or irregularity. Bowel movement is generally produced in ½ to 6 hours. Also for use as part of a bowel cleansing regimen in preparing the patients for surgery, or the colon for x-ray or endoscopic examination.

Directions: Adults (12 yrs. and older) ½ to 1 full bottle. Children (6 to 12 yrs.) ⅓ to ½ bottle. Children under 6 consult a physician. Drink a full glass (8 oz) of liquid with each dose. The dose may be taken as a single daily dose or in divided doses. Do not exceed maximum daily dose. Discard unused product within 24 hours after opening bottle.

Warnings: Frequent and continued use may cause dependence upon laxatives. Do not use in excess of ten days. Do not use this product if you are on a low salt diet or have kidney disease unless directed by a physician. Do not use when abdominal pain, nausea or vomiting are present. Rectal blood or failure to have a bowel movement after use of a laxative may indicate a serious condition. Discontinue use and consult a physician. As with any drug, if you are pregnant or nursing a baby, seek the advice of a health professional before using this product.

Warning: KEEP THIS AND ALL DRUGS OUT OF THE REACH OF CHILDREN.

Continued on next page

Cumberland-Swan—Cont.

In case of accidental overdose, consult a physician or contact a Poison Control Center immediately.

Caution: (CHERRY FLAVOR ONLY) May cause a red color in the feces.

How Supplied: Bottles of 10 fluid ounces.

Shown in Product Identification Section, page 408

Daywell Laboratories Corporation
78 UNQUOWA PLACE
FAIRFIELD, CT 06430

VERGO® Cream

Composition: Vergo contains Pancin®, a special formulation of calcium pantothenate, ascorbic acid and starch.

Action and Uses: Vergo is a conservative, painless and safe treatment of warts. Vergo is very gentle, even for diabetics. It is not liquid. It is not caustic. It can be used on all parts of the body, even on the face. Vergo will not burn, blister, scar or injure surrounding tissue. Vergo is easily applied by finger. The ingredients are essential to the soundness of tissues and skin and will relieve the pain of warts and promote healing. Vergo is not irritating and there are no contraindications to its use. The average treatment time is from 2 to 8 weeks depending on the size of the wart and the response of the patient. It is important that the directions be carefully followed and that treatment be continued without interruption as long as necessary. Mosaic-type warts are more resistant and usually require longer treatment for relief.

Administration and Dosage: Cleanse area with soap and water; rinse thoroughly. Apply Vergo liberally to wart. Do not massage or rub in. Cover with plain Band-Aid® or gauze and adhesive tape. Change dressing and apply Vergo twice a day, morning and evening.

Side Effects: None known.

How Supplied: In one-half ounce tubes.

Product Identification Mark: Vergo®.

Literature Available: Yes.

Vergo
Painless and safe treatment for the removal of warts.

Products are cross-indexed by generic and chemical names in the
YELLOW SECTION

Dermik Laboratories, Inc.
790 PENLLYN PIKE
BLUE BELL, PA 19422

HYTONE® CREAM ½%
[hi 'tōne]
(hydrocortisone ½%)

Active Ingredient: Hydrocortisone 0.5%.

Indications: For the temporary relief of minor skin irritations, itching, and rashes due to eczema, dermatitis, insect bites, poison ivy, poison oak, poison sumac, soaps, detergents, cosmetics, jewelry, and for itchy genital and anal areas.

Actions: Provides temporary relief of itching and minor skin irritations.

Warnings: For External Use Only. Avoid contact with eyes. If condition worsens, or if symptoms persist for more than 7 days, discontinue use of this product and consult a physician. Do not use on children under 2 years of age except under the advice and supervision of a physician. KEEP OUT OF THE REACH OF CHILDREN.

Dosage and Administration: For adults and children 2 years of age and older: Apply to affected area not more than 3 or 4 times daily, or as directed by physician.

How Supplied: Tube, 1 ounce.

SHEPARD'S CREAM LOTION
Skin Lubricant—Moisturizer

Composition: Water, sesame oil, SD alcohol 40-B, stearic acid, propylene glycol, ethoxydiglycol, glycerin, triethanolamine, glyceryl stearate, cetyl alcohol, may contain fragrance ("scented" only), simethicone, methylparaben, propylparaben, vegetable oil, monoglyceride citrate, BHT and citric acid.

Indications: For generalized dryness and itching, sunburn, "winter-itch", dry skin, heat rash.

Actions and Uses: Shepard's Cream Lotion is a rich lotion containing soothing Oil of Sesame.

Dosage and Administration: Apply as often as needed. Use particularly after bathing and exposure to sun, water, soaps and detergents.

How Supplied: Scented and Unscented 8 oz bottle and 16 oz pump bottle.

SHEPARD'S SKIN CREAM
Concentrated
Moisturizer—Non-greasy Emollient

Composition: Water, glyceryl stearate, ethoxydiglycol, propylene glycol, glycerin, stearic acid, isopropyl myristate, cetyl alcohol, urea, lecithin, may contain fragrance ("scented" only) methylparaben and propylparaben.

Indications: For problem dry skin of the hands, face, elbows, feet, legs. Helps resist effects of soaps, detergents and chemicals.

Actions: Soothing, rich lubricant containing glyceryl stearate in a non-greasy or sticky base containing no lanolin or mineral oil. Shepard's Skin Cream helps retain moisture that makes skin feel soft, smooth, supple.

Dosage and Administration: A small amount is rubbed into dry skin areas as needed.

How Supplied: Scented and Unscented, 4 oz jars.

SHEPARD'S MOISTURIZING SOAP
Cleanser for Dry Skin

Composition: Sodium Tallowate, Sodium Cocoate, Water, Fragrance, Lanolin, Mineral Oil, Titanium Dioxide, Pentasodium Penetate, Tetrasodium Etidronate.

Indications: As a daily cleanser of dry skin of the face, hands, or in the bath or shower. Shepard's Soap helps to give the skin an overall smoothness.

Actions: A lightly scented, non-detergent moisturizing soap containing lanolin that cleanses the skin while helping to minimize the excessive drying inherent in most detergent-type soaps.

Dosage and Administration: Use regularly to cleanse face and hands as well as in the bath or shower.

How Supplied: 4 oz bars.

VANOXIDE® ACNE LOTION
[van 'ox-īd]
(Dries Clear)
LOROXIDE® ACNE LOTION
[lor 'ox-īd]
(Flesh Tinted)

Description: Vanoxide® Lotion contains (as dispensed) benzoyl peroxide 5%, incorporated in a lotion that dries on clear. Loroxide® Lotion contains (as dispensed) benzoyl peroxide 5.5%, incorporated in a flesh-tinted lotion.

Actions: Provides keratolytic, peeling and drying action.

Indications: An aid in the treatment of acne and oily skin.

Contraindications: These products are contraindicated for use by patients having known hypersensitivity to benzoyl peroxide or any other component of these preparations.

Precautions: For external use only. Keep away from eyes. Do not add any other medicaments or substances to these lotions unless specifically directed by physician to do so. Patients should be observed carefully for possible local irritation or sensitivity during long-term topical therapy. If any irritation or sensitivity is observed, discontinue use and consult physician. Apply with caution on neck and/or other sensitive areas. There may be a slight, transitory stinging or burning sensation on initial application which invariably disappears on contin-

ued use. Ultraviolet and cold quartz light should be employed in lesser amounts as these lotions are keratolytic and drying. Harsh, abrasive cleansers should not be used simultaneously with these lotions. Colored or dyed garments may be bleached by the oxidizing action of benzoyl peroxide. Occurrence of excessive redness or peeling indicates that the amount and frequency of application should be reduced. Keep out of the reach of children.

Adverse Reactions: The sensitizing potential of benzoyl peroxide is low; but it can, on occasion, produce allergic reaction.

Directions: Shake well before using. Apply a thin film to affected areas with light massaging to blend in each application 1 or 2 times daily or in accordance with the physician's directions.

How Supplied: Vanoxide® Lotion—Bottles 25 grams (0.88 oz) and 50 grams (1.76 oz) net weights as dispensed. Loroxide® Lotion—Bottles, 25 grams (0.88 oz) net weight as dispensed. A "Dermik Color Blender™" is provided with Loroxide® Lotion which enables the patient to alter the basic shade of the lotion to match the skin color.

VLEMASQUE®
[vle 'mask]
Acne Mask Treatment

Active Ingredient: Contains sulfurated lime topical solution 6%, S.D. alcohol 7% in a drying clay mask.

Indications: For the treatment of acne.

Warnings: Keep away from eyes. In case of contact, flush eyes thoroughly. For external use only. If any irritation appears, stop treatment immediately and consult physician.

Dosage and Administration: Daily, apply generous layer over entire face and neck, or as directed by physician. Avoid eyes, nostrils and lips. Leave on for 20–25 minutes. Remove with lukewarm water, using a gentle circular motion. Pat dry. U.S. Pat. No. 4,388,301

How Supplied: 4 oz Jars

ZETAR® SHAMPOO
[ze 'tar]
(Antidandruff Shampoo)

Active Ingredients: WHOLE Coal Tar (as Zetar®) 1.0%, in a golden foam shampoo which produces soft, fluffy abundant lather.

Actions and Indications: Antiseptic, antibacterial, antiseborrheic. Loosens and softens scales and crusts. Indicated in psoriasis, seborrhea, dandruff, cradlecap and other oily, itchy conditions of the body and scalp.

Contraindications: Acute inflammation, open or infected lesions.

Precautions: If undue skin irritation develops or increases, discontinue use

and consult physician. In rare instances, temporary discoloration of blond, bleached or tinted hair may occur. Avoid contact with eyes.

Dosage and Administration: Massage into moistened scalp. Rinse. Repeat; leave on 5 minutes. Rinse thoroughly.

How Supplied: 6 oz plastic bottles.

Fisons
Consumer Health Div.
Fisons Pharmaceuticals
P.O. BOX 1212
ROCHESTER, NY 14603

AMERICAINE® HEMORRHOIDAL OINTMENT
[a-mer 'i-kān]

Active Ingredient: Benzocaine 20%

Other Ingredients: Benzethonium Chloride; Polyethylene Glycol 300; Polyethylene Glycol 3350.

Indications: For the temporary relief of pain, itching and soreness of hemorrhoids and other minor anorectal irritation.

Warnings: For external use only. If condition worsens, or if symptoms persist for more than 7 days, consult a physician. Some people are allergic to benzocaine. Discontinue use and consult a physician if rash or irritation develops. In case of rectal bleeding, consult a physician promptly. Keep this and all drugs out of the reach of children. In case of accidental ingestion, seek professional assistance or contact a Poison Control Center immediately.

Directions: Adults and children over 12 years of age: Apply externally to the anorectal area not more than 6 times daily. Children 12 years of age and under: Consult a physician.

How Supplied: Hemorrhoidal Ointment —1 oz. tube.

AMERICAINE® TOPICAL ANESTHETIC SPRAY AND OINTMENT
[a-mer 'i-kān]

Active Ingredient: Benzocaine 20%

Other Ingredients: Spray —Butane (propellant); Isobutane (propellant); Polyethylene Glycol 200; Propane (propellant). Ointment —Benzethonium chloride; Polyethylene Glycol 300; Polyethylene Glycol 3350.

Indications: For the temporary relief of pain and itching associated with minor cuts, scrapes, burns, sunburn, insect bites, or minor skin irritations.

Warnings: For external use only. Avoid contact with the eyes. If condition worsens, or if symptoms persist for more than 7 days or clear up and occur again within a few days, discontinue use of this product and consult a physician. Keep this and all drugs out of the reach of children. In case of accidental ingestion, seek

professional assistance or contact a Poison Control Center immediately. *For Spray only* —Contents under pressure. Do not puncture or incinerate. Flammable mixture; do not use near fire or flame. Do not store at temperature above 120°F. Use only as directed. Intentional misuse by deliberately concentrating and inhaling the contents can be harmful or fatal.

Directions: Adults and children 2 years of age and older: Apply liberally to affected area not more than 3 to 4 times daily. Children under 2 years of age: Consult a physician.

How Supplied: *Topical Anesthetic Spray* —⅔ oz., 2 oz. and 4 oz. aerosol containers. *Topical Anesthetic Ointment* —¾ oz. tube.

ALLEREST® TABLETS, CHILDREN'S CHEWABLE TABLETS, HEADACHE STRENGTH TABLETS, SINUS PAIN FORMULA TABLETS, 12 HOUR CAPLETS AND NO DROWSINESS ALLEREST™ TABLETS
[al 'e-rest]

Active Ingredients:
acetaminophen
  Headache Strength, 325 mg
  No Drowsiness, 325 mg
  Sinus Pain Formula, 500 mg
chlorpheniramine maleate
  Tablets, 2 mg
  Children's Chewables, 1 mg
  Sinus Pain Formula, 2 mg
  Headache Strength, 2 mg
  12 Hour Caplets, 12 mg
phenylpropanolamine HCl
  Tablets, 18.7 mg
  Children's Chewables, 9.4 mg
  Sinus Pain Formula, 18.7 mg
  Headache Strength, 18.7 mg
  12 Hour Caplets, 75 mg
pseudoephedrine HCl
  No Drowsiness, 30 mg

Other Ingredients:
Allerest Tablets — Blue 1; Dibasic Calcium Phosphate; Magnesium Stearate; Microcrystalline Cellulose; Povidone; Pregelatinized Starch; Sodium Starch Glycolate.
Children's Chewable Tablets —Blue 1; Calcium Stearate; Citric Acid; Flavor; Magnesium Trisilicate Mannitol; Red 3; Saccharin Sodium; Sorbitol.
Headache Strength and No Drowsiness Tablets —Magnesium Stearate; Microcrystalline Cellulose; Povidone; Pregelatinized Starch.
Sinus Pain Formula Tablets —Magnesium Stearate; Microcrystalline Cellulose; Povidone; Pregelatinized Starch; Sodium Starch Glycolate.
12 Hour Caplets —Carnauba Wax; Colloidal Silicon Dioxide; Lactose; Methylcellulose; Polyethylene Glycol; Povidone; Red 30; Stearic Acid; Titanium Dioxide; Yellow 6.

Indications: Allerest is indicated for symptomatic relief of hay fever, pollen allergies, upper respiratory allergies (pe-

Continued on next page

Fisons—Cont.

rennial allergic rhinitis), allergic colds, sinusitis and nasal passage congestion. Those symptoms include headache pain, sneezing, runny nose, itchy/watery eyes, and itching nose and throat.

Actions: Allerest contains the antihistamine chlorpheniramine maleate which acts to suppress the symptoms of allergic rhinitis. In addition, it contains the decongestant phenylpropanolamine hydrochloride which acts to reduce swelling of the upper respiratory tract mucosa. Headache Strength and Sinus Pain Formula also contain acetaminophen to relieve headache pain.
No Drowsiness Allerest contains the decongestant pseudoephedrine hydrochloride and the analgesic acetaminophen to relieve headache pain and nasal congestion without causing drowsiness.

Contraindications: Known hypersensitivity to the ingredients in this drug.

Warnings: Allerest should be used with caution in patients with high blood pressure, heart disease, diabetes, thyroid disease, asthma, glaucoma, or difficulty in urination due to enlargement of the prostate gland. Since antihistamines may cause drowsiness, patients should be instructed not to operate a car or machinery. Products containing analgesics should not be taken for more than 10 days in adults and 5 days in children under 12.

Drug Interaction Precautions: Not to be taken by patients currently taking a prescription antihypertensive or antidepressant drug containing a monoamine oxidase inhibitor except under the advice and supervision of a physician.
Antihistamines and oral nasal decongestants have additive effects with alcohol and other CNS depressants.

Adverse Reactions: Drowsiness; excitability, especially in children; nervousness; and dizziness.

Overdosage: Acetaminophen in massive overdosage may cause hepatotoxicity.

Dosage and Administration:
Tablets and Headache Strength —Adults, 2 tablets every 4 hours. Not to exceed 8 tablets in 24 hours. Children (6–12)—half the adult dose. Dosage for children under 6 should be individualized under the supervision of a physician. *Children's Chewable Tablets* —Children (6–12) 2 tablets every 4 hours. Not to exceed 8 tablets in 24 hours. Children under 6 consult a physician. Adults double the children's dose. *Sinus Pain Formula* —Adults, 2 tablets every 6 hours. Not to exceed 8 tablets in 24 hours. Not recommended for children 12 and under. *12 Hour Caplets* —Adults and children over 12 years of age, one caplet every 12 hours. Do not exceed 2 caplets in 24 hours.

How Supplied: *Tablets* —packaged on blister cards in 24, 48 and 72 count cartons. *Children's Chewable Tablets* —packaged on blister cards in 24 count cartons. *Headache Strength Tablets* —packaged on blister cards in 24 count cartons. *Sinus Pain Formula Tablets* —packaged on blister cards in 20 count cartons. *12 Hour Caplets* —packaged on blister cards in 10 count cartons. *No Drowsiness Tablets* —packaged on blister cards in 20 count cartons.

CaldeCORT® ANTI-ITCH CREAM AND SPRAY; CaldeCORT Light™ CREME
[kal 'de-kort]

Active Ingredient: *Cream, Light Creme* —Hydrocortisone Acetate (equivalent to Hydrocortisone 0.5%). *Spray* —Hydrocortisone 0.5%.

Other Ingredients: *Cream* —Glyceryl Monostearate; Lanolin Alcohol; Methylparaben; Mineral Oil; Polyoxyl 40 Stearate; Propylparaben; Sodium Metabisulfite; Sorbitol Solution; Stearyl Alcohol; Water; White Petrolatum; White Wax. *Light Creme* —Aloe Vera Gel; Isopropyl Myristate; Methylparaben; Polysorbate 60; Propylparaben; Sorbitan Monostearate; Sorbitol Solution; Stearic Acid; Water. *Spray* —Isobutane (propellant); Isopropyl Myristate; SD Alcohol 40-B 89.5% by volume.

Indications: For the temporary relief of itching associated with minor skin irritations, inflammation and rashes due to eczema, insect bites, poison ivy, poison oak, poison sumac, soaps, detergents, cosmetics and jewelry; and for external genital and anal itching.

Actions: Antidermatitis cream and spray for the temporary relief from itching and minor skin irritations.

Warnings: For external use only. Avoid contact with the eyes. If condition worsens, or if symptoms persist for more than 7 days or clear up and occur again within a few days, discontinue use and consult a doctor. Do not use if you have a vaginal discharge. Consult a doctor. Keep this and all drugs out of the reach of children. In case of accidental ingestion, seek professional assistance or contact a Poison Control Center immediately. *For Spray only* —Avoid spraying in eyes or on other mucous membranes. Contents under pressure. Do not puncture or incinerate. Flammable mixture, do not use near fire or flame. Do not store at temperature above 120°F. Use only as directed. Intentional misuse by deliberately concentrating and inhaling the contents can be harmful or fatal.

Directions: Adults and children 2 years of age and older: Apply to affected area not more than 3 to 4 times daily. Children under 2 years of age: Consult a doctor.

How Supplied: *Anti-Itch Cream* —½ and 1 oz. tubes. *Anti-Itch Spray* —1½ oz. can. *Light Creme* —½ oz. tubes.

CALDESENE® MEDICATED POWDER AND OINTMENT
[kal 'de-sēn]

Active Ingredients: *Powder* —Calcium Undecylenate 10%. *Ointment* —Petrolatum 53.9%; Zinc Oxide 15%.

Other Ingredients: *Powder* — Fragrance; Talc. *Ointment* —Cod Liver Oil; Fragrance; Lanolin Oil; Methylparaben; Propylparaben; Talc.

Indications: Caldesene Medicated Powder is indicated to help heal, relieve and prevent diaper rash, prickly heat and chafing. Medicated Ointment helps prevent diaper rash and soothe minor skin irritations.

Actions: Antifungal and antibacterial Medicated Powder inhibits the growth of bacteria and fungi which cause diaper rash. Also, forms a protective coating to repel moisture, soothe and comfort minor skin irritations, helps heal and prevent chafing and prickly heat. Medicated Ointment forms a protective skin coating to repel moisture and promote healing of diaper rash, while its natural ingredients protect irritated skin against wetness. Soothes minor skin irritations, superficial wounds and burns.

Warnings: For external use only. Avoid contact with eyes. If condition worsens or does not improve within 7 days, consult a doctor. Do not apply ointment over deep or puncture wounds, infections and lacerations. Keep this and all drugs out of the reach of children. In case of accidental ingestion, seek professional assistance or contact a Poison Control Center immediately.

Directions: Cleanse and thoroughly dry affected area. Smooth on Caldesene 3–4 times daily, after every bath or diaper change, or as directed by a physician.

How Supplied: *Medicated Powder* —2.0 oz. and 4.0 oz. shaker containers. *Medicated Ointment* —1.25 oz. collapsible tubes.

CRUEX® ANTIFUNGAL POWDER, SPRAY POWDER AND CREAM
[kru 'ex]

Active Ingredients: *Powder* —Calcium Undecylenate 10%. *Spray Powder* —Total Undecylenate 19%, as Undecylenic Acid and Zinc Undecylenate. *Cream* —Total Undecylenate 20%, as Undecylenic Acid and Zinc Undecylenate.

Other Ingredients: *Powder* —Colloidal Silicon Dioxide; Fragrance; Isopropyl Myristate; Talc. *Spray Powder* —Fragrance; Isobutane (propellant); Isopropyl Myristate; Menthol; Talc; Trolamine. *Cream* —Anhydrous Lanolin; Fragrance; Glycol Stearate SE; Methylparaben; PEG-6 Stearate; PEG-8 Laurate; Propylparaben; Sorbitol Solution; Stearic Acid; Trolamine; Water; White Petrolatum.

Indications: For the treatment of Jock Itch (tinea cruris) and relief of itching, chafing, burning rash and irritation in the groin area. Cruex powders also absorb perspiration.

Actions: Antifungal Powder, Spray Powder and Cream are proven clinically effective in the treatment of superficial fungus infections of the skin.

Warnings: Do not use on children under 2 years of age except under the advice and supervision of a doctor. For external use only. If irritation occurs, or if there is no improvement within 2 weeks, discontinue use and consult a doctor or pharmacist. Keep this and all drugs out of the reach of children. In case of accidental ingestion, seek professional assistance or contact a Poison Control Center immediately. *For Spray Powder only* —Avoid spraying in eyes or on other mucous membranes. Contents under pressure. Do not puncture or incinerate. Flammable mixture, do not use near a fire or flame. Do not store at temperature above 120° F. Use only as directed. Intentional misuse by deliberately concentrating and inhaling the contents can be harmful or fatal.

Directions: Cleanse skin with soap and water and dry thoroughly. Apply Cruex to affected area morning and night, before and after athletic activity, or as directed by a doctor. Best results are usually obtained with 2 weeks' use of this product. If satisfactory results have not occurred within this time, consult a doctor or pharmacist. Children under 12 years of age should be supervised in the use of this product. This product is not effective on the scalp or nails.

How Supplied: *Powder* —1.5 oz. plastic squeeze bottle. *Spray Powder* —1.8 oz., 3.5 oz. and 5.5 oz. aerosol containers. *Cream* —½ oz. tube.

DESENEX® ANTIFUNGAL POWDER, SPRAY POWDER, CREAM, OINTMENT, LIQUID AND PENETRATING FOAM; SOAP; FOOT & SNEAKER SPRAY
[dess 'i-nex]

Active Ingredients: *Powder, Spray Powder* —Total Undecylenate 19%, as Undecylenic Acid and Zinc Undecylenate. *Cream* —Total Undecylenate 20%, as Undecylenic Acid and Zinc Undecylenate. *Ointment* —Total Undecylenate 22%, as Undecylenic Acid and Zinc Undecylenate. *Liquid, Penetrating Foam* —Undecylenic Acid 10%. *Foot & Sneaker Spray* —Aluminum Chlorohydrex.

Other Ingredients: *Powder* — Fragrance; Talc. *Spray Powder* —Fragrance; Isobutane (propellant); Isopropyl Myristate; Menthol; Talc; Trolamine. *Cream, Ointment* —Anhydrous Lanolin; Fragrance; Glycol Stearate SE; Methylparaben; PEG-6 Stearate; PEG-8 Laurate; Propylparaben; Sorbitol Solution; Stearic Acid; Trolamine; Water; White Petrolatum. *Liquid* —Fragrance; Isopropyl Alcohol 47.1% by volume; Polysorbate 80; Propylene Glycol; Trolamine; Water. *Penetrating Foam* —Emulsifying Wax; Fragrance; Isobutane (propellant); Isopropyl Alcohol 35.2% by volume; Sodium Benzoate; Trolamine; Water. *Foot & Sneaker Spray* —Colloidal Silicon Dioxide; Diisopropyl Adipate; Fragrance; Isobutane (propellant); Menthol; SD Alcohol 40-B 89.3% by volume; Talc; Tartaric Acid.

Indications: Desenex Antifungal Products cure athlete's foot (tinea pedis) and body ringworm (tinea corporis) exclusive of the nails and scalp. Relieves itching and burning. With daily use, prevents athlete's foot from coming back. Desenex Foot & Sneaker Spray helps stop odor and reduces wetness.

Actions: Desenex Antifungal Powders, Cream, Ointment, Liquid and Penetrating Foam are proven effective in the treatment of superficial fungus infections of the skin caused by the three major types of dermatophytic fungi (T. rubrum, T. mentagrophytes, E. floccosum). Penetrating Foam quickly dissolves into a highly concentrated liquid. Foot & Sneaker Spray is a formulated liquid that dries to a fine powder to protect feet from odor causing perspiration. Powder also helps keep feet dry and comfortable.

Warnings: Do not use on children under 2 years of age except under the advice and supervision of a doctor. For external use only. If irritation occurs, or if there is no improvement within 4 weeks, discontinue use and consult a doctor or pharmacist. Keep this and all drugs out of the reach of children. In case of accidental ingestion, seek professional assistance or contact a Poison Control Center immediately. *For Spray Powder, Penetrating Foam and Foot & Sneaker Spray only* —Avoid spraying in eyes or on other mucous membranes. Contents under pressure. Do not puncture or incinerate. Flammable mixture, do not use near fire or flame. Do not store at temperature above 120° F. Use only as directed. Intentional misuse by deliberately concentrating and inhaling the contents can be harmful or fatal.

Directions: *Powder, Spray Powder, Cream, Ointment, Liquid and Penetrating Foam* —Cleanse skin with soap and water and dry thoroughly. Apply over affected area morning and night or as directed by a doctor, paying special attention to the spaces between the toes. It is also helpful to wear well-fitting, ventilated shoes and to change shoes and socks at least once daily. Best results are usually obtained with 4 weeks' use of this product. If satisfactory results have not occurred within this time, consult a doctor or pharmacist. Children under 12 years of age should be supervised in the use of this product. This product is not effective on the scalp or nails. To prevent athlete's foot from coming back, use Desenex Powder or Spray Powder daily. For persistent cases of athlete's foot, use Desenex Ointment or Cream at night and Desenex Powder or Spray Powder during the day. *Soap* —Use in conjunction with Desenex Antifungal Products. *Foot & Sneaker Spray* —Spray on soles of feet and between toes daily. To fight offensive odor, spray liberally over entire inside area of shoes and sneakers before and after wearing.

How Supplied: *Powder* —1.5 oz. and 3.0 oz. shaker containers. *Spray Powder* —2.7 oz. and 5.5 oz. aerosol containers. *Cream* —½ oz. and 1 oz. tubes. *Ointment* —0.9 oz. and 1.8 oz. tubes. *Liquid* —1.5 oz. plastic squeeze bottle. *Penetrating Foam* —1.5 oz. aerosol container. *Soap* —3.25 oz. bar. *Foot & Sneaker Spray* —2.7 oz. aerosol container.

SINAREST® TABLETS, EXTRA STRENGTH TABLETS AND NO DROWSINESS SINAREST™ TABLETS
[sīn 'a-rest]

Active Ingredients:
acetaminophen:
  Tablets, 325 mg
  Extra Strength, 500 mg
  No Drowsiness, 500 mg
chlorpheniramine maleate
  Tablets 2 mg
  Extra Strength, 2 mg
phenylpropanolamine HCl
  Tablets, 18.7 mg
  Extra Strength, 18.7 mg
pseudoephedrine HCl
  No Drowsiness, 30 mg

Other Ingredients: *All Tablets* — Magnesium Stearate; Microcrystalline Cellulose; Povidone; Pregelatinized Starch. *Extra Strength Tablets and No Drowsiness Tablets only* —Sodium Starch Glycolate. *Sinarest Tablets and Extra Strength Tablets only* —Yellow 10; Yellow 6.

Indications: Sinarest is indicated for symptomatic relief from the headache pain, pressure and congestion associated with sinusitis, allergic rhinitis or the common cold.

Actions: Sinarest Tablets and Extra Strength Sinarest contain an antihistamine (chlorpheniramine maleate) and a decongestant (phenylpropanolamine) for the relief of sinus and nasal passage congestion as well as an analgesic (acetaminophen) to relieve pain and discomfort. No Drowsiness Sinarest contains a decongestant (pseudoephedrine hydrochloride) and an analgesic (acetaminophen) for the relief of headache pain, sinus pressure and nasal congestion without causing drowsiness.

Contraindications: Known hypersensitivity to any of the ingredients in this compound.

Warnings: Sinarest should be used with caution in patients with high blood pressure, heart disease, diabetes, thyroid disease, asthma, glaucoma, or difficulty in urination due to enlargement of the prostate gland. Since antihistamines may cause drowsiness, patients should be instructed not to operate a car or machinery. Products containing analgesics should not be taken for more than 10 days in adults and 5 days in children under 12.

Drug Interaction Precautions: Not to be taken by patients currently taking

Continued on next page

Fisons—Cont.

a prescription antihypertensive or anti-depressant drug containing a monoamine oxidase inhibitor except under the advice and supervision of a physician. Antihistamines and oral nasal decongestants have additive effects with alcohol and other CNS depressants.

Adverse Reactions: Drowsiness; excitability, especially in children; nervousness; and dizziness.

Overdosage: Acetaminophen in massive overdosage may cause hepatotoxicity.

Dosage and Administration: *Tablets*—Adults—take 2 tablets every 4 hours. Not to exceed 8 tablets in 24 hours. Children (6–12 years)—One half of adult dosage. Dosage for children under 6 should be individualized under the supervision of a physician. *Extra Strength Tablets*—Adults and Children over 12—take 2 tablets every 6 hours. Not to exceed 8 tablets in 24 hours. Not recommended for children 12 and under. *No Drowsiness Tablets*—Adults and Children 12 years of age and over—take 2 tablets every 6 hours. Not to exceed 8 tablets in 24 hours. Not recommended for children under 12.

How Supplied: *Tablets*—Blister packages of 20, 40 and 80 tablets. *Extra Strength tablets*—package of 24 tablets. *No Drowsiness tablets*—blister package of 20 tablets.

Fleming & Company
1600 FENPARK DR.
FENTON, MO 63026

CHLOR-3
Medicinal Condiment

Active Ingredients: A troika of sodium chloride (50% 24.3 mEq/half tsp. iodized); potassium chloride (30% 11.5 mEq/half tsp.); magnesium chloride (20% 5.6 mEq/half tsp.).

Indications: The first medicinal condiment to restore needed K^+ & Mg^{++} lost during diuresis, at the expense of Na^+. To restore electrolytes lost by overcooking foods, or to add to diets that lack green vegetables, bananas, etc. And to replace conventional salting of foods in culinary and gourmet arts.

Symptoms and Treatment of Oral Overdosage: Hyperkalemia and hypermagnesemia are not end-stage results of usage.

How Supplied: In 8-oz plastic shaker, tamper-evident bottles.

IMPREGON Concentrate

Active Ingredient: Tetrachloro-salicylanilide 2%

Indications: Diaper Rash Relief, 'Staph' control, Mold inhibitor.

Actions: This is a bacteriostatic/fungistatic agent for home usage and hospital usage.

Warnings: Impregon should not be exposed to direct sunlight for long periods after applications.

Precaution: Addition of bleach prior to diaper treatment negates application effects.

Dosage and Administration: One capful (5ml) per gallon of water to impregnate diapers in the diaper pail. Dilutions for many home areas accompany the full package.

Note: For disposable-type diapers, add one teaspoonful to 8 oz of water to a 'Windex-type' sprayer. Spray middle half area of diapers until damp, and allow to dry before using, to prevent rashes.

How Supplied: Four ounce amber plastic bottles.

MAGONATE TABLETS
Magnesium Gluconate (Dihydrate)

Active Ingredients: Magnesium gluconate (dihydrate) 500mg (27mg of Mg^{++})

Indications: Alcoholism; digitalis toxicity; cardiac arrhythemias; extrinsic asthma; dysmenorrhea; eclampsia; hypertension; insomnia; muscle twitching; tremors; anxiety; pancreatitis, and toxicity of chemotherapy.

Precaution: Excessive dosage may cause loose stools.

Dosage and Administration: Magonate is recommended during and three weeks after a course in chemotherapy, then monitored regularly.
Adults and children over 12 yrs.—one or two tablets t.i.d. Under 12 yrs. one tablet t.i.d. Dosage may be increased in severe cases.

How Supplied: Bottles of 100 & 1000 tablets.

MARBLEN Suspensions and Tablet

Composition: A modified 'Sippy Powder' antacid containing magnesium and calcium carbonates;

Action and Uses: The peach/apricot (pink) or unflavored (green) antacid suspensions are sugar-free and neutralize 18 mEq acid per teaspoonful with a low sodium content of 18mg per fl. oz. Each pink tablet consumes 18.0 mEq acid.

Administration and Dosage: One teaspoonful rather than a tablespoonful or one tablet to reduce patient cost by ⅔.

How Supplied: Plastic pints and bottles of 100 and 1000.

NEPHROX SUSPENSION
(aluminum hydroxide)
Antacid Suspension

Composition: A watermelon flavored aluminum hydroxide (320mg as gel)/

mineral oil (10% by volume) antacid per teaspoonful.

Action and Uses: A sugar-free/saccharin-free pink suspension containing no magnesium and low sodium (19mg/oz). Extremely palatable and especially indicated in renal patients. Each teaspoon consumes 9 mEq acid.

Administration and Dosage: Two teaspoonfuls or as directed by a physician.

Caution: To be taken only at bedtime. Do not use at any other time or administer to infants, expectant women, and nursing mothers except upon the advice of a physician as this product contains mineral oil.

How Supplied: Plastic pints and gallons.

NICOTINEX Elixir
nicotinic acid

Composition: Contains niacin 50 mg./tsp. in a sherry wine base (amber color).

Action and Uses: Produces flushing when tablets fail. To increase micro-circulation of inner-ear in Meniere's, tinnitus and labyrinthine syndromes. For 'cold hands & feet', and as a vehicle for additives.

Administration and Dosage: One or two teaspoonful on fasting stomach.

Side Effects: Patients should be warned of dermal flush. Ulcer and gout patients may be affected by 14% alcoholic content.

Contraindications: Severe hypotension and hemorrhage.

How Supplied: Plastic pints and gallons.

OCEAN MIST
(buffered saline)

Composition: Special isotonic saline, buffered with sodium bicarbonate to proper pH so as not to irritate the nose.

Action and Uses: Rhinitis medicamentosa, rhinitis sicca and atrophic rhinitis. For patients 'hooked on nose drops' and glaucoma patients on diuretics having dry nasal capillaries. OCEAN may be used as a mist or drop.

Administration and Dosage: One or two squeezes in each nostril.

Supplied: Plastic 45cc spray bottles and pints.

PURGE
(flavored castor oil)

Composition: Contains 95% castor oil (USP) in a sweetened lemon flavored base that completely masks the odor and taste of the oil.

Indications: Preparation of the bowel for x-ray, surgery and proctological procedures, IVPs, and constipation.

Dosage: Infants—1–2 teaspoonfuls. Children—adjust between infant and adult dose. Adult—2–4 tablespoonfuls.

Precaution: Not indicated when nausea, vomiting, abdominal pain or symptoms of appendicitis occur. Pregnancy, use only on advice of physician.

Supplied: Plastic 1 oz. & 2 oz. bottles.

Glenbrook Laboratories
Division of Sterling Drug Inc.
90 PARK AVENUE
NEW YORK, NY 10016

CHILDREN'S BAYER® CHEWABLE ASPIRIN
Aspirin (Acetylsalicylic Acid)

Active Ingredients: Bayer Children's Chewable Aspirin-Aspirin 1¼ grains (81 mg) per orange flavored chewable tablet.

Inactive Ingredients: Dextrose excipient FD&C Yellow #6, flavor, saccharin sodium, starch.

Actions and Uses: Analgesic, antipyretic, anti-inflammatory, antiplatelet. For effective, gentle relief of painful discomforts, sore throat, fever of colds, headache, teething pain, toothache and other minor aches and pains.

Warnings: Children and teenagers should not use this medicine for chicken pox or flu symptoms before a doctor is consulted about Reye Syndrome, a rare but serious illness reported to be associated with aspirin. Keep this and all drugs out of the reach of children. In case of accidental overdose, seek professional assistance or contact a poison control center immediately. As with any drug, if you are pregnant or nursing a baby, seek the advise of a health professional before using this product.

Administration and Dosage: The following dosages are those provided in the packaging, as appropriate for self-medication.
Children's Dose: To be administered only under adult supervision. For children under 3 consult physician.

Age (Years)	Weight (Lbs.)	Dosage
Under 3 consult a physician		
3 up to 4	32 to 35	2 tablets
4 up to 6	36 to 45	3 tablets
6 up to 9	46 to 65	4 tablets
9 up to 11	66 to 76	5 tablets
11 up to 12	77 to 83	6 tablets
12 and over	84 and over	8 tablets

Indicated dosage may be repeated every four hours up to but not more than five times a day. Larger dosage may be prescribed by a physician.

Ways to Administer: CHEW then follow with a half glass of water, milk or fruit juice.
SWALLOW WHOLE with a half a glass of water, milk or fruit juice.
DISSOLVE ON TONGUE follow with a half a glass of water, milk or fruit juice.
DISSOLVE TABLET in a little water, milk or fruit juice and drink the solution.

CRUSHED in a teaspoonful of water—followed with part of a glass of water.

How Supplied: Bayer Children's Chewable Aspirin 1¼ grains (81 mg)—NDC 12843-131-05, bottle of 36 tablets with child resistant safety closure.
Shown in Product Identification Section, page 409

BAYER® CHILDREN'S COLD TABLETS

Active Ingredients: Each tablet contains phenylpropanolamine HCl 3.125 mg, aspirin 1¼ gr. (81 mg). The tablets are orange flavored and chewable.

Inactive Ingredients: Colloidal Silicon Dioxide, Compressible Sugar, Ethylcellulose, FD&C Red #3, Red #40 and FD&C Yellow #6, Flavor, Mannitol, Microcrystalline Cellulose, Povidone, Saccharin Sodium, Starch, Stearic Acid.

Action and Uses: Bayer Children's Cold Tablets combine two effective ingredients: a gentle decongestant to relieve nasal congestion and ease breathing, and Genuine Bayer Aspirin to reduce fever and relieve minor aches and pains of colds.

Administration and Dosage: The following dosage is provided in the packaging:

Age (yrs)	Weight (lbs)	Dosage
3 up to 6	32–45	2 tabs
6 up to 12	46–83	4 tabs
12 & over	84+	8 tabs

Indicated dosage may be repeated every four hours up to but not more than five times a day. Larger dosage may be prescribed by your physician. For easy administration, tablets may be chewed, dissolved or swallowed whole. Follow with liquid.

Contraindications: Side effects at higher doses may include nervousness, dizziness, sleeplessness. To be used with caution in presence of high blood pressure, heart disease, diabetes, asthma, or thyroid disease.

Caution: Do not exceed recommended dosage. For larger or more frequent doses, or for children under 3, consult physician. If symptoms persist or are accompanied by high fever or vomiting, consult your physician before continuing use.

Warnings: Children and teenagers should not use this medicine for chicken pox or flu symptoms before a doctor is consulted about Reye Syndrome, a rare but serious illness reported to be associated with aspirin. Keep this and all drugs out of the reach of children. In case of accidental overdose, seek professional assistance or contact a poison control center immediately. As with any drug, if you are pregnant or nursing a baby, seek the advice of a health professional before using this product.

How Supplied: NDC-12843-181-01, bottles of 30 tablets with child-resistant safety closure.
Shown in Product Identification Section, page 409

BAYER® CHILDREN'S COUGH SYRUP

Active Ingredients: Each 5 ml (1 tsp.) contains phenylpropanolamine HCl 9 mg and dextromethorphan hydrobromide 7.5 mg.

Inactive Ingredients: Alcohol 5%, Caramel, Flavor, Glycerin, Liquid Glucose, Parabens, Purified Water, Saccharin Sodium, Sorbitol Solution. May also contain Sodium Chloride. Cherry flavored.

Action and Uses: Bayer Children's Cough Syrup combines two effective ingredients in a syrup with a very appealing cherry flavor: a gentle nasal decongestant and a cough suppressant. It is non-narcotic, and contains no chloroform or red dyes.

Administration and Dosage: The following dosage is provided on the packaging:
Dosage: For children under 2 consult physician.

Age (yrs)	Weight (lbs)	Dosage
2 up to 6	27–45	1 tsp.
6 up to 12	46–83	2 tsp.
12 & over	84+	4 tsp.

Dose may be repeated every 4 hrs., not more than 4 times/day.

Contraindications and Precautions: To be used with caution in presence of high blood pressure, heart disease, diabetes, asthma, or thyroid disease.
Caution: Consult your physician if cough persists for more than 7 days or if cough is accompanied by high fever since either may be signs of a serious condition.

Warnings: Do not give this product to children under 2 years of age or exceed recommended dosage, unless directed by a physician. Keep this and all drugs out of the reach of children. In case of accidental overdose, seek professional assistance or contact a poison control center immediately. As with any drug, if you are pregnant or nursing a baby, seek the advice of a health professional before using this product.

How Supplied: NDC–12843-401-02, 3.0 oz. bottles.
Shown in Product Identification Section, page 409

GENUINE BAYER® ASPIRIN
Aspirin (Acetylsalicylic Acid)
Tablets and Caplets

Active Ingredients: Each Bayer Aspirin contains Aspirin 5 grains (325 mg) in a thin, inert, hydroxypropyl methylcellulose coating for easier swallowing. This is not an enteric coating and does not alter the onset of action of Genuine Bayer Aspirin.

Inactive Ingredients: Starch and Triacetin.

Continued on next page

Glenbrook—Cont.

Actions and Uses: Analgesic, antipyretic, anti-inflammatory, antiplatelet. For relief of headache; painful discomfort, and fever of colds and flu; sore throats; muscular aches and pains; temporary relief of minor pains of arthritis, rheumatism, bursitis, lumbago, sciatica; toothache, teething pains, and pain following dental procedures; neuralgia and neuritic pain; functional menstrual pain; sleeplessness when caused by minor painful discomfort; painful discomfort and fever accompanying immunizations.

Caution: If pain persists for more than 10 days, or redness is present, or in conditions affecting children under 12 years of age, consult a physician immediately.

Warnings: Children and teenagers should not use this medicine for chicken pox or flu symptoms before a doctor is consulted about Reye Syndrome, a rare but serious illness reported to be associated with aspirin. Keep this and all drugs out of the reach of children. In case of accidental overdose, seek professional assistance or contact a poison control center immediately. As with any drug, if you are pregnant or nursing a baby, seek the advice of a health professional before using this product.

Administration and Dosage: The following dosages are those provided in the packaging, as appropriate for self-medication. Larger or more frequent dosage may be necessary as appropriate to the condition or needs of the patient.
The hydroxypropyl methylcellulose coating makes Genuine Bayer Aspirin particularly appropriate for those who must take frequent doses of aspirin and for those who have difficulty in swallowing uncoated tablets and caplets.

Usual Adult Dose: One or two tablets/caplets with water. May be repeated every four hours as necessary up to 12 tablets/caplets a day.

For Antiplatelet Use:
Recurrent TIA: There is evidence that aspirin is safe and effective for reducing the risk of recurrent transient ischemic attacks or stroke in men who have had transient ischemia of the brain due to fibrin platelet emboli:
There is no evidence that aspirin is effective in reducing TIA's in women, or is of benefit in the treatment of completed strokes in men or women. Patients presenting with signs and symptoms of TIA's should have a complete medical and neurologic evaluation. Consideration should be given to other disorders which resemble TIA's.
It is important to evaluate and treat, if appropriate, other diseases associated with TIA's and stroke, such as hypertension and diabetes.
DOSAGE: The recommended dosage for this new indication is 1,300 mg/day (650 mg twice/day or 325 mg four times a day).

Precautions: A complete medical and neurologic evaluation should be performed on the male patient with recurrent TIA prior to instituting antiplatelet therapy with aspirin. The differential diagnosis should include consideration of disorders that resemble TIA's. An assessment of the presence and need for treatment of other diseases associated with TIA's or stroke, such as diabetes and hypertension, should be made.

IN MI PROPHYLAXIS
Aspirin is indicated to reduce the risk of death and/or non-fatal myocardial infarction in patients with a previous infarction or unstable angina pectoris.

Clinical Trials: The indication is supported by the results of six, large, randomized multicenter, placebo-controlled studies 1–6 by the word-studies involving 10,816, predominantly male, post-myocardial infarction (MI) patients and one randomized placebo-controlled study of 7 by the word study 1,266 men with unstable angina. Therapy with aspirin was begun at intervals after the onset of acute MI varying from less than 3 days to more than 5 years and continued for periods of from less than one year to four years. In the unstable angina study, treatment was started within 1 month after the onset of unstable angina and continued for 12 weeks and complicating conditions, such as congestive heart failure, were not included in the study.
Aspirin therapy in MI patients was associated with about a 20 percent reduction in the risk of subsequent death and/or non-fatal reinfarction, a median absolute decrease of 3 percent from the 12 to 22 percent event rates in the placebo groups. In the aspirin-treated unstable angina patients the reduction in risk was about 50 percent, a reduction in the event rate of 5 percent from the 10 percent rate in the placebo group over the 12 weeks of the study.
Daily dosage of aspirin in the post-myocardial infarction studies was 300 mg in one study and 900–1500 mg in five studies. A dose of 325 mg was used in the study of unstable angina.

Adverse Reactions: Gastrointestinal Reactions: Doses of 1000 mg per day of aspirin caused gastrointestinal symptoms and bleeding that in some cases were clinically significant. In the largest post-infarction study (the Aspirin Myocardial Infarction Study (AMIS) trial with 4,500 people), the percentage incidences of gastrointestinal symptoms for the aspirin (1000 mg of a standard, solid-tablet formulation) and placebo-treated subjects, respectively, were: stomach pain (14.3%; 4.4%); heartburn (11.9%; 4.3%); nausea and/or vomiting (7.3%; 2.1%); hospitalization for GI disorder (4.9%; 3.3%). In the AMIS and other trials, aspirin treated patients had increased rates of gross gastrointestinal bleeding. Symptoms and signs of gastrointestinal irritation were not significantly increased in subjects treated for unstable angina with buffered aspirin in solution.

Cardiovascular and Biochemical: In the AMIS trial, the dosage of 1000 mg per day of aspirin was associated with small increases in systolic blood pressure (BP) (average 1.5 to 2.1 mm) and diastolic BP (0.5 to 0.6 mm), depending upon whether maximal or last available readings were used. Blood urea nitrogen and uric acid levels were also increased, but by less than 1.0 mg%. Subjects with marked hypertension or renal insufficiency had been excluded from the trial so that the clinical importance of these observations for such subjects or for any subjects treated over more prolonged periods is not known. It is recommended that patients placed on long-term aspirin treatment, even at doses of 300 mg per day, be seen at regular intervals to assess changes in these measurements.

Sodium in Buffered Aspirin for Solution Formulations: One tablet daily of buffered aspirin in solution adds 553 mg of sodium to that in the diet and may not be tolerated by patients with active sodium-retaining states such as congestive heart or renal failure. This amount of sodium adds about 30 percent to the 70 to 90 meq intake suggested as appropriate for dietary treatment of essential hypertension in the 1984 Report of the Joint National Committee on Detection, Evaluation, and Treatment of High Blood Pressure.[8]

Dosage and Administration: Although most of the studies used dosages exceeding 300 mg, two trials used only 300 mg daily and pharmacologic data indicate that this dose inhibits platelet function fully. Therefore, 300 mg or a conventional 325 mg aspirin dose, daily is a reasonable routine dose that would minimize gastrointestinal adverse reactions. This use of aspirin applies to both solid, oral dosage forms (buffered and plain aspirin) and buffered aspirin in solution.

References:
(1) Elwood, P.C., et al., A Randomized Controlled Trial of Acetylsalicylic Acid in the Secondary Prevention of Mortality from Myocardial Infarction, *British Medical Journal*, 1:436–440, 1974.
(2) The Coronary Drug Project Research Group, "Aspirin in Coronary Heart Disease," *Journal of Chronic Disease*, 29:625–642, 1976.
(3) Breddin, K., et al., "Secondary Prevention of Myocardial Infarction: A Comparison of Acetylsalicylic Acid, Phenprocoumon or Placebo," *Homeostasis*, 470:263–258, 1979.
(4) Aspirin Myocardial Infarction Study Research Group, "A Randomized, Controlled Trial of Aspirin in Persons Recovered from Myocardial Infarction," *Journal American Medical Association* 245:661–669, 1980.
(5) Elwood, P.C., and Sweetnam P.M., "Aspirin and Secondary Mortality after Myocardial Infarction," *Lancet*, pp. 1313–1315, December 22–29, 1979.
(6) The Persantine-Aspirin Reinfarction Study Research Group, "Persantine and Aspirin in Coronary Heart Disease," *Circulation*, 62: 449–460, 1980.

(7) Lewis, H.D., et al., "Protective Effects of Aspirin Against Acute Myocardial Infarction and Death in Men with Unstable Angina. Results of a Veterans Administration Cooperative Study," *New England Journal of Medicine*, 309:396–403, 1983.

(8) "1984 Report of the Joint National Committee on Detection, Evaluation and Treatment of High Blood Pressure," U.S. Department of Health and Human Services and United States Public Health Service, National Institutes of Health.

How Supplied: Genuine Bayer Aspirin 5 grains (325 mg)—
NDC 12843-101-10, packs of 12 tablets
NDC 12843-101-11, bottles of 24 tablets
NDC 12843-101-17, bottles of 50 tablets
NDC 12843-101-12, bottles of 100 tablets
NDC 12843-101-20, bottles of 200 tablets
NDC 12843-101-13, bottles of 300 tablets
NDC 12843-102-40, calendar pack of 28 caplets
NDC 12843-102-38, bottles of 50 caplets
NDC 12843-102-39, bottles of 100 caplets
Child resistant safety closures on 12's, 24's, 50's, 200's, 300's, tablets and 50's caplets. Bottles of 100's tablets and caplets available without safety closure for households without small children.

Shown in Product Identification Section, page 408

MAXIMUM BAYER® ASPIRIN
Aspirin (Acetylsalicylic Acid)
Tablets and Caplets

Active Ingredients: Maximum Bayer Aspirin—Aspirin 500 mg (7.7 grains) contains a thin, inert, hydroxypropyl methylcellulose coating for easier swallowing. This is not an enteric coating and does not alter the onset of action of Bayer Aspirin.

Inactive Ingredients: Starch and Triacetin.

Actions and Uses: Analgesic, antipyretic, anti-inflammatory. For relief of headache; painful discomfort and fever of colds and flu; sore throats; muscular aches and pains; temporary relief of minor pains of arthritis, rheumatism, bursitis, lumbago, sciatica, toothache, teething pains, and pain following dental procedures; neuralgia and neuritic pain; functional menstrual pain; sleeplessness when caused by minor painful discomforts; painful discomfort and fever accompanying immunizations.

Caution: If pain persists for more than 10 days, or redness is present, or in conditions affecting children under 12 years of age, consult a physician immediately.

Warnings: Children and teenagers should not use this medicine for chicken pox or flu symptoms before a doctor is consulted about Reye Syndrome, a rare but serious illness reported to be associated with aspirin. Keep this and all drugs out of the reach of children. In case of accidential overdose, seek professional assistance or contact a poison control center immediately. As with any drug, if you are pregnant or nursing a baby, seek the advice of a health professional before using this product.

Administration and Dosage: The following dosages are those provided on the packaging, as appropriate for self-medication. Larger or more frequent dosage may be necessary as appropriate to the condition or needs of the patient.
The hydroxypropyl methylcellulose coating makes Maximum Bayer Aspirin particularly appropriate for those who must take frequent doses of aspirin and for those who have difficulty in swallowing uncoated tablets/caplets.
Maximum Bayer Aspirin—500 mg (7.7 grains) tablets/caplets.
Usual Adult Dose: One or two tablets/caplets with water. May be repeated every four hours as necessary up to 8 tablets/caplets a day.

How Supplied: Maximum Bayer Aspirin 500 mg (7.7 grains)
NDC 12843-161-51 tube of 10 tablets
NDC 12843-161-53 bottles of 30 tablets
NDC 12843-161-56 bottles of 60 tablets
NDC 12843-161-58 bottles of 100 tablets
NDC 12843-202-56 bottles of 60 caplets
Child-resistant safety closures on 30's and 100's bottles of tablets and 60's bottles of caplets. Bottle of 60's tablets available without safety closure for households without small children.

Shown in Product Identification Section, page 408

8 HOUR BAYER®
TIMED–RELEASE ASPIRIN
(aspirin)

Active Ingredients: Each oblong white scored tablet contains 10 grains (650 mg) of aspirin in microencapsolated form.

Inactive Ingredients: Guar Gum, Microcrystalline Cellulose, Starch and other ingredients.

Indications: 8 Hour Bayer Timed-Release Aspirin is indicated for the temporary relief of low grade pain amenable to relief with salicylates, such as in rheumatoid arthritis, osteoarthritis, spondylitis, bursitis and other forms of rheumatism, as well as in many common musculoskeletal disorders. It possesses the same advantages for other types of prolonged aches and pains, such as minor injuries, dental pain and dysmenorrhea. Its long-lasting effectiveness should also make it valuable as an analgesic in simple headache, colds, grippe, flu and other similar conditions in which aspirin is indicated for symptomatic relief, either by itself or as an adjunct to specific therapy.

Caution: If pain persists for more than 10 days, or redness is present, or in conditions affecting children under 12 years, consult a physician immediately.

Warnings: Children and teenagers should not use this medicine for chicken pox or flu symptoms before a doctor is consulted about Reye Syndrome, a rare but serious illness reported to be associated with aspirin. Keep this and all drugs out of the reach of children. In case of ac-cidental overdose, seek professional assistance or contact a poison control center immediately. As with any drug, if you are pregnant or nursing a baby, seek the advice of a health professional before using this product.

Administration and Dosage: Two 8 Hour Bayer Timed-Release Aspirin tablets q. 8 h. provide effective long-lasting pain relief. This two-tablet (20 grain or 1300 mg) dose of timed-release aspirin promptly produces salicylate blood levels greater than those achieved by a 10-grain (650 mg) dose of regular aspirin, and in the second 4 hour period produces a salicylate blood level curve which approximates that of two successive 10-grain (650 mg) doses of regular aspirin at 4 hour intervals. The 10-grain (650 mg) scored 8 Hour Bayer Timed-Release Aspirin tablets permit administration of aspirin in multiples of 5 grains (325 mg), allowing individualization of dosage to meet the specific needs of the patient. For the convenience of patients on a regular aspirin dosage schedule, two 10-grain (650 mg) 8 Hour Bayer Timed-Release Aspirin tablets may be administered with water every 8 hours. Whenever necessary, two tablets (20 grains or 1300 mg) should be given before retiring to provide effective analgesic and anti-inflammatory action—for relief of pain throughout the night and lessening of stiffness upon arising. Do not exceed 6 tablets in 24 hours. 8 Hour Bayer Timed-Release Aspirin has been made in a special capsule-shaped tablet to permit easy swallowing. However, for patients who do have difficulty, 8 Hour Bayer Timed-Release Aspirin tablets may be gently crumbled in the mouth and swallowed with water without loss of timed-release effect. There is no bitter "aspirin" taste. For children under 12, consult physician.

Side Effects: Side effects encountered with regular aspirin may be encountered with 8 Hour Bayer Timed-Release Aspirin. Tinnitus and dizziness are the ones most frequently encountered.

Contraindications and Precautions: 8 Hour Bayer Timed-Release Aspirin is contraindicated in patients with marked aspirin hypersensitivity, and should be given with extreme caution to any patient with a history of adverse reaction to salicylates. It may cautiously be tried in patients intolerant to aspirin because of gastric irritation, but the usual precautions for any form of aspirin should be observed in patients with gastric ulcers, bleeding tendencies, asthma, or hypoprothrombinemia.

Supplied:
Tablets in Bottle of 30's
NDC-12843-191-72
Tablets in Bottle of 72's
NDC-12843-191-74
Tablets in Bottle of 125's
NDC-12843-191-76
All sizes packaged in child-resistant safety closure except 72's which is a size recommended for households without young children.

Shown in Product Identification Section, page 408

Continued on next page

Glenbrook—Cont.

DIAPARENE® BABY POWDER

Description: Powder comprised of corn starch, magnesium carbonate, methylbenzethonium chloride 0.055% and fragrance.

Action and Uses: Diaparene Baby Powder has a corn starch base for high absorbency to help keep baby's skin dry and for soothing diaper rash, prickly heat and chafing.

Administration and Dosage: Apply liberally to baby's skin after bath and with each diaper change.

How Supplied: Available in 4 oz, 9 oz, 14 oz containers.

*Shown in Product Identification
Section, page 409*

DIAPARENE

[See table below].

*Shown in Product Identification
Section, page 409*

DIAPARENE® SUPERS BABY WASH CLOTHS

Description: Wash cloths are impregnated with a cleansing solution containing water, SD alcohol-40, propylene glycol, PEG/60, lanolin, sodium nonoxynol-9-phosphate, sorbic acid, citric acid, disodium phosphate, oleth-20, and fragrance.

Action and Uses: Diaparene Baby Wash Cloths contain lanolin and a mild cleansing solution to clean and condition baby's skin.

Administration and Dosage: Wipe baby's skin with solution-impregnated wash cloths as required.

How Supplied: Available in canisters of 70 and 150 wash cloths.

*Shown in Product Identification
Section, page 409*

HALEY'S M-O®

Active Ingredients: A suspension of magnesium hydroxide in purified water plus mineral oil. Haley's M-O contains 304 mg per teaspoon (5 ml) of Magnesium Hydroxide and 1.25 ml of Mineral Oil.

Inactive Ingredients: Purified water. For flavored Haley's M-O only, D&C #28, flavor, purified water, saccharin sodium.

Indications: For the relief of occasional constipation or irregularity accompanied by hemorrhoids.

Action at Laxative Dosage: Haley's M-O is a mild saline laxative which acts by drawing water into the gut, increasing intraluminal pressure, and increasing intestinal motility. This product generally produces bowel movement in $\frac{1}{2}$ to 6 hours.

Administration and Dosage: As a laxative, especially for hemorrhoid sufferers, adults 1–2 tbsp. at bedtime and upon arising. For constipation relief, adults 2 tbsp. at bedtime and upon arising; children 6–12, minimum single dose: 1 tsp. maximum daily dose: 1 tbsp. For adults and children, as bowel function improves reduce dose gradually.

Caution: Do not take this product if you are presently taking a stool softener laxative unless directed by a doctor. Do not take with meals.

Warnings: Do not use laxative products when abdominal pain, nausea or vomiting are present unless directed by a doctor. If you have noticed a sudden change in bowel habits that persists over a period of 2 weeks, consult a doctor before using a laxative. Laxative products should not be used for a period longer than 1 week unless directed by a doctor. Rectal bleeding, or failure to have a bowel movement after use of a laxative may indicate a serious condition; discontinue use and consult your doctor. Do not administer to children under 6 years of age, to pregnant women, to bedridden patients, or to persons with difficulty swallowing. As with any drug, if you are nursing a baby, seek the advice of a health professional before using this product. Keep this and all drugs out of the reach of children. In case of accidental overdose, seek professional assistance or contact a poison control center immediately.

How Supplied: Haley's M-O is available in regular and flavored liquids:
Regular
4 fl. oz. NDC 12843-350-45; 12 fl. oz. NDC 12843-350-46; 26 fl. oz. NDC 12843-350-47.
Flavored
4 fl. oz. NDC 12843-360-67; 12 fl. oz. NDC 12843-260-68; 26 fl. oz. NDC 12843-360-69.

*Shown in Product Identification
Section, page 409*

ORIGINAL MIDOL®
MULTI-SYMPTOM FORMULA

Active Ingredients: Each Caplet contains: Acetaminophen 325 mg and Pyrilamine Maleate 12.5 mg.

Inactive Ingredients: Croscarmellose Sodium Type A, Hydroxypropyl Methylcellulose, Magnesium Stearate, Microcrystalline Cellulose, Pregelatinized Starch and Triacetin.

Action and Uses: For relief of multi-symptoms suffered during menstrual cycle: cramps, bloating, headache, tension, irritability, and backache caused by menstrual discomfort.
Its combination of ingredients safely relieves menstrual cramps as well as the menstrual headache, breast and leg pain that often accompany cramps.

Caution: May cause drowsiness. Use caution when driving or operating machinery. Alcohol, sedatives or tranquilizers may increase drowsiness.

	Diaparene® Medicated Cream	Diaparene® Peri-Anal® Medicated Ointment	Diaparene® Cradol®
Description:	Special lotion formula to soothe and protect baby's skin.	Ointment that soothes and helps heal diaper rash, helps protect against wetness and irritation.	Medicated lotion scalp treatment for "cradle cap" developed by babies.
	Contains: Methylbenzethonium Chloride 0.1% (w/w) Also contains: Dibasic Sodium Phosphate, Fragrance, Glycerine, Mineral Oil, Parabens, Polysorbate 60, Purified Water, Sorbitan Monostearate, Stearyl Alcohol, White Petrolatum.	Contains: Cod Liver Oil (vitamins A & D), Zinc Oxide, Methylbenzethonium Chloride 0.1% (w/w) Also contains: Calcium Caseinate, Fragrance, Lanolin, Lanolin Alcohol, Mineral Oil, Starch, Paraffin, White Petrolatum, Yellow Wax.	Contains: Methylbenzethonium Chloride 0.07%. Also contains: Anhydrous Lanolin, Fragrance, Glyceryl Sterate, Lanolin, Lanolin Alcohol, Light Mineral Oil, Mineral Oil, Parabens, Paraffin, PEG-6 Stearate, Purified Water, Stearamidoethyl Diethylamine, Yellow Wax.

Action and Uses:	Nonstaining cream formula soothes and protects diaper area, knees, elbows— anywhere baby's skin needs comfort.	The antibacterial action of methyl-benzethonium chloride combats ammonia-forming bacteria that can cause diaper rash and odor. Provides a water repellent shield to keep out wetness, and to protect skin from irritating urine, stool and perspiration.	Gently softens and separates crust and scales from the scalp. Helps prevent and treat local infection.
Administration and Dosage:	Directions: Apply anywhere skin chafing or irritation may develop. Use liberally, taking care to include skin folds where moisture collects.	Directions: At the first sign of redness or diaper rash, apply liberally to diaper area three times daily as needed. To help prevent diaper rash, apply to diaper area after each diaper change. Especially important at bedtime, or anytime that exposure to wet diapers may be prolonged. For minor skin irritations, apply a thin layer, using a gauze dressing if necessary.	Directions for "cradle cap" and scalp infection: Massage into wet or dry scalp 3 times daily for 3 days. Do not wash off or shampoo between applications. After 3 days, shampoo with mild soap and use a fine comb or scalp brush to gently brush away crusts and scales from baby's scalp. To prevent reoccurrence: Massage into wet or dry scalp 3 times weekly.
How Supplied:	NDC 12843-246-21 1 ounce tube NDC 12843-246-22 2 ounce tube NDC 12843-246-24 4 ounce tube	NDC 12843-236-10 1 ounce tube NDC 12843-236-20 2 ounce tube NDC 12843-236-40 4 ounce tube	NDC 12843-070-21 3 ounce bottle

Warnings: Keep this and all drugs out of the reach of children. In case of accidental overdose, seek professional assistance or contact a poison control center immediately. As with any drug, if you are pregnant or nursing a baby, seek the advice of a health professional before using this product.

Dosage: Take 2 caplets with water. Repeat every four hours as needed, up to a maximum of 12 caplets per day. Under age 12; consult your physician.

How Supplied: White, capsule-shaped Caplets.
NDC 12843-156-16, professional dispenser, 250 2-caplet Packets for sample use.
NDC 12843-156-17, bottles of 12 caplets
NDC-12843-156-18, bottles of 30 caplets
NDC-12843-156-19, bottles of 60 caplets
Child-resistant safety closures on bottles of 12 and 60 Caplets.
Shown in Product Identification Section, page 409

MAXIMUM STRENGTH MIDOL® PMS
Caplets

Active Ingredients: Each caplet contains: Acetaminophen 500 mg, Pamabrom 25 mg, Pyrilamine Maleate 15 mg.

Inctive Ingredients: Croscarmellose Sodium, Hydrogenated Vegetable Oil, Hydroxypropyl Methylcellulose, Magnesium Stearate, Microcrystalline Cellu-

lose, Pregelatinized Starch, Talc and Triacetin.

Action and Uses: Relieves the symptoms of Premenstrual Syndrome (PMS). Contains maximum strength medication for all these premenstrual symptoms: tension, irritability, anxiety, bloating, water-weight gain, cramps, backache and headache. Unlike general pain relievers, which contain only analgesics, Midol PMS contains a combination of ingredients (an analgesic, diuretic and a tension reliever) for the physical and emotional symptoms associated with PMS.

Dosage: Take 2 caplets with water. Repeat every 4 hours as needed, up to 2 maximum of 8 caplets per day. Under age 12: Take under the advice of your physician.

Caution: May cause drowsiness. Use caution when driving or operating machinery. Alcohol, sedatives or tranquilizers may increase drowsiness.

Warnings: Keep this and all drugs out of the reach of children. In case of accidental overdose, seek professional assistance or contact a poison control center immediately. As with any drug, if you are pregnant or nursing a baby, seek the advice of a health professional before using this product.

How Supplied: White capsule shaped caplets.

NDC 12843-163-46 bottles of 16 caplets.
NDC 12843-163-47 bottles of 32 caplets.
Child-resistant safety closure on bottles of 32 caplets.
Shown in Product Identification Section, page 409

MIDOL® 200 ADVANCED PAIN FORMULA
Ibuprofen Tablets, USP
Pain Reliever/Fever Reducer

Warning
ASPIRIN SENSITIVE PATIENTS. Do not take this product if you have had a severe allergic reaction to aspirin, e.g.—asthma, swelling, shock or hives, because even though this product contains no aspirin or salicylates cross-reactions may occur in patients allergic to aspirin.

Indications: For the temporary relief of minor aches and pains associated with the common cold, headache, toothache, muscular aches, backache, for the minor pain of arthritis, for the pain of menstrual cramps, and for reduction of fever.

Directions: Adults: Take 1 tablet every 4 to 6 hours while symptoms persist. If pain or fever does not respond to 1 tablet, 2 tablets may be used but do not exceed 6 tablets in 24 hours, unless directed by a doctor. The smallest effective dose should be used. Take with food or milk if occasional and mild heartburn, upset

Continued on next page

Glenbrook—Cont.

stomach, or stomach pain occurs with use. Consult a doctor if these symptoms are more than mild or if they persist. Children: Do not give this product to children under 12 except under the advice and supervision of a doctor.

Warnings: Do not take for pain for more than 10 days or for fever for more than 3 days unless directed by a doctor. If pain or fever persists or gets worse, if new symptoms occur, or if the painful area is red or swollen, consult a doctor. These could be signs of serious illness. If you are under a doctor's care for any serious condition, consult a doctor before taking this product. As with aspirin and acetaminophen, if you have any condition which requires you to take prescription drugs or if you have had any problems or serious side effects from taking any non-prescription pain relievers, do not take this product without first discussing it with your doctor. If you experience any symptoms which are unusual or seem unrelated to the condition for which you took ibuprofen, consult a doctor before taking any more of it. Although ibuprofen is indicated for the same conditions as aspirin and acetaminophen, it should not be taken with them except under a doctor's direction. As with any drug, if you are pregnant or nursing a baby, seek the advice of a health professional before using this product. IT IS ESPECIALLY IMPORTANT NOT TO USE IBUPROFEN DURING THE LAST 3 MONTHS OF PREGNANCY UNLESS SPECIFICALLY DIRECTED TO DO SO BY A DOCTOR BECAUSE IT MAY CAUSE PROBLEMS IN THE UNBORN CHILD OR COMPLICATIONS DURING DELIVERY. Keep this and all drugs out of the reach of children. In case of accidental overdose, seek professional assistance or contact a poison control center immediately.

Active Ingredients: Each tablet contains ibuprofen 200 mg. Store at room temperature; avoid excessive heat—40°C (104°F).

Inactive Ingredients: Calcium Phosphate, Cellulose, Magnesium Stearate, Silicon Dioxide, Sodium Lauryl Sulfate, Sodium Starch Glycolate, Stearic Acid, Titanium Dioxide.

How Supplied: White tablets NDC 12843-154-50 bottles of 16 tablets NDC 12843-154-51 bottles of 32 tablets Child resistant safety closure on bottles of 32 tablets.

Shown in Product Identification Section, page 409

MAXIMUM STRENGTH MIDOL® MULTI-SYMPTOM FORMULA

Active Ingredients: Each caplet contains Acetaminophen 500 mg and Pyrilamine Maleate 15 mg.

Inactive Ingredients: Croscarmellose Sodium Type A. Hydroxypropyl Methylcellulose, Magnesium Stearate, Micro-

crystalline Cellulose, Pregelatinized Starch and Triacetin.

Action and Uses: For maximum strength relief of multi-symptoms suffered during menstrual cycle: cramps, bloating, headache, tension, irritability and backache caused by menstrual discomfort.

Caution: May cause drowsiness. Use caution when driving or operating machinery. Alcohol, sedatives or tranquilizers may increase drowsiness.

Warnings: Keep this and all drugs out of the reach of children. In case of accidental overdose, seek professional assistance or contact a poison control center immediately. As with any drug, if you are pregnant or nursing a baby, seek the advice of a health professional before using this product.

Dosage: Two caplets with water as needed up to a maximum of 8 caplets per day. Under age 12; consult your physician.

How Supplied: White capsule-shaped Caplets.
NDC 12843-157-16, professional dispenser, 250 2-caplet Packets for sample use.
NDC 12843-157-17, bottles of 8 caplets
NDC 12843-157-18, bottles of 16 caplets
NDC 12843-157-19, bottles of 32 caplets
Child-resistant safety closures on bottles of 8 and 32 caplets.

Shown in Product Identification Section, page 409

CHILDREN'S PANADOL®
Acetaminophen Chewable Tablets, Liquid, Drops

Description: Each Children's PANADOL Chewable Tablet contains 80 mg acetaminophen in a fruit flavored sugar free tablet. Children's PANADOL Acetaminophen Liquid is fruit flavored, red in color, and is alcohol free, sugar free and aspirin-free. Each ½ teaspoon contains 80 mg of acetaminophen. Infant's PANADOL Drops are fruit flavored, red in color, and are alcohol free, sugar free and aspirin-free. Each 0.8 ml (one calibrated dropper full) contains 80 mg acetaminophen.

Actions and Indications: Acetaminophen, the active ingredient in PANADOL, is the analgesic/antipyretic most widely recommended by pediatricians for fast, effective relief of children's fevers. It also relieves the aches and pains of colds and flu, earaches, headaches, teething, immunizations, tonsillectomy, and childhood illnesses.
Children's PANADOL Tablets, Liquid, and Drops are aspirin free and contain no alcohol or sugar. The pleasant tasting formulations are not likely to upset or irritate children's stomachs.

Usual Dosage: Dosing is based on single doses in the range of 10–15 mg/kg body weight. Doses may be repeated every four hours up to 4 or 5 times daily, but not to exceed 5 doses in 24 hours. The

package labeling states that for children under 2 years to "consult a physician".
Children's PANADOL Chewable Tablets: Children under 2 yrs., under 24 lbs., contact a physician; 2–3 yrs., 24–35 lbs., 2 tablets; 4–5 yrs., 36–47 lbs., 3 tablets; 6–8 yrs., 48–59 lbs., 4 tablets; 9–10 yrs., 60–71 lbs., 5 tablets; 11–12 yrs., 72–95 lbs., 6 tablets. Dosage may be repeated every four hours, no more than 5 times in 24 hours.
Children's PANADOL Liquid: (a special 3 teaspoon cup for accurate measurement is provided). Under 2 yrs., under 24 lbs., consult a physician; 2–3 yrs., 24–35 lbs., 1 teaspoonful; 4–5 yrs., 36–47 lbs., 1½ teaspoonfuls; 6–8 yrs., 48–59 lbs., 2 teaspoonfuls; 9–10 yrs., 60–71 lbs., 2½ teaspoonfuls; 11–12 yrs., 72–95 lbs., 3 teaspoonfuls. Repeat every 4 hours up to 5 times in a 24 hour period. Children's PANADOL Liquid may be administered alone or mixed with formula, milk, juice, cereal, etc.
Infant's PANADOL Drops: Under 2 yrs., under 24 lbs., consult a physician; 2–3 yrs., 24–35 lbs., 2 dropperfuls (1.6 ml); 4–5 yrs., 36–47 lbs., 3 dropperfuls (2.4 ml); 6–8 yrs., 48–59 lbs., 4 dropperfuls (3.2 ml). May be repeated every 4 hours, up to 5 times in a 24 hour period.

Warnings: Since Children's PANADOL Acetaminophen Chewable Tablets, Liquid, and Drops are available without a prescription as an analgesic/antipyretic, the following appears on the package labels: "WARNINGS: Do not take this product for more than 5 days. If symptoms persist or new ones occur, consult a physician. If fever persists for more than 3 days, or recurs, consult a physician. Keep this and all drugs out of the reach of children. In case of accidental overdose, seek professional assistance or contact a poison control center immediately. High fever, severe or persistent sore throat, cough, headache, nausea or vomiting may be serious; consult a physician."

Tamper Resistant: Children's PANADOL Acetaminophen Chewable Tablets packaging provides tamper resistant features on both the outer carton and bottle. The following copy appears on the end flaps of this carton—"Purchase only if carton end flaps are sealed." The following copy appears on the bottle—"Use only if printed seal under cap is intact." Children's PANADOL Liquid and Drops provide tamper resistant features on the carton. The following copy appears on the carton—"Purchase only if Red Tear Tape and Plastic Overwrap are intact," and bottle—"Use only if Carton Overwrap and Red Tear Tape Are Intact."

Composition:
Tablets: Active Ingredients: Acetaminophen. Inactive Ingredients: FD&C Red #3, Flavor, Mannitol, Saccharin Sodium, Starch, Stearic Acid and other ingredients.
Liquid: Active Ingredients: Acetaminophen. Inactive Ingredients: Benzoic Acid, FD&C Red #40, Flavor, Glycerin, Polyethylene Glycol, Potassium Sorbate, Propylene Glycol, Purified Water, Sac-

charin Sodium, Sorbitol Solution. May also contain Sodium Chloride or Sodium Hydroxide.

Drops: Active Ingredients: Acetaminophen. Inactive Ingredients: Citric Acid, FD&C Red #40, Flavors, Glycerin, Parabens, Polyethylene Glycol, Propylene Glycol, Purified Water, Saccharin Sodium, Sodium Chloride, Sodium Citrate.

How Supplied: Chewable Tablets (colored pink and scored)—bottles of 30. Liquid (colored red)—bottles of 2 fl. oz. and 4 fl. oz. Drops (colored red)—bottles of ½ oz. (15 ml).

All packages listed above have child resistant safety caps and tamper resistant features.

Shown in Product Identification Section, page 409

JUNIOR STRENGTH PANADOL®

Description: Each Junior Strength PANADOL® Caplet contains 160 mg of acetaminophen.

Actions and Indications: Acetaminophen, the active ingredient in Junior Strength PANADOL®, is the analgesic/antipyretic most widely recommended by pediatricians for fast, effective relief of children's fevers. It also relieves the aches and pains of colds and flu, earaches, headaches, teething, immunizations, tonsillectomy, menstrual discomfort, and childhood illness.

Junior Strength PANADOL® Caplets are aspirin free, sugar free.

Usual Dosage: Under 6 yrs., under 48 lbs., contact a physician. 6–8 yrs., 48–59 lbs., 2 Caplets. 9–10 yrs., 60–71 lbs., 2½ Caplets. 11–12 yrs., 72–95 lbs., 3 Caplets. Over 12 yrs., 96 lbs. and over, 4 Caplets.

Inactive Ingredients: Hydroxypropyl Methylcellulose, Potassium Sorbate, Povidone, Pregelatinized Starch, Starch, Stearic Acid, Talc, Triacetin.

Warnings: If symptoms persist or new ones occur, consult physician. If fever persists for more than 3 days, or recurs, consult a physician. Do not take this product for more than 5 days. Keep this and all drugs out of the reach of children. In case of accidental overdose, seek professional assistance or contact a poison control center immediately. As with any drug, if you are pregnant, or nursing a baby, seek the advice of a health professional before using this product.

How Supplied: Swallowable caplets (white)—blister-pack of 30. Package has child resistant and tamper resistant features.
NDC 12843-216-14

MAXIMUM STRENGTH PANADOL®
Tablets and Caplets

Description: Active Ingredients: Each Maximum Strength PANADOL micro-thin coated Tablet and Caplet contains acetaminophen 500 mg. Inactive Ingredients: Hydroxypropyl Methylcellulose,

Potassium Sorbate, Povidone, Pregelatinized Starch, Starch, Stearic Acid, Talc, Triacetin.

Actions: PANADOL acetaminophen has been clinically proven as a fast, effective analgesic (pain reliever) and antipyretic (fever reducer). PANADOL acetaminophen is a non-aspirin product designed to provide relief without stomach upset. Its patented micro-thin coating makes each 500 mg tablet or caplet easy to swallow.

Indications: For the temporary relief from pain of headaches, colds or flu, sinusitis, bachaches, muscle aches, and menstrual discomfort. Also to reduce fever and for temporary relief of minor arthritis pain and headache.

Precautions: If a rare sensitivity reaction occurs, the drug should be stopped. PANADOL acetaminophen has rarely been found to produce any side effects. It is usually well tolerated by aspirin sensitive patients.

Severe recurrent pain or high continued fever may indicate a serious condition. Under these circumstances consult a physician.

Warning: As with other products available without prescription, the following appears on the label of PANADOL acetaminophen: "Do not give to children under 12 or use for more than 10 days unless directed by a physician. Keep this and all drugs out of the reach of children. In case of accidental overdose, seek professional assistance or contact a poison control center immediately. As with any drug, if you are pregnant or nursing a baby, seek the advice of a health professional before using this product.

Usual Dosage: *Adults:* Two tablets or caplets every 4 hours as needed. Do not exceed 8 tablets or caplets in 24 hours unless directed by a physician.

Overdosage: In massive overdosage acetaminophen may cause hepatic toxicity in some patients. Clinical and laboratory evidence of overdosage may be delayed up to 7 days. Under circumstances of suspected overdose, contact your regional poison control center immediately.

How Supplied: Tablets and caplets (white, micro-thin coated, imprinted "PANADOL" and "500"). Tablets packaged in tamper-evident bottles of 10, 30, 60 and 100. Caplets packaged in tamper-evident bottles of 24, 50.

Shown in Product Identification Section, page 409

PHILLIPS'® LAXCAPS®

Active Ingredients: A combination of phenolphthalein (90 mg) and Docusate Sodium (83 mg) per gelatin capsule.

Inactive Ingredients: FD&C Blue #1, Red #3, Red #40 and Yellow #6, Gelatin, Glycerin, PEG 400 and 3350, Propylene Glycol and Sorbitol.

Indications: For relief of occasional constipation (irregularity).

Action: Phenolphthalein is a stimulant laxative which increases the peristaltic activity of the intestine. Docusate Sodium is a stool softener which allows easier passage of the stool. This product generally produces bowel movement in 6 to 12 hours.

Administration and Dosage: Adults and children 12 and over take one (1) or two (2) capsules daily with a full glass (8 ounce) of liquid, or as directed by a physician. For children under 12, consult your physician.

Warnings: Do not take any laxative if abdominal pain, nausea, vomiting, change in bowel habits persisting for over 2 weeks, rectal bleeding or kidney disease are present. Laxative products should not be used for a period longer than one week, unless directed by a physician. If there is a failure to have a bowel movement after use, discontinue and consult your doctor. If a skin rash appears do not take this or any other preparation which contains phenolphthalein. Keep this and all drugs out of the reach of children. In case of accidental overdose, seek professional assistance or contact a Poison Control Center immediately. As with any drug, if you are pregnant or nursing a baby, seek the advice of a health professional before using this product.

How Supplied: Blister packs for safety of:
8's NDC 12843-384-18
24's NDC 12843-384-19

Shown in Product Identification Section, page 410

PHILLIPS'® MILK OF MAGNESIA

Active Ingredients: A suspension of magnesium hydroxide in purified water meeting all USP specifications. Phillips' Milk of Magnesia contains 405 mg per teaspoon (5 ml) of Magnesium Hydroxide.

Inactive Ingredients: Purified water. For Mint Flavored Phillips' Milk of Magnesia only: Flavor, Mineral Oil and Saccharin Sodium.

Indications: For relief of occasional constipation (irregularity), relief of acid indigestion, sour stomach and heartburn.

Action At Laxative Dosage: Phillips' Milk of Magnesia is a mild saline laxative which acts by drawing water into the gut, increasing intraluminal pressure, and increasing intestinal motility. This product generally produces bowel movement in ½ to 6 hours.

At Antacid Dosage: Phillips' Milk of Magnesia is an effective acid neutralizer.

Administration and Dosage: As a laxative, adults and children 12 years and older, 2–4 tbsp.: children 6–11, 1–2 tbsp.; children 2–5, 1–3 tsp. followed by a full glass (8 oz) of liquid. Children under 2, consult a physician.

Continued on next page

Glenbrook—Cont.

As an antacid, 1–3 tsps with a little water, up to four times a day, or as directed by your physician.

Cautions: Antacids may interact with certain prescription drugs. If you are taking a prescription drug do not take this product without checking with your physician.

Laxative Warnings: Do not take any laxative if abdominal pain, nausea, vomiting, change in bowel habits persisting for over 2 weeks, rectal bleeding, or kidney disease are present. Laxative products should not be used for a period longer than 1 week, unless directed by a doctor. If there is a failure to have a bowel movement after use, discontinue and consult your doctor.

Antacid Warnings: Do not take more than the maximum recommended daily dosage in a 24 hour period (See Directions), or use the maximum dosage of this product for more than two weeks, or use this product if you have kidney disease, except under the advice and supervision of a physician. May have laxative effect.

General Warnings: As with any drug, if you are pregnant or nursing a baby, seek the advice of a health professional before using this product. Keep this and all drugs out of reach of children. In case of accidental overdose, seek professional assistance or contact a poison control center immediately.

How Supplied: Phillips' Milk of Magnesia is available in regular and mint flavor in bottles of:
Regular
4 fl. oz. NDC-12843-353-01, 12 fl. oz. NDC-12843-353-02, 26 fl. oz. NDC-12843-353-03.
Mint
4 fl. oz. NDC-12843-363-04, 12 fl. oz. NDC-12843-363-05, 26 fl. oz. NDC-12843-363-06.
Also available in tablet form.
Shown in Product Identification Section, page 409

PHILLIPS® MILK OF MAGNESIA TABLETS

Active Ingredients: Each Tablet contains 311 mg of Magnesium Hydroxide.

Inactive Ingredients: Flavor, Starch, Sucrose. Product description not USP.

Indications: For relief of acid indigestion, sour stomach, heartburn and occasional constipation (irregularity).

Actions: At Laxative Dosage: Phillips' Milk of Magnesia Tablets offer the same mild saline laxative ingredient as liquid Phillips' Milk of Magnesia in a convenient, chewable tablet form. It acts by drawing water into the gut, increasing intraluminal pressure, and increasing intestinal motility. This product generally produces bowel movement in ½ to 6 hours.

At Antacid Dosage: Phillips' Milk of Magnesia Tablets are effective acid neutralizers.

Administration and Dosage: As an Antacid, adults chew thoroughly 2 to 4 tablets up to 4 times a day. Children 7 to 14 years, 1 tablet up to 4 times a day or as directed by a physician.
As a laxative, adults and children 12 years of age and older chew thoroughly 6 to 8 tablets. Children 6 to 11, 3 to 4 tablets; children 2 to 5, 1 to 2 tablets, preferably before bedtime and follow with a full glass (8 oz.) of liquid. Children under 2, consult a physician.

Laxative Warnings: Do not take any laxative if abdominal pain, nausea, vomiting, change in bowel habits (that persists for over 2 weeks), rectal bleeding, or kidney disease are present. Laxative products should not be used for a period longer than 1 week, unless directed by a doctor. If there is a failure to have a bowel movement after use, discontinue and consult your doctor.

Antacid Warnings: Do not take more than the maximum recommended daily dosage in a 24 hour period (See Directions), or use the maximum dosage of this product for more than two weeks, or use this product if you have kidney disease, except under the advice and supervision of a physician. May have laxative effect.

General Warnings: As with any drug, if you are pregnant or nursing a baby, seek the advice of a health professional before using this product. Keep this and all drugs out of reach of children. In case of accidental overdose, seek professional assistance or contact a poison control center immediately.

STRI-DEX® REGULAR STRENGTH PADS and
STRI-DEX® MAXIMUM STRENGTH PADS

Active Ingredients: Stri-Dex® Regular Strength: Salicylic Acid 0.5%, Alcohol 28% by volume.

Inactive Ingredients: Citric Acid, Fragrance, Purified Water, Simethicone Emulsion, Sodium Carbonate, Sodium Dodecylbenzenesulfonate, Sodium Xylenesulfonate.

Stri-Dex® Maximum Strength: Salicylic Acid 2.0%, SD Alcohol 40 44% by volume.

Inactive Ingredients: Ammonium Xylenesulfonate, Citric Acid, Fragrance, Purified Water, Simethicone Emulsion, Sodium Carbonate, Sodium Dodecylbenzenesulfonate.

Indications: For the treatment of acne. Reduces the number of acne pimples and blackheads, and allows the skin to heal. Helps prevent new acne pimples from forming.

Directions: Cleanse the skin thoroughly before using medicated pad. Use the pad to wipe the entire affected area one to three times daily. Because excessive drying of the skin may occur, start

with one application daily, then gradually increase to two or three times daily if needed or as directed by a doctor.

Warning:
FOR EXTERNAL USE ONLY. Using other topical acne medications at the same time or immediately following use of this product may increase dryness or irritation of the skin. If this occurs, only one medication should be used unless directed by a doctor.
Persons with very sensitive skin or known allergy to salicylic acid should not use this medication. If irritation or excessive dryness and/or peeling occurs, reduce frequency of use or dosage. If excessive itching, dryness, redness, or swelling occurs, discontinue use. If these symptoms persist, consult a physician promptly.
Keep away from eyes, lips and other mucous membranes.
Keep this and all drugs out of reach of children. In the case of accidental ingestion, seek professional assistance or contact a Poison Control Center immediately.

Dosage and Administration: See labeling instructions for use.

How Supplied:
Stri-Dex Regular Strength is available in NDC 12843-087-13—Porta-Pak Refillable Plastic container consisting of 12 pads, 2″ in diameter.
NDC 12843-087-07—Plastic jar consisting of 42 pads, 2″ in diameter.
NDC 12843-087-08—Plastic jar consisting of 75 pads, 2″ in diameter.
NDC 12843-087-04—Stri-Dex Big Pads in a plastic jar consisting of 42 pads, 2⅞″ in diameter.
Stri-Dex Maximum Strength is available in:
NDC 12843-097-12—Porta-Pak Refillable Plastic container consisting of 12 pads, 2″ in diameter.
NDC 12843-097-09—Plastic jar consisting of 42 pads, 2″ in diameter.
NDC 12843-097-11—Plastic jar consisting of 75 pads, 2″ in diameter.
NDC 12843-097-03—Stri-Dex Big Pads in a plastic jar consisting of 42 pads, 2⅞″ in diameter.
Shown in Product Identification Section, page 410

VANQUISH® Analgesic Caplets

Active Ingredients: Each Caplet contains aspirin 227 mg, acetaminophen 194 mg, caffeine 33 mg, dried aluminum hydroxide gel 25 mg, magnesium hydroxide 50 mg.

Inactive Ingredients: Acacia, Colloidal Silicon Dioxide, Hydrogenated Vegetable Oil, Microcrystalline Cellulose, Powdered Cellulose, Sodium Lauryl Sulfate, Starch, Talc.

Action and Uses: A buffered analgesic, antipyretic for relief of headache; muscular aches and pains; neuralgia and neuritic pain; toothache; pain following dental procedures; for painful discomforts and fever of colds and flu; sinusitis; functional menstrual pain, headache

and pain due to cramps; temporary relief from minor pains of arthritis, rheumatism, bursitis, lumbago, sciatica.

Caution: If pain persists for more than 10 days, or redness is present, or in conditions affecting children under 12 years of age, consult a physician immediately.

Warnings: Children and teenagers should not use this medicine for chicken pox or flu symptoms before a doctor is consulted about Reye Syndrome, a rare but serious illness reported to be associated with aspirin. Keep this and all drugs out of the reach of children. In case of accidental overdose, seek professional assistance or contact a poison control center immediately. As with any drug, if you are pregnant or nursing a baby, seek the advice of a health professional before using this product.

Usual Adult Dosage: Two caplets with water. May be repeated every four hours if necessary up to 12 tablets per day. Larger or more frequent doses may be prescribed by physician if necessary.

Contraindications: Hypersensitivity to salicylates and acetaminophen. (To be used with caution during anticoagulant therapy or in asthmatic patients.)

How Supplied: White, capsule-shaped Caplets in bottles of:
  30 Caplets NDC 12843-171-44
  60 Caplets NDC 12843-171-46
100 Caplets NDC 12843-171-48
  Shown in Product Identification Section, page 410

Gulf Bio-Systems, Inc.
**5310 HARVEST HILL ROAD
DALLAS, TX 75230**

SUPERCHAR®
Highly Activated Charcoal
Poison Adsorbent
SuperChar® Liquid with Sorbitol—suspension in sorbitol solution and water
SuperChar® Aqueous—suspension in water
SuperChar® Powder—Add water for suspension

Highly activated poison adsorbent/antidote, liquid; significantly greater adsorptive capacity per gram vs all other regular USP activated charcoals; pleasant taste for children and adults.

Active Ingredients: Highly activated charcoal, 30 grams and 50 grams per bottle, suspended in sorbitol solution (62 grams of sorbitol) or in water only.

Indication: For the emergency treatment of acute poisoning.

Action: Adsorbent.

Warning: If possible call a poison control center, emergency medical facility, or health professional for help before using the product. If help cannot be reached quickly, follow the directions. Read the warnings and directions as soon as you buy this product. Have emergency phone numbers accessible. Do not use in

poisonings involving corrosives or petroleum distillates. If patient has been given ipecac syrup, do not give activated charcoal until after patient has vomited, except on the advice of a physician. Do not administer orally to a semiconscious or unconscious person.

Precaution: May turn stool dark or black. Formulation with sorbitol added may cause a laxative effect which should particularly be monitored in small children. Do not give more than one bottle of the suspension containing sorbitol in a 24 hour period.

Dosage and Administration: Shake vigorously and drink entire contents of bottle. When administering via lavage tube, shake vigorously and immediately snip spout cap and squeeze entire contents into tube. A repeat dose may be indicated.

How Supplied:
Premixed Liquid: 30 grams (8 fl oz) or 50 grams (10 fl oz) highly activated charcoal in sorbitol and water suspension or in plain aqueous suspension.
Powder: 30 grams highly activated charcoal in 8 oz bottle or 50 grams highly activated charcoal in 10 oz bottle. Add water directly to bottle to form aqueous suspension.

EDUCATIONAL MATERIAL

1) ***At Last, A Revolutionary Breakthrough in Activating Charcoal***
Brochure describing the use of and greater efficacy of SuperChar® highly activated charcoal for acute toxic ingestion.
2) ***SuperChar® Highly Activated Charcoal Is the Recognized Leader***
Brochure comparing efficacy of adsorption per gram of SuperChar® to all other activated charcoal products.
3) ***Some Reference Studies on SuperChar® Highly Activated Charcoal***
Bibliography of various published studies showing the superior efficacy of SuperChar® versus all other activated charcoal adsorbents.
4) ***Superiority of SuperChar Including Its Use In Treatment of Drug Overdose and Accidental Poisoning***
Bibliography of published studies showing superior efficacy of SuperChar® versus all other activated charcoal adsorbents.

Products are cross-indexed by generic and chemical names in the **YELLOW SECTION**

Herald Pharmacal, Inc.
**6503 WARWICK ROAD
RICHMOND, VA 23225**

AQUA GLYCOLIC LOTION

Description: Aqua Glycolic lotion is a high potency moisturizer containing 5 per cent Glycolic Acid in an unscented lanolin-free lotion base.

How Supplied: 8 oz. bottles.

AQUA GLYCOLIC SHAMPOO

Description: Cosmetically elegant shampoo, non-irritating, containing Glycolic Acid, leaves hair soft, manageable, helps eliminate itching, leaves scalp free from scale.

How Supplied: 8 oz. bottles.

AQUA GLYDE CLEANSER

Description: A cleanser for acne and other oily skin conditions. Contains special denatured alcohol #40, purified water, fragrance, salcylic and Glycolic Acid.

How Supplied: 8 oz. plastic bottles.

CAM LOTION

Description: Lipid free, soap free skin cleanser for atopic dermatitis and other diseases aggravated by oily, greasy substances of animal and vegetable origin.

How Supplied: 8 and 16 oz. bottles.

Herbert Laboratories
**2525 DUPONT DRIVE
IRVINE, CA 92715**

AQUATAR®
Therapeutic Tar Gel

Contains: BioTar™ (coal tar extract —biologically active) 2.5% with: DEA-oleth-3 phosphate; glycerin; imidurea; methylparaben; mineral oil; oleth-3; oleth-10; oleth-20; poloxamer 407; polysorbate 80; propylparaben; and purified water.

How Supplied: 3 oz tube.

BLUBORO® Powder
Astringent Soaking Solution

Contains: Aluminum sulfate 53.9% and calcium acetate 43% with: boric acid and FD&C Blue #1.

How Supplied: 12 packet carton, 100 packet carton (0.06 oz/packet)

DANEX®
Protein Enriched Dandruff Shampoo

Active Ingredient: Pyrithione zinc 1%.

How Supplied: 4 oz bottle.

Continued on next page

Herbert—Cont.

VANSEB® Cream and Lotion
Dandruff Shampoos

Active Ingredients: Salicylic acid 1% and sulfur 2% with cocamide DEA.

How Supplied: 3 oz tube, 4 oz bottle.

VANSEB-T® Cream and Lotion
Tar Dandruff Shampoos

Active Ingredients: Coal tar solution USP 5%; salicylic acid 1% and sulfur 2% with cocamide DEA.

How Supplied: 3 oz tube, 4 oz bottle.

EDUCATIONAL MATERIAL

HERBERT LABORATORIES
Immediate Relief Begins with Bluboro® Powder Astringent Soaking Solution
A pad containing physician instructions plus tear-off sheets for customized patient instructions for the use of Bluboro®.

Instructions For Use of Fluoroplex® (fluorouracil) 1%
Pamphlet explains what actinic keratosis is and how Fluoroplex® works, containing color photos of before, during and after treatment.

Patient Instructions for Treatment of Tinea Versicolor
Fact sheets describing tinea versicolor and how to apply Excel® (selenium sulfide) 2.5% Lotion. (English & Spanish)

The Causes and Treatment of Itching . . . and the Use of Temaril® (trimeprazine tartrate) the Oral Anti-Itch Medication
A 10-page booklet designed for adults on the causes and treatment of itching and the use of Temaril®.

Why We Itch . . . And What To Do About It
Booklet designed for parents to use in explaining the cause and treatment of itching and the use of Temaril® (trimeprazine tartrate) to their children.

What You Should Know About Psoriasis
Patient instruction sheets discussing psoriasis and its treatment with AquaTar® Therapeutic Tar Gel.

What You Should Know About Your Fungal Infection and Your Prescription Drug Gris-PEG® (griseofulvin ultramicrosize) Tablets, USP
A booklet describing certain fungal infections, how griseofulvin works, what the patient can do to speed recovery and prevent recurrence.

Griseofulvin: Clinical Considerations in Current Treatment of Superficial Fungal Infections
A monograph focusing on current concepts of how most effectively to use griseofulvin in therapy.

Hoechst-Roussel Pharmaceuticals Inc.
SOMERVILLE, NJ 08876

DOXIDAN®
Stimulant/Stool Softener Laxative

Ingredients: Each Liquigel™ contains 65 mg yellow phenolphthalein USP, 60 mg docusate calcium USP, and the following inactive ingredients: alcohol USP up to 1.5% (w/w), corn oil NF, FD&C Blue #1 and Red #40, gelatin NF, glycerin USP, hydrogenated vegetable oil NF, lecithin NF, parabens NF, sorbitol NF, titanium dioxide USP, vegetable shortening, yellow wax NF, and other ingredients.

Indications: Doxidan is a safe, reliable laxative for the relief of occasional constipation. The combination of a stimulant/stool softener laxative allows positive laxative action on a softened stool for gentle evacuation without straining. Doxidan generally produces a bowel movement in 6 to 12 hours. Doxidan may be of particular benefit when stool softening alone is insufficient and as an adjunct to bowel retraining.
SURGICAL AFTERCARE: Doxidan is useful in both pre- and post-operative conditions that require gentle peristaltic stimulation.
OBSTETRICS: The gentle, effective laxative action of Doxidan is useful in prenatal and postpartum patients where straining at stool is to be avoided.
GERIATRICS: Dietary changes, decreased physical activity and the use of certain drugs often contribute to constipation in the elderly patient.
Doxidan promotes a gentle laxation and eliminates the need for harsh cathartics.
ANORECTAL CONDITIONS: Doxidan contains an effective stool softener laxative that facilitates the passage of softened stools and their elimination from the rectum in patients with proctologic problems.

Warnings: Do not use when abdominal pain, nausea, or vomiting is present unless directed by a doctor. If you have noticed a sudden change in bowel habits that persists over a period of 2 weeks, consult a doctor before using a laxative. Do not use for a period longer than 1 week unless directed by a doctor. Rectal bleeding or failure to have a bowel movement after use may indicate a serious condition. Discontinue use and consult your doctor. Occasional cramping may occur. If skin rash appears, do not use this product or any other preparation containing phenolphthalein. As with any drug, if you are pregnant or nursing a baby, seek the advice of a health professional before using this product.
Keep this and all medication out of the reach of children. In case of accidental overdose, seek professional assistance or contact a poison control center immediately.

Usual Dosage: Adults and children 12 years of age and over, one or two Liquigels by mouth daily. For use in children

under 12 consult a physician. Store at controlled room temperature (59°–86°F) in a dry place.

How Supplied: Packages of 10, 30, 100 and 1,000 maroon Liquigels, and Unit Dose 100s (10 × 10 strips).
Liquigel TM R. P. Scherer
Doxidan REG TM Hoechst-Roussel
Manufactured by R. P. Scherer, Clearwater, FL, expressly for Hoechst-Roussel Pharmaceuticals Inc.
Shown in Product Identification Section, page 410

FESTAL® II
Digestive Aid

Composition: Each enteric sugar-coated tablet contains lipase 6,000 USP units, amylase 30,000 USP units, protease 20,000 USP units and the following inactive ingredients: acacia NF, calcium carbonate USP, castor oil USP, cellulose acetate phthalate NF, gelatin NF, FD&C Blue #2, flavors, microcrystalline cellulose NF, parabens NF, povidone USP, sodium chloride USP, sucrose NF, talc USP and titanium dioxide USP.

Actions and Uses: Festal® II provides a high degree of protected digestive activity in a formula of standardized enzymes. Enteric coating of the tablet prevents release of ingredients in the stomach so that high enzymatic potency is delivered to the site in the intestinal tract where digestion normally takes place.
Festal® II is indicated in any condition where normal digestion is impaired by insufficiency of natural digestive enzymes, or when additional digestive enzymes may be beneficial. These conditions often manifest complaints of discomfort due to excess intestinal gas, such as bloating, cramps and flatulence. The following are conditions or situations where Festal® II may be helpful: pancreatic insufficiency, chronic pancreatitis, pancreatic necrosis, and removal of gas prior to x-ray examination.
Keep this and all medication out of the reach of children.

Dosage: Usual adult dose is one or two tablets with each meal, or as directed by a physician. Store at controlled room temperature (59°–86°F).

Contraindications: Festal® II should not be given to patients sensitive to protein of porcine origin.

How Supplied: Bottles of 100 and 500 white, enteric sugar-coated tablets for oral use.
Festal REG TM Hoechst AG
Shown in Product Identification Section, page 410

SURFAK®
Stool Softener

Ingredients: Each 240 mg Liquigel™ contains 240 mg docusate calcium USP, alcohol USP up to 3% (w/w) and the following inactive ingredients: corn oil NF, FD&C Blue #1 and Red #40 gelatin NF, glycerin USP, parabens NF, sorbitol NF and other ingredients.

Each 50 mg Liquigel™ contains 50 mg docusate calcium USP, alcohol USP up to 1.3% (w/w) and the following inactive ingredients: corn oil NF, FD&C Red #3, and Red #40, gelatin NF, glycerin USP, parabens NF, sorbitol NF, soybean oil USP and other ingredients.

Actions: Surfak provides homogenization and formation of soft, easily evacuated stools without disturbance of body physiology, discomfort of bowel distention or oily leakage. Surfak is non-habit forming.

Indications: Surfak is indicated for the prevention and treatment of constipation in conditions in which hard stools may cause discomfort. Surfak is useful in patients who require only stool softening without propulsive action to accomplish defecation. Surfak does not cause peristaltic stimulation, and because of its safety it may be effectively used in patients with heart conditions, anorectal conditions, obstetrical patients, following surgical procedures, ulcerative colitis, diverticulitis and bedridden patients.

Warnings: Surfak has no known side effects or disadvantages, except for the unusual occurrence of mild, transitory cramping pains. If cramping pain occurs, discontinue the medication. As with any drug, if you are pregnant or nursing a baby, seek the advice of a health professional before using this product. Keep this and all medication out of reach of children.

Overdosage: Overdosage does not lead to systemic toxicity.

Dosage and Administration: Adults —one red 240 mg Liquigel by mouth daily for several days or until bowel movements are normal. Children and adults with minimal needs—one to three orange 50 mg Liquigels daily. For use in children under 6, consult a physician.

How Supplied: 240 mg red Liquigels—packages of 7 and 30, bottles of 100 and 500, and Unit Dose 100s (10 × 10 strips); 50 mg orange Liquigels—bottles of 30 and 100.
Store at controlled room temperature (59°–86°F) in a dry place.
Liquigel REG TM R.P. Scherer
Manufactured by R.P. Scherer, Clearwater, FL, expressly for Hoechst-Roussel Pharmaceuticals Inc.
Shown in Product Identification Section, page 410

EDUCATIONAL MATERIAL

Changes, Cycles and Constipation
Pamphlet describing constipation and its causes, with instructions on prevention and self-treatment, and when to consult a physician. (English and Spanish)
What You Should Know About Hemorrhoids and Fissures
Pamphlet describing these conditions, with instructions on self-care and when to consult a physician. (English and Spanish)

Hynson, Westcott & Dunning Products
Becton Dickinson Microbiology Systems
250 SCHILLING CIRCLE
COCKEYSVILLE, MD 21030

LACTINEX® TABLETS AND GRANULES
[lak 'tĕ-neks]

Composition: A viable mixed culture of *Lactobacillus acidophilus* and *L. bulgaricus* with the naturally occurring metabolic products that are produced by these organisms.

Action and Uses: Lactinex has been found to be useful in the treatment of uncomplicated diarrhea (including that due to antibiotic therapy).

Indications and Dosage: (for adults and children):
Gastrointestinal Disturbances—4 tablets or 1 packet of granules added to or taken with cereal, food, milk, fruit juice or water; three or four times a day.
   Lactinex Must Be Refrigerated
Individuals sensitive to milk products should not use Lactinex.

How Supplied: Tablets—bottles of fifty (NDC 0011-8368-50). Granules, boxes of twelve, 1 gram packets (unit dose dispensing), (NDC 0011-8367-12).

Literature Available: On request.
Shown in Product Identification Section, page 410

Inter-Cal Corporation
421 MILLER VALLEY RD.
PRESCOTT, AZ 86301

ESTER–C®
(Calcium Ascorbate)

Description: Each Ester-C tablet contains 500 mg Vitamin C in the form of Calcium Ascorbate 550 mg, vegetable-derived cellulose, stearic acid, and magnesium stearate. Ester-C contains no preservatives, sugars, artificial colorings, or flavorings.
As the calcium salt of L-ascorbic acid, Ester-C has an empirical formula of $CaC_{12}H_{14}O_{12}$ and a formula weight of 390.3.

Actions: Vitamin C has been found to be essential for the prevention of scurvy. In humans, an exogenous source of the vitamin is required for collagen formation and tissue repair. Ascorbate ion is reversibly oxidized to dehydroascorbate ion in the body. Both of these are active forms of the vitamin and are considered to play important roles in biochemical oxidation-reduction reactions. The vitamin is involved in tyrosine metabolism, carbohydrate metabolism, iron metabolism, folic acid-folinic acid conversion, synthesis of lipids and proteins, resistance to infections, and cellular respiration.

Indications and Usage: Vitamin C and its salts, such as Calcium Ascorbate, are recommended as nutritional supplements in the prevention of scurvy. In scurvy, collagenous structures are primarily affected, and lesions develop in blood vessels and bones. Symptoms of mild deficiency may include faulty development of teeth and bones, bleeding gums, gingivitis, and loose teeth. An increased need for the vitamin exists in febrile states, chronic illness and infection, e.g., rheumatic fever, pneumonia, tuberculosis, whooping cough, diphtheria, sinusitis, etc. Additional increases in the daily intake of ascorbate are indicated in burns, delayed healing of bone fractures and wounds, and hemovascular disorders. Immature and premature infants require relatively larger amounts of Vitamin C.

Contraindications: Because of its calcium content, Ester-C is contraindicated in hypercalcemic states, e.g., from dosing with parathyroid hormone or overdosage of Vitamin D.
Diabetics, persons prone to recurrent renal calculi, those undergoing stool occult blood tests, and those on anticoagulant therapy should not take excessive doses of Vitamin C over extended periods of time.

Precautions: Because of its calcium content, Ester-C should be used with caution by those undergoing treatment with digitalis or cardiotonic glycosides such as digitoxin and digoxin.
Laboratory Tests—Diabetics taking more than 500 mg of Vitamin C may generate false readings in their urinary glucose tests. To avoid false-negative results, forms of the vitamin should not be taken as supplements for 48 to 72 hours before amine-dependent stool occult blood tests are conducted.
Drug Interactions—There is limited evidence suggesting that Vitamin C may influence the intensity and duration of action of bishydroxycoumarin.
Usage in Pregnancy—Pregnancy Category C—Animal reproduction studies have not been carried out with Ester-C tablets. It is also not known whether Ester-C can cause fetal harm when administered to a pregnant woman or can affect reproductive capacity.
Nursing Mothers—Caution should be exercised when Ester-C tablets are recommended for nursing mothers.

Adverse Reactions: There are no known adverse reactions following ingestion of Ester-C tablets. The gastric disturbances characteristic of large doses of ascorbic acid are absent or greatly diminished when the pH-neutral form of calcium ascorbate present in Ester-C tablets is utilized as the source of Vitamin C supplementation.

Dosage and Administration: The minimum U.S. Recommended Daily Allowance for Vitamin C for the prevention of diseases such as scurvy is 60 mg per day. Optimum daily allowances, e.g., for

Continued on next page

Inter-Cal—Cont.

the maintenance of increased plasma and cellular reserves, are significantly greater. For adults, the recommended average preventative dose of the vitamin is 70 to 150 mg daily. The recommended average optimum dose of Ester-C is 550 to 1650 mg (1 to 3 tablets) daily.

For frank scurvy, doses of 300 mg to one gram of Vitamin C daily have been recommended. Normal adults, however, have received as much as six grams of the vitamin without evidence of toxicity.

For enhancement of wound healing, doses of the vitamin approximating two Ester-C tablets daily for a week or ten days both preoperatively and postoperatively are generally considered adequate, although considerably larger amounts may be recommended. In the treatment of burns, the daily number of Ester-C tablets recommended is governed by the extent of tissue injury. For severe burns, daily doses of 2 to 4 tablets (approximately one to two grams of Vitamin C) are recommended.

In other conditions in which the need for increased Vitamin C is recognized, three to five times the optimum allowance appears to be adequate.

How Supplied: 550 mg tablets of Ester-C in plastic bottles of 100 or 250 tablets.

Store at room temperature.
Literature revised: July, 1987.
Mfd. by Inter-Cal Corp.
Prescott, AZ 86301

Jackson-Mitchell Pharmaceuticals, Inc.
P.O. BOX 5425
SANTA BARBARA, CA 93150

MEYENBERG GOAT MILK
[my 'en-berg]
Concentrated liquid • powder

Composition: A natural, mammalian milk more closely related to the structure of human milk than cow milk. Does not contain alpha S_1 casein. More easily digested.

Normal dilution (adults and babies over 1 year) supplies 20 calories/fl oz). EVAPORATED supplemented with folic acid and Vitamin D. POWDER, folic acid only.

NOTE: **Not a complete formula.** Vitamin supplement recommended if sole source of nutrition.

Action and Uses: For cow milk and/or soy milk sensitive adults and children.

Preparation: Adults—20 calories/fl oz with concentrated liquid—1 part to 1 part water. Refrigerate. Baby Formula—should be refrigerated & used within 48 hours.

MEYENBERG Evaporated GOAT MILK Fortified with Folic Acid and Vitamin D

	Evap. Milk	Water	Calories Fl. Oz.*
First or transitional dilution	1 part	2 parts	14
Standard dilution	1 part	1 part	20

*Increase calorie value as desired by the addition of a carbohydrate.

MEYENBERG Powdered GOAT MILK Fortified with Folic Acid

RECOMMENDED FOR BABIES OVER 1 YEAR BECAUSE OF FLAVOR

	Pwdr. Milk	Water	Calories Fl. Oz.*
Standard dilution	1 Tbsp.	2 Fl. Oz.	20

EDUCATIONAL MATERIAL

Is It Really Milk Allergy?
Brochure.
Meyenberg Story
Brochure.

Johnson & Johnson
Baby Products Company
GRANDVIEW ROAD
SKILLMAN, NJ 08558

JOHNSON'S BABY SUNBLOCK
Ultra Sunblock (SPF 15) Cream
Ultra Sunblock (SPF 15) Lotion

Active Ingredients: Octyl Methoxycinnamate, Octyl Salicylate, Oxybenzone, Titanium Dioxide.

Inactive Ingredients: Barium Sulfate, Benzyl Alcohol, Carbomer 941, Cetyl Alcohol, Dimethicone, Dioctyl Maleate, Disodium EDTA, Fragrance, Glycerin, Isopropyl Isostearate Acid, Methyl Glucose Sesquistearate, Methylparaben, Propylene Glycol, Propylparaben, PVP/Eicosene Copolymer, Quaternium-15, Stearic Acid, Triethanolamine, Water.

Indications: JOHNSON'S BABY SUNBLOCK products provide gentle effective protection. The PABA-free lotion and cream formulas each provide 15 times a child's natural sunburn protection. Both are waterproof providing protection for at least 80 minutes in water and resist removal by sweating. Liberal and regular use may help reduce the change of skin cancer due to overexposure to the sun.

Actions: Screens out ultraviolet rays (UVA and UVB).

Warning: For external use only. AVOID CONTACT WITH EYES. Should temporary stinging and tearing occur through accidental contact, thoroughly rinse eyes with water. Discontinue use if signs of irritation or rash appear. Use on children under six months of age only with the advise of a physician. Keep out of reach of children.

Dosage and Administration: Apply generously and evenly to all exposed areas before going in the sun. Both formulas are waterproof but should be reapplied after 80 minutes in water or excessive perspiration.

How Supplied: Lotion in 4 fl. oz. plastic bottle; Cream in 2 oz. tube.
Shown in Product Identification Section, page 410

PURPOSE® Dry Skin Cream

Ingredients: Water, White petrolatum, Propylene glycol, Glyceryl stearate, Sodium Lactate, Sweet almond oil, Steareth-20, Cetyl alcohol, Cetyl esters wax, Mineral oil, Steareth-2, Xanthan gum, Sorbic acid, Lactic acid and fragrance.

Indications: PURPOSE Dry Skin Cream is formulated especially to meet the need for an effective dry skin cream that dermatologists can recommend. PURPOSE Dry Skin Cream moisturizes dry, chapped and irritated skin and provides effective, lasting relief from drying and scaling. PURPOSE Dry Skin Cream smoothes easily into skin for over-all body care.

Administration and Dosage: Instruct patients to use PURPOSE Dry Skin Cream as any other dry skin cream.

How Supplied: 3 oz. tube.

PURPOSE™ Dual Treatment Moisturizer (SPF 12)

Active Ingredients: Octyl methoxycinnamate, oxybenzone.

Inactive Ingredients: Water, Glycerin, Cetyl Phosphate, DEA-Cetyl Phosphate, Cetyl Palmitate, Dimethicone, Stearoxytrimethylsilane, Octyl Stearate, Mineral Oil, Stearyl Alcohol, Cetyl Alcohol, Glyceryl Cocoate, Hydrogenated Coconut Oil, Ceteareth-25, Carbomer 941, Benzyl Alcohol, Methylparaben, Propylparaben, Disodium EDTA, Quaternium 15, Fragrance, BHT.

Indications: PURPOSE Dual Treatment Moisturizer is a light, greaseless facial moisturizer with the added benefit of PABA-free sunscreens. This formula was created to allow for everyday sun protection as a part of a morning facial moisturizing routine. To this end, the PURPOSE formula is exceptionally cosmetically elegant, and is particularly acceptable for under makeup base.

Warnings: For external use only. Avoid contact with eyes. Keep out of reach of children. Discontinue use if signs of irritation or rash appear.

Administration and Dosage: Apply daily under makeup or by itself.

How Supplied: Lotion in a 4 fluid ounce glass bottle (fragrance-free and lightly scented).

PURPOSE® Soap

Ingredients: Sodium tallowate, Sodium cocoate, Water, Glycerin, Fragrance, Sodium chloride, BHT, Trisodium HEDTA, D&C Yellow No. 10, D&C Orange No. 4.

Indications: Extraordinary mild PURPOSE Soap was created to wash tender, sensitive skin. Formulated especially to meet the need for a mild soap that dermatologists can recommend. This translucent washing bar is non-medicated and completely free of harsh detergents or other ingredients that might dry or irritate skin.

Administration and Dosage: Wash face with PURPOSE Soap two or three times a day or as directed by your physician. Rinse with warm water. For complete skin care, use it also for bath and shower.

How Supplied: 3.6 oz. and 6 oz. bars.

SUNDOWN® BROAD SPECTRUM
Ultra Sunblock (SPF 15) LOTION
Ultra Sunblock (SPF 25) LOTION
Ultra Sunblock (SPF 30) CREAM

Active Ingredients: SPF 15, 25 and 30: Octyl Methoxycinnamate, Octyl Salicylate, Oxybenzone, Titanium Dioxide

Inactive Ingredients: SPF 15 and 25: Barium Sulfate, Benzyl Alcohol, C12-15 Alcohols Benzoate, Carbomer 941, Dimethicone, Disodium EDTA, Fragrance, Glycerin, Glyceryl Stearate, Isostearic Acid, Mineral Oil, Quaternium-15, Stearic Acid, Stearoxytrimethysilane, Stearyl Alcohol, Tocopheryl Acetate, Water and Other Ingredients.
SPF 30: Barium Sulfate, Benzyl Alcohol, C12-15 Alcohols Benzoate, Carbomer 934, Dimethicone, Disodium EDTA, Fragrance, Glycerin, Glyceryl Stearate, Isostearic Acid, Mineral Oil, Polysorbate 21, Quaternium-15, Stearic Acid, Stearoxytrimethysilane, Stearyl Alcohol, Tocopheryl Acetate, Water and Other Ingredients.

Indications: The SUNDOWN® BROAD SPECTRUM products provide your skin with a broad spectrum barrier to the harmful ultraviolet sunlight rays that contribute to premature aging. These sunblock products block a broader range of UVA rays than ordinary sunscreens. Liberal and regular use may help reduce the chance of premature skin aging, skin wrinking and skin cancer due to overexposure to the sun. These products are also PABA-free and therefore suitable for those sensitive to PABA and its related compounds.

Actions: Screens out ultraviolet rays (UVA and UVB).

Warnings: For external use only. AVOID CONTACT WITH EYES. Should temporary stinging and tearing occur through accidental contact, discontinue use if signs of irritation or rash appear. Use on children under six months of age only with the advice of a physician. Keep out of reach of children.

Dosage and Administration: CREAM and LOTION: Apply generously and evenly to all exposed areas. All formulas are waterproof but should be reapplied after 80 minutes in water or excessive perspiration.

How Supplied: LOTIONS in 4 fl. oz. plastic bottles; CREAM in 3.5 oz. tube.
Shown in Product Identification Section, page 410

SUNDOWN® SUNSCREENS
Moderate Protection (SPF 4) LOTION
Extra Protection (SPF 6) LOTION
Maximal Protection (SPF 8) LOTION and STICK
Ultra Protection (SPF 15) LOTION and STICK
Ultra Protection (SPF 20) LOTION and STICK
Ultra Protection (SPF 24) CREAM

LOTIONS AND CREAM
Active Ingredients:
SPF 4, 6, 8 and 24: Octyl Dimethyl PABA, Oxybenzone
SPF 15: Octyl Dimethyl PABA, Octyl Methoxycinnamate, Oxybenzone
SPF 20: Octyl Dimethyl PABA, Octyl Methoxycinnamate, Oxybenzone, Titanium Dioxide

Inactive Ingredients:
SPF 4, 6, 8 and 15: Benzyl Alcohol, Carbomer 934, Carbomer 941, Dimethicone, Disodium EDTA, Fragrance, Glyceryl Stearate, Isostearic Acid, Mineral Oil, Quaternium-15, Stearyl Alcohol, Water, and Other Ingredients.
SPF 20: Barium Sulfate, Benzyl Alcohol, Carbomer 941, Dimethicone, Disodium EDTA, Fragrance, Glyceryl Stearate, Isostearic Acid, Mineral Oil, Quaternium-15, Stearic Acid, Stearyl Alcohol, Water, and Other Ingredients.
SPF 24: Beeswax, Fragrance, Imidazolidinyl Urea, Isopropyl Myristate, Methylparaben, Mineral Oil, Polyethylene, Polyglyceryl-3 Diisostearate, Propylparaben, Quaterium-18 Hectorite, Sodium Borate, Sorbitol, Water

STICKS
Active Ingredients:
SPF 8 and 15: Octyl Dimethyl PABA, Oxybenzone
SPF 20: Octyl Dimethyl PABA, Octyl Methoxycinnamate, Oxybenzone, Titanium Dioxide

Inactive Ingredients:
SPF 8 and 15: Beeswax, C18–36 Acid Glycol Ester, D18–36 Acid Triglyceride, Petrolatum, Propylparaben
SPF 20: Barium Sulfate, C18–36 Acid Glycol Ester, C18–36 Acid Triglyceride, Petrolatum, Propylparaben, Stearic Acid and Synthetic Beeswax.

Indications: Sunscreens help prevent harmful effects from the sun. The SPF values designate that the products provide 4, 6, 8, 15, 20 and 24, times your natural sunburn protection, respectively. SPF 4 and 6 permit tanning, SPF 8 permits minimal tanning and SPF 15, 20 and 24 permit no tanning. Liberal and regular use may help reduce the chance of premature skin aging, skin wrinkling and skin cancer due to overexposure to the sun.

Actions: Screens out ultraviolet rays (UVA and UVB).

Warning: For external use only. AVOID CONTACT WITH EYES. Should temporary stinging and tearing occur through accidental contact, thoroughly rinse eyes with water. If sensitive to PABA or its related compounds such as aniline dyes, benzocaine, PABA esters or sulfonamides, consult your physician before using. Discontinue use if signs of irritation or rash appear. Use on children under six months of age only with the advice of a physician. Keep out of reach of children.

Dosage and Administration:
CREAM and LOTION: Apply generously and evenly to all exposed areas.
STICK: For spot applications, apply generously and evenly to nose, lips, face, ears and shoulders.
All formulas are waterproof but should be reapplied after 80 minutes in water or excessive perspiration.
How Supplied: LOTIONS in 4 fl. oz. plastic bottles; STICKS in 0.35 oz. sticks; SPF 20 STICK in 0.40 oz. stick; CREAM in 3.5 oz. tube.
Shown in Product Identification Section, page 410

Johnson & Johnson Consumer Products, Inc.
501 GEORGE STREET
NEW BRUNSWICK, NJ 08903

K-Y® BRAND LUBRICATING JELLY

Description: K-Y® Brand Lubricating Jelly is a greaseless, water-soluble jelly which is clear, spreads easily and is non-irritating.

Indications: K-Y® Brand Jelly is indicated as a greaseless sexual lubricant which is safe and non-irritating for both men and women. It may also be used for easy insertion of rectal thermometers, enemas, applicator tampons and other devices inserted into body cavities. (K-Y® will not harm rubber, plastic, diaphrams or glass surfaces.)

Actions: Helps lubricate body cavities for easier insertion. When used as a sexual lubricant, K-Y® Jelly helps overcome vaginal dryness caused by menopause, postnatal and psychological reasons.

Warnings: KEEP OUT OF EYES AND EARS. For External Use Only. IT IS NOT A CONTRACEPTIVE, DOES NOT CONTAIN SPERMACIDE. Store at room temperature.

Directions: Apply to the area of insertion the desired amount of jelly and

Continued on next page

Johnson & Johnson Products—Cont.

spread smoothly over the area. Repeat applications may be used.

How Supplied: Brand K-Y® Jelly is available in 2 and 4 oz. tubes and single-use foil packs.

Shown in Product Identification Section, page 410

EDUCATIONAL MATERIAL

A Woman's Guide to Condoms
A fact sheet informing women of the proper use of condoms and the important reasons for using them.
What Every Woman Should Know About Vaginal Lubrication
Brochure for women about the causes of and treatment for vaginal dryness.
Following Childbirth: A New Mother's Guide to Her Body
An easy-to-understand brochure which explains typical new mother experiences and offers helpful advice on coping with the many discomforts experienced after childbirth (i.e., fatigue, vaginal dryness, post-partum depression)

Kremers Urban Company

See SCHWARZ PHARMA

Laclede Research Laboratories
**15011 STAFF CT.
GARDENA, CA 90248**

BIOTENE™
DENTAL CHEWING GUM

Description: Converts sugar into hydrogen peroxide. Controls bacterial plaque and neutralizes oral acids. The only sugar-free gum that will not stick to dentures.

BIOTENE™
DRY MOUTH RELIEF TOOTHPASTE

Active Ingredients: Lactoperoxidase and Glucose Oxidase. Also contains 0.76 Sodium Monofluorophosphate in a gentle mild-flavored dentifrice.

Action and Uses: Biotene is the only anti-Xerostomia dentifrice formulated to reduce caries, gum bleeding and oral inflammation resulting from dry mouth caused by over 300 saliva-reducing prescription drugs, age, extreme stress, radiation therapy, Sjorgren's Syndrome, or diabetes. The dentifrice contains glucose oxidase and lactoperoxidase that activate an intraoral antibacterial system similar to the one normally found in saliva. The dentifrice is also recommended for the mentally and physically disabled who find it difficult to maintain good proper home oral hygiene. Biotene Dry Mouth Toothpaste is formulated so that rinsing out is not necessary.

ORAL BALANCE™
Long Lasting Moisturizing Gel

Description: Contains BIOTENE Toothpaste antibacterial system. Helps prevent yeast infections and inhibit gram-negative bacteria. Non-drying gel formula coats tender tissues to provide prompt relief of irritations, itching and soreness due to dry mouth.

Lakeside Pharmaceuticals
**Division of Merrell Dow Pharmaceuticals Inc.
CINCINNATI, OH 45242-9553**

CĒPACOL®/CĒPACOL MINT
[sē 'pə-cŏl]
Mouthwash/Gargle

Description: Cēpacol Mouthwash contains: Ceepryn® (cetylpyridinium chloride) 0.05%. Also contains: Alcohol 14%, Edetate Disodium, FD&C Yellow No. 5 (tartrazine) as a color additive, Flavors, Glycerin, Polysorbate 80, Saccharin, Sodium Biphosphate, Sodium Phosphate, and Water.
Cēpacol Mint Mouthwash contains: Ceepryn® (cetylpyridinium chloride) 0.05%. Also contains: Alcohol 14.5%, D&C Yellow No. 10, FD&C Green No. 3, Flavor, Glucono Delta-Lactone, Glycerin, Poloxamer 407, Saccharin Sodium, Sodium Gluconate, and Water.

Actions: Cēpacol/Cēpacol Mint is a soothing, pleasant tasting mouthwash/gargle. It kills germs that cause bad breath and plaque buildup when used with daily brushing and flossing.
Cēpacol/Cēpacol Mint has a low surface tension, approximately ½ that of water. This property is the basis of the spreading action in the oral cavity as well as its foaming action. Cēpacol/Cēpacol Mint leaves the mouth feeling fresh and clean and helps provide soothing, temporary relief of dryness and minor mouth irritations.

Uses: Recommended as a mouthwash and gargle for daily oral care, as an antibacterial plaque-fighter; as an aromatic mouth freshener to provide a clean feeling in the mouth; as a soothing, foaming rinse to freshen the mouth.
Used routinely before dental procedures, helps give patient confidence of not offending with mouth odor. Often employed as a foaming and refreshing rinse before, during, and after instrumentation and dental prophylaxis. Convenient as a mouth-freshening agent after taking dental impressions. Helpful in reducing the unpleasant taste and odor in the mouth following gingivectomy.
Used in hospitals as a mouthwash and gargle for daily oral care. Also used to refresh and soothe the mouth following emesis, inhalation therapy, and intubations, and for swabbing the mouths of patients incapable of personal care.

Warning: Keep out of the reach of children.

Directions for Use: Rinse vigorously before or after brushing or any time to freshen the mouth. Particularly useful after meals or before social engagements. Cēpacol/Cēpacol Mint leaves the mouth feeling refreshingly clean.
Use full strength every two or three hours as a soothing, foaming gargle, or as directed by a physician or dentist. May also be mixed with warm water.
Product label directions are as follows: Use full strength. Rinse mouth thoroughly before or after brushing or whenever desired or use as directed by a physician or dentist.

How Supplied:
Cēpacol Mouthwash: 12 oz, 18 oz, 24 oz, and 32 oz
4 oz Hospital Bedside Bottles (not for retail sale), 4 oz trial size
Cēpacol Mint Mouthwash: 12 oz, 18 oz, and 24 oz
4 oz trial size

Shown in Product Identification Section, page 410

CĒPACOL®
[sē 'pə-cŏl]
Throat Lozenges

Description: Each lozenge contains Ceepryn® (cetylpyridinium chloride) 0.07%, Benzyl Alcohol 0.3%. Also contains: FD&C Yellow No. 5 (tartrazine) as a color additive, Flavor, Glucose, and Sucrose.

Actions: Cetylpyridinium chloride (Ceepryn) is a cationic quaternary ammonium compound, which is a surface-active agent. Aqueous solutions of cetylpyridinium chloride have a surface tension lower than that of water.
Cetylpyridinium chloride in the concentration used in Cēpacol is non-irritating to tissues.

Indications: Cēpacol Lozenges stimulate salivation to help provide soothing temporary relief of dryness and minor irritations of mouth and sore throat and resulting cough.

Warnings: Severe sore throat or sore throat accompanied by high fever, headache, nausea, or vomiting, or any sore throat or mouth irritations persisting more than 2 days may be serious. Consult a physician promptly. Persons with a high fever or persistent cough should not use this preparation unless directed by a physician. Do not administer to children under 6 years of age unless directed by a physician or dentist. If sensitive to any of the ingredients, do not use. Keep this and all drugs out of the reach of children. In case of accidental overdose, seek professional assistance or contact a Poison Control Center immediately. As with any drug, if you are pregnant or nursing a baby, seek the advice of a health professional before using this product.

Dosage and Administration: Adults and children 6 years and older, dissolve 1 lozenge in the mouth every 2 hours, if needed. For children under 6 years, consult a physician or dentist.

How Supplied:
Trade Package: 18 lozenges in 2 pocket packs of 9 each.
Professional Package: 648 lozenges in 72 blisters of 9 each.
Store at room temperature, below 86°F (30°C). Protect contents from humidity.
Shown in Product Identification Section, page 410

CĒPACOL®
[sē'pə-cŏl]
Anesthetic Lozenges (Troches)

Description: Each lozenge contains Benzocaine 10 mg, Ceepryn® (cetylpyridinium chloride) 0.07%. Also contains: FD&C Blue No. 1, FD&C Yellow No. 5 (tartrazine) as a color additive, Flavors, Glucose, and Sucrose.

Actions: Cetylpyridinium chloride (Ceepryn) is a cationic quaternary ammonium compound, which is a surface-active agent. Aqueous solutions of cetylpyridinium chloride have a surface tension lower than that of water.
Cetylpyridinium chloride in the concentration used in Cēpacol is non-irritating to tissues.
Cēpacol Anesthetic Lozenges stimulate salivation to relieve dryness of the mouth and provide a mild anesthetic effect for pain relief.

Indications: *Sore Throat:* For prompt, temporary relief of pain and discomfort due to minor sore throat. For temporary relief of minor pain and discomfort associated with tonsillitis and pharyngitis. *Mouth Irritations:* For prompt, temporary relief of pain and discomfort due to minor mouth irritations. For temporary relief of discomfort associated with stomatitis. For adjunctive, temporary relief of minor pain and discomfort following periodontal procedures and minor surgery of the mouth.

Warnings: Severe sore throat or sore throat accompanied by high fever, headache, nausea, or vomiting, or any sore throat or mouth irritation persisting more than 2 days may be serious. Consult a physician promptly. Persons with a high fever or persistent cough should not use this preparation unless directed by a physician. Do not administer to children under 6 years of age unless directed by physician or dentist. If sensitive to any of the ingredients, do not use. As with any drug, if you are pregnant or nursing a baby, seek the advice of a health professional before using this product. Keep this and all drugs out of the reach of children. In case of accidental overdose, seek professional assistance or contact a Poison Control Center immediately.

Dosage and Administration: Adults and children 6 years and older, dissolve 1 lozenge in the mouth every 2 hours, if needed. For children under 6 years, consult a physician or dentist.

How Supplied:
Trade Package: 18 troches in 2 pocket packs of 9 each.
Professional Package: 324 troches in 36 blisters of 9 each.
Store at room temperature, below 86°F (30°C). Protect contents from humidity.
Shown in Product Identification Section, page 410

CĒPASTAT®
[sē'pə-stăt]
Sore Throat Lozenges

Description: Each cherry flavor lozenge contains: Phenol 14.5 mg, Menthol 2.4 mg. Also contains: Antifoam Emulsion, D&C Red No. 33, FD&C Yellow No. 6, Flavor, Gum Crystal, Mannitol, Saccharin Sodium, and Sorbitol.
Each regular flavor lozenge contains: Phenol 29 mg, Menthol 2.4 mg. Also contains: Antifoam Emulsion, Caramel, Eucalyptus Oil, Gum Crystal, Mannitol, Saccharin Sodium, and Sorbitol.

Indications:
1. Sore throat:
   For prompt temporary relief of minor sore throat or discomfort associated with pharyngitis or tonsillitis or following tonsillectomy.
2. Mouth or gum irritation:
   For prompt temporary relief of minor pain or discomfort associated with pericoronitis or periodontitis or with dental procedures such as extractions, gingivectomies, and other minor oral surgery.

Actions: Phenol is a recognized topical anesthetic. Menthol provides a cooling sensation to aid in symptomatic relief and adds to the lozenge effect in stimulating salivary flow. The sugar-free formula should not promote tooth decay as sugar-based lozenges can.

Warnings*: Do not exceed recommended dosage. If soreness is severe, persists for more than 2 days, or is accompanied by high fever, headache, nausea, or vomiting, consult your physician or dentist promptly. Do not give to children under 6 years of age unless directed by a physician or dentist. Do not use for more than 10 days at a time. As with any drug, if you are pregnant or nursing a baby, seek the advice of a health professional before using this product.
KEEP THIS AND ALL DRUGS OUT OF THE REACH OF CHILDREN.
In case of accidental overdose, seek professional assistance or contact a Poison Control Center immediately.

Note to Diabetics*: Each lozenge contains approximately 8 calories from 2 grams of sorbitol.

Dosage and Administration:
Lozenges–cherry flavor
ADULTS AND CHILDREN 12 YEARS AND OLDER: Dissolve 1 lozenge in the mouth, followed by another if needed, every 2 hours. Do not use more than 2 lozenges in 2 hours or more than 18 daily. CHILDREN 6 to UNDER 12 YEARS:

Dissolve 1 lozenge in the mouth, followed by another if needed, every 3 hours. Do not exceed 2 lozenges in 3 hours or more than 10 daily. CHILDREN UNDER 6 YEARS: Consult a physician or dentist.
Lozenges–regular flavor
ADULTS AND CHILDREN 12 YEARS AND OLDER: Dissolve 1 lozenge in the mouth every 2 hours. Do not exceed 9 lozenges per day. CHILDREN 6 TO UNDER 12 YEARS: Dissolve 1 lozenge in the mouth every 3 hours. Do not exceed 4 lozenges per day. CHILDREN UNDER 6 YEARS: Consult a physician or dentist.

How Supplied:
Lozenges–cherry flavor
Trade package: Boxes of 18 lozenges as 2 pocket packs of 9 lozenges each. Professional package: 648 lozenges in 72 blisters of 9 lozenges each.
Lozenges–regular flavor
Trade package: Boxes of 18 lozenges as 2 pocket packs of 9 lozenges each. Professional package: 648 lozenges in 72 blisters of 9 lozenges each.
Store at room temperature, below 86°F (30°C). Protect contents from humidity.
Shown in Product Identification Section, page 410

---

*This section appears on the label for the consumer.

Regular Flavor
CITRUCEL®
[sĭt'rə-sĕl]
(Methylcellulose)
Bulk-forming Fiber Laxative

Description: Each 5.50 g adult dose (approximately one level measuring tablespoonful) contains Methylcellulose 2 g. Each 2.75 g child's dose (approximately one rounded measuring teaspoonful) contains Methylcellulose 1 g. Also contains: Malic Acid, Maltodextrin, Natural Citrus Flavor, Potassium Citrate, Riboflavin, Sucrose, and Other Ingredients. Each 5.50 g dose contains approximately 3 mg of sodium, 80 mg of potassium, and contributes 12 calories (from Maltodextrin and Sucrose).

Actions: Promotes elimination by providing additional fiber (bulk) to the diet. This product generally produces bowel movement in 12 to 72 hours.

Indications: For relief of constipation (irregularity). May also be used for relief of constipation associated with other bowel disorders such as irritable bowel syndrome, diverticular disease, and hemorrhoids as well as for bowel management during postpartum, postsurgical, and convalescent periods.

Contraindications: Intestinal obstruction, fecal impaction, known hypersensitivity to formula ingredients.

Precautions: Patients should be instructed to consult their physician before using any laxative if they have noticed a sudden change in bowel habits which persists for two weeks. Unless directed by a physician, patients should be advised not to use laxative products when

Continued on next page

Lakeside—Cont.

abdominal pain, nausea, or vomiting is present. Patients should also be advised to discontinue use and consult a physician if rectal bleeding or failure to have a bowel movement occurs after use of any laxative product.

Dosage and Administration: Adults and children 12 years and older: *one level measuring* tablespoonful stirred briskly into 8 ounces of cold water or fruit juice, one to three times a day and administered promptly. Children 6 to under 12 years: *one rounded measuring* teaspoonful stirred briskly into 4 ounces of cold water or fruit juice, one to three times a day and administered promptly. Children under 6 years: use only as directed by a physician.
Continued use for two or three days may be necessary for full benefit.
Administering additional water is helpful.

How Supplied: 7 oz and 10 oz containers
Store below 86°F (30°C). Protect contents from humidity; keep tightly closed.
Shown in Product Identification Section, page 410

Orange Flavor
CITRUCEL®
[sĭt ′rə-sĕl]
(Methylcellulose)
Bulk-forming Fiber Laxative

Description: Each 19 g adult dose (approximately one heaping measuring tablespoonful) contains Methylcellulose 2 g. Each 9.5 g child's dose (approximately 1 level measuring tablespoonful) contains Methylcellulose 1 g. Also contains: Citric Acid, FD&C Yellow No. 6, Orange Flavors (Natural and Artificial), Potassium Citrate, Riboflavin, Sucrose, and Other Ingredients. Each adult dose contains approximately 3 mg of sodium, 105 mg of potassium, and contributes 60 calories from 15 g of Sucrose.

Actions: Promotes elimination by providing additional fiber (bulk) to the diet. This product generally produces bowel movement in 12 to 72 hours.

Indications: For relief of constipation (irregularity). May also be used for relief of constipation associated with other bowel disorders such as irritable bowel syndrome, diverticular disease, and hemorrhoids as well as for bowel management during postpartum, postsurgical, and convalescent periods.

Contraindications: Intestinal obstruction, fecal impaction, known hypersensitivity to formula ingredients.

Precautions: Patients should be instructed to consult their physician before using any laxative if they have noticed a sudden change in bowel habits which persists for two weeks. Unless directed by a physician, patients should be advised not to use laxative products when abdominal pain, nausea, or vomiting is present. Patients should also be advised

to discontinue use and consult a physician if rectal bleeding or failure to have a bowel movement occurs after use of any laxative product.

Dosage and Administration: Adults and children 12 years and older: *one heaping measuring* tablespoonful stirred briskly into 8 ounces of cold water, one to three times a day and administered promptly. Children 6 to under 12 years: *one level measuring* tablespoonful stirred briskly into 4 ounces of cold water, one to three times a day and administered promptly. Children under 6 years: use only as directed by a physician.
Continued use for two or three days may be necessary for full benefit.
Administering additional water is helpful.

How Supplied: 16 oz and 30 oz containers
Store below 86°F (30°C). Protect contents from humidity; keep tightly closed.
Shown in Product Identification Section, page 410

NOVAHISTINE® DMX
[nō ″vă-hĭs ′tēn]
Cough/Cold Formula & Decongestant

Description: Each 5 ml teaspoonful of NOVAHISTINE DMX contains: Dextromethorphan Hydrobromide 10 mg, Guaifenesin 100 mg, Pseudoephedrine Hydrochloride 30 mg. Also contains: Alcohol 10%, FD&C Red No. 40, FD&C Yellow No. 6, Flavors, Glycerin, Hydrochloric Acid, Invert Sugar, Saccharin Sodium, Sodium Chloride, Sorbitol, and Water. Dextromethorphan hydrobromide, a synthetic non-narcotic antitussive, is the dextrorotatory isomer of 3-methoxy-N-methylmorphinan. Guaifenesin is the glyceryl ether of guaiacol. Pseudoephedrine hydrochloride is the salt of a pharmacologically active stereoisomer of ephedrine (1-phenyl-2-methylamino-1-propanol).

Actions: Dextromethorphan hydrobromide suppresses the cough reflex by a direct effect on the cough center in the medulla of the brain. Although it is chemically related to morphine, it produces no analgesia or addiction. Its antitussive activity is about equal to that of codeine.
Pseudoephedrine hydrochloride is an orally effective nasal decongestant. It is a sympathomimetic amine with peripheral effects similar to epinephrine and central effects similar to, but less intense than, amphetamines. Therefore, it has the potential for excitatory side effects. Pseudoephedrine hydrochloride at the recommended oral dosage has little or no pressor effect in normotensive adults. Patients taking pseudoephedrine orally have not been reported to experience the rebound congestion sometimes experienced with frequent, repeated use of topical decongestants. Pseudoephedrine is not known to produce drowsiness.
Guaifenesin acts as an expectorant by increasing respiratory tract fluid which

reduces the viscosity of tenacious secretions, thus making expectoration easier.

Indications: NOVAHISTINE DMX is indicated when exhausting, nonproductive cough accompanies respiratory tract congestion. It is useful in the symptomatic relief of upper respiratory congestion associated with the common cold, influenza, bronchitis, and sinusitis.

Contraindications: NOVAHISTINE DMX is contraindicated in patients with severe hypertension, severe coronary artery disease, and in patients on MAO inhibitor therapy. Patient idiosyncrasy to adrenergic agents may be manifested by insomnia, dizziness, weakness, tremor, or arrhythmias.
Nursing mothers: Pseudoephedrine is contraindicated in nursing mothers because of the higher than usual risk for infants from sympathomimetic amines.
Hypersensitivity: NOVAHISTINE DMX is contraindicated in patients with hypersensitivity or idiosyncrasy to sympathomimetic amines, dextromethorphan, or to other formula ingredients.

Warnings: At dosages higher than the recommended dose, nervousness, dizziness, sleeplessness, nausea, or headache may occur. Do not take for more than 7 days. If symptoms do not improve, recur, or are accompanied by fever, rash, or persistent headache, patients should be advised to consult their physician before continuing use. Sympathomimetic amines should be used judiciously and sparingly in patients with hypertension, diabetes mellitus, ischemic heart disease, increased intraocular pressure, hyperthyroidism, or prostatic hypertrophy. Sympathomimetics may produce central nervous system stimulation with convulsions or cardiovascular collapse with accompanying hypotension. See Contraindications.
Use in elderly: The elderly (60 years and older) are more likely to have adverse reactions to sympathomimetics. Overdosage of sympathomimetics in this age group may cause hallucinations, convulsions, CNS depression, and death.
Use in children: Novahistine DMX should not be used in children under 2 years except under the advice and supervision of a physician.
Use in pregnancy: Safety for use during pregnancy has not been established. As with any drug, if you are pregnant or nursing a baby, seek the advice of a health professional before using this product.
If sensitive to any of the ingredients, do not use.
Keep this and all drugs out of the reach of children. In case of accidental overdose, seek professional assistance or contact a Poison Control Center immediately.

Precautions: Drugs containing pseudoephedrine should be used with caution in patients with diabetes, hypertension, cardiovascular disease, and hyperreac-

tivity to ephedrine. See Contraindications.

Adverse Reactions: Adverse reactions occur infrequently with usual oral doses of NOVAHISTINE DMX. When they occur, adverse reactions may include gastrointestinal upset and nausea. Because of the pseudoephedrine in NOVAHISTINE DMX, hyperreactive individuals may display ephedrine-like reactions such as tachycardia, palpitations, headache, dizziness or nausea. Sympathomimetic drugs have been associated with certain untoward reactions including fear, anxiety, tenseness, restlessness, tremor, weakness, pallor, respiratory difficulty, dysuria, insomnia, hallucinations, convulsions, CNS depression, arrhythmias, and cardiovascular collapse with hypotension.

Note: Guaifenesin interferes with the colorimetric determination of 5-hydroxyindoleacetic acid (5-HIAA) and vanillylmandelic acid (VMA).

Drug Interactions: Novahistine DMX should not be used in patients taking a prescription drug for hypertension or depression without the advice of a physician. MAO inhibitors and beta-adrenergic blockers increase the effects of pseudoephedrine (sympathomimetics). Sympathomimetics may reduce the antihypertensive effects of methyldopa, mecamylamine, reserpine, and veratrum alkaloids.

Dosage and Administration: Adults and children 12 years and older, 2 teaspoonfuls every 4 to 6 hours. Children 6 to under 12 years, 1 teaspoonful every 4 to 6 hours. Children 2 to under 6 years, ½ teaspoonful every 4 to 6 hours. Not more than 4 doses every 24 hours. For children under 2 years of age, give only as directed by a physician.

How Supplied: As a red syrup in 4 fluid ounce bottles.
Keep tightly closed. Protect from excessive heat and light. Avoid freezing.

NOVAHISTINE® Elixir
[nō"vă-hĭs'tēn]
Cold & Hay Fever Formula

Description: Each 5 ml teaspoonful of NOVAHISTINE Elixir contains: Chlorpheniramine Maleate 2 mg, Phenylephrine Hydrochloride 5 mg. Also contains: Alcohol 5%, D&C Yellow No. 10, FD&C Blue No. 1, Flavors, Glycerin, Sodium Chloride, Sorbitol, and Water. Although considered sugar-free, each 5 ml contributes approximately 7 calories from sorbitol.

Actions: Phenylephrine is a nasal decongestant. Its effects are similar to epinephrine, but it is less potent on a weight basis, and has a longer duration of action. Phenylephrine produces peripheral effects similar to epinephrine, but has little or no central nervous system stimulation. After oral administration, nasal decongestion may occur within 15 or 20 minutes and persist for 2 to 4 hours. Chlorpheniramine maleate, an antihistaminic effective for the symptomatic relief of allergic rhinitis, possesses anticholinergic and sedative effects. Chlorpheniramine antagonizes many of the pharmacologic actions of histamine. It prevents released histamine from dilating capillaries and causing edema of the respiratory mucosa.

Indications: For the temporary relief of nasal congestion and eustachian tube congestion associated with the common cold, sinusitis, and hay fever (allergic rhinitis). Also provides temporary relief of runny nose, sneezing, itching of nose or throat, and itchy, watery eyes due to the common cold, hay fever (allergic rhinitis) or other upper respiratory allergies. May be given concomitantly, when indicated, with analgesics and antibiotics.

Contraindications: NOVAHISTINE Elixir is contraindicated in patients with severe hypertension, severe coronary artery disease, and in patients on MAO inhibitor therapy. Patient idiosyncrasy to adrenergic agents may be manifested by insomnia, dizziness, weakness, tremor, or arrhythmias.
NOVAHISTINE Elixir is also contraindicated in patients with narrow-angle glaucoma, urinary retention, peptic ulcer, asthma, emphysema, chronic pulmonary disease, shortness of breath, or difficulty in breathing.
Nursing mothers: Phenylephrine is contraindicated in nursing mothers.
Hypersensitivity: NOVAHISTINE Elixir is also contraindicated in patients with hypersensitivity or idiosyncrasy to sympathomimetic amines, antihistamines or to other formula ingredients.

Warnings: At dosages higher than the recommended dose, nervousness, dizziness, sleeplessness, nausea, or headache may occur. If symptoms do not improve within 7 days or are accompanied by high fever, patients should be advised to consult their physician before continuing use. Sympathomimetic amines should be used judiciously and sparingly in patients with hypertension, diabetes mellitus, ischemic heart disease, increased intraocular pressure, hyperthyroidism, or prostatic hypertrophy. Sympathomimetics may produce central nervous system stimulation with convulsions or cardiovascular collapse with accompanying hypotension. See Contraindications.
Use in elderly: The elderly (60 years and older) are more likely to have adverse reactions to sympathomimetics. Overdosage of sympathomimetics in this age group may cause hallucinations, convulsions, CNS depression, and death.
Use in children: May cause excitability. Novahistine Elixir should not be used in children under 6 years except under the advice and supervision of a physician.
Use in pregnancy: Safety for use during pregnancy has not been established. As with any drug, if you are pregnant or nursing a baby, seek the advice of a health professional before using this product.
If sensitive to any of the ingredients, do not use.
Keep this and all drugs out of the reach of children. In case of accidental overdose, seek professional assistance or contact a Poison Control Center immediately.

Precautions: Caution should be exercised if used in patients with high blood pressure, heart disease, diabetes or thyroid disease. The antihistamine may cause drowsiness, and ambulatory patients who operate machinery or motor vehicles should be cautioned accordingly.

Adverse Reactions: Drugs containing sympathomimetic amines have been associated with certain untoward reactions, including fear, anxiety, tenseness, restlessness, tremor, weakness, pallor, respiratory difficulty, dysuria, insomnia, hallucinations, convulsions, CNS depression, arrhythmias, and cardiovascular collapse with hypotension. Individuals hyperreactive to phenylephrine may display ephedrine-like reactions such as tachycardia, palpitation, headache, dizziness, or nausea.
Phenylephrine is considered safe and relatively free of unpleasant side effects when taken at recommended dosage. Patients sensitive to antihistamine drugs may experience mild sedation. Other side effects from antihistamines may include dry mouth, dizziness, weakness, anorexia, nausea, vomiting, headache, nervousness, polyuria, heartburn, diplopia, dysuria, and, very rarely, dermatitis.

Drug Interactions: Novahistine Elixir should not be used in patients taking a prescription drug for hypertension or depression without the advice of a physician. MAO inhibitors and beta-adrenergic blockers increase the effects of sympathomimetics. Sympathomimetics may reduce the antihypertensive effects of methyldopa, mecamylamine, reserpine, and veratrum alkaloids. Antihistamines have been shown to enhance one or more of the effects of tricyclic antidepressants, barbiturates, alcohol, and other central nervous system depressants.

Dosage and Administration: Adults and children 12 years and older, 2 teaspoonfuls every 4 hours; children 6 to under 12 years, 1 teaspoonful every 4 hours; children 2 to under 6 years, ½ teaspoonful every 4 hours.
For children under 2 years, at the discretion of the physician.
Product label dosage is as follows: Adults and children 12 years and older, 2 teaspoonfuls every 4 hours. Children 6 to under 12 years, 1 teaspoonful every 4 hours. Not more than 6 doses every 24 hours. For children under 6 years, give only as directed by a physician.

How Supplied: NOVAHISTINE Elixir, as a green liquid in 4 fluid ounce bottles. Keep tightly closed. Protect from excessive heat and light. Avoid freezing.

Continued on next page

Lakeside—Cont.

SINGLET®
[sĭng-lət]
**Decongestant/Antihistamine/
Analgesic**

Description: Each pink Singlet tablet contains Pseudoephedrine Hydrochloride 60 mg, Chlorpheniramine Maleate 4 mg, and Acetaminophen 650 mg. Also contains: FD&C Red No. 3, Hydroxypropyl Cellulose, Hydroxypropyl Methylcellulose 2910, Magnesium Stearate, Microcrystalline Cellulose, Pregelatinized Corn Starch, Sodium Starch Glycolate, Talc and Titanium Dioxide. May also contain: Ethylcellulose, Glycerin, Polyethylene Glycol 8000, and Sucrose.

Indications: For the temporary relief of nasal congestion, runny nose, occasional sinus headache, fever, sneezing, watery eyes or itching of the nose, throat, and eyes due to colds, hay fever, or other upper respiratory allergies.

Warnings: Do not take this product for more than 7 days. Do not take this product for the treatment of arthritis except under the advice and supervision of a physician. Unless directed by a physician, do not take this product if you have asthma, glaucoma, emphysema, chronic pulmonary disease, heart disease, high blood pressure, thyroid disease, diabetes, shortness of breath, difficulty in breathing, difficulty in urination due to enlargement of the prostate gland, or if you are presently taking a prescription drug for high blood pressure or depression. Do not exceed recommended dosage because severe liver damage, nervousness, dizziness, or sleeplessness may occur. May cause excitability. Consult your physician if symptoms persist or if new symptoms occur. Consult your physician if fever persists for more than 3 days (72 hours) or recurs. May cause drowsiness; alcohol, sedatives, and tranquilizers may increase the drowsiness effect. Avoid alcoholic beverages while taking this product. Do not take this product if you are taking sedatives or tranquilizers without first consulting your physician. Use caution when driving a motor vehicle or operating machinery. If sensitive to any of the ingredients, do not use.
As with any drug, if you are pregnant or nursing a baby, seek the advice of a health professional before using this product. KEEP THIS AND ALL DRUGS OUT OF THE REACH OF CHILDREN. In case of accidental overdose, seek professional assistance or contact a Poison Control Center immediately.

Dosage and Administration: Adults and children 12 years and older: one tablet 3 to 4 times a day, taken with water, while symptoms persist. Do not take more than 1 tablet within a 4 hour period. Do not exceed 4 tablets in 24 hours. Children under 12 years of age: consult a physician.

Storage: Protect from excessive heat and moisture.

How Supplied: Bottles of 100.

Lavoptik Company, Inc.
**661 WESTERN AVENUE N.
ST. PAUL, MN 55103**

LAVOPTIK® Eye Wash

Description: Isotonic LAVOPTIK Eye Wash is a buffered solution designed to help physically remove contaminants from the surface of the eye and lids. Formulated to buffer contaminants toward the safe range and help restore normal salts and water ratios in the tears.

Contents: Each 100 ml

Sodium Chloride	0.49 grams
Sodium Biphosphate	0.40 grams
Sodium Phosphate	0.45 grams
Preservative Agent	
Benzalkonium Chloride	0.005 grams

Precautions: If you experience severe eye pain, headache, rapid change in vision (side or straight ahead); sudden appearance of floating objects, acute redness of the eyes, pain on exposure to light or double vision consult a physician at once. If symptoms persist or worsen after use of this product, consult a physician. If solution changes color or becomes cloudy do not use. Keep this and all medicines out of reach of children. Keep container tightly closed. Do not use if safety seal is broken at time of purchase.

Administration: 6 ounce size with Eye Cup.
Rinse cup with clean water immediately before and after each use, avoid contamination of rim and inside surfaces of cup. Apply cup, half-filled with LAVOPTIK Eye Wash tightly to the eye. Tilt head backward. Open eyelids wide, rotate eyeball and blink several times to insure thorough washing. Discard washings. Repeat other eye. Tightly cap bottle. 32 ounce size.
Break seal as you remove cap and pour directly on contaminated area.

How Supplied: 6 ounce bottle with eyecup, NDC 10651-01040.
32 ounce bottle, NDC 10651-01019.

IDENTIFICATION PROBLEM?
Consult the
Product Identification Section
where you'll find
products pictured
in full color.

Lederle Laboratories
**A Division of American
Cyanamid Co.
ONE CYANAMID PLAZA
WAYNE, NJ 07470**

LEDERMARK®
Product Identification Code

Many Lederle tablets and capsules bear an identification code. A current listing appears in the Product Information Section of the 1988 PDR for Prescription Drugs.

CALTRATE®, JR.
[căl-trāte]
**Calcium Supplement For Children
Chewable Orange Flavored**

- Nature's most concentrated form of calcium
- Made with pure calcium carbonate
- No lactose, no salt, no starch

ONE TABLET DAILY CONTAINS:

	Children 4+ % U.S. RDA
750 mg Calcium Carbonate which provides 300 mg elemental calcium	30%
60 I.U. Vitamin D	15%

Inactive Ingredients: Dextrose, dl-Alpha Tocopheryl, FD&C Yellow No. 6*, Gelatin, Magnesium Stearate, Malto Dextrin, Mannitol, Orange Flavor, Silica Gel, Sorbitol, Stearic Acid, Sucrose and other ingredients.
*FD&C Yellow No. 6 (Sunset Yellow) as a color additive.
- Great orange taste. Nonchalky.
- Plus Vitamin D to help absorb calcium.
- Children 4–10 years old need 1000 mg of calcium (U.S. RDA) everyday to help keep teeth and bones strong.

Recommended Intake: One or two tablets daily or as directed by a physician.
Keep out of the reach of children.

How Supplied: Bottles of 60—NDC 0005-5516-19
Store at Room Temperature.   D1
*Shown in Product Identification
Section, page 411*

CALTRATE® 600
[căl-trāte]
**Smaller Tablet
High Potency Calcium Supplement
Nature's Most Concentrated Form of
Calcium®
No Sugar, No Salt, No Lactose, No
Cholesterol, No Preservatives,
Film-Coated for easy swallowing**

Inactive Ingredients: Croscarmellose Sodium, Hydroxypropyl Methylcellulose, Magnesium Stearate, Microcrystalline Cellulose, PVPP, Sodium Lauryl Sulfate, Titanium Dioxide, and other ingredients.

TWO TABLETS DAILY PROVIDE: 3000

mg CALCIUM CARBONATE which provides 1200 mg elemental calcium

For Adults—
Percentage of U.S.
Recommended Daily
Allowance (U.S. RDA)

120%

Recommended Intake: One or two tablets daily or as directed by the physician.

Warnings: Keep this and all medications out of the reach of children.

How Supplied: Bottles of 60—NDC 0005-5510-19

Store at Room Temperature.   D10

Shown in Product Identification Section, page 411

CALTRATE® 600+Iron & Vitamin D

[căl-trāte]

High Potency Calcium Supplement Nature's Most Concentrated Form of Calcium®

No Sugar, No Salt, No Lactose, No Cholesterol, Film-Coated for Easy Swallowing

ONE TABLET DAILY CONTAINS:

Adults—
% U.S. RDA

1500 mg Calcium Carbonate which provides 600 mg elemental calcium.	60%
18 mg elemental Iron in the Exclusive Optisorb® Time-Release System. (as ferrous fumarate)	100%
125 I.U. Vitamin D	31%

Inactive Ingredients: Diethyl Phthalate, Ethylcellulose, Hydroxypropyl Cellulose, Magnesium Stearate, Microcrystalline Cellulose, Pharmaceutical Glaze, Povidone, Red 40, Silica Gel, Sodium Lauryl Sulfate, Sodium Starch Glycolate, Stearic Acid, Talc, Titanium Dioxide and other ingredients.

- CALTRATE + Iron contains pure calcium and time-release iron for diets deficient in both minerals.
- Plus Vitamin D to help absorb calcium.

Recommended Intake: One or two tablets daily or as directed by the physician.

Keep out of the reach of children.

How Supplied: Bottles of 60—NDC 0005-5523-19

Store at Room Temperature.   D5

Shown in Product Identification Section, page 411

CALTRATE® 600 + Vitamin D

[căl-trāte]

Smaller Tablet
High Potency Calcium Supplement Nature's Most Concentrated Form of Calcium®

No Sugar, No Salt, No Lactose, No Cholesterol, Film-Coated for easy swallowing

Inactive Ingredients: Colloidal Silicon Dioxide, Diethyl Phthalate, Ethylcellulose, Hydroxypropyl Methylcellulose, Magnesium Stearate, Microcrystalline Cellulose, Pharmaceutical Glaze, Povidone, Sodium Lauryl Sulfate, Sodium Starch Glycolate, Stearic Acid, Talc, Titanium Dioxide.

TWO TABLETS DAILY PROVIDE:

Adults—
% U.S. RDA

3000 mg Calcium Carbonate which provides 1200 mg elemental calcium	120%
Vitamin D 250 I.U.	62%

Recommended Intake: Minimum dosage one tablet daily; two or more if directed by the physician.

Keep out of the reach of children.

How Supplied: Bottles of 60—
NDC-0005-5509-19   D6

Store at Room Temperature.

Shown in Product Identification Section, page 411

CENTRUM®

[sĕn-trŭm]

High Potency Multivitamin/Multimineral Formula, Advanced Formula From A to Zinc®

Each tablet contains:

For Adults
Percentage of U.S.
Recommended Daily
Allowance (U.S. RDA)

Vitamin A	5000 I.U.	(100%)
(as Acetate and Beta Carotene)		
Vitamin E	30 I.U.	(100%)
(as dl-Alpha Tocopheryl Acetate)		
Vitamin C	60 mg	(100%)
(as Ascorbic Acid)		
Folic Acid	400 mcg	(100%)
Vitamin B$_1$	1.5 mg	(100%)
(as Thiamine Mononitrate)		
Vitamin B$_2$	1.7 mg	(100%)
(as Riboflavin)		
Niacinamide	20 mg	(100%)
Vitamin B$_6$	2 mg	(100%)
(as Pyridoxine Hydrochloride)		
Vitamin B$_{12}$	6 mcg	(100%)
(as Cyanocobalamin)		
Vitamin D	400 I.U.	(100%)
Biotin	30 mcg	(10%)
Pantothenic Acid	10 mg	(100%)
(as Calcium Pantothenate)		
Calcium	162 mg	(16%)
(as Dibasic Calcium Phosphate)		
Phosphorus	125 mg	(13%)
(as Dibasic Calcium Phosphate)		
Iodine	150 mcg	(100%)
(as Potassium Iodide)		
Iron	18 mg	(100%)
(as Ferrous Fumarate)		
Magnesium	100 mg	(25%)
(as Magnesium Oxide)		
Copper	2 mg	(100%)
(as Cupric Oxide)		
Zinc	15 mg	(100%)
(as Zinc Oxide)		
Manganese	2.5 mg*	
(as Manganese Sulfate)		
Potassium	40 mg*	
(as Potassium Chloride)		
Chloride	36.3 mg*	
(as Potassium Chloride)		
Chromium	25 mcg*	
(as Chromium Chloride)		
Molybdenum	25 mcg*	
(as Sodium Molybdate)		
Selenium	25 mcg*	
(as Sodium Selenate)		
Vitamin K$_1$	25 mcg*	
(as Phytonadione)		
Nickel	5 mcg*	
(as Nickelous Sulfate)		
Tin	10 mcg*	
(as Stannous Chloride)		
Silicon	10 mcg*	
(as Sodium Metasilicate)		
Vanadium	10 mcg*	
(as Sodium Metavanadate)		

*No U.S. RDA established.

Inactive Ingredients: Acacia Gum, Dextrose, Hydroxypropyl Methylcellulose, Lactose, Magnesium Stearate, Microcrystalline Cellulose, Methylparaben, Modified Food Starch, Mono- and Diglycerides, Potassium Sorbate, Propylparaben, PVPP, Silica Gel, Sodium Aluminum Silicate, Sodium Benzoate, Sorbic Acid, Stearic Acid, Sucrose, and Yellow 6.

Recommended Intake: Adults, 1 tablet daily.

How Supplied:
Light peach, engraved CENTRUM C1.
Bottle of 60—NDC 0005-4239-19
Combopack*—NDC 0005-4239-30
*Bottles of 100 plus 30
Store at Room Temperature.   D27

Shown in Product Identification Section, page 411

CENTRUM, JR.®

[sĕn-trŭm]

Children's Chewable Vitamin/Mineral Formula+Extra C Tablets

[See table on next page].

Inactive Ingredients: Acacia, Artificial Flavorings, Blue 1, Blue 2, Colloidal Silicon Dioxide, Dextrins, Dextrose, Gelatin, Hydrogenated Vegetable Oil, Hydrolyzed Protein, Lactose, Magnesium Stearate, Methylparaben, Microcrystalline Cellulose, Modified Food Starch, Mono- and Di-glycerides, Potassium Sorbate, Povidone, Propylparaben, Red 40, Sodium Benzoate, Sorbic Acid, Stearic Acid, Sucrose, Yellow 6.

Warnings: CONTAINS IRON, WHICH CAN BE HARMFUL IN LARGE DOSES. CLOSE TIGHTLY AND KEEP OUT OF THE REACH OF CHILDREN. IN CASE OF ACCIDENTAL OVERDOSE, CONTACT A PHYSICIAN OR POISON CONTROL CENTER IMMEDIATELY.

How Supplied: Bottles of 60—
NDC 0005-4249-19   D6
Store at Room Temperature.

Shown in Product Identification Section, page 411

Continued on next page

Lederle—Cont.

CENTRUM, JR.®
[sĕn-trŭm]
**Children's Chewable
Vitamin/Mineral Formula+Extra
Calcium**

[See table on next page].

Inactive Ingredients:
Acacia, Artificial Flavorings, BHA, BHT, Dextrins, Dextrose, Gelatin, Hydrogenated Vegetable Oil, Hydrolyzed Protein, Lactose, Magnesium Stearate, Methylparaben, Microcrystalline Cellulose, Modified Food Starch, Mono- and Di-glycerides, Potassium Sorbate, Propylparaben, Red 40, Silica Gel, Sodium Benzoate, Sodium Starch Glycolate, Sorbic Acid, Stearic Acid, Sucrose.

Warnings: CONTAINS IRON, WHICH CAN BE HARMFUL IN LARGE DOSES. CLOSE TIGHTLY AND KEEP OUT OF THE REACH OF CHILDREN. IN CASE OF ACCIDENTAL OVERDOSE, CONTACT A PHYSICIAN OR POISON CONTROL CENTER IMMEDIATELY.

Recommended Intake: 2 to 4 years of age: chew one-half tablet daily. Over 4 years of age: chew one tablet daily.

How Supplied: Bottles of 60—NDC 0005-4222-19, engraved: C60.   D2
Store at Room Temperature.
*Shown in Product Identification
Section, page 411*

CENTRUM, JR.®
[sĕn-trŭm]
**Children's Chewable
Vitamin/Mineral Formula + Iron
Tablets**

[See table on page 570]

Inactive Ingredients: Acacia, Artificial Flavorings, Blue 1, Blue 2, Colloidal Silicon Dioxide, Dextrins, Dextrose, Gelatin, Hydrogenated Vegetable Oil, Hydrolyzed Protein, Lactose, Magnesium Stearate, Methylparaben, Microcrystalline Cellulose, Modified Food Starch, Mono- and Di-glycerides, Potassium Sorbate, Propylparaben, Red 40, Sodium Benzoate, Sodium Starch Glycolate, Sorbic Acid, Stearic Acid, Sucrose, Yellow 6.

Recommended Intake: 2 to 4 years of age: Chew one-half tablet daily. Over 4 years of age: Chew one tablet daily.

Warnings: CONTAINS IRON, WHICH CAN BE HARMFUL IN LARGE DOSES. CLOSE TIGHTLY AND KEEP OUT OF THE REACH OF CHILDREN. IN CASE OF ACCIDENTAL OVERDOSE, CONTACT A PHYSICIAN OR POISON CONTROL CENTER IMMEDIATELY.

How Supplied: Assorted Flavors— Uncoated Tablet—Partially Scored —Engraved Lederle C2 and CENTRUM, JR. Bottles of 60 NDC 0005-4234-19 Store at room temperature.   D8
*Shown in Product Identification
Section, page 411*

**Dual Action
FERRO–SEQUELS®**
[fĕrrō-sēēquals]
**High Potency Iron Supplement
Time-Release Iron Plus
Clinically Proven Anticonstipant
Easy-to-Swallow Tablets
Low Sodium, No Sugar, No Lactose**

Active Ingredients: Each tablet contains 150 mg of ferrous fumarate equivalent to 50 mg of elemental iron and 100 mg of docusate sodium (DSS).

Inactive Ingredients: Blue 1, Colloidal Silicon Dioxide, Corn Starch, Diethyl Phthalate, Ethylcellulose, Hydroxypropyl Cellulose, Magnesium Stearate, Microcrystalline Cellulose, Pharmaceutical Glaze, Povidone, Sodium Benzoate, Talc, Titanium Dioxide, Yellow 10 and other ingredients.

Warning: As with any drug, if you are pregnant or nursing a baby, seek the advice of a health professional before using this product. Keep this and all medications out of the reach of children. In case of accidental overdose, seek professional assistance or contact a Poison Control Center immediately.

Recommended Intake: One tablet, once or twice daily or as prescribed by a physician.

How Supplied: Boxes of 30—NDC 0005-5267-68
Bottle of 30—NDC 0005-5267-13
Bottle of 100—NDC 0005-5267-23
Green, Capsule-shaped, film coated tablets
Engraved LL and F2   D2
Store at Room Temperature.
*Shown in Product Identification
Section, page 411*

FIBERCON®
[fī-bĕr-cŏn]
**Calcium Polycarbophil
Bulk-Forming Fiber Laxative
Concentrated Fiber In A Tablet**

Safe and effective, Less than one calorie per tablet, Sodium free, No preservatives, Film coated for easy swallowing, Calcium rich, No chemical stimulants.

Active Ingredient: Each tablet contains 625 mg calcium polycarbophil equivalent to 500 mg polycarbophil.

Inactive Ingredients: Magnesium Stearate, Microcrystalline Cellulose, Silica Gel, Stearic Acid and other ingredients.

Indications: Relief of constipation (irregularity).

Actions: Increases bulk volume and water content of the stool.

Warnings: If you have noticed a sudden change in bowel habits that persists over a period of 2 weeks, consult a physician before using a laxative. If the recommended use of this product for 1 week has no effect, discontinue use and consult a physician.
Do not use laxative products when abdominal pain, nausea or vomiting is present except under the direction of a phy-

---

CENTRUM, JR.®
**Children's Chewable
Vitamin/Mineral Formula+Extra C**

EACH TABLET CONTAINS: VITAMINS	Quantity per tablet	Percentage of U.S. Recommended Daily Allowance (U.S. RDA) For Children 2 to 4 (½ tablet)	For Children Over 4 (1 tablet)
Vitamin A (as Acetate)	5,000 I.U.	(100%)	(100%)
Vitamin D	400 I.U.	(50%)	(100%)
Vitamin E (as Acetate)	30 I.U.	(150%)	(100%)
Vitamin C (as Ascorbic Acid and Sodium Ascorbate)	300 mg	(375%)	(500%)
Folic Acid	400 mcg	(100%)	(100%)
Biotin	45 mcg	(15%)	(15%)
Thiamine (as Thiamine Mononitrate)	1.5 mg	(107%)	(100%)
Pantothenic Acid (as Calcium Pantothenate)	10 mg	(100%)	(100%)
Riboflavin	1.7 mg	(107%)	(100%)
Niacinamide	20 mg	(111%)	(100%)
Vitamin B$_6$ (as Pyridoxine Hydrochloride)	2 mg	(143%)	(100%)
Vitamin B$_{12}$ (as Cyanocobalamin)	6 mcg	(100%)	(100%)
Vitamin K$_1$ (as Phytonadione)	10 mcg*		
MINERALS			
Iron (as Ferrous Fumarate)	18 mg	(90%)	(100%)
Magnesium (as Magnesium Oxide)	40 mg	(10%)	(10%)
Iodine (as Potassium Iodide)	150 mcg	(107%)	(100%)
Copper (as Cupric Oxide)	2 mg	(100%)	(100%)
Phosphorous (as Tribasic Calcium Phosphate)	50 mg	(3.12%)	(5.0%)
Calcium (as Tribasic Calcium Phosphate)	108 mg	(6.75%)	(10.8%)
Zinc (as Zinc Oxide)	15 mg	(93%)	(100%)
Manganese (as Manganese Sulfate)	1 mg*		
Molybdenum (as Sodium Molybdate)	20 mcg*		
Chromium (as Chromium Chloride)	20 mcg*		

*Recognized as essential in human nutrition but no U.S. RDA established.

CENTRUM, JR.®
Children's Chewable
Vitamin/Mineral Formula + Extra Calcium

EACH TABLET CONTAINS: VITAMINS	Quantity per tablet	Percentage of U.S. Recommended Daily Allowance (U.S. RDA)	
		For Children 2 to 4 (½ tablet)	For Children Over 4 (1 tablet)
Vitamin A (as Acetate)	5,000 I.U.	(100%)	(100%)
Vitamin D	400 I.U.	(50%)	(100%)
Vitamin E (as Acetate)	30 I.U.	(150%)	(100%)
Vitamin C (as Ascorbic Acid)	60 mg	(75%)	(100%)
Folic Acid	400 mcg	(100%)	(100%)
Biotin	45 mcg	(15%)	(15%)
Thiamine (as Thiamine Mononitrate)	1.5 mg	(107%)	(100%)
Pantothenic Acid (as Calcium Pantothenate)	10 mg	(100%)	(100%)
Riboflavin	1.7 mg	(107%)	(100%)
Niacinamide	20 mg	(111%)	(100%)
Vitamin B_6 (as Pyridoxine Hydrochloride)	2 mg	(143%)	(100%)
Vitamin B_{12} (as Cyanocobalamin)	6 mcg	(100%)	(100%)
Vitamin K_1 (as Phytonadione)	10 mcg*		
MINERALS			
Iron (as Ferrous Fumarate)	18 mg	(90%)	(100%)
Magnesium (as Magnesium Oxide)	40 mg	(10%)	(10%)
Iodine (as Potassium Iodide)	150 mcg	(107%)	(100%)
Copper (as Cupric Oxide)	2 mg	(100%)	(100%)
Phosphorus (as Dibasic Calcium Phosphate)	50 mg	(6.25%)	(5.0%)
Calcium (as Dibasic Calcium Phosphate and Calcium Carbonate)	160 mg	(20%)	(16%)
Zinc (as Zinc Oxide)	15 mg	(93%)	(100%)
Manganese (as Manganese Sulfate)	1 mg*		
Molybdenum (as Sodium Molybdate)	20 mcg*		
Chromium (as Chromium Chloride)	20 mcg*		

*Recognized as essential in human nutrition but no U.S. RDA established.

sician. Discontinue use and consult a physician if rectal bleeding occurs after use of any laxative product.

Interaction Precaution: Contains calcium. Take this product at least one hour before or two hours after taking an oral dose of a prescription antibiotic containing any form of tetracycline.
KEEP THIS AND ALL MEDICINES OUT OF THE REACH OF CHILDREN. STORE AT CONTROLLED ROOM TEMPERATURE 15–30°C (59–86°F). PROTECT CONTENTS FROM MOISTURE.

Recommended Intake: Adults and children 12 years and older: swallow 2 tablets one to four times a day. Children 6 to 12 years: swallow 1 tablet one to three times a day. Children under 6 years: consult a physician. See package insert for additional information.
A FULL GLASS (8 fl. oz.) OF LIQUID SHOULD BE TAKEN WITH EACH DOSE.

How Supplied: Engraved LL and F66 (60 tabs) NDC 0005-2500-86, engraved: F66
(36 tabs) NDC 0005-2500-02   D3
(90 tabs) NDC 0005-2500-33
Shown in Product Identification Section, page 411

FILIBON®
[fĭ-lĭ-bōn]
prenatal tablets

Each tablet contains:

	For Pregnant or Lactating Women Percentage of U.S. Recommended Daily Allowance (U.S. RDA)
Vitamin A (as Acetate)	5000 I.U. (63%)
Vitamin D_2	400 I.U. (100%)
Vitamin E (as dl-Alpha Tocopheryl Acetate)	30 I.U. (100%)
Vitamin C (Ascorbic Acid)	60 mg (100%)
Folic Acid	0.4 mg (50%)
Vitamin B_1 (as Thiamine Mononitrate)	1.5 mg (88%)
Vitamin B_2 (as Riboflavin)	1.7 mg (85%)
Niacinamide	20 mg (100%)
Vitamin B_6 (as Pyridoxine Hydrochloride)	2 mg (80%)
Vitamin B_{12} (as Cyanocobalamin)	6 mcg (75%)
Calcium (as Calcium Carbonate)	125 mg (10%)
Iodine (as Potassium Iodide)	150 mcg (100%)
Iron (as Ferrous Fumarate)	18 mg (100%)
Magnesium (as Magnesium Oxide)	100 mg (22%)

Inactive Ingredients: BHA, BHT, Dextrose, Ethylcellulose, Gelatin, Hydrolyzed Protein, Hydroxypropyl Methylcellulose, Lactose, Magnesium Stearate, Methylparaben, Modified Food Starch, Mono- and Di-glycerides, Polacrilin, Polysorbate 60, Povidone, Propylparaben, Red 40, Silica Gel, Sodium Benzoate, Sodium Bisulfite, Sodium Lauryl Sulfate, Sorbic Acid, Stearic Acid, Sucrose, Titanium Dioxide, Tricalcium Phosphate, and other ingredients.

Recommended Intake: 1 daily, or as prescribed by the physician.

How Supplied: Capsule-shaped tablets (film-coated, pink) engraved LL F4—bottles of 100 NDC-0005-4294-23 Store at Room Temperature.   D10

GEVRABON®
[jĕv-ra băn]
vitamin-mineral supplement

Composition: Each fluid ounce (30 ml.) contains:

	For Adults Percentage of U.S. Recommended Daily Allowance (U.S. RDA)
Vitamin B_1 (as Thiamine Hydrochloride)	5 mg (333%)
Vitamin B_2 (as Riboflavin-5-Phosphate Sodium)	2.5 mg (147%)
Niacinamide	50 mg (250%)
Vitamin B_6 (Pyridoxine Hydrochloride)	1 mg (50%)
Vitamin B_{12} (as Cyanocobalamin)	1 mcg (17%)
Pantothenic Acid (as D-Pantothenyl Alcohol)	10 mg (100%)
Iodine (as Potassium Iodide)	100 mcg (67%)
Iron (as Ferrous Gluconate)	15 mg (83%)
Magnesium (as Magnesium Chloride)	2 mg (0.5%)
Zinc (as Zinc Chloride)	2 mg (13%)
Choline (as Tricholine Citrate)	100 mg.*
Manganese (as Manganese Chloride)	2 mg.*

*Recognized as essential in human nutrition but no U.S. RDA established.

| Alcohol | 18% |

Inactive Ingredients: Alcohol, citric acid, glycerin, sherry wine, sucrose.

Indications: For use as a nutritional supplement. Shake well.

Warning: As with any drug, if you are pregnant or nursing a baby, seek the ad-

Continued on next page

Lederle—Cont.

vice of a health professional before using this product. Keep this preparation out of the reach of children.

Administration and Dosage: Adult: One ounce (30 ml) daily or as prescribed by the physician as a nutritional supplement.

Important Note: In time a slight natural deposit, characteristic of the sherry wine base, may occur. This does not indicate in any way a loss of quality.

How Supplied: Syrup (sherry flavor) decanters of 16 fl. oz. NDC 0005-5250-35
Keep Out of Direct Sunlight
Store at Room Temperature, 15°–30°C (59°–86°F).
DO NOT FREEZE   D4

GEVRAL®
[jĕv-ral]
Multivitamin and Multimineral Supplement
TABLETS

Composition: Each tablet contains:
For Adults
Percentage of U.S.
Recommended Daily
Allowance (U.S. RDA)

Vitamin A (as Acetate)	5000 I.U. (100%)
Vitamin E (as dl-Alpha Tocopheryl Acetate)	30 I.U. (100%)
Vitamin C (as Ascorbic Acid)	60 mg (100%)
Folic Acid	0.4 mg (100%)
Vitamin B₁ (as Thiamine Mononitrate)	1.5 mg (100%)
Vitamin B₂ (as Riboflavin)	1.7 mg (100%)

Niacinaminde	20 mg (100%)
Vitamin B₆ (as Pyridoxine Hydrochloride)	2 mg (100%)
Vitamin B₁₂ (as Cyanocobalamin)	6 mcg (100%)
Calcium (as Dibasic Calcium Phosphate)	162 mg (16%)
Phosphorus (as Dibasic Calcium Phosphate)	125 mg (13%)
Iodine (as Potassium Iodide)	150 mcg (100%)
Iron (as Ferrous Fumarate)	18 mg (100%)
Magnesium (as Magnesium Oxide)	100 mg (25%)

Inactive Ingredients: Blue 2, Ethylcellulose, FD&C Yellow No. 6,* Gelatin, Hydrolyzed Protein, Hydroxypropyl Methylcellulose, Lactose, Magnesium Stearate, Methylparaben, Microcrystalline Cellulose, Modified Food Starch, Mono- and Di-glycerides, Polacrilin, Potassium Sorbate, Propylparaben, PVPP, Red 30, Silica Gel, Sodium Benzoate, Sorbic Acid, Stearic Acid, Sucrose, Titanium Dioxide, and other ingredients.
*Contains FD&C Yellow No. 6 (Sunset Yellow) as a color additive.

Indications: Supplementation of the diet.

Administration and Dosage: One tablet daily or as prescribed by the physician.
Keep this and all medications out of the reach of children.

How Supplied: Capsule-shaped tablets (film-coated, brown) engraved LL G1—bottles of 100 NDC 0005-4289-23
Store at Room Temperature.
A SPECTRUM® Product   D14

GEVRAL® T
[jĕv-ral t]
High Potency
Multivitamin and Multimineral Supplement
TABLETS

Each tablet contains:
For Adults
Percentage of U.S.
Recommended Daily
Allowance (U.S. RDA)

Vitamin A (as Acetate)	5000 I.U. (100%)
Vitamin E (as dl-Alpha Tocopheryl Acetate)	45 I.U. (150%)
Vitamin C (as Ascorbic Acid)	90 mg (150%)
Folic Acid	0.4 mg (100%)
Vitamin B₁ (as Thiamine Mononitrate)	2.25 mg (150%)
Vitamin B₂ (as Riboflavin)	2.6 mg (153%)
Niacinamide	30 mg (150%)
Vitamin B₆ (as Pyridoxine Hydrochloride)	3 mg (150%)
Vitamin B₁₂ (as Cyanocobalamin)	9 mcg (150%)
Vitamin D₂	400 I.U. (100%)
Calcium (as Dibasic Calcium Phosphate)	162 mg (16%)
Phosphorus (as Dibasic Calcium Phosphate)	125 mg (13%)
Iodine (as Potassium Iodide)	225 mcg (150%)
Iron (as Ferrous Fumarate)	27 mg (150%)
Magnesium (as Magnesium Oxide)	100 mg (25%)
Copper (as Cupric Oxide)	1.5 mg (75%)
Zinc (as Zinc Oxide)	22.5 mg (150%)

Inactive Ingredients: BHA, BHT, Blue 2, Gelatin, Hydrolyzed Protein, Hy-

CENTRUM, JR.®
Children's Chewable
Vitamin/Mineral Formula + Iron

EACH TABLET CONTAINS:	Quantity per tablet	Percentage of U.S. Recommended Daily Allowance (U.S. RDA) For Children 2 to 4 (½ tablet)	For Children Over 4 (1 tablet)
VITAMINS			
Vitamin A (as Acetate)	5,000 I.U.	(100%)	(100%)
Vitamin D	400 I.U.	(50%)	(100%)
Vitamin E (as Acetate)	30 I.U.	(150%)	(100%)
Vitamin C (as Ascorbic Acid)	60 mg	(75%)	(100%)
Folic Acid	400 mcg	(100%)	(100%)
Biotin	45 mcg	(15%)	(15%)
Thiamine (as Thiamine Mononitrate)	1.5 mg	(107%)	(100%)
Pantothenic Acid (as Calcium Pantothenate)	10 mg	(100%)	(100%)
Riboflavin	1.7 mg	(107%)	(100%)
Niacinamide	20 mg	(111%)	(100%)
Vitamin B₆ (as Pyridoxine Hydrochloride)	2 mg	(143%)	(100%)
Vitamin B₁₂ (as Cyanocobalamin)	6 mcg	(100%)	(100%)
Vitamin K₁ (as Phytonadione)	10 mcg*		
MINERALS			
Iron (as Ferrous Fumarate)	18 mg	(90%)	(100%)
Magnesium (as Magnesium Oxide)	40 mg	(10%)	(10%)
Iodine (as Potassium Iodide)	150 mcg	(107%)	(100%)
Copper (as Cupric Oxide)	2 mg	(100%)	(100%)
Phosphorus (as Dibasic Calcium Phosphate)	50 mg	(3.12%)	(5.0%)
Calcium (as Dibasic Calcium Phosphate and Calcium Carbonate)	108 mg	(6.75%)	(10.8%)
Zinc (as Zinc Oxide)	15 mg	(93%)	(100%)
Manganese (as Manganese Sulfate)	1 mg*		
Molybdenum (as Sodium Molybdate)	20 mcg*		
Chromium (as Chromium Chloride)	20 mcg*		

*Recognized as essential in human nutrition but no U.S. RDA established.

droxypropyl Methylcellulose, Lactose, Magnesium Stearate, Methylparaben, Microcrystalline Cellulose, Modified Food Starch, Mono- and Di-glycerides, Polacrilin, Polysorbate 60, Potassium Sorbate, Propylparaben, PVPP, Red 40, Silica Gel, Sodium Benzoate, Sodium Lauryl Sulfate, Sorbic Acid, Stearic Acid, Sucrose, Titanium Dioxide, and other ingredients.

Indications: For the treatment of vitamin and mineral deficiencies.

Dosage: 1 tablet daily or as prescribed by physician.
Keep this and all medications out of the reach of children.
Store at Room Temperature.

How Supplied: Tablets (film coated, maroon). Printed LL G2—bottle of 100 NDC 0005-4286-23
A SPECTRUM® Product   D7

INCREMIN®
[*ĭn-cre-mĭn*]
WITH IRON SYRUP
Vitamins + Iron
DIETARY SUPPLEMENT
(Cherry Flavored)

Composition: Each teaspoonful (5 ml.) contains:
Elemental Iron
  (as Ferric Pyrophosphate)..........30 mg
L-Lysine HCl ....300 mg
Thiamine HCl (B₁)...........................10 mg
Pyridoxine HCl (B₆)...........................5 mg
Vitamin B₁₂
  (Cyanocobalamin)......................25 mcg
Sorbitol ....3.50 gm
Alcohol..0.75%

Inactive Ingredients: Alcohol, Flavorings, Red 33, Sodium Benzoate, Sorbic Acid.

Each teaspoonful (5 ml) supplies the following Minimum Daily Requirements:

	Child under 6	Child over 6	Adults
Vitamin B₁	20 MDR	13⅓ MDR	10 MDR
Iron	4 MDR	3 MDR	3 MDR

Indications: For the prevention and treatment of iron deficiency anemia in children and adults.

Warning: As with any drug, if you are pregnant or nursing a baby, seek the advice of a health professional before using this product.
Keep this and all medications out of the reach of children.

Administration and Dosage: or as prescribed by a physician.
Children: One teaspoonful (5 ml) daily for the prevention of iron deficiency anemia.
Adults: One teaspoonful (5 ml) daily for the prevention of iron deficiency anemia.

Notice: To protect from light always dispense in this container or in an amber bottle.

Store at Room Temperature.

How Supplied: Syrup (cherry flavor)—bottles of 4 fl. oz—NDC 0005-5604-58 and 16 fl. oz—NDC 0005-5604-65
                                        D10

NEOLOID®
[*nēē-o-loid*]
emulsified castor oil
Peppermint Flavored

Composition: NEOLOID Emulsified Castor Oil USP 36.4% (w/w) with 0.1% (w/w) Sodium Benzoate and 0.2% (w/w) Potassium Sorbate added as preservatives, emulsifying and flavoring agents in water. Also contains the following inactive ingredients: Citric Acid, Glyceryl Monostearate, Polysorbate 80, Propylene Glycol, Sodium Alginate, Sodium Saccharin, Stearic Acid, Tenox II. NEOLOID is an emulsion with an exceptionally bland, pleasant taste.

Indications: For the treatment of isolated bouts of constipation.
SHAKE WELL

Administration and Dosage:
Infants —½ to 1½ teaspoonfuls
Children —Adjust between infant and adult dose.
Adult —Average dose, 2 to 4 tablespoonfuls or as prescribed by a physician.

Precautions: Not to be used when abdominal pain, nausea, vomiting, or other symptoms of appendicitis are present. Frequent or continued use of this preparation may result in dependence on laxatives. Do not use during pregnancy except on a physician's advice. Keep this and all drugs out of the reach of children.

Warning: As with any drug, if you are pregnant or nursing a baby, seek the advice of a health professional before using this product. In case of accidental overdose, seek professional assistance or contact a Poison Control Center immediately.

How Supplied: Bottles of 4 fl. oz. (118 ml) (peppermint flavor)
NDC-0005-5442-58
Store at Room Temperature.
DO NOT FREEZE   D4

PERITINIC®
[*perĭ-tĭn-ĭc*]
hematinic with vitamins and fecal softener
Tablets

Each tablet contains:
Elemental Iron
  (as Ferrous Fumarate)..............100 mg
Docusate Sodium U.S.P. (DSS)
  (to counteract the
  constipating effect of iron).......100 mg
Vitamin B₁
  (as Thiamine Mononitrate).......7.5 mg
  (7½ MDR)
Vitamin B₂ (Riboflavin).................7.5 mg
  (6¼ MDR)
Vitamin B₆
  (Pyridoxine Hydrochloride).......7.5 mg
Vitamin B₁₂
  (Cyanocobalamin) ....50 mcg
Vitamin C (Ascorbic Acid)...........200 mg

(6⅔ MDR)
Niacinamide....................................30 mg
  (3 MDR)
Folic Acid ....0.05 mg
Pantothenic Acid
  (as D-Pantothenyl Alcohol)........15 mg
MDR—Adult Minimum Daily Requirement

Inactive Ingredients: Alginic Acid, Amberlite Resin, Blue 2, Ethyl Cellulose, FD&C Yellow No. 6,* Hydroxypropyl Methylcellulose, Lactose, Magnesium Stearate, Modified Food Starch, Povidone, Red 40, Silica Gel, Titanium Dioxide, and other ingredients.
*Contains FD&C Yellow No. 6 (Sunset Yellow) as a color additive.

Warning: As with any drug, if you are pregnant or nursing a baby, seek the advice of a health professional before using this product. In case of accidental overdose, seek professional assistance or contact a Poison Control Center immediately. Keep out of the reach of children.

Action and Uses: In the prevention of nutritional anemias, certain vitamin deficiencies, and iron-deficiency anemias.

Administration and Dosage:
Adults: 1 or 2 tablets daily.

How Supplied: Tablets (maroon, capsule-shaped, film coated) P8—bottles of 60 NDC 0005-5124-19   D15

STRESSTABS® 600 Advanced
Formula
[*strĕss-tăbs*]
High Potency
Stress Formula Vitamins

Each tablet contains:

	For Adults- Percentage of U.S. Recommended Daily Allowance (U.S. RDA)
Vitamin E (as *dl*-Alpha Tocopheryl Acetate) 30 I.U.	(100%)
Vitamin C (as Ascorbic Acid) ....600 mg	(1000%)
B VITAMINS	
Folic Acid ....400 mcg	(100%)
Vitamin B₁ (as Thiamine Mononitrate) ....15 mg	(1000%)
Vitamin B₂ (as Riboflavin) ....10 mg	(588%)
Niacinamide.................100 mg	(500%)
Vitamin B₆ (as Pyridoxine Hydrochloride) ....5 mg	(250%)
Vitamin B₁₂ (as Cyanocobalamin) 12 mcg	(200%)
Biotin ....45 mcg	(15%)
Pantothenic Acid (as Calcium Pantothenate USP) ... 20 mg	(200%)

Inactive Ingredients: Dextrose, Dibasic Calcium Phosphate, Hydrolyzed Protein, Hydroxypropyl Methylcellulose, Lactose, Magnesium Stearate, Microcrystalline Cellulose, Modified Food Starch, Polacrilin, Silica Gel, Sodium Benzoate, Sorbic Acid, Stearic Acid, Titanium Dioxide, Yellow 6 and other ingredients.

Continued on next page

Lederle—Cont.

Store at Room Temperature.

Recommended Intake: Adults, 1 tablet daily or as directed by the physician.

How Supplied:
Bottles of 30—NDC 0005-4124-13
Bottles of 60—NDC 0005-4124-19
Unit Dose 10 × 10's —NDC 0005-4124-60
D14

*Shown in Product Identification
Section, page 411*

STRESSTABS® 600 + IRON
Advanced Formula
[strĕss-tăbs]
High Potency
Stress Formula Vitamins

Each tablet contains:

	For Adults-Percentage of U.S. Recommended Daily Allowance (U.S. RDA)
Vitamin E (as dl-Alpha Tocopheryl Acetate) 30 I.U.	(100%)
Vitamin C (as Ascorbic Acid) ....600 mg	(1000%)
B VITAMINS	
Folic Acid .... 400 mcg	(100%)
Vitamin B$_1$ (as Thiamine Mononitrate) .... 15 mg	(1000%)
Vitamin B$_2$ (as Riboflavin) .... 10 mg	(588%)
Niacinamide ....100 mg	(500%)
Vitamin B$_6$ (as Pyridoxine Hydrochloride) .... 5 mg	(250%)
Vitamin B$_{12}$ (as Cyanocobalamin) 12 mcg	(200%)
Biotin ....45 mcg	(15%)
Pantothenic Acid (as Calcium Pantothenate USP) ... 20 mg	(200%)
Iron (as Ferrous Fumarate) .... 27 mg	(150%)

Inactive Ingredients: Dextrose, Dibasic Calcium Phosphate, Ethylcellulose, Hydrolyzed Protein, Hydroxypropyl Methylcellulose, Lactose, Magnesium Stearate, Microcrystalline Cellulose, Modified Food Starch, Polacrilin, Silica Gel, Sodium Benzoate, Sorbic Acid, Stearic Acid, Titanium Dioxide, Yellow 6 and other ingredients. May also contain Sodium Lauryl Sulfate and Red 3 or Red 40.

Recommended Intake: Adults, 1 tablet daily or as directed by physician.

How Supplied: Capsule-shaped tablets (film-coated, orange-red, scored) Engraved LL S2—
Bottles of 30—NDC 0005-4126-13
Bottles of 60—NDC 0005-4126-19
Store at Room Temperature.   D12

*Shown in Product Identification
Section, page 411*

STRESSTABS® 600 + ZINC
Advanced Formula
[strĕss-tăbs]
High Potency
Stress Formula Vitamins

Each tablet contains:

	For Adults-Percentage of U.S. Recommended Daily Allowance (U.S. RDA)
Vitamin E (as dl-Alpha Tocopheryl Acetate) 30 IU	(100%)
Vitamin C (as Ascorbic Acid) ...600 mg	(1000%)
B VITAMINS	
Folic Acid ....400 mcg	(100%)
Vitamin B$_1$ (as Thiamine Mononitrate)....15 mg	(1000%)
Vitamin B$_2$ (as Riboflavin)............10 mg	(588%)
Niacinamide.................100 mg	(500%)
Vitamin B$_6$ (as Pyridoxine Hydrochloride)......5 mg	(250%)
Vitamin B$_{12}$ (as Cyanocobalamin).................12 mcg	(200%)
Biotin..............................45 mcg	(15%)
Pantothenic Acid (as Calcium Pantothenate USP) 20 mg	(200%)
Copper (as Cupric Oxide)...........................3 mg	(150%)
Zinc (as Zinc Sulfate)23.9 mg	(159%)

Inactive Ingredients: Dextrose, Dibasic Calcium Phosphate, Hydrolyzed Protein, Hydroxypropyl Methylcellulose, Lactose, Magnesium Stearate, Microcrystalline Cellulose, Modified Food Starch, Polacrilin, Silica Gel, Sodium Benzoate, Sodium Lauryl Sulfate, Sorbic Acid, Stearic Acid, Titanium Dioxide, Yellow 6 and other ingredients.

Recommended Intake: Adults, 1 tablet daily or as directed by the physician.

How Supplied: Capsule-shaped Tablet (film coated, peach color) Engraved LL S3—
Bottles of 30—NDC 0005-4125-13
Bottles of 60—NDC 0005-4125-19
Store at Room Temperature.   D14

*Shown in Product Identification
Section, page 411*

ZINCON®
[zinc-ŏn]
Dandruff Shampoo

Contains: Pyrithione zinc (1%), water, sodium methyl cocoyl taurate, cocamide MEA, sodium chloride, magnesium aluminum silicate, sodium cocoyl isethionate, fragrance, glutaraldehyde, D&C green #5, citric acid or sodium hydroxide to adjust pH if necessary.

Indications: Relieves the itching and scalp flaking associated with dandruff. Relieves the itching, irritation, and skin flaking associated with seborrheic dermatitis of the scalp.

Directions: For best results use twice a week. Wet hair, apply to scalp and massage vigorously. Rinse and repeat. Shake Well Before Using.

Warnings: Keep this and all drugs out of the reach of children. For external use only. Avoid contact with the eyes—if this happens, rinse thoroughly with water. If condition worsens or does not improve after regular use of this product as directed, consult a doctor. Do not use on children under 2 years of age except as directed by a doctor.

How Supplied:
4 oz. Bottles—NDC 0005-5455-58
8 oz. Bottles—NDC 0005-5455-61
D4

*Shown in Product Identification
Section, page 411*

If desired, additional information on any Lederle product will be provided by contacting Lederle Professional Services Dept.

EDUCATIONAL MATERIAL

Are Our Children Getting Enough Calcium?
4-page pamphlet describing why children need to get enough calcium in their diets.
Calcium Supplements: The Differences Are Real
8-page pamphlet describing why today's women need to supplement their diet with calcium.
Fiber Action—The Secret to Healthy Regularity
8-page pamphlet describing the role of fiber in maintaining good digestive health.
Write to: Lederle Promotional Center
2200 Bradley Hill Road
Blauvelt, NY 10913

Leeming Division
Pfizer, Inc.
**100 JEFFERSON ROAD
PARSIPPANY, NJ 07054**

BEN–GAY® External Analgesic Products

Description: Ben-Gay is a combination of methyl salicylate and menthol in a suitable base for topical application. In addition to the Original Ointment (methyl salicylate, 18.3%; menthol, 16%), Ben-Gay is offered as a Greaseless/Stainless Ointment (methyl salicylate, 15%; menthol, 10%), an Extra Strength Arthritis Rub (methyl salicylate, 30%; menthol, 8%), a Lotion and a Clear Gel (both of which contain methyl salicylate, 15%; menthol, 7%) and Ben Gay Warming Ice (2.5% methol in an alcohol base gel). Ben-Gay Sports-Gel (methyl salicylate 15%; menthol 10%) and Extra Strength Ben-Gay Sports-Balm (methyl salicylate 28%; menthol 10%) are available for use before and after exercise.

Action and Uses: Methyl salicylate and menthol are external analgesics which stimulate sensory receptors of warmth and cold. This produces a counter-irritant response which alleviates the more severe pain in the joints and muscles to

provide transient, temporary symptomatic relief.

Several double blind clinical studies of Ben-Gay products have shown the effectiveness of the menthol-methyl salicylate combination in counteracting minor pain of skeletal muscle stress and arthritis.

Three studies involving a total of 102 normal subjects in which muscle soreness was experimentally induced showed statistically significant beneficial results from use of the active product vs. placebo for lowered Muscle Action Potential (spasms), greater rise in threshold of muscular pain and greater reduction in perceived muscular pain.

Six clinical studies of a total of 207 subjects suffering from minor pain and skeletal muscular spasms due to osteoarthritis and rheumatoid arthritis showed the active product to give statistically significant beneficial results vs. placebo for lowered Muscle Action Potential (spasm), greater relief of perceived pain, increased range of motion of the affected joints and increased digital dexterity.

In two studies designed to measure the effect of topically applied Ben-Gay vs. Placebo on muscular endurance, discomfort, onset of exercise pain and fatigue, and cardiovascular efficiency, 30 subjects performed a submaximal three-hour run and another 30 subjects performed a maximal treadmill run. Ben-Gay was found to significantly decrease the discomfort during the submaximal and maximal run, and increase the time before onset of fatigue during the maximal run. It did not improve cardiovascular function or affect recovery. Applied before workouts, Ben-Gay exercise rubs relax tight muscles and increase circulation to make exercising more comfortable, longer.

To help reduce muscle ache and soreness after exercise, a Ben-Gay exercise rub can be applied and allowed to work before taking a shower.

Directions: Rub generously into painful area, then massage gently until Ben-Gay disappears. Repeat as necessary.

Warning: Use only as directed. Do not use with a heating pad. Keep away from children to avoid accidental poisoning. Do not swallow. If swallowed, induce vomiting, call a physician. Keep away from eyes, mucous membrane, broken or irritated skin. If skin irritation develops, pain lasts 10 days or more, redness is present, or with arthritis-like conditions in children under 12, call a physician.

BONINE®
(meclizine hydrochloride)
Chewable Tablets

Actions: BONINE is an antihistamine which shows marked protective activity against nebulized histamine and lethal doses of intravenously injected histamine in guinea pigs. It has a marked effect in blocking the vasodepressor response to histamine, but only a slight blocking action against acetylcholine. Its activity is relatively weak in inhibiting the spasmogenic action of histamine on isolated guinea pig ileum.

Indications: BONINE is effective in the management of nausea, vomiting and dizziness associated with motion sickness.

Contraindications: Asthma, glaucoma, emphysema, chronic pulmonary disease, shortness of breath, difficulty in breathing, or difficulty in urination due to enlargement of the prostate gland unless directed by a doctor.

Warnings: May cause drowsiness; alcohol, sedatives and tranquilizers may increase the drowsiness effect. Avoid alcoholic beverages while taking this product. Do not take this product if you are taking sedatives or tranquilizers without first consulting your doctor. Do not drive or operate dangerous machinery while taking this medication.

Usage in Children: Clinical studies establishing safety and effectiveness in children have not been done; therefore, usage is not recommended in children under 12 years of age.

Usage in Pregnancy: As with any drug, if you are pregnant or nursing a baby, seek advice of a health care professional before taking this product.

Adverse Reactions: Drowsiness, dry mouth, and on rare occasions, blurred vision have been reported.

Dosage and Administration: For motion sickness 1 or 2 tablets of BONINE should be taken one hour prior to embarkation. Thereafter, the dose may be repeated every 24 hours for the duration of the journey.

How Supplied: BONINE (meclizine HCl) is available in convenient packets of 8 chewable tablets of 25 mg. meclizine HCl.

Inactive Ingredients: Cornstarch, FD&C Red #40, Lactose, Magnesium Stearate, Purified Siliceous Earth, Raspberry Flavor, Sodium Saccharin, Talc.

DESITIN® OINTMENT

Description: Desitin Ointment combines Zinc Oxide (40%) with Cod Liver Oil (high in Vitamins A & D), and Talc in a petrolatum-lanolin base suitable for topical application.

Actions and Uses: Desitin Ointment is designed to provide relief of diaper rash, superficial wounds and burns, and other minor skin irritations. It helps prevent incidence of diaper rash, protects against urine and other irritants, soothes chafed skin and promotes healing.

Relief and protection is afforded by Zinc Oxide, Cod Liver Oil, Lanolin and Petrolatum. They provide a physical barrier by forming a protective coating over skin or mucous membrane which serves to reduce further effects of irritants on the affected area and relieves burning, pain or itch produced by them. In addition to its protective properties, Zinc Oxide acts as an astringent that helps heal local irritation and inflammation by lessening the flow of mucus and other secretions. Several studies have shown the effectiveness of Desitin Ointment in the relief and prevention of diaper rash.

Two clinical studies involving 90 infants demonstrated the effectiveness of Desitin Ointment in curing diaper rash. The diaper rash area was treated with Desitin Ointment at each diaper change for a period of 24 hours, while the untreated site served as controls. A significant reduction was noted in the severity and area of diaper dermatitis on the treated area.

Ninety-seven (97) babies participated in a 12-week study to show that Desitin Ointment helps prevent diaper rash. Approximately half of the infants (49) were treated with Desitin Ointment on a regular daily basis. The other half (48) received the ointment as necessary to treat any diaper rash which occurred. The incidence as well as the severity of diaper rash was significantly less among the babies using the ointment on a regular daily basis.

In a comparative study of the efficacy of Desitin Ointment vs. a baby powder, forty-five babies were observed for a total of eight weeks. Results support the conclusion that Desitin Ointment is a better prophylactic against diaper rash than the baby powder.

In another study, Desitin was found to be dramatically more effective in reducing the severity of medically diagnosed diaper rash than a commercially available diaper rash product in which only anhydrous lanolin and petrolatum are listed as ingredients. Fifty infants participated in the study, half of whom were treated with Desitin and half with the other product. In the group (25) treated with Desitin, seventeen infants showed significant improvement within 10 hours which increased to twenty-three improved infants within 24 hours. Of the group (25) treated with the other product, only three showed improvement at ten hours with a total of four improved within twenty-four hours. These results are statistically valid to conclude that Desitin Ointment reduces severity of diaper rash within ten hours.

Several other studies show that Desitin Ointment helps relieve other skin disorders, such as contact dermatitis.

Directions: Prevention: To prevent diaper rash, apply Desitin Ointment to the diaper area—especially at bedtime when exposure to wet diapers may be prolonged.

Treatment: If diaper rash is present, or at the first sign of redness, minor skin irritation or chafing, simply apply Desitin Ointment three or four times daily as needed. In superficial noninfected surface wounds and minor burns, apply a thin layer of Desitin Ointment, using a gauze dressing, if necessary. For external use only.

Continued on next page

Leeming—Cont.

How Supplied: Desitin Ointment is available in 1 ounce (28g), 2 ounce (57g), 4 ounce (113g), 8 ounce (226g) tubes, and 1-lb. (452g) jar.

Shown in Product Identification Section, page 412

RHEABAN® Maximum Strength TABLETS
[rē'ăban]
(attapulgite)

Description: Maximum Strength Rheaban is an anti-diarrheal medication containing activated attapulgite and is offered in tablet form.
Each white Rheaban tablet contains 750 mg. of colloidal activated attapulgite. Rheaban provides the maximum level of medication when taken as directed. Rheaban contains no narcotics, opiates or other habit-forming drugs.

Actions and Uses: Rheaban is indicated for relief of diarrhea and the cramps and pains associated with it. Attapulgite, which has been activated by thermal treatment, is a highly sorptive substance which absorbs nutrients and digestive enzymes as well as noxious gases, irritants, toxins and some bacteria and viruses that are common causes of diarrhea.
In clinical studies to show the effectiveness in relieving diarrhea and its symptoms, 100 subjects suffering from acute gastroenteritis with diarrhea participated in a double-blind comparison of Rheaban to a placebo. Patients treated with the attapulgite product showed significantly improved relief of diarrhea and its symptoms vs. the placebo.

Dosage and Administration:
TABLETS
Adults—2 tablets after initial bowel movement, 2 tablets after each subsequent bowel movement.
Children 6 to 12 years—1 tablet after initial bowel movement, 1 tablet after each subsequent bowel movement.

Warnings: Do not exceed 12 tablets in 24 hours. Do not use for more than two days, or in the presence of high fever. Tablets should not be used for children under 6 years of age unless directed by physician. If diarrhea persists consult a physician.

How Supplied:
Tablets—Boxes of 12 tablets.

Inactive Ingredients: Colloidal Silicon Dioxide, Croscarmellose Sodium, Ethylcellulose, Hydroxypropyl Methylcellulose 2910, Pectin, Pharmaceutical Glaze, Sucrose, Talc, Titanium Dioxide, Zinc Stearate.

RID® Spray
Lice Control Spray

THIS PRODUCT IS NOT FOR USE ON HUMANS OR ANIMALS

Active Ingredient:
(5-Benzyl-3-Furyl) methyl 2, 2-dimethyl-3-(2-methylpropenyl) cyclopropanecarboxylate
      0.500%

Related Compounds	0.068%
Aromatic petroleum hydrocarbons	0.664%
Inert Ingredients	98.768%
	100.000%

Actions: A highly active synthetic pyrethroid for the control of lice and louse eggs on garments, bedding, furniture and other inanimate objects.

Warnings: Avoid contamination of feed and foodstuffs. Cover or remove fishbowls. HARMFUL IF SWALLOWED. This product is not for use on humans or animals. If lice infestations should occur on humans, consult either your physician or pharmacist for a product for use on humans.

Physical and Chemical Hazards: Contents under pressure. Do not use or store near heat or open flame. Do not puncture or incinerate container. Exposure to temperatures above 130° F may cause bursting.
CAUTION: Avoid spraying in eyes. Avoid breathing spray mist. Use only in well ventilated areas. Avoid contact with skin. In case of contact wash immediately with soap and water. Vacate room after treatment and ventilate before reoccupying.

Statement of Practical Treatment: If inhaled: Remove affected person to fresh air. Apply artificial respiration if indicated.
If in eyes: Flush with plenty of water. Contact physician if irritation persists.
If on skin: Wash affected areas immediately with soap and water.

Direction For Use: It is a violation of Federal law to use this product in a manner inconsistent with its labeling.
Shake well before each use. Remove protective cap. Aim spray opening away from person. Push button to spray.
To kill lice and louse eggs: Spray in an inconspicuous area to test for possible staining or discoloration. Inspect again after drying, then proceed to spray entire area to be treated.
Hold container upright with nozzle away from you. Depress valve and spray from a distance of 8 to 10 inches.
Spray each square foot for 3 seconds.
Spray only those garments, parts of bedding, including mattresses and furniture that cannot be either laundered or dry cleaned.
Allow all sprayed articles to dry thoroughly before use. Repeat treatment as necessary.
Buyer assumes all risks of use, storage or handling of this material not in strict accordance with direction given herewith.
DISPOSAL OF CONTAINER
Wrap container and dispose of in trash. Do not incinerate.

How Supplied: 5 oz. aerosol can. Also available in combination with RID® Lice Treatment Kit as the RID® Lice Elimination System.

RID®
Lice Treatment Kit

Description: Rid contains a liquid pediculicide whose active ingredients are: pyrethrins 0.3% and piperonyl butoxide, technical 3.00%, equivalent to 2.4% (butylcarbityl) (6-propylpiperonyl) ether and to 0.6% related compounds. Also contains petroleum distillate 1.20% and benzyl alcohol 2.4%. Inert ingredients 93.1%.

Actions: RID kills head lice (Pediculus humanus capitis), body lice (Pediculus humanus humanus), and pubic or crab lice (Phthirus pubis), and their eggs.
The pyrethrins act as a contact poison and affect the parasite's nervous system, resulting in paralysis and death. The efficacy of the pyrethrins is enhanced by the synergist, piperonyl butoxide. Rid rinses out completely after treatment and is not designed to leave long-acting residues.
The active ingredients in RID are poorly absorbed through the skin. Of the relatively minor amounts that are absorbed, they are rapidly metabolized to water-soluble compounds and eliminated from the body without ill effects. RID works faster than other OTC pediculicides.

Indications: RID is indicated for the treatment of infestations of head lice, body lice and pubic (crab) lice, and their eggs.

Warning: RID should be used with caution by ragweed sensitized persons.

Precautions: This product is for external use only. It is harmful if swallowed. It should not be inhaled. It should be kept out of the eyes and contact with mucous membranes should be avoided. If accidental contact with eyes occurs, flush immediately with water. In case of infection or skin irritation, discontinue use and consult a physician. Consult a physician if infestation of eyebrows or eyelashes occurs. Avoid contamination of feed or foodstuffs.

Storage and Disposal: Do not store below 32°F (0°C). Do not reuse empty container. Wrap in several layers of newspaper and discard in trash.

Dosage and Administration: (1) Shake well. Apply undiluted RID to dry hair and scalp or to any other infested area until entirely wet. Do not use on eyelashes or eyebrows. (2) Allow RID to remain on area for 10 minutes but no longer. (3) Wash thoroughly with warm water and soap or shampoo. (4) Dead lice and eggs should be removed with the special nit comb provided. (5) Repeat treatment in 7 to 10 days to kill any newly hatched lice. Do not exceed two consecutive applications within 24 hours.
Since lice infestations are spread by contact, each family member should be examined carefully. If infested, he or she should be treated promptly to avoid spread or reinfestation of previously treated individuals. Contaminated clothing and other articles, such as hats, etc. should be dry cleaned, boiled or otherwise treated until decontaminated to prevent reinfestation or spread.

How Supplied: In 2, 4 and 8 fl. oz. plastic bottles. Exclusive nit removal comb that removes all the nits and patient instruction booklet (English and Spanish) are included in each package of RID. Also available in combination with RID Lice Control Spray as the RID Lice Elimination System.

UNISOM® DUAL RELIEF™

Description: Unisom® Dual Relief™ is a pale blue, capsule-shaped, coated tablet.

Active ingredients: 650 mg. acetaminophen and 50 mg. diphenhydramine HCl per tablet.

Inactive Ingredients: Corn starch, FD&C Blue #1, FD&C Blue #2, hydroxypropyl methylcellulose, magnesium stearate, polyethylene glycol, polysorbate 80, titanium dioxide.

Indications: Unisom Dual Relief (diphenhydramine sleep aid formula) is indicated to help reduce difficulty in falling asleep while relieving accompanying minor aches and pains such as headache, muscle ache or menstrual discomfort. If there is difficulty in falling asleep, but pain is not being experienced at the same time, regular Unisom sleep aid is indicated which contains doxylamine succinate as its active ingredient.

Administration and Dosage: One tablet 30 minutes before retiring. Take once daily or as directed by a physician.

Warnings: DO NOT TAKE THIS PRODUCT IF YOU HAVE ASTHMA, GLAUCOMA OR ENLARGEMENT OF THE PROSTATE GLAND EXCEPT UNDER THE ADVICE AND SUPERVISION OF A PHYSICIAN.
Do not take this product for treatment of arthritis except under the advice and supervision of a physician. Do not exceed recommended dosage because severe liver damage may occur. If symptoms persist continuously for more than ten days, consult your physician. Insomnia may be a symptom of serious underlying medical illness. Take this product with caution if alcohol is being consumed. Do not take this product if pregnant or nursing a baby. For adults only. Do not give to children under 12 years of age. Keep this and all medications out of reach of children. IN CASE OF ACCIDENTAL OVERDOSE SEEK PROFESSIONAL ADVICE OR CONTACT A POISON CONTROL CENTER IMMEDIATELY.

Caution: This product contains an antihistamine and will cause drowsiness. It should be used only at bedtime.

Drug Interaction: Monoamine oxidase (MAO) inhibitors prolong and intensify the anticholinergic effects of antihistamines. The CNS depressant effect is heightened by alcohol and other CNS depressant drugs.

Attention: Use only if tablet blister seals are unbroken. Child resistant packaging.

How Supplied: Boxes of 8 and 16 tablets in child resistant blisters.

UNISOM® NIGHTTIME SLEEP AID
[yu 'nä-som]
(doxylamine succinate)

Description: Pale blue oval scored tablets containing 25 mg. of doxylamine succinate, 2-(α-(2-dimethylaminoethoxy)α-methylbenzyl) pyridine succinate.

Action and Uses: Doxylamine succinate is an antihistamine of the ethanolamine class, which characteristically shows a high incidence of sedation. In a comparative clinical study of over 20 antihistamines on more than 3000 subjects, doxylamine succinate 25 mg. was one of the three most sedating antihistamines, producing a significantly reduced latency to end of wakefulness and comparing favorably with established hypnotic drugs such as secobarbital and pentobarbital in sedation activity. It was chosen as the antihistamine, based on dosage, causing the earliest onset of sleep. In another clinical study, doxylamine succinate 25 mg. scored better than secobarbital 100 mg. as a nighttime hypnotic. Two additional, identical clinical studies involving a total of 121 subjects demonstrated that doxylamine succinate 25 mg. reduced the sleep latency period by a third, compared to placebo. Duration of sleep was 26.6% longer with doxylamine succinate, and the quality of sleep was rated higher with the drug than with placebo. An EEG study of 6 subjects confirmed the results of these studies. In yet another study, no statistically significant difference was found between doxylamine succinate and flurazepam in the average time required for 200 patients with mild to moderate insomnia to fall asleep over 5 nights following a nightly dose of doxylamine succinate 25 mg. or flurazepam 30 mg., nor was any statistically significant difference found in the total time the 200 patients slept. Patients on doxylamine succinate awoke an average of 1.2 times per night while those on flurazepam awoke an average of 0.9 times per night. In either case the patients awoke rested the following morning. On a rating scale of 1 to 5, doxylamine succinate was given a 3.0, flurazepam a 3.4 by patients rating the degree of restfulness provided by their medication (5 represents "very well rested"). Although statistically significant, the difference between doxylamine succinate 25 mg. and flurazepam 30 mg. in the number of awakenings and degree of restfulness are clinically insignificant.

Administration and Dosage: One tablet 30 minutes before retiring. Not for children under 12 years of age.

Side Effects: Occasional anticholinergic effects may be seen.

Precautions: Unisom® should be taken only at bedtime.

Contraindications: This product should not be taken by pregnant women, or those who are nursing a baby. This product is also contraindicated for asthma, glaucoma, enlargment of the prostate gland.

Warnings: Should be taken with caution if alcohol is being consumed. Product should not be taken if patient is concurrently on any other drug, without prior consultation with physician. Should not be taken for longer than two weeks unless approved by physician.

How Supplied: Boxes of 8, 16, 32 or 48 tablets in child resistant blisters.

Inactive Ingredients: Dibasic Calcium Phosphate, FD&C Blue #1 Aluminum Lake, Magnesium Stearate, Microcrystalline Cellulose, Sodium Starch Glycolate.

VISINE®
Tetrahydrozoline Hydrochloride
Redness Reliever Eye Drops

Description: Visine is a sterile, isotonic, buffered ophthalmic solution containing tetrahydrozoline hydrochloride 0.05%, boric acid, sodium borate, sodium chloride and water. It is preserved with benzalkonium chloride 0.01% and edetate disodium 0.1%. Visine is a decongestant ophthalmic solution designed to provide symptomatic relief of conjunctival edema and hyperemia secondary to minor irritations, due to conditions such as smoke, dust, other airborne pollutants, swimming etc. and so called non-specific or catarrhal conjunctivitis. Relief is afforded by tetrahydrozoline hydrochloride, a sympathomimetic agent, which brings about decongestion by vasoconstriction. Reddened eyes are rapidly whitened by this effective vasoconstrictor, which limits the local vascular response by constricting the small blood vessels. The onset of vasoconstriction becomes apparent within minutes.
The effectiveness of Visine in relieving conjunctival hyperemia has been demonstrated by numerous clinicals, including several double blind studies, involving more than 2,000 subjects suffering from acute or chronic hyperemia induced by a variety of conditions. Visine was found to be efficacious in providing relief from conjunctival hyperemia.

Indications: Relieves redness of the eye due to minor eye irritations.

Directions: Place 1 to 2 drops in the affected eye(s) up to four times daily.

Warning: To avoid contamination, do not touch tip of container to any surface. Replace cap after using. If you experience eye pain, changes in vision, continued redness or irritation of the eye, or if the condition worsens or persists for more than 72 hours, discontinue use and consult a doctor. If you have glaucoma, do not use this product except under the advice and supervision of a doctor. Overuse of this product may produce increased redness of the eye. If solution changes color or becomes cloudy, do not use. Remove contact lenses before using.

Continued on next page

Leeming—Cont.

How Supplied: In 0.5 fl. oz., 0.75 fl. oz., and 1.0 fl. oz. plastic dispenser bottle and 0.5 fl. oz. plastic bottle with dropper.
Shown in Product Identification Section, page 412

VISINE a.c.®
Astringent/Redness Reliever Eye Drops

Description: Visine a.c. is a sterile, isotonic, buffered ophthalmic solution containing tetrahydrozoline hydrochloride 0.05%, zinc sulfate 0.25%, boric acid, sodium chloride, sodium citrate and purified water. It is preserved with benzalkonium chloride 0.01% and edetate disodium 0.1%. Visine a.c. is an ophthalmic solution combining the effects of the vasoconstrictor tetrahydrozoline hydrochloride with the astringent effects of zinc sulfate. The vasoconstrictor provides symtomatic relief of conjunctival edema and hyperemia secondary to minor irritation due to conditions such as dust and airborne pollutants as well as so called non-specific or catarrhal conjunctivitis, while zinc sulfate provides relief from hayfever, allergies, etc. Beneficial effects include amelioration of burning, irritation, pruritis, and removal of mucous from the eye. Relief is afforded by both ingredients, tetrahydrozoline hydrochloride and zinc sulfate.
Tetrahydrozoline hydrochloride is a sympathomimetic agent, which brings about decongestion by vasoconstriction. Reddened eyes are rapidly whitened by this effective vasoconstrictor, which limits the local vascular response by constricting the small blood vessels. The onset of vasoconstriction becomes apparent within minutes. Zinc sulfate is an ocular astringent which, by precipitating protein, helps to clear mucous from the outer surface of the eye.
The effectiveness of Visine a.c. in relieving conjunctival hyperemia and associated symptoms induced by allergies has been clinically demonstrated. In one double blind study allergy sufferers experienced acute episodes of minor eye irritation. Visine a.c. produced statistically significant beneficial results versus a placebo of normal saline solution in relieving irritation of bulbar conjunctiva, irritation of palpebral conjunctiva, and mucous build-up. Treatment with Visine a.c. containing zinc sulfate also significantly improved burning and itching symptoms.

Indications: For temporary relief of discomfort and redness due to minor eye irritations.

Directions: Place 1 to 2 drops in the affected eye(s) up to 4 times daily.

Warning: To avoid contamination, do not touch tip of container to any surface. Replace cap after using. If you experience eye pain, changes in vision, continued redness or irritation of the eye, or if the condition worsens or persists for more than 72 hours, discontinue use and consult a doctor. If you have glaucoma, do not use this product except under the advice and supervision of a doctor. Overuse of this product may produce increased redness of the eye. If solution changes color or becomes cloudy, do not use. Remove contact lenses before using.

How Supplied: In 0.5 fl. oz. and 1.0 fl. oz. plastic dispenser bottle.
Shown in Product Identification Section, page 412

VISINE® EXTRA
Redness Reliever/Lubricant Eye Drops

Description: Visine Extra is a sterile, isotonic, buffered ophthalmic solution containing tetrahydrozoline hydrochloride 0.05%, polyethylene glycol 400 1.0%, boric acid, sodium borate, sodium chloride and water. It is preserved with benzalkonium chloride 0.013% and edetate disodium 0.1%.
Visine Extra is an ophthalmic solution combining the effects of the decongestant tetrahydrozoline hydrochloride with the demulcent effects of polyethylene glycol. It provides symptomatic relief of conjunctival edema and hyperemia secondary to ocular allergies, minor irritations and so called non-specific or catarrhal conjunctivitis. Tetrahydrozoline hydrochloride is a sympathomimetic agent, which brings about decongestion by vasoconstriction. Reddened eyes are rapidly whitened by this effective vasoconstrictor, which limits the local vascular response by constricting the small blood vessels. The onset of vasoconstriction becomes apparent within minutes. Additional effects include amelioration of burning, irritation, pruritus, soreness, and excessive lacrimation. Relief is afforded by polyethylene glycol.
Polyethylene glycol is an ophthalmic demulcent which has been shown to be effective for the temporary relief of discomfort of minor irritations of the eye due to exposure to wind or sun. It is effective as a protectant and lubricant against further irritation or to relieve dryness of the eye.
The effectiveness of tetrahydrozoline hydrochloride in relieving conjunctival hyperemia and associated symptoms has been demonstrated by numerous clinicals, including several double blind studies, involving more than 2000 subjects suffering from acute or chronic hyperemia induced by a variety of conditions. Visine Extra is a product that combines the redness relieving effects of a vasoconstrictor and the soothing moisturizing and protective effects of a demulcent.

Indications: Relieves redness of the eye due to minor eye irritations. For use as a protectant against further irritation or to relieve dryness.

Directions: Place 1 to 2 drops in the affected eye(s) up to 4 times daily.

Warning: To avoid contamination, do not touch tip of container to any surface. Replace cap after using. If you experience eye pain, changes in vision, continued redness or irritation of the eye, or if the condition worsens or persists for more than 72 hours, discontinue use and consult a doctor. If you have glaucoma, do not use this product except under the advice and supervision of a doctor. Overuse of this product may produce increased redness of the eye. If solution changes color or becomes cloudy, do not use. Remove contact lenses before using.

How Supplied: In 0.5 fl. oz. and 1.0 fl. oz. plastic dispenser bottle.
Shown in Product Identification Section, page 412

WART–OFF™
Liquid

Active Ingredient: Salicylic Acid, U.S.P., 17%.

Inactive Ingredients: Alcohol, 18.1%, Camphor, Castor Oil, Ether 47.7%, Lactic Acid, Pyroxylin.

Indications: Removal of Warts

Warnings: Keep this and all medications out of reach of children to avoid accidental poisoning.
Flammable—Do not use near fire or flame. For external use only. In case of accidental ingestion, contact a physician or a Poison Control Center immediately. Do not use near eyes or on mucous membranes. Diabetics or other people with impaired circulation should not use Wart-Off™. Do not use on moles, birthmarks or unusual warts with hair growing from them. If wart persists, see your physician. If pain should develop, consult your physician. **Do not apply to surrounding skin.**

Instructions For Use: Read warning and enclosed instructional brochure. Apply Wart-Off™ to warts only. Do not apply to surrounding skin. Make sure that surrounding skin is protected from accidental application. Before applying, soak affected area in hot water for several minutes. If any tissue has been loosened, remove by rubbing surface of wart gently with cleaning brush enclosed in Wart-Off™ package. Dry thoroughly. Warts are contagious, so don't share your towel. Apply once or twice daily. Using pinpoint applicator attached to cap, apply one drop at a time until entire wart is covered. Lightly cover with small adhesive bandage. Replace cap tightly to avoid evaporation. This treatment may be used daily for three to four weeks if necessary.

How Supplied: 0.5 fluid ounce bottle with special pinpoint plastic applicator, cleaning brush and instructional brochure.

Products are
indexed alphabetically
in the
PINK SECTION

Lever Brothers Company
390 PARK AVENUE
NEW YORK, NY 10022

DOVE BAR

Active Ingredients: Sodium Cocoyl Isethionate, Stearic Acid, Sodium Tallowate, Water, Sodium Isethionate, Coconut Acid, Sodium Stearate, Sodium Dodecylbenzenesulfonate, Sodium Cocoate, Fragrance, Sodium Chloride, Titanium Dioxide.

Actions and Uses: Dove is specially formulated to be predictably gentle to all kinds of skin—dry, oily, normal skin, as well as sensitive pediatric or senescent skin. Dove is not a soap but a neutral cleansing bar with a pH of 7 that leaves skin soft, moist, and healthy looking.

Directions: Instruct patients to use Dove Bar as they would any other cleansing bar or soap.

How Supplied: Original Dove 3.5 oz. and 4.75 oz. bars; Unscented Dove 4.75 oz.

Shown in Product Identification Section, page 412

EDUCATIONAL MATERIAL

The Delicate Facts About Your Baby's Skin
A 12-page booklet instructing parents about the care of a baby's skin.
A Healthier Outlook For Your Skin
A 12-page booklet on proper skin care for adults.

Loma Linda Foods Inc.
11503 PIERCE STREET
RIVERSIDE, CA 92515

SOYALAC®   K PAREVE

Description: A milk free nutritionally balanced formula for infants. Liquid products are packed in solderless cans, eliminating lead from this source. Soyalac has a high polyunsaturated to saturated fatty acid ratio together with a liberal supply of Vitamin E. When prepared as directed, one quart of Soyalac daily contains essential nutrients in balanced combination and sufficient quantities to provide adequate nutrition for infants.

Action and Uses: Soyalac provides a highly satisfactory alternative or supplement for infants when breast milk is not available or the supply is inadequate. It is especially valuable for all infants, children, and adults - who may be sensitive to dairy milk, or who prefer a vegetarian diet. It may also be prescribed successfully for use in hypocholestrogenic diets; for pre-operative and post-operative diets; for fortifying any milk free diet; for geriatric cases, etc.

Preparation: Standard dilution is—
Ready to Serve—as canned
Concentrate—one part mixed with an equal part of water
Powder (can)—four scoops to one cup of water (scoop supplied in can).

Ingredients: Water, Soybean Solids, Corn Syrup, Sucrose, Soy Oil, Calcium Carbonate, Soy Lecithin, Sodium Citrate, Calcium Citrate, Salt, Potassium Phosphate, Calcium Phosphate, Vitamins (Ascorbic Acid, Alpha Tocopheryl Acetate, Niacinamide, Calcium Pantothenate, Vitamin A Palmitate, Thiamine Hydrochloride, Riboflavin, Pyridoxine Hydrochloride, Biotin, Phytonadione, Folic Acid, Cholecalciferol, Cyanocobalamin), Calcium Carrageenan, L-Methionine, Potassium Chloride, Ferrous Sulfate, Taurine, Zinc Sulfate, L-Carnitine, Calcium Chloride, Cupric Sulfate, Potassium Iodide.

Typical Analysis: Standard Dilution

SOYALAC

	NUTRIENTS	
	PER 100 CALORIES	PER LITER
Protein (g)	3.1	21
Fat (g)	5.5	37
Carbohydrate (g)	10	68
Calories		690
Calories Per Fluid Ounce 20		
Essential Fatty Acids (linoleate) (g)	2.8	19.0
Vitamins:		
A (IU)	312	2110
D (IU)	62	420
K (mcg)	7.8	53
E (IU)	2.3	16
C (Ascorbic Acid) (mg)	12	80
B_1 (Thiamine) (mcg)	78	530
B_2 (Riboflavin) (mcg)	94	640
B_6 (Pyridoxine) (mcg)	70	480
B_{12} (mcg)	0.31	2.1
Niacin (mcg)	1250	8400
Folic Acid (mcg)	23	160
Pantothenic Acid (mcg)	469	3200
Biotin (mcg)	9.4	65
Choline (mg)	16	105
Inositol (mg)	16	105
Minerals:		
Calcium (mg)	94	635
Phosphorus (mg)	55	370
Magnesium (mg)	12	80
Iron (mg)	1.9	13
Iodine (mcg)	7.8	53
Zinc (mg)	0.78	5.3
Copper (mcg)	78	530
Manganese (mcg)	156	1100
Sodium (mg)	44	295
Potassium (mg)	117	795
Chloride (mg)	65	445

Supply:
Soyalac Ready to Serve liquid:
32 fl. oz. cans, 6 cans per case
Soyalac Double Strength Concentrate:
13 fl. oz. cans, 12 cans per case
Soyalac Powder—Cans:
14 oz. cans, 6 cans per case

I-SOYALAC   K PAREVE

Description: A corn free, milk free nutritionally balanced formula for infants. i-Soyalac contains a negligible amount of soy carbohydrates and has a high polyunsaturated to saturated fatty acid ratio together with a liberal supply of Vitamin E. In every respect except for the absence of corn derivatives and its negligible content of soy carbohydrates, i-Soyalac conforms to the description given on the page for Soyalac.

Action and Uses: Same as Soyalac, with the added advantage that it may be used with confidence by infants, children and adults who may be sensitive to corn and corn products.

Preparation: Standard dilution is—
Ready to Serve—as canned
Concentrate—one part mixed with an equal part water

Ingredients: Water, Sucrose, Soy Oil, Soy Protein Isolate, Tapioca Dextrin, Calcium Phosphate, Potassium Citrate, Soy Lecithin, Calcium Carbonate, Potassium Chloride, Calcium Carrageenan, L-Methionine, Magnesium Phosphate, Vitamins (Ascorbic Acid, Alpha Tocopheryl Acetate, Niacinamide, Calcium Pantothenate, Vitamin A Palmitate, Thiamine Hydrochloride, Riboflavin, Pyridoxine Hydrochloride, Folic Acid, Biotin, Phytonadione, Cholecalciferol, Cyanocobalamin), Calcium Citrate, Magnesium Chloride, Salt, Choline Chloride, Ferrous Sulfate, Inositol, Taurine, Zinc Sulfate, L-Carnitine, Cupric Sulfate, Potassium Iodide.

Typical Analysis: Standard Dilution

i-SOYALAC

	NUTRIENTS	
	PER 100 CALORIES	PER LITER
Protein (g)	3.1	21
Fat (g)	5.5	37
Carbohydrate (g)	10.0	68
Calories		690
Calories Per Fluid Ounce 20		
Essential Fatty Acids (linoleate) (g)	2.8	19.0
Vitamins:		
A (IU)	312	2110
D (IU)	63	420
K (mcg)	7.8	53
E (IU)	2.3	16
C (Ascorbic Acid) (mg)	12	80
B_1 (Thiamine) (mcg)	94	630
B_2 (Riboflavin) (mcg)	94	630
B_6 Pyridoxine (mcg)	86	580
B_{12} (mcg)	0.31	2.1
Niacin (mcg)	1250	8400
Folic Acid (mcg)	23	160
Pantothenic Acid (mcg)	469	3200
Biotin (mcg)	7.8	53
Choline (mg)	20	130
Inositol (mg)	17	120
Minerals:		
Calcium (mg)	102	690
Phosphorus (mg)	70	480

Continued on next page

Loma Linda—Cont.

Magnesium (mg)	11	74
Iron (mg)	1.9	13
Iodine (mcg)	7.8	53
Zinc (mg)	0.78	5.3
Copper (mcg)	117	790
Manganese (mcg)	47	320
Sodium (mg)	42	285
Potassium (mg)	117	790
Chloride (mg)	78	530

Supply:
i-Soyalac RTS liquid
  32 fl. oz. cans, 6 cans per case
i-Soyalac Double Strength Concentrate
  13 fl. oz. cans, 12 cans per case

EDUCATIONAL MATERIAL

Compare The Facts
Four-color 4-page brochure giving a comparison chart of Ingredients and Nutrition per 100 calories on all the leading soy-based infant formulas.
Congratulations on Your New Baby
New, updated version of the booklet on infant feeding.
Milk Allergy and Milk Substitutes
Booklet on milk allergies—diagnosis, symptoms, defense and course of action.
Milk Free Recipes
Booklet of milk-free recipes

Luyties Pharmacal Company
P.O. BOX 8080
ST. LOUIS, MO 63156

YELLOLAX
[yel'o-laks]

Description: YELLOLAX is a combination of time proven Yellow-phenolphthalein, and the Homeopathic ingredients, Bryonia and Hydrastis. Clinically YELLOLAX is an oral laxative. Each tablet contains two grains of yellow phenolphthalein and the Bryonia and Hydrastis approximately one fortieth grain each.

Action: Yellow-phenolphthalein is an effective and safe laxative, which is not contraindicated in pregnancy. Homeopathic Bryonia is used to treat constipation and the pain associated with constipation. Homeopathic Bryonia tends to increase mucous membrane moisture. Homeopathic Hydrastis is also included in the treatment of constipation because, the Homeopathic Hydrastis provides some relief of constipation and the associated pain and headaches by relaxing mucous membranes and encouraging their secretion. YELLOLAX has been safely used in pregnancy, children, and as conjunctive treatment with hemorrhoidal complications.

Indications: YELLOLAX is indicated in the management of simple constipation. YELLOLAX is also indicated in those conditions which require a gentle laxative.

Contraindications: YELLOLAX and all laxatives are contraindicated in appendicitis. All laxatives containing phenolphthalein are contraindicated in patients who have hypersensitivity to phenolphthalein.

Warnings: Do not use laxatives in cases of severe colic, nausea and other symptoms of appendicitis. Do not use laxatives habitually nor continually. If condition persists consult physician. Keep this and all medication out of the reach of children. DO NOT exceed the recommended dosage.

Caution: Frequent or prolonged use may result in laxative dependence. If skin rash appears, discontinue use.

Side Effects: The phenolphthalein may impart a red color to the urine, (phenolphthalein is also used as a pH indicator), this is normal.

Dosage: For adults one or two tablets chewed before retiring. For children over six a quarter tablet to half tablet before retiring. Tablets should be well chewed. For younger children consult physician.

Supplied: Compressed tablets packed in glass bottles of 36 (NDC 0618-0832-55) and 100 (NDC 0618-0832-12), and in repackers of 1000 tablets.

Homoeopathic
Luyties also manufactures a complete line of homoeopathic products. If more information is needed contact them direct.

EDUCATIONAL MATERIAL

Packets are available containing descriptive literature on products manufactured by Luyties Pharmacal Company, company history, and pricing information.

3M Company
Personal Care Products
Consumer Specialties
Division/3M
3M CENTER
ST. PAUL, MN 55144-1000

TITRALAC® Antacid Tablets
[tī'trəlăk]
(calcium carbonate)

Description: Titralac tablets are an effective antacid with a pleasant taste to help increase patient compliance. They are also an additional source of necessary calcium and are dietetically sodium free, aluminum free and sugar free. Each white, spearmint-flavored tablet contains calcium carbonate 0.42 gm. and glycine for a smooth, pleasant taste. This equates to 168 mg. of elemental calcium per tablet.

Indications: An antacid for the relief of heartburn, sour stomach, acid indigestion and upset stomach associated with these symptoms. Titralac antacid also provides symptomatic relief of hyperacidity associated with the diagnosis of peptic ulcer, gastritis, peptic esophagitis, gastric hyperacidity, and hiatal hernia.

Warnings: Do not take more than 19 tablets in a 24-hour period or use maximum dosage for more than two weeks, except under the advice and supervision of a physician. Keep this and all medications out of the reach of children.

Dosage and Administration: Two tablets every two or three hours as symptoms occur or as directed by a physician.

Neutralizing Capacity: 15 mEq. per 2 tablets. This neutralization equivalent is expressed as milliequivalents of acid neutralized in 15 minutes when tested in accordance with USP antacid effectiveness test as prescribed in the Code of Federal Regulations for OTC antacid products.
Pleasant Taste
Calcium Rich
Aluminum Free
Sugar Free
Dietetically Sodium Free
Not more than 0.3 mg (0.01 mEq.) sodium per tablet

Availability: Bottles of 40 (NDC 00890-35504-5), 100 (NDC 00890-35510-6) and 1000 (NDC 00890-35580-9).

TITRALAC® PLUS
Antacid/Anti-Gas Tablets and Liquid
[tī'trəlăk]
(calcium carbonate with simethicone)

Description: Titralac Plus tablets and liquid are an effective antacid/antiflatulent with a pleasant taste to help increase patient compliance. They are also an additional source of necessary calcium and are dietetically sodium free, aluminum free and sugar free. Liquid: Two teaspoons (10 ml.) of white, pleasant tasting, spearmint-flavored liquid contains calcium carbonate 1.0 gm with simethicone 40 mg. This equates to 400 mg. of elemental calcium per two teaspoons. Tablets: Each white, peppermint-flavored tablet contains calcium carbonate 0.42 gm., simethicone 21 mg. and glycine for a smooth, pleasant taste. This equates to 168 mg. of elemental calcium per tablet.

Indications: An antacid/antiflatulent for the relief of heartburn, sour stomach, acid indigestion and gas which can accompany these symptoms. Titralac Plus tablets and liquid also provide symptomatic relief of hyperacidity associated with the diagnosis of peptic ulcer, gastritis, peptic esophagitis, gastric hyperacidity, and hiatal hernia.

Warnings: Do not take more than 19 tablets or 16 teaspoons in a 24-hour period or use maximum dosage for more than two weeks, except under the advice and supervision of a physician. Keep this and all medications out of the reach of children.

Dosage and Administration:
Liquid: Two teaspoons between meals and at bedtime or as directed by a physician.
Tablets: Two tablets every two or three hours as symptoms occur or as directed by a physician.

Neutralizing Capacity: Titralac Plus Liquid: 22 mEq. per 10 ml. Titralac Plus Tablets: 15 mEq. per 2 tablets. These neutralization equivalents are expressed as milliequivalents of acid neutralized in 15 minutes when tested in accordance with USP antacid effectiveness test as prescribed in the Code of Federal Regulations for OTC antacid products.
Pleasant Taste
Calcium Rich
Aluminum Free
Sugar Free
Dietetically Sodium Free
Titralac Plus Liquid: Not more than 0.0005 mg. (0.00002) mEq.) sodium per teaspoon (5 ml.).
Titralac Plus Tablets: Not more than 0.03 mg. (0.001 mEq.) sodium per tablet.

Availability:
Tablets: bottles of 100 (NDC 017518-013-01)
Liquid: bottles of 12 fl. oz. (NDC 00890-95012-7).

Macsil, Inc.
1326 FRANKFORD AVENUE
PHILADELPHIA, PA 19125

BALMEX® BABY POWDER

Composition: Contains: Active Ingredients—zinc oxide; Inactive Ingredients—corn starch, calcium carbonate, BALSAN®, (especially purified balsam Peru).

Action and Uses: Absorbent, emollient, soothing—for diaper irritation, intertrigo, and other common dermatological conditions. In acute, simple miliaria, itching ceases in minutes and lesions dry promptly. For routine use after bathing and each diaper change.

How Supplied: 8 oz. shaker-top plastic containers.

BALMEX® EMOLLIENT LOTION

Gentle and effective scientifically compounded infant's skin conditioner.

Composition: Contains a special lanolin oil (non-sensitizing, dewaxed, moisturizing fraction of lanolin), BALSAN® (specially purified balsam Peru) and silicone.

Action and Uses: The special Lanolin Oil aids nature lubricate baby's skin to keep it smooth and supple. Balmex Emollient Lotion is also highly effective as a physiologic conditioner on adult's skin.

How Supplied: Available in 6 oz. dispenser-top plastic bottles.

BALMEX® OINTMENT

Composition: Contains: Active Ingredients—Bismuth Subnitrate, Zinc Oxide; Inactive Ingredients—Balsan (Specially Purified Balsam Peru), Benzoic Acid, Beeswax, Mineral Oil, Silicone, Synthetic White Wax, Purified Water, and other ingredients.

Action and Uses: Emollient, protective, anti-inflammatory, promotes healing—for diaper rash, minor burns, sunburn, and other simple skin conditions; also decubitus ulcers, skin irritations associated with ileostomy and colostomy drainage. Nonstaining, readily washes out of diapers and clothing.

How Supplied: 1, 2, 4 oz. tubes; 1 lb. plastic jars (½ oz. tubes for Hospitals only). Balmex Ointment-All Commercial Sizes-Safety Sealed.

Marion Laboratories, Inc.
Pharmaceutical Products Division
MARION INDUSTRIAL PARK
MARION PARK DRIVE
KANSAS CITY, MO 64137

DEBROX® Drops
[dē 'brŏx]

Description: Carbamide peroxide 6.5%. Also contains citric acid, glycerin, propylene glycol, sodium stannate, water, and other ingredients.

Actions: DEBROX®, used as directed, cleanses the ear with sustained microfoam. DEBROX Drops foam on contact with earwax due to the release of oxygen.

Indications: DEBROX Drops provide a safe, nonirritating method of softening and removing earwax.

Directions: FOR USE IN THE EAR ONLY. Adults and children over 12 years of age: tilt head sideways and place 5 to 10 drops into ear. Tip of applicator should not enter ear canal. Keep drops in ear for several minutes by keeping head tilted or placing cotton in the ear. Use twice daily for up to four days if needed, or as directed by a doctor. Any wax remaining after treatment may be removed by gently flushing the ear with warm water, using a soft rubber bulb ear syringe. Children under 12 years of age: consult a doctor.

Warnings: Do not use if you have ear drainage or discharge, ear pain, irritation or rash in the ear, or are dizzy, unless directed by a physician. Do not use if you have an injury or perforation (hole) of the eardrum or after ear surgery unless directed by a physician. Do not use for more than four consecutive days. If excessive earwax remains after use of this product, consult a physician. Consult a physician prior to use in children under 12.

Cautions: Avoid exposing bottle to excessive heat and direct sunlight. Keep color tip on bottle when not in use. Avoid contact with eyes. Keep this and all drugs out of the reach of children. In case of accidental ingestion, seek professional assistance or contact a poison control center immediately.

How Supplied: DEBROX Drops are available in ½- or 1-fl-oz plastic squeeze bottles with applicator spouts.
Issued 12/86
Shown in Product Identification Section, page 412

GAVISCON® Antacid Tablets
[găv 'ĭs-kŏn]

Composition: Each chewable tablet contains the following active ingredients:
Aluminum hydroxide dried gel... 80 mg
Magnesium trisilicate .... 20 mg
and the following inactive ingredients: alginic acid, calcium stearate, flavor, sodium bicarbonate, starch (may contain cornstarch), and sucrose.

Actions: Unique formulation produces soothing foam which floats on stomach contents. Foam containing antacid precedes stomach contents into the esophagus when reflux occurs to help protect the sensitive mucosa from further irritation. GAVISCON® acts locally without neutralizing entire stomach contents to help maintain integrity of the digestive process. Endoscopic studies indicate that GAVISCON Antacid Tablets are equally as effective in the erect or supine patient.

Indications: GAVISCON is specifically formulated for the temporary relief of heartburn (acid indigestion) due to acid reflux. GAVISCON is not indicated for the treatment of peptic ulcers.

Directions: Chew two to four tablets four times a day or as directed by a physician. Tablets should be taken after meals and at bedtime or as needed. For best results follow by a half glass of water or other liquid. DO NOT SWALLOW WHOLE.

Warnings: Do not take more than 16 tablets in a 24-hour period or 16 tablets daily for more than 2 weeks, except under the advice and supervision of a physician. Do not use this product except under the advice and supervision of a physician if you are on a sodium-restricted diet. Each GAVISCON Tablet contains approximately 0.8 mEq sodium.

Drug Interaction Precautions: Do not take this product if you are presently taking a prescription antibiotic drug containing any form of tetracycline.
Store at a controlled room temperature in a dry place.
Keep this and all drugs out of the reach of children. In case of accidental overdose, seek professional assistance or contact a poison control center immediately.

How Supplied: Available in bottles of 100 tablets and in foil-wrapped 2s in boxes of 30 tablets.
Issued 2/87
Shown in Product Identification Section, page 412

Continued on next page

Marion—Cont.

GAVISCON® EXTRA STRENGTH RELIEF FORMULA Antacid Tablets
[găv 'ĭs-kŏn]

Composition: Each chewable tablet contains the following active ingredients:
Aluminum hydroxide .... 160 mg
Magnesium carbonate .... 105 mg
and the following inactive ingredients: alginic acid, calcium stearate, flavor, mannitol, sodium bicarbonate, stearic acid, and sucrose.

Directions: Chew 2 to 4 tablets four times a day or as directed by a physician. Tablets should be taken after meals and at bedtime or as needed. For best results follow by a half glass of water or other liquid. DO NOT SWALLOW WHOLE.

> **FDA Approved Uses:** For the relief of heartburn, sour stomach, and/or acid indigestion, and upset stomach associated with heartburn, sour stomach, and/or acid indigestion.

Warnings: Do not take more than 16 tablets in a 24-hour period or 16 tablets daily for more than 2 weeks, except under the advice and supervision of a physician. Do not use this product except under the advice and supervision of a physician if you are on a sodium-restricted diet. Each tablet contains approximately 1.3 mEq sodium.

Drug Interaction Precautions: Do not take this product if you are presently taking a prescription antibiotic drug containing any form of tetracycline.
Store at a controlled room temperature in a dry place.
Keep this and all drugs out of the reach of children.
In case of accidental overdose, seek professional assistance or contact a poison control center immediately.

How Supplied: Available in bottles of 100 tablets.

Issued 4/87

Shown in Product Identification Section, page 412

GAVISCON® Liquid Antacid
[găv 'ĭs-kŏn]

Composition: Each tablespoonful (15 ml) contains the following active ingredients:
Aluminum hydroxide .... 95 mg
Magnesium carbonate .... 412 mg
And the following inactive ingredients: D&C Yellow #10, edetate disodium, FD&C Blue #1, flavor, glycerin, paraben preservatives, saccharin sodium, sodium alginate, sorbitol solution, water, and xanthan gum.

> **FDA Approved Uses:** For the relief of heartburn, sour stomach and/or acid indigestion, and upset stomach associated with heartburn, sour stomach and/or acid indigestion.

Directions: SHAKE WELL BEFORE USING. Take 1 or 2 tablespoonfuls four times a day or as directed by a physician. GAVISCON Liquid should be taken after meals and at bedtime, followed by half a glass of water. Dispense product only by spoon or other measuring device.

Warnings: Except under the advice and supervision of a physician, do not take more than 8 tablespoonfuls in a 24-hour period or 8 tablespoonfuls daily for more than 2 weeks. May have laxative effect. Do not use this product if you have a kidney disease; do not use this product if you are on a sodium-restricted diet. Each tablespoonful of GAVISCON Liquid contains approximately 1.7 mEq sodium.

Drug Interaction Precautions: Do not take this product if you are presently taking a prescription antibiotic drug containing any form of tetracycline.
Keep tightly closed. Avoid freezing. Store at a controlled room temperature.
Keep this and all drugs out of the reach of children.
In case of accidental overdose, seek professional assistance or contact a poison control center immediately.

How Supplied: Bottles of 12 fluid ounce (355 ml) and 6 fluid ounce (177 ml).

Issued 2/87

Shown in Product Identification Section, page 412

GAVISCON®-2 Antacid Tablets
[găv 'ĭs-kŏn]

Composition: Each chewable tablet contains the following active ingredients:
Aluminum hydroxide dried gel...160 mg
Magnesium trisilicate .... 40 mg
and the following inactive ingredients: alginic acid, calcium stearate, flavor, sodium bicarbonate, starch (may contain cornstarch), and sucrose.

Indications: GAVISCON® is specifically formulated for the temporary relief of heartburn (acid indigestion) due to acid reflux. GAVISCON is not indicated for the treatment of peptic ulcers.

Directions: Chew one to two tablets four times a day or as directed by a physician. Tablets should be taken after meals and at bedtime or as needed. For best results follow by a half glass of water or other liquid. DO NOT SWALLOW WHOLE.

Warnings: Do not take more than eight tablets in a 24-hour period or eight tablets daily for more than 2 weeks, except under the advice and supervision of a physician. Do not use this product except under the advice and supervision of a physician if you are on a sodium-restricted diet. Each GAVISCON-2 Tablet contains approximately 1.6 mEq sodium.

Drug Interaction Precautions: Do not take this product if you are presently taking a prescription antibiotic drug containing any form of tetracycline.
Store at a controlled room temperature in a dry place.
Keep this and all drugs out of the reach of children. In case of accidental over-

dose, seek professional assistance or contact a poison control center immediately.

How Supplied: Boxes of 48 foil-wrapped tablets.

Issued 2/87

Shown in Product Identification Section, page 412

GLY–OXIDE® Liquid
[glī-ok 'sīd]

Description: GLY-OXIDE® Liquid contains carbamide peroxide 10%. Also contains citric acid, flavor, glycerin, propylene glycol, sodium stannate, water, and other ingredients.

Actions: GLY-OXIDE® Liquid has an oxygen-rich formula that works to relieve the pain of canker sores by cleaning and debriding damaged tissue so natural healing can occur.

Administration: Do not dilute. Apply directly from bottle. Replace color tip on bottle when not in use.

Indications: For local treatment and hygienic prevention of minor oral inflammation such as canker sores, denture irritation, and postdental procedure irritation. Place several drops on affected area four times daily, after meals and at bedtime, or as directed by a dentist or physician; expectorate after two or three minutes. Or place 10 drops onto tongue, mix with saliva, swish for several minutes, and expectorate.
As an adjunct to oral hygiene (orthodontics, dental appliances) after regular brushing, swish 10 or more drops vigorously. Continue for two to three minutes; expectorate.
When normal oral hygiene is inadequate or impossible (total care geriatrics, etc), swish 10 or more drops vigorously after meals and expectorate.

Precautions: Severe or persistent oral inflammation, denture irritation, or gingivitis may be serious. If these conditions or unexpected side effects occur, consult a dentist or physician immediately.
Avoid contact with eyes. Protect from heat and direct light. Keep this and all drugs out of the reach of children. In case of accidental overdose, seek professional assistance or contact a poison control center immediately.

How Supplied: GLY-OXIDE® Liquid is available in ½-fl-oz and 2-fl-oz nonspill, plastic squeeze bottles with applicator spouts.

Issued 2/86

Shown in Product Identification Section, page 412

OS-CAL® 500 Chewable Tablets
[ăhs 'kăl]
(calcium supplement)

Each Tablet Contains: 1,250 mg of calcium carbonate.
Elemental calcium........................ 500 mg
Ingredients: calcium carbonate, dextrose monohydrate, maltodextrin, microcrystalline cellulose, magnesium stea-

rate, Bavarian cream flavor, sodium chloride, and coconut cream flavor.

Directions: One tablet two to three times a day with meals, or as recommended by your physician.

Two Tablets Provide: 1,000 mg calcium, 100% of U.S. RDA for adults and children 12 or more years of age.

Three Tablets Provide: 1,500 mg calcium, 115% of U.S. RDA for pregnant and lactating women.

Store at room temperature. Keep out of reach of children.

How Supplied: OS-CAL® 500 Chewable Tablets is available in bottles of 60 tablets.

Issued 10/87

Shown in Product Identification Section, page 412

OS-CAL® 500 Tablets
[ăhs'kăl]
(calcium supplement)

Each Tablet Contains: 1,250 mg of calcium carbonate from oyster shell, an organic calcium source.
Elemental calcium .... 500 mg
Ingredients: oyster shell powder, corn syrup solids, talc, hydroxypropyl methylcellulose, cornstarch, sodium starch glycolate, calcium stearate, polysorbate 80, pharmaceutical glaze, titanium dioxide, methyl propyl paraben, polyethylene glycol, polyvinylpyrrolidone, carnauba wax, D&C Yellow #10, acetylated monoglyceride, edetate disodium, FD&C Blue #1, and simethicone emulsion.

Directions: One tablet two or three times a day with meals, or as recommended by your physician.

Two Tablets Provide: 1,000 mg calcium, 100% of U.S. RDA for adults and children 12 or more years of age.

Three Tablets Provide: 1,500 mg calcium, 115% of U.S. RDA for pregnant and lactating women.

Store at room temperature. Keep out of reach of children.

How Supplied: OS-CAL® 500 is available in bottles of 60 and 120 tablets.

Issued 10/87

Shown in Product Identification Section, page 412

OS-CAL® 250+D Tablets
[ăhs'kăl]
(calcium supplement with vitamin D)

Each Tablet Contains: 625 mg of calcium carbonate from oyster shell, an organic calcium source.
Elemental calcium .... 250 mg
Vitamin D .... 125 USP Units

Ingredients: oyster shell powder, corn syrup solids, talc, cornstarch, hydroxypropyl methylcellulose, calcium stearate, polysorbate 80, titanium dioxide, methyl propyl paraben, polyethylene glycol, pharmaceutical glaze, vitamin D, polyvinylpyrrolidone, carnauba wax, D&C Yellow #10, acetylated mono-

glyceride, edetate disodium, FD&C Blue #1, simethicone emulsion, and edible gray ink.

Directions: One tablet three times a day with meals, or as recommended by your physician.

Three Tablets Provide:

	% U.S. RDA for Adults
Calcium .... 750 mg	75%
Vitamin D ..... 375 Units	94%

Store at room temperature. Keep out of reach of children.

How Supplied: OS-CAL® 250+D is available in bottles of 100, 240, 500, and 1,000 tablets.

Issued 10/87

Shown in Product Identification Section, page 412

OS-CAL® 500+D Tablets
[ăhs'kăl]
(calcium supplement with vitamin D)

Each Tablet Contains: 1,250 mg of calcium carbonate from oyster shell, an organic calcium source.
Elemental calcium .... 500 mg
Vitamin D .... 125 USP Units

Ingredients: oyster shell powder, corn syrup solids, talc, hydroxypropyl methylcellulose, cornstarch, sodium starch glycolate, calcium stearate, polysorbate 80, pharmaceutical glaze, titanium dioxide, methyl propyl paraben, polyethylene glycol, polyvinylpyrrolidone, vitamin D, carnauba wax, D&C Yellow #10, acetylated monoglyceride, edetate disodium, FD&C Blue #1, and simethicone emulsion.

Directions: One tablet two or three times a day with meals, or as recommended by your physician.

Two Tablets Provide: 1,000 mg calcium, 100% of U.S. RDA for adults and children 12 or more years of age and 64% of vitamin D.

Three Tablets Provide: 1,500 mg calcium, 115% of U.S. RDA for pregnant and lactating women and 94% of vitamin D.

Store at room temperature. Keep out of reach of children.

How Supplied: OS-CAL® 500+D is available in bottles of 60.

Issued 10/87

Shown in Product Identification Section, page 412

OS-CAL FORTE® Tablets
[ăhs'kăl fŏr'tā]
(multivitamin and mineral supplement)

Each Tablet Contains:
Vitamin A (palmitate) 1668 USP Units
Vitamin D .... 125 USP Units
Thiamine mononitrate
(vitamin B₁)................................. 1.7 mg
Riboflavin (vitamin B₂)................ 1.7 mg
Pyridoxine hydrochloride
(vitamin B₆)................................. 2.0 mg
Ascorbic acid (vitamin C).......... 50.0 mg

dl-alpha-tocopherol acetate
(vitamin E)................................. 0.8 IU
Niacinamide .... 15.0 mg
Calcium (from oyster shell) .... 250.0 mg
Iron (as ferrous fumarate)........... 5.0 mg
Magnesium (as oxide)................... 1.6 mg
Manganese (as sulfate)............... 0.3 mg
Zinc (as sulfate)............................. 0.5 mg

Ingredients: oyster shell powder, ascorbic acid, corn syrup solids, niacinamide, D&C Yellow #10 Aluminum Lake, ferrous fumarate, calcium stearate, FD&C Blue #1 Aluminum Lake, cornstarch, vitamin A palmitate, polysorbate 80, magnesium oxide, pyridoxine, thiamine, riboflavin, vitamin E, pharmaceutical glaze, methyl paraben, zinc sulfate, manganese sulfate, propylparaben, povidone, vitamin D, hydroxypropyl methylcellulose, carnauba wax, titanium dioxide, ethylcellulose, and acetylated monoglyceride.

Indication: Multivitamin and mineral supplement.

Dosage: One tablet three times daily or as directed by physician. In case of accidental overdose, seek professional assistance or contact a poison control center immediately.

Keep out of reach of children.
Store at room temperature.

How Supplied: Bottles of 100 tablets.

Issued 7/87

Shown in Product Identification Section, page 412

OS-CAL® PLUS Tablets
[ăhs'kăl]
(multivitamin and multimineral supplement)

Each Tablet Contains:
Elemental calcium (from oyster shell).. 250 mg
Vitamin D .... 125 USP Units
Vitamin A (palmitate) 1666 USP Units
Vitamin C (ascorbic acid)....... 33.0 mg
Vitamin B₂ (riboflavin)........... 0.66 mg
Vitamin B₁ (thiamine
mononitrate) .... 0.5 mg
Vitamin B₆ (pyridoxine HCl) 0.5 mg
Niacinamide.............................. 3.33 mg
Iron (as ferrous fumarate) ..... 16.6 mg
Zinc (as the sulfate)................ 0.75 mg
Manganese (as the sulfate).... 0.75 mg

Ingredients: oyster shell powder, corn syrup solids, ferrous fumarate, ascorbic acid, calcium stearate, cornstarch, hydroxypropyl methylcellulose, polysorbate 80, titanium dioxide, vitamin A palmitate, niacinamide, ethylcellulose, manganese sulfate, methyl propyl paraben, zinc sulfate, pharmaceutical glaze, acetylated monoglyceride, riboflavin, thiamine mononitrate, pyridoxine hydrochloride, povidone, vitamin D, carnauba wax, and D&C Red #33.

Indications: As a multivitamin and multimineral supplement.

Dosage: One (1) tablet three times a day before meals or as directed by a physi-

Continued on next page

Marion—Cont.

cian. For children under 4 years of age, consult a physician.

Store at room temperature.

Keep out of reach of children. In case of accidental overdose, seek professional assistance or contact a poison control center immediately.

How Supplied: Bottles of 100 tablets.
Issued 5/87

Shown in Product Identification Section, page 413

THROAT DISCS® Throat Lozenges
[*thrōt dĭsks*]

Description: Each lozenge contains sucrose, starch (may contain cornstarch), acacia, glycyrrhiza extract (licorice), gum tragacanth, anethole, linseed, cubeb oleoresin, anise oil, peppermint oil, capsicum, and mineral oil.

Indications: Effective for soothing, temporary relief of minor throat irritations from hoarseness and coughs due to colds.

Precautions: For severe or persistent cough or sore throat, or sore throat accompanied by high fever, headache, nausea, and vomiting, consult physician promptly. Not recommended for children under 3 years of age.

Directions: Allow lozenge to dissolve slowly in mouth. One or two should give the desired relief.

How Supplied: Boxes of 60 lozenges.
Issued 5/85

Shown in Product Identification Section, page 413

Marlyn Health Care
6324 FERRIS SQUARE
SAN DIEGO, CA 92121

4 HAIR

Composition: L-Cysteine, L-Cystine, Biotin, Silicon (Amino Acid Chelate), Choline, Methionine, Inositol, L-Tyrosine, Para Aminobenzoic Acid, Niacin, Vitamin B$_{12}$, B$_6$, C, E, Folic Acid, Beta Carotene, Magnesium, Zinc, Iron, Iodine, Boron, Copper, Manganese, Gelatin, Collagen Protein, Mucopolysaccharides, Sulfur, D-Pantothenol.

Indications: A nutritional supplement to help maintain attractive, fuller, thicker, healthier looking hair.

Actions: Supplies vitamins, minerals, and other factors present in hair.

Dosage and Administration: Take 2 capsules daily, one in the morning and one at night, or as recommended by a healthcare professional.

How Supplied: Soft gelatin capsules in bottles of 90.

4 NAILS

Composition: Bonemeal Calcium, Gelatine, Hydrolized Collagen, Silicon, Boron,

Vitamin A, C, B-1, B-2, D, E, B-6, B-12, Niacin, Iron, Iodine, Magnesium, Zinc, Copper, Biotin, Pantothenic Acid, Paba, Potassium, Manganese, Chromium, Selenomethionine, Choline, Methionine, Inositol, L-Cysteine, Sulfur, Phosphorus, Mucopolysaccharides.

Indications: Nutritional building blocks to maintain stronger and healthier nail growth.

Actions: Supplies minerals, proteins, amino acids, and other factors present in healthy nails.

Dosage and Administration: Take two capsules daily or as recommended by a healthcare professional.

How Supplied: Soft gelatin capsules in bottles of 90.

PRO SKIN-E (Face Capsule)

Composition: Vitamin E, A (Retinol), Benzophenone 3, Padimate, Myristate, Rice Bran Oil, Natural Fragrance.

Indications: This topical formula helps to maintain youthful looking skin.

Actions: The active ingredients in PRO SKIN E twist off face capsules are an effective skin care protection to filter out damaging UV light rays and which help to neutralize free radical compounds caused by the environment.

Dosage and Administration: Each topical capsule is an individual dose for easy application.

How Supplied: Soft gelatin twist off capsules in bottles of 60.

PRO-SKIN NUTRIBLOXX

Composition: Vitamin A (Retinol), E, and C, Zinc, Collagen Protein, Mucopolysaccharides, Unsaturated Fatty Acids, Acidophilus, Chlorophyll, Aloe Vera, Proline, Lysine, Cysteine, Cystine, Niacinamide, Selenomethionine, Aminobenzoic Acid, Apricot, Avocado, Peppermint, Dandelion and Wheat Germ Oil, d-Pantothenol.

Indication: A nutritional supplement to help maintain youthful looking skin.

Actions: Scientifically balanced to provide vitamins, minerals, amino acids, polyunsaturated fatty acids and other essential nutritional factors designed to give a feeling of soft, smooth, youthfulness.

Dosage and Administration: Take two capsules daily or as recommended by a healthcare professional.

How Supplied: Soft gelatin capsules in bottles of 90.

Products are cross-indexed by generic and chemical names in the **YELLOW SECTION**

McNeil Consumer Products Company
FORT WASHINGTON, PA 19034

CHILDREN'S CoTYLENOL®
Chewable Cold Tablets and Liquid Cold Formula

PRODUCT OVERVIEW

Key Facts: Children's CoTYLENOL® Products are formulated to relieve a child's fever, aches and pains, congestion and runny nose. The products are aspirin free and formulated for accurate dosing by age and weight.

Major Uses: Children's CoTYLENOL Products contain the same amount of acetaminophen as comparable Children's TYLENOL Products (80mg per tablet, 160mg per 5ml) for relief of fever and pain resulting from a cold in children ages 11 and under. Additionally, Children's CoTYLENOL Products contain pseudoephedrine hydrochloride (7.5mg per tablet, 15mg per 5ml) for treatment of nasal congestion and chlorpheniramine maleate (0.5mg per tablet, 1mg per 5ml) for treatment of runny noses and sneezing.

PRODUCT INFORMATION
CHILDREN'S CoTYLENOL®
Chewable Cold Tablets and Liquid Cold Formula

Description: Each Children's CoTYLENOL Chewable Cold Tablet contains acetaminophen 80 mg, chlorpheniramine maleate 0.5 mg and pseudoephedrine hydrochloride 7.5 mg. Children's CoTYLENOL Liquid Cold Formula is stable, cherry-flavored, red in color and contains no alcohol. Each teaspoon (5 ml) contains acetaminophen 160 mg, chlorpheniramine maleate 1 mg, and pseudoephedrine hydrochloride 15 mg.

Actions and Indications: Children's CoTYLENOL Chewable Cold Tablets and Liquid Cold Formula combine the analgesic-antipyretic acetaminophen with the decongestant pseudoephedrine hydrochloride and the antihistamine chlorpheniramine maleate to help relieve nasal congestion, dry runny noses and prevent sneezing as well as to relieve the fever, aches, pains and general discomfort associated with colds and upper respiratory infections.

While acetaminophen is equal to aspirin in analgesic and antipyretic effectiveness, it is unlikely to produce the side effects often associated with aspirin or aspirin-containing products.

Dosage: Administer to children under 6 years only on the advice of a physician. Children's CoTYLENOL Chewable Cold Tablets: 2–5 years—2 tablets, 6–11 years—4 tablets.
Children's CoTYLENOL Liquid Cold Formula: 2–5 years—1 teaspoonful; 6–11 years—2 teaspoonsful. Measuring cup is provided and marked for accurate dosing.

Doses may be repeated every 4-6 hours as needed, not to exceed 4 doses in 24 hours.

Note: Since Children's CoTYLENOL Chewable Cold Tablets and Liquid Cold Formula are available without prescription, the following information appears on the package labels. The Warnings are identical for the two dosage forms except the Liquid Cold Formula does not contain the phenylketonurics statement since the product does not contain aspartame.

Warning: Do not use if carton is opened, or if printed plastic bottle wrap or printed foil inner seal is broken.
Keep this and all medication out of the reach of children. In case of accidental overdosage, contact a physician or poison control center immediately. Phenylketonurics: contains phenylalanine, 4 mg per tablet. Do not exceed the recommended dosage because nervousness, dizziness or sleeplessness may occur. If fever persists for more than three days, or if symptoms do not improve or new ones occur within five days or are accompanied by high fever, consult a physician before continuing use. This preparation may cause drowsiness, or in some cases, excitability. Do not give this product to children who have heart disease, high blood pressure, thyroid disease, diabetes, glaucoma or asthma or are taking a prescription drug for high blood pressure or depression, except under the advice and supervision of a physician.

Overdosage: Acetaminophen in massive overdosage may cause hepatic toxicity in some patients. In adults and adolescents, hepatic toxicity has rarely been reported following ingestion of acute overdosage of less than 10 grams. Fatalities are infrequent (less than 3–4% of untreated cases) and have rarely been reported with overdoses of less than 15 grams. In children, an acute overdosage of less than 150 mg/kg has not been associated with hepatic toxicity.
Early symptoms following a potentially hepatotoxic overdose may include: nausea, vomiting, diaphoresis and general malaise. Clinical and laboratory evidence of hepatic toxicity may not be apparent until 48 to 72 hours postingestion. In adults and adolescents, regardless of the quantity of acetaminophen reported to have been ingested, administer MUCOMYST® acetylcysteine immediately if 24 hours or less have elapsed from the reported time of ingestion. For full prescribing information, refer to the MUCOMYST package insert. Do not await the results of assays for acetaminophen level before initiating treatment with MUCOMYST acetylcysteine. The following additional procedures are recommended: The stomach should be emptied promptly by lavage or by induction of emesis with syrup of ipecac. A serum acetaminophen assay should be obtained as early as possible, but no sooner than four hours following ingestion. Liver function studies should be obtained initially and repeated at 24-hour intervals.
Serious toxicity or fatalities are extremely infrequent in children, possibly due to differences in the way they metabolize acetaminophen. In children, the maximum potential amount ingested can be more easily estimated. If more than 150 mg/kg or an unknown amount was ingested, obtain an acetaminophen plasma level. The acetaminophen plasma level should be obtained as soon as possible, but no sooner than 4 hours following the ingestion. Induce emesis using syrup of ipecac. If the plasma level is obtained and falls above the broken line on the nomogram, the MUCOMYST acetylcysteine therapy should be initiated and continued for a full course of therapy. If acetaminophen plasma assay capability is not available, and the estimated acetaminophen ingestion exceeds 150 mg/kg, MUCOMYST acetylcysteine therapy should be initiated and continued for a full course of therapy.
For additional emergency information, call your regional poison center or toll-free (1-800-525-6115) to the Rocky Mountain Poison Center for assistance in diagnosis and for directions in the use of MUCOMYST acetylcysteine as an antidote.
Chlorpheniramine toxicity should be treated as you would an antihistamine/anticholinergic overdose and is likely to be present within a few hours after acute ingestion.
Pseudoephedrine may produce central nervous system stimulation and sympathomimetic effects on the cardiovascular system which are likely to be manifested within a few hours following ingestion.

Inactive Ingredients: Chewable Tablets—Aspartame, cellulose, citric acid, dextrose, ethylcellulose, flavors, magnesium stearate, mannitol, starch, sucrose and Yellow #6 (Sunset Yellow).
Liquid—Benzoic acid, citric acid, flavors, glycerin, polyethylene glycol, propylene glycol, sodium benzoate, sorbitol, sucrose, purified water and Red #40.

How Supplied: Chewable Tablets (colored orange, scored, imprinted "CoTYLENOL")—bottles of 24. Cold Formula—bottles (colored red) of 4 fl. oz.

Shown in Product Identification Section, page 414

DELSYM®
[del 'sim]
(dextromethorphan polistirex)

Description: Provides 12-hour relief of coughs due to minor throat and bronchial irritation. Each teaspoonful (5 ml) contains dextromethorphan polistirex equivalent to 30 mg dextromethorphan hydrobromide.

Indications: For temporary relief of cough due to minor throat and bronchial irritation as may occur with the common cold or with inhaled irritants.

Contraindications: Hypersensitivity to dextromethorphan.
Note: Since DELSYM dextromethorphan polistirex syrup is available without prescription, the following appears on the package labels.

Warnings: Do not give this product to children under 2 years except under the advice and supervision of a physician. Do not take this product for persistent or chronic cough such as occurs with smoking, asthma, or emphysema, or where cough is accompanied by excessive phlegm (mucus) unless directed by a physician.
As with any drug, if you are pregnant or nursing a baby, seek the advice of a health professional before using this product.

Caution: A persistent cough may be a sign of a serious condition. If cough persists for more than 1 week, tends to recur or is accompanied by fever, rash or persistent headache, consult a physician. Keep this and all drugs out of reach of children. In case of accidental overdose, seek professional assistance or contact a Poison Control Center immediately. Do not use if carton is opened, or break-away ring is separated or missing.

Directions: Shake well before using. Adults: 2 teaspoonsful every 12 hours; do not exceed 4 teaspoonsful in 24 hours. Children 6–12: 1 teaspoonful every 12 hours; do not exceed 2 teaspoonsful in 24 hours. Children 2–5: ½ teaspoonful every 12 hours: do not exceed 1 teaspoonful in 24 hours. Children under 2: Use only under the advice and supervision of a physician.

Overdosage: Acute dextromethorphan overdose usually does not result in serious signs and symptoms unless a massive amount has been ingested. Signs and symptoms of a substantial overdose may include nausea and vomiting, visual disturbance, CNS disturbances, and urinary retention. Because of the sustained action of DELSYM, the onset of symptoms may be delayed, and the duration of symptoms may be prolonged.

How Supplied: 3 fl. oz. bottles (NDC 0045-0288-03)

Inactive Ingredients: Citric Acid; Ethylcellulose; Flavor; High Fructose Corn Syrup; Methylparaben; Polyethylene Glycol 3350; Polysorbate 80; Propylene Glycol; Propylparaben; Sucrose; Tragacanth; Vegetable Oil; Purified Water; Xanthan Gum, Yellow #6 (Sunset Yellow).

Shown in Product Identification Section, page 414

IMODIUM® A–D
(loperamide hydrochloride)

Active Ingredients: Each 5 ml (teaspoon) of Imodium A-D liquid contains loperamide hydrochloride 1 mg. Imodium A-D liquid is stable, cherry flavored, and clear in color.

Inactive Ingredients: Alcohol (5.25%), citric acid, flavors, glycerin, methylparaben, propylparaben and purified water.

Indication: Imodium A-D is indicated for the control and symptomatic relief of acute nonspecific diarrhea.

Continued on next page

McNeil Consumer—Cont.

Actions: Imodium A-D contains a clinically proven antidiarrheal medication. Loperamide HCl acts by slowing intestinal motility and by affecting water and electrolyte movement through the bowel.

Warnings: Since Imodium A-D liquid is available without a prescription, the following information appears on the package label: "WARNINGS: DO NOT USE FOR MORE THAN TWO DAYS UNLESS DIRECTED BY A PHYSICIAN. Do not use if diarrhea is accompanied by high fever (greater than 101°F), or if blood is present in the stool, or if you have had a rash or other allergic reaction to loperamide HCl. If you are taking antibiotics or have a history of liver disease, consult a physician before using this product. As with any drug, if you are pregnant or nursing a baby, seek the advice of a physician before using this product. Keep this and all drugs out of the reach of children. In case of accidental overdose, seek professional assistance or contact a poison control center immediately. Store at room temperature."

Drug Interaction: There was no evidence in clinical trials of drug interactions with concurrent medications.

Precautions: In acute diarrhea, if improvement is not observed in 48 hours, the administration of Imodium A-D should be discontinued.

Symptoms and Treatment of Oral Overdosage: Overdosage of loperamide HCl in man may result in constipation, CNS depression and nausea. A slurry of activated charcoal administered promptly after ingestion of loperamide hydrochloride can reduce the amount of drug which is absorbed. If vomiting occurs spontaneously upon ingestion, a slurry of 100 grams of activated charcoal should be administered orally as soon as fluids can be retained. If vomiting has not occurred, gastric lavage should be performed followed by administration of 100 gms of the activated charcoal slurry through the gastric tube. In the event of overdosage, patients should be monitored for signs of CNS depression for at least 24 hours. Children may be more sensitive to central nervous system effects than adults. If CNS depression is observed, naloxone may be administered. If responsive to naloxone, vital signs must be monitored carefully for recurrence of symptoms of drug overdose for at least 24 hours after the last dose of naloxone.

Dosage and Administration: Adults: Take four teaspoonfuls after first loose bowel movement. If needed, take two teaspoonfuls after each subsequent loose bowel movement. Do not exceed eight teaspoonfuls in any 24 hour period, unless directed by a physician.
9–11 years old (60–95 lbs.): Two teaspoonfuls after first loose bowel movement, followed by one teaspoonful after each subsequent loose bowel movement. Do not exceed six teaspoonfuls a day.

6–8 years old (48–59 lbs.): Two teaspoonfuls after first loose bowel movement, followed by one teaspoonful after each subsequent loose bowel movement. Do not exceed four teaspoonfuls a day.
Under six years old (up to 47 lbs.): Consult a physician

How Supplied: Cherry flavored liquid (clear) 2 fl. oz., 3 fl. oz., and 4 fl. oz. tamper resistant bottles with child resistant safety caps and special dosage cups. BK403

Shown in Product Identification Section, page 414

MEDIPREN®
Ibuprofen Caplets and Tablets
Pain Reliever/Fever Reducer

WARNING: ASPIRIN SENSITIVE PATIENTS. Do not take this product if you have had a severe allergic reaction to aspirin (e.g., asthma, swelling, shock or hives) because even though this product contains no aspirin or salicylates, cross-reactions may occur in patients allergic to aspirin.

Indications: For the temporary relief of minor aches and pains associated with the common cold, headache, toothaches, muscular aches, backache, for the minor pain of arthritis, for the pain of menstrual cramps, and for reduction of fever.

Directions: Adults: One Caplet or Tablet every 4 to 6 hours while symptoms persist. If pain or fever does not respond to 1 Caplet or Tablet, 2 Caplets or Tablets may be used but do not exceed 6 Caplets or Tablets in 24 hours, unless directed by a doctor. The smallest effective dose should be used. Take with food or milk if occasional and mild heartburn, upset stomach, or stomach pain occurs with use. Consult a doctor if these symptoms are more than mild or if they persist. Children: Do not give this product to children under 12 except under the advice and supervision of a doctor.

Warnings: Do not take for pain for more than 10 days or for fever for more than 3 days unless directed by a doctor. If pain or fever persists or gets worse, if new symptoms occur, or if the painful area is red or swollen, consult a doctor. These could be signs of serious illness. If you are under a doctor's care for any serious condition, consult a doctor before taking this product. As with aspirin and acetaminophen, if you have any condition which requires you to take prescription drugs or if you have had any problems or serious side effects from taking any non-prescription pain reliever, do not take this product without first discussing it with your doctor. If you experience any symptoms which are unusual or seem unrelated to the condition for which you took ibuprofen, consult a doctor before taking any more of it. Although ibuprofen is indicated for the same conditions as aspirin and acetaminophen, it should not be taken with them except under a doctor's direction. Do not combine this product with any other ibuprofen containing product. As with any drug, if you are pregnant or nursing a

baby, seek the advice of a health professional before using this product. IT IS ESPECIALLY IMPORTANT NOT TO USE IBUPROFEN DURING THE LAST 3 MONTHS OF PREGNANCY UNLESS SPECIFICALLY DIRECTED TO DO SO BY A DOCTOR BECAUSE IT MAY CAUSE PROBLEMS IN THE UNBORN CHILD OR COMPLICATIONS DURING DELIVERY. Keep this and all drugs out of the reach of children.

Overdosage: In case of accidental overdose, contact a physician or poison control center.

Active Ingredient: Each MEDIPREN Caplet or Tablet contains ibuprofen 200 mg.

Inactive Ingredients: Colloidal silicon dioxide, glyceryl triacetate, hydroxypropyl methylcellulose, microcrystalline cellulose, pregelatinized starch, sodium lauryl sulfate, sodium starch glycolate, titanium dioxide, Red Dye #40.

Storage: Store at room temperature; avoid excessive heat 40°C (104°F).

How Supplied: Coated Caplets (colored white, imprinted "MEDIPREN")— bottles of 24's, 50's, 100's. Coated Tablets (colored white, imprinted "MEDIPREN")—bottles of 24's, 50's, 100's.

Shown in Product Identification Section, page 413

PEDIACARE® Cold Formula Liquid
PEDIACARE® Cough-Cold Formula Liquid and Chewable Tablets
PEDIACARE® Infants' Oral Decongestant Drops

PRODUCT OVERVIEW

Key Facts: PediaCare® Cold Relief Products are formulated specifically for relief of pediatric cold and cough symptoms. These products are formulated to allow accurate dosing by age and weight, especially when using the enclosed dropper or dosage cup.

Major Uses: PediaCare Infants' Oral Decongestant Drops provide 0.8ml per dropperful of pseudoephedrine hydrochloride for treatment of congestion in infants ages 3 and under. PediaCare Cold Formula Liquid provides 15mg of pseudoephedrine hydrochloride and 1mg of chlorphemiramine maleate per 5ml for treatment of congestion, runny nose and sneezing resulting from a cold or allergies in children ages 11 and under. PediaCare Cough-Cold Formula Liquid and Chewables treat all the above symptoms plus they contain 5mg of dextromethorphan hydrobromide per 5ml (or 2 tablets) for additional relief of coughs in children ages 11 and under. Recommended dosage schedules for PediaCare Infants' Drops, Cold Formula and Cough-Cold Formula are the same as recommended dosage schedules for Children's TYLENOL Infants' Drops, Elixir and Chewable Tablets, respectively.

Age Group	0–3 mos	4–11 mos	12–23 mos	2–3 yrs	4–5 yrs	6–8 yrs	9–10 yrs	11 yrs	Dosage
Weight (lbs)	6–11 lb	12–17 lb	18–23 lb	24–35 lb	36–47 lb	48–59 lb	60–71 lb	72–95 lb	
PEDIACARE Infants' Drops*	½ dropper (0.4 ml)	1 dropper (0.8 ml)	1½ droppers (1.2 ml)	2 droppers (1.6 ml)					q4–6h
PEDIACARE Cold Formula Liquid**				1 tsp	1½ tsp	2 tsp	2½ tsp	3 tsp	q4–6h
PEDIACARE Cough-Cold Formula Liquid**				1 tsp	1½ tsp	2 tsp	2½ tsp	3 tsp	q4–6h
Chewable Tablets**				2 tabs	3 tabs	4 tabs	5 tabs	6 tabs	q4–6h

*administer to children under 2 years only on the advice of a physician
**administer to children under 6 years only on the advice of a physician

PRODUCT INFORMATION

PEDIACARE® Cold Formula Liquid
PEDIACARE® Cough-Cold Formula Liquid and Chewable Tablets
PEDIACARE® Infants' Oral Decongestant Drops

Description: Each 5 ml of PEDIACARE Cold Formula Liquid contains pseudoephedrine hydrochloride 15 mg and chlorpheniramine maleate 1 mg. Each 5 ml of PEDIACARE Cough-Cold Formula Liquid contains pseudoephedrine hydrochloride 15 mg, chlorpheniramine maleate 1 mg and dextromethorphan hydrobromide 5 mg. Each PEDIACARE Cough-Cold Formula Chewable Tablet contains pseudoephedrine hydrochloride 7.5 mg, chlorpheniramine maleate 0.5 mg and dextromethorphan hydrobromide 2.5 mg. Each 0.8 ml oral dropper of PEDIACARE Infants' Oral Decongestant Drops contains pseudoephedrine hydrochloride 7.5 mg. PEDIACARE Liquid Products and Infants' Drops are stable, cherry flavored and red in color. PEDIACARE Cough-Cold Formula Chewable Tablets are fruit flavored and pink in color.

Actions and Indications: PEDIACARE Cold Products are available in three different formulas, allowing you to select the ideal cold product to temporarily relieve the patient's cold symptoms. PEDIACARE Cold Formula Liquid contains a decongestant, pseudoephedrine hydrochloride, and an antihistamine, chlorpheniramine maleate, to provide temporary relief of nasal congestion, runny nose and sneezing due to the common cold, hay fever or other upper respiratory allergies. PEDIACARE Cough-Cold Formula Liquid and Chewable Tablets contain both of the above ingredients plus a cough suppressant, dextromethorphan hydrobromide, to provide temporary relief of nasal congestion, runny nose, sneezing and coughing due to the common cold, hay fever or other upper respiratory allergies. PEDIACARE Infants' Oral Decongestant Drops contain a decongestant, pseudoephedrine hydrochloride, to provide temporary relief of nasal congestion due to the common cold, hay fever or other upper respiratory allergies.

Professional Dosage: A calibrated dosage cup is provided for accurate dosing of the PEDIACARE Liquid formulas. A calibrated oral dropper is provided for accurate dosing of PEDIACARE Infants' Drops. All doses of PEDIACARE Cold Formula Liquid, PEDIACARE Cough-Cold Formula Liquid and Chewable Tablets and PEDIACARE Infants' Drops may be repeated every 4–6 hours, not to exceed 4 doses in 24 hours.
[See table above].

Note: Since PEDIACARE cold products are available without prescription, the following information appears on the package labels: "WARNINGS: Do not use if carton is opened, or if printed plastic bottle wrap or foil inner seal is broken. Keep this and all medication out of the reach of children. In case of accidental overdosage, contact a physician or poison control center immediately."
The following information appears on the appropriate package labels:
PEDIACARE Cold Formula Liquid: "Do not exceed the recommended dosage because nervousness, dizziness or sleeplessness may occur. If symptoms do not improve within seven days or are accompanied by fever, consult a physician before continuing use. This preparation may cause drowsiness, or in some cases, excitability. Do not give this product to children who have heart disease, high blood pressure, thyroid disease, diabetes, glaucoma or asthma, or are taking a prescription drug for high blood pressure or depression, except under the advise and supervision of a physician."
"Inactive Ingredients: Benzoic acid, citric acid, flavors, glycerin, polyethylene glycol, propylene glycol, sodium benzoate, sorbitol, sucrose, purified water, Red #33, Blue #1 and Red #40.
PEDIACARE Cough-Cold Formula Liquid and Chewable Tablets: "Do not exceed the recommended dosage because nervousness, dizziness or sleeplessness may occur. A persistent cough may be a sign of a serious condition. If symptoms do not improve within seven days, tend to recur, or are accompanied by fever, rash, excessive mucus, persistent cough or headache, consult a physician before continuing use. This preparation may cause drowsiness or, in some cases, excitability. Do not give this product to children who have heart disease, high blood pressure, thyroid disease, diabetes, glaucoma or asthma, or are taking a prescription drug for high blood pressure or depression, except under the advice and supervision of a physician."
PEDIACARE Cough-Cold Formula Liquid: Inactive Ingredients: Benzoic acid, citric acid, flavors, glycerin, polyethylene glycol, propylene glycol, sodium benzoate, sorbitol, sucrose, purified water, Red #33, Blue #1 and Red #40.
PEDIACARE Cough-Cold Formula Chewable Tablets also contain the warning, "Phenylketonurics: contains phenylalanine 3 mg per tablet", and the inactive ingredient listing, "Inactive Ingredients: Aspartame, cellulose, citric acid, dextrose, flavors, magnesium stearate, magnesium trisilicate, mannitol, starch, sucrose and Red #3."
PEDIACARE Infants' Oral Decongestant Drops: "Do not exceed the recommended dosage because at higher doses nervousness, dizziness or sleeplessness may occur. Do not give this product to children who have heart disease, high blood pressure, thyroid disease or diabetes unless directed by a physician. Do not give this product to children for more than seven days. If symptoms do not improve or are accompanied by fever, consult a physician. Do not give this product to children who are taking a prescription drug for high blood pressure or depression without first consulting a physician. Take by mouth only. Not for nasal use."
"Inactive Ingredients: Benzoic acid, citric acid, flavors, glycerin, polyethylene glycol, propylene glycol, purified water, sodium benzoate, sorbitol, sucrose and Red #40."

Overdosage: Acute dextromethorphan overdose usually does not result in serious signs and symptoms unless massive amounts have been ingested. Signs and symptoms of a substantial overdose may include nausea and vomiting, visual disturbances, CNS disturbances, and urinary retention. Symptoms from pseudoephedrine overdose consist most often of mild anxiety, tachycardia and/or mild hypertension. Symptoms usually appear within 4 to 8 hours of ingestion and are transient, usually requiring no treatment. Chlorpheniramine toxicity should be treated as you would an antihistamine/anticholinergic overdose and is likely to be present within a few hours after acute ingestion.

How Supplied: PEDIACARE Liquid products (colored red)—bottles of 4 fl. oz with child-resistant safety cap and calibrated dosage cup. PEDIACARE Cough-Cold Formula Chewable Tablets (pink, scored)—bottles of 24 with child-resistant safety cap. PEDIACARE Infants' Drops (colored red)—bottles of ½ fl. oz with calibrated dropper.

Shown in Product Identification Section, page 413

Continued on next page

McNeil Consumer—Cont.

SINE–AID®
Sinus Headache Tablets

Description: Each SINE-AID® Tablet contains acetaminophen 325 mg and pseudoephedrine hydrochloride 30 mg.

Actions: SINE-AID® Tablets contain a clinically proven analgesic-antipyretic and a decongestant. Acetaminophen produces analgesia by elevation of the pain threshold and antipyresis through action on the hypothalamic heat-regulating center. Pseudoephedrine hydrochloride is a sympathomimetic amine which promotes sinus cavity drainage by reducing nasopharyngeal mucosal congestion.

Indications: SINE-AID® Tablets provide effective symptomatic relief from sinus headache pain and pressure caused by sinusitis.

Adverse Reactions: While acetaminophen is equal to aspirin in analgesic and antipyretic effectiveness, it is unlikely to produce many of the side effects associated with aspirin and aspirin-containing products. Since the product contains no antihistamine, SINE-AID® Tablets will not produce the drowsiness that may interfere with work, driving an automobile or operating dangerous machinery. SINE-AID® is particularly well-suited in patients with aspirin allergy, hemostatic disturbances (including anticoagulant therapy), and bleeding diatheses (e.g. hemophilia) and upper gastrointestinal disease (e.g. ulcer, gastritis, hiatus hernia). If a rare sensitivity occurs, the drug should be discontinued. Although pseudoephedrine is virtually without pressor effect in normotensive patients, it should be used with caution in hypertensives.

Usual Dosage: Adult dosage: Two tablets every four to six hours. Do not exceed eight tablets in any 24 hour period. **Note:** Since SINE-AID® tablets are available without a prescription, the following appears on the package labels: "**WARNING:** Do not exceed the recommended dosage because at higher doses nervousness, dizziness or sleeplessness may occur. Do not administer to children under 12. If you have high blood pressure, heart disease, diabetes, thyroid disease, difficulty in urination due to enlargement of the prostate gland, or are presently taking a prescription drug for the treatment of high blood pressure or depression, do not take except under the advice and supervision of a physician. Do not take this product for more than 7 days. If symptoms do not improve or are accompanied by high fever, consult a physician. **Do not use if carton is opened, or printed foil inner seal is broken. Keep this and all medication out of the reach of children. As with any drug, if you are pregnant or nursing a baby, seek the advice of a health professional before using this product. In case of accidental overdosage, contact a physician or poison control center immediately.**"

Overdosage: Acetaminophen in massive overdosage may cause hepatic toxicity in some patients. In adults and adolescents, hepatic toxicity has rarely been reported following ingestion of acute overdoses of less than 10 grams. Fatalities are infrequent (less than 3–4% of untreated cases) and have rarely been reported with overdoses of less than 15 grams. In children, an acute overdosage of less than 150 mg/kg has not been associated with hepatic toxicity.

Early symptoms following a potentially hepatotoxic overdose may include: nausea, vomiting, diaphoresis and general malaise. Clinical and laboratory evidence of hepatic toxicity may not be apparent until 48 to 72 hours postingestion. In adults and adolescents, regardless of the quantity of acetaminophen reported to have been ingested, administer MUCOMYST® acetylcysteine immediately if 24 hours or less have elapsed from the reported time of ingestion. For full prescribing information, refer to the MUCOMYST package insert. Do not await results of assays for acetaminophen level before initiating treatment with MUCOMYST acetylcysteine. The following additional procedures are recommended: The stomach should be emptied promptly by lavage or by induction of emesis with syrup of ipecac. A serum acetaminophen assay should be obtained as early as possible, but no sooner than four hours following ingestion. Liver function studies should be obtained initially and repeated at 24-hour intervals.

Serious toxicity or fatalities are extremely infrequent in children, possibly due to differences in the way they metabolize acetaminophen. In children, the maximum potential amount ingested can be more easily estimated. If more than 150 mg/kg or an unknown amount was ingested, obtain an acetaminophen plasma level. The acetaminophen plasma level should be obtained as soon as possible, but no sooner than 4 hours following the ingestion. Induce emesis using syrup of ipecac. If the plasma level is obtained and falls above the broken line on the nomogram, the MUCOMYST acetylcysteine therapy should be initiated and continued for a full course of therapy. If acetaminophen plasma assay capability is not available, and the estimated acetaminophen ingestion exceeds 150 mg/kg, MUCOMYST acetylcysteine therapy should be initiated and continued for a full course of therapy.

For additional emergency information, call your regional poison center or toll-free (1-800-525-6115) to the Rocky Mountain Poison Center for assistance in diagnosis and for directions in the use of MUCOMYST acetylcysteine as an antidote.

Symptoms from pseudoephedrine overdose consist most often of mild anxiety, tachycardia and/or mild hypertension. Symptoms usually appear within 4 to 8 hours of ingestion and are transient, usually requiring no treatment.

Inactive Ingredients: Cellulose, Sodium Lauryl Sulfate, Starch, Magnesium Stearate.

How Supplied: Tablets (colored white, imprinted "SINE-AID®")—tamper-resistant bottles of 24, 50 and 100.

Shown in Product Identification Section, page 413

MAXIMUM STRENGTH SINE–AID®
Sinus Headache Caplets

Description: Each MAXIMUM STRENGTH SINE-AID® Caplet contains acetaminophen 500 mg and pseudoephedrine hydrochloride 30 mg.

Actions: MAXIMUM STRENGTH SINE-AID® Caplets contain a clinically proven analgesic-antipyretic and a decongestant. Maximum allowable nonprescription levels of acetaminophen and pseudophedrine provide temporary relief of sinus congestion and pain. Acetaminophen produces analgesia by elevation of the pain threshold and antipyresis through action on the hypothalamic heat-regulating center. Pseudoephedrine hydrochloride is a sympathomimetic amine which promotes sinus cavity drainage by reducing nasopharyngeal mucosal congestion.

Indications: MAXIMUM STRENGTH SINE-AID® Caplets provide effective symptomatic relief from sinus headache pain and pressure caused by sinusitis.

Adverse Reactions: While acetaminophen is equal to aspirin in analgesic and antipyretic effectiveness, it is unlikely to produce many of the side effects associated with aspirin and aspirin-containing products. Since the product contains no antihistamine, MAXIMUM STRENGTH SINE-AID® Caplets will not produce the drowsiness that may interfere with work, driving an automobile or operating dangerous machinery. SINE-AID® is particularly well-suited in patients with aspirin allergy, hemostatic disturbances (including anticoagulant therapy), and bleeding diatheses (e.g. hemophilia) and upper gastrointestinal disease (e.g. ulcer, gastritis, hiatus hernia). If a rare sensitivity occurs, the drug should be discontinued. Although pseudoephedrine is virtually without pressor effect in normotensive patients, it should be used with caution in hypertensives.

Usual Dosage: Adult dosage: Two caplets every four to six hours. Do not exceed eight caplets in any 24 hour period. **Note:** Since MAXIMUM STRENGTH SINE-AID® Caplets are available without a prescription, the following appears on the package labels: "**WARNING:** Do not exceed the recommended dosage because at higher doses nervousness, dizziness or sleeplessness may occur. Do not administer to children under 12. If you have high blood pressure, heart disease, diabetes, thyroid disease, difficulty in urination due to enlargement of the prostate gland, or are presently taking a pre-

scription drug for the treatment of high blood pressure or depression, do not take except under the advice and supervision of a physician. Do not take this product for more than 7 days. If symptoms do not improve or are accompanied by high fever, consult a physician. **Do not use if carton is opened, or if printed red neck wrap or printed foil inner seal is broken. Keep this and all medication out of the reach of children. As with any drug, if you are pregnant or nursing a baby, seek the advice of a health professional before using this product. In case of accidental overdosage, contact a physician or poison control center immediately."**

Overdosage: Acetaminophen in massive overdosage may cause hepatic toxicity in some patients. In adults and adolescents, hepatic toxicity has rarely been reported following ingestion of acute overdoses of less than 10 grams. Fatalities are infrequent (less than 3–4% of untreated cases) and have rarely been reported with overdoses of less than 15 grams. In children, an acute overdosage of less than 150 mg/kg has not been associated with hepatic toxicity.

Early symptoms following a potentially hepatotoxic overdose may include: nausea, vomiting, diaphoresis and general malaise. Clinical and laboratory evidence of hepatic toxicity may not be apparent until 48 to 72 hours postingestion. In adults and adolescents, regardless of the quantity of acetaminophen reported to have been ingested, administer MUCOMYST® acetylcysteine immediately if 24 hours or less have elapsed from the reported time of ingestion. For full prescribing information, refer to the MUCOMYST package insert. Do not await results of assays for acetaminophen level before initiating treatment with MUCOMYST acetylcysteine. The following additional procedures are recommended: The stomach should be emptied promptly by lavage or by induction of emesis with syrup of ipecac. A serum acetaminophen assay should be obtained as early as possible, but no sooner than four hours following ingestion. Liver function studies should be obtained initially and repeated at 24-hour intervals.

Serious toxicity or fatalities are extremely infrequent in children, possibly due to differences in the way they metabolize acetaminophen. In children, the maximum potential amount ingested can be more easily estimated. If more than 150 mg/kg or an unknown amount was ingested, obtain an acetaminophen plasma level. The acetaminophen plasma level should be obtained as soon as possible, but no sooner than 4 hours following the ingestion. Induce emesis using syrup of ipecac. If the plasma level is obtained and falls above the broken line on the nomogram, the MUCOMYST acetylcysteine therapy should be initiated and continued for a full course of therapy. If acetaminophen plasma assay capability is not available, and the estimated acetaminophen ingestion exceeds 150 mg/kg, MUCOMYST acetylcysteine

therapy should be initiated and continued for a full course of therapy.

For additional emergency information, call your regional poison center or toll-free (1-800-525-6115) to the Rocky Mountain Poison Center for assistance in diagnosis and for directions in the use of MUCOMYST acetylcysteine as an antidote.

Symptoms from pseudoephedrine overdose consist most often of mild anxiety, tachycardia and/or mild hypertension. Symptoms usually appear within 4 to 8 hours of ingestion and are transient, usually requiring no treatment.

Inactive Ingredients: Cellulose, hydroxypropyl methylcellulose, magnesium stearate, polyethylene glycol, sodium starch glycolate, starch, titanium dioxide, Blue #1 and Red #40.

How Supplied: Caplets (colored white imprinted "Maximum SINE-AID") —tamper-resistant bottles of 24 and 50.

Shown in Product Identification Section, page 413

CHILDREN'S TYLENOL®
acetaminophen
Chewable Tablets, Elixir, Drops

Description: Each Children's TYLENOL Chewable Tablet contains 80 mg. acetaminophen in a fruit or grape flavored tablet. Children's TYLENOL acetaminophen Elixir is stable and alcohol free, cherry flavored is red in color grape flavored purple in color. Infants' TYLENOL Drops are stable, fruit flavored, orange in color and are alcohol free.
Children's TYLENOL Elixir: Each 5 ml. contains 160 mg. acetaminophen.
Infant's TYLENOL Drops: Each 0.8 ml. (one calibrated dropperful) contains 80 mg. acetaminophen.

Actions: Acetaminophen is a clinically proven analgesic/antipyretic. Acetaminophen produces analgesia by elevation of the pain threshold and antipyresis through action on the hypothalamic heat regulating center.

Indications: Children's TYLENOL Chewable Tablets, Elixir and Drops are designed for treatment of infants and children with conditions requiring reduction of fever or relief of pain—such as mild upper respiratory infections (tonsillitis, common cold, "grippe"), headache, myalgia, post-immunization reactions, post-tonsillectomy discomfort and gastroenteritis. TYLENOL acetaminophen is useful as an analgesic and antipyretic in many bacterial or viral infections, such as bronchitis, pharyngitis, tracheobronchitis, sinusitis, pneumonia, otitis media, and cervical adenitis.

Adverse Reactions: While acetaminophen is equal to aspirin in analgesic and antipyretic effectiveness, it is unlikely to produce many of the side effects associated with aspirin and aspirin containing products. If a rare sensitivity reaction occurs, the drug should be stopped.

Usual Dosage: Doses may be repeated 4 or 5 times daily, but not to exceed 5

doses in 24 hours. Administer to children under 2 years only on the advice of a physician. Children's TYLENOL Chewable Tablets: 2–3 years: two tablets. 4–5 years: three tablets, 6–8 years: four tablets. 9–10 years: five tablets. 11–12 years: six tablets.
Children's TYLENOL Elixir: (special cup for measuring dosage is provided) 4–11 months: one-half teaspoon. 12–23 months: three-quarters teaspoon, 2–3 years: one teaspoon. 4–5 years: one and one-half teaspoons. 6–8 years: 2 teaspoons. 9–10 years: two and one-half teaspoons. 11–12 years: three teaspoons.
Infants' TYLENOL Drops: 0–3 months: 0.4 ml. 4–11 months: 0.8 ml. 12–23 months: 1.2 ml. 2–3 years: 1.6 ml. 4–5 years: 2.4 ml.

Warning: Keep this and all medication out of reach of children. In case of accidental overdose, contact a physician or poison control center immediately. Consult your physician if fever persists for more than 3 days or if pain continues for more than 5 days. See bottom panel of carton for expiration date. Store at room temperature.
NOTE: In addition to the above:
Children's TYLENOL® Drops—Do not use if printed carton overwrap or printed plastic bottle wrap is broken or missing or if carton is opened.
Children's TYLENOL Elixir—Do not use if printed carton overwrap is broken or missing or if carton is opened. Do not use if printed plastic bottle wrap or printed foil inner seal is broken. Not a USP elixir.
Children's TYLENOL Chewables—Do not use if carton is opened or if printed plastic bottle wrap or printed foil inner seal is broken. Phenylketonurics: contains phenylalanine 3mg per tablet.

Overdosage: Acetaminophen in massive overdosage may cause hepatic toxicity in some patients. In adults and adolescents, hepatic toxicity has rarely been reported following ingestion of acute overdoses of less than 10 grams. Fatalities are infrequent (less than 3–4% of untreated cases) and have rarely been reported with overdoses of less than 15 grams. In children, an acute overdosage of less than 150 mg/kg has not been associated with hepatic toxicity.

Early symptoms following a potentially hepatotoxic overdose may include: nausea, vomiting, diaphoresis and general malaise. Clinical and laboratory evidence of hepatic toxicity may not be apparent until 48 to 72 hours postingestion. In adults and adolescents, regardless of the quantity of acetaminophen reported to have been ingested, administer MUCOMYST® acetylcysteine immediately if 24 hours or less have elapsed from the reported time of ingestion. For full prescribing information, refer to the MUCOMYST package insert. Do not await results of assays for acetaminophen level before initiating treatment with MUCOMYST acetylcysteine. The following additional procedures are

Continued on next page

McNeil Consumer—Cont.

recommended: The stomach should be emptied promptly by lavage or by induction of emesis with syrup of ipecac. A serum acetaminophen assay should be obtained as early as possible, but no sooner than four hours following ingestion. Liver function studies should be obtained initially and repeated at 24-hour intervals.

Serious toxicity or fatalities are extremely infrequent in children, possibly due to differences in the way they metabolize acetaminophen. In children, the maximum potential amount ingested can be more easily estimated. If more than 150 mg/kg or an unknown amount was ingested, obtain an acetaminophen plasma level. The acetaminophen plasma level should be obtained as soon as possible, but no sooner than 4 hours following the ingestion. Induce emesis using syrup of ipecac. If the plasma level is obtained and falls above the broken line on the nomogram, the MUCOMYST acetylcysteine therapy should be initiated and continued for a full course of therapy. If acetaminophen plasma assay capability is not available, and the estimated acetaminophen ingestion exceeds 150 mg/kg, MUCOMYST acetylcysteine therapy should be initiated and continued for a full course of therapy.

For additional emergency information, call your regional poison center or toll-free (1-800-525-6115) to the Rocky Mountain Poison Center for assistance in diagnosis and for directions in the use of MUCOMYST acetylcysteine as an antidote.

Inactive Ingredients: Children's Tylenol Chewable Tablets—Aspartame, Cellulose, Citric Acid, Ethylcellulose, Flavors, Hydroxypropyl Methylcellulose, Mannitol, Starch, Magnesium Stearate, Red #7 and Blue #1 (Grape only). Children's Tylenol Elixir—Benzoic Acid, Citric Acid, Flavors, Glycerin, Polyethylene Glycol, Propylene Glycol, Sodium Benzoate, Sorbitol, Sucrose, Purified Water, Red #40. In addition to the above ingredients cherry flavored elixir contains Red #33 and grape flavored elixir contains malic acid and Blue #1. Infant's Tylenol Drops—Flavors, Propylene Glycol, Saccharin, Purified Water, Yellow #6.

How Supplied: Chewable Tablets (pink colored fruit, purple colored grape, scored, imprinted "TYLENOL")—Bottles of 30 and child resistant blister packs of 48 (fruit only). Elixir (cherry colored red and grape colored purple)—bottles of 2 and 4 fl. oz. Drops (colored orange)—bottles of ½ oz. (15 ml.) with calibrated plastic dropper.

All packages listed above have child resistant safety caps.

Shown in Product Identification Section, page 413

Junior Strength TYLENOL®
acetaminophen
Coated Caplets

Description: Each Junior Strength Caplet contains 160mg acetaminophen in a small, coated, capsule shaped tablet.

Actions: Acetaminophen is a clinically proven analgesic/antipyretic. Acetaminophen produces analgesia by elevation of the pain threshold and antipyresis through action on the hypothalamic heat-regulating center.

Indications: Junior Strength TYLENOL Caplets are designed for older children and young adults with conditions requiring reduction of fever or relief of pain—such as mild upper respiratory infections (tonsillitis, common cold, "grippe"), headache, myalgia, post-immunization reactions, post-tonsillectomy discomfort and gastroenteritis. TYLENOL acetaminophen is useful as an analgesic and antipyretic in many bacterial or viral infections, such as bronchitis, pharyngitis, tracheobronchitis, sinusitis, pneumonia, otitis media and cervical adenitis.

Adverse Reactions: While acetaminophen is equal to aspirin in analgesic and antipyretic effectiveness, it is unlikely to produce many of the side effects associated with aspirin and aspirin-containing products. If a rare sensitivity reaction occurs, the drug should be stopped.

Usual Dosage: Doses may be repeated 4 or 5 times daily, but not to exceed 5 doses in 24 hours each. For ages: 6–8 years: two Caplets, 9–10 years: two and one-half Caplets, 11 years: three Caplets, 12–14 years: four Caplets.
Note: Since Junior Strength TYLENOL acetaminophen Caplets are available without a prescription as an analgesic, the following appears on the package labels:

Warnings: Do not use if carton is opened or if a blister unit is broken. Keep this and all medications out of the reach of children. In case of accidental overdosage, contact a physician or poison control center immediately. Consult your physician if fever persists for more than three days or if pain continues for more than five days. As with any drugs, if you are pregnant or nursing a baby, seek the advice of a health professional before using this product. Not for children who have difficulty swallowing tablets.

Overdosage: Acetaminophen in massive overdosage may cause hepatic toxicity in some patients. In adults and adolescents, hepatic toxicity has rarely been reported following ingestion of acute overdosage of less than 10 grams. Fatalities are infrequent (less than 3–4% of untreated cases) and have rarely been reported with overdoses of less than 15 grams. In children, an acute overdosage of less than 150 mg/kg has not been associated with hepatic toxicity.
Early symptoms following a potentially hepatotoxic overdose may include: nausea, vomiting, diaphoresis and general malaise. Clinical and laboratory evidence of hepatic toxicity may not be ap-

parent until 48 to 72 hours postingestion. In adults and adolescents, regardless of the quantity of acetaminophen reported to have been ingested, administer MUCOMYST® acetylcysteine immediately if 24 hours or less have elapsed from the reported time of ingestion. For full prescribing information, refer to the MUCOMYST package insert. Do not await the results of assays for acetaminophen level before initiating treatment with MUCOMYST acetylcysteine. The following additional procedures are recommended: The stomach should be emptied promptly by lavage or by induction of emesis with syrup of ipecac. A serum acetaminophen assay should be obtained as early as possible, but no sooner than four hours following ingestion. Liver function studies should be obtained initially and repeated at 24-hour intervals.

Serious toxicity or fatalities are extremely infrequent in children, possibly due to differences in the way they metabolize acetaminophen. In children, the maximum potential amount ingested can be more easily estimated. If more than 150 mg/kg or an unknown amount was ingested, obtain an acetaminophen plasma level. The acetaminophen plasma level should be obtained as soon as possible, but no sooner than 4 hours following the ingestion. Induce emesis using syrup of ipecac. If the plasma level is obtained and falls above the broken line on the nomogram, the MUCOMYST acetylcysteine therapy should be initiated and continued for a full course of therapy. If acetaminophen plasma assay capability is not available, and the estimated acetaminophen ingestion exceeds 150 mg/kg, MUCOMYST acetylcysteine therapy should be initiated and continued for a full course of therapy.

For additional emergency information, call your regional poison center or toll-free (1-800-525-6115) to the Rocky Mountain Poison Center for assistance in diagnosis and for directions in the use of MUCOMYST acetylcysteine as an antidote.

Inactive Ingredients: Cellulose, Ethylcellulose, Magnesium Stearate, Sodium Lauryl Sulfate, Sodium Starch Glycolate, Starch.

How Supplied: Coated Caplets, (colored white, coated, scored, imprinted "TYLENOL 160"). Package of 30. All packages are safety sealed and use child resistant blister packaging.

Shown in Product Identification Section, page 413

Regular Strength
TYLENOL® acetaminophen
Tablets and Caplets

Description: Each Regular Strength TYLENOL Tablet or Caplet contains acetaminophen 325 mg.

Actions: Acetaminophen is a clinically proven analgesic and antipyretic. Acetaminophen produces analgesia by elevation of the pain threshold and antipyre-

sis through action on the hypothalamic heat-regulating center.

Indications: Acetaminophen provides effective analgesia in a wide variety of arthritic and rheumatic conditions involving musculoskeletal pain, as well as in other painful disorders such as headache, dysmenorrhea, myalgias and neuralgias. In addition, Acetaminophen is indicated as an analgesic and antipyretic in diseases accompanied by discomfort and fever, such as the common cold and other viral infections. Acetaminophen is particularly well suited as an analgesic-antipyretic in the presence of aspirin allergy, hemostatic disturbances (including anticoagulant therapy), and bleeding diatheses (e.g., hemophilia) and upper gastrointestinal disease (e.g., ulcer, gastritis, hiatus hernia).

Precautions and Adverse Reactions: While acetaminophen is equal to aspirin in analgesic and antipyretic effectiveness, it is unlikely to produce many of the side effects associated with aspirin and aspirin-containing products. If a rare sensitivity reaction occurs, the drug should be discontinued.

Usual Dosage: Adults: One to two tablets or caplets every 4–6 hours. Not to exceed 12 tablets or caplets per day. Children (6 to 12): One-half to one tablet 3 or 4 times daily. (Junior Strength TYLENOL acetaminophen Swallowable Tablets, Chewable Tablets, Elixir and Drops are available for greater convenience in younger patients).
Note: Since TYLENOL acetaminophen tablets and caplets are available without prescription as an analgesic, the following appears on the package labels: "Caution: If pain persists for more than 10 days, or redness is present, or in arthritic or rheumatic conditions affecting children under 12 years, consult a physician immediately."
"WARNING: Do not use if printed red neck wrap or printed foil inner seal is broken. Keep this and all medications out of the reach of children. As with any drug, if you are pregnant or nursing a baby, seek the advice of a health professional before using this product. In case of accidental overdosage, contact a physician or poison control center immediately."

Overdosage: Acetaminophen in massive overdosage may cause hepatic toxicity in some patients. In adults and adolescents, hepatic toxicity has rarely been reported following ingestion of acute overdoses of less than 10 grams. Fatalities are infrequent (less than 3–4% of untreated cases) and have rarely been reported with overdoses of less than 15 grams. In children, an acute overdosage of less than 150 mg/kg has not been associated with hepatic toxicity.
Early symptoms following a potentially hepatotoxic overdose may include: nausea, vomiting, diaphoresis and general malaise. Clinical and laboratory evidence of hepatic toxicity may not be apparent until 48 to 72 hours postingestion. In adults and adolescents, regardless of the quantity of acetaminophen reported to have been ingested, administer MUCOMYST® acetylcysteine immediately if 24 hours or less have elapsed from the reported time of ingestion. For full prescribing information, refer to the MUCOMYST package insert. Do not await results of assays for acetaminophen level before initiating treatment with MUCOMYST acetylcysteine. The following additional procedures are recommended: The stomach should be emptied promptly by lavage or by induction of emesis with syrup of ipecac. A serum acetaminophen assay should be obtained as early as possible, but no sooner than four hours following ingestion. Liver function studies should be obtained initially and repeated at 24-hour intervals.
Serious toxicity or fatalities are extremely infrequent in children, possibly due to differences in the way they metabolize acetaminophen. In children, the maximum potential amount ingested can be more easily estimated. If more than 150 mg/kg or an unknown amount was ingested, obtain an acetaminophen plasma level. The acetaminophen plasma level should be obtained as soon as possible, but no sooner than 4 hours following the ingestion. Induce emesis using syrup of ipecac. If the plasma level is obtained and falls above the broken line on the nomogram, the MUCOMYST acetylcysteine therapy should be initiated and continued for a full course of therapy. If acetaminophen plasma assay capability is not available, and the estimated acetaminophen ingestion exceeds 150 mg/kg, MUCOMYST acetylcysteine therapy should be initiated and continued for a full course of therapy.
For additional emergency information, call your regional poison center or toll-free (1-800-525-6115) to the Rocky Mountain Poison Center for assistance in diagnosis and for directions in the use of MUCOMYST acetylcysteine as an antidote.

Inactive Ingredients: Tablets—Calcium Stearate or Magnesium Stearate, Cellulose, Docusate Sodium and Sodium Benzoate or Sodium Lauryl Sulfate, and Starch. Caplets—Cellulose, Hydroxpropyl Methylcellulose, Magnesium Stearate, Polyethylene Glycol, Sodium Starch Glycolate and Starch.

How Supplied: Tablets (colored white, scored, imprinted "TYLENOL")—tins and vials of 12, and tamper-resistant bottles of 24, 50, 100 and 200. Caplets (colored white, "TYLENOL")—tamper-resistant bottles of 24, 50, 100.

Also Available: For additional pain relief, Extra-Strength TYLENOL® Tablets and Caplets, 500 mg, and Extra-Strength TYLENOL® Adult Liquid Pain Reliever (colored green; 1 fl. oz. = 1000 mg.)

Shown in Product Identification Section, page 413

**Extra-Strength
TYLENOL® acetaminophen
Caplets, Gelcaps, Tablets**

Description: Each Extra-Strength TYLENOL Caplet, Gelcap or Tablet contains acetaminophen 500 mg.

Actions: Acetaminophen is a clinically proven analgesic and antipyretic. Acetaminophen produces analgesia by elevation of the pain threshold and antipyresis through action on the hypothalamic heat-regulating center.

Indications: For relief of pain and fever. Extra-Strength TYLENOL acetaminophen provides increased analgesic strength for minor conditions when the usual doses of mild analgesics are insufficient.

Precautions and Adverse Reactions: While acetaminophen is equal to aspirin in analgesic and antipyretic effectiveness, it is unlikely to produce many of the side effects associated with aspirin and aspirin-containing products. If a rare sensitivity reaction occurs, the drug should be discontinued.

Usual Dosage: Adults: Two Caplets, Gelcaps or Tablets 3 or 4 times daily. No more than a total of eight Caplets, Gelcaps or Tablets in any 24-hour period.
Note: Since Extra-Strength TYLENOL acetaminophen is available without a prescription, the following appears on the package labels: "Severe or recurrent pain or high or continued fever may be indicative of serious illness. Under these conditions, consult a physician. **WARNING: Do not use if printed red neck wrap or printed foil inner seal is broken. Keep this and all medication out of the reach of children. As with any drug, if you are pregnant or nursing a baby, seek the advice of a health professional before using this product. In case of accidental overdosage, contact a physician or poison control center immediately."**

Overdosage: Acetaminophen in massive overdosage may cause hepatic toxicity in some patients. In adults and adolescents, hepatic toxicity has rarely been reported following ingestion of acute overdosage of less than 10 grams. Fatalities are infrequent (less than 3–4% of untreated cases) and have rarely been reported with overdoses of less than 15 grams. In children, an acute overdosage of less than 150 mg/kg has not been associated with hepatic toxicity.
Early symptoms following a potentially hepatotoxic overdose may include: nausea, vomiting, diaphoresis and general malaise. Clinical and laboratory evidence of hepatic toxicity may not be apparent until 48 to 72 hours postingestion. In adults and adolescents, regardless of the quantity of acetaminophen reported to have been ingested, administer MUCOMYST® acetylcysteine immediately if 24 hours or less have elapsed from the reported time of ingestion. For full prescribing information, refer to the MUCOMYST package insert. Do not

Continued on next page

McNeil Consumer—Cont.

await the results of assays for acetaminophen level before initiating treatment with MUCOMYST acetylcysteine. The following additional procedures are recommended: The stomach should be emptied promptly by lavage or by induction of emesis with syrup of ipecac. A serum acetaminophen assay should be obtained as early as possible, but no sooner than four hours following ingestion. Liver function studies should be obtained initially and repeated at 24-hour intervals.

Serious toxicity or fatalities are extremely infrequent in children, possibly due to differences in the way they metabolize acetaminophen. In children, the maximum potential amount ingested can be more easily estimated. If more than 150 mg/kg or an unknown amount was ingested, obtain an acetaminophen plasma level. The acetaminophen plasma level should be obtained as soon as possible, but no sooner than 4 hours following the ingestion. Induce emesis using syrup of ipecac. If the plasma level is obtained and falls above the broken line on the nomogram, the MUCOMYST acetylcysteine therapy should be initiated and continued for a full course of therapy. If acetaminophen plasma assay capability is not available, and the estimated acetaminophen ingestion exceeds 150 mg/kg, MUCOMYST acetylcysteine therapy should be initiated and continued for a full course of therapy.

For additional emergency information, call your regional poison center or toll-free (1-800-525-6115) to the Rocky Mountain Poison Center for assistance in diagnosis and for directions in the use of MUCOMYST acetylcysteine as an antidote.

Inactive Ingredients: Tablets—Calcium Stearate or Magnesium Stearate, Cellulose, Docusate Sodium and Sodium Benzoate or Sodium Lauryl Sulfate and Starch. Caplets—Cellulose, Hydroxypropyl Methylcellulose, Magnesium Stearate, Polyethylene Glycol, Sodium Starch Glycolate, Starch and Red #40. Gelcaps—Benzyl Alcohol, Butylparaben, Castor Oil, Cellulose, Edetate Calcium Disodium, Gelatin, Hydroxypropyl Methylcellulose, Magnesium Stearate, Methylparaben, Propylparaben, Sodium Lauryl Sulfate, Sodium Propionate, Sodium Starch Glycolate, Starch, Titanium Dioxide, Blue #1 and #2, Red #40 and Yellow #10.

How Supplied: Tablets (colored white, imprinted "TYLENOL" and "500")—vials of 10 and tamper-resistant bottles of 30, 60, 100, and 200. Caplets (colored white, imprinted "TYLENOL 500 mg")—vials of 10 and tamper-resistant bottles of 24, 50, 100, 175, and 250's. Gelcaps (colored yellow and red, imprinted "Tylenol 500" tamper-resistant bottles of 24, 50 and 100.

Also Available: For adults who prefer liquids or can't swallow solid medication, Extra-Strength TYLENOL® Adult Liquid Pain Reliever (colored green; 1 fl. oz. = 1000 mg.).

Shown in Product Identification Section, page 413

Extra-Strength TYLENOL® acetaminophen Adult Liquid Pain Reliever

Description: Each 15 ml. (½ fl. oz. or one tablespoonful) contains 500 mg. acetaminophen (alcohol 7%).

Actions: TYLENOL acetaminophen is a clinically proven analgesic and antipyretic. Acetaminophen produces analgesia by elevation of the pain threshold and antipyresis through action on the hypothalamic heat-regulating center.

Indications: TYLENOL acetaminophen provides fast, effective relief of pain and/or fever for adults who prefer liquids or can't swallow solid medication, e.g., the aged, patients with easily triggered gag reflexes, extremely sore throats, or those on liquid diets.

Precautions and Adverse Reactions: While acetaminophen is equal to aspirin in analgesic & antipyretic effectiveness, it is unlikely to produce many of the side effects associated with aspirin and aspirin-containing products. If a rare sensitivity reaction occurs, the drug should be discontinued.

Usual Dosage: Extra-Strength TYLENOL Adult Liquid Pain Reliever is an adult preparation. Not for use in children under 12. Measuring cup is marked for accurate dosage. Extra-Strength Dose—1 fl. oz. (30 ml or 2 tablespoonsful, 1000 mg), which is equivalent to two 500 mg Extra-Strength TYLENOL Tablets or Caplets. Take every 4–6 hours, no more than 4 doses in any 24-hour period.

Note: Since Extra-Strength TYLENOL Adult Liquid Pain Reliever is available without a prescription, the following appears on the package labels: "Severe or recurrent pain or high or continued fever may be indicative of serious illness. Under these conditions, consult a physician. **WARNING: Do not use if printed plastic overwrap or printed foil inner seal is broken. Keep this and all medication out of the reach of children. As with any drug, if you are pregnant or nursing a baby, seek the advice of a health professional before using this product. In case of accidental overdosage, contact a physician or poison control center immediately."**

Overdosage: Acetaminophen in massive overdosage may cause hepatic toxicity in some patients. In adults and adolescents, hepatic toxicity has rarely been reported following ingestion of acute overdosage of less than 10 grams. Fatalities are infrequent (less than 3–4% of untreated cases) and have rarely been reported with overdoses of less than 15 grams. In children, an acute overdosage of less than 150 mg/kg has not been associated with hepatic toxicity. Early symptoms following a potentially hepatotoxic overdose may include: nausea, vomiting, diaphoresis and general malaise. Clinical and laboratory evidence of hepatic toxicity may not be apparent until 48 to 72 hours postingestion. In adults and adolescents, regardless of the quantity of acetaminophen reported to have been ingested, administer MUCOMYST® acetylcysteine immediately if 24 hours or less have elapsed from the reported time of ingestion. For full prescribing information, refer to the MUCOMYST package insert. Do not await the results of assays for acetaminophen level before initiating treatment with MUCOMYST acetylcysteine. The following additional procedures are recommended: The stomach should be emptied promptly by lavage or by induction of emesis with syrup of ipecac. A serum acetaminophen assay should be obtained as early as possible, but no sooner than four hours following ingestion. Liver function studies should be obtained initially and repeated at 24-hour intervals.

Serious toxicity or fatalities are extremely infrequent in children, possibly due to differences in the way they metabolize acetaminophen. In children, the maximum potential amount ingested can be more easily estimated. If more than 150 mg/kg or an unknown amount was ingested, obtain an acetaminophen plasma level. The acetaminophen plasma level should be obtained as soon as possible, but no sooner than 4 hours following the ingestion. Induce emesis using syrup of ipecac. If the plasma level is obtained and falls above the broken line on the nomogram, the MUCOMYST acetylcysteine therapy should be initiated and continued for a full course of therapy. If acetaminophen plasma assay capability is not available, and the estimated acetaminophen ingestion exceeds 150 mg/kg, MUCOMYST acetylcysteine therapy should be initiated and continued for a full course of therapy.

For additional emergency information, call your regional poison center or toll-free (1-800-525-6115) to the Rocky Mountain Poison Center for assistance in diagnosis and for directions in the use of MUCOMYST acetylcysteine as an antidote.

Inactive Ingredients: Alcohol, Citric Acid, Flavors, Glycerin, Polyethylene Glycol, Purified Water, Sodium Benzoate, Sorbitol, Sucrose, Yellow #6 (Sunset Yellow), Yellow #10 and Blue #1.

How Supplied: Mint-flavored liquid (colored green), 8 fl. oz. tamper-resistant bottle with child resistant safety cap and special dosage cup.

TYLENOL® Cold Medication Liquid

Description: Each 30 ml (1 fl. oz.) contains acetaminophen 650 mg., chlorpheniramine maleate 4 mg., pseudoephedrine hydrochloride 60 mg., and dextromethorphan hydrobromide 30 mg. (alcohol 7%).

Actions: TYLENOL Cold Medication Liquid contains a clinically proven

analgesic - antipyretic, decongestant, cough suppressant and antihistamine. Acetaminophen produces analgesia by elevation of the pain threshold and antipyresis through action on the hypothalamic heat-regulating center. Pseudoephedrine hydrochloride is a sympathomimetic amine which provides temporary relief of nasal congestion. Dextromethorphan is a cough suppressant which provides temporary relief of coughs due to minor throat irritations that may occur with the common cold. Chlorpheniramine is an antihistamine which helps provide temporary relief of runny nose, sneezing and watery and itchy eyes.

Indications: TYLENOL Cold Medication Liquid provides effective temporary relief of the symptoms associated with common colds and other upper respiratory infections including: fever, aches, pains, general discomfort, nasal and sinus congestion, cough, runny nose, sneezing, minor sore throat pain, headache, watery eyes.

Adverse Reactions: While the acetaminophen component is equal to aspirin in analgesic and antipyretic effectiveness, it is unlikely to produce many of the side effects associated with aspirin and aspirin-containing products. If a rare sensitivity reaction occurs, the drug should be stopped. Although pseudoephedrine is virtually without pressor effect in normotensive patients, it should be used with caution in hypertensives.

Usual Dosage: Measuring cup is provided and marked for accurate dosing. Adults: 1 fluid ounce (2 tbsp.) every 6 hours as needed, not to exceed 4 doses in 24 hours. Children (6–12 yrs): ½ the adult dose (1 tbsp.) as indicated on the measuring cup provided, not to exceed 4 doses in 24 hours.

Note: Since TYLENOL Cold Medication Liquid is available without a prescription, the following appears on the package label: "WARNING: Do not administer to children under 6 or exceed the recommended dosage because nervousness, dizziness or sleeplessness may occur. May cause excitability especially in children. A persistent cough may be a sign of a serious condition. If fever persists for more than three days, or if symptoms do not improve or new ones occur within five days or are accompanied by high fever, rash, excessive mucus, persistent cough or headache, consult a physician before continuing use. This preparation may cause drowsiness; alcohol may increase the drowsiness effect. Avoid alcoholic beverages when taking this product. Use caution when driving a motor vehicle or operating machinery. Do not take this product if you have heart disease, high blood pressure, thyroid disease, diabetes, asthma, glaucoma, emphysema, chronic pulmonary disease, shortness of breath, difficulty in breathing, or difficulty in urination due to enlargement of the prostate gland or are taking a prescription drug for high blood pressure or depression, unless directed by a doctor. **Do not use if carton is opened, or if printed plastic overwrap**

or printed foil inner seal is broken. Keep this and all medication out of the reach of children. As with any drug, if you are pregnant or nursing a baby, seek the advice of a health professional before using this product. In case of accidental overdosage, contact a physician or poison control center immediately."

Overdosage: Acetaminophen in massive overdosage may cause hepatic toxicity in some patients. In adults and adolescents, hepatic toxicity has rarely been reported following ingestion of acute overdosage of less than 10 grams. Fatalities are infrequent (less than 3–4% of untreated cases) and have rarely been reported with overdoses of less than 15 grams. In children, an acute overdosage of less than 150 mg/kg has not been associated with hepatic toxicity.

Early symptoms following a potentially hepatotoxic overdose may include: nausea, vomiting, diaphoresis and general malaise. Clinical and laboratory evidence of hepatic toxicity may not be apparent until 48 to 72 hours postingestion. In adults and adolescents, regardless of the quantity of acetaminophen reported to have been ingested, administer MUCOMYST® acetylcysteine immediately if 24 hours or less have elapsed from the reported time of ingestion. For full prescribing information, refer to the MUCOMYST package insert. Do not await results of assays for acetaminophen level before initiating treatment with MUCOMYST acetylcysteine. The following additional procedures are recommended: The stomach should be emptied promptly by lavage or by induction of emesis with syrup of ipecac. A serum acetaminophen assay should be obtained as early as possible, but no sooner than four hours following ingestion. Liver function studies should be obtained initially and repeated at 24-hour intervals.

Serious toxicity or fatalities are extremely infrequent in children, possibly due to differences in the way they metabolize acetaminophen. In children, the maximum potential amount ingested can be more easily estimated. If more than 150 mg/kg or an unknown amount was ingested, obtain an acetaminophen plasma level. The acetaminophen plasma level should be obtained as soon as possible, but no sooner than 4 hours following the ingestion. Induce emesis using syrup of ipecac. If the plasma level is obtained and falls above the broken line on the nomogram, the MUCOMYST acetylcysteine therapy should be initiated and continued for a full course of therapy. If acetaminophen plasma assay capability is not available, and the estimated acetaminophen ingestion exceeds 150 mg/kg, MUCOMYST acetylcysteine therapy should be initiated and continued for a full course of therapy.

For additional emergency information, call your regional poison center or toll-free (1-800-525-6115) to the Rocky Mountain Poison Center for assistance in diagnosis and for directions in the use of

MUCOMYST acetylcysteine as an antidote.

Chlorpheniramine toxicity should be treated as you would an antihistamine/anticholinergic overdose and is likely to be present within a few hours after acute ingestion.

Symptoms from pseudoephedrine overdose consist most often of mild anxiety, tachycardia and/or mild hypertension. Symptoms usually appear within 4 to 8 hours of ingestion and are transient, usually requiring no treatment.

Acute dextromethorphan overdose usually does not result in serious signs and symptoms unless massive amounts have been ingested. Signs and symptoms of a substantial overdose may include nausea and vomiting, visual disturbances, CNS disturbances, and urinary retention.

Inactive Ingredients: Alcohol (7%), Citric Acid, Flavors, Glycerin, Liquid Polyethylene Glycol, Saccharin, Sodium Benzoate, Sorbitol, Sucrose, Purified Water, Yellow #6 (sunset yellow) and Blue #1.

How Supplied: Cherry/mint mentholated flavored (colored amber) in 5 oz. bottles with child-resistant safety cap, special dosage cup graded in ounces and tablespoons, and tamper-resistant packaging.

Shown in Product Identification Section, page 414

TYLENOL® Cold Medication Tablets and Caplets

Description: Each TYLENOL Cold Tablet or Caplet contains acetaminophen 325 mg., chlorpheniramine maleate 2 mg., pseudoephedrine hydrochloride 30 mg. and dextromethorphan hydrobromide 15 mg.

Actions: TYLENOL Cold Medication Tablets and Caplets contain a clinically proven analgesic-antipyretic, decongestant, cough suppressant and antihistamine. Acetaminophen produces analgesia by elevation of the pain threshold and antipyresis through action on the hypothalamic heat-regulating center. Pseudoephedrine hydrochloride is a sympathomimetic amine which provides temporary relief of nasal congestion. Dextromethorphan is a cough suppressant which provides temporary relief of coughs due to minor throat irritations that may occur with the common cold. Chlorpheniramine is an antihistamine which helps provide temporary relief of runny nose, sneezing and watery and itchy eyes.

Indications: TYLENOL Cold Medication provides effective temporary relief of the symptoms associated with common colds and other upper respiratory infections including: fever, aches, pains, general discomfort, nasal and sinus congestion, cough, runny nose, sneezing, minor sore throat pain, headache, watery eyes.

Adverse Reactions: While the acetaminophen component is equal to aspirin

Continued on next page

McNeil Consumer—Cont.

in analgesic and antipyretic effectiveness, it is unlikely to produce many of the side effects associated with aspirin and aspirin-containing products. If a rare sensitivity reaction occurs, the drug should be stopped. Although pseudoephedrine is virtually without pressor effect in normotensive patients, it should be used with caution in hypertensives.

Usual Dosage: Adults: Two tablets or caplets every 6 hours, not to exceed 8 tablets or caplets in 24 hours. Children (6–12 years): One caplet or tablet every 6 hours, not to exceed 4 tablets or caplets in 24 hours for 5 days.

Note: Since TYLENOL Cold Medication Tablets and Caplets are available without prescription, the following appears on the package label: "WARNING: Do not administer to children under 6 or exceed the recommended dosage because nervousness, dizziness or sleeplessness may occur. May cause excitability especially in children. A persistent cough may be a sign of a serious condition. If fever persists for more than three days, or if symptoms do not improve or new ones occur within five days or are accompanied by high fever, rash, excessive mucus, persistent cough or headache, consult a physician before continuing use. This preparation may cause drowsiness; alcohol may increase the drowsiness effect. Avoid alcoholic beverages when taking this product. Use caution when driving a motor vehicle or operating machinery. Do not take this product if you have heart disease, high blood pressure, thyroid disease, diabetes, asthma, glaucoma, emphysema, chronic pulmonary disease, shortness of breath, difficulty in breathing, or difficulty in urination due to enlargement of the prostate gland or are taking a prescription drug for high blood pressure or depression, unless directed by a doctor. **Do not use if carton is opened, or if printed green neck wrap or printed foil inner seal is broken. Keep this and all medication out of the reach of children. As with any drug, if you are pregnant or nursing a baby, seek the advice of a health professional before using this product. In case of accidental overdosage, contact a physician or poison control center immediately."**

Overdosage: Acetaminophen in massive overdosage may cause hepatic toxicity in some patients. In adults and adolescents, hepatic toxicity has rarely been reported following ingestion of acute overdosage of less than 10 grams. Fatalities are infrequent (less than 3–4% of untreated cases) and have rarely been reported with overdoses of less than 15 grams. In children, an acute overdosage of less than 150 mg/kg has not been associated with hepatic toxicity.
Early symptoms following a potentially hepatotoxic overdose may include: nausea, vomiting, diaphoresis and general malaise. Clinical and laboratory evidence of hepatic toxicity may not be ap-

parent until 48 to 72 hours postingestion. In adults and adolescents, regardless of the quantity of acetaminophen reported to have been ingested, administer MUCOMYST® acetylcysteine immediately if 24 hours or less have elapsed from the reported time of ingestion. For full prescribing information, refer to the MUCOMYST package insert. Do not await results of assays for acetaminophen level before initiating treatment with MUCOMYST acetylcysteine. The following additional procedures are recommended: The stomach should be emptied promptly by lavage or by induction of emesis with syrup of ipecac. A serum acetaminophen assay should be obtained as early as possible, but no sooner than four hours following ingestion. Liver function studies should be obtained initially and repeated at 24-hour intervals.
Serious toxicity or fatalities are extremely infrequent in children, possibly due to differences in the way they metabolize acetaminophen. In children, the maximum potential amount ingested can be more easily estimated. If more than 150 mg/kg or an unknown amount was ingested, obtain an acetaminophen plasma level. The acetaminophen plasma level should be obtained as soon as possible, but no sooner than 4 hours following the ingestion. Induce emesis using syrup of ipecac. If the plasma level is obtained and falls above the broken line on the nomogram, the MUCOMYST acetylcysteine therapy should be initiated and continued for a full course of therapy. If acetaminophen plasma assay capability is not available, and the estimated acetaminophen ingestion exceeds 150 mg/kg, MUCOMYST acetylcysteine therapy should be initiated and continued for a full course of therapy.
For additional emergency information, call your regional poison center or toll-free (1-800-525-6115) to the Rocky Mountain Poison Center for assistance in diagnosis and for directions in the use of MUCOMYST acetylcysteine as an antidote.
Chlorpheniramine toxicity should be treated as you would an antihistamine/anticholinergic overdose and is likely to be present within a few hours after acute ingestion.
Symptoms from pseudoephedrine overdose consist most often of mild anxiety, tachycardia and/or mild hypertension. Symptoms usually appear within 4 to 8 hours of ingestion and are transient, usually requiring no treatment.
Acute dextromethorphan overdose usually does not result in serious signs and symptoms unless massive amounts have been ingested. Signs and symptoms of a substantial overdose may include nausea and vomiting, visual disturbances, CNS disturbances, and urinary retention.

Inactive Ingredients: Tablets: Cellulose, Starch, Magnesium Stearate, Yellow #6 and Yellow #10. Caplets: Cellulose, Glyceryl, Triacetate, Hydroxypropyl Methylcellulose, Magnesium Stearate, Sodium Starch Glycolate, Starch,

Titanium Dioxide, Blue #1 and Yellow #6 & #10.

How Supplied: Tablets (colored yellow, imprinted "TYLENOL Cold")—blister packs of 24, tamper-resistant bottles of 50 and 100. Caplets (light yellow, imprinted "TYLENOL Cold")—blister packs of 24 and tamper-resistant bottles of 50.
Shown in Product Identification Section, page 414

TYLENOL® Cold Medication No Drowsiness Formula Caplets

Description: Each TYLENOL Cold Medication No Drowsiness Formula Caplet contains acetaminophen 325 mg., pseudoephedrine hydrochloride 30 mg. and dextromethorphan hydrobromide 15 mg.

Actions: TYLENOL Cold Medication No Drowsiness Formula Caplets contain a clinically proven analgesic-antipyretic, decongestant and cough suppressant. Acetaminophen produces analgesia by elevation of the pain threshold and antipyresis through action on the hypothalamic heat-regulating center. Pseudoephedrine hydrochloride is a sympathomimetic amine which provides temporary relief of nasal congestion. Dextromethorphan is a cough suppressant which provides temporary relief of coughs due to minor throat irritations that may occur with the common cold.

Indications: TYLENOL Cold Medication No Drowsiness Formula provides effective temporary relief of the symptoms associated with common colds and other upper respiratory infections including: fever, aches, pains, general discomfort, nasal and sinus congestion, cough, sneezing, minor sore throat pain, headache.

Adverse Reactions: While acetaminophen is equal to aspirin in analgesic and antipyretic effectiveness, it is unlikely to produce many of the side effects associated with aspirin and aspirin-containing products. If a rare sensitivity reaction occurs, the drug should be stopped. Although pseudoephedrine is virtually without pressor effect in normotensive patients, it should be used with caution in hypertensives.

Usual Dosage: Adults: Two caplets every 6 hours, not to exceed 8 caplets in 24 hours. Children (6–12 years): One caplet every 6 hours, not to exceed 4 tablets or caplets in 24 hours for 5 days.

Note: Since TYLENOL Cold Medication No Drowsiness Formula Caplets are available without prescription, the following appears on the package label: "WARNING: Do not administer to children under 6 or exceed the recommended dosage because nervousness, dizziness or sleeplessness may occur. May cause excitability especially in children. A persistent cough may be a sign of a serious condition. If fever persists for more than three days, or if symptoms do not improve or new ones occur within five days

or are accompanied by fever, rash, excessive mucus, persistent cough or headache, consult a physician before continuing use. Avoid alcoholic beverages when taking this product. Use caution when driving a motor vehicle or operating machinery. Do not take this product if you have heart disease, high blood pressure, thyroid disease, diabetes, asthma, glaucoma, emphysema, chronic pulmonary disease, shortness of breath, difficulty in breathing, or difficulty in urination due to enlargement of the prostate gland or are taking a prescription drug for high blood pressure or depression, unless directed by a doctor. Do not use if carton is opened, or if printed green neck wrap or printed foil inner seal is broken. Keep this and all medication out of the reach of children. As with any drug, if you are pregnant or nursing a baby, seek the advice of a health professional before using this product. In case of accidental overdosage, contact a physician or poison control center immediately."

Overdosage: Acetaminophen in massive overdosage may cause hepatic toxicity in some patients. In adults and adolescents, hepatic toxicity has rarely been reported following ingestion of acute overdosage of less than 10 grams. Fatalities are infrequent (less than 3–4% of untreated cases) and have rarely been reported with overdosage of less than 15 grams. In children, an acute overdosage of less than 150 mg/kg has not been associated with hepatic toxicity.

Early symptoms following a potentially hepatotoxic overdose may include: nausea, vomiting, diaphoresis and general malaise. Clinical and laboratory evidence of hepatic toxicity may not be apparent until 48 to 72 hours postingestion. In adults and adolescents, regardless of the quantity of acetaminophen reported to have been ingested, administer MUCOMYST® acetylcysteine immediately if 24 hours or less have elapsed from the reported time of ingestion. For full prescribing information, refer to the MUCOMYST package insert. Do not await results of assays for acetaminophen level before initiating treatment with MUCOMYST acetylcysteine. The following additional procedures are recommended: The stomach should be emptied promptly by lavage or by induction of emesis with syrup of ipecac. A serum acetaminophen assay should be obtained as early as possible, but no sooner than four hours following ingestion. Liver function studies should be obtained initially and repeated at 24–hour intervals.

Serious toxicity or fatalities are extremely infrequent in children, possibly due to differences in the way they metabolize acetaminophen. In children, the maximum potential amount ingested can be more easily estimated. If more than 150 mg/kg or an unknown amount was ingested, obtain an acetaminophen plasma level. The acetaminophen plasma level should be obtained as soon as possible, but no sooner than 4 hours following the ingestion. Induce emesis using syrup of ipecac. If the plasma level

is obtained and falls above the broken line on the nomogram, the MUCOMYST acetylcysteine therapy should be initiated and continued for a full course of therapy. If acetaminophen plasma assay capability is not available, and the estimated acetaminophen ingestion exceeds 150 mg/kg. MUCOMYST acetylcysteine therapy should be initiated and continued for a full course of therapy.

For additional emergency information, call your regional poison center or toll–free (1-800-525-6115) to the Rocky Mountain Poison Center for assistance in diagnosis and for direction in the use of MUCOMYST acetylcysteine as an antidote.

Symptoms from pseudoephedrine overdose consist most often of mild anxiety, tachycardia and/or mild hypertension. Symptoms usually appear within 4 to 8 hours of ingestion and are transient, usually requiring no treatment.

Acute dextromethorphan overdose usually does not result in serious signs and symptoms unless massive amounts have been ingested. Signs and symptoms of a substantial overdose may include nausea and vomiting, visual disturbances, CNS disturbances, and urinary retention.

Inactive Ingredients: Cellulose, Glyceryl, Triacetate, Hydroxypropyl Methylcellulose, Magnesium Stearate, Sodium Starch Glycolate, Starch, Titanium Dioxide, Blue #1 and Yellow #10.

How Supplied: Caplets (colored white, imprinted TYLENOL "cold")—blister packs of 24, tamper–resistant bottles of 50.

Maximum-Strength TYLENOL® Sinus Medication Tablets and Caplets

Description: Each Maximum-Strength TYLENOL® Sinus Medication tablet or caplet contains acetaminophen 500 mg and pseudoephedrine hydrochloride 30 mg.

Actions: TYLENOL Sinus Medication contains a clinically proven analgesic-antipyretic and a decongestant. Maximum allowable non-prescription levels of acetaminophen and pseudoephedrine provide temporary relief of sinus congestion and pain.

Acetaminophen produces analgesia by elevation of the pain threshold and antipyresis through action on the hypothalamic heat-regulating center. Pseudoephedrine hydrochloride is a sympathomimetic amine which promotes sinus cavity drainage by reducing nasopharyngeal mucosal congestion.

Indications: Maximum-Strength TYLENOL Sinus Medication provides effective symptomatic relief from sinus headache pain and pressure caused by sinusitis.

Adverse Reactions: While acetaminophen is equal to aspirin in analgesic and antipyretic effectiveness, it is unlikely to produce many of the side effects associated with aspirin and aspirin-containing products. Since it contains no antihistamine, TYLENOL Sinus Medication will

not produce the drowsiness that may interfere with work, driving an automobile or operating dangerous machinery. Maximum-Strength TYLENOL Sinus Medication is particularly well-suited in patients with aspirin allergy, hemostatic disturbances (including anticoagulant therapy), and bleeding diatheses (e.g. hemophilia) and upper gastrointestinal disease (e.g. ulcer, gastritis, hiatus hernia). If a rare sensitivity occurs, the drug should be discontinued. Although pseudoephedrine is virtually without pressor effect in normotensive patients, it should be used with caution in hypertensives.

Usual Dosage: Adult dosage: Two tablets or caplets every four to six hours. Do not exceed eight tablets or caplets in any 24 hour period. **Note:** Since TYLENOL Sinus Medication tablets and caplets are available without a prescription, the following appears on the package labels: "WARNING: Do not exceed the recommended dosage because at higher doses nervousness, dizziness, or sleeplessness may occur. Do not administer to children under 12. If you have high blood pressure, heart disease, diabetes, thyroid disease, difficulty in urination due to enlargement of the prostate gland, or are presently taking a prescription drug for the treatment of high blood pressure or depression, do not take except under the advice and supervision of a physician. Do not take this product for more than 7 days. If symptoms do not improve or are accompanied by high fever, consult a physician. **Do not use if carton is opened or if printed green neck wrap or printed foil inner seal is broken. Keep this and all medication out of the reach of children. As with any drug, if you are pregnant or nursing a baby, seek the advice of a health professional before using this product. In case of accidental overdosage, contact a physician or poison control center immediately.**

Overdosage: Acetaminophen in massive overdosage may cause hepatic toxicity in some patients. In adults and adolescents, hepatic toxicity has rarely been reported following ingestion of acute overdosage of less than 10 grams. Fatalities are infrequent (less than 3–4% of untreated cases) and have rarely been reported with overdoses of less than 15 grams. In children, an acute overdosage of less than 150 mg/kg has not been associated with hepatic toxicity.

Early symptoms following a potentially hepatotoxic overdose may include: nausea, vomiting, diaphoresis and general malaise. Clinical and laboratory evidence of hepatic toxicity may not be apparent until 48 to 72 hours postingestion. In adults and adolescents, regardless of the quantity of acetaminophen reported to have been ingested, administer MUCOMYST® acetylcysteine immediately if 24 hours or less have elapsed from the reported time of ingestion. For full prescribing information, refer to the MUCOMYST package insert. Do not

Continued on next page

McNeil Consumer—Cont.

await the results of assays for acetaminophen level before initiating treatment with MUCOMYST acetylcysteine. The following additional procedures are recommended: The stomach should be emptied promptly by lavage or by induction of emesis with syrup of ipecac. A serum acetaminophen assay should be obtained as early as possible, but no sooner than four hours following ingestion. Liver function studies should be obtained initially and repeated at 24-hour intervals.

Serious toxicity or fatalities are extremely infrequent in children, possibly due to differences in the way they metabolize acetaminophen. In children, the maximum potential amount ingested can be more easily estimated. If more than 150 mg/kg or an unknown amount was ingested, obtain an acetaminophen plasma level. The acetaminophen plasma level should be obtained as soon as possible, but no sooner than 4 hours following the ingestion. Induce emesis using syrup of ipecac. If the plasma level is obtained and falls above the broken line on the nomogram, the MUCOMYST acetylcysteine therapy should be initiated and continued for a full course of therapy. If acetaminophen plasma assay capability is not available, and the estimated acetaminophen ingestion exceeds 150 mg/kg, MUCOMYST acetylcysteine therapy should be initiated and continued for a full course of therapy.

For additional emergency information, call your regional poison center or toll-free (1-800-525-6115) to the Rocky Mountain Poison Center for assistance in diagnosis and for directions in the use of MUCOMYST acetylcysteine as an antidote.

Symptoms from pseudoephedrine overdose consist most often of mild anxiety, tachycardia and/or mild hypertension. Symptoms usually appear within 4 to 8 hours of ingestion and are transient, usually requiring no treatment.

Inactive Ingredients: Caplets—Cellulose, Hydroxypropyl Methylcellulose, Magnesium Stearate, Polysorbate 80, Sodium Starch Glycolate, Starch, Titanium Dioxide, Blue #1, Red #40 and Yellow #10. Tablets—Cellulose, Magnesium Stearate, Sodium Lauryl Sulfate, Starch, Yellow #6 (Sunset Yellow), Yellow #10 and Blue #1.

How Supplied: Tablets (colored light green, imprinted "Maximum-Strength TYLENOL Sinus")—tamper-resistant bottles of 24 and 50. Caplets (light green coating, printed "TYLENOL Sinus" in dark green) tamper resistant bottles of 24 and 50.

Shown in Product Identification Section, page 413

Mead Johnson Nutritionals
A Bristol-Myers Company
2400 W. LLOYD EXPRESSWAY
EVANSVILLE, IN 47721

CASEC® powder
[kā'sek]
Calcium caseinate

Composition: Consists of dried, soluble calcium caseinate (88% protein) derived from skim milk curd and lime water (calcium carbonate) by a special process. Contains only 43 mg sodium per 6 packed level tbsp (1 ounce).

Action and Uses: Supplementing diets of children and adults, including sodium restricted diets and diets low in fat or cholesterol.

Precautions: When Casec is used to modify tube feedings, water intake should be monitored to assure the patient's daily water requirement is met. This is particularly important for comatose or semicomatose patients.

Preparation: Casec powder may be mixed with cereals, vegetables, meat dishes, or blended into milk drinks. For protein supplementation—give as needed.

How Supplied: Casec® powder
0087-0390-07   Cans of 2½ oz

CE-VI-SOL®
[see 'vĭ-sahl'']
Vitamin C drops

Ingredients: Glycerin, water, alcohol (5% v/v), sodium carbonate, disodium EDTA, artificial flavor, and ascorbic acid. Each 0.6 mL supplies 35 mg vitamin C.

Action and Uses: Dietary supplement of vitamin C for infants.

Administration and Dosage: 0.6 mL (35 mg) or as indicated. Dropper calibrated for doses of 0.6 and 0.3 mL (35 and 17.5 mg ascorbic acid).

How Supplied: Ce-Vi-Sol® drops (with calibrated dropper)
0087-0400-01 Bottles of 1⅔ fl oz (50 mL)

CRITICARE HN®
[crĭ'tĭ-care hn']
High nitrogen elemental diet

Composition: Water, maltodextrin, enzymatically hydrolyzed casein, modified corn starch, safflower oil, potassium citrate, calcium gluconate, calcium glycerophosphate, magnesium chloride, choline bitartrate, L-methionine, polyglycerol esters of fatty acids, carrageenan, L-tyrosine, magnesium oxide, L-tryptophan, diacetyl tartaric acid esters of mono- and diglycerides, vitamins (vitamin A palmitate, cholecalciferol, dl-alpha-tocopheryl acetate, sodium ascorbate, folic acid, thiamine hydrochloride, riboflavin, niacinamide, pyridoxine hydrochloride, cyanocobalamin, biotin, calcium pantothenate and phytonadione) and minerals (potassium iodide, ferrous gluconate, copper gluconate, zinc gluconate and manganese gluconate).

Criticare HN provides 14% of the calories as protein, 3% as fat and 83% as carbohydrate.

Actions and Uses: Criticare HN is the first complete, high nitrogen, elemental nutrition in a commercially sterile, ready-to-use liquid form for patients with impaired digestion and absorption. Under physician supervision, it is intended for use in patients with inflammatory bowel disease, chronic pancreatitis, short gut syndrome, cystic fibrosis, non-specific malabsorption/maldigestion states, and transitions from TPN to enteral nutrition.

Criticare HN contains at least 100% of the U.S. RDA's for all vitamins and minerals in 2000 Calories with extra amounts of vitamin C and B-complex vitamins to meet the increased requirements for these vitamins in the critically ill patient.

Criticare HN is lactose-free and has a moderate osmolality (650 mOsm/kg H_2O) to assure rapid patient adaptation and good patient tolerance.

Preparation: It is recommended that Criticare HN be tube fed and that tube feeding be initiated as follows:

Day 1—1:1 dilution of Criticare HN with water at 50 ml/hour (or full strength at 25 ml/hr).

Day 2—full strength at 50 ml/hour.

Day 3—full strength up to 100–125 ml/hour.

Opened bottles of unused Criticare HN should be covered, kept refrigerated and used within 48 hours of opening. Do not freeze or refrigerate unopened bottles of Criticare HN.

If used with an oral feeding, it is advisable to counsel patients that the flavor of Criticare HN differs significantly from other liquid diets because of the special characteristics of the protein.

Tube Feeding Precaution: Additional water should be given as needed to meet the patient's requirements. Particular attention should be given to water supply for comatose and unconscious patients and others who cannot express the usual sensation of thirst.

Additional water is important also when renal concentrating ability is impaired, when there is extensive breakdown of tissue protein, or when water requirements are high, as in fever, burns or under dry atmospheric conditions.

Criticare HN provides 830 ml of water per 1000 ml of formula.

How Supplied: Criticare HN® liquid
0087-0563-41 Bottles of 8 fl oz

ENFAMIL®
[en 'fah-mil"]
**Concentrated liquid • powder •
ready-to-use
Low iron infant formula**

Composition: A whey-predominant infant formula that is nutritionally closer to breast milk than casein-predominant formulas. Caloric distribution: 9% from protein, 50% from fat, 41% from carbohydrate.
Each quart of Enfamil formula (normal dilution, 20 Calories/fl oz) supplies 640 Calories.
[See table right].
NOTE: Fer-In-Sol® iron supplement drops are a convenient source of added iron.

Action and Uses: For feeding of full term and premature infants during the first twelve months of life and a supplementary formula for breast-fed babies.

Preparation: Concentrated liquid and powder: For 20 Calories/fl oz: With concentrated liquid—1 part to 1 part water. With powder—1 level scoop to each 2 fl oz water; or 1 level cup to water sufficient to make a quart of formula.
Formula prepared from Enfamil concentrated liquid and opened cans of this liquid should be refrigerated and used within 48 hours. Formula prepared from Enfamil powder should be refrigerated and used within 24 hours. Opened cans of powder should be kept in a cool, dry place and used within 30 days. Ready-to-use: Pour liquid into sterilized nursing bottle without diluting. No refrigeration is necessary for the unopened cans. The formula need not be heated before feeding baby. Interchangeable with formulas in normal dilution (20 Calories/fl oz) prepared from Enfamil concentrated liquid or powder and Enfamil Nursette® in filled formula bottles.

Precautions: Opened cans of Enfamil ready-to-use formula should be stored in refrigerator and used within 48 hours.

How Supplied: Powder, 16-oz (1-lb) cans with measuring scoop. Concentrated liquid, 40 Calories/fl oz 13-fl oz cans. Ready-to-use, 8-fl oz cans in an easy to carry handy six-can pack, and 32-fl oz (1 qt) cans.
Also available, Enfamil with iron at 40 Calories/fl oz concentrated liquid, 13-fl oz cans. Powder, 16-oz (1-lb) cans with scoop. Ready-to-use, 8-fl oz cans in an easy to carry handy six-can pack, and 32-fl oz (1 qt) cans.
Shown in Product Identification Section, page 414

ENFAMIL® with Iron
[en 'fah-mil"]
**Concentrated liquid • powder •
ready-to-use
Iron fortified infant formula**

Composition: A whey-predominant infant formula which is nutritionally closer to breast milk than casein-predominant formulas, with added iron (12 mg/qt). Caloric distribution: 9% from

ENFAMIL®

NUTRIENTS	Per 100 Calories (5 fl oz)	Per Quart
Protein, g	2.2	14.4
Fat, g	5.6	36
Carbohydrate, g	10.3	66
Water, g	134	860
Linoleic acid, mg	1100	7000
Vitamins:		
Vitamin A, IU	310	2000
Vitamin D, IU	62	400
Vitamin E, IU	3.1	20
Vitamin K, µg	8.6	55
Thiamine (Vitamin B_1), µg	78	500
Riboflavin (Vitamin B_2), µg	156	1000
Vitamin B_6, µg	62	400
Vitamin B_{12}, µg	0.23	1.5
Niacin, µg	1250	8000
Folic acid (Folacin), µg	15.6	100
Pantothenic acid, µg	470	3000
Biotin, µg	2.3	15
Vitamin C (Ascorbic acid), mg	8.1	52
Choline, mg	15.6	100
Inositol, mg	4.7	30
Minerals:		
Calcium, mg	69	440
Phosphorus, mg	47	300
Magnesium, mg	7.8	50
Iron, mg	0.16	1
Zinc, mg	0.78	5
Manganese, µg	15.6	100
Copper, µg	94	600
Iodine, µg	10.2	65
Sodium, mg	27	175
Potassium, mg	108	690
Chloride, mg	62	400

Supplemental iron should be considered.

protein, 50% from fat, 41% from carbohydrate. Except for the higher iron content, the normal dilution (20 Calories/fl oz) has the same vitamin and mineral content as Enfamil (see Enfamil).

Action and Uses: Enfamil with Iron supplies a daily intake of iron for full term and premature infants during the first twelve months of life. Feeding of infants with special needs for exogenous iron, such as: premature infants, offspring of anemic mothers, infants of multiple births, infants with low birth weights and those who grow rapidly, infants who have minor losses of blood at birth or in surgery. As a supplementary formula for breast-fed infants. For older infants the formula provides an easily digestible "beverage milk" with supplemental iron. One quart (32 fl oz) of formula supplies 12 mg of iron.

Preparation: See Enfamil section.

Precautions: If therapeutic or larger supplementary amounts of iron are indicated, the iron content of the formula should be taken into account (12 mg iron per qt) in calculating the total iron dosage. Opened cans of Enfamil with Iron ready-to-use formula should be stored in refrigerator and used within 48 hours.

How Supplied: Powder, 16-oz (1-lb) cans with measuring scoop. Concentrated liquid, 40 Calories/fl oz 13-fl oz cans. Ready-to-use, 8-fl oz cans in an easy to carry handy six-can pack, and 32-fl oz (1 qt) cans.
Also available, Enfamil at 40 Calories/fl oz concentrated liquid, 13-fl oz cans. Pow-

der, 16-oz (1-lb) cans with scoop. Ready-to-feed Enfamil® infant formula, 8-fl oz cans in an easy to carry handy six-can pack, and 32-fl oz (1 qt) cans.
Shown in Product Identification Section, page 414

ENFAMIL NURSETTE®
[en 'fah-mil" nur-set']
Infant formula (Low iron and iron fortified)

Composition: Glass formula bottle filled with ready-to-feed Enfamil® infant formula (20 Calories/fl oz) (See Enfamil concentrated liquid and powder for nutrient values.) A whey-predominant infant formula which is nutritionally closer to breast milk than casein-predominant formulas.

Action and Uses: A very convenient form of Enfamil for routine formula feeding for the first twelve months of life. Especially useful for feeding for first weeks at home, infants of working mothers, infant travel, emergency feedings, or as a supplementary formula for breast-fed babies.

Preparation: Remove cap, attach any standard sterilized nipple unit and feed baby. The Nursette bottle needs no refrigeration until opened and can be fed at room temperature. Interchangeable with Enfamil Ready-To-Use liquid in cans and formulas in normal dilution (20 Calories/fl oz) prepared from Enfamil concentrated liquid or powder.

Continued on next page

Mead Johnson Nutr.—Cont.

Note: Contents remaining in bottle after feeding should be discarded. Nipples and collar rings should be washed, rinsed and sterilized before reuse; bottle not for reuse.

How Supplied: Available in convenient 4 fl oz, 6 fl oz, and 8 fl oz Nursette® bottles, packed four bottles to a sealed carton, six 4-packs per case.
Enfamil Nursette with Iron also available in 6-fl oz bottles.

FER-IN-SOL®
[fair 'in-sahl "]
Iron supplement
● drops
● syrup
● capsules
Ferrous sulfate, Mead Johnson

Composition:

Fer-In-Sol	Ferrous Sulfate	As Iron	Alcohol
	mg	mg	%
Drops (per 0.6 mL dose)	75	15	.02
Syrup (per 5 mL teaspoonful)	90	18	5
Capsule (1 capsule)	190 (dried)	60	—

Action and Uses: Source of supplemental iron.

Administration and Dosage:
drops
0.6 mL daily supplies 15 mg of iron, 100% of the U.S. RDA for infants and 150% of the U.S. RDA for children under 4 years of age.
Give in water or in fruit or vegetable juice.
Fer-In-Sol should be given immediately after meals. When an infant or child is taking iron, stools may appear darker in color. This is to be expected and should be no cause for concern. When drops containing iron are given to young babies, some darkening of the membrane covering the baby's teeth may occur. This is not serious or permanent. The enamel of the teeth is not affected. Should this darkening or staining occur, it may be removed by rubbing the baby's teeth with a little baking soda on a small cloth once a week.
syrup
1 teaspoon (5 mL) daily supplies 18 mg of iron, 100% of the U.S. RDA for adults and children 4 or more years of age.
capsules
1 capsule daily supplies 60 mg of iron, 333% of the U.S. RDA for pregnant or lactating women.

How Supplied: Fer-In-Sol® drops (with calibrated 'Safti-Dropper')
    0087-0740-02 Bottles of 1-⅔ fl oz (50 mL)
    6505-00-664-0856 (1-⅔ fl oz, 50 mL) Defense

Fer-In-Sol® syrup
    0087-0741-01 Bottles of 16 fl oz
Fer-In-Sol® capsules
    0087-0742-01 Bottles of 100

ISOCAL®
[ī 'sō-cal "]
Complete liquid diet
Tube-feeding formulation

Composition:

Isocal: Water, maltodextrin, soy oil, calcium caseinate, sodium caseinate, medium chain triglycerides (fractionated coconut oil), soy protein isolate, lecithin, potassium citrate, potassium chloride, magnesium phosphate, calcium citrate, calcium carbonate, choline chloride, sodium citrate, magnesium chloride, carrageenan, vitamins (vitamin A palmitate, cholecalciferol, dl-alpha-tocopheryl acetate, sodium ascorbate, folic acid, thiamine hydrochloride, riboflavin, niacinamide, pyridoxine hydrochloride, cyanocobalamin, biotin, calcium pantothenate and phytonadione) and minerals (potassium iodide, ferrous sulfate, cupric sulfate, zinc sulfate and manganese sulfate).

Actions and Uses: Isocal is a complete liquid diet specifically formulated to provide well-balanced nutrition for tube-fed patients when used as the sole source of nourishment. Isocal is lactose-free, has an osmolality of 300 mOsm/kg water and provides at least 100% of the U.S. RDA for vitamins and minerals in 2000 Calories.

Preparation and Administration: Isocal is ready to feed and require no additional water; shake well before use. Isocal comes in cans or bottles and, unopened, can be stored at room temperature. After opening, Isocal should be covered and refrigerated if not used immediately.
Nasogastric tube feedings with Isocal may be given using a standard tube feeding set. Feedings may be given by continuous drip or by intervals. The rate should be adjusted for the best comfort and needs of the patient.
Isocal has a bland, unsweetened taste because it is specifically formulated for tube feedings. However, patients on long-term oral diet may prefer the taste of Isocal to the sweet taste of some oral liquid nutritional supplements.

Precautions: Additional water may be needed to meet the patient's requirements. Particular attention should be given to water needs of comatose and unconscious patients and others who cannot express the usual sensations of thirst. Additional water is important also when renal-concentrating ability is impaired, when there is extensive breakdown of tissue protein, or when water requirements are high, as in fever. Isocal provides 843 ml of water per 1000 ml. Tube feeding preparations should be at room temperature during administration.

How Supplied: Isocal® Complete Liquid Diet

    0087-0355-01 Cans of 8 fl oz
    0087-0355-02 Cans of 12 fl oz
    0087-0355-44 Cans of 32 fl oz (1 quart)
    0087-0356-01 Bottles of 8 fl oz
    VA 8940-00-609-2636 (8-fl-oz bottles)

Also Available:
    0087-0357-01 Isocal Tube Feeding Set

ISOCAL® HCN
[ī 'sō-cal " hcn ']
High calorie and nitrogen
nutritionally complete liquid
tube-feeding formula

Composition: Water, corn syrup, soybean oil, calcium caseinate, medium chain triglycerides (fractionated coconut oil), sodium caseinate, lecithin, potassium citrate, magnesium chloride, magnesium phosphate, potassium carbonate, salt, calcium phosphate, carrageenan, potassium chloride, vitamins (vitamin A palmitate, cholecalciferol, dl-alpha-tocopheryl acetate, sodium ascorbate, folic acid, thiamine hydrochloride, riboflavin, niacinamide, pyridoxine hydrochloride, cyanocobalamin, biotin, calcium pantothenate, phytonadione and choline bitartrate) and minerals (potassium iodide, ferrous gluconate, cupric sulfate, zinc sulfate and manganese sulfate).

Indication: Isocal HCN is a complete, concentrated liquid tube feeding diet specifically formulated to provide patients with generous calorie (2.0 Cal/ml) and protein levels (75 g protein/1000 ml). Isocal HCN provides 15% of the calories as protein, 45% as fat, 40% as carbohydrate and 100% of the U.S. RDA of all essential vitamins and minerals in 1000 ml. This lactose-free formulation has an osmolality of 690 mOsm/kg water.

Actions and Uses: Isocal HCN is of particular value to patients who are fluid-restricted (neurosurgery, congestive heart failure, etc.) or are volume-restricted (cardiac or cancer cachexia, chronic obstructive lung disease) and require tube feeding.
Isocal HCN may be used as a nutritional supplement in situations: where taste perceptions have been altered by therapy and illness; where variety is indicated during long-term full liquid diet use; during the transition from tube feedings to conventional supplements and normal diets. Flavorings may be added to Isocal HCN to suit individual preferences.

Preparation: Isocal HCN is ready to feed; shake well before opening. Unopened Isocal HCN should be stored at room temperature. Unused Isocal HCN should be covered, kept refrigerated and used within 48 hours of opening.
It is recommended that Isocal HCN be tube fed and that tube feeding be initiated as follows:
Day 1—1:1 dilution of Isocal HCN to water at 50 ml/hour (or full strength at 25 ml/hr).
Day 2—full strength at 50 ml/hour.
Day 3—full strength up to 100–125 ml/hour.
Administration via infusion pump is recommended.

Precaution: Additional water may be given as needed to meet the patient's requirements. Particular attention should be given to water needs of comatose and unconscious patients, those who cannot express the usual sensation of thirst and patients with impaired renal concentrating capacity, extensive breakdown of tissue protein, or when water requirements are high, e.g. fever, burns, and dry atmospheric conditions. Isocal HCN provides 700 ml of water per 1000 ml of formula.

How Supplied: Isocal® HCN liquid
0087-0462-42 Cans of 8 fl oz
VA 8940-01-124-7909 (8-fl-oz cans)

LOFENALAC®
[lō-fen 'ah-lak "]
Iron fortified low phenylalanine diet powder

Ingredients: Corn syrup solids, casein enzymatically hydrolyzed and specially treated to reduce phenylalanine, corn oil, modified tapioca starch, vitamins (vitamin A palmitate, vitamin D_3, dl-alpha-tocopheryl acetate, phytonadione, thiamine hydrochloride, riboflavin, pyridoxine hydrochloride, vitamin B_{12}, niacinamide, folic acid, calcium pantothenate, biotin, ascorbic acid, choline chloride, and inositol), minerals (calcium citrate, calcium hydroxide, calcium phosphate, magnesium oxide, ferrous sulfate, zinc sulfate, manganese sulfate, cupric sulfate, sodium iodide, potassium citrate, and potassium phosphate), L-tyrosine, L-tryptophan, L-histidine hydrochloride, L-methionine, taurine (38 mg/qt 20 Calorie dilution), and L-carnitine.
Phenylalanine content of Lofenalac powder is approximately 0.08% (not more than 0.1% nor less than 0.06%). Each 100 g of powder supplies about 460 Calories and 80 mg phenylalanine. One packed level scoop contains 9.6 g.
[See table above].
*The protein is incomplete since it contains an inadequate amount of the essential amino acid, phenylalanine, for normal growth. With added phenylalanine, the PER is greater than that of casein.

Action and Uses: For use as basic food in dietary management of infants and children with phenylketonuria. Provides essential nutrients without the high phenylalanine content (approx. 5%) present in natural food proteins. Except for its low and carefully limited phenylalanine content, Lofenalac is nutritionally complete.

Preparation: 20 Calories/fl oz Formula for Infants: To make a quart of formula, add one packed level cup (139 g) of Lofenalac powder to 29 fl oz water. For smaller amounts of formula, add 1 packed level measuring scoop (9.6 g) of powder to each 2 fluid ounces of water. To prepare as a beverage (about 30 Calories/fl oz) for older children and adults, add one packed level cup (139 g) of powder to 20 fl oz of warm water; mix with beater until smooth, then store in refrigerator. Prescribe a specific amount of this mixture daily, and carefully add spe-

LOFENALAC®

NUTRIENTS (20 Calories/fl oz dilution):	Per 100 Calories (5 fl oz)	Per Quart
Protein, g*	3.3	21
Fat, g	3.9	25
Carbohydrate, g	13	83
Water, g	134	860
Linoleic acid, mg	2000	12800
Vitamins:		
Vitamin A, IU	310	2000
Vitamin D, IU	62	400
Vitamin E, IU	3.1	20
Vitamin K, mcg	15.6	100
Thiamine (Vitamin B_1), mcg	78	500
Riboflavin (Vitamin B_2), mcg	94	600
Vitamin B_6, mcg	62	400
Vitamin B_{12}, mcg	0.31	2
Niacin, mcg	1250	8000
Folic acid (Folacin), mcg	15.6	100
Pantothenic acid, mcg	470	3000
Biotin, mcg	7.8	50
Vitamin C (Ascorbic acid), mg	8.1	52
Choline, mg	13.3	85
Inositol, mg	4.7	30
Minerals:		
Calcium, mg	94	600
Phosphorus, mg	70	450
Magnesium, mg	10.9	70
Iron, mg	1.88	12
Zinc, mg	0.78	5
Manganese, mcg	31	200
Copper, mcg	94	600
Iodine, mcg	7	45
Sodium, mg	47	300
Potassium, mg	102	650
Chloride, mg	70	450

cific amounts of other foods to the diet. Lofenalac contains approximately 110 mg of phenylalanine per quart of formula (17 mg/100 Calories). This low level does not provide sufficient phenylalanine to meet total daily requirements of the growing infant. Other foods should be given as required to bring phenylalanine intake to adequate, but not excessive, level. The diet and the phenylalanine intake must be adapted to individual needs.
Store bottled formula in refrigerator and use within 24 hours.

Contraindications: Lofenalac (low phenylalanine food) should not be used for normal infants and children, but should be used only as part of the diet of patients with phenylketonuria. Continued usage must be carefully and frequently supervised by the physician and the diet periodically adjusted on the basis of frequent tests of urine and blood.

How Supplied: Lofenalac® powder
Cans of 40 oz (2½ lb). List # 340-26
Consult PKU—A Guide for Dietary Management for details.

LONALAC® powder
[lōn 'ah-lack "]
Low sodium, high protein beverage mix

Composition: Lactose, casein, coconut oil, calcium phosphate, potassium carbonate, calcium citrate, potassium citrate, calcium hydroxide, calcium chloride, potassium chloride, magnesium ox-

ide, calcium carbonate, vitamin A palmitate, thiamine hydrochloride, riboflavin, niacinamide, artificial color and flavor. Each 100 g of Lonalac powder supplies 27 g protein, 28 g fat and 38 g carbohydrate. Each quart (30 Cal/fl oz) contains the following:

Vitamin A, IU	1440
Thiamine, mg	0.6
Riboflavin, mg	2.6
Niacin, mg	1.2
Calcium, mg	1690
Phosphorus, mg	1500
Magnesium, mg	135
Chloride, mg	750
Potassium, mg	1880
Sodium, mg	38

It contains only 38 mg sodium per quart of normal dilution, in contrast to 480 mg sodium in a quart of milk.

Action and Uses: A substitute for milk when dietary sodium restriction is prescribed, as in congestive heart failure, hypertension, nephrosis, acute nephritis, toxemia of pregnancy, hepatic cirrhosis with ascites, and therapy with certain drugs.

Preparation: For 30 Cal/fl oz: add 1½ cups (188 g) Lonalac powder to 27 fl oz of water. Concentrated preparation: ½ cup Lonalac powder to 1 cup water.
Store bottled formula in refrigerator and use within 24 hours.

Precautions: Care should be taken to avoid additional sodium intake from other dietary or non-dietary sources.

Continued on next page

Mead Johnson Nutr.—Cont.

Subjects receiving low sodium diets must be observed for signs of sodium deprivation such as weakness, exhaustion and abdominal cramps. In long term management (using Lonalac), additional sources of sodium must be given since Lonalac is almost void of the essential nutrient sodium.

How Supplied: Lonalac® powder
0087-0391-01 Cans of 16 oz (1 lb)
VA 8940-00-191-6565 (1 lb can)

LYTREN®
[lī'tren]
Oral electrolyte solution

Lytren provides important electrolytes plus carbohydrate in a balanced formulation. It is designed for oral administration when food intake is discontinued.

Composition: Water, dextrose (D-glucose), potassium citrate, salt (sodium chloride), sodium citrate, citric acid.

Concentrations of Electrolytes:

Electrolyte	mEq/L
Sodium	50
Chloride	45
Citrate	30
Potassium	25
Total*	150

*NOTE: Lytren oral electrolyte solution has an osmolality of approximately 220 mOsm per kilogram of water and contains 20 grams of D-glucose per liter.

Indications: When intake of the usual foods and liquids is discontinued, oral feedings of Lytren solution may be used:
• To supply water and electrolytes for maintenance.
• To replace mild to moderate fluid losses.
Such oral electrolyte feedings have particular application in mild and moderate diarrheas, to forestall dehydration,[1-6] and in postoperative states.

Intake and Administration: Feed by nursing bottle, glass or straw.
Administration of Lytren should be begun as soon as intake of usual foods and liquids is discontinued, and before serious fluid losses or deficits develop.
Intake of Lytren should approximate the patient's calculated daily water require-ments, for maintenance and for replacement of losses. The prescribed quantity may be divided and used throughout the day as desired or appropriate. (Note: No more than this amount of Lytren should be given. Additional liquid to satisfy thirst should be water or other non-electrolyte-containing fluids.)

●For infants and young children. The water requirement should be calculated on the basis of body surface area. Estimated daily water requirements such as the following may be used as a general guide:
    For maintenance in illness—1500 mL (50 fl oz) per square meter.[7]
    For maintenance plus replacement of moderate losses (as in diarrhea or vomiting)—2400 mL (80 fl oz) per square meter.[7]
Daily amount of Lytren solution based on these estimated requirements is shown in the Intake Guide table. Intake should be adjusted according to the size of the individual patient and the clinical conditions.

●For older children and adults. When fluid losses are mild to moderate, amounts such as the following may be given daily: Children 5 to 10 years—1 to 2 quarts. Older children and adults—2 to 3 quarts.[7]
Intake should be adjusted on the basis of clinical indications, amount of fluid loss, patient's usual water intake and other relevant factors.
[See table below].

●Lytren in conjunction with other fluids. When severe fluid losses or accumulated deficits require parenteral fluid therapy, Lytren by mouth may be given simultaneously to supply part of the estimated fluid requirement. After emergency needs have been met, Lytren solution alone may be used.

Contraindications:
Lytren should not be used:
●In the presence of severe, continuing diarrhea or other critical fluid losses requiring parenteral fluid therapy.
●In intractable vomiting, adynamic ileus, intestinal obstruction or perforated bowel.
●When renal function is depressed (anuria, oliguria) or homeostatic mechanisms are impaired.

Precautions: Lytren oral electrolyte solution should only be used in the recommended volume intakes in order to avoid excessive electrolyte ingestion. Do not mix with, or give with, other electrolyte-containing liquids, such as milk or fruit juices.
Urgent needs in severe fluid imbalances must be met parenterally. When Lytren solution by mouth is used in addition to parenteral fluids, do not exceed total water and electrolyte requirements.
Intake of Lytren should be discontinued upon reintroduction of other electrolyte-containing foods into the diet. Should be administered on physician's orders only.

How Supplied:
Lytren is available in the hospital in an 8-fl oz Nursette® Disposable Bottle. List # 292-04

References:
1. Darrow DC: Pediatrics, (1952); (May) 9:519–533. 2. Harrison HE: Pediatr Clin North America, 1954; (May), pp 335–348. 3. Vaughan VC, III, in Nelson WE: Textbook of Pediatrics, ed 7, Philadelphia, WB Saunders Company, 1959, pp 187–189. 4. Brooke CE, Anast CS: JAMA 1962; (March), 179:148–153. 5. Darrow DC, Welsh JS: J Pediatr 1960; (Feb) 56:204–210. 6. Cooke RE: JAMA 1958; (July 5) 167:1243–1246. 7. Worthen HG, Raile RB: Minnesota Med 1954; (Aug) 37:558–564. 8. McLester JS, Darby WJ: Nutrition and Diet in Health and Disease, ed 6, Philadelphia, WB Saunders Company, 1952, pp 32–34.

MCT Oil
[mct oyl]
Medium chain triglycerides

Composition: MCT Oil contains triglycerides of medium chain fatty acids which are more easily digested and absorbed than conventional food fat.
MCT Oil is bland tasting and light yellow in color. It provides 8.3 Cal/g. One tablespoon (15 ml) weighs 14 g and contains 115 Cal. It is a lipid fraction of coconut oil and consists primarily of the triglycerides of C_8 and C_{10} saturated fatty acids. MCT Oil does not provide essential fatty acids.
Approximate percentages are:

Fatty Acid	%
Shorter than C_8	<6
C_8 (Octanoic)	67
C_{10} (Decanoic)	23
Longer than C_{10}	<4

Actions and Uses: MCT Oil is a special dietary supplement for use in the nutritional management of children and adults who cannot efficiently digest and absorb conventional long chain food fats. One tablespoonful 3 to 4 times per day or as recommended by the physician. MCT oil may soften or break certain types of plastic containers and utensils. Therefore, non-plastic containers and utensils should be used. MCT Oil should be mixed with fruit juices, used on salads and vegetables, incorporated into sauces for use on fish, chicken, or lean meat, or used

LYTREN INTAKE GUIDE
for infants and young children

(Adjust to meet individual needs)

LYTREN SOLUTION DAILY INTAKE

*Averages of Benedict-Talbot estimated surface areas for boys and girls.[8]	Body Weight Kg	Body Weight Lb	Average Surface Area Sq Meter*	Maintenance Approx. Fl Oz†	Maintenance plus Replacement of Moderate Losses Approx. Fl Oz‡
†Based on water requirement of 1500 mL (50 fl oz) per sq meter.[7]	3	6–7	0.2	10	16
	5	11	0.29	15	23
	7	15	0.38	19	30
‡Based on water requirement of 2400 mL (80 fl oz) per sq meter.[7]	10	22	0.49	25	40
	12	26	0.55	28	44
	15	33	0.64	32	51
	18	40	0.76	38	61

in cooking or baking. Recipes or professional literature available upon request.

Precaution: In persons with advanced cirrhosis of the liver, large amounts of medium chain triglycerides in the diet may result in elevated blood and spinal fluid levels of medium chain fatty acids (MCFA), due to impaired hepatic clearance of these fatty acids, which are rapidly absorbed via the portal vein. These elevated levels have been reported to be associated with reversible coma and precoma in certain subjects with advanced cirrhosis, particularly with portacaval shunts. Therefore, diets containing high levels of medium chain triglyceride fat should be used with caution in persons with hepatic cirrhosis and complications thereof, such as portacaval shunts or tendency to encephalopathy.

Use of MCT Oil-containing products in abetalipoproteinemia is not indicated.

How Supplied: MCT Oil
0087-0365-03 Bottles of 1 quart

NUTRAMIGEN®
[nū-tram 'ĭ-jen]
Powder • ready-to-use • concentrate
Iron fortified protein hydrolysate
formula
Lactose-free, sucrose-free

Composition: 52% corn syrup solids, 18% corn oil, 16.3% casein enzymically hydrolyzed, 10.5% modified corn starch, and less than 2% of each of the following: vitamins (vitamin A palmitate, vitamin D₃, dl-alpha-tocopheryl acetate, phytonadione, thiamine hydrochloride, riboflavin, pyridoxine hydrochloride, vitamin B₁₂, niacinamide, folic acid, calcium pantothenate, biotin, ascorbic acid, choline chloride, and inositol), minerals (calcium citrate, calcium hydroxide, calcium phosphate, magnesium oxide, ferrous sulfate, zinc sulfate, manganese sulfate, cupric sulfate, sodium iodide, potassium citrate, and potassium chloride), L-cystine, L-tyrosine, L-tryptophan, taurine and L-carnitine.
[See table above].

Action and Uses: Provides virtually non-antigenic protein for feeding of infants and children allergic or intolerant to cow milk or soy protein in infant formulas, or to proteins in other foods. Provides a formula with extensively predigested protein for infants with diarrhea, colic or other gastrointestinal disturb-

NUTRAMIGEN®

NUTRIENTS (Normal Dilution)	Per 100 Calories (5 fl oz)	Per Quart
Protein, g	2.8	18
Fat, g	3.9	25
Carbohydrate, g	13.4	86
Water, g	134	860
Linoleic acid, mg	2000	12800
Vitamins:		
Vitamin A, IU	310	2000
Vitamin D, IU	62	400
Vitamin E, IU	3.1	20
Vitamin K, µg	15.6	100
Thiamine (Vitamin B₁), µg	78	500
Riboflavin (Vitamin B₂), µg	94	600
Vitamin B₆, µg	62	400
Vitamin B₁₂, µg	0.31	2
Niacin, µg	1250	8000
Folic acid (Folacin), µg	15.6	100
Pantothenic acid, µg	470	3000
Biotin, µg	7.8	50
Vitamin C (Ascorbic acid), mg	8.1	52
Choline, mg	13.3	85
Inositol, mg	4.7	30
Minerals:		
Calcium, mg	94	600
Phosphorus, mg	62	400
Magnesium, mg	10.9	70
Iron, mg	1.88	12
Zinc, mg	0.78	5
Manganese, µg	31	200
Copper, µg	94	600
Iodine, µg	7	45
Sodium, mg	47	300
Potassium, mg	109	700
Chloride, mg	86	550

ances. Provides lactose-free feedings in galactosemia.

Nutritionally complete. Appropriate as the sole source of infant nutrition.

Precautions: Nutramigen is not recommended for routine use in highly stressed low birthweight infants. Some of these infants may be at increased risk of developing gastrointestinal complications.

Preparation: Powder: For 20 Calories/fl oz: 1 packed level scoop powder (9.6 g) to 2 fl oz water, or 1 level cup (139 g) to water sufficient to make a quart of formula.
Ready-to-Use: Shake well, open, and pour into bottle.
Concentrate: Mix formula with equal amounts of sterilized water. Store bottled formula in refrigerator and use within 24 hours (Powder), or 48 hours (Ready-to-Use and Concentrate).

How Supplied: Nutramigen®
List #338-21 Cans of 16 oz (1 lb) powder, with scoop
List #499-11 Cans of 32 fl oz ready-to-use
List #498-11 Cans of 13 fl oz concentrate

POLY-VI-SOL®
[pahl-ē-vī-sahl '']
Vitamin drops • chewable tablets

Composition: Usual daily doses supply: [See table below].

Action and Uses: Daily vitamin supplementation for infants and children. Chewable tablets useful also for adults.

Administration and Dosage: Usual doses or as indicated.

How Supplied: Poly-Vi-Sol® vitamin drops: (with 'Safti-Dropper' marked to deliver 1.0 mL)
0087-0402-02 Bottles of 1 fl oz (30 mL)
0087-0402-03 Bottles of 1⅔ fl oz (50 mL)
6505-00-104-8433 (50 mL) (Defense)
Poly-Vi-Sol® chewable vitamins tablets:
0087-0412-03 Bottles of 100
Poly-Vi-Sol® chewable vitamins tablets in Circus Shapes:
0087-0414-02 Bottles of 100
0087-0414-06 Bottles of 60
Shown in Product Identification Section, page 414

POLY-VI-SOL® Vitamin drops, chewable tablets	Drops 1.0 mL	% U.S. RDA for Infants	Chewable Tablets 1 tablet	% U.S. RDA	
				Children Age 2–3 Years	Adults and Children Age 4 Years or more
Vitamin A, IU	1500	100	2500	100	50
Vitamin D, IU	400	100	400	100	100
Vitamin E, IU	5	100	15	150	50
Vitamin C, mg	35	100	60	150	100
Folic acid, mg	—	—	0.3	150	75
Thiamine, mg	0.5	100	1.05	150	70
Riboflavin, mg	0.6	100	1.2	150	70
Niacin, mg	8	100	13.5	150	68
Vitamin B₆, mg	0.4	100	1.05	150	53
Vitamin B₁₂, µg	2	100	4.5	150	75

Continued on next page

Mead Johnson Nutr.—Cont.

POLY-VI-SOL® with Iron
[pahl-ē-vī'sahl"]
Vitamin and Iron drops

Composition: Each 1.0 mL supplies:

		% U.S. RDA Infants
Vitamin A, IU	1500	100
Vitamin D, IU	400	100
Vitamin E, IU	5	100
Vitamin C, mg	35	100
Thiamine, mg	0.5	100
Riboflavin, mg	0.6	100
Niacin, mg	8	100
Vitamin B₆, mg	0.4	100
Iron, mg	10	67

Action and Uses: Daily vitamin and iron supplement for infants.

Administration and Dosage: Drop into mouth with 'Safti-Dropper.' Dose: 1.0 mL daily, or as indicated.

When an infant or child is taking iron, stools may appear darker in color. This is to be expected and should be no cause for concern. When drops containing iron are given to infants or young children, some darkening of the plaque on the teeth may occur. This is not serious or permanent as it does not affect the enamel. The stains can be removed or prevented by rubbing the teeth with a little baking soda or powder on a toothbrush or small cloth once or twice a week.

How Supplied: Poly-Vi-Sol® vitamin and iron drops (with dropper marked to deliver 1 mL)
0087-0405-01 Bottles of 1⅔ fl oz (50 mL)

Shown in Product Identification Section, page 414

POLY-VI-SOL® with Iron
[pahl-ē-vī-sahl"]
Chewable vitamins and minerals

Composition: Each tablet supplies same vitamins as Poly-Vi-Sol tablets [See

preceding page] plus 12 mg iron, 8 mg zinc, and 0.8 mg copper.
[See table below].

Action and Uses: Daily vitamin and mineral supplement for adults and children.

Administration and Dosage: 1 tablet daily.

How Supplied: Poly-Vi-Sol® chewable vitamins with Iron tablets.
0087-0455-02 Bottles of 100
Poly-Vi-Sol® chewable vitamins with Iron tablets in Circus Shapes.
0087-0456-02 Bottles of 100
0087-0456-06 Bottles of 60
Shown in Product Identification Section, page 414

PORTAGEN®
[port 'ă-jen]
Iron fortified nutritionally complete powder with
Medium Chain Triglycerides
U.S. Patent No. 3,450,819

Composition: Corn syrup solids, medium chain triglycerides (fractionated coconut oil), sodium caseinate, sugar (sucrose), corn oil, lecithin, vitamins (vitamin A palmitate, vitamin D₃, dl-alpha-tocopheryl acetate, phytonadione, thiamine hydrochloride, riboflavin, pyridoxine hydrochloride, vitamin B₁₂, niacinamide, folic acid, calcium pantothenate, biotin, ascorbic acid, choline chloride, and inositol), minerals (calcium citrate, calcium phosphate, magnesium phosphate, ferrous sulfate, zinc sulfate, manganese sulfate, cupric sulfate, sodium iodide, potassium citrate, and potassium chloride), taurine (38 mg/qt 20 Calories dilution), and L-carnitine.
Portagen powder provides 14% of the calories as protein, 41% as fat (87% of the fat is Medium Chain Triglycerides) and 45% as carbohydrate. One quart of prepared Portagen at 20 Cal/fl oz supplies 640 Calories; one quart at 30 Cal/fl oz supplies 960 Calories; one quart at 60 Cal/fl oz supplies 1920 Calories.

Action and Uses: A nutritionally complete dietary is prepared by adding Portagen powder to water. Portagen may be used where conventional food fats are not well digested or absorbed such as in patients with cystic fibrosis, pancreatic

or hepatic disease, lymphatic system disorders and in some patients with "fat storage" disorders.
This dietary may be used, according to physician recommendation, as the major or sole constituent of the diet. Or, it may be used as a beverage to be consumed with each meal, or it may be incorporated in various recipes. Recipes or professional literature available upon request.

Preparation: *To Prepare as a Beverage (30 Calories per fluid ounce):* Add 1½ packed level cups of Portagen powder (203 g) to 3 cups of water. Mix with electric mixer, egg beater or fork until smooth. Then stir in enough water to make 1 quart of beverage.
To Prepare as an Infant Formula (in normal dilution of 20 Calories per fluid ounce): Add 1 packed level cup (136 g) of Portagen powder to 3 cups of water. Mix with electric mixer, egg beater or fork until smooth. Then stir in enough water to make 1 quart of formula.
Store bottled formula in refrigerator and use within 24 hours.

Precautions: Recent studies indicate that, contrary to earlier recommendations, Portagen should not be used in cases of abetalipoproteinemia (faulty chylomicron formation). The usual intake of water should be maintained when Portagen beverage is used as the sole article or major part of the diet.

How Supplied: Portagen® powder
0087-0387-01 Cans of 16 oz (1 lb)

PREGESTIMIL®
[prē-jest 'ĭ-mĭl"]
Iron fortified protein hydrolysate formula with medium chain triglycerides
Lactose-free, sucrose-free

Composition: 52% corn syrup solids, 15.5% casein enzymatically hydrolyzed, 10.5% corn oil, 10.3% modified tapioca starch, 7.7% medium chain triglycerides (fractionated coconut oil), and less than 2% of each of the following: vitamins (vitamin A palmitate, vitamin D₃, dl-alpha-tocopheryl acetate, phytonadione, thiamine hydrochloride, riboflavin, pyridoxine hydrochloride, vitamin B₁₂, niacinamide, folic acid, calcium pantothenate, biotin, sodium ascorbate, choline chloride, and inositol), minerals (calcium citrate, calcium phosphate, magnesium oxide, ferrous sulfate, zinc sulfate, manganese sulfate, cupric sulfate, sodium iodide, potassium citrate, and potassium chloride), soy lecithin, L-cystine, L-tyrosine, L-tryptophan, taurine, and L-carnitine.
[See table on next page].

Action and Uses: Provides very easily digestible and assimilable fat, carbohydrate, and extensively hydrolyzed protein for feeding of infants and children with severe problems of diarrhea and those infants and children with fat absorption problems:

POLY-VI-SOL® with Iron Chewable Tablets	Chewable Tablets 1 tablet	% U.S. RDA		
		Children 2–3 Years	Adults and Children Age 4 Years or more	
Vitamin A, IU	2500	100	50	
Vitamin D, IU	400	100	100	
Vitamin E, IU	15	150	50	
Vitamin C, mg	60	150	100	
Folic acid, mg	0.3	150	75	
Thiamine, mg	1.05	150	70	
Riboflavin, mg	1.2	150	70	
Niacin, mg	13.5	150	68	
Vitamin B₆, mg	1.05	150	53	
Vitamin B₁₂, μg	4.5	150	75	
Iron, mg	12	120	67	
Copper, mg	0.8	80	40	
Zinc, mg	8	100	53	

- cystic fibrosis
- steatorrhea
- short gut syndrome

Since the protein source in casein hydrolysate, Pregestimil may be used when fat absorption problems occur concurrently with protein allergy or intolerance.

Since Pregestimil contains protein hydrolysate, it may be used for malabsorption problems complicated by protein allergies. Pregestimil is isotonic (300 mOsm per kg H_2O formula) to avoid problems associated with hyperosmolar formulas; and contains protective levels of important micronutrients to offset increased losses of these nutrients due to a malabsorption disorder. In infants with severe malabsorption problems of non-specific etiologies, such as intractable diarrhea, nutritional maintenance with Pregestimil permits trial of specific disaccharides, milk protein or regular dietary fats to determine if the dietary intolerance is due to a component of conventional feedings.

Nutritionally complete. Appropriate as the sole source of infant nutrition.

Precautions: Initial feedings of Pregestimil should be diluted to 10 Calories/fl oz or less and gradually increased to 20 Calories/fl oz over a period of 3 to 5 days. This product is not recommended for routine use in highly stressed low birthweight infants. Some of these infants may be at increased risk of developing gastrointestinal complications.

Preparation: For 10 Calories/fl oz: add one packed level scoop (enclosed) (9.7 g) of Pregestimil powder to each 4 fl oz (120 mL) of water. Always add powder to water. To make a quart of 10 Calories/fl oz formula, add 1/2 packed level cup (70 g) of powder to 29 fl oz (860 mL) of water. For 20 Calories/fl oz: add one packed level scoop (9.7 g) of Pregestimil powder to each 2 fl oz (60 mL) of water. To make a quart of 20 Calories/fl oz formula, add one packed level cup (140 g) of powder to 29 fl oz (860 mL) of water.

Feed immediately, or cover and refrigerate until needed.

Caution: Store remaining liquid formula in refrigerator in a covered container and use within 24 hours after mixing.

Caution: Use within 24 hours after mixing. After opening can, keep tightly covered and use contents within one month.

Caution: Unless medically indicated to manage fat malabsorption problems, medium chain triglycerides may be digested too rapidly and may cause cramping, bloating, and even projectile diarrhea.

How Supplied: Pregestimil® powder Cans of 16 oz (1 lb) with measuring scoop. Makes 3.5 quarts at standard dilution. List # 367-21

PREGESTIMIL®

NUTRIENTS (Normal Dilution):	Per 100 Calories (5 fl oz)	Per Quart
Protein equivalent, g	2.8	18
Fat, g	4.1	26
Carbohydrate, g	13.4	86
Water, g	127	810
Linoleic acid, mg	1360	8700
Vitamins:		
Vitamin A, IU	310	2000
Vitamin D, IU	62	400
Vitamin E, IU	2.3	15
Vitamin K, μg	15.6	100
Thiamine (Vitamin B_1), μg	78	500
Riboflavin (Vitamin B_2), μg	94	600
Vitamin B_6, μg	62	400
Vitamin B_{12}, μg	0.31	2
Niacin, μg	1250	8000
Folic acid (Folacin), μg	15.6	100
Pantothenic acid, μg	470	3000
Biotin, μg	7.8	50
Vitamin C (Ascorbic acid), mg	8.1	52
Choline, mg	13.3	85
Inositol, mg	4.7	30
Minerals:		
Calcium, mg	94	600
Phosphorus, mg	62	400
Magnesium, mg	10.9	70
Iron, mg	1.88	12
Zinc, mg	0.62	4
Manganese, μg	31	200
Copper, μg	94	600
Iodine, μg	7	45
Sodium, mg	47	300
Potassium, mg	109	700
Chloride, mg	86	550

PROSOBEE® concentrated liquid
[prō-sō 'bee]
- ready-to-use liquid • powder
Iron fortified milk-free soy protein formula

ProSobee Concentrated Liquid

Ingredients: 75% water, 13.2% corn syrup solids, 4.1% soy protein isolate, 3.6% coconut oil, 3% soy oil, and less than 1% of each of the following: soy lecithin, mono- and diglycerides, carrageenan, vitamins (vitamin A palmitate, vitamin D_3, dl-alpha-tocopheryl acetate, phytonadione, thiamine hydrochloride, riboflavin, pyridoxine hydrochloride, vitamin B_{12}, niacinamide, folic acid, calcium pantothenate, biotin, sodium ascorbate, choline chloride, inositol), minerals (calcium phosphate, magnesium chloride, ferrous sulfate, zinc sulfate, cupric sulfate, potassium iodide, salt, potassium citrate, potassium hydroxide, potassium chloride, sodium selenite), L-methionine, taurine and L-carnitine.

ProSobee Ready-To-Use

Ingredients: 87% water, 6.8% corn syrup solids, 2.1% soy protein isolate, 1.9% coconut oil, 1.5% soy oil, and less than 1% of each of the following: soy lecithin, mono- and diglycerides, carrageenan, vitamins (vitamin A palmitate, vitamin D_3, dl-alpha-tocopheryl acetate, phytonadione, thiamine hydrochloride, riboflavin, pyridoxine hydrochloride, vitamin B_{12}, niacinamide, folic acid, calcium pantothenate, biotin, sodium ascorbate, choline chloride, inositol), minerals (calcium phosphate, magnesium chlo-

ride, ferrous sulfate, zinc sulfate, cupric sulfate, potassium iodide, salt, potassium citrate, potassium hydroxide, potassium chloride, sodium selenite), L-methionine, taurine, L-carnitine).

ProSobee Powder

Ingredients: 51% corn syrup solids, 17.4% soy protein isolate, 15.3% coconut oil, 12.5% corn oil, and less than 2% of each of the following: vitamins (vitamin A palmitate, vitamin D_3, dl-alpha-tocopheryl acetate, phytonadione, thiamine hydrochloride, riboflavin, pyridoxine hydrochloride, vitamin B_{12}, niacinamide, folic acid, calcium pantothenate, biotin, sodium ascorbate, choline chloride, inositol), minerals (calcium phosphate, calcium carbonate, magnesium phosphate, ferrous sulfate, zinc sulfate, cupric sulfate, potassium iodide, potassium citrate, potassium hydroxide, potassium chloride, sodium selenite), L-methionine, taurine, L-carnitine.
[See table on next page].

Action and Uses: Milk-free, lactose-free and sucrose-free formula with soy protein for infants with common feeding problems associated with milk sensitivity, such as: mild diarrhea, fussiness, spitting up, rash and eczema. ProSobee should be considered for infants sensitive to milk, with lactose or sucrose intolerance, or with galactosemia. As a milk substitute for children and adults with poor tolerance to milk. Its sucrose-free

Continued on next page

Mead Johnson Nutr.—Cont.

formulation avoids the unnecessary sweetness of other soy formulas.

Preparation: *Concentrated Liquid:* For 20 Calories/fl oz, 1 part ProSobee Concentrated Liquid to 1 part water. ProSobee may be used to replace milk as a beverage or in cooking.

An opened can of ProSobee liquid should be covered, refrigerated and used within 48 hours.

Powder: To make a quart of formula, add 1 unpacked level cup of powder to 29 fl oz of water; for single bottle feeding, add 1 unpacked level scoop of powder to each 2 fl oz of water. Mix vigorously. Reconstituted powder should be covered, kept refrigerated and used within 24 hours. ProSobee powder needs no refrigeration.

How Supplied: ProSobee®
List 308-01 Cans of 13 fl oz concentrated liquid (40 Calories/fl oz)
List 309-01 Cans of 32 fl oz (1 qt) ready-to-use (20 Calories/fl oz)
List 309-42 Cans of 8 fl oz ready-to-use (20 Calories/fl oz)
List 3101-21 Cans of 14 oz powder

SMURF™
[smerf]
chewable vitamins

Composition: Usual daily dose supplies: [See table above].

Action and Uses: Daily vitamin supplementation for children and adults.

PROSOBEE® NUTRIENTS	Per 100 Calories (5 fl oz)	Per Quart
Protein, g	3	19.2
Fat, g	5.3	34
Carbohydrate, g	10	64
Water, g	134	860
Linoleic acid, mg	1000	6400
Vitamins:		
Vitamin A, IU	310	2000
Vitamin D, IU	62	400
Vitamin E, IU	3.1	20
Vitamin K, μg	15.6	100
Thiamine (Vitamin B_1), μg	78	500
Riboflavin (Vitamin B_2), μg	94	600
Vitamin B_6, μg	62	400
Vitamin B_{12}, μg	0.31	2
Niacin, μg	1250	8000
Folic acid (Folacin), μg	15.6	100
Pantothenic acid, μg	470	3000
Biotin, μg	7.8	50
Vitamin C (Ascorbic acid), mg	8.1	52
Choline, mg	7.8	50
Inositol, mg	4.7	30
Minerals:		
Calcium, mg	94	600
Phosphorus, mg	74	475
Magnesium, mg	10.9	70
Iron, mg	1.88	12
Zinc, mg	0.78	5
Manganese, μg	25	160
Copper, μg	94	600
Iodine, μg	10.2	65
Sodium, mg	36	230
Potassium, mg	122	780
Chloride, mg	83	530

SMURF™

		Percentage of U.S. Recommended Daily Allowance	
		Children Age 2–3 Years	Adults & Children Age 4 Years or More
Vitamin A, IU	2500	100	50
Vitamin D, IU	400	100	100
Vitamin E, IU	15	150	50
Vitamin C, mg	60	150	100
Folic acid, mg	0.3	150	75
Thiamine, mg	1.05	150	70
Riboflavin, mg	1.2	150	70
Niacin, mg	13.5	150	68
Vitamin B_6, mg	1.05	150	53
Vitamin B_{12}, μg	4.5	150	75

Administration and Dosage: 1 tablet daily.

How Supplied: Smurf™ chewable vitamins:
0087-0484-01 Bottles of 60

SMURF™
[smerf]
chewable vitamins with Iron and Zinc

Composition: Each tablet supplies same vitamins as Smurf™ chewable vitamins (see above) plus 12 mg iron and 8 mg zinc.

Action and Uses: Daily vitamin and mineral supplement for children and adults.

Administration and Dosage: 1 tablet daily.

How Supplied: Smurf™ chewable vitamins with Iron and Zinc:
0087-0485-01 Bottles of 60

SUSTACAL®
[sŭs'tă-cal"]
● liquid (ready to use)
● powder (mix with milk)
● pudding (ready-to-eat)
Nutritionally complete food

Composition: (Vanilla Liquid)
Water, sugar (sucrose), corn syrup, calcium caseinate, partially hydrogenated soy oil, soy protein isolate, sodium caseinate, potassium citrate, magnesium phosphate, salt (sodium chloride), potassium chloride, calcium carbonate, artificial flavor, calcium phosphate, lecithin, carrageenan, vitamins (vitamin A palmitate, cholecalciferol, dl-alpha-tocopheryl acetate, sodium ascorbate, folic acid, thiamine hydrochloride, riboflavin, niacinamide, pyridoxine hydrochloride, cyanocobalamin, biotin, calcium pantothenate, phytonadione and choline bitartrate) and minerals (sodium iodide, ferric pyrophosphate, ferrous sulfate, cupric sulfate, zinc sulfate and manganese sulfate). (In addition to the above, Chocolate liquid contains Dutch process cocoa [alkalized], and artificial color.) Eggnog flavored liquid contains artificial color.
Each 12-fl-oz can of Sustacal supplies 21.7 g protein, 8.3 g fat, 49.6 g carbohydrate, 360 Calories (1 Calorie per ml) and 33% of the U.S. RDA for all essential vitamins and minerals. Sustacal liquid is lactose free.

Vanilla Powder—Nonfat milk, sugar, corn syrup solids, artificial flavor, magnesium phosphate, vitamins (vitamin A palmitate, cholecalciferol, dl-alpha-tocopheryl acetate, sodium ascorbate, folic acid, thiamine hydrochloride, niacinamide, pyridoxine hydrochloride, cyanocobalamin, biotin and calcium pantothenate) and minerals (ferrous sulfate, cupric carbonate, zinc sulfate, and manganese sulfate). (In addition to the above, Chocolate Powder contains Dutch process cocoa [alkalized], and lecithin.)
With the exception of lactose, one pouch of Sustacal powder mixed with 8-fl oz whole milk provides essentially the same nutritional value as a 12 fl oz can of Sustacal.

Vanilla Pudding—Water, nonfat milk, sugar, partially hydrogenated soy oil,

modified food starch, magnesium phosphate, sodium stearoyl lactylate, natural and artificial flavor, sodium phosphate, carrageenan, artificial color (includes FD&C Yellow No. 5), and vitamins and minerals (vitamin A palmitate, sodium ascorbate, thiamine hydrochloride, riboflavin, niacinamide, ferric pyrophosphate, cholecalciferol, dl-alpha-tocopheryl acetate, pyridoxine hydrochloride, folic acid, cyanocobalamin, zinc sulfate, cupric sulfate, biotin and calcium pantothenate).

In addition to the above, Chocolate contains Dutch process cocoa (alkalized) but no FD&C Yellow No. 5. Butterscotch does not contain FD&C Yellow No. 5.

Sustacal Pudding provides 11% of Calories as protein, 36% as fat, 53% as carbohydrate and 15% of the U.S. RDA for all essential vitamins and minerals in a 5 oz serving.

Action and Uses: Sustacal liquid and powder are ideally formulated to provide for the nutritional needs of the broad range of patients requiring an oral supplement or high protein diet (21.7 g protein in one 12 fl oz serving).

Sustacal liquid is of particular value to patients who require a supplement and can be used effectively for anorectic cancer patients, hypermetabolic patients (as in burn or multiple trauma patients) and elderly patients. It is also recommended to be used as the sole source of diet in the above mentioned patients and in those patients who require less than 1500 Cal per day (Sustacal liquid is designed to provide 100% of the daily nutrient needs in less than 1500 Cal.)

Sustacal Pudding is a convenient and well-accepted means of providing supplemental nutrition and is especially appropriate to help avoid taste fatigue and monotony associated with liquid supplements.

Preparation: Liquid: ready to serve in 30 Cal/fl oz dilution (one Cal per milliliter). Powder: mix contents of one packet with 8-fl oz whole milk to prepare a 40 Calorie per fluid ounce dilution. To prepare powder in 30 Calorie per fluid ounce dilution, add 90 ml (3 fl oz) of water to the above mixture to yield approximately 12 fl oz. Both forms may be used orally or by tube. Vanilla flavor is recommended for tube feeding if chocolate allergy is suspected.

In initiating tube feeding, particularly for malnourished patients, feedings should be diluted to half-strength on Day 1; increase volume and concentration gradually over a period of several days.

Precautions: When Sustacal liquid is used as the sole food, give additional water as needed for adequate daily intake. This is particularly important for unconscious or semiconscious patients. Do not begin postoperative tube feedings until peristalsis is reestablished. Electrolyte content of Sustacal should be considered for cardiac patients and others who tend to have edema. Sustacal liquid supplies 840 ml of water per 1000 ml.

Store bottled formula in refrigerator and use within 48 hours.

How Supplied: Sustacal® Vanilla liquid and powder.
0087-0351-42 Cans of 8 fl oz
0087-0351-01 Cans of 12 fl oz
0087-0351-44 Cans of 32 fl oz (1 quart)
0087-0353-01 Packets of 1.9 oz, 4 packets per carton
0087-0353-04 Cans of 1 lb
VA 8940-01-024-6421 (8 fl oz, van.)
Sustacal® Chocolate liquid and powder.
0087-0350-42 Cans of 8 fl oz
0087-0350-01 Cans of 12 fl oz
0087-0350-44 Cans of 32 fl oz (1 quart)
0087-0352-01 Packets of 1.9 oz, 4 packets per carton
VA 8940-01-048-3360 (8 fl oz, choc.)
Sustacal® Eggnog liquid.
0087-0457-42 Cans of 8 fl oz, 12 cans per case
0087-0457-44 Cans of 32 fl oz, 6 cans per case
VA 8940-01-087-2875 (8 fl oz, eggnog)
Sustacal® Pudding
0087-0409-41 Vanilla, 5 oz cans, 4 cans per carton, 12 cartons per case
0087-0410-41 Chocolate, 5 oz cans, 4 cans per carton, 12 cartons per case
0087-0415-41 Butterscotch, 5 oz cans, 4 cans per carton, 12 cartons per case
VA8940-01-074-3125 (Vanilla, 5 oz cans)
VA8940-01-074-3124 (Chocolate, 5 oz cans)
VA8940-01-074-3123 (Butterscotch, 5 oz cans)

SUSTACAL® HC
[sŭs'tă-cal' hc']
High calorie nutritionally complete food

Composition: (Vanilla Flavored Liquid) Water, corn syrup solids, corn oil, sugar, calcium caseinate, sodium caseinate, lecithin, potassium chloride, magnesium phosphate, calcium carbonate, artificial flavor, sodium citrate, carrageenan, potassium citrate, vitamins (vitamin A palmitate, cholecalciferol, dl-alpha-tocopheryl acetate, sodium ascorbate, folic acid, thiamine hydrochloride, riboflavin, niacinamide, pyridoxine hydrochloride, cyanocobalamin, biotin, calcium pantothenate, phytonadione and choline bitartrate) and minerals (sodium iodide, ferric pyrophosphate, ferrous sulfate, cupric sulfate, zinc sulfate and manganese sulfate).

Sustacal HC is available in vanilla, chocolate, and eggnog flavors. (In addition to the above, chocolate flavored liquid contains Dutch process cocoa [alkalized], and artificial color. Eggnog flavored liquid also contains artificial color.)

Each 8-fl oz can of Sustacal HC supplies 14.4 g protein, 13.6 g fat, 45 g carbohydrate, 360 Calories (1.5 Cal/ml) and at least 20% of the U.S. RDA for all essential vitamins and minerals.

Actions and Uses: Sustacal HC liquid is formulated to meet the supplemental or total nutritional needs of patients requiring generous calorie and protein intake (1.5 Cal/ml; 14.4 g protein/8 fl oz)

while limiting total fluid volume. Sustacal HC is of particular value to patients in these situations: hypermetabolic states (burn, major trauma, thyrotoxicosis, etc.); fluid restrictions (neurosurgery, congestive heart failure, etc.); volume restrictions (cardiac or cancer cachexia, chronic obstructive lung disease); and lactose intolerance.

Preparation: Sustacal HC is ready to drink. Shake well before opening. Unopened Sustacal HC should be stored at room temperature. Refrigerate unused Sustacal HC and use within 48 hours. Acceptance by some patients is enhanced if Sustacal HC liquid is chilled before serving. Very ill patients should be directed to sip the liquid slowly.

Preparation for Tube Feeding: If Sustacal HC is used for this purpose, initial feedings should be diluted to half strength (0.75 Cal/ml) on the first day and three-fourths strength (1.12 Cal/ml) on the second day. This will allow the body to adjust to the osmolality of Sustacal HC Liquid. As tolerance is established, Sustacal HC Liquid can be fed full strength—1.5 Cal/ml.

Tube Feeding Precaution: Additional water should be given as needed to meet the patient's requirements. Particular attention should be given to water supply for comatose and unconscious patients and others who cannot express the usual sensation of thirst. Additional water is important also when renal concentrating ability is impaired, when there is extensive breakdown of tissue protein, or when water requirements are high, as in fever, burns or under dry atmospheric conditions. Sustacal HC provides 775 ml of water per 1000 ml of formula.

How Supplied: Sustacal® HC vanilla flavored liquid.
0087-0460-42 Cans of 8 fl oz
Sustacal HC chocolate flavored liquid
0087-0466-42 Cans of 8 fl oz
Sustacal HC eggnog flavored liquid
0087-0461-42 Cans of 8 fl oz

SUSTAGEN® powder
[sŭs'tă-djen"]
Nutritional supplement

Composition: Corn syrup solids, nonfat milk, powdered whole milk, calcium caseinate, dextrose, artificial vanilla flavor, vitamins (vitamin A palmitate, cholecalciferol, dl-alpha-tocopheryl acetate, ascorbic acid, folic acid, thiamine hydrochloride, riboflavin, niacinamide, pyridoxine hydrochloride, cyanocobalamin, biotin, calcium pantothenate, phytonadione, and choline bitartrate), and minerals (ferrous sulfate, dibasic magnesium phosphate, cupric carbonate, zinc sulfate, and manganese sulfate).

Chocolate-flavored Sustagen also contains sugar and cocoa. High in protein, low in fat; generous in vitamins, calcium and iron. Easily mixed with water to make a pleasant-tasting beverage or a feeding via nasogastric tube.

Continued on next page

Mead Johnson Nutr.—Cont.

One quart of prepared Sustagen supplies 107 g protein, 300 g carbohydrate, 15.9 g fat and at least 100% of the U.S. RDA for all essential vitamins and minerals.

Actions and Uses: Orally or by tube, provides extra nutritional support for ill, injured, surgical, and convalescent patients and those with impediments to eating or swallowing. Useful in peptic ulcer for buffering effect plus nutrition.

Preparation: Oral dilution: Mix equal parts (by volume) of Sustagen powder and water. This yields about 50 Cal/fl oz. One pound (3 packed level cups) Sustagen powder and 3 cups water make about a quart. ⅔ packed level cup Sustagen powder and ⅔ cup water make a single serving.
Refrigerate reconstituted Sustagen and use within 24 hours.

Tube-feeding dilution: Use 400 g Sustagen powder to 800 ml water for 1 liter. This mixture yields about 45 Cal/fl oz. More dilute mixtures may be utilized if desired. **In initiating tube feeding,** particularly for malnourished patients, feedings should be diluted to half-strength on Day 1; increase volume and concentration gradually over a period of several days. Vanilla flavor is recommended for tube feeding if chocolate allergy is suspected.

Precautions: When Sustagen is used as the sole food, give additional water as needed for adequate daily intake. This is particularly important for unconscious or semiconscious patients. Do not begin post-operative tube feedings until peristalsis is reestablished. Electrolyte content of Sustagen should be considered for cardiac patients and others who tend to have edema.

How Supplied: Sustagen® vanilla
0087-0393-01 Cans of 16 oz (1 lb)
0087-0393-03 Cans of 5 lb
Sustagen chocolate
0087-0394-01 Cans of 16 oz (1 lb)

TEMPRA®
[tem'prah]
Acetaminophen

**Drops • syrup • chewable tablets
For infants and children**

Composition: Tempra is acetaminophen, a safe and effective analgesic-antipyretic. It is not a salicylate. It contains no phenacetin or caffeine. It has no effect on prothrombin time. Tempra offers prompt, non-irritating therapy. Because it provides significant freedom from side effects, it is particularly valuable for patients who do not tolerate aspirin well. Tempra drops contain no alcohol. Tempra syrup contains no alcohol. Tempra chewable tablets are sugar-free.

Action and Uses: Tempra drops, syrup and chewable tablets are useful for reducing fever and for the temporary relief of minor aches, pains and discomfort associated with the common cold or "flu," inoculations or vaccination. Tempra syrup is valuable in reducing pain following tonsillectomy and adenoidectomy. When Tempra is used by pregnant or nursing women, there are no known adverse effects upon fetal development or nursing infants.

Administration and Dosage:
Every 4 hours as needed but not more than 5 times daily.
[See table below]

Drops are given with calibrated 'Safti-Dropper' or mixed with water or fruit juices. Syrup is given by teaspoon.

Precaution: Acetaminophen has been reported to potentiate the effect of orally administered anticoagulants and may enhance the elimination of chloramphenicol. Therapeutic drug monitoring should be considered whenever these drugs are used concurrently.

Side Effects: Infrequent, nonspecific side effects have been reported with the therapeutic use of acetaminophen.

Overdosage: Acetaminophen in overdosage may cause hepatic toxicity in some patients. In all cases of suspected overdose, **immediately** contact a Poison Control Center for assistance in diagnosis and for information on the antidotes used to treat acetaminophen overdosage. The Rocky Mountain Poison Center toll-free number is (800) 525-6115.
Following the ingestion of a large quantity of acetaminophen, patients may be asymptomatic for several days. Likewise, clinical laboratory evidence of hepatotoxicity may be delayed for up to a week. Parents' estimates of the quantity of a drug ingested are often also unreliable. Therefore, any report of the ingestion of an overdose should be corroborated by assaying for the acetaminophen plasma concentration. Since plasma levels at specific time points following an overdose correlate closely with the potential occurrence and probable severity of hepatotoxicity, it is important to accurately determine the elapsed time from ingestion of an overdose to the time of plasma acetaminophen determination.
Close clinical monitoring and serial hepatic enzyme studies are recommended for patients who delay presentation until several days following a reported acetaminophen overdose.

Note: A prescription is not required for Tempra drops, syrup or tablets as an analgesic. To prevent its misuse by the layman, the following information appears on the package label:

Warning: If fever persists for more than 3 days (72 hours) or if pain continues for more than 5 days, consult your physician.
Phenylketonurics: Each 80 mg tablet contains 3.3 mg phenylalanine. Each 160 mg tablet contains 6.6 mg phenylalanine.

How Supplied: Tempra® (acetaminophen) drops: (with calibrated 'Safti-Dropper') grape-flavored
NDC 0087-0730-01 Bottles of 15 mL
Tempra® (acetaminophen) syrup: cherry-flavored
NDC 0087-0733-04 Bottles of 4 fl oz
NDC 0087-0733-03 Bottles of 16 fl oz
Tempra chewables: grape-flavored, no sucrose
NDC 0087-0738-01 Bottles of 30 (80 mg) tablets

Age	Approximate Weight Range*	Dosage			
		Drops	Syrup	Chewables 80 mg	Chewables 160 mg
Under 3 mo	Under 13 lb	½ dropper	¼ tsp	—	—
3 to 9 mo	13–20 lb	1 dropper	½ tsp	—	—
10 to 24 mo	21–26 lb	1½ dropper	¾ tsp	—	—
2 to 3 yr	27–35 lb	2 droppers	1 tsp	2 tablets	—
4 to 5 yr	36–43 lb	3 droppers	1½ tsp	3 tablets	1½ tablets
6 to 8 yr	44–62 lb	—	2 tsp	4 tablets	2 tablets
9 to 10 yr	63–79 lb	—	2½ tsp	5 tablets	2½ tablets
11 yr	80–89 lb	—	3 tsp	6 tablets	3 tablets
12 yr and older	90 lb & over	—	3–4 tsp	6–8 tablets	3–4 tablets

Dosage may be given every 4 hours as needed but not more than 5 times daily.
HOW SUPPLIED:
DROPS: Each 0.8 mL dropper contains 80 mg (1.23 grains) acetaminophen.
SYRUP: Each 5 mL teaspoon contains 160 mg (2.46 grains) acetaminophen.
CHEWABLES: Each 80 mg tablet contains 1.23 grains acetaminophen. Each 160 mg tablet contains 2.46 grains acetaminophen.
*If child is significantly under- or overweight, dosage may need to be adjusted accordingly.

NDC 0087-0749-01 Bottles of 30 (160 mg) tablets
No ℞ required.
Shown in Product Identification Section, page 414

TRAUMACAL®
[tră'mă-cal"]
High nitrogen and high calorie nutritionally complete formula for traumatized patients
Liquid (ready-to-use)

Composition: Water, corn syrup, calcium caseinate, soybean oil, sodium caseinate, sugar, medium chain triglycerides (fractionated coconut oil), lecithin, potassium citrate, magnesium chloride, salt, artificial flavor, potassium chloride, calcium carbonate, carrageenan, vitamins (vitamin A palmitate, cholecalciferol, dl-alpha-tocopheryl acetate, sodium ascorbate, folic acid, thiamine hydrochloride, riboflavin, niacinamide, pyridoxine hydrochloride, cyanocobalamin, biotin, calcium pantothenate, phytonadione and choline bitartrate) and minerals (potassium iodide, ferrous sulfate, cupric sulfate, zinc sulfate and manganese sulfate).

Indication: TraumaCal is a nutritionally complete ready-to-use liquid specifically formulated for patients requiring high nitrogen and calorie intake in limited volume (multiple trauma, moderate to severe burns). This formula may be fed orally or as a tube-feeding.

Actions: TraumaCal provides 22% of the total calories as protein, 40% as fat and 38% as carbohydrate in a 1.5 Cal/ml formula. TraumaCal is lactose-free with an osmolality of 490 mOsm/kg water.

Preparation: TraumaCal liquid is ready to feed; shake well before opening. Unused TraumaCal should be covered, refrigerated and used within 48 hours of opening. -
It is recommended that TraumaCal be tube fed and that tube feeding be initiated as follows: Day 1—1:1 dilution of TraumaCal to water at 50 ml/hour (or full strength at 25 ml/hour). Day 2—full strength at 50 ml/hour. Day 3—full strength up to 100–125 ml/hour. Administration via infusion pump is recommended. If gravity feeding is utilized, larger diameter indwelling tubes are recommended to facilitate flow rate (12 French or larger.)

Precaution: Additional water should be given as needed to meet the patient's requirements. Particular attention should be given to water supply for comatose and unconscious patients and others who cannot express the usual sensation of thirst. Additional water is important also when renal concentrating ability is impaired, when there is extensive breakdown of tissue protein, or when water requirements are high, as in fever, burns or under dry atmospheric conditions. TraumaCal provides 780 ml of water per 1000 ml of formula.

How Supplied: TraumaCal liquid 0087-0464-42 Cans of 8 fl oz

TRIND® liquid
[trĭnd]
Antihistamine • nasal decongestant
Sugar-free

Description:
Active Ingredients: Each teaspoon (5 mL) contains 12.5 mg phenylpropanolamine HCl and 2 mg chlorpheniramine maleate.
Inactive Ingredients: Alcohol (5% V/V), citric acid, edetate disodium, FD&C Yellow No. 6, glycerin, orange flavor (artificial), sodium benzoate, sodium citrate, sorbitol, water.

Indications: Pleasant tasting, orange-flavored liquid temporarily suppresses cough, relieves runny nose, sneezing, nasal congestion and itchy, watery eyes due to the common cold or hay fever. When Trind is used by pregnant or nursing women according to the recommended dosage schedule, there are no known adverse effects upon fetal development or nursing infants.

Directions: One dose every 4 hours as needed but not more than 6 times daily.

Age (yrs)	Approximate Weight Range*	Dosage
Under 3 months	Under 13 lb	As directed by physician
3–9 months	13–20 lb	⅛ tsp
10–24 months	21–26 lb	¼ tsp
2–5	27–43 lb	½ tsp
6–12	44–90 lb	1 tsp
Adult	91 lb and over	2 tsp

*If child is significantly under or overweight, consult a physician for appropriate dosage.

Warnings: If symptoms do not improve within 7 days or are accompanied by high fever, consult a doctor before continued use. Exceeding recommended dosage may cause nervousness, dizziness, or sleeplessness. May cause excitability in children. Do not take this product if you have asthma, glaucoma, emphysema, difficulty in breathing, high blood pressure, heart disease, diabetes, thyroid disease, prostatitis, or are taking sedatives or transquilizers without first consulting your doctor. May cause drowsiness. Avoid alcoholic beverages. Use caution when driving a motor vehicle or operating machinery. As with any drug, if you are pregnant or nursing a baby, seek the advice of a health professional before using this product.

How Supplied: Trind® liquid (available without prescription)
NDC 0087-0750-44 Bottles of 5 fl oz

TRIND-DM® liquid
[trĭnd-dm']
Cough suppressant • antihistamine • nasal decongestant
Sugar-free

Description:
Active Ingredients: Each teaspoon (5 mL) contains 12.5 mg phenylpropanolamine HCl, 7.5 mg dextromethorphan HBr, and 2 mg chlorpheniramine maleate.
Inactive Ingredients: Alcohol (5% V/V), citric acid, D&C Red No. 33, edetate disodium, fruit flavor (artificial), glycerin, sodium benzoate, sodium citrate, sorbitol, water.

Indications: Pleasant tasting, fruit-flavored liquid temporarily suppresses cough, relieves runny nose, sneezing, nasal congestion and itchy, watery eyes due to the common cold or hay fever. When Trind-DM is used by pregnant or nursing women according to the recommended dosage schedule, there are no known adverse effects on fetal development or nursing infants.

Dosage: One dose every 4 hours as needed but not more than 6 times daily.

Age (yrs)	Approximate Weight Range*	Dosage
Under 3 months	Under 13 lb	As directed by physician
3–9 months	13–20 lb	⅛ tsp
10–24 months	21–26 lb	¼ tsp
2–5	27–43 lb	½ tsp
6–12	44–90 lb	1 tsp
Adult	91 lb and over	2 tsp

*If child is significantly under or overweight, consult a physician for appropriate dosage.

Warnings: A persistent cough may be a sign of a serious condition. If cough or other symptoms persists for more than 7 days, tends to recur, or is accompanied by fever, rash or persistent headaches, consult a doctor. Do not take this product for persistent cough such as occurs with smoking or if cough is accompanied by excessive phlegm (mucus) unless directed by a doctor. Exceeding recommended dosage may cause nervousness, dizziness, or sleeplessness. May cause excitability in children. Do not take this product if you have asthma, glaucoma, emphysema, difficulty in breathing, high blood pressure, heart disease, diabetes, thyroid disease, prostatitis, or are taking sedatives or tranquilizers without first consulting your doctor. May cause drowsiness. Avoid alcoholic beverages. Use caution when driving a motor vehicle or operating machinery. As with any drug, if you are pregnant or nursing a baby, seek the advice of a health professional before using this product.

How Supplied: Trind-DM® liquid: (Available without prescription.)
NDC 0087-0753-44 Bottles of 5 fl oz

TRI-VI-SOL®
[trī-vī-sahl"]
Vitamins A, D and C drops

	Drops 1.0 mL	% U.S. RDA for Infants
Vitamin A, IU	1500	100

Continued on next page

Mead Johnson Nutr.—Cont.

Vitamin D, IU	400	100
Vitamin C, mg	35	100

Action and Uses: Tri-Vi-Sol drops provide vitamins A, D and C.

How Supplied: Tri-Vi-Sol® drops: (with 'Safti-Dropper' marked to deliver 1 mL)
0087-0403-02 Bottles of 1 fl oz (30 mL)
0087-0403-03 Bottles of 1⅔ fl oz (50 mL)

Shown in Product Identification Section, page 414

TRI-VI-SOL® with Iron
[*trī-vī-sahl* ʺ]
Vitamins A, D, C and Iron drops

Composition: Each 1.0 mL supplies same vitamins as in Tri-Vi-Sol® vitamin drops (see above) plus 10 mg iron.

Action and Uses: Tri-Vi-Sol with Iron vitamins A, D, C and Iron for infants and children.

Administration and Dosage: Drop into mouth with 'Safti-Dropper'. Dose: 1.0 mL daily, or as indicated.

How Supplied: Tri-Vi-Sol® vitamin drops with Iron (with dropper marked to deliver 1 mL)
0087-0453-03 Bottles of 1⅔ fl oz (50 mL)

Shown in Product Identification Section, page 414

Mead Johnson Pharmaceuticals
**A Bristol-Myers Company
2400 W. LLOYD EXPRESSWAY
EVANSVILLE, IN 47721**

COLACE®
[*kōlās*]
**Docusate sodium, Mead Johnson
capsules • syrup • liquid (drops)**

Description: Colace (Docusate sodium) is a stool softener.
Colace Capsules, 50 mg, contain the following inactive ingredients: citric acid, D&C Red No. 33, FD&C Red No. 40, non-porcine gelatin, edible ink, polyethylene glycol, propylene glycol, and purified water.
Colace Capsules, 100 mg, contain the following inactive ingredients: citric acid, D&C Red No. 33, FD&C Red No. 40, FD&C Yellow No. 6, non-porcine gelatin, edible ink, polyethylene glycol, propylene glycol, titanium dioxide, and purified water.
Colace Liquid, 1%, contains the following inactive ingredients: citric acid, D&C Red No. 33, methylparaben, poloxamer, polyethylene glycol, propylene glycol, propylparaben, sodium citrate, vanillin, and purified water.
Colace Syrup contains the following inactive ingredients: alcohol, citric acid, D&C Red No. 33, FD&C Red No. 40, flavor (natural), menthol, methylparaben, peppermint oil, poloxamer, polyethylene glycol, propylparaben, sodium citrate, sucrose, and purified water.

Actions and Uses: Colace, a surface-active agent, helps to keep stools soft for easy, natural passage. Not a laxative, thus not habit-forming. Useful in constipation due to hard stools, in painful anorectal conditions, in cardiac and other conditions in which maximum ease of passage is desirable to avoid difficult or painful defecation, and when peristaltic stimulants are contraindicated. *Note:* When peristaltic stimulation is needed due to inadequate bowel motility, see Peri-Colace® (laxative and stool softener).

Contraindications: There are no known contraindications to Colace.

Side Effects: The incidence of side effects—none of a serious nature—is exceedingly small. Bitter taste, throat irritation, and nausea (primarily associated with the use of the syrup and liquid) are the main side effects reported. Rash has occurred.

Administration and Dosage: *Orally* —Suggested daily Dosage: *Adults and older children:* 50 to 200 mg *Children 6 to 12:* 40 to 120 mg *Children 3 to 6:* 20 to 60 mg. *Infants and children under 3:* 10 to 40 mg. The higher doses are recommended for initial therapy. Dosage should be adjusted to individual response. The effect on stools is usually apparent one to three days after the first dose. Give Colace liquid in half a glass of milk or fruit juice or in infant formula, to mask bitter taste. *In enemas* —Add 50 to 100 mg Colace (5 to 10 mL Colace liquid) to a retention or flushing enema.

Warning: As with any drug, if you are pregnant or nursing a baby, seek the advice of a health professional before using this product.

How Supplied: Colace capsules, 50 mg
NDC 0087-0713-01 Bottles of 30
NDC 0087-0713-02 Bottles of 60
NDC 0087-0713-03 Bottles of 250
NDC 0087-0713-05 Bottles of 1000
NDC 0087-0713-07 Cartons of 100 single unit packs
Colace capsules, 100 mg
NDC 0087-0714-01 Bottles of 30
NDC 0087-0714-02 Bottles of 60
NDC 0087-0714-03 Bottles of 250
NDC 0087-0714-05 Bottles of 1000
NDC 0087-0714-07 Cartons of 100 single unit packs
Note: Colace capsules should be stored at controlled room temperature (59°–86°F or 15°–30°C)
Colace liquid, 1% solution; 10 mg/mL (with calibrated dropper)
NDC 0087-0717-04 Bottles of 16 fl oz
NDC 0087-0717-02 Bottles of 30 mL.
6505-00-045-7786 (Bottle of 30 mL) Defense
Colace syrup, 20 mg/5-mL teaspoon; contains not more than 1% alcohol
NDC 0087-0720-01 Bottles of 8 fl oz
NDC 0087-0720-02 Bottles of 16 fl oz
Shown in Product Identification Section, page 414

PERI-COLACE® capsules • syrup
Casanthranol and docusate sodium

Description: Peri-Colace is a combination of the mild stimulant laxative casanthranol, and the stool-softener Colace® (docusate sodium). Each capsule contains 30 mg of casanthranol and 100 mg of Colace; the syrup contains 30 mg of casanthranol and 60 mg of Colace per 15-mL tablespoon (10 mg of casanthranol and 20 mg of Colace per 5-mL teaspoon) and 10% alcohol.
Peri-Colace Capsules contain the following inactive ingredients: D&C Red No. 33, FD&C Red No. 40, non-porcine gelatin, edible ink, polyethylene glycol, propylene glycol, titanium dioxide, and purified water.
Peri-Colace Syrup contains the following inactive ingredients: alcohol, citric acid, flavors, methyl salicylate, methylparaben, poloxamer, polyethylene glycol, propylparaben, sodium citrate, sorbitol solution, sucrose, and purified water.

Action and Uses: Peri-Colace provides gentle peristaltic stimulation and helps to keep stools soft for easier passage. Bowel movement is induced gently—usually overnight or in 8 to 12 hours. Nausea, griping, abnormally loose stools, and constipation rebound are minimized. Useful in management of chronic or temporary constipation.
Note: To prevent hard stools when laxative stimulation is not needed or undesirable, see Colace (stool softener).

Side Effects: The incidence of side effects—none of a serious nature—is exceedingly small. Nausea, abdominal cramping or discomfort, diarrhea, and rash are the main side effects reported.

Administration and Dosage:
Adults —1 or 2 capsules, or 1 or 2 tablespoons syrup at bedtime, or as indicated. In severe cases, dosage may be increased to 2 capsules or 2 tablespoons twice daily, or 3 capsules at bedtime. *Children* —1 to 3 teaspoons of syrup at bedtime, or as indicated.

Warnings: Do not use when abdominal pain, nausea, or vomiting are present. Frequent or prolonged use of this preparation may result in dependence on laxatives. As with any drug, if you are pregnant or nursing a baby, seek the advice of a health professional before using this product.

Overdosage: In addition to symptomatic treatment, gastric lavage, if timely, is recommended in cases of large overdosage.

How Supplied: Peri-Colace® Capsules
NDC 0087-0715-01 Bottles of 30
NDC 0087-0715-02 Bottles of 60
NDC 0087-0715-03 Bottles of 250
NDC 0087-0715-05 Bottles of 1000
NDC 0087-0715-07 Cartons of 100 single unit packs
Note: Peri-Colace capsules should be stored at controlled room temperatures (59°–86°F or 15°–30°C).
Peri-Colace® Syrup
NDC 0087-0721-01 Bottles of 8 fl oz
NDC 0087-0721-02 Bottles of 16 fl oz
Shown in Product Identification Section, page 414

Medicone Company
225 VARICK ST.
NEW YORK, NY 10014

MEDICONE® DERMA Ointment

Composition: Each gram contains: Benzocaine 2%; 8-Hydroxyquinoline Sulfate 1.05%; Menthol .48%; Zinc Oxide 13.73%; Ichthammol 1%; Lavender Perfume .08%; Petrolatum—Lanolin Base 79.87%.

Action and Uses: For prompt, temporary relief of intolerable itching, burning and pain associated with minor skin irritations. A bland, well balanced formula in a non-drying base which will not disintegrate or liquefy at body temperature and is not washed away by urine, perspiration or exudate. Exerts a soothing, cooling influence on irritated skin surfaces by affording mild anesthesia to control the scratch reflex, promotes healing of the affected area and checks the spread of infection. Useful for symptomatic relief in a wide variety of pruritic skin irritations resulting from insect bites, prickly heat, eczema, chafed and raw skin surfaces, sunburn, fungus infections, plant poisoning, pruritus ani and pruritus vulvae—mouth sores, cracked lips, under dentures.

Administration and Dosage: Apply liberally directly to site of irritation and gently rub into affected area for better penetration and absorption. Cover area with gauze if necessary.

Precautions: Do not use in the eyes. If the condition for which this preparation is used persists, or if rash or irritation develops, discontinue use and consult physician.

How Supplied: 1½ ounce tubes.
Shown in Product Identification Section, page 414

MEDICONE® DRESSING Cream

Composition: Each gram contains: Benzocaine .50%; 8-Hydroxyquinoline Sulfate .05%; Cod Liver Oil 12.50%; Zinc Oxide 12.50%; Menthol .18%; Talcum 2.99%; Paraffin 1.66%; Petrolatum-Lanolin Base 65.53%; Lavender Perfume .10%.

Action and Uses: Meets the first requisite in the treatment of minor burns, wounds and other denuded skin lesions by exerting mild, cooling anesthetic action for the prompt temporary relief of pain, burning and itching. A stable, anesthetic dressing which does not liquefy or wash off at body temperature, nor is it decomposed by exudate, urine or perspiration. Promotes granulation and aids epithelization of affected tissue. The anesthetic, antipruritic, antibacterial properties make Medicone Dressing ideal for the treatment of 1st and 2nd degree burns, minor wounds, abrasions, diaper rashes and a wide variety of pruritic skin irritations.

Administration and Dosage: The smooth, specially formulated consistency allows comfortable application directly to the painful, irritated affected area. It may be spread on gauze before application or covered with gauze as desired.

Precautions: Do not use in the eyes. If the condition for which this preparation is used persists or if a rash or irritation develops, discontinue use and consult physician.

How Supplied: Tubes of 1½ ounce.
Shown in Product Identification Section, page 414

MEDICONE® RECTAL OINTMENT

Composition: Each gram contains: Benzocaine, 2.01%; 8-Hydroxyquinoline Sulfate .5%; Menthol .4%; Zinc Oxide 10.04%; Balsam Peru 1.26%; Castor Oil 1.26%; Petrolatum—Lanolin Base 83.61%; Certified Color Added.

Action and Uses: A soothing, effective formulation which affords prompt, temporary relief of pain, burning and itching by exerting surface anesthetic action on the affected area in minor internal-external hemorrhoids and anorectal disorders. The active ingredients promote healing and protect against irritation, aiding inflamed tissue to retrogress to normal. The emollient petrolatum-lanolin base provides lubrication making bowel movements easier and more comfortable. Accelerates the normal healing process. Medicone Rectal Ointment and Medicone Rectal Suppositories are excellent for concurrent management of internal-external irritations.

Administration and Dosage: For internal use—attach pliable applicator and lubricate tip with a small amount of Ointment to ease insertion. Apply liberally into affected area morning and night and after each stool or as directed. When used externally, cover area with gauze. When used with Medicone Rectal Suppositories, insert a small amount of Ointment into the rectum before inserting suppository.

Precautions: If a rash or irritation develops or rectal bleeding occurs, discontinue use and consult physician.

How Supplied: 1½ ounce tubes with pliable rectal applicator.
Shown in Product Identification Section, page 415

MEDICONE® RECTAL SUPPOSITORIES

Composition: Each suppository contains:

Benzocaine	2 gr.
8-Hydroxyquinoline sulfate	¼ gr.
Zinc oxide	3 gr.
Menthol	⅟₇ gr.
Balsam Peru	1 gr.

Cocoa butter—vegetable & petroleum oil base; Certified color added ....q.s.

Action and Uses: A soothing, comprehensive formula carefully designed to meet the therapeutic requirements in adequately treating simple hemorrhoids and minor anorectal disorders. Performs the primary function of promptly alleviating pain, burning and itching temporarily by exerting satisfactory local anesthesia. The muscle spasm, present in many cases of painful anal and rectal conditions, is controlled and together with the emollients provided, helps the patient to evacuate the bowel comfortably and normally. The active ingredients reduce congestion and afford antisepsis, accelerating the normal healing process. Used pre- and post-surgically in hemorrhoidectomy, in prenatal and postpartum care and whenever surgery is contraindicated for the comfort and well-being of the patient during treatment of an underlying cause.

Administration and Dosage: One suppository in the morning and one at night and after each stool, or as directed. Use of the suppositories should be continued for 10 to 15 days after cessation of discomfort to help protect against recurrence of symptoms. See Medicone Rectal Ointment for concurrent internal-external use.

Precautions: If a rash or irritation develops, or bleeding from the rectum occurs, discontinue use and consult physician.

How Supplied: Boxes of 12 and 24 individually foil-wrapped green suppositories.
Shown in Product Identification Section, page 415

MEDICONET®
(medicated rectal wipes)

Composition: Each cloth wipe medicated with Benzalkonium chloride, 0.02%; Ethoxylated lanolin, 0.5%; Methylparaben, 0.15%; Hamamelis water, 50%; Glycerin, 10%; Alkylaryl Polyether, Purified water, USP and Perfume, q.s.

Action and Uses: Soft disposable cloth wipes which fulfill the important requisite in treating anal discomfort by providing the facility for gently and thoroughly cleansing the affected area. For the temporary relief of intolerable pain, itching and burning in minor external hemorrhoidal, anal and outer vaginal discomfort. Lanolized, delicately scented, durable and delightfully soft. Antiseptic, antipruritic, astringent. Useful as a substitute for harsh, dry toilet tissue. May also be used as a compress in the pre- and post-operative management of anorectal discomfort. The hygienic Mediconet pad is generally useful in relieving pain, burning and itching in diaper rash, sunburn, heat rash, minor burns and insect bites.

Continued on next page

Medicone—Cont.

How Supplied: Boxes of 20 individually packaged, pre-moistened cleansing cloths.

Shown in Product Identification Section, page 415

EDUCATIONAL MATERIAL

Clinical Evaluation Fact Cards and Samples
Medical study in the usage of our rectal suppositories.
The Latest Approach in Early Detection and Evaluation of Rectal Bleeding
A 16-page symposium for physicians of a medical mediconference.
Medical Mediconference
A discussion by experts on the latest approaches in Early Detection and Evaluation of Rectal Bleeding.

Mericon Industries, Inc.
8819 N. PIONEER RD.
PEORIA, IL 61615

DELACORT
(hydrocortisone USP ½%)

Active Ingredient: Hydrocortisone USP ½%.

Indications: For the temporary relief of minor skin irritations, itching and rashes due to eczema, dermatitis, insect bites, poison ivy, poison oak, poison sumac, soaps; detergents, cosmetics, and jewelry, and for itchy genital and anal areas.

Warnings: For external use only. Avoid contact with the eyes. If condition worsens, or if symptoms persist for more than 7 days discontinue use (of this product) and consult a physician. Do not use on children 2 years of age except under the advice and supervision of a physician.

Precaution: KEEP OUT OF REACH OF CHILDREN.

Dosage and Administration: For adults and children 2 years of age and older: Apply to affected area 3 or 4 times daily.

How Supplied: 2 oz. and 4 oz. squeeze bottle.

ORAZINC®
(zinc sulfate)

Active Ingredient: Zinc Sulfate U.S.P. 220 mg. and 110 mg. Capsules.

Indications: A Dietary Supplement containing Zinc.

Warnings: Should be taken with milk or meals to alleviate possible gastric distress.

Symptoms and Treatment of Oral Overdosage: Nausea, mild diarrhea or rash—to control, reduce dosage or discontinue.

Dosage and Administration: One capsule daily or as recommended by physician.

How Supplied: Bottles of 100 and 1000 Capsules each.

ORAZINC® LOZENGES
(zinc gluconate)

Active Ingredient: Zinc (Zinc Gluconate) 10 mg. Contains no starch, no artificial colors, flavors or preservatives. Sweetened with sorbitol and fructose.

Directions: As a dietary supplement, slowly dissolve one or two lozenges in mouth. To alleviate possible gastric distress, do not take on empty stomach.

Warnings: Keep this and all medications out of the reach of children.

How Supplied: Bottles of 100 Lozenges (NDC 0394-0495-02).

Miles Inc.
P. O. BOX 340
ELKHART, IN 46515

ALKA–MINTS® Chewable Antacid Rich in Calcium

Active Ingredient: Each ALKA-MINTS Chewable Antacid tablet contains calcium carbonate 850 mg. (340 mg of elemental calcium). Each tablet contains less than .5 mg sodium per tablet, and is dietarily sodium free.

Inactive Ingredients: Dioctyl sodium sulfosuccinate, flavor, hydrolyzed cereal solids, polyethylene glycol, sugar (compressible), magnesium stearate, sorbitol.

Indications: ALKA-MINTS is an antacid for occasional use for relief of acid indigestion, heartburn and sour stomach.

Actions: ALKA-MINTS has a natural, clean, spearmint taste that leaves the mouth feeling refreshed. Measured by the in-vitro standard established by the Food and Drug Administration, one ALKA-MINTS tablet neutralizes 15.9 mEq of acid.

Warnings: Do not take more than 9 tablets in a 24 hour period, or use the maximum dosage of this product for more than 2 weeks, except under the advice and supervision of a physician. May cause constipation. As with any drug, if you are pregnant or nursing a baby, seek the advice of a health professional before using this product. Keep this and all drugs out of the reach of children.

Dosage and Administration: Chew 1 tablet every 2 hours or as directed by a physician.

How Supplied: Cartons of 30's. Each carton contains convenient pocket-sized packs with individually sealed tablets so ALKA-MINTS stay fresh wherever you go.

Product Identification Mark:
ALKA-MINTS embossed on each tablet.
Shown in Product Identification Section, page 415

ALKA–SELTZER® Effervescent Antacid & Pain Reliever With Specially Buffered Aspirin

Active Ingredients: Each tablet contains: aspirin 325 mg., heat treated sodium bicarbonate 1916 mg., citric acid 1000 mg. ALKA-SELTZER® in water contains principally the antacid sodium citrate and the analgesic sodium acetylsalicylate. Buffered pH is between 6 and 7.

Inactive Ingredients: None.

Indications: ALKA-SELTZER® Effervescent Antacid & Pain Reliever is an analgesic and an antacid and is indicated for relief of sour stomach, acid indigestion or heartburn with headache or body aches and pains. Also for fast relief of upset stomach with headache from overindulgence in food and drink—especially recommended for taking before bed and again on arising. Effective for pain relief alone: headache or body and muscular aches and pains.

Actions: When the ALKA-SELTZER® Effervescent Antacid & Pain Reliever tablet is dissolved in water, the acetylsalicylate ion differs from acetylsalicylic acid chemically, physically and pharmacologically. Being fat insoluble, it is not absorbed by the gastric mucosal cells. Studies and observations in animals and man including radiochrome determinations of fecal blood loss, measurement of ion fluxes and direct visualization with gastrocamera, have shown that, as contrasted with acetylsalicylic acid, the acetylsalicylate ion delivered in the solution does not alter gastric mucosal permeability to permit back-diffusion of hydrogen ion, and gastric damage and acute gastric mucosal lesions are therefore not seen after administration of the product. ALKA-SELTZER® Effervescent Antacid & Pain Reliever has the capacity to neutralize gastric hydrochloric acid quickly and effectively. In-vitro, 154 ml. of 0.1 N hydrochloric acid are required to decrease the pH of one tablet of ALKA-SELTZER® Effervescent Antacid & Pain Reliever in solution to 4.0. Measured against the in vitro standard established by the Food and Drug Administration one tablet neutralizes 17.2 mEq of acid. In vivo, the antacid activity of two ALKA-SELTZER® Antacid & Pain Reliever tablets is comparable to that of 10 ml. of milk of magnesia. ALKA-SELTZER® Effervescent Antacid & Pain Reliever is able to resist pH changes caused by the continuing secretion of acid in the normal individual and to maintain an elevated pH until emptying occurs. ALKA-SELTZER® Effervescent Antacid & Pain Reliever provides highly water soluble acetylsalicylate ions which are fat insoluble. Acetylsalicylate ions are not absorbed from the stomach. They

empty from the stomach and thereby become available for absorption from the duodenum. Thus, fast drug absorption and high plasma acetylsalicylate levels are achieved. Plasma levels of salicylate following the administration of ALKA-SELTZER® Effervescent Antacid & Pain Reliever solution (acetylsalicylate ion equivalent to 648 mg. acetylsalicylic acid) can reach 29 mg./liter in 10 minutes and rise to peak levels as high as 55 mg./liter within 30 minutes.

Warnings: Children and teenagers should not use this medicine for chicken pox or flu symptoms before a doctor is consulted about Reye Syndrome, a rare but serious illness reported to be associated with aspirin. As with any drug, if you are pregnant or nursing a baby, seek the advice of a health professional before using this product. Except under the advice and supervision of a physician, do not take more than, Adults: 8 tablets in a 24 hour period. (60 years of age or older: 4 tablets in a 24 hour period), or use the maximum dosage for more than 10 days. Do not use if you are allergic to aspirin or have asthma, if you have a coagulation (bleeding) disease, or if you are on a sodium restricted diet. Each tablet contains 567 mg. of sodium.
Keep this and all drugs out of the reach of children.

Dosage and Administration:
ALKA-SELTZER® Effervescent Antacid & Pain Reliever is taken in solution, approximately three ounces of water per tablet is sufficient.
Adults: 2 tablets every 4 hours. CAUTION: If symptoms persist or recur frequently, or if you are under treatment for ulcer, consult your physician.

Professional Labeling:

ASPIRIN FOR MYOCARDIAL INFARCTION

Indication: The Aspirin contained in ALKA-SELTZER is indicated to reduce the risk of death and/or non-fatal myocardial infarction in patients with a previous infarction or unstable angina pectoris.

Clinical Trials: The indication is supported by the results of six, large, randomized multicenter, placebo-controlled studies[1-7] involving 10,816, predominantly male, post-myocardial infarction (MI) patients and one randomized placebo-controlled study of 1,266 men with unstable angina. Therapy with aspirin was begun at intervals after the onset of acute MI varying from less than 3 days to more than 5 years and continued for periods of from less than one year to four years. In the unstable angina study, treatment was started within 1 month after the onset of unstable angina and continued for 12 weeks and complicating conditions such as congestive heart failure were not included in the study.
Aspirin therapy in MI patients was associated with about a 20 percent reduction in the risk of subsequent death and/or non-fatal reinfarction, a median absolute decrease of 3 percent from the 12 to 22 percent event rates in the placebo groups. In aspirin-treated unstable angina patients the reduction in risk was about 50 percent, a reduction in event rate of 5 percent from the 10 percent rate in the placebo group over the 12 weeks of the study.
Daily dosage of aspirin in the post-myocardial infarction studies was 300 mg in one study and 900 to 1500 mg in five studies. A dose of 325 mg was used in the study of unstable angina.

Adverse Reactions: Gastrointestinal Reactions: Symptoms and signs of gastrointestinal irritation were not significantly increased in subjects treated for unstable angina with buffered aspirin in solution. (ALKA-SELZER®.) Doses of 1000 mg per day of aspirin tablets caused gastrointestinal symptoms and bleeding that in some cases were clinically significant. In the largest post-infarction study (the Aspirin Myocardial Infarction Study (AMIS) with 4,500 people), the percentage incidences of gastrointestinal symptoms for the aspirin (1000 mg of a standard, solid-tablet formulation) and placebo-treated subjects, respectively, were: stomach pain (14.5%; 4.4%); heartburn (11.9%; 4.8%); nausea and/or vomiting (7.6%; 2.1%); hospitalization for gastrointestinal disorder (4.9%; 3.5%). In the AMIS and other trials, aspirin treated patients had increased rates of gross gastrointestinal bleeding. As with all aspirin products ALKA-SELTZER is contraindicated in patients with aspirin sensitivity, with asthma, or with coagulation disease.

Cardiovascular and Biochemical: In the AMIS trial, the dosage of 1000 mg per day of aspirin was associated with small increases in systolic blood pressure (BP) (average 1.5 to 2.1 mm) and diastolic BP (0.5 to 0.6 mm), depending upon whether maximal or last available readings were used. Blood urea nitrogen and uric acid levels were also increased, but by less than 1.0 mg%. Subjects with marked hypertension or renal insufficiency had been excluded from the trial so that the clinical importance of these observations for such subjects or for any subjects treated over more prolonged periods is not known. It is recommended that patients placed on long-term aspirin treatment, even at doses of 300 mg per day, be seen at regular intervals to assess changes in these measurements.

Sodium in Buffered Aspirin for Solution Formulations: One tablet daily of buffered aspirin in solution adds 567 mg of sodium to that in the diet and may not be tolerated by patients with active sodium-retaining states such as congestive heart or renal failure. This amount of sodium adds about 30 percent to the 70 to 90 meq intake suggested as appropriate for dietary treatment of essential hypertension in the 1984 Report of the Joint National Committee on Detection, Evaluation, and Treatment of High Blood Pressure[8].

Dosage and Administration: Although most of the studies used dosages exceeding 300 mg, daily, two trials used only 300 mg and pharmacologic data indicate that this dose inhibits platelet function fully. Therefore, 300 mg or a conventional 325 mg aspirin dose daily is a reasonable, routine dose that would minimize gastrointestinal adverse reactions. This use of aspirin applies to both solid, oral dosage forms (buffered and plain aspirin) and buffered aspirin in solution.

References:
(1) Elwood, P. C., et al., A Randomized Controlled Trial of Acetysalicylic Acid in the Secondary Prevention of Mortality from Myocardial Infarction," *British Medical Journal* 1:436–440, 1974.
(2) The Coronary Drug Project Research Group, "Aspirin in Coronary Heart Disease," *Journal of Chronic Diseases,* 29:625–642, 1976.
(3) Breddin K., et al., "Secondary Prevention of Myocardial Infarction: A Comparison of Acetylsalicylic Acid, Phenprocoumon or Placebo," *International Congress Series* 470:263–268, 1979.
(4) Aspirin Myocardial Infarction Study Research Group, "A Randomized, Controlled Trial of Aspirin in Persons Recovered from Myocardial Infarction," *Journal American Medical Association* 245:661–669, 1980.
(5) Elwood, P. C., and P. M. Sweetnam, "Aspirin and Secondary Mortality after Myocardial Infarction," *Lancet* pp. 1313–1315, December 22–29, 1979.
(6) The Persantine-Aspirin Reinfarction Study Research Group, "Persantine and Aspirin in Coronary Heart Disease," *Circulation,* 62: 449–460, 1980.
(7) Lewis, H. D., et al., "Protective Effects of Aspirin Against Acute Myocardial Infarction and Death in Men with Unstable Angina, Results of a Veterans Administration Cooperative Study," *New England Journal of Medicine* 309:396–403, 1983.
(8) "1984 Report of the Joint National Committee on Detection, Evaluation, Treatment of High Blood Pressure," U.S. Department of Health and Human Services and United States Public Health Service, National Institutes of Health.

How Supplied: Tablets: foil sealed; box of 12 in 6 foil twin packs; box of 24 in 12 foil twin packs; box of 36 tablets in 18 foil twin packs; 100 tablets in 50 foil twin packs; carton of 72 tablets in 36 foil twin 96's card packs. Product Identification Mark: "ALKA-SELTZER" embossed on each tablet.
Shown in Product Identification Section, page 415

Flavored ALKA-SELTZER® Effervescent Antacid & Pain Reliever

Active Ingredients: Each tablet contains: Aspirin 325 mg, heat treated sodium bicarbonate 1710 mg, citric acid 1220 mg. Alka-Seltzer in water contains

Continued on next page

Miles—Cont.

principally the antacid sodium citrate and the analgesic sodium acetylsalicylate.

Inactive Ingredients: Flavors, Saccharin Sodium.

Indications: SPARKLING FRESH TASTE!

Flavored Alka-Seltzer®

For speedy relief of ACID INDIGESTION, SOUR STOMACH or HEARTBURN with HEADACHE, or BODY ACHES AND PAINS. Also for fast relief of UPSET STOMACH with HEADACHE from overindulgence in food and drink —especially recommended for taking before bed and again on arising. EFFECTIVE FOR PAIN RELIEF ALONE: HEADACHE or BODY and MUSCULAR ACHES and PAINS.

Warnings: Children and teenagers should not use this medicine for chicken pox or flu symptoms before a doctor is consulted about Reye Syndrome, a rare but serious illness reported to be associated with aspirin.

As with any drug, if you are pregnant or nursing a baby, seek the advice of a health professional before using this product.

Except under the advice and supervision of a physician: Do not take more than, ADULTS: 6 tablets in a 24-hour period, (60 years of age or older: 4 tablets in a 24-hour period), or use the daily maximum dosage for more than 10 days. Do not use if you are allergic to aspirin or have asthma, if you have a coagulation (bleeding) disease, or if you are on a sodium restricted diet. Each tablet contains 506 mg of sodium.

Keep this and all drugs out of the reach of children.

Directions: Alka-Seltzer must be dissolved in water before taking. ADULTS: 2 tablets every 4 hours. CAUTION: If symptoms persist or recur frequently or if you are under treatment for ulcer, consult your physician.

Professional Labeling:

ASPIRIN FOR MYOCARDIAL INFARCTION

Indication: The Aspirin contained in Alka-Seltzer is indicated to reduce the risk of death and/or non-fatal myocardial infarction in patients with a previous infarction or unstable angina pectoris.

Clinical Trials: The indication is supported by the results of six, large, randomized multicenter, placebo-controlled studies[1-7] involving 10,816, predominantly male, post-myocardial infarction (MI) patients and one randomized placebo-controlled study of 1,266 men with unstable angina. Therapy with aspirin was begun at intervals after the onset of acute MI varying from less than 3 days to more than 5 years and continued for periods of from less than one year to four years. In the unstable angina study, treatment was started within 1 month

after the onset of unstable angina and continued for 12 weeks and complicating conditions such as congestive heart failure were not included in the study.

Aspirin therapy in MI patients was associated with about a 20 percent reduction in the risk of subsequent death and/or non-fatal reinfarction, a median absolute decrease of 3 percent from the 12 to 22 percent event rates in the placebo groups. In aspirin-treated unstable angina patients the reduction in risk was about 50 percent, a reduction in event rate of 5 percent from the 10 percent rate in the placebo group over the 12 weeks of the study.

Daily dosage of aspirin in the post-myocardial infarction studies was 300 mg in one study and 900 to 1500 mg in five studies. A dose of 325 mg was used in the study of unstable angina.

Adverse Reactions: Gastrointestinal Reactions: Symptoms and signs of gastrointestinal irritation were not significantly increased in subjects treated for unstable angina with buffered aspirin in solution (ALKA-SELZER®). Doses of 1000 mg per day of aspirin tablets caused gastrointestinal symptoms and bleeding that in some cases were clinically significant. In the largest post-infarction study (the Aspirin Myocardial Infarction Study (AMIS) with 4,500 people), the percentage incidences of gastrointestinal symptoms for the aspirin (1000 mg of a standard, solid-tablet formulation) and placebo-treated subjects, respectively, were: stomach pain (14.5%; 4.4%); heartburn (11.9%; 4.8%); nausea and/or vomiting (7.6%; 2.1%); hospitalization for gastrointestinal disorder (4.9%; 3.5%). In the AMIS and other trials, aspirin treated patients had increased rates of gross gastrointestinal bleeding. As with all aspirin products Alka-Seltzer is contraindicated in patients with aspirin sensitivity, with asthma, or with coagulation disease.

Cardiovascular and Biochemical: In the AMIS trial, the dosage of 1000 mg per day of aspirin was associated with small increases in systolic blood pressure (BP) (average 1.5 to 2.1 mm) and diastolic BP (0.5 to 0.6 mm), depending upon whether maximal or last available readings were used. Blood urea nitrogen and uric acid levels were also increased, but by less than 1.0 mg%. Subjects with marked hypertension or renal insufficiency had been excluded from the trial so that the clinical importance of these observations for such subjects or for any subjects treated over more prolonged periods is not known. It is recommended that patients placed on long-term aspirin treatment, even at doses of 300 mg per day, be seen at regular intervals to assess changes in these measurements.

Sodium in Buffered Aspirin for Solution Formulations: One tablet daily of flavored buffered aspirin in solution adds 506 mg of sodium to that in the diet and may not be tolerated by patients with active sodium-retaining states such as congestive heart or renal failure. This amount of sodium adds about 30 percent

to the 70 to 90 meq intake suggested as appropriate for dietary treatment of essential hypertension in the 1984 Report of the Joint National Committee on Detection, Evaluation, and Treatment of High Blood Pressure[8].

Dosage and Administration: Although most of the studies used dosages exceeding 300 mg, daily, two trials used only 300 mg and pharmacologic data indicate that this dose inhibits platelet function fully. Therefore, 300 mg or a conventional 325 mg aspirin dose daily is a reasonable, routine dose that would minimize gastrointestinal adverse reactions. This use of aspirin applies to both solid, oral dosage forms (buffered and plain aspirin) and buffered aspirin in solution.

References:
(1) Elwood, P. C., et al., A Randomized Controlled Trial of Acetysalicylic Acid in the Secondary Prevention of Mortality from Myocardial Infarction," *British Medical Journal* 1:436–440, 1974.
(2) The Coronary Drug Project Research Group, "Aspirin in Coronary Heart Disease," *Journal of Chronic Diseases*, 29:625–642, 1976.
(3) Breddin K., et al., "Secondary Prevention of Myocardial Infarction: A Comparison of Acetylsalicylic Acid, Phenprocoumon or Placebo," *International Congress Series* 470:263–268, 1979.
(4) Aspirin Myocardial Infarction Study Research Group, "A Randomized, Controlled Trial of Aspirin in Persons Recovered from Myocardial Infarction," *Journal American Medical Association* 245:661–669, 1980.
(5) Elwood, P. C., and P. M. Sweetnam, "Aspirin and Secondary Mortality after Myocardial Infarction," *Lancet* pp. 1313–1315, December 22–29, 1979.
(6) The Persantine-Aspirin Reinfarction Study Research Group, "Persantine and Aspirin in Coronary Heart Disease," *Circulation*, 62: 449–460, 1980.
(7) Lewis, H. D., et al., "Protective Effects of Aspirin Against Acute Myocardial Infarction and Death in Men with Unstable Angina, Results of a Veterans Administration Cooperative Study," *New England Journal of Medicine* 309:396–403, 1983.
(8) "1984 Report of the Joint National Committee on Detection, Evaluation, Treatment of High Blood Pressure," U.S. Department of Health and Human Services and United States Public Health Service, National Institutes of Health.

How Supplied: Foil sealed effervescent tablets in cartons of 12's and 36's; 12's in 6 foil twin packs; 24's in 12 foil twin packs; 36's in 18 foil twin packs.

Shown in Product Identification Section, page 415

ALKA–SELTZER® Effervescent Antacid

Active Ingredients: Each tablet contains heat treated sodium bicarbonate

958 mg., citric acid 832 mg., potassium bicarbonate 312 mg. ALKA-SELTZER® Effervescent Antacid in water contains principally the antacids sodium citrate and potassium citrate.

Inactive Ingredients: A tableting aid.

Indications: ALKA-SELTZER® Effervescent Antacid is indicated for relief of acid indigestion, sour stomach or heartburn.

Actions: The ALKA-SELTZER® Effervescent Antacid solution provides quick and effective neutralization of gastric acid. Measured by the in vitro standard established by the Food and Drug Administration one tablet will neutralize 10.6 mEq of acid.

Warnings: Except under the advice and supervision of a physician, do not take more than: Adults: 8 tablets in a 24 hour period (60 years of age or older: 7 tablets in a 24 hour period), Children: 4 tablets in a 24 hour period; or use the maximum dosage of this product for more than 2 weeks.
Do not use this product if you are on a sodium restricted diet. Each tablet contains 311 mg. of sodium.
Keep this and all drugs out of the reach of children. As with any drug, if you are pregnant or nursing a baby, seek the advice of a health professional before using this product.

Dosage and Administration:
ALKA-SELTZER® Effervescent Antacid is taken in solution; approximately 3 oz. of water per tablet is sufficient. Adults: one or two tablets every 4 hours as needed. Children: ½ the adult dosage.

How Supplied: Boxes of 20 tablets in 10 foil twin packs; 36 tablets in 18 foil twin packs.
Shown in Product Identification Section, page 415

ALKA-SELTZER® Extra Strength Antacid & Pain Reliever

Active Ingredients: Each tablet contains: Aspirin 500mg, heat treated sodium bicarbonate 1985mg, citric acid 1000mg. Alka-Seltzer in water contains principally the antacid sodium citrate and the analgesic sodium acetylsalicylate.

Inactive Ingredients: Flavors

Indications: For speedy relief of acid indigestion, sour stomach or heartburn with headache or body aches and pains. Also, for fast relief of upset stomach with headache from overindulgence in food and drink—especially recommended for taking before bed and again on arising. Effective for pain relief alone. Headache or body and muscular aches and pains.

Warnings: Children and teenagers should not use this medicine for chicken pox or flu symptoms before a doctor is consulted about Reye Syndrome, a rare but serious illness reported to be associated with aspirin. As with any drug, if you are pregnant or nursing a baby, seek the advice of a health professional before

using this product. Except under the advice and supervision of a physician, do not take more than, Adults: 7 tablets in a 24-hour period (60 years of age or older, 4 tablets in a 24-hour period), or use the daily maximum dosage for more than 10 days. Do not use if you are allergic to aspirin or have asthma, if you have a coagulation (bleeding) disease, or if you are on a sodium restricted diet. Each tablet contains 588mg of sodium. Keep this and all drugs out of the reach of children.

Dosage and Administration: Extra Strength Alka-Seltzer must be dissolved in water before taking. Adults: 2 tablets every 4 hours. Caution: If symptoms persist, or recur frequently, or if you are under treatment for ulcer, consult your physician.

How Supplied: Foil sealed effervescent tablets in cartons of 12's and 24's; 12's in 6 foil twin packs; 24's in 12 foil twin packs.
Shown in Product Identification Section, page 415

ALKA-SELTZER PLUS® Cold Medicine

Active Ingredients:
Each dry ALKA-SELTZER PLUS® Cold Tablet contains the following active ingredients: Phenylpropanolamine bitartrate 24.08 mg., chlorpheniramine maleate 2 mg., aspirin 325 mg. The product is dissolved in water prior to ingestion and the aspirin is converted into its soluble ionic form, sodium acetylsalicylate.

Inactive Ingredients: Citric acid, flavors, sodium bicarbonate.

Indications: For relief of the symptoms of head colds, common flu, sinus congestion and hay fever.

Actions: Each tablet contains: A decongestant which helps restore free breathing, shrink swollen nasal tissue and relieve sinus congestion due to head colds or hay fever. An antihistamine which helps relieve the runny nose, sneezing, sniffles, itchy watering eyes that accompany colds or hay fever. Specially buffered aspirin which relieves headache, scratchy sore throat, general body aches and the feverish feeling of a cold and common flu.

Warnings: Children and teenagers should not use this medicine for chicken pox or flu symptoms before a doctor is consulted about Reye Syndrome, a rare but serious illness reported to be associated with aspirin.
Do not use if you are allergic to aspirin, have asthma, or if you have a coagulation (bleeding) disease. If symptoms do not improve within 7 days or are accompanied by high fever or if fever persists for more than 3 days, consult a physician before continuing use. Do not take this product if you have glaucoma or difficulty in urination due to enlargement of the prostate gland except under the advice and supervision of a physician. Avoid alcoholic beverages while taking this product. As with any drug, if you are

pregnant or nursing a baby, seek the advice of a health professional before using this product.

Caution: Individuals with high blood pressure, diabetes, heart or thyroid disease, or on a sodium restricted diet should use only as directed by a physician. Each tablet contains 506 mg of sodium. Product may cause drowsiness: Use caution if operating heavy machinery or driving a vehicle. Keep this and all drugs out of the reach of children.

Dosage and Administration:
ALKA-SELTZER PLUS® is taken in solution; approximately 3 ounces of water per tablet is sufficient. Adults: two tablets every 4 hours up to 8 tablets in 24 hours.

How Supplied: Tablets: carton of 12 tablets in 6 foil twin packs; 20 tablets in 10 foil twin packs; carton of 36 tablets in 18 foil twin packs.
Product Identification Mark: "Alka-Seltzer Plus" embossed on each tablet.
Shown in Product Identification Section, page 415

ALKA-SELTZER PLUS® Night-Time Cold Medicine

Active Ingredients: Each tablet contains phenylpropanolamine bitartrate 24.08 mg, diphenhydramine citrate 38.33 mg, acetylsalicylic acid (aspirin) 325 mg. In water the aspirin is converted into its soluble ionic form, sodium acetylsalicylate.

Inactive Ingredients: Citric acid, flavors, heat-treated sodium bicarbonate, tableting aids.

Indications: For relief of the symptoms of head colds, common flu, sinus congestion and hay fever so you can get the rest you need.

Actions: Temporarily restores freer breathing through the nose, relieves runny nose, itching of the nose or throat, itchy watery eyes, and headache and minor body aches and pain due to common colds, hay fever, or common flu.

Warnings: Children and teenagers should not use this medicine for chicken pox or flu symptoms before a doctor is consulted about Reye Syndrome, a rare but serious illness reported to be associated with aspirin. Do not use if you are allergic to aspirin, have asthma or if you have a coagulation (bleeding) disease. If symptoms do not improve within 7 days or are accompanied by high fever or if fever persists for more than 3 days, consult a physician before continuing use. Do not take this product if you have glaucoma or difficulty in urination due to enlargement of the prostate gland except under the advice and supervision of a physician. Product may cause marked drowsiness: alcohol may increase the drowsiness effect. Avoid alcoholic beverages while taking this product. Use caution when driving a motor vehicle or op-

Continued on next page

Miles—Cont.

erating machinery. As with any drug, if you are pregnant or nursing a baby, seek the advice of a health professional before using this product.

Caution: Individuals with high blood pressure, diabetes, heart or thyroid disease, or on a sodium restricted diet should use only as directed by a physician. Each tablet contains 506 mg of sodium. Keep this and all drugs out of the reach of children.

Dosage and Administration: Adults: Take 2 tablets dissolved in water every 4 to 6 hours, not to exceed 8 tablets daily.

How Supplied: Tablets: carton of 20 tablets in 10 child-resistant foil twin packs; carton of 36 tablets in 18 child-resistant foil twin packs.

Product Identification Mark: "A/S PLUS NIGHT-TIME" etched on each tablet
Shown in Product Identification Section, page 415

BACTINE® Antiseptic · Anesthetic First Aid Spray

Active Ingredients: Benzalkonium Chloride 0.13% w/w, Lidocaine HCl. 2.5% w/w.
Aerosol ingredients are % w/w of concentrate.

Inactive Ingredients:
Liquid—Edetate Disodium, Fragrances, Octoxynol 9, Propylene Glycol, Purified Water. Alcohol 3.17% w/w
Aerosol—Dimethyl Polysiloxane Fluid 1000, Edetic Acid, Fragrances, Isobutane, Malic Acid, Povidone, Propylene Glycol, Purified Water, Sorbitol, and Emulsifier System

Indications: Antiseptic/anesthetic for helping prevent infection, cleanse wounds, and for the temporary relief of pain and itching due to insect bites, minor burns, sunburn, minor cuts and minor skin irritations.

Warnings: (Aerosol Spray and Liquid Spray)
For external use only. Do not use in large quantities, particularly over raw surfaces or blistered areas. Avoid spraying in eyes, mouth, ears or on sensitive areas of the body. This product is not for use on wild or domestic animal bites. If you have an animal bite or puncture wound, consult your physician immediately. If condition worsens or if symptoms persist for more than 7 days, discontinue use of this product and consult a physician. Do not bandage tightly. Keep this and all drugs out of reach of children. In case of accidental ingestion, seek professional assistance or contact a Poison Control Center immediately.
(Aerosol Only): Contents under pressure. Do not puncture or incinerate. Do not store at temperature above 120° F. Use only as directed. Intentional misuse by deliberately concentrating and inhaling the contents can be harmful or fatal.

Dosage and Administration: For adults and children 2 years of age or older. For superficial skin wounds, cuts, scratches, scrapes, cleanse affected area thoroughly.

Directions: (Liquid) First Aid Spray
To apply, hold bottle 2 to 3 inches from injured area and squeeze repeatedly. To aid in removing foreign particles, dab injured area with clean gauze saturated with product. For sunburn, minor burns, insect bites, and minor skin irritations, apply to affected area of skin for temporary relief. Product can be applied to affected area with clean gauze saturated with product.
(Aerosol First Aid Spray)
Shake well. For adults and children 2 years of age and older. For superficial skin wounds, cuts, scratches, scrapes, cleanse affected area thoroughly. Hold can upright 2 to 3 inches from injured area and spray until wet. To aid in removing foreign particles, dab injured area with clean gauze saturated with product. For sunburn, minor burns, insect bites, and minor skin irritations, hold can upright 4 to 6 inches from injured area and spray until wet. Product can be applied to affected area with clean gauze saturated with product.

How Supplied: 2 oz., 4 oz. liquid spray, 16 oz. liquid, 3 oz. aerosol.
Shown in Product Identification Section, page 415

BACTINE® First Aid Antibiotic Ointment

Active Ingredients: Each gram contains Polymyxin B Sulfate 5000 units; Bacitracin 500 units; Neomycin Sulfate 5 mg (equivalent to 3.5 mg Neomycin base).

Inactive Ingredients: Mineral Oil, White Petrolatum.

Indications: First aid to help prevent infection in minor cuts, scrapes and burns. Decreases the number of bacteria on the treated area and helps prevent bacterial contamination in minor cuts, scrapes and burns.

Warning: For external use only. Do not use in the eyes or apply over large areas of the body. In case of deep or puncture wounds, animal bites or serious burns, consult a physician. Stop use and consult a physician if the condition persists or gets worse. Do not use longer than one (1) week unless directed by a physician. Keep this and all medicines out of children's reach. In case of accidental ingestion, seek professional assistance or contact a Poison Control Center immediately.

Directions: Clean the affected area. Apply a small amount of this product one to three times daily. May be covered with a sterile bandage.

How Supplied: ½ oz. tube.
Shown in Product Identification Section, page 415

BACTINE® Brand Hydrocortisone Skin Care Cream Antipruritic (Anti-Itch)

Active Ingredient: Hydrocortisone 0.5%

Inactive Ingredients: Butylated Hydroxyanisole, Butylated Hydroxytoluene, Butylparaben, Carbomer, Cetyl Alcohol, Colloidal Silicon Dioxide, Corn oil (and) Gylceryl Oleate (and) Propylene Glycol (and) (BHA) (and) BHT (and) Propyl Gallate (and) Citric Acid, DEA-Oleth-3 Phosphate, Diisopropyl Sebacate, Edetate Disodium, Glycerin, Hydroxypropyl Methylcellulose 2906, Lanolin Alcohol, Methylparaben, Mineral Oil (and) Lanolin Alcohol, Propylene Glycol Stearate SE, Propylparaben, Purified Water.

Indications: For the temporary relief of minor skin irritations, itching, and rashes due to eczema, dermatitis, insect bites, poison ivy, poison oak, poison sumac, soaps, detergents, cosmetics, and jewelry.

Warnings: For external use only. Avoid contact with the eyes. If condition worsens or if symptoms persist for more than seven days, discontinue use and consult a physician.
Do not use on children under 2 years of age except under the advice and supervision of a physician.
Keep this and all drugs out of the reach of children. In case of accidental ingestion, seek professional assistance or contact a Poison Control Center immediately.

Directions: For adults and children 2 years of age and older. Gently massage into affected skin area not more than 3 or 4 times daily.

How Supplied: ½ oz. plastic tube.
Shown in Product Identification Section, page 415

BIOCAL™ 500 mg Tablets Calcium Supplement

Each Tablet Contains: 1250 mg of calcium carbonate, U.S.P. which provides elemental calcium 500 mg.

Indications: Calcium supplementation.

Description: BIOCAL™ 500 mg Tablets are white, capsule-shaped tablets containing pure calcium carbonate. No sugar, salt, preservatives, artificial colors or flavors added.

Directions: Two tablets daily provide:

Elemental Calcium	For Adults % U.S. RDA	For Pregnant or Lactating Women % U.S. RDA
1000 mg	100%	77%

Take one or two tablets daily or as recommended by a physician.
Keep out of reach of children.

How Supplied: Bottles of 60 tablets in tamper-resistant package.
Shown in Product Identification Section, page 415

BUGS BUNNY® Children's Chewable Vitamins (Sugar Free)
BUGS BUNNY® Children's Chewable Vitamins Plus Iron (Sugar Free)
FLINTSTONES® Children's Chewable Vitamins
FLINTSTONES® Children's Chewable Vitamins Plus Iron

Vitamin Ingredients: Each multivitamin supplement with iron contains the ingredients listed in the chart below: [See table right].
BUGS BUNNY® Children's Chewable Vitamins and FLINTSTONES® Children's Chewable Vitamins provide the same quantities of vitamins, but do not provide iron.

Indication: Dietary supplementation.

Dosage and Administration: One chewable tablet daily. For adults and children two years and older; tablet must be chewed.

Warning For Bugs Bunny Only: Phenylketonurics: Contains Phenylalanine.

Precaution:
IRON SUPPLEMENTS ONLY.
Contains iron, which can be harmful in large doses. Close tightly and keep out of reach of children. In case of overdose contact a Poison Control Center immediately.

How Supplied: Flintstones are supplied in bottles of 60 and 100, Bugs Bunny in bottles of 60 with child resistant caps.
Shown in Product Identification Section, page 415

FLINTSTONES® With Extra C Children's Chewable Vitamins
BUGS BUNNY® With Extra C Children's Chewable Vitamins (Sugar Free)

Vitamin Ingredients: Each multivitamin supplement contains the ingredients listed in the chart above: [See table below].

Indication: Dietary supplementation.

Dosage and Administration: One chewable tablet daily for adults and chil-

BUGS BUNNY® Children's Chewable Vitamins Plus Iron (Sugar Free)
FLINTSTONES® Children's Chewable Vitamins Plus Iron

One Tablet Provides		% of U.S. RDA	
Vitamins	Quantity	For Children 2 to 4 Years of Age	For Adults and Children over 4 Years of Age
Vitamin A	2500 I.U.	100	50
Vitamin D	400 I.U.	100	100
Vitamin E	15 I.U.	150	50
Vitamin C	60 mg.	150	100
Folic Acid	0.3 mg.	150	75
Thiamine	1.05 mg.	150	70
Riboflavin	1.20 mg.	150	70
Niacin	13.50 mg.	150	67
Vitamin B_6	1.05 mg.	150	52
Vitamin B_{12}	4.5 mcg.	150	75
Mineral:			
Iron (Elemental)	15 mg.	150	83

dren two years and older; tablet must be chewed.

Warning For Bugs Bunny Only: Phenylketonurics: Contains Phenylalanine.

How Supplied: Flintstones in bottles of 60's & 100's, Bugs Bunny in bottles of 60 with child resistant caps.
Shown in Product Identification Section, page 415

FLINTSTONES® COMPLETE With Iron, Calcium & Minerals Children's Chewable Vitamins
BUGS BUNNY® Children's Chewable Vitamins + Minerals With Iron and Calcium (Sugar Free)

Ingredients: Each supplement provides the ingredients listed in the chart below: [See table on next page].

Indication: Dietary Supplementation

Dosage and Administration: 2–4 years of age: Chew one-half tablet daily. Over 4 years of age: Chew one tablet daily.

Warning: Phenylketonurics: Contains Phenylalanine.

Precaution: Contains iron, which can be harmful in large doses. Close tightly and keep out of reach of children. In case of overdose, contact a physician or poison control center immediately.

How Supplied: Bottles of 60's with child resistant caps.
Shown in Product Identification Section, pages 415 & 416

MILES® Nervine Nighttime Sleep–Aid

Active Ingredient: Each capsule-shaped tablet contains diphenhydramine HCl 25 mg.

Inactive Ingredients: Calcium Phosphate Dibasic, Calcium Sulfate, Carboxymethylcellulose Sodium, Corn Starch, Magnesium Stearate, Microcrystalline Cellulose.

Indications: Miles® Nervine helps you fall asleep and relieves occasional sleeplessness.

Actions: Antihistamines act on the central nervous system and produce drowsiness.

Warnings: Use only as directed. Do not give to children under 12 years of age. Take this product with caution if alcohol is being consumed. As with any drug, if you are pregnant or nursing a baby, seek the advice of a health professional before using this product. NOT FOR PROLONGED USE. If sleeplessness persists continuously for more than 2 weeks, consult your physician. Insomnia may be a symptom of serious underlying medical illness. Keep this and all drugs out of the reach of children. In case of accidental overdose, seek professional assistance or contact a Poison Control Center immediately. DO NOT TAKE THIS PRODUCT IF YOU HAVE ASTHMA, GLAUCOMA OR ENLARGEMENT OF THE PROSTATE GLAND EXCEPT UNDER THE ADVICE AND SUPERVISION OF A PHYSICIAN.

Dosage and Administration: Two tablets once daily at bedtime or as directed by a physician.

How Supplied: Blister pack 12's, bottles of 30's and 50's with child resistant caps.
Shown in Product Identification Section, page 416

BUGS BUNNY® With Extra C Children's Chewable Vitamins (Sugar Free)
FLINTSTONES® With Extra C Children's Chewable Vitamins

One Tablet Provides		% of U.S. RDA	
Vitamins	Quantity	For Children 2 To 4 Years of Age	For Adults and Children Over 4 Years of Age
Vitamin A	2500 I.U.	100	50
Vitamin D	400 I.U.	100	100
Vitamin E	15 I.U.	150	50
Vitamin C	250 mg.	625	417
Folic Acid	0.3 mg.	150	75
Thiamine	1.05 mg.	150	70
Riboflavin	1.20 mg.	150	70
Niacin	13.50 mg.	150	67
Vitamin B_6	1.05 mg.	150	52
Vitamin B_{12}	4.5 mcg.	150	75

Continued on next page

Miles—Cont.

ONE-A-DAY® Essential Vitamins
11 Essential Vitamins

Ingredients: One tablet daily of ONE-A-DAY® Essential provides:

Vitamins	Quantity	U.S. RDA
Vitamin A	5,000 I.U.	100
Vitamin C	60 mg.	100
Thiamine (B₁)	1.5 mg.	100
Riboflavin (B₂)	1.7 mg.	100
Niacin	20 mg.	100
Vitamin D	400 I.U.	100
Vitamin E	30 I.U.	100
Vitamin B₆	2 mg.	100
Folic Acid	0.4 mg.	100
Vitamin B₁₂	6 mcg.	100
Pantothenic Acid	10 mg.	100

Indication: Dietary supplementation.

Dosage and Administration: One tablet daily for adults and teens.

How Supplied: ONE-A-DAY® Essential, bottles of 60 and 100.

Shown in Product Identification Section, page 416

ONE-A-DAY® Maximum Formula
Vitamins and Minerals
Supplement for adults
The most complete ONE-A-DAY® brand.

Ingredients:
One tablet daily of ONE-A-DAY® Maximum Formula provides:

Vitamins	Quantity	% of U.S. RDA
Vitamin A	5,000 I.U.	100
(as Beta Carotene)		
Vitamin A	1,500 I.U.	30
(as Acetate)		
Vitamin C	60 mg.	100
Thiamine (B₁)	1.5 mg.	100
Riboflavin (B₂)	1.7 mg.	100
Niacin	20 mg.	100
Vitamin D	400 I.U.	100
Vitamin E	30 I.U.	100
Vitamin B₆	2 mg.	100
Folic Acid	0.4 mg.	100
Vitamin B₁₂	6 mcg.	100
Biotin	30 mcg.	10
Pantothenic Acid	10 mg.	100

Minerals	Quantity	% of U.S. RDA
Iron (Elemental)	18 mg.	100
Calcium	130 mg.	13
Phosphorus	100 mg.	10
Iodine	150 mcg.	100
Magnesium	100 mg.	25
Copper	2 mg.	100
Zinc	15 mg.	100
Chromium	10 mcg.	*
Selenium	10 mcg.	*
Molybdenum	10 mcg.	*
Manganese	2.5 mg.	*
Potassium	37.5 mg.	*
Chloride	34 mg.	*

*No U.S. RDA established

Indication: Dietary supplementation.

Dosage and Administration: One tablet daily for adults.

Precaution: Contains iron, which can be harmful in large doses. Close tightly and keep out of reach of children. In case of overdose, contact a physician or Poison Control Center immediately.

How Supplied: Bottles of 30, 60, and 100 with child-resistant caps.

Shown in Product Identification Section, page 416

FLINESTONES® COMPLETE
Children's Chewable Vitamins
BUGS BUNNY®
Children's Chewable
Vitamins + Minerals
(Sugar Free)

Vitamins	Quantity Per Tablet	For Children 2 to 4 Years of Age (½ tablet)	For Adults & Children Over 4 Years of Age (1 tablet)
		Percentage of U.S. Recommended Daily Allowance (U.S. RDA)	
Vitamin A	5000 I.U.	100	100
Vitamin D	400 I.U.	50	100
Vitamin E	30 I.U.	150	100
Vitamin C	60 mg	75	100
Folic Acid	0.4 mg	100	100
Vitamin B-1 (Thiamine)	1.5 mg	107	100
Vitamin B-2 (Riboflavin)	1.7 mg	106	100
Niacin	20 mg	111	100
Vitamin B-6 (Pyridoxine)	2 mg	143	100
Vitamin B-12 (Cyanocobalamin)	6 mcg	100	100
Biotin	40 mcg	13	13
Pantothenic Acid	10 mg	100	100

Minerals	Quantity	Percent U.S. RDA	
Iron (elemental)	18 mg	90	100
Calcium	100 mg	6	10
Copper	2 mg	100	100
Phosphorus	100 mg	6	10
Iodine	150 mcg	107	100
Magnesium	20 mg	5	5
Zinc	15 mg	94	100

ONE-A-DAY® Plus Extra C
Vitamins. For adults and teens.

Vitamin ingredients: One tablet daily of ONE-A-DAY® Plus Extra C provides:

Vitamins	Quantity	% of U.S. RDA
Vitamin A	5,000 I.U.	100
Vitamin C	300 mg.	500
Thiamine (B₁)	1.5 mg.	100
Riboflavin (B₂)	1.7 mg.	100
Niacin	20 mg.	100
Vitamin D	400 I.U.	100
Vitamin E	30 I.U.	100
Vitamin B₆	2 mg.	100
Folic Acid	0.4 mg.	100
Vitamin B₁₂	6 mcg.	100
Pantothenic Acid	10 mg.	100

Indication: Dietary supplementation.

Dosage and Administration: One tablet daily.

How Supplied: Bottles of 60's with child resistant caps.

Shown in Product Identification Section, page 416

STRESSGARD®
High Potency B Complex and C plus A, D, E, Iron and Zinc
The most complete stress product.
Multivitamin/Multimineral Supplement For Adults

Ingredients:

Vitamins	Quantity	% of U.S. RDA
Vitamin A	5000 I.U.	100
Vitamin C	600 mg.	1000
Thiamine (B₁)	15 mg.	1000
Riboflavin (B₂)	10 mg.	588
Niacin	100 mg.	500
Vitamin D	400 I.U.	100
Vitamin E	30 I.U.	100
Vitamin B₆	5 mg.	250
Folic Acid	400 mcg.	100
Vitamin B₁₂	12 mcg.	200
Pantothenic Acid	20 mg.	200

Minerals	Quantity	% of U.S. RDA
Iron (Elemental)	18 mg.	100
Zinc	15 mg.	100
Copper	2 mg.	100

Indication: Dietary supplementation.

Dosage and Administration: Adults —one tablet daily with food.

Precaution: Contains iron, which can be harmful in large doses. Close tightly and keep out of reach of children. In case of overdose, contact a physician or Poison Control Center immediately.

How Supplied: Bottles of 60 with child-resistant caps.

Shown in Product Identification Section, page 416

WITHIN® Advanced Multivitamin
for women with calcium, extra iron, zinc and Beta Carotene.
Provides calcium and extra iron
Plus the daily nutritional support of
11 essential vitamins.

Ingredients: One tablet daily of WITHIN® provides:

Vitamins	Quantity	% of U.S. RDA
Vitamin A (as Beta Carotene)	2,500 I.U.	100
Vitamin A (as Acetate)	2,500 I.U.	100
Vitamin C	60 mg.	100
Thiamine (B₁)	1.5 mg.	100
Riboflavin (B₂)	1.7 mg.	100
Niacin	20 mg.	100
Vitamin D	400 I.U.	100
Vitamin E	30 I.U.	100
Vitamin B₆	2 mg.	100
Folic Acid	0.4 mg.	100
Vitamin B₁₂	6 mcg.	100
Pantothenic Acid	10 mg.	100

Mineral	Quantity	% of U.S. RDA
Iron (Elemental)	27 mg.	150
Calcium	450 mg.	45
Zinc (Elemental)	15 mg.	100

Indication: Dietary supplementation.

Dosage and Administration: One tablet daily.

Precaution: Contains iron, which can be harmful in large doses. Close tightly and keep out of reach of children. In case of overdose, contact a physician or Poison Control Center immediately.

How Supplied: Bottles of 60 and 100 with child resistant caps.

Shown in Product Identification Section, page 416

More Direct Response, Inc.
6351-E YARROW DRIVE
CARLSBAD, CA 92009

CigArrest™
Smoking Deterrent Tablets

Active Ingredient: Lobeline sulfate 2 mg.

Indications: A temporary aid to breaking the cigarette habit. The effectiveness of the tablet is directly related to the user's motivation to stop smoking.

Use: Lobeline sulfate resembles nicotine both chemically and pharmacologically which aids the smoker in developing a sense of satiety for smoking almost identical to that obtained from tobacco. Not habit forming.

Warnings: As with any drug, if you are pregnant or nursing a baby, seek the advice of a health professional before using CigArrest.™ Keep this and all drugs out of the reach of children.

Symptoms and Treatment of Overdosage: In case of accidental overdose, seek the advice of a physician immediately.

Dosage and Administration: Take 1 (one) tablet at or after each meal, 3 (three) tablets per day. Recommended usage not to exceed six weeks.

How Supplied: Consumer packages of 15 (fifteen) blister packed tablets.

Muro Pharmaceutical, Inc.
890 EAST STREET
TEWKSBURY, MA 01876-9987

BROMFED® SYRUP
Antihistamine-Decongestant
(alcohol free)
ORANGE-LEMON FLAVOR

Each 5 mL (1 teaspoonful) contains: 2 mg brompheniramine maleate and 30 mg pseudoephedrine hydrochloride; also contains citric acid, FD & C Yellow #6, flavor, glycerin, methyl paraben, sodium benzoate, sodium citrate, sodium saccharin, sorbitol, sucrose, purified water.

Indications: For temporary relief of nasal congestion, sneezing, itchy and watery eyes and running nose due to common cold, hay fever or other upper respiratory allergies.

Directions: Adults and children 12 years of age and over: 2 teaspoonfuls every 4–6 hours. Children 6 to 12 years of age: 1 teaspoonful every 4–6 hours. Do not exceed 4 doses in 24 hours. Children under 6 years of age, consult a physician.

Warnings: If symptoms do not improve within 7 days or are accompanied by high fever, consult a physician before continuing use. May cause drowsiness. May cause excitability especially in children. DO NOT exceed recommended daily dosage because at higher doses nervousness, dizziness, or sleeplessness may occur. **Except under the advice and supervision of a physician:** DO NOT give this product to children under 6 years. DO NOT take this product if you have asthma, glaucoma, difficulty in urination due to enlargement of the prostate gland, high blood pressure, heart disease, diabetes, or thyroid disease. As with any drug, if you are pregnant or nursing a baby, seek the advice of a health professional before using this product.

Caution: Avoid operating a motor vehicle or heavy machinery and alcoholic beverages while taking this product. Keep this and all drugs out of the reach of children.

Drug Interaction Precaution: Do not take this product if you are presently taking a prescription antihypertensive or antidepressant drug containing a monoamine oxidase inhibitor except under the advice and supervision of a physician.

Overdosage: In case of accidental overdose, seek professional assistance or contact a Poison Control Center immediately.

Store between 15° and 30°C (59° and 86°F). Dispense in tight, light resistant containers as defined in USP.

How Supplied: NDC 0451-4201-16—16 fl. oz. (480 mL), NDC 0451-4201-04—4 fl. oz. (120 mL).

SALINEX NASAL MIST AND DROPS
Buffered Isotonic Saline Solutions

Ingredients: Sodium Chloride 0.4%. Also contains disodium phosphate, edetate disodium, hydroxypropyl methylcellulose, monosodium phosphate, polyethylene glycol, propylene glycol and purified water. Preservative used is benzalkonium chloride 0.01%.

Indications: Rhinitis Medicamentosa and Rhinitis Sicca. For relief of nasal congestion associated with overuse of nasal sprays, drops and inhalers.
To alleviate crusting due to nose bleeds; to compensate for nasal stuffiness and dryness due to lack of humidity.

Directions: Squeeze twice in each nostril as needed.

How Supplied: SPRAY: 50 ml plastic spray bottle. DROPS: 15 ml plastic dropper bottle.

Natren Inc.
10935 CAMARILLO STREET
NORTH HOLLYWOOD, CA 91602

BIFIDO FACTOR™
(Bifidobacterium bifidum)

Predominant probiotic in healthy adult large intestines.

Ingredients: Active—Bifidobacterium bifidum, strain Malyoth. Inactive—Whey and milk solids.

How Supplied:
2.5 oz. Powder NDC 53983-200-25
4.5 oz. Powder NDC 53983-200-45

BULGARICUM I.B.™
(Lactobacillus bulgaricus)

Major transient probiotic in healthy adult intestines.

Ingredients: Active—L. bulgaricus, strain LB-51. Inactive—Whey and milk solids.

How Supplied:
2.5 oz. Powder—NDC 53983-300-50
4.5 oz. Powder—NDC 53983-300-55

LIFE START®
(Bifidobacterium infantis)

Predominant intestinal probiotic in healthy, breast-fed infants and small children.

Ingredients: Active—Bifidobacterium infantis, special strain. Inactive—Whey and milk solids.

How Supplied:
2.5 oz. Powder—NDC 53983-500-70
4.5 oz. Powder—NDC 53983-500-75

M.F.A.™—Milk Free Acidophilus
(Dairy free Lactobacillus acidophilus)

A milk free source of the predominant probiotic in healthy adult small intestines.

Continued on next page

Natren—Cont.

Ingredients: Active—Lactobacillus acidophilus, strain DDS-1. Inactive—Banana concentrate, rice flour, rice protein, rice bran, rice bran oil, rice syrup, barley grass, spirulina, lecithin.

How Supplied:
2.5 oz. Powder—NDC 53983-400-60
4.5 oz. Powder—NDC 53983-400-65

SUPERDOPHILUS™
(Lactobacillus acidophilus)

Predominant probiotic in the healthy adult small intestines.

Ingredients: Active—Lactobacillus acidophilus, strain DDS-1. Inactive—Whey and milk solids.

How Supplied:
2.5 oz. Powder—NDC 53983-100-15
4.5 oz. Powder—NDC 53983-100-25

Educational materials and professional samples available to qualified health practitioners while supplies last.
National (800) 992-3323
California (800) 992-9393

Nature's Bounty, Inc.
90 ORVILLE DRIVE
BOHEMIA, NY 11716

ENER–B™
Vitamin B-12 Nasal Gel
Dietary Supplement

Description: ENER-B™ is the first intra-nasal application for Vitamin B-12. Each delivery supplies 400 mcg. of Vitamin B-12. This method of delivery provides the highest Vitamin B-12 blood levels that can be obtained without a prescription. Clinical tests show that ENER-B produced 8.4 to 10 times more Vitamin-B-12 in the blood than tablets.

Measured Vitamin B-12 Increase in Blood Levels

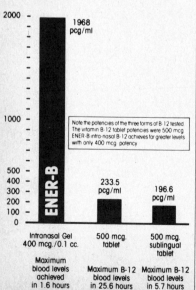

Clinical Tests results are available by writing Nature's Bounty.

Potency and Administration: Each nasal applicator delivers $\frac{1}{10}$ cc of gel into the nose which adheres to the mucous membranes providing 400 mcg. of Vitamin B-12. Odorless and non-irritating to the nose.

Directions: As a dietary supplement, one unit every two to three days.

How Supplied: Packages of 12 unit doses. Supplies 400 mcg. of B-12 each.

Norcliff Thayer Inc.
303 SOUTH BROADWAY
TARRYTOWN, NY 10591

A–200® Pediculicide Shampoo Concentrate
A–200® Pediculicide Gel Concentrate

Description: Active ingredients: Pyrethrins 0.33%, piperonyl butoxide technical 4% (equivalent to 3.2% (butylcarbityl) (6-propylpiperonyl) ether and 0.8% related compounds.

Inert ingredients: 95.67%

Indications: A-200 is indicated for the treatment of human pediculosis—head lice, body lice and pubic lice, and their eggs. A-200 Gel is specially formulated for public lice and head lice in children, where control of application is desirable.

Actions: A-200 is an effective pediulicide for control of head lice (Pediculus humanus capitis), pubic lice (Phthirus pubis) and body lice (Pediculus humanus corporis), and their nits.

Warnings: May cause eye injury. Do not get in eyes or permit contact with mucous membranes. Harmful if swallowed. Wash thoroughly after handling. Do not leave children unattended with product on their heads.

Drug Interaction: **NOT TO BE USED BY PERSONS ALLERGIC TO RAGWEED.** If skin irritation or infection is present or develops, discontinue use and consult a physician.

Precaution: If in Eyes: Flush with plenty of water. Get medical attention.

Symptoms and Treatment of Oral Overdosage: If swallowed: Call a physician or Poison Control Center. Drink 1 or 2 glasses of water and induce vomiting by touching the back of throat with finger. Do not induce vomiting or give anything by mouth to an unconscious person.

Dosage and Administration: It is a violation of Federal law to use this product in a manner inconsistent with its labeling.

Directions For Use: 1. Apply A-200 Shampoo to **dry** hair and scalp or other infested areas. Use enough to completely wet area being treated. Massage in. (For

---

head lice, avoid getting product into eyes. Helpful hint: When shampooing a child's head, place towel across forehead.) 2. Allow product to remain for 10 minutes, but no longer. 3. Add small quantities of water, and work rich lather into hair and scalp. 4. Rinse thoroughly with warm water. Towel dry. 5. Comb hair with special A-200 precision comb to remove dead lice and eggs. (See left side panel for combing suggestions.) Repeat treatment in 7–10 days or earlier if reinfestation has occurred. Do not use more than 2 applications of A-200 Shampoo in 24 hours. When used on children, adult supervision is recommended.

Additional Control Measures: At time of shampoo treatment, all infested clothing, bed linen and other articles should be laundered in hot water or dry cleaned. Carpets, upholstery and mattresses should be vacuumed thoroughly. Combs and brushes should be soaked in hot water (above 130°) for 5 to 10 minutes.

Storage and Disposal: Store at room temperature. Do not re-use empty bottle. Wrap and put in trash.

How Supplied: A-200 Shampoo Concentrate in 2 and 4 fl. oz. unbreakable plastic bottles and A-200 Gel Concentrate in 1 oz. tubes, all with special comb and bilingual patient insert.

Literature Available: Additional patient literature available upon request.
Shown in Product Identification Section, page 416

ASTHMAHALER® Mist
epinephrine bitartrate bronchodilator
Alcohol Free Formula

Active Ingredients: Contains epinephrine bitartrate 7 mg per ml in inert propellant.

Inactive Ingredients: Cetylpyridinium Chloride, Propellants 11, 12, & 114, Sorbitan Trioleate.

Indications: For temporary relief of shortness of breath, tightness of chest, and wheezing due to bronchial asthma.

Warnings: Do not use this product unless a diagnosis of asthma has been made by a doctor. Do not use this product if you have heart disease, high blood pressure, thyroid disease, diabetes, or difficulty in urination due to enlargement of the prostate gland unless directed by a doctor. Do not use this product if you have ever been hospitalized for asthma or if you are taking any prescription drug for asthma unless directed by a doctor. **DO NOT USE THIS PRODUCT MORE FREQUENTLY OR AT HIGHER DOSES THAN RECOMMENDED UNLESS DIRECTED BY A DOCTOR.** Excessive use may cause nervousness and rapid heart beat, and possibly, adverse effects on the heart. **DO NOT CONTINUE TO USE THIS PRODUCT, BUT SEEK MEDICAL ASSISTANCE IMMEDIATELY IF SYMPTOMS ARE NOT RELIEVED WITHIN 20 MINUTES OR BECOME WORSE.**

Drug Interaction Precaution: Do not use this product if you are presently taking a prescription drug for high blood pressure or depression, without first consulting your doctor.

As with any drug, if you are pregnant or nursing a baby, seek the advice of a health professional before using this product.

Keep this and all medication out of the reach of children. In case of accidental overdose, consult a physician immediately.

Contents under pressure. Do not puncture or incinerate container. Do not expose to heat or store at temperature above 120°F.

Dosage and Administration: For oral inhalation only. Each inhalation contains the equivalent of 0.16 milligram of epinephrine base.

Dosage: Inhalation dosage for adults and children 4 years of age and older: Start with one inhalation, then wait at least 1 minute. If not relieved, use once more. Do not use again for at least 3 hours. Use of this product by children should be supervised by an adult. Children under 4 years of age: consult a doctor.

Directions: Shake well before each use.
1. Remove plastic dust cap, take mouthpiece off metal vial and fit other end of mouthpiece onto top of vial, turn vial upside down. Shake well.
2. Breathe out fully and place mouthpiece well into mouth, aimed at the back of the throat.
3. As you begin to breathe in deeply, press the vial firmly down into the adapter with the index finger. This releases one dose.
4. Release pressure on vial and remove unit from mouth. Hold the breath as long as possible, then breathe out slowly.

The plastic mouthpiece should be cleaned daily. Remove metal vial and wash adapter with soap and hot water and rinse thoroughly. Dry and replace with vial.

How Supplied: ½ fl. oz. (15 ml). Available as combination package metal vial plus plastic mouthpiece, or as refill metal vial only.

ASTHMANEFRIN®
Solution "A" Bronchodilator

Active Ingredients: Racepinephrine hydrochloride equivalent to 2.25% epinephrine base.

Inactive Ingredients: Benzoic acid, Chlorobutanol, Glycerin, Hydrochloric Acid, Sodium Bisulfite, Sodium Chloride, Water.

Indications: For temporary relief of shortness of breath, tightness of chest, and wheezing due to bronchial asthma.

Warnings: Do not use this product unless a diagnosis of asthma has been made by a doctor. Do not use this product if you have heart disease, high blood pressure, thyroid disease, diabetes, or difficulty in urination due to enlargement of the prostate gland unless directed by a doctor. Do not use this product if you have ever been hospitalized for asthma or if you are taking any prescription drug for asthma unless directed by a doctor. **DO NOT USE THIS PRODUCT MORE FREQUENTLY OR AT HIGHER DOSES THAN RECOMMENDED UNLESS DIRECTED BY A DOCTOR.** Excessive use may cause nervousness and rapid heart beat, and possibly, adverse effects on the heart. **DO NOT CONTINUE TO USE THIS PRODUCT, BUT SEEK MEDICAL ASSISTANCE IMMEDIATELY IF SYMPTOMS ARE NOT RELIEVED WITHIN 20 MINUTES OR BECOME WORSE.**

Do not use this product if it is brown in color or cloudy.

Drug Interaction Precaution: Do not use this product if you are presently taking a prescription drug for high blood pressure or depression, without first consulting your doctor.

As with any drug, if you are pregnant or nursing a baby, seek the advice of a physician before using this product.

Keep this and all medication out of the reach of children.

Store at room temperature; avoid excessive heat.

Dosage and Administration: Inhalation dosage for adults and children 4 years of age and older: 1 to 3 inhalations not more often than every 3 hours. The use of this product by children should be supervised by an adult. Children under 4 years of age: consult a doctor.

Directions: For use in hand-held rubber bulb nebulizer. Pour at least 8 drops of solution into AsthmaNefrin Nebulizer.

Care of Solution: Refrigerate once bottle has been opened.

How Supplied: ½ fl. oz. (15 ml) and 1 fl. oz. (30 ml) Solutions. FOR USE WITH ASTHMANEFRIN® NEBULIZER.

AVAIL™

Ingredients:
One Avail™ tablet daily provides:

Vitamins	Quantity		% U.S. RDA
Vitamin A	5000	I.U.	100%
Vitamin D	400	I.U.	100%
Vitamin E	30	I.U.	100%
Vitamin C	90	mg	150%
Folic Acid	0.4	mg	100%
Vitamin B1	2.25	mg	150%
Vitamin B2	2.55	mg	150%
Niacinamide	20	mg	100%
Vitamin B6	3.0	mg	150%
Vitamin B12	9.0	mcg	150%
Minerals			
Magnesium	100	mg	25%
Calcium	400	mg	40%
Zinc	22.5	mg	150%
Iodine	150	mcg	100%
Chromium	15	mcg	*
Selenium	15	mcg	*
Iron	18	mg	100%

*Recognized as essential in human nutrition, but no U.S. RDA established.

Indications: Dietary Supplement.

Dosage and Directions: One tablet daily or as directed by a physician.

Precaution: Contains Iron which can be harmful in large doses. Close tightly and keep out of the reach of children. In case of accidental overdose contact a physician or Poison Control Center immediately.

How Supplied: Bottles of 60 tablets with child resistant closures.

Shown in Product Identification Section, page 416

ESOTÉRICA® MEDICATED FADE CREAM
Regular
Facial with Sunscreen
Fortified Scented with Sunscreen
Fortified Unscented with Sunscreen

Description:
Regular:
Active Ingredient: Hydroquinone 2%.
Other Ingredients: Water, glyceryl stearate, isopropyl palmitate, propylene glycol, ceresin, mineral oil, stearyl alcohol, propylene glycol stearate, PEG-6-32 stearate, poloxamer 188, steareth-20, laureth-23, dimethicone, sodium lauryl sulfate, citric acid, sodium bisulfite, methylparaben, propylparaben, trisodium EDTA, BHA.
Facial with Sunscreen:
Active Ingredients: Hydroquinone 2.0%, padimate O 3.3%, oxybenzone 2.5%. **Other Ingredients:** Water, isopropyl myristate, stearyl alcohol, glyceryl stearate, propylene glycol, ceresin, poloxamer 188, steareth-20, ceteareth-3, dimethicone, sodium lauryl sulfate, citric acid, fragrance, trisodium EDTA, BHA, sodium bisulfite, methylparaben, propylparaben.
Fortified Scented and Unscented with Sunscreen:
Active Ingredients: Hydroquinone 2%, padimate O 3.3%, oxybenzone 2.5%. **Other Ingredients:** Water, glyceryl stearate, isopropyl palmitate, ceresin, propylene glycol, stearyl alcohol, PEG-6-32 stearate, poloxamer 188, mineral oil, steareth-20, laureth-23, steareth-10, allantoin ascorbate, dimethicone, sodium lauryl sulfate, methylparaben, propylparaben, sodium bisulfite, BHA, trisodium EDTA.
Fragrance in all except Fortified Unscented with Sunscreen.

Indications: Regular and Fortified Scented and Unscented with Sunscreen: Indicated for helping fade darkened skin areas including age spots, liver spots, freckles and melasma on the face, hands, legs and body and when used as directed helps prevent their recurrence. Facial with Sunscreen: Specially designed to help fade darkened skin areas including age spots, liver spots, freckles and melasma on the face and when used as directed helps prevent their recurrence. It has emollients to help moisturize while it

Continued on next page

Norcliff Thayer—Cont.

lightens, so it makes an excellent night cream as well.

Actions: Esotérica Medicated helps bleach and lighten hyperpigmented skin.

Contraindications: Should not be used by persons with known sensitivity to hydroquinone.

Warnings: Do not use if skin is irritated. Some individuals may be sensitive to the active ingredient(s) in this cream. Discontinue use if irritation appears. Avoid contact with eyes. Excessive exposure to the sun should be avoided. For external use only.
Facial and Fortified Scented and Unscented with Sunscreen: Not for use in the prevention of sunburn.

Directions: Apply Esotérica to areas you wish to lighten and rub in well. Use cream in the morning and at bedtime for at least six weeks for maximum results. Esotérica is greaseless and may be used under makeup.

How Supplied: 3 oz. plastic jars.

LIQUIPRIN®
Infants' Drops and Children's Elixir (acetaminophen)

Description: Liquiprin is a nonsalicylate analgesic and antipyretic particularly suitable for infants and children. Liquiprin Drops is a raspberry flavored, reddish pink solution. Liquiprin Elixir is a cherry flavored, reddish solution. Neither contain alcohol.

Active Ingredient:
Liquiprin Drops: Acetaminophen 80 mg per 1.66 ml (top mark on dropper).
Liquiprin Elixir: Acetaminophen 80 mg per ½ teaspoon.

Inactive Ingredients:
Liquiprin Drops: Artificial Raspberry and other artificial and natural flavors, citric acid, D&C Red No. 33, dextrose, FD&C Red No. 40, fructose, glycerin, methylparaben, polyethylene glycol, propylparaben, sodium citrate, sodium gluconate, water.
Liquiprin Elixir: Artificial cherry and other artificial and natural flavors, citric acid, D&C Red No. 33, FD&C Red No. 40, dextrose, fructose, glycerin, methylparaben, polyethylene glycol, propylparaben, sodium citrate, sodium gluconate, sucrose, water.

Actions: Liquiprin Children's Elixir and Infants' Drops safely and effectively reduces fever and pain in infants and children without the hazards of salicylate therapy (e.g., gastric mucosal irritation).

Indications: Liquiprin is indicated for use in the treatment of infants and children with conditions requiring reduction of fever and/or relief of pain such as mild upper respiratory infections (tonsillitis, common cold, flu), teething, headache, myalgia, postimmunization reactions, post-tonsillectomy discomfort and gas-

troenteritis. As adjunctive therapy with antibiotics or sulfonamides, Liquiprin may be useful as an analgesic and antipyretic in bacterial or viral infections, such as bronchitis, pharyngitis, tracheobronchitis, sinusitis, pneumonia, otitis media and cervical adenitis.

Precautions and Adverse Reactions: If a sensitivity reaction occurs, the drug should be discontinued. Liquiprin has rarely been found to produce side effects. It is usually well tolerated by patients who are sensitive to products containing aspirin.

Usual Dosage:
Liquiprin Drops and Elixir may be given alone or mixed with milk, juices, applesauce or other beverages and foods. All dosages may be repeated every 4 hours, if pain and fever persist, but not to exceed 5 times daily or as directed by physician.
Liquiprin Drops should be administered in the following dosages:
Under 2 years, under 24 lbs.: Consult physician
2–3 years, 24–35 lbs.: 160 mg—2 dropperfuls
4–5 years, 36–47 lbs.: 240 mg—3 dropperfuls
Liquiprin Elixir should be administered in the following dosages:
Under 2 years, under 24 lbs.: Consult physician
2–3 years, 24–35 lbs.: 1 teaspoonful
4–5 years, 36–47 lbs.: 1½ teaspoonfuls
6–8 years, 48–59 lbs.: 2 teaspoonfuls
9–10 years, 60–71 lbs.: 2½ teaspoonfuls
11–12 years, 72–95 lbs.: 3 teaspoonfuls

How Supplied: Liquiprin Drops is available in a 1.16 fl. oz. (35 ml) plastic bottle with a calibrated dropper and child-resistant cap, and safety sealed package.
Liquiprin Elixir is available in a 4 fl. oz. plastic bottle with a pre-marked measuring cup and child-resistant cap, and safety sealed package.
Shown in Product Identification Section, page 416

NATURE'S REMEDY®
Natural Vegetable Laxative

Active Ingredients: Cascara sagrada 150 mg, aloe 100 mg.

Inactive Ingredients: Calcium stearate, cellulose, lactose, coating, colors (contains FD&C Yellow No. 6).

Indications: For gentle, overnight relief of constipation.

Actions: Nature's Remedy has two natural active ingredients that give gentle, overnight relief of constipation. These ingredients, cascara sagrada and aloe, gently stimulate the body's natural function.

Warnings: Do not take any laxative when nausea, vomiting, abdominal pain, or other symptoms of appendicitis are present. Frequent or prolonged use of laxatives may result in dependence on them. If pregnant or nursing, consult

your physician before using this or any medicine.

Dosage and Administration: Adults, swallow two tablets daily along with a full glass of water; children (8–15 yrs.), one tablet daily; or as directed by a physician.

How Supplied: Beige, film-coated tablets with foil-backed blister packaging in boxes of 12s, 30s and 60s.
Shown in Product Identification Section, page 416

NOSALT®
Salt Alternative Regular and Seasoned

Description: Food seasoning to be used as an alternative or substitute for salt (NaCl) at the table and in cooking to help regulate dietary sodium intake.

Regular Ingredients: Contains potassium chloride, potassium bitartrate, adipic acid, mineral oil, fumaric acid. Looks, sprinkles and tastes like salt. Each ¼ teaspoon contains less than 5 mg of sodium which is considered dietetically sodium free. Contains 625 mg potassium, 563 mg chloride, 60 mg flavor enhancers.

Seasoned Ingredients: Potassium chloride, dextrose, onion and garlic, spices and other natural flavors, lactose, cream of tartar, paprika, silica, disodium inosinate and disodium guanylate, turmeric and extratives of paprika. Contains less than 5 mg sodium per teaspoon which is considered dietetically sodium free. Contains approximately 664 mg potassium (17 mEq) per ½ level teaspoon.

Uses: Sprinkled on food or in cooking, in the same proportion or less than regular salt, gives food salt flavor while helping to reduce sodium intake. Appropriate for persons on low sodium diets, as for example, those whose sodium intake has been restricted for medical reasons.

Caution to Physicians: The potassium intake of persons receiving potassium-sparing diuretics or potassium supplementation should be evaluated. Potassium chloride should not be used in patients with hyperkalemia, oliguria, and severe kidney disease.

Consumer Warning: Persons having diabetes, heart or kidney disease, or persons receiving medical treatment should consult a physician before using a salt alternative or substitute.

How Supplied: Regular: 11 oz. container with shaker top. **Seasoned:** 8 oz. container with shaker top.
Shown in Product Identification Section, page 416

OXY CLEAN®
Lathering Facial Scrub

Description: Oxy Clean Scrub is a skin cleanser containing dissolving abradant granules and is useful for opening plugged pores and for removing excess oil. Oxy Clean Scrub can't over-abrade as

can cleansers with non-dissolving abradant particles.

Composition: Contains dissolving abradant granules (sodium tetraborate decahydrate) in a base containing a unique combination of surface active soapless cleaning agents.

Directions: Use in place of your usual soap or cleanser. Wet face with warm water. Squeeze Oxy Clean Scrub onto fingertips and gently massage into face. Continue massaging and adding water until abradant granules are completely dissolved. (About one minute.) Rinse thoroughly with warm water and dry. Use once or twice daily, or as required.

Caution: Avoid contact with eyes. If particles get into eyes, flush thoroughly with water and avoid rubbing eyes. Discontinue use if skin irritation or excessive dryness develops. Not to be used on infants or children under 3 years of age. Do not use on inflamed skin. Keep out of reach of children.

How Supplied: 2.65 oz. plastic tubes.
Shown in Product Identification Section, page 416

OXY CLEAN®
Medicated Cleanser, Regular and Maximum Strength Pads, Soap

Active Ingredient:
Oxy Clean® Medicated Cleanser: Salicylic Acid* 0.5%, SD Alcohol 40B 40%
Oxy Clean® Medicated Pads Regular Strength: Salicylic Acid* 0.5%, SD Alcohol 40B 40%.
Oxy Clean® Medicated Pads Maximum Strength: Salicylic Acid* 2.0%, SD Alcohol 40B 50%.
Oxy Clean® Medicated Soap: Salicylic Acid* 3.5%
*Salicylic Acid (2-Hydroxybenzoic Acid)

Inactive Ingredients:
Oxy Clean® Medicated Cleanser: Water, propylene glycol, sodium lauryl sulfate, citric acid, menthol.
Oxy Clean® Medicated Pads Regular Strength: Water, propylene glycol, sodium lauryl sulfate, citric acid, fragrance, menthol.
Oxy Clean® Medicated Pads Maximum Strength: Water, PEG-8, propylene glycol, sodium lauryl sulfate, citric acid, fragrance, menthol.

Other Ingredients:
Oxy Clean® Medicated Soap: Sodium tallowate, sodium cocoate, water, triethanolamine, fragrance, iron oxides, trisodium HEDTA, sodium borate, D&C Green No. 5.

Indications: These medicated skin products are useful for opening plugged pores and for removing excess dirt and oil. Also helps remove and prevent blackheads.

Additional Benefits: When used regularly cleanses acne prone skin and removes dirt, grime and excess skin oil. For a complete anti-acne program, after using Oxy Clean® follow use with Oxy-5® Tinted and Vanishing, or Oxy-10® Tinted and Vanishing acne pimple medications.

Caution: For external use only. If skin irritation develops, discontinue use and consult a physician. May be irritating to eyes or mucous membranes. If contact occurs, flush thoroughly with water. Keep this and all drugs out of reach of children. Store at room temperature. Keep away from flame, fire and heat.

Dosage and Administration: See labeling instructions for use.

How Supplied:
Medicated Liquid Cleanser—4 fl. oz.
Medicated Pads Regular Strength—Plastic Jar/50 pads or 90 pads
Medicated Pads Maximum Strength—Plastic Jar/50 pads or 90 pads
Medicated Soap—3.25 oz. soap bar.
Shown in Product Identification Section, page 416

OXY-5® and OXY-10®
with SORBOXYL®
Benzoyl peroxide lotions 5% and 10%
with silica oil absorber
Tinted Formula

Description: Active Ingredient: Oxy-5: Benzoyl peroxide 5%. Oxy-10: Benzoyl peroxide 10%.

Inactive Ingredients: Oxy-5: Water, titanium dioxide, sodium PCA, cetyl alcohol, silica (Sorboxyl®), iron oxides, propylene glycol, citric acid, sodium lauryl sulfate, stearyl alcohol, methylparaben, propylparaben.
Oxy-10: Water, titanium dioxide, silica (Sorboxyl®), cetyl alcohol, glyceryl stearate, propylene glycol, stearic acid, iron oxides, sodium lauryl sulfate, citric acid, sodium citrate, methylparaben, propylparaben.

Indications: Topical medications for the treatment of acne vulgaris.

Action: Provides antibacterial activity against Propionibacterium acnes.

Additional Benefits: Absorbs excess skin oil up to 12 hours. Flesh tone, odorless, greaseless lotions that cover up acne pimples while they treat them.

Directions for Use: Wash skin thoroughly and dry well. Shake well before using. Dab on smoothing into oily acne pimple areas of face, neck and body (see Caution). Apply once a day initially, then two or three times a day, or as directed by a physician.

Caution: Those with known sensitivity to benzoyl peroxide or especially sensitive skin should not use this medication. Before using, determine if you are sensitive by applying to a small affected area once a day for two days. Follow label instructions and continue use if no discomfort occurs. If, during treatment, irritation, redness, burning, itching or excessive drying and peeling occur, reduce dosage or frequency of use. Discontinue if irritation is severe and if it persists, consult a doctor. Keep away from eyes, lips, and mouth. Keep this and all drugs out of the reach of children. This product may bleach hair or dyed fabrics. Keep tightly closed. Store at room temperature, avoid excessive heat. For external use only.

How Supplied: 1 fl. oz. plastic bottles.
Shown in Product Identification Section, page 416

OXY-5® and OXY-10®
with SORBOXYL®
Benzoyl peroxide lotion 5% and 10%
with silica oil absorber
Vanishing Formula

Description: Active Ingredient: Oxy-5: Benzoyl peroxide 5%. Oxy-10: Benzoyl peroxide 10%.

Inactive Ingredients: Oxy-5: Water, sodium PCA, cetyl alcohol, silica (Sorboxyl®), propylene glycol, citric acid, sodium lauryl sulfate, methylparaben, propylparaben.
Oxy-10: Water, silica (Sorboxyl®), cetyl alcohol, propylene glycol, citric acid, sodium citrate, sodium lauryl sulfate, methylparaben and propylparaben.

Indications: Topical medications for the treatment of acne vulgaris.

Action: Provides antibacterial activity against Propionibacterium acnes.

Additional Benefits: Absorbs excess skin oil up to 12 hours. Colorless, odorless, greaseless lotions that vanish upon application.

Directions for Use: Wash skin thoroughly and dry well. Shake well before using. Dab on smoothing into oily acne pimple areas of face, neck and body (see Caution). Apply once a day initially, then two or three times a day, or as directed by a physician.

Caution: Those with known sensitivity to benzoyl peroxide or especially sensitive skin should not use this medication. Before using, determine if you are sensitive by applying to a small affected area once a day for two days. Follow label instructions and continue use if no discomfort occurs. If, during treatment, irritation, redness, burning, itching or excessive drying and peeling occur, reduce dosage or frequency of use. Discontinue if irritation is severe and if it persists, consult a doctor. Keep away from eyes, lips, and mouth. Keep this and all drugs out of the reach of children. This product may bleach hair or dyed fabrics. Keep tightly closed. Store at room temperature, avoid excessive heat. For external use only.

How Supplied: 1 fl. oz. plastic bottles.
Shown in Product Identification Section, page 416

OXY 10® WASH Antibacterial Skin Wash

Active Ingredient: Benzoyl peroxide 10%.

Inactive Ingredients: Cetyl alcohol, citric acid, methylparaben, propylene glycol, propylparaben, sodium citrate, sodium lauryl sulfate, water.

Continued on next page

Norcliff Thayer—Cont.

Indications: Antibacterial skin wash used as an aid in the treatment of acne vulgaris.

Actions: Promotes antibacterial activity against Propionibacterium acnes.

Additional Benefits: When used instead of regular soap, cleanses acne-prone skin and removes dirt, grime and excess skin oil.
For a complete anti-acne program, follow Oxy 10® Wash with Oxy-5® acne-pimple medication. Or for stubborn and adult acne, use Oxy-10® maximum strength acne-pimple medication.

Contraindications: Should not be used by persons with known sensitivity to benzoyl peroxide.

Caution: Persons with sensitive skin or known allergy to benzoyl peroxide should not use this medication. First test on a small affected area by applying this product as directed once a day for two days. If discomforting irritation or undue dryness occurs during treatment, reduce frequency of use or dosage. If excessive itching, redness, burning, swelling, irritation or dryness occurs, discontinue use and consult a physician. Avoid contact with eyes, lips and mouth. May bleach hair or dyed fabrics. **For external use only.**

Directions: Shake well. Wet area to be washed. Apply Oxy 10® Wash massaging gently for 1 to 2 minutes. Rinse thoroughly. Use 2 to 3 times daily or as directed by physician.

How supplied: 4 fl. oz. plastic bottles.
Shown in Product Identification Section, page 416

TUMS® Antacid Tablets
TUMS E–X® Antacid Tablets

Description: Tums: Active Ingredient: Calcium Carbonate, precipitated U.S.P. 500 mg.
Tums Original Flavor: Inactive Ingredients: Flavor, mineral oil, sodium polyphosphate, starch, sucrose, talc.
Tums Assorted Flavors: Inactive Ingredients: Adipic acid, colors (contains FD&C Yellow No. 6), flavors, mineral oil, sodium polyphosphate, starch, sucrose, talc.
An antacid composition providing liquid effectiveness in a low cost, pleasant-tasting tablet. Tums tablets are free of the chalky aftertaste usually associated with calcium carbonate therapy and remain pleasant tasting even during long-term therapy. Each TUMS tablet contains not more than 2 mg of sodium and is considered to be dietetically sodium free. Non-laxative/non-constipating.
Tums E-X: Active Ingredient: Calcium Carbonate, 750 mg.
Tums E-X Wintergreen Flavor Inactive Ingredients: Colors (contains FD&C Yellow No. 6), flavor, mineral oil, sodium polyphosphate, starch, sucrose, talc.

Tums E-X Assorted Flavors Inactive Ingredients: Adipic acid, colors (contains FD&C Yellow No. 6), flavors, mineral oil, sodium polyphosphate, starch, sucrose, talc.
Each tablet contains not more than 2 mg of sodium and is considered to be dietetically sodium free. Non-laxative/non-constipating.

Indications: For fast relief of acid indigestion, heartburn, sour stomach and upset stomach associated with these symptoms.

Actions: Tums lowers the upper limit of the pH range without affecting the innate antacid efficiency of calcium carbonate. One tablet, when tested *in vitro* according to the *Federal Register* procedure (*Fed. Reg.* 39-19862, June 4, 1974), neutralizes 10 mEq of 0.1N HCl. This high neutralization capacity combined with a rapid rate of reaction makes Tums an ideal antacid for management of conditions associated with hyperacidity. It effectively neutralizes free acid yet does not cause systemic alkalosis in the presence of normal renal function. A double-blind placebo controlled clinical study demonstrated that calcium carbonate taken at a dosage of 16 Tums tablets daily for a two-week period was non-constipating/non-laxative.

Warnings: Tums: Do not take more than 16 tablets in a 24-hour period or use the maximum dosage of this product for more than 2 weeks, except under the advice and supervision of a physician.
Tums E-X: Do not take more than 10 tablets in a 24 hour period or use the maximum dosage of this product for more than two weeks, except under the advice and supervision of a physician. Keep this and all drugs out of the reach of children.

Dosage and Administration: Chew 1 or 2 TUMS tablets as symptoms occur. Repeat hourly if symptoms return, or as directed by a physician. No water is required. Simulated Drip Method: The pleasant-tasting TUMS tablet may be kept between the gum and cheek and allowed to dissolve gradually by continuous sucking to prolong the effective relief time.

Important Dietary Information—As a Source of Extra Calcium—Chew 1 or 2 tablets after meals or as directed by a physician.
Tums Original and Assorted Flavors: The 500 mg of calcium carbonate in each tablet provide 200 mg of elemental calcium which is 20% of the adult U.S. RDA for calcium. Five tablets provide 100% of the daily calcium needs for adults.
Tums E-X: The 750 mg of calcium carbonate in each tablet provide 300 mg of elemental calcium which is 30% of the adult U.S. RDA for calcium. Four tablets provide 120% of the daily calcium needs for adults.

Professional Labeling: Indicated for the symptomatic relief of hyperacidity associated with the diagnosis of peptic

ulcer, gastritis, peptic esophagitis, gastric hyperacidity, and hiatal hernia.

How Supplied: Tums: Peppermint and Assorted Flavors of Cherry, Lemon, Orange and Lime are available in 12-tablet rolls, 3-roll wraps, and bottles of 75 and 150 tablets. **Tums E-X Wintergreen and Assorted Flavors of Cherry, Lemon, Lime and Orange:** 8-tablet rolls, 3-roll wraps and bottles of 48 and 96 tablets.
Shown in Product Identification Section, page 416

TUMS® Liquid Extra-Strength Antacid
TUMS® Liquid Extra-Strength Antacid with Simethicone

Description: Tums Liquid and Tums Liquid with Simethicone is an extra-strength antacid with a fresh, minty flavor.

Tums Liquid Extra-Strength Antacid

Active Ingredient: 1,000 mg Calcium Carbonate per teaspoon.

Inactive Ingredients: Carboxymethyl-cellulose Sodium, Citric Acid, Glycerin, Magnesium Aluminum Silicate, Methylparaben, Peppermint Oil, Potassium Pyrophosphate, Propylparaben, Sorbitol, Sucrose, Water.

Indications: For the relief of acid indigestion, heartburn, sour stomach and the symptoms of upset stomach associated with these conditions.

Tums Liquid Extra-Strength Antacid with Simethicone

Active Ingredients: 1,000 mg Calcium Carbonate and 30 mg Simethicone per teaspoon.

Inactive Ingredients: Carboxymethyl-cellulose Sodium, Citric Acid, Glycerin, Magnesium Aluminum Silicate, Methylparaben, Peppermint Oil, Potassium Pyrophosphate, Propylparaben, Sorbitol, Sucrose, Water.

Indications: For the relief of acid indigestion, heartburn, sour stomach and the symptoms of upset stomach and gas associated with these conditions.

Sodium Content: Tums Liquid and Tums Liquid with Simethicone: Each teaspoonful contains less than 5 mg of sodium which is considered dietetically sodium free.
Calcium Rich: Tums Liquid and Tums Liquid with Simethicone: Each teaspoonful contains 400 mg of elemental calcium which is 40% of the adult U.S. RDA for calcium.
Acid Neutralizing Capacity: Tums Liquid and Tums Liquid with Simethicone: 20.0 mEq/5 ml

Directions: Tums Liquid and Tums Liquid with Simethicone: Take one or two teaspoonfuls as symptoms occur. Repeat hourly if symptoms return, or as directed by a physician.

Warnings: Tums Liquid and Tums Liquid with Simethicone: Do not take more than 8 teaspoonfuls in a 24 hour

period or the maximum dosage of this product for more than 2 weeks except under the advice and supervision of a physician. Store at room temperature. Keep this and all drugs out of the reach of children.

How Supplied: Tums Liquid and Tums Liquid with Simethicone are available in 12 oz. bottles.

Shown in Product Identification Section, pages 416 & 417

Noxell Corporation
**11050 YORK ROAD
HUNT VALLEY, MARYLAND
21030-2098**

NOXZEMA®
**Antiseptic Skin Cleanser
Regular Formula**

Active Ingredient: SD Alcohol 40 (63%)

Inactive Ingredients: Water, PPG-11 Stearyl Ether, Menthol, Camphor, Clove Oil, Eucalyptus Oil, Fragrance, FD&C Blue No. 1.

Indications: To deep clean oily, acne-prone skin without leaving skin dry and flaky.

Actions: Anti-bacterial skin cleanser specially formulated to remove dirt and oil without leaving skin dry.

Warnings: For external use only, avoid use around eyes and mucous membranes. Discontinue use if excessive irritation develops.

Precaution: Flammable until dry. Keep away from flame, fire and heat. Keep out of reach of children.

Dosage and Administration: Wash as you normally do. Moisten cotton pad. Scrub face and neck thoroughly. Repeat with fresh pads until no trace of dirt is visible. Don't rinse after use.

How Supplied: Noxzema Antiseptic Skin Cleanser Regular Formula is available in 4 oz. and 8 oz. bottles.

Shown in Product Identification Section, page 417

NOXZEMA®
**Antiseptic Skin Cleanser
Extra Strength Formula**

Active Ingredients: SD Alcohol 40 (36%), Isopropyl Alcohol (34%)

Inactive Ingredients: Water, Disodium Oleamido Peg-2 Sulfosuccinate, Menthol, Camphor, Clove Oil, Eucalyptus Oil, Fragrance, Yellow No. 5, Blue No. 1.

Indications: To deep clean oily, acne-prone skin.

Actions: Anti-bacterial skin cleanser specially formulated to deep clean and remove dirt and oil while leaving a refreshing feeling.

Warnings: For external use only. Avoid use around eyes and mucous mem-

branes. Discontinue use if excessive irritation develops.

Precaution: Flammable until dry. Keep away from flame, fire and heat. Keep out of reach of children.

Dosage and Administration: Wash as you normally do. Moisten cotton pad. Scrub face and neck thoroughly. Repeat with fresh pads until no trace of dirt is visible. Don't rinse after use.

How Supplied: Noxzema Antiseptic Skin Cleanser Extra Strength Formula is available in 4 oz. and 8 oz. bottles.

Shown in Product Identification Section, page 417

NOXZEMA®
**Antiseptic Skin Cleanser
Sensitive Skin Formula**

Active Ingredient: Benzalkonium Chloride—0.13%

Inactive Ingredient: Water, SD Alcohol 40, Oleth 20, Phenoxyethanol, PPG-10 Methyl Glucose Ether, Menthol, Camphor, Clove Oil, Eucalyptus Oil, Fragrance, DMDM Hydantoin, Citric Acid, Sodium Citrate, Red No. 33, Red No. 4.

Indications: To gently deep clean oil and dirt from sensitive skin.

Actions: Anti-bacterial skin cleanser specially formulated to clean without being irritating. Leaves the skin fresh and soft.

Warnings: For external use only. Avoid use around eyes and mucous membranes. Discontinue use if excessive irritation develops.

Precaution: Flammable until dry. Keep away from flame, fire and heat. Keep out of reach of children.

Dosage and Administration: Wash as you normally do. Moisten cotton pad. Stroke over face and neck thoroughly. Repeat with fresh pads until no trace of dirt is visible. Don't rinse after use.

How Supplied: Noxzema Antiseptic Skin Cleanser Sensitive Skin Formula is available in 4 oz. and 8 oz. bottles.

Shown in Product Identification Section, page 417

NOXZEMA CLEAR–UPS®
Anti-Acne Gel

Active Ingredient: Salicylic Acid 0.5%

Inactive Ingredients: Carbomer 940, DMDM Hydantoin, Glycerin, Methylparaben, Phenoxyethanol, Polyglycerylmethacrylate, Propylene Glycol, Tetrahydroxypropyl Ethylenediamine, Water.

Indications: Topical medication for treatment of acne vulgaris. Designed for effective treatment of pimples on sensitive or easily irritated skin.

Warnings: For external use only. Avoid use around eyes and mucous membranes. Discontinue use if excessive skin irritation develops.

How Supplied: Available in 0.50 ounce squeeze container.

Shown in Product Identification Section, page 417

NOXZEMA CLEAR–UPS®
**MAXIMUM STRENGTH LOTION
Vanishing
10% Benzoyl Peroxide**

Active Ingredient: 10% Benzoyl Peroxide

Inactive Ingredients: DMDM Hydantoin, Glyceryl Stearate, Isopropyl Palmitate, Magnesium Aluminum Silicate, Methylparaben, Peg-20 Stearate, PPG-11 Stearyl Ether, Propylene Glycol, Propylparaben, Stearic Acid, Water, Xanthan Gum, Zinc Stearate.

Indications: Topical Medication for the treatment of acne vulgaris in vanishing base.

Actions: Noxzema Clear-Ups Maximum Strength Lotion contains benzoyl peroxide, which provides an anti-bacterial and keratolytic action. The product helps heal and prevent acne, helps eliminate blackheads and dries up excess oils.

Warnings: Persons with a known sensitivity to Benzoyl Peroxide should not use this medication. For external use only. Avoid contact with eyes, lips, mouth, or other sensitive areas. If swelling, itching, redness, or undue dryness occurs, discontinue use. Call physician if symptoms persist. Store at room temperature; avoid excess heat. Avoid contact with hair, fabrics and clothing since the oxidizing action of Benzoyl Peroxide may bleach colored or dyed fabrics.

Dosage and Administration: SHAKE WELL BEFORE USING. Wash skin thoroughly. For best results use Noxzema Skin Cream. Towel dry. Some people are sensitive to benzoyl peroxide so the first day of use, apply lotion lightly on a pimple or small affected area. If no discomfort occurs, apply Clear-Ups Maximum Strength Lotion directly on pimples and around affected areas twice daily. To help prevent pimples, apply lotion twice daily to areas where pimples and oily skin normally occur. Smooth in lotion with figertips until it disappears. Re-cap tightly after use. See Caution.

How Supplied: Available in a 1 fluid ounce bottle.

Shown in Product Identification Section, page 417

NOXZEMA CLEAR–UPS®
**Medicated Pads
Regular Strength**

Active Ingredients: Salicylic Acid 0.5%, Alcohol 63%.

Other Ingredients: Camphor, clove oil, eucalyptus oil, fragrance, menthol, PPG-11 stearyl ether, water.

Indications: Topical medication for the treatment of acne vulgaris. The abra-

Continued on next page

Noxell—Cont.

sive pads provide astringency and deep-down cleaning. The salicylic acid works to clear acne and to prevent new pimples from forming. The product helps clear blackheads and absorbs excess oils.

Warnings: For external use only. Avoid use around eyes and mucous membranes. Discontinue use if excessive skin irritation develops.

How Supplied: In a safety-sealed jar of 50 pads.
Shown in Product Identification Section, page 417

NOXZEMA CLEAR–UPS®
Medicated Pads
Maximum Strength

Active Ingredients: Salicylic Acid 2.0%, Alcohol 64%.

Other Ingredients: Camphor, clove oil, eucalyptus oil, fragrance, menthol, PEG 4, PPG-11 stearyl ether, water.

Indications: Topical medication for the treatment of acne vulgaris. The abrasive pads provide astringency and deep-down cleaning. The salicylic acid works to clear acne and to prevent new pimples from forming. The product helps clear blackheads and absorbs excess oils.

Warnings: For external use only. Avoid use around eyes and mucous membranes. Discontinue use if excessive skin irritation develops.

How Supplied: In a safety-sealed jar of 50 pads.
Shown in Product Identification Section, page 417

NOXZEMA CLEAR–UPS®
ON-THE-SPOT TREATMENT
Tinted and Vanishing

Active Ingredient: 10% Benzoyl Peroxide

Inactive Ingredients: DMDM Hydantoin, Glyceryl Stearate, Iron Oxides (tinted only), Isopropyl Palmitate, Magnesium Aluminum Silicate, Methylparaben, Peg-20 Stearate, Peg-100 Stearate (tinted only), PPG-11 Stearyl Ether, Propylene Glycol, Propylparaben, Stearic Acid, Titanium Dioxide (tinted only), Water, Xanthan Gum, Zinc Stearate (vanishing only).

Indications: Topical medication for the treatment of acne vulgaris in one skin-toned shade to hide blemishes while they heal and 1 vanishing formulation to work invisibly. Comes in a unique, easy-to-use applicator to target problem areas.

Actions: Noxzema On-The-Spot contains benzoyl peroxide which provides an anti-bacterial and keratolytic action. The product helps heal and prevent acne and blackheads and comes in a unique, portable container with an easy-to-use applicator.

Warnings: Persons with a known sensitivity to Benzoyl Peroxide should not

use this medication. For external use only. Avoid contact with eyes, lips, mouth or other sensitive areas. If swelling, itching, redness, or undue dryness occurs, discontinue use. Call physician if symptoms persist. Store at room temperature; avoid excess heat. Avoid contact with hair, fabrics and clothing since the oxidizing action of Benzoyl Peroxide may bleach colored or dyed fabrics.

Dosage and Administration:
1. SHAKE WELL BEFORE USING. Wash skin thoroughly. For best results use Noxzema Skin Cream. Towel dry.
2. Some people are sensitive to benzoyl peroxide, so for the first two days of use, apply lotion lightly on a pimple, or small affected area.
3. If no discomfort occurs, apply Clear-Ups On-The-Spot Treatment directly on pimples and around affected areas twice daily.
4. To help prevent pimples, smooth Clear-Ups On-The-Spot Treatment twice daily to areas where pimples and oily skin normally occur. Recap tightly after use. See caution.

How Supplied: Available in a .25 oz. unique container with an easy-to-use applicator. Clear-Ups On-The-Spot is available in one skin-tone, covering shade and one vanishing formulation.
Shown in Product Identification Section, page 417

NOXZEMA®
Medicated Skin Cream

Active Ingredients: Camphor, Phenol (less than 0.5%), Clove Oil, Eucalyptus Oil, Menthol.

Other Ingredients: Water, Stearic Acid, Linseed Oil, Soybean Oil, Fragrance, Propylene Glycol, Gelatin, Ammonium Hydroxide, Calcium Hydroxide.

Actions: Antipruritic, counterirritant and antiseptic.

Indications: This medicated skin product is an effective facial cleanser and has been demonstrated to be more effective than soap in an acne washing regimen. When used on sunburned skin, this medicated cream actually reduces the surface temperature of the skin to relieve pain almost instantly.

Additional Benefits: Noxzema is also an effective moisturizer. For an effective anti-acne program: instead of soap, wash with Noxzema and treat acne prone areas with Noxzema Acne 12.

Directions: (Wash) Morning and night wash your face with Noxzema Skin Cream. Scoop or pump out some Noxzema and spread over your face with a wet washcloth, gently work in using a circular motion. Rinse. (Sunburn) Apply Noxzema Skin Cream liberally to areas of burn or discomfort.

Contraindications: None.

Cautions: For persistent skin problems or serious burn, consult physician. Keep out of the reach of children.
Shown in Product Identification Section, page 417

NuAge Laboratories, Ltd.
4200 LACLEDE AVENUE
ST. LOUIS, MO 63108

BIOCHEMIC TISSUE SALTS
[bī̄o "kem 'ik tish 'u sawlt]

Ingredients: Each tissue salt tablet provides Schuessler homoeopathic ingredients as the recommended triturated tablet in the required Lactose base per U.S.H.P.

Action: Biochemic Tissue Salts (or Cell Salts) work homoeopathically to help the body achieve relief and maintain health and fitness by stimulating the body's healing process.

History: The NuAge Biochemic Tissue Tablets were developed over one hundred years ago by Dr. Wm. Schuessler. Their use is explained in THE BIOCHEMIC HANDBOOK and many other publications. The Tissue Salts are "official" when made in accordance with the United States Homoeopathic Pharmacopoeia.

Contraindications: None

Warning: As with any drug, if nursing or pregnant seek the advice of a professional before using. Keep this and all medicine out of the reach of children. If symptoms persist or recur, consult a licensed medical practitioner.

Instructions: Use according to standard Homoeopathic indications.

EDUCATIONAL MATERIAL

The Biochemic Handbook
Published by Formur, Inc., a paperback pocket edition giving complete description of biochemic tissue salts and proper applications for noted symptoms. ($1.50)
Product Description Charts
Color sheet, 8½ × 11, describing each biochemic tissue salt and its proper application.

Numark Laboratories, Inc.
P.O. BOX 6321
EDISON, NJ 08818

CERTAN–DRI® ANTIPERSPIRANT

Active Ingredient: Aluminum Chloride

Inactive Ingredient: Aloe Vera

Actions: Antiperspirant protection—helps solve, control and lessen underarm perspiration.

Warnings: Do not apply after shaving, on broken skin, or immediately after bathing. If rash develops, discontinue use. Keep out of reach of children.

Directions: Must be applied <u>sparingly</u> on dry skin <u>at bedtime</u> only. Recommended for underarm use only.

How Supplied: 1.1-oz. and 2-oz. unscented roll-on.
For more information contact NUMARK Laboratories, Inc., PO Box 6321, Edison, NJ 08818 for a free booklet, "Facts About Perspiration & Perspiration Problems". From outside New Jersey call 1-800-331-0221, in New Jersey 1-201-417-1870.

Oral-B Laboratories
ONE LAGOON DRIVE
REDWOOD CITY, CA 94065

AMOSAN®
[ăm′ō-săn]

Active Ingredients: Sodium Peroxyborate Monohydrate derived from Sodium Perborate

Inactive Ingredients: Sodium Bitartrate, Sodium Saccharin, Flavors (Peppermint oil USP, Menthol USP, Imitation Vanilla)

Indication: For cleansing minor oral wounds and gum inflammation resulting from dental procedures, dentures, orthodontic appliances, accidental injury, and canker sores. Amosan is effective as an aid to oral hygiene in physically handicapped patients and as an adjunct to professional care in the treatment of gingivitis and other gum diseases.

Actions: When mixed with water and introduced as a rinse, oxygen is liberated upon contact with the mouth fluids and blood. The liberated oxygen provides both a chemical and mechanical cleansing action.

Warnings: If symptoms do not improve in seven days; if irritation, pain or redness persists or worsens, or if swelling or fever develops, a dentist or doctor should be seen promptly.

Drug Interactions: There are no known drug interactions with Amosan.

Precaution: Do not swallow. Consult a dentist or doctor before administering Amosan to children under six years of age. Children under twelve years of age should be supervised in the use of this product.

Symptoms and Treatment of Oral Overdosage: In cases of accidental ingestion of large amounts (6 grams in children, 20 grams in adults) symptoms of toxicity such as nausea, vomiting, and diarrhea may occur. Seek professional assistance or contact a poison control center.

Dosage and Administration: "Dissolve contents of one envelope of Amosan in 1 ounce (30 milliliters) of warm water. Use immediately. Swish solution around in the mouth over the affected area for at least 1 minute and then spit out. Do not swallow. Use up to four times daily after meals and at bedtime or as directed by a dentist or doctor. Children under 6 years of age: consult a dentist or doctor."

Professional Labeling: Amosan is effective as adjunctive therapy in the treatment of gingivitis, periodontitis, stomatitis and generalized inflammation of the oral cavity.

How Supplied: Amosan is supplied in boxes of 20 and 40 single use packets. Each packet contains 0.06 ounces (1.7 g) of powder.
Shown in Product Identification Section, page 417

Ortho Pharmaceutical Corporation
Advanced Care Products Division
RARITAN, NJ 08869

CONCEPTROL® Single Use Contraceptives

Description: An unscented, unflavored, colorless, greaseless and non-staining gel in convenient, easy-to-use disposable plastic applicators. Each applicator is filled with a single, pre-measured dose containing the active spermicide Nonoxynol-9—4.0%, (100 mg) at pH 4.5.

Indication: Contraception

Actions and Uses: A spermicidal gel for use whenever control of conception is desirable.

Warning: Occasional burning and/or irritation of the vagina or penis have been reported. If this occurs, discontinue use and consult a physician as necessary. Not effective if taken orally. Keep out of reach of children. When pregnancy is contraindicated, the contraceptive program should be discussed with a health care professional.

Dosage and Administration: One applicatorful of CONCEPTROL should be inserted deeply into the vagina just before intercourse. An additional applicatorful is required each time intercourse is repeated. If intercourse has not occurred within one hour after the application of CONCEPTROL, repeat the application of CONCEPTROL before intercourse.
Douching is not recommended after using CONCEPTROL Gel. However, if desired for cleansing purposes, wait at least six hours following last intercourse to allow for full spermicidal activity of CONCEPTROL Gel.
While no method of contraception can provide an absolute guarantee against becoming pregnant, for maximum protection, CONCEPTROL Gel must be used according to directions.

Inactive Ingredients: Lactic Acid, Methylparaben, Povidone, Propylene Glycol, Purified Water, Sodium Carboxymethylcellulose, Sorbic Acid, Sorbitol Solution.

How Supplied: CONCEPTROL Gel is available in packages of 6 and 10 easy to use applicators, premeasured, prefilled, prewrapped.

Storage: Conceptrol Gel should be stored at room temperature.
Shown in Product Identification Section, page 417

DELFEN®
Contraceptive Foam

Description: A contraceptive foam in an aerosol dosage formulation containing 12.5% Nonoxynol-9 and buffered to normal vaginal pH 4.5.

Indication: Contraception.

Action and Uses: A spermicidal foam for intravaginal contraception.

Warning: Occasional burning and/or irritation of the vagina or penis have been reported. In such cases, the medication should be discontinued and a physician consulted as necessary. Not effective if taken orally. Keep out of reach of children.
When pregnancy is contraindicated, the contraceptive program should be discussed with a health care professional.

Dosage and Administration: Insert DELFEN Contraceptive Foam just prior to each intercourse. You may have intercourse any time up to one hour after you have inserted the foam. If you repeat intercourse, insert another applicatorful of DELFEN Foam. After shaking the vial, place the measured-dose (5cc) applicator over the top of the vial, then press applicator down very gently. Fill to the top of the barrel threads. Remove applicator to stop flow of foam. Insert the filled applicator well into the vagina and depress the plunger. Remove the applicator with the plunger in depressed position. If a douche is desired for cleansing purposes, wait at least six hours after intercourse. Refer to directions and diagrams for detailed instructions. DELFEN Foam is a reliable method of birth control. While no method of birth control can provide an absolute guarantee against becoming pregnant, for maximum protection, DELFEN Foam must be used according to directions.

How Supplied: DELFEN Contraceptive Foam 0.70 oz. Starter vial with applicator. Also available in 0.70 oz. and 1.75 oz. Refill vials without applicator.

Inactive Ingredients: Benzoic Acid, Cetyl Alcohol, Diethylaminoethyl Stearamide, Glacial Acetic Acid, Methylparaben, Perfume, Phosphoric Acid, Polyvinyl Alcohol, Propellant 12, Propellant 114, Propylene Glycol, Purified Water, Sodium Carboxymethylcellulose, Stearic Acid.

Storage: Contents under pressure. Do not puncture or incinerate container. Do not expose to heat or store at temperatures above 120°F.
Shown in Product Identification Section, page 417

Continued on next page

Ortho Pharm.—Cont.

GYNOL II®
Contraceptive Jelly

Description: A colorless, unscented, unflavored, greaseless and non-staining contraceptive jelly containing the active spermicide Nonoxynol-9 (2%) and having a pH of 4.5.

Indication: Contraception.

Actions and Uses: An aesthetically pleasing spermicidal jelly to be used in conjunction with a diaphragm whenever control of conception is desired.

Warning: Occasional burning and/or irritation of the vagina or penis have been reported. In such cases, the medication should be discontinued and a physician consulted as necessary. Not effective if taken orally. Keep out of reach of children. When pregnancy is contraindicated, the contraceptive program should be discussed with a health care professional.

Dosage and Administration: Used in conjunction with a vaginal diaphragm. Prior to insertion, put about a teaspoonful of GYNOL II Contraceptive Jelly into the cup of the dome of the diaphragm and spread a small amount around the edge with your fingertip. This will aid in insertion and provide protection.
It is also important to remember that if intercourse occurs more than six hours after insertion, or if repeated intercourse takes place, an additional application of GYNOL II is necessary. DO NOT REMOVE THE DIAPHRAGM—simply add more GYNOL II with the applicator provided in the applicator package, being careful not to dislodge the diaphragm.
Remember, another application of GYNOL II is required each time intercourse is repeated, regardless of how little time has transpired since the diaphragm has been in place.
IMPORTANT—For contraceptive effectiveness, the diaphragm should remain in place for six hours after intercourse and should be removed as soon as possible thereafter. Continuous wearing of the diaphragm for more than 24 hours is not recommended. Retention of the diaphragm for prolonged periods may encourage the growth of certain bacteria in the vaginal tract. It has been suggested that under certain as yet unestablished conditions overgrowth of these bacteria may lead to symptoms of toxic shock syndrome (TSS). For further information, consult your physician.
If a douche is desired for cleansing purposes, wait at least six hours after intercourse. While no method of contraception can provide an absolute guarantee against becoming pregnant, for maximum protection, GYNOL II must be used according to directions.

Inactive Ingredients: Lactic Acid, Methylparaben, Povidone, Propylene Glycol, Purified Water, Sodium Carboxymethylcellulose, Sorbic Acid, Sorbitol Solution.

How Supplied: 2.5 oz Starter tube with measured dose applicator. Regular size 2.5 oz tube only. Large size 3.8 oz tube only.

Storage: Gynol II should be stored at room temperature.
Shown in Product Identification Section, page 417

INTERCEPT®
Contraceptive Inserts

Description: An effervescent, single dose vaginal contraceptive insert containing the active spermicide Nonoxynol-9—5.56%, (100 mg) at pH 4.5.

Indication: Contraception

Action: A spermicidal insert for intravaginal contraception.

Warning: Occasional burning and/or irritation of the vagina or penis have been reported. Should sensitivity to the ingredients or irritation of the vagina or penis develop, discontinue use and consult a physician as necessary. Not effective if taken orally. Keep out of reach of children. When pregnancy is contraindicated, the contraceptive program should be discussed with a health care professional.

Dosage and Administration: INTERCEPT should be inserted into the vagina at least ten minutes prior to male penetration to insure proper dispersion. INTERCEPT provides protection from ten minutes to one hour after product insertion. Insert a new INTERCEPT Contraceptive Insert each time intercourse is repeated. If a douche is desired for cleansing purposes, wait at least six hours following intercourse.
INTERCEPT is an effective method of contraception. While no method of birth control can provide an absolute guarantee against becoming pregnant, for maximum protection, Intercept must be used according to directions.

How Supplied: INTERCEPT Contraceptive Inserts are available in two packages, package containing 12 inserts with applicator and in a 12 insert package.

Inactive Ingredients: Citric Acid, Lauroamphodiacetate Sodium Trideceth Sulfate, Polyethylene Glycol 1000, Polyethylene Glycol 1450, Povidone, Sodium Bicarbonate.

Storage: Avoid exposing Intercept to excessive heat (over 86°F or 30°C).
Shown in Product Identification Section, page 417

MASSÉ®
Breast Cream

Composition: MASSE Breast Cream.

Action and Uses: MASSE Breast Cream is especially designed for care of the nipples of pregnant and nursing women.

Administration and Dosage:
BEFORE BIRTH
During the last two or three months of pregnancy, it is often desirable to prepare the nipple and the nipple area of the breast for eventual nursing. In these cases, MASSE is used once or twice daily in the following manner: Carefully cleanse the breast with a soft, clean cloth and plain water and dry. Squeeze a ribbon of MASSE, approximately an inch long, and lightly massage into the nipple and immediate surrounding area. Do so until the cream has completely disappeared. The massage motion should be gentle and outward.
AFTER BABY IS BORN
During the nursing period MASSE is used as follows: BEFORE AND AFTER EACH NURSING cleanse the breasts with a clean cloth and water. After drying squeeze a ribbon of MASSE, approximately an inch long, and gently massage into the nipple and the immediate surrounding area.

Contraindications: MASSE should not be used in cases of acute mastitis or breast abscess.

Caution: In cases of excessive tenderness or irritation of any kind, consult your physician.

How Supplied: MASSE Breast Cream is available in a 2 oz. tube.

Inactive Ingredients: Water, Glyceryl Monostearate, Glycerin, Cetyl Alcohol, Lanolin, Peanut Oil, Span-60, Stearic Acid, Tween-60, Sodium Benzoate, Propylparaben, Methylparaben, Potassium Hydroxide.

Storage: Massé should be stored at room temperature.
Shown in Product Identification Section, page 417

MICATIN®
['mī-kə-tin]
Antifungal For Athlete's Foot

Description: An antifungal containing the active ingredient miconazole nitrate 2%, clinically proven to cure athlete's foot, jock itch and ringworm.

Indications: Athlete's foot (tinea pedis), jock itch (tinea cruris), and ringworm (tinea corporis).

Actions and Uses: Proven clinically effective in the treatment of athlete's foot (tinea pedis), jock itch (tinea cruris), and ringworm (tinea corporis). For effective relief of the itching, scaling, burning and discomfort that can accompany these conditions.

Directions: Cleanse skin with soap and water and dry thoroughly. Apply a thin layer of MICATIN over affected area morning and night or as directed by a doctor. For athlete's foot, pay special attention to the spaces between the toes. It is also helpful to wear well-fitting, ventilated shoes and to change shoes and socks at least once daily. Best results in athlete's foot and ringworm are usually obtained with 4 weeks' use of this product and in jock itch with 2 weeks' use. If satisfactory results have not occurred within these times, consult a doctor or pharmacist. Children under 12 years of

age should be supervised in the use of this product. This product is not effective on the scalp or nails.

Do not use on children under 2 years of age except under the advice and supervision of a doctor. For external use only. If irritation occurs, or if there is no improvement within 4 weeks (for athlete's foot or ringworm) or within 2 weeks (for jock itch), discontinue use and consult a doctor or pharmacist. Keep this and all drugs out of the reach of children. In case of accidental ingestion, seek professional assistance or contact a Poison Control Center immediately.

How Supplied:
MICATIN® Antifungal Cream is available in a 0.5 oz. tube and a 1.0 oz. tube.
MICATIN Antifungal Spray Powder is available in a 3.0 oz. aerosol can.
MICATIN Antifungal Deodorant Spray Powder is available in a 3.0 oz. aerosol can.
MICATIN Antifungal Powder is available in a 1.5 oz. plastic bottle.
MICATIN Antifungal Spray Liquid is available in a 3.5 oz. aerosol can.

Inactive Ingredients:
MICATIN Antifungal Cream: Benzoic Acid, BHA, Mineral Oil, Peglicol 5 Oleate, Pegoxol 7 Stearate, Purified Water.
MICATIN Antifungal Spray Powder: Alcohol, Propellant A-46, Sorbitan Sesquioleate, Stearalkonium Hectorite, Talc.
MICATIN Antifungal Deodorant Spray Powder: Alcohol, Propellant A-46, Talc, Stearalkonium Hectorite, Sorbitan Sesquioleate, Fragrance.
MICATIN Antifungal Powder: Talc.
MICATIN Antifungal Spray Liquid: Alcohol, Benzyl Alcohol, Cocamide DEA, Propellant A-46, Sorbitan Sesquioleate, Tocopherol.

Storage: Store at room temerature.
Shown in Product Identification Section, page 418

MICATIN®
['mī-kə-tin]
Antifungal For Jock Itch

Description: An antifungal containing the active ingredient miconazole nitrate 2%, clinically proven to cure jock itch.

Indications: Jock itch (tinea cruris).

Actions and Uses: Proven clinically effective in the treatment of jock itch (tinea cruris). For effective relief of the itching, scaling, burning and discomfort that can accompany this condition.

Directions: Cleanse skin with soap and water and dry thoroughly. Apply a thin layer of product over affected area morning and night or as directed by a doctor. Best results are usually obtained within 2 weeks' use of this product. If satisfactory results have not occurred within this time, consult a doctor or pharmacist. Children under 12 years of age should be supervised in the use of this product. This product is not effective on the scalp or nails.

Warnings: Do not use on children under 2 years of age except under the advice and supervision of a doctor. For external use only. If irritation occurs, or if there is no improvement of jock itch within 2 weeks, discontinue use and consult a doctor or pharmacist. Keep this and all drugs out of the reach of children. In case of accidental ingestion, seek professional assistance or contact a Poison Control Center immediately.

How Supplied:
MICATIN® Jock Itch Cream is available in a 0.5 oz. tube.
MICATIN Jock Itch Spray Powder is available in a 3.0 oz. aerosol can.

Inactive Ingredients:
MICATIN Jock Itch Cream: Benzoic Acid, BHA, Mineral Oil, Peglicol 5 Oleate, Pegoxol 7 Stearate, Purified Water.
MICATIN Jock Itch Spray Powder: Alcohol, Propellant A-46, Sorbitan Sesquioleate, Stearalkonium Hectorite, Talc.

Storage: Store at room temperature.
Shown in Product Identification Section, page 418

ORTHO–CREME®
Contraceptive Cream

Description: ORTHO-CREME Contraceptive Cream is a white, pleasantly scented cream of cosmetic consistency. ORTHO-CREME is a greaseless, non-staining and non-irritating spermicidal cream containing the active spermicide Nonoxynol-9 (2%), at pH 4.5.

Indication: Contraception.

Action and Uses: An aesthetically pleasing spermicidal vaginal cream for use with a vaginal diaphragm when control of conception is desirable.

Warning: Occasional burning and/or irritation of the vagina or penis have been reported. In such cases, the medication should be discontinued and a physician consulted as necessary. Not effective if taken orally. Keep out of reach of children. When pregnancy is contraindicated the contraceptive program should be discussed with a health care professional.

Dosage and Administration: Used in conjunction with a vaginal diaphragm. Prior to insertion, put about a teaspoonful of ORTHO-CREME Contraceptive Cream into the cup of the dome of the diaphragm and spread a small amount around the edge with the fingertip. This will aid in insertion and provide protection.
It is also important to remember that if intercourse occurs more than six hours after insertion, or if repeated intercourse takes place, an additional application of ORTHO-CREME is necessary. DO NOT REMOVE THE DIAPHRAGM—simply add more ORTHO-CREME being careful not to dislodge the diaphragm.
Remember, another application of OR-THO-CREME is required each time intercourse is repeated, regardless of how little time has transpired since the diaphragm has been in place.

IMPORTANT—For contraceptive effectiveness, the diaphragm should remain in place for six hours after intercourse and should be removed as soon as possible thereafter. Continuous wearing of the diaphragm for more than 24 hours is not recommended. Retention of the diaphragm for prolonged periods may encourage the growth of certain bacteria in the vaginal tract. It has been suggested that under certain as yet unestablished conditions overgrowth of these bacteria may lead to symptoms of toxic shock syndrome (TSS). For further information, consult your physician.
If a douche is desired for cleansing purposes, wait at least 6 hours after intercourse. Refer to directions and diagrams for detailed instructions. While no method of contraception can provide an absolute guarantee against becoming pregnant, for maximum protection, OR-THO-CREME must be used according to directions.

How Supplied: 2.15 oz and 3.45 oz tube only packages.

Inactive Ingredients: Benzoic Acid, Castor Oil, Cetyl Alcohol, Fragrance, Glacial Acetic Acid, Methylparaben, Potassium Hydroxide, Propylene Glycol, Propylparaben, Purified Water, Sodium Carboxymethylcellulose, Sodium Lauryl Sulfate, Sorbic Acid, Stearic Acid, Trolamine.

Storage: Ortho-Creme should be stored at room temperature.
Shown in Product Identification Section, page 418

ORTHO–GYNOL®
Contraceptive Jelly

Description: ORTHO-GYNOL Contraceptive Jelly is a water dispersible spermicidal jelly having a pH of 4.5 and contains the active spermicide Octoxynol-9 (1%).

Indication: Contraception.

Action and Uses: An aesthetically pleasing spermicidal vaginal jelly for use with a vaginal diaphragm whenever the control of conception is desirable.

Warning: Occasional burning and/or irritation of the vagina or penis have been reported. In such cases, the medication should be discontinued and a physician consulted as necessary. Not effective if taken orally. Keep out of reach of children. When pregnancy is contraindicated, the contraceptive program should be discussed with a health care professional.

Dosage and Administration: Used in conjunction with a vaginal diaphragm. Prior to insertion, put about a teaspoonful of ORTHO-GYNOL Contraceptive Jelly into the cup of the dome of the diaphragm and spread a small amount around the edge with the fingertip. This will aid in insertion and provide protection.

Continued on next page

Ortho Pharm.—Cont.

It is also important to remember that if intercourse occurs more than six hours after insertion, or if repeated intercourse takes place, an additional application of ORTHO-GYNOL is necessary. DO NOT REMOVE THE DIAPHRAGM—simply add more ORTHO-GYNOL with the applicator provided in the applicator package, being careful not to dislodge the diaphragm.

Remember, another application of OR-THO-GYNOL is required each time intercourse is repeated, regardless of how little time has transpired since the diaphragm has been in place.

IMPORTANT—For contraceptive effectiveness, the diaphragm should remain in place for six hours after intercourse and should be removed as soon as possible thereafter. Continuous wearing of the diaphragm for more than 24 hours is not recommended. Retention of the diaphragm for prolonged periods may encourage the growth of certain bacteria in the vaginal tract. It has been suggested that under certain as yet unestablished conditions overgrowth of these bacteria may lead to symptoms of toxic shock syndrome (TSS). For further information, consult your physician.

If a douche is desired for cleansing purposes, wait at least 6 hours after intercourse. Refer to directions and diagrams for complete instructions. While no method of contraception can provide an absolute guarantee against becoming pregnant, for maximum protection OR-THO-GYNOL must be used according to directions.

How Supplied: 2.5 oz Starter tube with measured-dose applicator. Regular size 2.5 oz tube only. Large size 3.8 oz. tube only.

Inactive Ingredients: Benzoic Acid, Castor Oil, Fragrance, Glacial Acetic Acid, Methylparaben, Potassium Hydroxide, Propylene Glycol, Purified Water, Sodium Carboxymethylcellulose, Sorbic Acid.

Storage: Ortho-Gynol should be stored at room temperature.

Shown in Product Identification Section, page 418

ORTHO® PERSONAL LUBRICANT

Description: ORTHO PERSONAL LUBRICANT is a non-staining, water soluble lubricating jelly that is safe for delicate tissues.

Indications: ORTHO PERSONAL LUBRICANT is especially formulated as a sexual lubricant that is designed to be gentle and non-irritating for both women and men. It may also be used for easy insertion of rectal thermometers, tampons, douche nozzles and enema nozzles.

Dosage and Administration: Apply a one (1″) to two (2″) inch ribbon of product, or desired amount, to external vaginal area and/or penis. Repeat applications may be used by one or both partners. If desired, this product may be used inside the vagina.

Precaution: ORTHO PERSONAL LUBRICANT does not contain spermicide. It is not a contraceptive.

How Supplied: ORTHO PERSONAL LUBRICANT is available in 2 oz. and 4 oz. tubes.

Inactive Ingredients: Glycerin, Methylparaben, Propylene Glycol, Purified Water, Sodium Alginate, Sodium Carboxymethylcellulose, Sorbic Acid.

Storage: Store at room temperature (59–86°F). Do not freeze.

Shown in Product Identification Section, page 418

Paddock Laboratories, Inc.
3101 LOUISIANA AVE. NORTH MINNEAPOLIS, MN 55427

ACTIDOSE–AQUA
(Highly Activated Charcoal Suspension)

Supplied in bottles containing 25 grams per 120ml and 50 grams per 240ml highly activated charcoal suspension. Each milliliter contains 208mg (0.208 grams) highly activated charcoal in aqueous suspension. Detailed blue color-coded attached package insert.

ACTIDOSE with SORBITOL
(Highly Activated Charcoal Suspension with Sorbitol)

Supplied in bottles containing 25 grams per 120ml and 50 grams per 240ml highly activated charcoal suspension. Each milliliter contains 208mg (0.208 grams) highly activated charcoal and 400mg (0.4 grams) sorbitol. Detailed red color-coded attached package insert.

EMULSOIL®
[*ē-muls-oil*]
Castor Oil

Emulsoil is a self-emulsifying, flavored castor oil formulated to instantly mix with any beverage.

Active Ingredient: Each 2-ounce bottle contains 95% w/w Castor Oil, USP with self-emulsifying and natural sugarless flavoring agents.

Indications: Emulsoil is used in the preparation of the small and large bowel for radiography, colonoscopy, surgery, proctologic procedures and exploratory IVP use. Can also be used for isolated bouts of constipation.

Warnings: Not to be used when abdominal pain, nausea, vomiting or other symptoms of appendicitis are present. Frequent or prolonged use may result in dependence on laxatives. Do not use during pregnancy except under competent advice.

Dosage and Administration: Adults: 1–4 tablespoonfuls. Children: 1–2 teaspoonfuls.

How Supplied: Available in 2-ounce bottles. Packaged 12 and 48 bottles per case.

GLUTOSE®
[*glū-tose*]
Dextrose Gel

Active Ingredient: Dextrose 40%, Each 80-gram bottle contains 32 grams dextrose in a dye free jel base.

Indications: Glutose is a concentrated glucose (40% Dextrose) used for insulin reactions and hypoglycemic states.

Dosage and Administration: Usual dose is ⅓ bottle Glutose (10 grams dextrose) orally, which can be repeated in 10 minutes if necessary. Response should be noticed in 10 minutes. The physician should then be notified when a hypoglycemic reaction occurs so that the insulin dose can be accurately adjusted. Glutose should not be given to children under 2 years of age unless otherwise directed by physician.

How Supplied: 80-gram squeeze bottle, 6 bottles/case. 25-gram unit-dose tube, 3 tubes/box.

IPECAC SYRUP
[*ĭp-ĕ-kak*]

Active Ingredients: Ipecac Syrup, USP contains in each 30 ml, not less than 36.9 mg and not more than 47.1 mg of the total ether soluble alkaloids of ipecac. The content of emetine and cephaeline together is not less than 90.0% of the amount of the total ether-soluble alkaloids.

Indications: Ipecac Syrup is indicated for emergency use to cause vomiting in poisoning.

Warnings: Do not use in unconscious persons. Ordinarily, this drug should not be used if strychnine, corrosives such as alkalies, lye and strong acids, or petroleum distillates such as kerosene, gasoline, coal oil, fuel oil, paint thinners, or cleaning fluids have been ingested.

Dosage and Administration: Usual Dosage: One tablespoonful (15 ml) followed by one to two glasses of water, in persons over 1 year of age. Repeat dosage in 20 minutes if vomiting does not occur.

How Supplied: Available in 1-ounce bottles. Packaged 12 bottles per case.

IDENTIFICATION PROBLEM?
Consult the
Product Identification Section
where you'll find
products pictured
in full color.

Parke-Davis
**Consumer Health Products Group
Division of Warner-Lambert
    Company
201 TABOR ROAD
MORRIS PLAINS, NJ 07950
(See also Warner-Lambert)**

AGORAL® Plain
[ă 'gō-răl "]
AGORAL® Raspberry
AGORAL® Marshmallow

Description: Each tablespoonful (15 mL) of Agoral Plain contains 4.2 grams mineral oil in a thoroughly homogenized emulsion.
Also contains acacia; agar; benzoic acid; egg albumin; flavors; glycerin; sodium benzoate; tragacanth; citric acid; or sodium hydroxide; to adjust pH; water.
Each tablespoonful (15 ml) of Agoral Raspberry (pink) or of Agoral Marshmallow (white) contains 4.2 grams mineral oil and 0.2 gram phenolphthalein in a thoroughly homogenized emulsion.
Also contains acacia; agar; benzoic acid; egg albumin; flavors; glycerin; saccharin sodium; sodium benzoate; tragacanth; citric acid; or sodium hydroxide; to adjust pH; water. Agoral Raspberry Flavor also contains D&C Red No. 30 Lake.

Actions: Agoral, containing mineral oil, facilitates defecation by lubricating the fecal mass and softening the stool. More effective than nonemulsified oil in penetrating the feces, Agoral thereby greatly reduces the possibility of oil leakage at the anal sphincter. Phenolphthalein gently stimulates motor activity of the lower intestinal tract. Agoral's combined lubricating-softening and peristaltic actions can help to restore a normal pattern of evacuation.

Indications: Relief of constipation. Agoral may be especially required when straining at stool is a hazard, as in hernia, cardiac, or hypertensive patients; during convalescence from surgery; before and after surgery for hemorrhoids or other painful anorectal disorders; for patients confined to bed.
The management of chronic constipation should also include attention to fluid intake, diet and bowel habits.

Contraindication: Sensitivity to phenolphthalein.

Warning: Do not use laxative products when abdominal pain, nausea, or vomiting are present unless directed by a physician. If you have noticed a sudden change in bowel habits that persists over a period of 2 weeks, consult a physician before using a laxative. Laxative products should not be used for a period longer than 1 week unless directed by a physician. Rectal bleeding or failure to have a bowel movement after use of a laxative may indicate a serious condition. Discontinue use and consult your physician. Do not administer to children under 6 years of age, to pregnant women, to bedridden patients or to persons with difficulty swallowing. As with any drug, if you are nursing a baby, seek the advice of a health professional before using this product. Do not take with meals. If skin rash appears, do not use this product or any other preparation containing phenolphthalein. Keep this and all drugs out of the reach of children. In case of accidental overdose, seek professional assistance or contact a Poison Control Center immediately. Drug interaction precaution: Do not take this product if you are presently taking a stool softener laxative.

Dosage: Agoral Plain—Adults—1 to 2 tablespoonfuls at bedtime only, unless other time is advised by physician. Children—Over 6 years, 2 to 4 teaspoonfuls at bedtime only, unless other time is advised by physician.
Agoral Raspberry and Marshmallow —Adults—½ to 1 tablespoonful at bedtime only, unless other time is advised by physician. Children—Over 6 years, ½ to ¾ teaspoonfuls at bedtime only, unless other time is advised by physician. This product generally produces bowel movement in 6 to 8 hours.

Supplied: Agoral Plain (without phenolphthalein), plastic bottles of 16 fl oz. Agoral (raspberry flavor), plastic bottles of 16 fl oz. Agoral (marshmallow flavor), plastic bottles of 8 fl oz and 16 fl oz.
Store between 15°–30° C (59°–86° F). Keep this and all drugs out of the reach of children.
In case of accidental overdose, seek professional assistance or contact a poison control center immediately.

ANUSOL®
[ă 'nū-sŏl "]
Suppositories/Ointment

Description:

	Anusol Suppositories each contains	Anusol Ointment each gram
Bismuth subgallate	2.25%	—
Bismuth Resorcin Compound	1.75%	—
Benzyl Benzoate	1.2 %	12 mg
Peruvian Balsam	1.8 %	18 mg
Zinc Oxide	11.0 %	110 mg
Analgine™ (pramoxine hydrochloride)	—	10 mg

Also contains the following inactive ingredients: calcium phosphate dibasic; coconut oil base, FD&C Blue No. 2 Lake and Red No. 40 Lake, hydrogenated fatty acid in a bland hydrogenated vegetable oil base.

Also contains the following inactive ingredients: calcium phosphate dibasic; cocoa butter; glyceryl monooleate; glyceryl monostearate; kaolin; mineral oil; polyethylene wax; Peruvian balsam.

Actions: Anusol Suppositories and Anusol Ointment help to relieve pain, itching and discomfort arising from irritated anorectal tissues. They have a soothing, lubricant action on mucous membranes. Analgine (pramoxine hydrochloride) in Anusol Ointment is a rapidly acting local anesthetic for the skin and mucous membranes of the anus and rectum. Analgine is also chemically distinct from procaine, cocaine, and dibucaine and can often be used in the patient previously sensitized to other surface anesthetics. Surface analgesia lasts for several hours.

Indications: For prompt, temporary symptomatic relief of minor pain, itching, burning and soreness of hemorrhoids and other simple anorectal irritation.

Contraindications: Anusol Suppositories and Anusol Ointment are contraindicated in those patients with a history of hypersensitivity to any of the components of the preparations.

Precautions: Symptomatic relief should not delay definitive diagnoses or treatment.
If irritation develops, these preparations should be discontinued. In case of rectal bleeding or persistence of the condition, consult your physician. Keep this and all drugs out of the reach of children. In case of accidental ingestion seek professional assistance or contact a Poison Control Center immediately. Do not use in the eyes or nose.

Adverse Reactions: Upon application of Anusol Ointment, which contains Analgine (pramoxine HCl), a patient may occasionally experience burning, especially if the anoderm is not intact. Sensitivity reactions have been rare; discontinue medication if suspected.

Dosage and Administration: Anusol Suppositories—Adults: Remove foil wrapper and insert suppository into the anus. Insert one suppository in the morning and one at bedtime, and one immediately following each evacuation.
Anusol Ointment—Adults: After gentle bathing and drying of the anal area, remove tube cap and apply freely to the exterior surface and gently rub in. Ointment should be applied every 3 or 4 hours.
NOTE: If staining from either of the above products occurs, the stain may be removed from fabric by hand or machine washing with household detergent.

How Supplied: Anusol Suppositories— boxes of 12, 24 and 48; in silver foil strips. Anusol Ointment—1-oz tubes and 2-oz tubes with plastic applicator.
Store between 15° and 30°C (59° and 86°F).
Shown in Product Identification Section, page 418

Continued on next page

This product information was prepared in November 1988. On these and other Parke-Davis Products, detailed information may be obtained by addressing PARKE-DAVIS, Consumer Health Products Group, Division of Warner-Lambert Company, Morris Plains, NJ 07950.

Parke-Davis—Cont.

BENADRYL Anti-Itch Cream

Active Ingredients: BENADRYL® (diphenhydramine hydrochloride USP) 1%.

Inactive Ingredients: Cetyl Alcohol, Methylparaben, Polyethylene Glycol Monostearate, Propylene Glycol and Water, Purified.

Indications: For the temporary relief of ITCHING and PAIN associated with minor skin irritations, allergic itches, rashes, insect bites and sunburn.

Actions: Benadryl, the most prescribed topical antihistamine, in a soothing, greaseless cream, is easily absorbed into the skin. It provides safe, effective, temporary relief from many different types of itching.

Warnings: For external use only. Do not use on chicken pox or measles unless supervised by a doctor. Do not use on extensive areas of the skin or for longer than 7 days except as directed by a doctor. Avoid contact with the eyes or other mucous membranes. If condition worsens, or if symptoms persist for more than 7 days, or clear up and occur again within a few days, discontinue use of this product and consult a physician. KEEP THIS AND ALL DRUGS OUT OF THE REACH OF CHILDREN. In case of accidental ingestion, seek professional assistance or contact a Poison Control Center immediately.

Dosage and Administration: For adults and children 6 years of age and older: Apply to the affected area not more than three to four times daily, or as directed by your physician. For children under 6 years of age: Consult a physician.

How Supplied: Benadryl Anti-Itch Cream is supplied in ½ oz. and 1 oz. tubes.

*Shown in Product Identification
Section page 418*

BENADRYL® Decongestant
[bĕ'nă-drĭl]
Decongestant Tablets and Kapseals®

Active Ingredients: Each tablet/Kapseal® contains: Benadryl® (diphenhydramine hydrochloride USP) 25 mg. and pseudoephedrine hydrochloride 60 mg.

Inactive Ingredients: Each tablet contains: Corn Starch, Croscarmelose Sodium, Dibasic Calcium Phosphate Dihydrate, FD&C Blue No. 1 Aluminum Lake, Hydroxypropyl Methylcellulose, Microcrystalline Cellulose, Polyethylene Glycol, Polysorbate 80, Stearic Acid, Titanium Dioxide and Zinc Stearate.
Each Kapseals® capsule contains: Calcium Stearate, Lactose (Hydrous), Syloid Silica Gel. The Kapseals® capsule shell contains: D&C Red No. 28, FD&C Red No. 1 and Red No. 3, Gelatin, Glyceryl Mono-Oleate, PEG-200 Ricinoleate and Titanium Dioxide.

Indications: Temporarily relieves nasal congestion, runny nose, sneezing, itching of the nose or throat, itchy, watery eyes due to hay fever or other upper respiratory allergies, and runny nose, sneezing and nasal congestion of the common cold.

Warning: Do not exceed recommended dosage because at higher doses nervousness, dizziness, or sleeplessness may occur. Do not take this product for more than 7 days. If symptoms do not improve or are accompanied by fever, consult a physician. Do not take this product if you have high blood pressure, heart disease, diabetes, thyroid disease, asthma, glaucoma, emphysema, chronic pulmonary disease, shortness of breath, difficulty in breathing or difficulty in urination due to enlargement of the prostate gland unless directed by a physician. May cause excitability, especially in children. May cause marked drowsiness: alcohol may increase the drowsiness effect. Avoid alcoholic beverages while taking this product. Use caution when driving a motor vehicle or operating machinery. Do not give this product to children under 12 years except under the advice and supervision of a physician. As with any drug, if you are pregnant or nursing a baby seek the advice of a health professional before using this product. Keep this and all drugs out of the reach of children. In case of accidental overdose, seek professional assistance or contact a poison control center immediately.

Drug Interaction Precaution: Do not take this product if you are presently taking a prescription drug for high blood pressure or depression without first consulting your physician.

Directions: Adults and children over 12 years of age: 1 tablet/Kapseal® every 4 to 6 hours not to exceed 4 tablets/Kapseals® in 24 hours. Benadryl Decongestant is not recommended for children under 12 years of age.

How Supplied: Benadryl Decongestant Tablets and Kapseals® are supplied in boxes of 24.
Store at room temperature 15–30° C (59–86° F).
Protect from moisture.

*Shown in Product Identification
Section, page 418*

BENADRYL®
[bĕ'nă-drĭl]
Decongestant Elixir

Description: Each teaspoonful (5 mL) contains: Benadryl (diphenhydramine hydrochloride) 12.5 mg; pseudoephedrine hydrochloride 30 mg; alcohol 5%. Also contains: FD&C Yellow No. 6; glucose, liquid; glycerin, USP; flavors; menthol, USP; saccharin sodium, USP; sodium citrate, USP; sucrose, NF; water, purified, USP.

Indications: Temporarily relieves nasal congestion, runny nose, sneezing, itching of the nose or throat, itchy, watery eyes due to hay fever or other upper respiratory allergies, and runny nose, sneezing and nasal congestion of the common cold.

Warnings: Do not exceed recommended dosage because at higher doses nervousness, dizziness, or sleeplessness may occur. Do not take this product for more than 7 days. If symptoms do not improve or are accompanied by fever, consult a physician. Do not take this product if you have high blood pressure, heart disease, diabetes, thyroid disease, asthma, glaucoma, emphysema, chronic pulmonary disease, shortness of breath, difficulty in breathing or difficulty in urination due to enlargement of the prostate gland unless directed by a physician. May cause excitability, especially in children. May cause marked drowsiness: alcohol may increase the drowsiness effect. Avoid alcoholic beverages while taking this product. Use caution when driving a motor vehicle or operating machinery. As with any drug, if you are pregnant or nursing a baby seek the advice of a health professional before using this product. Keep this and all drugs out of the reach of children. In case of accidental overdose, seek professional assistance or contact a poison control center immediately.

Drug Interaction Precaution: Do not take this product if you are presently taking a prescription drug for high blood pressure or depression without first consulting your physician.

Directions: Children 6 to under 12 years oral dosage is one teaspoonful every 4 to 6 hours not to exceed 4 teaspoonfuls in 24 hours, or as directed by a physician. For children under 6 years of age, consult a physician. Adult oral dosage is two teaspoonfuls every 4 to 6 hours not to exceed 8 teaspoonfuls in 24 hours, or as directed by a physician.

How Supplied: Benadryl Decongestant Elixir is supplied in 4-oz bottles. Store below 30° C (86°F). Protect from freezing.

*Shown in Product Identification
Section, page 418*

BENADRYL® Elixir

Active Ingredients: Each teaspoonful (5 mL) contains: Benadryl® (diphenhydramine hydrochloride USP) 12.5 mg. and Alcohol 14%.

Inactive Ingredients: Also contains: D&C Red No. 33, FD&C Red No. 40, Flavors, Sugar, and Water, Purified.

Indications: Temporarily relieves runny nose, sneezing, itching of the nose or throat and itchy, watery eyes due to hay fever or other upper respiratory allergies and runny nose and sneezing associated with the common cold.

Warnings: Do not take this product if you have asthma, glaucoma, emphysema, chronic pulmonary disease, shortness of breath, difficulty in breathing or difficulty in urination due to enlargement of the prostate gland unless directed by a physician. May cause excit-

ability especially in children. May cause marked drowsiness; alcohol may increase the drowsiness effect. Avoid alcoholic beverages while taking this product. Use caution when driving a motor vehicle or operating machinery. As with any drug if you are pregnant or nursing a baby seek the advice of a healthy professional before using this product. Keep this and all drugs out of the reach of children. In case of accidental overdose, seek professional assistance or contact a Poison Control Center immediately.

Dosage and Administration: Children 6 to under 12 years of age oral dosage is 12.5 to 25 mg. (1 to 2 teaspoonfuls) every 4 to 6 hours not to exceed 12 teaspoonfuls in 24 hours, or as directed by a physician. For children under 6 years your physician should be contacted for the recommended dosage. Adult oral dosage is 25 mg. (2 teaspoonfuls) to 50 mg. (4 teaspoonfuls) every 4 to 6 hours not to exceed 24 teaspoonfuls in 24 hours, or as directed by a physician.

How Supplied: Benadryl Elixir is supplied in 4 oz. and 8 oz. bottles.
Shown in Product Identification Section, page 418

BENADRYL® 25
[bĕ'nă-drĭl]
Tablets and Kapseals®

Active Ingredient: Each tablet/Kapseal® contains: Benadryl® (diphenhydramine hydrochloride USP) 25 mg.

Inactive Ingredients: Each tablet contains: Corn Starch, Croscarmelose Sodium, Dibasic Calcium Phosphate Dihydrate, FD&C Red No. 3 Aluminum Lake, Hydroxypropyl Methylcellulose, Microcrystalline Cellulose, Polyethylene Glycol, Polysorbate 80, Stearic Acid, Titanium Dioxide and Zinc Stearate.
Each Kapseals® capsule contains: Lactose (Hydrous) and Magnesium Stearate. The Kapseals® capsule shell contains: D&C Red No. 28, FD&C Blue No. 1, Red No. 3 and Red No. 40, Gelatin, Glyceryl Mono-Oleate, PEG-200 Ricinoleate and Titanium Dioxide.

Indications: Temporarily relieves runny nose, sneezing, itching of the nose or throat, itchy, watery eyes due to hay fever or other upper respiratory allergies and runny nose and sneezing of the common cold.

Warnings: Do not take this product if you have asthma, glaucoma, emphysema, chronic pulmonary disease, shortness of breath, difficulty in breathing or difficulty in urination due to enlargement of the prostate gland unless directed by physician. May cause excitability, especially in children. May cause marked drowsiness: alcohol may increase the drowsiness effect. Avoid alcoholic beverages while taking this motor vehicle or operating machinery. As with any drug if you are pregnant or nursing a baby seek the advice of a health professional before using this product. Keep this and all drugs out of the reach of chil-

dren. In case of accidental overdose, seek professional assistance or contact a poison control center immediately.

Directions: Adult oral dosage is 25–50 mg (1 to 2 tablets/Kapseals®) every 4 to 6 hours not to exceed 12 tablets/Kapseals® in 24 hours, or as directed by a physician. Children 6 to under 12 years oral dosage is 12.5 mg to 25 mg (1 tablet/-Kapseal®) every 4 to 6 hours, not to exceed 6 tablets/Kapseals® in 24 hours, or as directed by a physician. For children under 6 years your physician should be contacted for the recommended dosage.

How Supplied: Benadryl 25 Tablets and Kapseals® are supplied in boxes of 24 and 48.
Store at room temperature 15–30° C (59–86° F). Protect from moisture.
Shown in Product Identification Section, page 418

BENADRYL PLUS®
Tablets

Active Ingredients: Each tablet contains: Benadryl® (diphenhydramine hydrochloride USP) 12.5 mg., pseudoephedrine hydrochloride 30 mg., and acetaminophen 500 mg.

Inactive Ingredients: Each tablet contains: Carboxymethylcellulose, Croscarmelose Sodium, Hydroxypropyl Cellulose, Hydroxypropyl Methylcellulose, Magnesium Stearate, Microcrystalline Cellulose, Polyethylene Glycol, Propylene Glycol, Starch, Stearic Acid, Titanium Dioxide, and Zinc Stearate.

Indications: Temporarily relieves sneezing, running nose, nasal and sinus congestion, fever, minor sore throat pain, headache, sinus pressure, body aches and pain due to the common cold, and sneezing, runny nose, itching of the nose or throat, and itchy, watery eyes due to hay fever or other upper respiratory allergies.

Warnings: Do not exceed recommended dosage because at higher doses nervousness, dizziness, or sleeplessness may occur. Do not take this product if you have high blood pressure, heart disease, diabetes, thyroid disease, asthma, glaucoma, emphysema, chronic pulmonary disease, shortness of breath, difficulty in breathing, or difficulty in urination due to enlargement of the prostate gland unless directed by a physician. May cause excitability especially in children. May cause marked drowsiness; alcohol may increase the drowsiness effect. Avoid alcoholic beverages while taking this product. Use caution when driving a motor vehicle or operating machinery. If fever persists for more than 3 days (72 hours) or recurs, consult your physician. If sore throat persists for more than 2 days, is accompanied or followed by fever, headache, rash, nausea or vomiting, consult a physician promptly. As with any drug if you are pregnant or nursing a baby seek the advice of a health professional before using this product. Keep this and all drugs out of the reach of children. In case of accidental overdose, seek

professional assistance or contact a Poison Control Center immediately. Do not give this product to children under 12 years except under the advice and supervision of a physician.

Drug Interaction Precaution: Do not take this product if you are presently taking a prescription drug for high blood pressure or depression without consulting your physician.

Directions: Adults (12 years and over): Two tablets every 6 hours, not to exceed 8 tablets in a 24 hour period. Benadryl Plus is not recommended for children under 12 years of age.

How Supplied: Benadryl Plus Tablets are supplied in boxes of 24 and 48.
Store at room temperature 15–30°C (59–86°F). Protect from moisture.
Shown in Product Identification Section, page 418

BENADRYL® Spray

Active Ingredients: Benadryl® (diphenhydramine hydrochloride USP) 2% and Alcohol 90%.

Inactive Ingredients: Also contains: Acetylated Lanolin Alcohol, Povidone, Tris (Hydroxymethyl) Amino Methane, Water, Purified and Wheat Germ Glycerides.

Indications: For the temporary relief of ITCHING and PAIN associated with minor skin irritations, allergic itches, rashes, insect bites and sunburn.

Actions: Benadryl spray helps relieve itching. It forms an anti-itch "bandage" to protect and relieve affected areas. Its spray feature allows soothing relief without touching or rubbing the affected area. Benadryl spray is clear, won't stain clothing and won't rinse off (can be easily removed with soap and water).

Warnings: For external use only. Avoid contact with the eyes. Do not apply to blistered, raw or oozing areas of the skin. If condition worsens or if symptoms persist for more than 7 days, or clear up and occur again within a few days, discontinue use of this product and consult a physician. FLAMMABLE—Keep away from fire or flame. Keep this and all drugs out of the reach of children. In case of accidental ingestion, seek professional assistance or contact a Poison Control Center immediately.

Dosage and Administration: For adults and children over 2 years of age and older: Spray on affected area not more than three to four times daily, or as directed by your physician. For children under 2 years of age: Consult a physician.

Continued on next page

This product information was prepared in November 1988. On these and other Parke-Davis Products, detailed information may be obtained by addressing PARKE-DAVIS, Consumer Health Products Group, Division of Warner-Lambert Company, Morris Plains, NJ 07950.

Parke-Davis—Cont.

How Supplied: Benadryl® Spray is available in a 2 oz. pump spray bottle.
Shown in Product Identification Section, page 418

BENYLIN®
Cough Syrup

Description: Each teaspoonful (5 ml) contains:

Diphenhydramine
  Hydrochloride   12.5 mg
Also contains: Alcohol 5%; Ammonium Chloride; Caramel; Citric Acid; D&C Red No. 33; FD&C Red No. 40; Flavor; Glucose Liquid; Glycerin; Menthol; Purified Water; Sodium Citrate; Sodium Saccharin; Sucrose.

Indications: For the temporary relief of cough due to minor throat and bronchial irritation as may occur with the common cold or with inhaled irritants.

Warnings: May cause marked drowsiness. Keep this and all drugs out of the reach of children. In case of accidental overdose, seek professional assistance or contact a poison control center immediately. Do not give to children under 6 years of age except under the advice and supervision of a physician. May cause excitability, especially in children. Do not take this product for persistent or chronic cough such as occurs with smoking, asthma, emphysema, or when cough is accompanied by excessive secretions, or if you have glaucoma, or difficulty in urination due to enlargement of the prostate gland except under the advice and supervision of a physician. As with any drug, if you are pregnant or nursing a baby, seek the advice of a health professional before using this product.

Caution: Avoid driving a motor vehicle or operating heavy machinery, or drinking alcoholic beverages. A persistent cough may be a sign of a serious condition. If cough persists for more than one week, tends to recur, or is accompanied by high fever, rash, or persistent headache, consult a physician.

Directions for Use:
Adults: (12 years and older): Take 2 teaspoonfuls every 4 hours. Do not exceed 12 teaspoonfuls in 24 hours.
Children (6–12 years): Take 1 teaspoonful every 4 hours. Do not exceed 6 teaspoonfuls in 24 hours.
Children (under 6 years): Consult physician for recommended dosage.

How Supplied: Benylin Cough Syrup is supplied in 4-oz and 8-oz bottles. Store at 59°–86°F.
Shown in Product Identification Section, page 418

BENYLIN DM®
dextromethorphan cough syrup

Description: Each teaspoonful (5 ml) contains:
Dextromethorphan
Hydrobromide   10 mg
Also contains: Alcohol 5%; Ammonium Chloride; Caramel; Citric Acid; D&C Red No. 33; Flavor; Glucose Liquid; Glycerin; Menthol; Purified Water; Sodium Citrate; Sucrose.

Indications: For temporary relief of coughs due to colds, bronchial irritation or upper respiratory allergies.

Warnings: Do not take this product for persistent or chronic cough such as occurs with smoking, asthma, emphysema, or when cough is accompanied by excessive secretions except under the advice and supervision of a physician. A persistent cough may be a sign of a serious condition. If cough persists for more than one week, tends to recur, or is accompanied by high fever, rash or persistent headache, consult a physician. Do not give to children under 2 years of age except under the advice and supervision of a physician. As with any drug, if you are pregnant or nursing a baby, seek the advice of a health professional before using this product. Keep this and all drugs out of the reach of children. In case of accidental overdose, seek professional assistance or contact a poison control center immediately.

Directions for Use:
Adults (12 years and older): Take 1 to 2 teaspoonfuls every 4 hours or 3 teaspoonfuls every 6 to 8 hours. Do not exceed 12 teaspoonfuls in 24 hours.
Children (6–12 years): Take ½–1 teaspoonful every 4 hours or 1½ teaspoonfuls every 6 to 8 hours. Do not exceed 6 teaspoonfuls in 24 hours.
Children (2–6 years): Take ¼ to ½ teaspoonful every 4 hours or ¾ teaspoonful every 6 to 8 hours. Do not exceed 3 teaspoonfuls in 24 hours.
Children (under 2 years): Consult physician for recommended dosage.

How Supplied: 4-oz bottles. Store at 59°–86°F.
Shown in Product Identification Section, page 418

BENYLIN Decongestant

Description: Each teaspoonful (5 ml) contains:
Diphenhydramine
  Hydrochloride   12.5 mg
Pseudoephedrine
  Hydrochloride   30.0 mg
Also contains: Alcohol 5%; FD&C Yellow No. 6 (Sunset Yellow); Flavors; Glucose Liquid; Glycerin; Menthol; Purified Water; Saccharin Sodium; Sodium Citrate; Sucrose.

Indications: For the temporary relief of cough due to minor throat and bronchial irritations as may occur with the common cold or with inhaled irritants; and nasal congestion due to the common cold, hay fever, or other upper respiratory allergies.

Warnings: May cause marked drowsiness. Keep this and all drugs out of the reach of children. In case of accidental overdose, seek professional assistance or contact a poison control center immediately. Do not exceed recommended dosage because at higher doses nervousness, dizziness or sleeplessness may occur. Do not give to children under six years of age except under the advice and supervision of a physician. May cause excitability especially in children. Do not take this product for persistent or chronic cough such as occurs with smoking, asthma, emphysema or when cough is accompanied by excessive secretions, or if you have high blood pressure, heart disease, diabetes, thyroid disease, glaucoma or difficulty in urination due to enlargement of the prostate gland except under the advice and supervision of a physician. If symptoms do not improve within seven days or are accompanied by high fever, consult a physician before continuing use. As with any drug, if you are pregnant or nursing a baby, seek the advice of a health professional before using this product.

Caution: Avoid driving a motor vehicle or operating heavy machinery, or drinking alcoholic beverages. A persistent cough may be a sign of a serious condition. If cough persists for more than one week, tends to recur or is accompanied by high fever, rash, or persistent headache, consult a physician.

Drug Interaction Precaution: Do not take this product if you are presently taking a prescription drug for high blood pressure or depression without consulting your doctor.

Directions for Use:
Adults (12 years and older): Take 2 teaspoonfuls every 4 hours. Do not exceed 8 teaspoonfuls in 24 hours.
Children (6–12 years): Take 1 teaspoonful every 4 hours. Do not exceed 4 teaspoonfuls in 24 hours.
Children (under 6 years): Consult physician for recommended dosage.

How Supplied: 4-oz. bottles. Store at 59°–86°F.
Shown in Product Identification Section, page 418

BENYLIN® Expectorant

Description: Each 4 teaspoonfuls (20 ml) contains:
Dextromethorphan
  Hydrobromide   20.0 mg
Guaifenesin   400.0 mg
Also contains: Alcohol 5%; Citric Acid; FD&C Red No. 40; Flavors; Glycerin; Purified Water; Saccharin Sodium, Sodium Benzoate, Sodium Citrate; Sucrose.

Indications: For temporary relief of coughs plus accompanying upper chest congestion due to colds, bronchial irritation or upper respiratory allergies.

Warnings: Keep this and all drugs out of the reach of children. In case of accidental overdose, seek professional assistance or contact a poison control center immediately. Do not give to children under 2 years of age unless directed by a physician. Do not take this product for

persistent or chronic cough such as occurs with smoking, asthma, emphysema, or when cough is accompanied by excessive secretions unless directed by a physician. A persistent cough may be a sign of a serious condition. If cough persists for more than one week, tends to recur, or is accompanied by high fever, rash, or persistent headache, consult a physician. As with any drug, if you are pregnant or nursing a baby, seek the advice of a health professional before using this product.

Directions for Use:
Adults (12 years and older): Take 2–4 teaspoonfuls every 4 hours (or fill dosage cup to the corresponding teaspoon level indicated). Do not exceed 24 teaspoonfuls in 24 hours.
Children (6–12 years): Take 1–2 teaspoonfuls every 4 hours (or fill dosage cup to the corresponding teaspoon level indicated). Do not exceed 12 teaspoonfuls in 24 hours.
Children (2–6 years): Take ½–1 teaspoonful every 4 hours (or fill dosage cup to the corresponding teaspoon level indicated). Do not exceed 6 teaspoonfuls in 24 hours.
Children (under 2 years): Consult your physician for recommended dosage.

How Supplied: Benylin Expectorant is supplied in 4-oz and 8-oz bottles. Store at 59°–86°F.

Shown in Product Identification Section, page 418

CALADRYL® Lotion
[că 'lă drĭl "]
CALADRYL Cream

Description: Caladryl Lotion—A drying, calamine-antihistamine lotion containing Calamine 8%, Benadryl® (diphenhydramine hydrochloride), 1%. Also contains: Alcohol 2%; Camphor; Fragrances; Glycerin; Sodium Carboxymethylcellulose; and Water, Purified. Caladryl Cream—Calamine 8%, Benadryl (diphenhydramine hydrochloride) 1%. Also contains: Camphor; Cetyl Alcohol; Cresin White; Fragrance; Propylene Glycol; Proplyparaben; Polysorbate 60; Sorbitan Stearate; Water, Purified.

Indications: For relief of itching due to mild poison ivy or oak, insect bites, or other minor skin irritations, and soothing relief of mild sunburn

Warnings: For external use only. Do not apply to blistered, raw or oozing areas of the skin. Do not use on chicken pox or measles, unless supervised by a doctor. Do not use on extensive areas of the skin or for longer than 7 days except as directed by a doctor. Avoid contact with the eyes or other mucous membranes. Discontinue use if burning sensation or rash develops or condition persists. Remove by washing with soap and water.
KEEP THIS AND ALL DRUGS OUT OF THE REACH OF CHILDREN. In case of accidental ingestion seek professional assistance or contact a Poison Control Center immediately.

Directions: For adults and children 6 years or age and older: Apply sparingly to the affected area three to four times daily. Before each application cleanse skin with soap and water and dry affected area. Children under 6 years of age: Consult a doctor.

How Supplied: Caladryl Cream; 1½-oz tubes.
Caladryl Lotion—2½ fl.-oz. (75 ml) squeeze bottles and 6 fl.-oz. bottles.

Shown in Product Identification Section, page 418

GELUSIL®
[jĕl 'ū-sĭl "]
Antacid–Anti-gas
Liquid/Tablets
Sodium Free

Each teaspoonful (5 ml) or tablet contains:
200 mg aluminum hydroxide
200 mg magnesium hydroxide
25 mg simethicone
Also contains: Liquid: Citric Acid; Flavors; Hydroxypropyl Methylcellulose; Methylparaben; Propylparaben; Sodium Carboxymethyl Cellulose; Sodium Saccharin; Sorbitol Solution; Water; Xanthan Gum.
Tablets: Flavors; Magnesium Stearate; Mannitol; Sorbitol; Sugar.

Advantages:
● High acid-neutralizing capacity
● Sodium free
● Simethicone for antiflatulent activity
● Good taste for better patient compliance
● Fast dissolution of chewed tablets for prompt relief

Indications: For the relief of heartburn, sour stomach, acid indigestion and to relieve symptoms of gas.

Dosage and Administration: Two or more teaspoonfuls or tablets one hour after meals and at bedtime, or as directed by a physician.
Tablets should be chewed.

Warnings: Do not take more than 12 tablets or teaspoonfuls in a 24-hour period, or use this maximum dosage for more than two weeks, or use this product if you have kidney disease, except under the advice and supervision of a physician.
Keep this and all drugs out of the reach of children.

Drug Interaction Precaution: Do not take this product if you are presently taking a prescription antibiotic drug containing any form of tetracycline.

How Supplied:
Liquid—In plastic bottles of 12 fl oz.
Tablets—White, embossed Gelusil P-D 034—individual strips of 10 in boxes of 50 and 100.
Store between 59°–86°F (15°–30°C).
Shown in Product Identification Section, page 419

GELUSIL–II®
[jĕl 'ū-sĭl "]
Antacid–Anti-gas
Liquid/Tablets
High Potency
Sodium Free

Each teaspoonful (5 ml) or tablet contains:
400 mg aluminum hydroxide
400 mg magnesium hydroxide
30 mg simethicone
Also contains: Liquid: Citric Acid; Flavors; Hydroxypropyl Methylcellulose; Sodium Saccharin; Sorbitol Solution; Water; Xanthan Gum
Tablets: Artificial Orange Flavor; Calcium Stearate; FD&C Yellow No. 6; Fumaric Acid; Mannitol; Povidone; Saccharin Sodium; Sorbitol; Sugar, Syloid 244.

Advantages:
● High acid-neutralizing capacity
● Sodium free
● Simethicone for antiflatulent activity
● Good taste for better patient compliance
● Fast dissolution of chewed tablets for prompt relief
● Double strength antacid

Indications: For the relief of heartburn, sour stomach, acid indigestion and to alleviate or relieve symptoms of gas.

Dosage and Administration: Two or more teaspoonfuls or tablets one hour after meals and at bedtime, or as directed by a physician. Tablets should be chewed.

Warnings: Do not take more than 8 tablets or teaspoonfuls in a 24-hour period, or use this maximum dosage for more than two weeks, or use this product if you have kidney disease, except under the advice and supervision of a physician.
Keep this and all drugs out of the reach of children.

Drug Interaction Precaution: Do not take this product if you are presently taking a prescription antibiotic drug containing any form of tetracycline.

How Supplied:
Liquid—In plastic bottles of 12 fl oz.
Tablets—Double-layered white/orange, embossed P-D 043—individual strips of 10 in boxes of 80.
Store between 15–30°C (59°–86°F).

GERIPLEX-FS® KAPSEALS®
[jĕ 'rĭ-plĕx "]

Composition: Each Kapseal represents:
Vitamin A ....(1.5 mg) 5,000 IU*
(acetate)
Vitamin C.. 50 mg
(ascorbic acid)†

Continued on next page

This product information was prepared in November 1988. On these and other Parke-Davis Products, detailed information may be obtained by addressing PARKE-DAVIS, Consumer Health Products Group, Division of Warner-Lambert Company, Morris Plains, NJ 07950.

Parke-Davis—Cont.

Vitamin B₁	5 mg

Vitamin B$_1$ .... 5 mg
  (thiamine mononitrate)
Vitamin B$_2$ .... 5 mg
  (riboflavin)
Vitamin B$_{12}$, crystalline
  (cyanocobalamin)........................ 2 mcg
Choline dihydrogen
  citrate .... 20 mg
Nicotinamide .... 15 mg
  (niacinamide)
Vitamin E (dl -alpha tocoph-
  eryl acetate) .... (5 mg) 5 IU*
Iron‡ .... 6 mg
Copper sulfate.................................. 4 mg
Manganese sulfate
  (monohydrate).............................. 4 mg
Zinc sulfate .... 2 mg
Calcium phosphate, dibasic
  (anhydrous).................................. 200 mg
Taka-Diastase® (aspergillus
  oryzae enzymes)...........................2½ gr.
Docusate sodium .... 100 mg
Also contains magnesium stearate, NF.
The capsule shell contains FD&C Blue
#1, FD&C Red #3 and Gelatin.

* International Units
†Supplied as sodium ascorbate
‡Supplied as dried ferrous sulfate equivalent to the labeled amount of elemental
iron

Action and Uses: A preparation containing vitamins, minerals, and a fecal
softener for middle-aged and older individuals. The fecal softening agent, docusate sodium, acts to soften stools and
make bowel movements easier.

Administration and Dosage: USUAL
DOSAGE —One capsule daily, with or immediately after a meal.

How Supplied: Bottles of 100.
Store at controlled room temperature
15°–30°C (59° to 86°F). Protect from light
and moisture.

GERIPLEX-FS®
[jĕ 'rĭ-plĕx ″]
LIQUID
**Geriatric Vitamin Formula with
Iron and a Fecal Softener**

Composition: Each 30 ml represents
vitamin B$_1$ (thiamine hydrochloride), 1.2
mg; vitamin B$_2$ (as riboflavin-5'-
phosphate sodium), 1.7 mg; vitamin B$_6$
(pyridoxine hydrochloride), 1 mg; vitamin B$_{12}$ (cyanocobalamin) crystalline, 5
mcg; niacinamide, 15 mg; iron (as ferric
ammonium citrate, green), 15 mg; Plu-
ronic® F-68,* 200 mg; alcohol, 18%.
Also contains: Brandy, Caramel NF, Citric Acid Anhydrous NF, D&C Red No.
33, Flavors, FD&C Red No. 40, Glucono
Delta Lactone, Glucose Liquid USP,
Glycerin USP, Sodium Citrate USP, Sodium Saccharin NF, Sorbitol Solution
USP, Sugar, Water Purified.

Administration and Dosage: USUAL
ADULT DOSAGE—Two tablespoonfuls (30
ml) daily or as recommended by the physician.

How Supplied: 16-oz bottles.
Store below 30° (86°F). Protect from light
and freezing.

*Pluronic is a registered trademark of
BASF Wyandotte Corporation for polymers of ethylene oxide and propylene
oxide.

MEDIQUELL® Chewy Cough
Squares

Active Ingredient: Each cube con-
tains:
Dextromethorphan
  Hydrobromide   15 mg.
Also contains: Corn Syrup, FD&C Blue
No. 1, FD&C Red No. 40, Flavoring, Gela-
tin, Hydrolyzed Milk Protein, Partially
Hydrogenated Vegetable Oil, Sorbitol,
Starch, Sugar and other ingredients.

Indications: Mediquell® is a pleasant
tasting cough medicine concentrated
into soft, chewable cubes. Mediquell®
contains the maximum allowable dose of
dextromethorphan, a safe and effective
cough suppressant, so each dose relieves
coughs for up to 8 hours. Mediquell® is
non-narcotic, contains no alcohol, will
not cause drowsiness and is safe for children and adults.

Warnings: Do not use if cough persists
for more than one week or if high fever is
present since these may indicate the
presence of a serious condition. As with
any drug, if you are pregnant or nursing
a baby, seek the advice of a health professional before using this product.
Do not take this product for persistent or
chronic cough such as occurs with smoking, asthma or emphysema or where
cough is accompanied by excessive secretions except under the advice and supervision of a physician. Keep this and all
medicines out of the reach of children.

Directions for Use: Chew and swallow
every 6 to 8 hours as needed.
Not to exceed 4 doses per day.
Adult Dose:
  12 years and over ....2 cubes
Child Dose:
  6–12 years....................................1 cube
  2–6 years......................................½ cube
  Under 2 years:.....use only as directed
                       by a physician

How Supplied: Available in 12 and 24
tablet packages. Store at 59°–86°F
  *Shown in Product Identification
      Section, page 419*

MEDIQUELL® Decongestant
Formula

Active Ingredients: Each cube con-
tains:
Dextromethorphan
  Hydrobromide   15 mg
Pseudoephedrine Hydrochloride 30 mg
Also contains: Corn Syrup, FD&C Blue
No. 1, FD&C Red No. 40, Flavoring, Gela-
tin, Glycerin, Hydrolyzed Milk Protein,
Partially Hydrogenated Vegetable Oil,
Sorbitol, Starch, Sugar and other ingre-
dients.

Indications: Mediquell® Decongestant
Formula is a pleasant tasting cough and
nasal decongestant medicine concentrated into soft, chewable cubes. Medi-
quell® Decongestant Formula contains
the maximum allowable dose of dextromethorphan, a safe and effective cough
suppressant, to help relieve frequent and
annoying coughs. It also contains the
maximum allowable dose of pseudoephedrine to help relieve accompanying
nasal congestion and postnasal drip.
Each dose relieves coughs and nasal congestion for up to 6 hours. Mediquell®
Decongestant Formula is non-narcotic,
contains no alcohol, and is safe for children and adults.

Warnings: Do not exceed recommended dosage. Do not use if symptoms
persist for more than one week or if high
fever is present, since these may indicate
the presence of a serious condition. Persons with high blood pressure, heart disease, diabetes or thyroid disease should
only use as directed by a physician. Do
not take this product for persistent or
chronic cough such as occurs with smoking, asthma, or emphysema or where
cough is accompanied by excessive secretions except under the advice and supervision of a physician. As with any drug, if
you are pregnant or nursing a baby, seek
the advice of a health professional before
using this product. Keep this and all
drugs out of the reach of children.

Drug Interaction Precaution: Do not
take this product if you are presently
taking a prescription drug for high blood
pressure or depression without first consulting your physician.

Directions for Use: Chew and swallow
every 6 hours as needed.
Not to exceed 4 doses per day.
Adult Dose:
  12 years and over ....2 cubes
Child Dose:
  6–12 years ....1 cube
  2–6 years......................................½ cube
  Under 2 years......use only as directed
                       by a physician.

How Supplied: Available in packages
of 12 tablets. Store at 59°–86°F
  *Shown in Product Identification
      Section, page 419*

MYADEC
High Potency Multivitamin
Multimineral Formula

Each Tablet Represents:		% of US Recommended Daily Allowances (US RDA)
Vitamins		
Vitamin A	9,000 IU*	180%
Vitamin D	400 IU	100%
Vitamin E	30 IU	100%
Vitamin C	90 mg	150%
(ascorbic acid)		
Folic Acid	0.4 mg	100%
Thiamine	10 mg	667%
(vitamin B₁)		
Riboflavin	10 mg	588%
(vitamin B₂)		

Niacin**	20 mg	100%
Vitamin B$_6$	5 mg	250%
Vitamin B$_{12}$	10 mcg	167%
Pantothenic Acid	20 mg	200%
Vitamin K	25 mcg	***
Biotin	45 mcg	15%
MINERALS		
Iodine	150 mcg	100%
Iron	30 mg	167%
Magnesium	100 mg	25%
Copper	3 mg	150%
Zinc	15 mg	100%
Manganese	7.5 mg	***
Calcium	70 mg	7%
Phosphorus	54 mg	5%
Potassium	8 mg	***
Selenium	15 mcg	***
Molybdenum	15 mcg	***
Chromium	15 mcg	***

*   International Units
**   Supplied as niacinamide
*** No US Recommended Daily Allowance (US RDA) has been established for this nutrient.

Ingredients: Dicalcium phosphate, magnesium oxide, ferrous fumarate, niacinamide ascorbate, alcohol SD3A, dl-alpha tocopheryl acetate, microcrystalline cellulose, ascorbic acid, zinc sulfate, hydroxypropyl methylcellulose, calcium pantothenate, croscarmellose sodium, manganese sulfate, Vitamin A acetate, potassium chloride, purified water, povidone, FD&C Yellow No. 6 Al lake, thiamine mononitrate, riboflavin, silica gel, stearic acid, vitamin A and D crystalets, pyridoxine hydrochloride, titanium dioxide, FD&C Blue No. 2 Al lake, FD&C Red No. 40 Al lake, cupric sulfate, phytonadione, polyethylene glycol 3350, magnesium stearate, silicon dioxide, sterotex, citric acid, methyl paraben, folic acid, candelilla wax, hydroxypropyl cellulose, polysorbate 80, vanillin, potassium iodide, propyl paraben, chromium chloride, biotin, sodium molybdate, sodium selenate, cyanocobalamin.

Actions and Uses: High potency vitamin supplement with minerals for adults.

Dosage: One tablet daily with a full meal.

How Supplied: In bottles of 130. Store below 30°C (86°F). Protect from moisture.
Shown in Product Identification Section, page 419

NATABEC® KAPSEALS®

Each capsule represents:

Vitamins	
Vitamin A	4,000 IU*
Vitamin D	400 IU
Vitamin C	50 mg
Vitamin B$_1$	3 mg
Vitamin B$_2$	2.0 mg
Nicotinamide†	10 mg
Vitamin B$_6$	3 mg
Vitamin B$_{12}$	5 mcg
Minerals	
Precipitated Calcium carbonate	600 mg

Iron	30 mg

*IU = International Units
†Supplied as niacinamide

Action and Uses: A multivitamin and mineral supplement for use during pregnancy and lactation.

Dosage: One capsule daily, or as directed by physician.

How Supplied: In bottles of 100.
The color combination of the banded capsule is a Warner-Lambert trademark.

PROMEGA™
Natural Fish Oil Concentrate

Description: PROMEGA is a natural fish body oil concentrate which provides a rich dietary source of Omega-3 fatty acids, including eicosapentaenoic acid (EPA) and docosahexaenoic acid (DHA). Concentrated from certain oily cold water fish, not common in the American diet, these polyunsaturated fats can't be manufactured in the body. They must be obtained through the diet. If enough fish is not eaten, you may wish to include PROMEGA as part of a total dietary plan which includes reducing total fat and substituting polyunsaturated fats for some of the saturated animal fats in the diet to help lower the risk of heart disease. Other sensible steps such as regular exercise, smoking cessation, and weight control should be followed.
PROMEGA is cholesterol free (contains less than 1 mg cholesterol per softgel) and contains the highest percentage concentration of natural omega-3 available.

Recommended Adult Use: Take one to two softgels with each meal or together as a daily dietary supplement.
Each 1000 mg PROMEGA softgel supplies:

EPA (eicosapentaenoic acid)	280 mg
DHA (docosahexaenoic acid)	120 mg
Other Omega-3 fatty acids	100 mg
Vitamin E (d-alpha tocopherol)	1 IU

This and all dietary supplements should be kept out of reach of children.
MATERIALS IN THIS PRODUCT ARE DERIVED FROM ALL NATURAL SOURCES. PROMEGA contains no sugar, starch, wax, or artificial colors, flavors, preservatives. Excess saturated fats and environmental pollutants have been removed through the unique concentration process.

Ingredients: Fish oil concentrate, mixed tocopherols concentrate (antioxidant) in a softgel consisting of gelatin, glycerin and water.

Caution: If patients are taking anticoagulants or have bleeding problems a physician should be consulted before taking fish oil supplements.

How Supplied: Bottles of 30 or 60 softgels.

Storage: For maximum potency, store softgels at 59°F–86°F
Shown in Product Identification Section, page 419

PROMEGA™ PEARLS
Natural Fish Oil Concentrate

Description: PROMEGA Pearls is a natural fish body oil concentrate which provides a rich dietary source of Omega-3 fatty acids, including eicosapentaenoic acid (EPA) and docosahexaenoic acid (DHA). Concentrated from certain oily cold water fish, not common in the American diet, these polyunsaturated fats can't be manufactured in the body. They must be obtained through the diet. If enough fish is not eaten, you may wish to include Promega as part of a total dietary plan which includes reducing total fat and substituting polyunsaturated fats for some of the saturated animal fats in the diet to help lower the risk of heart disease. Other sensible steps such as regular exercise, smoking cessation, and weight control should be followed.
PROMEGA is cholesterol free (contains less than 1 mg cholesterol per softgel) and contains the highest percentage concentration of natural omega-3 available.

Recommended Adult Use: Take one to two softgels with each meal or together as a daily dietary supplement.
Each 600 mg PROMEGA softgel pearl supplies:

EPA (eicosapentaenoic acid)	168 mg
DHA (docosahexaenoic acid)	72 mg
Other Omega-3 fatty acids	60 mg
Vitamin E (d-alpha tocopherol)	1 IU

This and all dietary supplements should be kept out of reach of children.
MATERIALS IN THIS PRODUCT ARE DERIVED FROM ALL NATURAL SOURCES. PROMEGA contains no sugar, starch, wax, or artificial colors, flavors, preservatives. Excess saturated fats and environmental pollutants have been removed through the unique concentration process.

Ingredients: Fish oil concentrate, mixed tocopherols concentrate (antioxidant) in a softgel consisting of gelatin, glycerin and water.

Caution: If patients are taking anticoagulants or have bleeding problems a physician should be consulted before taking fish oil supplements.

How Supplied: Bottles of 60 or 90 softgel Pearls

Storage: For maximum potency, store softgels at 59°F–86°F
Shown in Product Identification Section, page 419

Continued on next page

This product information was prepared in November 1988. On these and other Parke-Davis Products, detailed information may be obtained by addressing PARKE-DAVIS, Consumer Health Products Group, Division of Warner-Lambert Company, Morris Plains, NJ 07950.

Parke-Davis—Cont.

SINUTAB® Tablets

Active Ingredients: Each tablet contains Acetaminophen 325 mg., Chlorpheniramine Maleate 2 mg., Pseudoephedrine Hydrochloride 30 mg.

Inactive Ingredients: Carboxymethyl Starch, Cellulose, Corn Starch, Croscarmellose Sodium, Hydroxypropyl Cellulose, Stearic Acid, Zinc Stearate, D&C Yellow No. 10 Aluminum Lake and FD&C Red No. 3 Aluminum Lake.

Indications: For temporary relief of sinus symptoms due to colds, flu, allergy and hay fever. Contains a non-aspirin analgesic to relieve headache pain, a decongestant to ease pressure and congestion and an antihistamine to dry up runny nose, watery eyes.

Actions: Sinutab® contains an analgesic (acetaminophen) to relieve pain, a decongestant (pseudoephedrine HCl) to reduce congestion of the nasopharyngeal mucosa, and an antihistamine (chlorpheniramine maleate) to help control allergic symptoms.
Acetaminophen is both analgesic and antipyretic. Because acetaminophen is not a salicylate, Sinutab® can be used by patients who are allergic to aspirin.
Pseudoephedrine HCl, a sympathomimetic drug provides vasoconstriction of the nasopharyngeal mucosa resulting in a nasal decongestant effect.
Chlorpheniramine maleate is an antihistamine to provide relief of running nose, sneezing, itching of the nose or throat, and itchy and watery eyes as may occur in allergic rhinitis.

Warnings: Do not exceed recommended dosage. If symptoms persist, do not improve within seven days, or are accompanied by high fever, or if new symptoms occur, see your doctor before continuing use. Do not take this product if you have high blood pressure, heart disease, diabetes, thyroid disease, asthma, glaucoma or difficulty in urination due to an enlarged prostate except under doctor's supervision. Do not take this product for more than ten days. As with any drug, if you are pregnant or nursing a baby, seek the advice of a health professional before using this product. This product may cause drowsiness. Avoid driving a motor vehicle or operating heavy machinery and avoid alcoholic beverages while taking this product.

Drug Interaction: Do not take this product if you are presently taking a prescription drug for high blood pressure or depression without first consulting your doctor.

Precaution: Keep this and all drugs out of the reach of children.

Symptoms and Treatment of Oral Overdosage: In case of accidental overdose, seek professional help or contact a Poison Control Center immediately.

Dosage and Administration: Adults 2 tablets every 4 hours, not to exceed 8 tablets in 24 hours, or as directed by physician. Children under 12 should use only as directed by physician.

How Supplied: Sinutab® tablets are pink, uncoated and scored so that tablets may be split in half. They are supplied in safety-capped bottles of 100 tablets, in child-resistant blister packs in boxes of 12 tablets and in easy-to-open (exempt) blister packs of 30 tablets.
Shown in Product Identification Section, page 419

SINUTAB® Maximum Strength Formula
Tablets and Caplets

Active Ingredients: Each tablet/Caplet contains: Acetaminophen 500 mg., Chlorpheniramine Maleate 2 mg., Pseudoephedrine Hydrochloride 30 mg.

Inactive Ingredients:
Tablets contain: Carboxymethyl Starch, Cellulose, Corn Starch, Croscarmellose Sodium, Hydroxypropyl Cellulose, Stearic Acid, Zinc Stearate, D&C Yellow No. 10 Aluminum Lake and FD&C Yellow No. 6 Aluminum Lake.
Caplets contain: Cellulose, Corn Starch, Croscarmellose Sodium, Hydroxypropyl Cellulose, Hydroxypropyl Methylcellulose, Magnesium Stearate, Polyethylene Glycol, Sodium Starch Glycolate, Stearic Acid, Titanium Dioxide, Zinc Stearate, D&C Yellow No. 10 Aluminum Lake, and FD&C Yellow No. 6 Aluminum Lake.

Indications: For temporary relief of sinus symptoms due to colds, flu, allergy and hay fever. Contains a non-aspirin analgesic to relieve headache pains, a decongestant to ease pressure and congestion and an antihistamine to dry up runny nose, watery eyes.

Actions: Sinutab® Maximum Strength Formula contains an analgesic (acetaminophen) to relieve pain, a decongestant (pseudoephedrine HCl) to reduce congestion of the nasopharyngeal mucosa, and an antihistamine (chlorpheniramine maleate) to help control allergic symptoms.
Acetaminophen is both analgesic and antipyretic. Because acetaminophen is not a salicylate, Sinutab® Maximum Strength Formula can be used by patients who are allergic to aspirin. Pseudoephedrine HCl, a sympathomimetic drug, provides vasoconstriction of the nasopharyngeal mucosa resulting in a nasal decongestant effect.
Chlorpheniramine maleate is an antihistamine incorporated to provide relief of running nose, sneezing, itching of the nose or throat, and itchy and watery eyes as may occur in allergic rhinitis.

Warnings: Do not exceed recommended dosage. If symptoms persist, do not improve within 7 days, or are accompanied by high fever or if new symptoms occur, see your doctor before continuing use. Do not take this product if you have high blood pressure, heart disease, diabe-

tes, thyroid disease, asthma, glaucoma, or difficulty in urination due to an enlarged prostate except under doctor's supervision. Do not take this product for more than 10 days. As with any drug, if you are pregnant or nursing a baby, seek the advice of a health professional before using this product. This product may cause drowsiness. Avoid driving a motor vehicle or operating heavy machinery and avoid alcoholic beverages while taking this product.

Drug Interaction: Do not take this product if you are presently taking a prescription drug for high blood pressure or depression without first consulting your doctor.

Precaution: Keep this and all drugs out of the reach of children.

Symptoms and Treatment of Oral Overdosage: In case of accidental overdose, seek professional help or contact a Poison Control Center immediately.

Dosage and Administration: Adults 2 tablets every 6 hours, not to exceed 8 tablets in 24 hours, or as directed by physician. Children under 12 should use only as directed by physician.

How Supplied: Sinutab® Maximum Strength Formula Caplets are yellow and coated. The tablets are yellow and uncoated. They are supplied in child-resistant blister packs in boxes of 24 tablets/capsules.
Shown in Product Identification Section, page 419

SINUTAB® Maximum Strength Without Drowsiness
Tablets and Caplets

Active Ingredients: Each tablet/Caplet contains: Acetaminophen 500 mg., Pseudoephedrine Hydrochloride 30 mg.

Inactive Ingredients:
Tablets contain: Carboxymethyl Starch, Cellulose, Corn Starch, Croscarmellose Sodium, Hydroxypropyl Cellulose, Stearic Acid, Zinc Stearate, D&C Yellow No. 10 Aluminum Lake and FD&C Yellow No. 6 Aluminum Lake.
Caplets contain: Cellulose, Corn Starch, Croscarmellose Sodium, Hydroxypropyl Cellulose, Hydroxypropyl Methylcellulose, Magnesium Stearate, Polyethylene Glycol, Sodium Starch Glycolate, Stearic Acid, Titanium Dioxide, Zinc Stearate, D&C Yellow No. 10 Aluminum Lake and FD&C Yellow No. 6 Aluminum Lake.

Indications: For temporary relief of sinus symptoms due to colds, flu, allergy and hay fever. Contains a non-aspirin analgesic to relieve headache pain and a decongestant to ease pressure and congestion.

Actions: Sinutab® Maximum Strength Without Drowsiness Formula tablets and Caplets contain: an analgesic (acetaminophen) to relieve pain, and a decongestant (pseudoephedrine HCl) to reduce congestion of the nasopharyngeal mucosa.

Acetaminophen is both analgesic and antipyretic. Because acetaminophen is not a salicylate Sinutab® Maximum Strength Without Drowsiness Formula can be used by patients who are allergic to aspirin.

Pseudoephedrine HCl, a sympathomimetic drug, provides vaso-constriction of the nasopharyngeal mucosa resulting in a nasal decongestant effect.

The absence of antihistamine in the formula provides the added benefit of reduced likelihood of drowsiness side effects.

Warnings: Do not exceed recommended dosage. If symptoms persist, do not improve within seven days, or are accompanied by high fever, or if new symptoms occur, see your doctor before continuing use. Do not take this product if you have high blood pressure, heart disease, diabetes, thyroid disease, or difficulty in urination due to an enlarged prostate except under doctor's supervision. Do not take this product for more than 10 days. As with any drug, if you are pregnant or nursing a baby, seek the advice of a health professional before using this product.

Drug Interaction: Do not take this product if you are presently taking a prescription drug for high blood pressure or depression without first consulting your doctor.

Precaution: Keep this and all drugs out of the reach of children.

Symptoms and Treatment of Oral overdosage: In case of accidental overdose, seek professional help or contact a Poison Control Center immediately.

Dosage and Administration: Adults 2 tablets every 6 hours, not to exceed 8 tablets in 24 hours or as directed by physician. Children under 12 should use only as directed by physician.

How Supplied: Sinutab® Maximum Strength Caplets are orange and coated. The tablets are orange and uncoated. They are supplied in child-resistant blister packs in boxes of 24 tablets/Caplets and in bottles of 50 tablets with child resistant caps.

Shown in Product Identification Section, page 419

THERA-COMBEX H-P®
High-Potency Vitamin B Complex with 500 mg Vitamin C

Composition: Each Kapseal contains:
Ascorbic acid
(vitamin C)................................. 500 mg
Thiamine (vitamin B₁)
mononitrate.............................. 25 mg
Riboflavin
(vitamin B₂)................................. 15 mg
Pyridoxine hydrochloride
(vitamin B₆)................................. 10 mg
Vitamin B₁₂
(cyanocobalamin)....................... 5 mcg

Niacinamide................................. 100 mg
dl-Panthenol .... 20 mg

Uses: For the prevention or treatment of vitamin B complex and vitamin C deficiencies.

Dosage: One or two capsules daily

How Supplied: Bottles of 100.

TUCKS®
Pre-moistened Hemorrhoidal/Vaginal Pads

Indications: For prompt, temporary relief of minor external itching, burning and irritation associated with hemorrhoids, rectal or vaginal surgical stitches and other minor rectal or vaginal irritation.
—Soothe, cool, and comfort itching, burning, and irritation of sensitive rectal and outer vaginal areas.
—As a compress, to help relieve discomfort from rectal/vaginal surgical stitches.
—Effective hygienic wipe to cleanse rectal area of irritation-causing residue.
—Solution buffered to help prevent further irritation.

Directions: For external use only. Use as a wipe following bowel movement, during menstruation, or after napkin or tampon change. Or, as a compress, apply to affected area 10 to 15 minutes as needed. Change compresses every 5 minutes.

Warnings: In case of rectal bleeding, consult physician promptly. In case of continued irritation, discontinue use and consult a physician. Keep this and all medication out of the reach of children. In case of accidental ingestion seek professional assistance or contact a Poison Control Center immediately.

Contains: Soft pads pre-moistened with a solution containing 50% Witch Hazel; 10% Glycerin USP; also contains: Benzalkonium Chloride NF 0.003%, Citric acid, USP ; Methylparaben NF 0.1%; sodium citrate, USP; water, purified USP. Buffered to acid pH.

How Supplied: Jars of 40 and 100. Also available as Tucks Take-Alongs®, individual, foil-wrapped, nonwoven wipes, 12 per box

Shown in Product Identification Section, page 419

TUCKS® OINTMENT, CREAM

Composition: Tucks Ointment and Cream contain a specially formulated aqueous phase of 50% Witch Hazel (hamamelis water). Tucks Ointment also contains: alcohol 7%; arlacel; benzethonium chloride; lanolin anhydrous; sorbitol solution; and white petrolatum.
Tucks Cream also contains: alcohol 7%; arlacel; benzethonium chloride; cetyl alcohol; lanolin anhydrous; polyethylene stearate; polysorbate; sorbitol solution; and white petrolatum.

Action and Uses: Both nonstaining Tucks Ointment and Tucks Cream exert

a temporary soothing, cooling, mildly astringent effect on such superficial irritations as simple hemorrhoids, vaginal and rectal area itch, postepisiotomy discomfort and anorectal surgical wounds. Neither the Ointment nor the Cream contains steroids or skin sensitizing "caine" type topical anesthetics.

Warning: If itching or irritation continue, discontinue use and consult your physician. In case of rectal bleeding, consult physician promptly. Keep this and all drugs out of the reach of children. In case of accidental ingestion seek professional assistance or contact a Poison Control Center immediately.

Directions: Apply locally 3 or 4 times daily to temporarily soothe anal or outer vaginal irritation and itching, hemorrhoids, postepisiotomy and posthemorrhoidectomy discomfort.

How Supplied: Tucks Ointment and Tucks Cream (water-washable) in 40-g tubes with rectal applicators.

ZIRADRYL® Lotion
[zĭ'rǎ-drĭl]

Description: A zinc oxide-antihistaminic lotion of 1% Benadryl® (diphenhydramine hydrochloride) and 2% zinc oxide; contains 2% alcohol. Also contains: camphor; chlorophylline sodium polysorbate; fragrances; glycerin; methocel; and water, purified.

Indications: For relief of itching due to mild poison ivy, poison oak or insect bites.

Directions: SHAKE WELL. For adults and children 6 years of age and older: Apply to the affected area not more than three to four times daily or as directed by your physician. Before each application, cleanse skin with soap and water and dry affected area. Temporary stinging sensation may follow application. Discontinue use if stinging persists. Removes easily with water. Children under 6 years of age: consult a physician.

Warnings: For external use only. Do not apply to blistered, raw or oozing areas of the skin. Do not use on chicken pox or measles unless supervised by a physician. Do not use on extensive areas of the skin or for longer than 7 days except as directed by a physician. Avoid contact with the eyes or other mucous membranes. If condition worsens or if symptoms persist for more than 7 days or clear up and occur again within a few days or if burning sensation or rash develops discontinue use of this product and consult a physician. KEEP THIS

Continued on next page

This product information was prepared in November 1988. On these and other Parke-Davis Products, detailed information may be obtained by addressing PARKE-DAVIS, Consumer Health Products Group, Division of Warner-Lambert Company, Morris Plains, NJ 07950.

Parke-Davis—Cont.

AND ALL DRUGS OUT OF REACH OF CHILDREN. In case of accidental ingestion, seek professional assistance or contact a Poison Control Center immediately.

How Supplied: 6-oz bottles. Protect from freezing.
Shown in Product Identification Section, page 419

Pharmafair, Inc.
**205-C KELSEY LANE
SILO BEND
TAMPA, FL 33619**

OPHTHALMICS

Boric Acid 5% Ointment
⅛oz tube
NDC 24208-850-55

Eye Drops 15ml
NDC 24208-595-73
(Tetrahydrozoline HCl)

Eye Wash 4oz
NDC 24208-835-80

Lubrifair Ointment ⅛oz
NDC 24208-480-55
(White Petroleum, Mineral Oil, Lanolin Ocular Emolient)

Lubrifair Solution 15ml
NDC 24208-840-64
(Dextran 70, Hydroxypropyl Methylcellulose)

Ocugestrin Solution 15ml
NDC 24208-765-04
(Phenylephrine HCl 0.12%)

Petrolatum Ointment ⅛oz
NDC 24208-870-55

Dry Eyes Solution (Tearfair) 15ml
NDC 24208-755-04
(Polyvinyl Alcohol)

Tearfair Ointment
(White Petrolatum, Mineral Oil, Lanolin)
⅛oz tube: NDC 24208-760-02
0.7gm unit dose (24 per box) NDC 24208-760-07

CONTACT LENS CARE PRODUCTS—HARD

Wetting Solution for Hard Contact Lenses 60ml
NDC 24208-610-77

CONTACT LENS CARE PRODUCTS—SOFT

Delicate Eyes Cleaning Solution 25ml
NDC 24208-995-25

Delicate Eyes Lubricating & Rewetting Solution 15ml
NDC 24208-990-73

Delicate Eyes Rinsing & Storage Solution 12oz
NDC 24208-516-71

Delicate Eyes Saline Solution (non-preserved) 2×4oz
NDC 24208-501-80

Delicate Eyes Saline Solution (preserved) 12oz
NDC 24208-511-71

EAR PREPARATIONS

Ear Drops 15ml
NDC 24208-531-73
(Carbamide Peroxide 6.5%)

DERMATOLOGICALS

Benzoyl Peroxide 5% Gel 45gm tube
NDC 24208-430-53

Benzoyl Peroxide 10% Gel 45gm tube
NDC 24208-435-53

Cortifair 0.5% Cream
(Hydrocortisone 0.5%)
15gm NDC 24208-510-82
30gm NDC 24208-510-84
120gm NDC 24208-510-88
425gm NDC 24208-510-90

Cortifair 0.5% Lotion
(Hydrocortisone 0.5%)
1oz NDC 24208-500-75
4oz NDC 24208-500-80

Tolnaftate 1% Cream 15gm
NDC 24208-985-52

Tolnaftate 1% Solution 10ml
NDC 24208-506-62

Topisporin Ointment
(Bacitracin Zinc, Neomycin Sulfate, Polymyxin B Sulfate)
15gm: NDC 24208-530-02
30gm: NDC 24208-530-04

TABLETS (ORAL PREPARATIONS)

Meclizine HCl Chewable Tablets 25mg
bottles of 100 NDC 24208-075-01
bottles of 1000 NDC 24208-075-10
unit dose 100's NDC 24208-075-11

Pseudoephedrine HCl 30mg sc
bottles of 1000 NDC 24208-170-10
unit dose 100's NDC 24208-170-11

Senna Tabs 217mg
bottles of 1000 NDC 24207-175-10
unit dose 100's NDC 24207-175-11

IDENTIFICATION PROBLEM?
Consult the
Product Identification Section
where you'll find
products pictured
in full color.

Plough, Inc.
**3030 JACKSON AVENUE
MEMPHIS, TN 38151**

**AFTATE® Antifungal
Aerosol Liquid
Aerosol Powder
Gel
Powder**

Active Ingredient: Tolnaftate 1% (Also contains: Aerosol Spray Liquid-36% alcohol; Aerosol Spray Powder-14% alcohol.)

How Supplied:
AFTATE for Athlete's Foot
Sprinkle Powder—2.25 oz. bottle
Aerosol Spray Powder—3.5 oz can
Gel—.5 oz. tube.
Aerosol Spray Liquid—4 oz. can.
AFTATE for Jock Itch
Aerosol Spray Powder—3.5 oz. can
Sprinkle Powder—1.5 oz. bottle.
Gel—.5 oz. tube.
Shown in Product Identification Section, page 419

COPPERTONE® Waterproof Sunscreens

COPPERTONE® Sunscreen Lotion SPF 6
COPPERTONE® Sunscreen Lotion SPF 8
COPPERTONE® Sunblock Lotion SPF 15
COPPERTONE® Sunblock Lotion SPF 25
COPPERTONE® Sunblock Lotion SPF 30
COPPERTONE Sunblock Lotion SPF 44

Active Ingredients: SPF 6, 8 & 15—Padimate O, Oxybenzone; SPF 25—Padimate O, Oxybenzone, Ethylhexyl-p-methoxycinnamate; SPF 30, and SPF 44—Ethylhexyl-p-methoxycinnamate, 2-Ethylhexyl salicylate, Padimate O, Oxybenzone.

How Supplied: 4 fl. oz. Plastic Bottles
Shown in Product Identification Section, page 420

COPPERTONE® Sun Spray Mist SPF 10

Active Ingredients: Ethylhexyl P-Methoxycinnamate, 2-Ethylhexyl Salicylate, Oxybenzone.

How Supplied: 7.25 oz. Plastic Bottle.

**CORRECTOL®
Laxative
Tablets**

Active Ingredients: Tablets—Yellow phenolphthalein, 65 mg. and docusate sodium, 100 mg. per tablet.

Inactive Ingredients: Butylparaben, calcium gluconate, calcium sulfate, carnauba wax, D&C No. 7 calcium lake, gelatin, magnesium stearate, sugar, talc, titanium dioxide, wheat flour, white wax, and other ingredients.

Indications: For relief of occasional constipation or irregularity. CORRECTOL generally produces bowel movement in 6 to 8 hours.

Actions: Yellow phenolphthalein—stimulant laxative; docusate sodium—fecal softener.

Warnings: Not to be taken in case of nausea, vomiting, abdominal pain, or signs of appendicitis. Take only as needed —as frequent or continued use of laxatives may result in dependence on them. If skin rash appears, do not use this or any other preparation containing phenolphthalein. As with any drug, if you are pregnant or nursing a baby, seek the advice of a health professional before using this product.

Dosage and Administration
Dosage: Adults—1 or 2 tablets daily as needed, at bedtime or on arising.
Children over 6 years—1 tablet daily as needed.

How Supplied: Tablets—Individual foil-backed safety sealed blister packaging in boxes of 15, 30, 60 and 90 tablets.
Shown in Product Identification Section, page 419

DI-GEL®
Antacid · Anti-Gas
Tablets/Liquid

DI-GEL Tablets: Active Ingredients: (Per Tablet)—Simethicone 20 mg., Calcium Carbonate 280 mg., Magnesium Hydroxide 128 mg. **Inactive Ingredients:** D & C yellow No. 10 aluminum lake, dextrin, FD&C yellow No. 6 aluminum lake, flavor, magnesium stearate, mannitol, polyvinyl-pyrrolidone, stearic acid, sucrose, talc.
Dietetically sodium free, calcium rich.

DI-GEL Liquid: Active Ingredients— per teaspoonful (5 ml): Simethicone 20 mg., aluminum hydroxide (equivalent to aluminum hydroxide dried gel USP) 200 mg., magnesium hydroxide 200 mg.
Also contains: Flavor, methylcellulose, methylparaben, propylparaben, sodium saccharin, sorbitol, water.
Sodium Content—Less than 5 mg. per teaspoonful.

Indications: For fast, temporary relief of acid indigestion, heartburn, sour stomach and accompanying painful gas symptoms.

Actions: The antacid system in DI-GEL relieves and soothes acid indigestion, heartburn and sour stomach. At the same time, the simethicone "defoamers" eliminate gas.
When air becomes entrapped in the stomach, heartburn and acid indigestion can result, along with sensations of fullness, pressure and bloating.

Warnings: Do not take more than 20 teaspoonfuls or 24 tablets in a 24 hour period, or use the maximum dosage of this product for more than 2 weeks, except under the advice and supervision of a physician. If you have kidney disease do not use this product except under the advice and supervision of a physician. May cause constipation or have a laxative effect.

Drug Interaction: (Liquid Only) This product should not be taken if patient is presently taking a prescription antibiotic drug containing any form of tetracycline.

Dosage and Administration: Two teaspoonfuls or tablets every 2 hours, or after or between meals and at bedtime, not to exceed 20 teaspoonfuls or 24 tablets per day, or as directed by a physician.

How Supplied:
DI-GEL Liquid in Mint and Lemon/Orange Flavors - 6 and 12 fl. oz. bottles, safety sealed.
DI-GEL Tablets in Mint and Lemon/Orange Flavors - In boxes of 30 and 90 in handy portable safety sealed blister packaging. Also available in Mint 3-roll (36 tablets) and in Mint 60-tablet bottles.
Shown in Product Identification Section, page 419

DURATION®
Long Acting Nasal Decongestant
Tablets

Active Ingredients: Pseudoephedrine Sulfate 120 mg.

Inactive Ingredients: Acacia, Butylparaben, Calcium Sulfate, Carnauba Wax, Corn Starch, Eiderdown Soap, FD&C Blue No. 1, FD&C Yellow No, 6, Gelatin, Lactose, Magnesium Stearate, Oleic Acid, Povidone, Rosin, Sugar, Talc, White Wax, Zein.

Indications: For temporary relief of nasal congestion due to cold, hay fever or other upper respiratory allergies, and nasal congestion associated with sinusitis; promotes nasal and/or sinus drainage.

Warnings: Do not exceed recommended dosage. Do not use if you have high blood pressure, heart disease, diabetes or thyroid disease except under the advice of a physician. If symptoms do not improve within 7 days or are accompanied by high fever, consult a physician before continuing use. If you are pregnant or nursing a baby, seek the advice of a health professional before using this product.

Drug Interaction: Do not take this product if you are presently taking a prescription antihypertensive or antidepressant drug containing a monoamine oxidase inhibitor, except under the advice and supervision of a physician.

Symptoms and Treatment of Oral Overdosage: In case of accidental overdose, seek professional assistance or contact a Poison Control Center immediately.

Dosage and Administration: Adults and children 12 years of age and over: One tablet every 12 hours. Not recommended for children under 12 years of age.

How Supplied: Available in packages of 10 and 20 individually sealed tablets.
Shown in Product Identification Section, page 419

DURATION®
12 Hour Nasal Spray
12 Hour Mentholated Nasal Spray
Topical Nasal Decongestant

Active Ingredient:
12 Hour Nasal Spray:
Oxymetazoline HCl 0.05%

Other Ingredients:
12 Hour Nasal Spray: Preservative Phenylmercuric Acetate (Mentholated Nasal Spray also contains the following aromatics: menthol, camphor, eucalyptol).

Indications: Temporary relief for up to 12 hours of nasal congestion due to colds, hay fever and sinusitis.

Actions: The sympathomimetic action of DURATION constricts the smaller arterioles of the nasal passages, producing a gentle and predictable decongesting effect.

Warnings: Do not exceed recommended dosage because symptoms may occur such as burning, stinging, sneezing, or increase of nasal discharge. Do not use this product for more than 3 days. If symptoms persist, consult a physician. The use of dispenser by more than one person may spread infection.

Dosage and Administration:
DURATION 12 Hour Nasal Spray—With head upright, spray 2 or 3 times in each nostril twice daily—morning and evening. To spray, squeeze bottle quickly and firmly. Not recommended for children under 6.

How Supplied:
DURATION 12 Hour Nasal Spray—½ and 1 fl. oz. plastic squeeze bottle.
DURATION 12 Hour Mentholated Nasal Spray—½ fl. oz. plastic squeeze bottle.
All bottles in safety sealed cartons.
Shown in Product Identification Section, page 419

DURATION®
12 Hour Nasal Spray Pump

Active Ingredients: Oxymetazoline Hydrochloride 0.05%

Inactive Ingredients: Aminoacetic Acid, Benzalkonium Chloride, Phenylmercuric Acetate (Preservative), Sorbitol, Water.

Indications: Delivers a measured dosage every time. Immediate relief of nasal congestion due to common cold, hay fever and sinusitis.

Warnings: Do not exceed recommended dosage because symptoms may occur such as burning, stinging, sneezing, or increase of nasal discharge. Do not use this product for more than 3 days. If symptoms persist, consult a physician. The use of dispenser by more than one person may spread infection. Keep this

Continued on next page

Plough—Cont.

and all medications out of the reach of children.

Symptoms and Treatment of Oral Overdosage: In case of accidental ingestion, seek professional assistance or contact a Poison Control Center immediately.

Dosage and Administration: Before using first time, remove protective cap. Prime the metered pump by depressing several times. Hold bottle with thumb at base and nozzle between first and second fingers. With head upright (do not tilt backward), insert metered pump-spray nozzle in nostril. Depress pump completely 2 or 3 times. Sniff deeply. Repeat in other nostil. Wipe tip clean after each use.

How Supplied: Available in ½ fl. oz. pump spray.
Shown in Product Identification Section, page 419

FEEN-A-MINT®
Laxative Gum/Pills

Active Ingredients: Gum—yellow phenolphthalein 97.2 mg. per tablet. Pills—yellow phenolphthalein, 65 mg., and docusate sodium 100 mg. per pill.

Indications: For relief of occasional constipation or irregularity. FEEN-A-MINT generally produces bowel movement in 6 to 8 hours.

Inactive Ingredients: Gum—Acacia, butylated hydroxyanisole, gelatin, glycerin, glucose, gum base, peppermint oil, sodium benzoate, starch, sugar, talc, water.
Pills—Butylparaben, calcium gluconate, calcium slufate, carnauba wax, gelatin, magnesium stearate, sugar, talc, titanium dioxide, wheat flour, white wax and other ingredients.

How Supplied: Gum—Individual foil-backed safety sealed blister packaging in boxes of 5, 16, and 40 tablets.
Pills—Safety sealed boxes of 15, 30, and 60 tablets.
Shown in Product Identification Section, page 420

REGUTOL®
Stool Softener Tablets

Active Ingredient: Each tablet contains 100 mg. docusate sodium.

Inactive Ingredients: Acacia, butylparaben, calcium sulfate, carnauba wax, D&C yellow No. 10 aluminum lake, FD&C yellow No. 6 aluminum lake, gelatin, lactose, magnesium stearate, povi-

done, sugar, talc, titanium dioxide, white wax.

How Supplied: REGUTOL tablets in boxes of 30, 60 and 90 individually safety sealed blister packaging.
Shown in Product Identification Section, page 420

ST. JOSEPH® Anti-Diarrheal

Active Ingredients: Non-fibrous attapulgite

Inactive Ingredients: Benzoic acid, citric acid, flavor, glycerin, magnesium aluminum silicate, methylparaben, polysorbate 80, propylene glycol, propylparaben, sodium saccharin, sorbitol, water, xanthan gum.

Indications: The product's simple non-systemic natural ingredient adsorbs the bacteria and toxins which cause diarrhea and works without entering the bloodstream.

Actions: Relieves diarrhea and cramping in children. Improves stool consistency and reduces number of bowel movements.

Warnings: Do not use for more than 2 days in the presence of high fever or in children under 3, unless directed by a physician. Keep this and all medications out of the reach of children.

Symptoms and Treatment of Oral Overdosage: In case of accidental overdose, seek professional assistance or contact a Poison Control Center immediately.

Dosage and Administration: For best results give full recommended dose at the first sign of diarrhea and after each bowel movement or every two hours, whichever comes first. Do not exceed recommended dose per day.
[See table below].

How Supplied: Cola flavored concentrated liquid in plastic 2 oz. bottle. In safety sealed packaging.
Shown in Product Identification Section, page 420

ST. JOSEPH® Aspirin–Free Fever Reducer
for Children
Chewable Tablets, Liquid, Drops

Active Ingredient: Each Children's St. Joseph Aspirin-Free Chewable Tablet contains 80 mg. acetaminophen in a fruit-flavored tablet. Children's St. Joseph Aspirin-Free Liquid is stable, cherry flavored, red in color and alcohol-free and sugar-free. Each 5 ml. contains 160 mg. acetaminophen. Infant's St. Joseph Aspirin-Free Drops are stable, fruit

flavored, orange in color and alcohol-free and sugar-free. Each 0.8 ml. (one calibrated dropperful) contains 80 mg. acetaminophen.

Inactive Ingredients: Tablets: Cellulose, D&C red No. 7 calcium lake, D&C red No. 30 aluminum lake, flavor, mannitol, silicon dioxide, sodium saccharin, zinc stearate.
Liquid: FD&C yellow No. 6, flavor, glycerin, maltol, polyethylene glycol, propylene glycol, saccharin, sodium benzoate, sodium chloride, sodium saccharin, water.
Drops: FD&C yellow No. 6, flavor, glycerin, maltol, polyethylene glycol, propylene glycol, saccharin, sodium benzoate, sodium chloride, sodium saccharin, water.

Indications: For temporary reduction of fever, relief of minor aches and pains of colds and flu.

Actions: Analgesic/Antipyretic

Warnings: Do not administer this product for more than 5 days. If symptoms persist or new ones occur, consult physician. If fever persists for more than three days, or recurs, consult physician. When using St. Joseph Aspirin-Free products do not give other medications containing acetaminophen unless directed by your physician. NOTE: SEVERE OR PERSISTENT SORE THROAT, HIGH FEVER, HEADACHES, NAUSEA OR VOMITING MAY BE SERIOUS. DISCONTINUE USE AND CONSULT PHYSICIAN IF NOT RELIEVED IN 24 HOURS. Do not exceed recommended dosage because severe liver damage may occur. As with any drug, if you are pregnant or nursing a baby, seek the advice of a health professional before using this product.

Dosage and Administration: [See table on page 639]
ST. JOSEPH Aspirin-Free Fever Reducer Tablets for Children may be given one of three ways. Always follow with ½ glass of water, milk or fruit juice.
1. Chewed, followed by liquid.
2. Crushed or dissolved in a teaspoon of liquid (for younger children).
3. Powdered for infant use, when so directed by physician.

How Supplied: Chewable fruit flavored tablets in plastic bottles of 30 tablets. Cherry tasting Liquid in 2 and 4 fl. oz. plastic bottles. Fruit flavored drops in ½ fl. oz. glass bottles, with calibrated plastic dropper.
All packages have child resistant safety caps and safety sealed packaging.
Shown in Product Identification Section, page 420

ST. JOSEPH® Cold Tablets for Children

Active Ingredients: Per tablet: Acetaminophen 80 mg and phenylpropanolamine hydrochloride 3.125 mg.

Inactive Ingredients: Cellulose, FD&C Yellow No. 6 aluminum lake, flavor,

Age/Weight Dosage Chart

Age	Weight	Dose	Maximum Dose Per 24 hours
Under 3 yrs.	Under 30 lbs.	Consult your physician	
3–5 yrs.	30–45 lbs.	1 teaspoon	3 teaspoons
6–12 yrs.	46–84 lbs.	2 teaspoons	6 teaspoons
Over 12 yrs.	Over 84 lbs.	4 teaspoons	12 teaspoons

ST. JOSEPH CHILDREN'S DOSAGE CHART

Age	0–3 (months)	4–11 (months)	12–23 (months)	2–3 (years)	4–5 (years)	6–8 (years)	9–10 (years)	11 (years)	12+ (years)
Weight (lbs.)	7–12	13–21	22–26	27–35	36–45	46–65	66–76	77–83	84+
Dose of St. Joseph Acetaminophen Drops Dropperfuls	½	1	1½	2	3	4	5	—	—
Acetaminophen Liquid Teaspoonfuls	—	½	¾	1	1½	2	2½	3	4
Chewable Tablets Acetaminophen (80 mg. each)	—	—	1½	2	3	4	5	6	8

All dosages may be repeated every 4 hours, but do not exceed 5 dosages daily.
Note: Since St. Joseph pediatric products are available without prescription, parents are advised on the package label to consult a physician for use in children under two years.

mannitol, silica, sodium saccharin, zinc stearate.

How Supplied: In bottle with 30 fruit flavored chewable tablets.
Shown in Product Identification Section, page 420

ST. JOSEPH® Cough Syrup for Children
Pediatric
Antitussive Syrup

Active Ingredient: Dextromethorphan hydrobromide 7.5 mg. per 5 cc.

Inactive Ingredients: Caramel, citric acid, flavor, glycerin, methylparaben, propylparaben, sodium benzoate, sodium citrate, sucrose, water.

How Supplied: Alcohol-Free Cherry tasting syrup in plastic bottle of 2 and 4 fl. ozs. In safety sealed packaging.
Shown in Product Identification Section, page 420

ST. JOSEPH® Measured Dose Nasal Decongestant

Active Ingredients: Phenylephrine Hydrochloride 0.125%

Inactive Ingredients: Cetyl pyridinium chloride, disodium phosphate, phenylmercuric acetate 0.002% (preservative), propylene glycol, sodium phosphate, sorbitol, water.

Indications: Gives temporary relief for up to 4 hours of nasal congestion due to colds, hay fever, sinusitis. The pump spray delivery system gives a measured dose every time (50 microliters).

Warnings: Do not exceed recommended dosage because symptoms may occur such as burning, stinging, sneezing, or increase of nasal discharge. Do not use this product for more than 3 days. If symptoms persist, consult a physician. Do not use in children under 2 years of age or who have heart disease, high blood pressure, thyroid disease or diabetes unless directed by a doctor. The use of the dispenser by more than one person may spread infection. Keep this and all medications out of the reach of children.

Symptoms and Treatment of Oral Overdosage: In case of accidental ingestion, seek professional assistance or contact a Poison Control Center immediately.

Dosage and Administration: For children 2 to under 6 years old. Before using first time, remove protective cap. Prime the metered pump by depressing several times. Hold bottle with thumb at base and nozzle between first and second fingers. With child's head upright (do not tilt child's head backward), insert metered pump spray nozzle in child's nostril. Depress pump completely 1 or 2 times. Have child sniff deeply. Repeat in other nostil. Repeat application every 4 hours needed. Wipe tip clean after each use.

How Supplied: Available in ½ fl. oz. measured dose pump spray.
Shown in Product Identification Section, page 420

ST. JOSEPH® Nighttime Cold Medicine

Active Ingredients: Chlorpheniramine maleate, pseudoephedrine hydrochloride, acetaminophen, dextromethorphan hydrobromide

Inactive Ingredients: Citric acid, FD&C red No. 40, flavor, methylparaben, polyethylene glycol, propylene glycol, propylparaben, sodium benzoate, sodium citrate, sucrose, water

Indications: Temporary relief of major cold and flu symptoms

Actions: Antihistamine for relief of runny nose, sneezing, itchy watery eyes, scratchy throat and post-nasal drip; nasal decongestant for relief of nasal and sinus congestion; analgesic for aspirin-free relief to reduce fever of colds and flu and relieve body aches and pain; and cough suppressant to calm and quiet coughing.

Warning: For children under 6 years or 48 pounds, consult physician. Do not give this product to children for more than 5 days. If symptoms do not improve, or if new ones occur, or are accompanied by fever for over 3 days, consult physician. Do not exceed recommended dosage because at higher doses nervousness, dizziness, sleeplessness or severe liver damage may occur. May cause drowsiness or excitability. Keep this and all drugs out of reach of children.

Symptoms and Treatment of Oral Overdosage: In case of accidental overdose, seek professional assistance or contact a Poison Control Center immediately.

Dosage and Administration: One dose every 4 to 6 hours, not to exceed 3 times daily. Use the enclosed dosage cup to measure the right dose for your child.

Age/Weight Dosage Chart

AGE	WEIGHT	DOSE
Under 6 yrs.	Under 48 lbs.	Consult Physician
6–8 yrs.	48–65 lbs.	2 tsp.
9–10 yrs.	66–76 lbs.	2½ tsp.
11–12 yrs.	77–85 lbs.	3 tsp.

How Supplied: Alcohol-Free Cherry tasting syrup in plastic 4 oz. bottle. In safety sealed packaging.
Shown in Product Identification Section, page 420

SOLARCAINE®
Antiseptic·Topical Anesthetic Lotion/Cream/Aerosol Spray Liquid

Active Ingredients:
SOLARCAINE Aloe Aerosol Spray—.5% lidocaine.
Also contains aloe vera and Vitamin E. Non-stinging and alcohol/fragrance free.
SOLARCAINE Aerosol Spray—to deliver benzocaine 20% (w/w), triclosan 0.13% (w/w). Also contains isopropyl alcohol 35% (w/w) in total contents.
SOLARCAINE Lotion—Benzocaine and triclosan.
SOLARCAINE Cream—Benzocaine and triclosan.

Indications: Medicated first aid to provide fast temporary relief of sunburn pain, minor burns, cuts, scrapes, chapping and skin injuries, poison ivy, detergent hands, insect bites (non-venomous). Aloe aerosol spray provides longer lasting/more cooling relief.

Continued on next page

Plough—Cont.

Actions: Lidocaine and benzocaine provide local anesthetic action to relieve itching and pain. Triclosan provides antimicrobial activity.

Caution: Not for use in eyes. Not for deep or puncture wounds or serious burns, nor for prolonged use. If condition persists, or infection, rash or irritation develops, discontinue use.

Warnings: For Aerosol Spray—Flammable—Do not spray while smoking or near fire. Do not spray into eyes or mouth. Avoid inhalation. Contents under pressure. For external use only.

Dosage and Administration: Lotion and Cream—Apply freely as needed. Sprays—Hold 3 to 5 inches from injured area. Spray until wet. To apply to face, spray on palm of hand. Use often for antiseptic protection.

How Supplied:
SOLARCAINE Aloe Aerosol Spray—4.5 oz. can.
SOLARCAINE Aerosol Spray—3- and 5-oz. cans.
SOLARCAINE Lotion—3- and 6-fl oz. bottles.
SOLARCAINE Cream—1-oz. tube.
Shown in Product Identification Section, page 420

SUPER SHADE® Sunscreens

SUPER SHADE® Sunblock Lotion SPF 15
SUPER SHADE® Sunblock Lotion SPF 25
SUPER SHADE® Sunblock Stick SPF 25
SUPER SHADE® Sunblock Lotion SPF 30
Also available in SPF 44 PABA based formula.
Also available in SPF-15 Paba based Oil-Free Clear Gel.

Active Ingredients: SPF 15, 25, and 30: Ethylhexyl p-methoxycinnamate, Oxybenzone. In addition, Super Shade 25 and 30 also has 2-Ethylhexyl salicylate, Homsalate. Super Shade Stick has Ethylhexyl p-methoxycinnamate, Homosalate, Menthyl anthranilate, Oxybenzone.

Indications: Waterproof Paba-free sunscreens to help prevent harmful effects from the sun. SHADE screens both UVB and UVA rays. SHADE Protection Formulas provide 15, 25 and 30 times your natural sunburn protection. Liberal and regular use may help reduce the chances of premature aging and wrinkling of skin, due to overexposure to the sun. All strengths are waterproof, maintaining sun protection for 80 minutes in water. Excellent for use on children.

Actions: Sunscreen

Warnings: For external use only. Avoid contact with eyes. Discontinue use if signs of irritation or rash appear.

Dosage and Administration: Apply evenly and liberally to all exposed skin.

Reapply after prolonged swimming or excessive perspiration.

How Supplied: 4 fl. oz. Plastic Bottles
Shown in Product Identification Section, page 420

Procter & Gamble
P. O. BOX 171
CINCINNATI, OH 45201

DENQUEL® Sensitive Teeth Toothpaste
Desensitizing Dentifrice

Each tube contains potassium nitrate (5%) in a low abrasion, pleasant mint flavored dentifrice.

Dentinal hypersensitivity is a condition in which pain or discomfort arises when various stimuli, such as hot, cold, sweet, sour or touch contact exposed dentin. Exposure of dentin often occurs as a result of either gingival recession or periodontal surgery.

Daily use of Denquel can provide, within the first 2 weeks of regular brushing, a significant decrease in hypersensitivity. As regular use continues, greater improvement will be noticed. The Council on Dental Therapeutics of the American Dental Association has given Denquel the ADA Seal of Acceptance as an effective desensitizing dentifrice for teeth sensitive to hot, cold or pressure (tactile) in otherwise normal teeth.

Contraindications: See a dentist if tooth sensitivity is not reduced after 4 weeks of regular use, as this may indicate a dental condition other than hypersensitivity.

Dosage: Use twice a day or as directed by a dentist.

How Supplied: Denquel Sensitive Teeth Toothpaste is supplied in tubes containing 1.6, 3.0, or 4.5 ounces.

HEAD & SHOULDERS® SHAMPOO
Antidandruff Shampoo

Head & Shoulders Lotion Shampoo contains the active ingredient pyrithione zinc (PTZ) in a patented platelet form. The PTZ platelets settle out of the shampoo lather and deposit directly onto the scalp, forming an antimicrobial barrier which remains after rinsing. Independently conducted clinical testing (double blind and dermatologist graded) has proven that Head & Shoulders significantly reduced dandruff. Head & Shoulders is pH balanced and gentle enough to use everyday for clean, manageable hair.

Active Ingredient: 1.0% pyrithione zinc suspended in an anionic detergent system. Cosmetic ingredients are also included.

Indications: For effective control of dandruff and seborrheic dermatitis of the scalp.

Actions: Pyrithione zinc is substantive to the scalp and remains after rinsing. Its mechanism of action has not been fully established, but it is believed to control

the microorganisms associated with dandruff flaking and itching.

Precautions: Not to be taken internally. Keep out of children's reach. Avoid getting shampoo in eyes—if this happens, rinse eyes with water.

Dosage and Administration: For best results, Head & Shoulders should be used regularly. Head & Shoulders can be used not only to treat dandruff, but also regular use will help control the recurrence of symptoms. It is gentle enough to use for every shampoo. In treating seborrheic dermatitis, a minimum of four shampooings are needed to achieve full effectiveness.

How Supplied: Normal-to-Oily and Normal-to-Dry lotions available in 4.0 fl. oz., 7.0 fl. oz., 11.0 fl. oz., and 15.0 fl. oz. unbreakable plastic bottles. Normal-to-Oily and Normal-to-Dry concentrate form available in 5.5 oz. tubes.

Composition: LOTION—Normal-to-Oily Formula: Pyrithione zinc in a shampoo base of water, ammonium laureth sulfate, ammonium lauryl sulfate, cocamide MEA, glycol distearate, ammonium xylenesulfonate, fragrance, citric acid, methylchloroisothiazolinone, methylisothiazolinone, and FD&C Blue No. 1.
LOTION:—Normal-to-Dry Formula: Pyrithione zinc in a shampoo base of water, ammonium laureth sulfate, ammonium lauryl sulfate, cocamide MEA, glycol distearate, ammonium xylenesulfonate, propylene glycol, fragrance, citric acid, methylchloroisothiazolinone, methylisothiazolinone, and FD&C Blue No. 1.
CONCENTRATE: Normal-to-Oily Formula: Pyrithione zinc in a shampoo base of water, sodium cocoglyceryl ether sulfonate, sodium chloride, sodium lauroyl sarcosinate, cocamide DEA, cocoyl sarcosine, fragrance, and FD&C Blue No. 1.
CONCENTRATE: Normal-to-Dry Formula: Pyrithione zinc in a shampoo base of water, sodium cocoglyceryl ether sulfonate, sodium chloride, sodium lauroyl sarcosinate, cocamide DEA, propylene glycol, cocoyl sarcosine, fragrance, and FD&C Blue No. 1.
Shown in Product Identification Section, page 420

Regular Flavor
METAMUCIL® Powder
[met "uh-mū 'sil]
(psyllium hydrophilic mucilloid)

Description: Regular Flavor Metamucil is a bulk forming natural therapeutic fiber for restoring and maintaining regularity. It contains refined hydrophilic mucilloid, a highly efficient dietary fiber derived from the husk of the psyllium seed *(Plantago ovata)*. Metamucil contains no chemical stimulants and is nonaddictive. Each dose contains approximately 3.4 g of psyllium hydrophilic mucilloid. Inactive ingredients include dextrose (a carbohydrate). Each dose contains less than 10 mg. of sodium, 31 mg of potassium, and 14 calories. Carbohydrate content is approximately 3.5 g.

Actions: Metamucil provides a bland, nonirritating bulk and promotes normal elimination. It is uniform, instantly miscible, palatable, and nonirritive in the gastrointestinal tract.

Indications: Metamucil is indicated in the management of chronic constipation, in irritable bowel syndrome, as adjunctive therapy in the constipation of duodenal ulcer and diverticular disease, in the bowel management of patients with hemorrhoids, and for constipation during pregnancy, convalescence, and senility.

Contraindications: Intestinal obstruction, fecal impaction.

Precaution: May cause allergic reaction in people sensitive to inhaled or ingested psyllium powder.

Dosage and Administration: The usual adult dosage is one rounded teaspoonful (7 g) stirred into a standard 8-oz glass of cool water, fruit juice, milk or other beverage. It can be taken orally one to three times a day, depending on the need and response. It may require continued use for 2 or 3 days to provide optimal benefit. An additional glass of liquid after each dose is helpful. For children (6 to 12 years old), use ½ the adult dose in 8 oz. of liquid. 1 to 3 times daily.

How Supplied: Powder, containers of 7 oz, 14 oz, 21 oz and 32 oz. (OTC); also available in cartons of 100 single-dose (7 g) packets.
Shown in Product Identification Section, page 420

Sugar Free Regular Flavor METAMUCIL® Powder
[met "uh-mū 'sil]
(psyllium hydrophilic mucilloid)

Description: Sugar Free Regular Flavor Metamucil is a bulk forming natural therapeutic fiber for restoring and maintaining regularity. It contains refined hydrophilic mucilloid, a highly efficient dietary fiber derived from the husk of the psyllium seed (*Plantago ovata*), which has been sweetened with NutraSweet®* brand sweetener (aspartame). It contains no chemical stimulants or sugar and is non-additive. Each dose contains approximately 3.4 g of psyllium hydrophilic mucilloid. Inactive ingredients include aspartame and maltodextrin. Each dose contains about 1 calorie, less than 10 mg. of sodium, 31 mg of potassium and 6 mg of phenylalanine. Carbohydrate content is 0.3 grams.

Actions: Metamucil provides a bland, nonirritating bulk and promotes normal elimination. It is uniform, instantly miscible, palatable, and nonirritive in the gastrointestinal tract.

Indications: Metamucil is indicated in the management of chronic constipation, in irritable bowel syndrome, as adjunctive therapy in the constipation of duodenal ulcer and diverticular disease, in the bowel management of patients with hemorrhoids, and for constipation during pregnancy, convalescence, and senility.

Contraindications: Intestinal obstruction, fecal impaction.

Warning: Phenylketonurics should be aware that Sugar Free Metamucil contains phenylalanine.

Precaution: May cause allergic reaction in people sensitive to inhaled or ingested psyllium powder.

Dosage and Administration: The usual adult dosage is one rounded teaspoonful (3.7 g) stirred into a standard 8-oz glass of cool water, fruit juice, milk or other beverage. It can be taken orally one to three times a day, depending on the need and response. It may require continued use for 2 or 3 days to provide optimal benefit. An additional glass of liquid after each dose is helpful. For children (6–12 years old), use ½ the adult dose in 8 oz. of liquid, 1 to 3 times daily.

How Supplied: Powder, containers of 3.7 oz, 7.4 oz, 11.1 oz, and 16.9 oz. (OTC); also available in cartons of 100 single-dose (3.7 g) packets.

*NutraSweet is a registered trademark of the NutraSweet Company.
Shown in Product Identification Section, page 420

Orange Flavor METAMUCIL® Powder
[met "uh-mū 'sil]
(psyllium hydrophilic mucilloid)

Description: Orange Flavor Metamucil is a bulk forming natural therapeutic fiber for restoring and maintaining regularity. It contains refined hydrophilic mucilloid, a highly efficient dietary fiber derived from the husk of the psyllium seed (*Plantago ovata*). Metamucil contains no chemical stimulants and is non-addictive. Each dose contains approximately 3.4 g of psyllium hydrophilic mucilloid. Inactive ingredients include citric acid, FD&C Yellow No. 6, flavoring, and sucrose (a carbohydrate). Each dose contains less than 10 mg. of sodium, 31 mg of potassium, and 30 calories. Carbohydrate content is approximately 7.1 g.

Actions: Metamucil provides a bland, nonirritating bulk and promotes normal elimination. It is uniform, instantly miscible, palatable, and nonirritative in the gastrointestinal tract.

Indications: Metamucil is indicated in the management of chronic constipation, in irritable bowel syndrome, as adjunctive therapy in the constipation of duodenal ulcer and diverticular disease, in the bowel management of patients with hemorrhoids, and for constipation during pregnancy, convalescence, and senility.

Contraindications: Intestinal obstruction, fecal impaction.

Precaution: May cause allergic reaction in people sensitive to inhaled or ingested psyllium powder.

Dosage and Administration: The usual adult dosage is one rounded tablespoonful (11 g) stirred into a standard 8-oz glass of cool water, fruit juice, milk or other beverage. It can be taken orally one to three times a day, depending on the need and response. It may require continued use for 2 or 3 days to provide optimal benefit. An additional glass of liquid after each dose is helpful. For children (6 to 12 years old), use ½ the adult dose in 8 oz. of liquid, 1 to 3 times daily.

How Supplied: Powder, containers of 7 oz, 14 oz, 21 oz, and 32 oz. (OTC)
Shown in Product Identification Section, page 420

Strawberry Flavor METAMUCIL® Powder
[met "uh-mū 'sil]
(psyllium hydrophilic mucilloid)

Description: Strawberry Flavor Metamucil is a bulk forming natural therapeutic fiber for restoring and maintaining regularity. It contains refined hydrophilic mucilloid, a highly efficient dietary fiber derived from the husk of the psyllium seed (*Plantago ovata*). Metamucil contains no chemical stimulants and is not addictive. Each dose contains approximately 3.4 g of psyllium hydrophilic mucilloid. Inactive ingredients include citric acid, FD&C Red No. 40, flavoring, and sucrose (a carbohydrate). Each dose contains less than 10 mg. of sodium, 31 mg of potassium, and 30 calories. Carbohydrate content is approximately 7.1 g.

Actions: Metamucil provides a bland, nonirritating bulk and promotes normal elimination. It is uniform, instantly miscible, palatable, and nonirritative in the gastrointestinal tract.

Indications: Metamucil is indicated in the management of chronic constipation, in irritable bowel syndrome, as adjunctive therapy in the constipation of duodenal ulcer and diverticular disease, in the bowel management of patients with hemorrhoids, and for constipation during pregnancy, convalescence, and senility.

Contraindications: Intestinal obstruction, fecal impaction.

Precaution: May cause allergic reaction in people sensitive to inhaled or ingested psyllium powder.

Dosage and Administration: The usual adult dose is one rounded tablespoonful (11 g) stirred into a standard 8-oz glass of cool water, fruit juice, milk or other beverage. It can be taken orally one to three times a day, depending on the need and response. It may require continued use for 2 or 3 days to provide optimal benefit. An additional glass of liquid after each dose is helpful. For children (6–12 years old), use ½ tablespoonful in 8 oz. of liquid, 1 to 3 times daily.

How Supplied: Powder, containers of 7 oz, 14 oz, and 21 oz. (OTC)
Shown in Product Identification Section, page 420

Continued on next page

Procter & Gamble—Cont.

Sugar Free Orange Flavor METAMUCIL® Powder
[met "uh-mū 'sil]
(psyllium hydrophilic mucilloid)

Description: Sugar Free Orange Flavor Metamucil is a bulk forming natural therapeutic fiber for restoring and maintaining regularity. It contains refined hydrophilic mucilloid, a highly efficient dietary fiber derived from the husk of the psyllium seed (Plantago ovata), which has been sweetened with NutraSweet®* brand sweetener (aspartame). It contains no chemical stimulants or sugar and is non-addictive. Each dose contains approximately 3.4 g of psyllium hydrophilic mucilloid. Inactive ingredients include aspartame, citric acid, FD&C Yellow No. 6, flavoring, maltodextrin, and silicon dioxide. Each dose contains about 5 calories, less than 10 mg. of sodium, 31 mg of potassium, and 30 mg of phenylalanine. Carbohydrate content is approximately 1.4 grams.

Actions: Metamucil provides a bland, nonirritating bulk and promotes normal elimination. It is uniform, instantly miscible, palatable, and nonirritative in the gastrointestinal tract.

Indications: Metamucil is indicated in the management of chronic constipation, in irritable bowel syndrome, as adjunctive therapy in the constipation of duodenal ulcer and diverticular disease, in the bowel management of patients with hemorrhoids, and for constipation during pregnancy, convalescence, and senility.

Contraindications: Intestinal obstruction, fecal impaction.

Warning: Phenylketonurics should be aware that Sugar Free Metamucil contains phenylalanine.

Precautions: May cause allergic reaction in people sensitive to inhaled or ingested psyllium powder.

Dosage and Administration: The usual adult dosage is one rounded teaspoonful (5.2 g) stirred into a standard 8-oz glass of cool water, fruit juice, milk or other beverage. It can be taken orally one to three times a day, depending on the need and response. It may require continued use for 2 or 3 days to provide optimal benefit. An additional glass of liquid after each dose is helpful. For children (6–12 years old), use ½ the adult dose in 8 oz. of liquid. 1 to 3 times daily.

How Supplied: Powder, containers of 4.7 oz, 8.7 oz, 12.9 oz, and 20.7 oz (OTC).

*NutraSweet is a registered trademark of the NutraSweet Company.
Shown in Product Identification Section, page 420

Sugar Free Lemon-Lime Flavor EFFERVESCENT METAMUCIL®
[met "uh-mū 'sil]
(psyllium hydrophilic mucilloid)

Description: Sugar Free Lemon-Lime Flavor Effervescent Metamucil is a bulk forming natural therapeutic fiber for restoring and maintaining regularity. It contains refined hydrophilic mucilloid, a highly efficient dietary fiber derived from the husk of the psyllium seed (Plantago ovata), which has been sweetened with NutraSweet®* brand sweetener (aspartame). It contains no chemical stimulants or sugar. Each dose contains approximately 3.4 g of psyllium hydrophilic mucilloid. Inactive ingredients include aspartame, calcium carbonate, citric acid, flavoring, potassium bicarbonate, silicon dioxide, and sodium bicarbonate. Each packet provides less than 1 calorie, 290 mg of potassium, less than 10 mg. of sodium, and 30 mg phenylalanine.

Actions: Effervescent Metamucil provides a bland, nonirritating bulk and promotes normal elimination. It is effervescent and requires no stirring. It is uniform, instantly miscible, palatable, and nonirritative in the gastrointestinal tract.

Indications: Effervescent Metamucil is indicated in the management of chronic constipation, in irritable bowel syndrome, as adjunctive therapy in the constipation of duodenal ulcer and diverticular disease, in the bowel management of patients with hemorrhoids, and for constipation during pregnancy, convalescence, and senility.

Contraindications: Intestinal obstruction, fecal impaction.

Warning: Phenylketonurics should be aware that Sugar Free Effervescent Metamucil contains phenylalanine.

Precaution: May cause allergic reaction in people sensitive to inhaled or ingested psyllium powder.

Dosage and Administration: The usual adult dosage is the contents of one packet (0.19 oz.) taken one to three times daily. The entire contents of a packet are poured into a standard 8-oz glass. The glass is slowly filled with cool water, fruit juice, milk or beverage. Drink promptly. An additional glass of liquid after each dose is helpful.

How Supplied: Cartons of 30 single-dose (0.19 oz.) packets (OTC); also available in cartons of 100 single-dose (0.19 oz.) packets.

*NutraSweet is a registered trademark of the NutraSweet Company.
Shown in Product Identification Section, page 420

Sugar Free Orange Flavor EFFERVESCENT METAMUCIL®
[met "uh-mū 'sil]
(psyllium hydrophilic mucilloid)

Description: Sugar Free Orange Flavor Effervescent Metamucil is a bulk forming natural therapeutic fiber for restoring and maintaining regularity. It contains refined hydrophilic mucilloid, a highly efficient dietary fiber derived from the husk of the psyllium seed (Plantago ovata), which has been sweetened with NutraSweet®* brand sweetener (aspartame). It contains no chemical stimulants or sugar and is non-addictive. Each dose contains approximately 3.4 g of psyllium hydrophilic mucilloid. Inactive ingredients include aspartame, citric acid, FD&C Yellow No. 6, flavoring, potassium bicarbonate, silicon dioxide, and sodium bicarbonate. Each packet provides less than 1 calorie, 310 mg of potassium, less than 10 mg. of sodium, and 30 mg phenylalanine.

Actions: Effervescent Metamucil provides a bland, nonirritating bulk and promotes normal elimination. It is effervescent and requires no stirring. It is uniform, instantly miscible, palatable, and nonirritative in the gastrointestinal tract.

Indications: Effervescent Metamucil is indicated in the management of chronic constipation, in irritable bowel syndrome, as adjunctive therapy in the constipation of duodenal ulcer and diverticular disease, in the bowel management of patients with hemorrhoids, and for constipation during pregnancy, convalescence, and senility.

Contraindications: Intestinal obstruction, fecal impaction.

Warning: Phenylketonurics should be aware that Sugar Free Effervescent Metamucil contains phenylalanine.

Precaution: May cause allergic reaction in people sensitive to inhaled or ingested psyllium powder.

Dosage and Administration: The usual adult dosage is the contents of one packet (0.18 oz.) taken one to three times daily. The entire contents of a packet are poured into a standard 8-oz glass. The glass is slowly filled with cool water, fruit juice, milk or beverage. Drink promptly. An additional glass of liquid after each dose is helpful.

How Supplied: Cartons of 30 single-dose (0.18 oz) packets OTC.

*NutraSweet is a registered trademark of the NutraSweet Company.
Shown in Product Identification Section, page 420

PEPTO–BISMOL®
LIQUID AND TABLETS
For diarrhea, heartburn, indigestion, upset stomach and nausea.

Description: Each Pepto-Bismol Tablet contains 262 mg bismuth subsalicylate and each tablespoonful (15 ml) of Pepto-Bismol Liquid contains 262 mg bismuth subsalicylate. Each tablet contains 102 mg salicylate and each tablespoonful of liquid contains 130 mg salicylate. Liquid and tablets contain no sugar. Tablets are sodium-free (less than 2 mg/tablet) and Liquid is low in sodium

(5 mg/tablespoonful). Inactive ingredients include (Tablets): calcium carbonate, FD&C Red. No. 3 aluminum lake, flavor, magnesium stearate, mannitol, povidone, saccharin sodium and talc; (Liquid): FD&C Red No. 3, FD&C Red No 40, flavor, magnesium aluminum silicate, methylcellulose, saccharin sodium, salicylic acid, sodium salicylate and water.

Indications: Pepto-Bismol controls diarrhea within 24 hours, relieving associated abdominal cramps; soothes heartburn and indigestion without constipating; and relieves nausea and upset stomach.

Caution: This product contains salicylates. If taken with aspirin and ringing of the ears occurs, discontinue use. This product does not contain aspirin, but should not be administered to those patients who have a known allergy to aspirin or salicylates. Caution is advised in the administration to patients taking medication for anticoagulation, diabetes and gout.

Warning: Consult a physician before giving this medication to children, including teenagers, during or after recovery from chicken pox or flu. As with any drug, if you are pregnant or nursing a baby, seek the advice of a health professional before taking this product. KEEP THIS AND ALL MEDICATIONS OUT OF THE REACH OF CHILDREN.
Note: This medication may cause a harmless darkening of the tongue and/or stool. Stool darkening should not be confused with melena.

Dosage and Administration:
Tablets:
Adults—Two tablets
Children (according to age)—
  9–12 yrs.   1 tablet
  6–9 yrs.   ⅔ tablet
  3–6 yrs.   ⅓ tablet
Chew or dissolve in mouth. Repeat every ½ to 1 hour as needed, to a maximum of 8 doses in a 24-hour period.
Liquid: Shake well before using.
Adults—2 tablespoonfuls
Children (according to age)—
  9–12 yrs.   1 tablespoonful
  6–9 yrs.   2 teaspoonfuls
  3–6 yrs.   1 teaspoonful
Repeat dosage every ½ to 1 hour, if needed, to a maximum of 8 doses in a 24-hour period.
For children under 3 years, dose according to weight.
  28+ lbs.   1 teaspoonful
  14–18 lbs.   ½ teaspoonful
Repeat every 4 hours, if needed, to a maximum of 6 doses in a 24-hour period.

How Supplied:
Pepto-Bismol Liquid is available in:
  NDC 37000-032-01   4 fl. oz. bottle
  NDC 37000-032-02   8 fl. oz. bottle
  NDC 37000-032-03   12 fl. oz. bottle
  NDC 37000-032-04   16 fl. oz. bottle
Pepto-Bismol Tablets are pink triangular chewable tablets imprinted with "Pepto-Bismol" on one side and "NE" on the other. Tablets are available in:

NDC 37000-033-03   box of 24
NDC 37000-033-04   box of 42
Shown in Product Identification Section, page 421

MAXIMUM STRENGTH PEPTO–BISMOL® LIQUID

For diarrhea, heartburn, indigestion, upset stomach and nausea.

Description: Each tablespoonful (15 ml) of Maximum Strength Pepto-Bismol Liquid contains 525 mg bismuth subsalicylate. Each tablespoonful of liquid contains 230 mg salicylate. Maximum Strength Pepto-Bismol Liquid contains no sugar and is low in sodium (less than 5 mg/tablespoonful). Inactive ingredients include: FD&C Red No. 3, FD&C Red No. 40, flavor, magnesium aluminum silicate, methylcellulose, saccharin sodium, salicylic acid, sodium salicylate, and water.

Indications: Maximum Strength Pepto-Bismol controls diarrhea within 24 hours, relieving associated abdominal cramps; soothes heartburn and indigestion without constipating; and relieves nausea and upset stomach.

Caution: This product contains salicylates. If taken with aspirin and ringing of the ears occurs, discontinue use. This product does not contain aspirin, but should not be administered to those patients who have a known allergy to aspirin or salicylates. Caution is advised in the administration to patients taking medication for anticoagulation, diabetes, and gout.

Warning: Consult a physician before giving this medication to children, including teenagers, during or after recovery from chicken pox or flu. As with any drug, if you are pregnant or nursing a baby, seek the advice of a health professional before taking this product. KEEP THIS AND ALL MEDICATION OUT OF THE REACH OF CHILDREN.
Note: This medication may cause a temporary and harmless darkening of the stool. Stool darkening should not be confused with melena.

Dosage and Administration: Shake well before using.
Adults—2 tablespoonfuls
Children (according to age)—
  9–12 yrs.   1 tablespoonful
  6–9 yrs.   2 teaspoonfuls
  3–6 yrs.   1 teaspoonful
Repeat dosage every hour, if needed, to a maximum of 4 doses in a 24 hour period.

How Supplied: Maximum Strength Pepto-Bismol is available in:
  NDC 37000-019-01   4 fl. oz. bottle
  NDC 37000-019-02   8 fl. oz. bottle
  NDC 37000-019-03   12 fl. oz. bottle
Shown in Product Identification Section, page 421

Reed & Carnrick
1 NEW ENGLAND AVENUE
PISCATAWAY, NJ 08855

PHAZYME® and PHAZYME®–95 Tablets

Description: A two-phase tablet. Contains specially-activated simethicone, both in the outer layer for release in the stomach and in the inner enteric-coated core for release in the small intestine.

Actions: PHAZYME is the only dual-approach to the problem of gastrointestinal gas. Simethicone minimizes gas formation and relieves gas entrapment in both the stomach and the lower G.I. tract. This action helps combat pain, due to gastrointestinal gas. Also, for relief of gas distress associated with other functional or organic conditions such as: diverticulitis, spastic colitis, hyperacidity, postcholecystectomy syndrome and chronic cholecystitis.

Indications: PHAZYME is indicated for the relief of occasional or chronic pain caused by gas entrapped in the stomach or in the lower gastrointestinal tract—resulting from aerophagia, postoperative distention, dyspepsia and food intolerance.

Contraindications: A known sensitivity to any ingredient.

PHAZYME
Contains: Active ingredient: Specially-activated simethicone, both in the outer layer for release in the stomach and in the inner enteric-coated core for release in the small intestine, a total of 60 mg.
Inactive ingredients: Acacia, Calcium Sulfate, Carnauba Wax, Crospovidone, D&C Red No. 7 Lake, FD&C Blue No. 1 Lake, Gelatin, Lactose, Microcrystalline, Cellulose, Polyoxyl-40 Stearate, Polyvinyl Acetate Phthalate, Povidone, Pregelatinized Starch, Rice Starch, Sodium Benzoate, Sucrose, Titanium Dioxide.

Dosage: One or two tablets with each meal and at bedtime, or as directed by a physician.

How Supplied: Pink coated two-phase tablet in bottles of 50 and 100.

PHAZYME-95
Contains: Active ingredient: Specially-activated simethicone, both in the outer layer for release in the stomach and in the inner enteric-coated core for release in the small intestine, a total of 95 mg.
Inactive ingredient: Acacia, Calcium Sulfate, Carnauba Wax, Crospovidone, FD&C Yellow No. 6 Lake, FD&C Red No. 40 Lake, Gelatin, Lactose, Microcrystalline Cellulose, Polyoxyl-40 Stearate, Pol-

Continued on next page

Reed & Carnrick—Cont.

yvinyl Acetate Phthalate, Povidone, Pregelatinized Starch, Rice Starch, Sodium Benzoate, Sucrose, Titanium Dioxide.

Dosage: One tablet with each meal and at bedtime, or as directed by a physician.

How Supplied: Red coated two-phase tablet in 10 pack, bottles of 50 and 100.
Shown in Product Identification Section, page 421

Maximum Strength PHAZYME®–125 Capsules

Description: A red softgel containing the highest dose of simethicone available in a single capsule.

Active Ingredients: Simethicone 125 mg.

Inactive Ingredients: Soybean oil, gelatin, glycerin, vegetable shortening, polysorbate 80, purified water, hydrogenated soybean oil, yellow wax, lecithin, titanium dioxide, FD&C Red #40, methylparaben, propylparaben.

Actions: Simethicone minimizes gas formation and relieves gas entrapment in both the stomach and the lower G.I. tract. This action combats pain, due to gastrointestinal gas. Also, for relief of gas distress associated with other functional or organic conditions such as diverticulitis, spastic colitis, hyperacidity, post-cholecystectomy syndrome and chronic cholecystitis.

Indications: PHAZYME-125 is indicated for the relief of acute severe lower intestinal pain due to gas—resulting from aerophagia, postoperative distention, dyspepsia and food intolerance.

Contraindications: A known sensitivity to any ingredient.

Dosage: One capsule with each meal and at bedtime, or as directed by a physician.

How Supplied: Red capsule in bottles of 50 and consumer 10 pack.
Rev. 8/87
Shown in Product Identification Section, page 421

proctoFoam®/non-steroid (pramoxine HCl 1%)

Description: proctoFoam is a foam for anal and perianal use.

Composition: Active ingredients: Pramoxine Hydrochloride 1%.

Inactive Ingredients: Butane, Cetyl Alcohol, Emulsifying Wax, Methylparaben, Mineral Oil, Polysorbate 60, Propane, Propylparaben, Sorbitan Seoquiolate, Trolamine, Water.

Actions: proctoFoam is an anesthetic mucoadhesive foam which medicates the anorectal mucosa, and provides prompt temporary relief from itching and pain. Its lubricating action helps make bowel evacuations more comfortable.

Indications: Prompt, temporary relief of anorectal inflammation, pruritus and pain associated with hemorrhoids, proctitis, cryptitis, fissures, postoperative pain and pruritus ani.

Contraindications: Contraindicated in persons hypersensitive to any of the ingredients.

Warning: Not for prolonged use. Do not use more than four consecutive weeks. If redness, pain, irritation or swelling persists or rectal bleeding occurs, discontinue use and consult a physician. Keep this and all medicines out of the reach of children.

Caution: Do not insert any part of the aerosol container into the anus. Contents of the container are under pressure, but not flammable. Do not burn or puncture the aerosol container. Store at room temperature not over 120° F.

Dosage:
One applicatorful two or three times daily and after bowel evacuation.
1. To fill—Shake foam container vigorously before use. Hold container upright and insert into opening of applicator tip. With applicator drawn out all the way, press down on container cap. When the foam reaches fill line in the applicator, it is ready to use.
CAUTION: The aerosol container should never be inserted directly into the anus.
2. To administer—Separate applicator from container. Hold applicator by barrel and gently insert tip into the anus. With applicator in place, push plunger in order to expel foam, then withdraw applicator. (Applicator parts should be pulled apart for thorough cleaning with warm water.)
Note: To relieve itching place some foam on a tissue and apply externally.

How Supplied: Available in 15 g aerosol container, with special plastic applicator. The aerosol supplies approximately 18 applications.

Literature Available: Instruction pads with directions for use available upon request.
Shown in Product Identification Section, page 421

R&C SHAMPOO®
Shampoo Pediculicide

Description: R&C SHAMPOO is a one-step pediculicide shampoo available without a prescription. Its active ingredients are: pyrethrins 0.30%, piperonyl butoxide technical 3.00%, equivalent to 2.40% (butycarbityl) (6-propylpiperonyl) ether and 0.60% related compounds, petroleum distillate 1.20%. Inert ingredients 95.50%.

Action: R&C SHAMPOO kills head lice (pediculus capitis), crab lice (phthirus pubis) and body lice (pediculus corporis) and their eggs.

Indications: R&C SHAMPOO is indicated for the treatment of infestations with head lice, crab lice and body lice.

Warning: R&C SHAMPOO should not be used by ragweed sensitized persons.

Caution: R&C SHAMPOO is for external use only. It can be harmful if swallowed or inhaled. It should be kept out of eyes and avoid contact with mucous membranes. If accidental contact with eyes occurs, flush immediately with water. In case of infection or skin irritation, discontinue use and consult a physician. Consult a physician if louse infestation of eyebrows and eyelashes occurs. Avoid contamination of feed or foodstuffs.

Storage and Disposal:
Storage: Store below 120°F.
Disposal: Do not reuse container. Rinse thoroughly before discarding in trash.

Dosage and Administration: (1) Apply a sufficient quantity of R&C SHAMPOO to throughly wet dry hair and skin, paying particular attention to the infested and adjacent hairy areas. (2) Allow R&C SHAMPOO to remain on the area for 10 minutes. (3) Add small quantities of water, working the shampoo into the hair and skin until a lather forms. (4) Rinse thoroughly. Dead lice and eggs will require removal with fine-tooth comb. If necessary, treatment may be repeated but do not exceed two consecutive applications within 24 hrs.
Since lice infestations are spread by contact, each family member should be examined carefully. If infested, he or she should be treated promptly to avoid spreading or reinfestation of previously treated individuals.
To eliminate infestation, it is important to wash all clothing, bedding, towels and combs and brushes, used by the infested person in hot water (130°). Dry clean nonwashable items.

How Supplied: In 2 and 4 fl oz. plastic bottles with pourable cap. Fine-tooth comb to aid in removal of dead lice and nits and patient booklet are included in each package of R&C SHAMPOO.

Literature Available: Patient information available on request.
Rev. 8/84
Shown in Product Identification Section, page 421

R&C SPRAY® III Lice Control Insecticide

Description: Active ingredients: 3-Phenoxybenzyl d-cis and trans 2,2-dimethyl-3-(2-methylpropenyl) cyclopropanecarboxylate

cyclopropanecarboxylate	0.382%
Other Isomers	0.018%
Petroleum Distillates	4.255%
Inert Ingredients:	95.345%
	100.000%

Actions: R&C SPRAY is specially formulated to kill lice and their nits on inanimate objects.

Indications: R&C SPRAY is recommended for use only on bedding, mattresses, furniture and other objects infested or possibly infested with lice

which cannot be laundered or dry cleaned.

Warnings: Contents under pressure. Do not use or store near heat or open flame. Do not puncture or incinerate container. Exposure to temperatures above 130°F may cause bursting. It is a violation of Federal law to use this product in a manner inconsistent with its labeling. NOT FOR USE ON HUMANS OR ANIMALS.

Caution: Avoid spraying in eyes. Avoid breathing spray mist. Avoid contact with the skin. May be absorbed through the skin. In case of contact, wash immediately with soap and water. Harmful if swallowed. Vacate room after treatment and ventilate before reoccupying. Avoid contamination of feed and foodstuffs. Remove pets, birds and cover fish aquariums before spraying.

Directions: SHAKE WELL BEFORE AND OCCASIONALLY DURING USE. Spray on an inconspicuous area to test for possible staining or discoloration. Inspect after drying, then proceed to spray entire area to be treated.
Hold container upright with nozzle away from you. Depress valve and spray from a distance of 8 to 10 inches.
Spray each square foot for about three seconds. For mattresses, furniture, or similar objects (that cannot be laundered or dry cleaned): Spray thoroughly. Do not use article until spray is dry. Repeat treatment as necessary. Do not use in commercial food processing, preparation, storage or serving areas.

Storage and Disposal:
Storage: Store in a cool area away from heat or open flame.
Disposal: Wrap container and put in trash.

How Supplied: In 5 oz. and 10 oz. aerosol container.
Shown in Product Identification Section, page 421

EDUCATIONAL MATERIAL

Brochures
Questions and Answers About Head Lice
Available in English and Spanish to physicians, pharmacists and patients.
Questions and Answers About Treating Lice That Can Live Off the Body
Available to physicians, pharmacists and patients.
Gas Pain
A brochure about what gas pain is, why it hurts, and how to control it. Available to physicians, pharmacists and patients.

Products are cross-indexed by generic and chemical names in the
YELLOW SECTION

Reid-Rowell
**901 SAWYER ROAD
MARIETTA, GA 30062
AND
210 MAIN STREET W.
BAUDETTE, MN 56623**

BALNEOL®
[băl′nē-ŏl]
Perianal cleansing lotion

Composition: Contains water, mineral oil, propylene glycol, glyceryl stearate/PEG-100 stearate, PEG-40 stearate, laureth-4, PEG-4 dilaurate, lanolin oil, sodium acetate, carbomer-934, triethanolamine, methylparaben, dioctyl sodium sulfosuccinate, fragrance, acetic acid.

Action and Uses: BALNEOL is a soothing, emollient cleanser for hygienic cleansing of irritated perianal and external vaginal areas. It helps relieve itching and other discomforts. BALNEOL gently yet thoroughly cleanses and provides a soothing, protecting film.

Administration and Dosage: For cleansing without discomfort after each bowel movement, a small amount of BALNEOL is spread on tissue or cotton and used to wipe the perianal area. Also used between bowel movements and at bedtime for additional comfort. For cleansing and soothing the external vaginal area: to be used on clean tissue or cotton as often as necessary.

Caution: In all cases of rectal bleeding, consult physician promptly. If irritation persists or increases, discontinue use and consult physician.

How Supplied: 3 fl oz (89 mL) plastic bottle.
Shown in Product Identification Section, page 421

HYDROCIL® INSTANT
[hī′dro-sĭl]

Description: A concentrated hydrophilic mucilloid containing 95% psyllium. Inactive ingredients: polyethylene glycol and povidone. Hydrocil Instant mixes instantly, is sugar-free, low in potassium and contains less than 10 mg of sodium per dose.

Indications: Hydrocil Instant is a natural bulk forming fiber useful in the treatment of constipation and other conditions as directed by a physician.

Directions: The usual adult dose is one packet or scoopful poured into an 8 oz glass. Add water, fruit juices or other liquid and stir. It mixes instantly. Drink immediately. Take in the morning and night or as directed by a physician. Follow each dose with another glass of liquid.

How Supplied: In unit-dose packets of 3.7 grams that are available in boxes of 30's or 500's. Also in 250 gram jars with a measuring scoop. Each packet or scoopful, 3.7 grams, contains one usual adult dose of psyllium hydrophilic mucilloid, 3.5 grams.
Rev. 8/88
Shown in Product Identification Section, page 421

Requa, Inc.
**BOX 4008
1 SENECA PLACE
GREENWICH, CT 06830**

CHARCOAID
Poison Adsorbent, liquid- has sweet, pleasant taste and feel; especially good for young patients.

Active Ingredient: Activated vegetable charcoal U.S.P., 30g per bottle, suspended in 70% sorbitol solution U.S.P., 110 g.

Indication: For the emergency treatment of acute poisoning.

Action: Adsorbent

Warnings: Before using call a poison control center, emergency room, or a physician for advice. If the patient has been given Ipecac Syrup, do not give activated charcoal until after patient has vomited. Do not use in a semi-conscious or unconscious person.

Precaution: May cause laxation. Careful attention to fluids and electrolytes is important, especially with young children and multiple dose therapy.

Dosage and Administration: Adults: Shake well and drink entire contents (add water if too sweet). To insure a full dose, rinse bottle with water and drink. For children, refer to Poison Control Center.

Professional Labeling: Some dilution may be necessary for administration via lavage tube. Add a small amount of water to bottle and shake.

How Supplied: 5 fl. oz. unit dose bottle, 30g activated charcoal U.S.P., suspended in 70% sorbitol solution U.S.P., 110 g.
U.S. Patent #4,122,169

CHARCOCAPS®
Activated Charcoal Capsules

Active Ingredient: Activated vegetable charcoal U.S.P., 260 mg per capsule.

Indications: Relief of intestinal gas, diarrhea, gastrointestinal distress associated with indigestion. Also to aid in the prevention of non-specific pruritus associated with kidney dialysis treatment.

Actions: Adsorbent, detoxicant, soothing agent. Reduces the volume of intestinal gas and allays related discomfort.

Warnings: As with all anti-diarrheals—not for children under 3 unless directed by physician. If diarrhea persists more than two days or is accompanied by high fever, consult physician.

Continued on next page

Requa—Cont.

Drug Interaction: Activated Charcoal USP can adsorb medication while they are in the digestive tract.

Precaution: General Guidelines— Take two hours before or one hour after medication including oral contraceptives.

Symptoms and Treatment of Oral Overdosage: Overdosage has not been encountered. Medical evidence indicates that high dosage or prolonged use does not cause side effect or harm the nutritional state of the patient.

Dosage and Administration: Two capsules after meals or at first sign of discomfort. Repeat as needed up to eight doses (16 capsules) per day.

Professional Labeling: None.

How Supplied: Bottles of 8, 36, 100 capsules

EDUCATIONAL MATERIAL

Questions & Answers
Brochure with questions and answers about the use of activated charcoal.
Trial Size
Professional sample of Charcocaps, which includes coupon for regular size for the patient.

Richardson-Vicks USA
**HEALTH CARE PRODUCTS DIVISION
TEN WESTPORT ROAD
WILTON, CT 06897**

CHILDREN'S CHLORASEPTIC® LOZENGES

Active Ingredients: Benzocaine 5 mg per lozenge in a grape flavored base.

Inactive Ingredients: Corn syrup, FD&C Blue #1, FD&C Red #4, flavor, glycerine, sucrose.

Indications: Children's Chloreseptic's Lozenges provide prompt, temporary relief of minor sore throat pain which may accompany conditions such as tonsillitis, pharyngitis and in posttonsillectomy soreness, and discomfort of minor mouth and gum irritations.

Dosage and Administration: Allow one lozenge to dissolve slowly in the mouth. Repeat hourly if needed. Do not take more than 12 lozenges per day.

Consumer labeling contains the following statements:
Warning: Severe or persistent sore throat accompanied by high fever, headache, nausea, and vomiting may be serious. Consult physician promptly. Do not use more than 2 days or administer to children under 3 years of age unless directed by a physician. In case of acciden-

tal overdose, seek professional assistance or contact a poison control center immediately. As with any drug, if you are pregnant or nursing a baby, seek the advice of a health professional before using this product.
Store at room temperature.
KEEP THIS AND ALL MEDICINES OUT OF THE REACH OF CHILDREN.

How Supplied: Cartons of 18.
Shown in Product Identification Section, page 421

CHLORASEPTIC® LIQUID (oral anesthetic, antiseptic) Cherry and Menthol Flavors

Active Ingredients: Phenol and sodium phenolate (total phenol 1.4%).

Inactive Ingredients:
CHERRY: FD&C Red #40, Flavor, Glycerine, Saccharin Sodium and Water.
MENTHOL: D&C Green #5, D&C Yellow #10, FD&C Green #3, Flavor, Glycerine, Saccharin Sodium, and Water.

Indications: Chloraseptic provides fast, temporary relief of occasional minor sore throat pain and irritations, and discomfort of minor mouth and gum irritations. It is also an effective deodorizing mouthwash for maintaining oral hygiene.
Chloraseptic's anesthetic and antiseptic formula is a valuable adjunct to systemic antibacterial therapy for prompt, temporary relief of minor oral pain and discomfort.
Chloraseptic is indicated for prompt, temporary relief of discomfort due to the following conditions: *Medical:* oropharyngitis and throat infections; acute tonsillitis; and post-tonsillectomy soreness; *Dental:* minor irritations or injury of soft tissue of the mouth; minor oral surgery or extractions; irritation caused by dentures or orthodontic appliances; and aphthous ulcers.

Administration and Dosage:
Chloraseptic Spray (Pump), Mouthwash and Gargle—*Irritated throat:* Spray 5 times (children 3–12 years of age, 3 times) and swallow. May be used as a gargle. Repeat every 2 hours if necessary. *After oral surgery:* Allow full-strength solution to run over affected areas for 15 seconds without swishing, then expel remainder. Repeat every 2 hours if necessary. *Oral Hygiene:* Dilute with equal parts of water and rinse thoroughly, or spray full strength, then expel remainder.
Chloraseptic Aerosol Spray: *Irritated throat:* Spray throat about 2 seconds (children 3–12 years about 1 second) and swallow. Repeat every 2 hours if necessary.
Consumer labeling contains the following statement:
Warning: Severe or persistent sore throat or sore throat accompanied by high fever, headache, nausea, and vomiting may be serious. Consult physician promptly. Do not use more than 2 days or administer to children under 3 years of age unless directed by physician. In case

of accidental overdose, seek professional assistance or contact a poison control center immediately. As with any drug, if you are pregnant or nursing a baby, seek the advice of a health professional before using this product.
Store at room temperature.
KEEP THIS AND ALL MEDICINES OUT OF THE REACH OF CHILDREN.

Warning: For 1.5 oz. Aerosol Spray— Avoid spraying in eyes. Contents under pressure. Do not puncture, incinerate or burn in fire.

How Supplied: Available in Menthol and Cherry flavor in 6 fl. oz. bottles with sprayer, 12 fl. oz. refill bottles and 1.5 oz. nitrogen propelled aerosol sprays.
Shown in Product Identification Section, page 421

CHLORASEPTIC® LOZENGES Cherry and Menthol Flavor

Active Ingredients: Phenol and Sodium Phenolate (total phenol 32.5 mg / Lozenge).

Inactive Ingredients:
CHERRY: Corn syrup, FD&C Blue #1, FD&C Red #40, Flavor, Sodium Hydroxide, and Sucrose.
MENTHOL: Corn Syrup, D&C Yellow #10, FD&C Blue #1, FD&C Yellow #6, Flavor and Sucrose.

Indications: Chloraseptic Lozenges provide temporary relief of discomfort due to minor sore throat and mouth and gum irritations. They also may be used for topical anesthesia as an adjunct to systemic antibacterial therapy. For prompt temporary relief of pain and discomfort associated with the following conditions: *Medical*—oropharyngitis and throat infections; acute tonsillitis; and post-tonsillectomy soreness; *Dental*—minor irritation or injury of soft tissue of the mouth; minor oral surgery; and aphthous ulcers.

Administration and Dosage: Adults and children over 3 years of age: Dissolve 1 lozenge in the mouth every 2 hours. Children under 12 years, do not exceed 8 lozenges per day.

Warning: Severe or persistent sore throat or sore throat accompanied by high fever, headache, nausea, and vomiting may be serious. Consult physician promptly. Do not use more than 2 days or administer to children under 3 years of age unless directed by a physician. In case of accidental overdose, seek professional assistance or contact a poison control center immediately. As with any drug, if you are pregnant or nursing a baby, seek the advice of a health professional before using this product.
Store at room temperature.
KEEP ALL MEDICINES OUT OF REACH OF CHILDREN.

How Supplied: Available in menthol or cherry flavor. In packages of 18 and 36.
Shown in Product Identification Section, page 421

DRAMAMINE® Liquid
[*dram'uh-meen*]
(dimenhydrinate syrup USP)
DRAMAMINE® Tablets
(dimenhydrinate USP)
DRAMAMINE® Chewable Tablets
(dimenhydrinate USP)

Description: Dimenhydrinate is the chlorotheophylline salt of the antihistaminic agent diphenhydramine. Dimenhydrinate contains not less than 53% and not more than 56% of diphenhydramine, and not less than 44% and not more than 47% of 8-chlorotheophylline, calculated on the dried basis.

Inactive Ingredients:
Dramamine Tablets: Acacia, Carboxymethylcellulose Sodium, Corn Starch, Magnesium Stearate, and Sodium Sulfate.
Dramamine Liquid: Cherry Flavor, FD&C Red #40, Ethyl Alcohol 5%, Glycerin, Methylparaben, Sucrose, and Water.
Dramamine Chewable Tablets: Aspartame, Citric Acid, FD&C Yellow #5, FD&C Yellow #6, Flavor, Magnesium Stearate, Methacrylic Acid Copolymer, Sorbitol.
Phenylketonurics: Contains Phenylalanine 1.5 mg per tablet.

Actions: While the precise mode of action of dimenhydrinate is not known, it has a depressant action on hyperstimulated labyrinthine function.

Indications: Dramamine is indicated for the prevention and treatment of the nausea, vomiting, dizziness or vertigo associated with motion sickness. Such an illness may arise from the motion of ships, planes, trains, automobiles, buses, swings, or even amusement park rides. Regardless of the cause of motion sickness, Dramamine has been found to be effective in its prevention or treatment.

Warnings: DRAMAMINE may cause marked drowsiness; alcohol, sedatives, and tranquilizers may increase the drowsiness effect. Avoid alcoholic beverages while taking this product. Do not take this product if you are taking sedatives or tranquilizers, without first consulting your doctor. Use caution when driving a motor vehicle or operating machinery. Do not take this product if you have asthma, glaucoma, emphysema, chronic pulmonary disease, shortness of breath, difficulty in breathing, or difficulty in urination due to enlargement of the prostate gland unless directed by a doctor. Do not give to children under 2 years of age unless directed by a doctor. In case of accidental overdose, seek professional assistance or consult a poison control center immediately. As with any drug, if you are pregnant or nursing a baby, seek the advice of a health professional before using this product. Keep this and all medications out of the reach of children.

Dosage and Administration
Dramamine Tablets: To prevent motion sickness, the first dose should be taken ½ to 1 hour before starting the activity. Additional medication depends on travel conditions. *Adults:* 1 to 2 tablets every 4 to 6 hours, not to exceed 8 tablets in 24 hours. *Children 6 to 12 years:* ½ to 1 tablet every 6 to 8 hours, not to exceed 3 tablets in 24 hours. *Children 2 to 6 years:* Up to ½ tablet every 6 to 8 hours, not to exceed 1½ tablets in 24 hours. Children may also be given Dramamine cherry-flavored liquid in accordance with directions for use. Not for frequent or prolonged use except on advice of a physician. Do not exceed recommended dosage.
Dramamine Liquid: To prevent motion sickness, the first dose should be taken ½ to 1 hour before starting the activity. Additional medication depends on travel conditions. *Adults:* 4 to 8 teaspoonfuls (4 ml per teaspoonful) every 4 to 6 hours, not to exceed 32 teaspoonfuls in 24 hours. *Children 6 to 12 years:* 2 to 4 teaspoonfuls every 6 to 8 hours, not to exceed 12 teaspoonfuls in 24 hours. *Children 2 to 6 years:* 1 to 2 teaspoonfuls every 6 to 8 hours, not to exceed 6 teaspoonfuls in 24 hours. *Children under 2 years:* Only on advice of a physician.
Not for frequent or prolonged use except on advice of a physician. Do not exceed recommended dosage. Use of a measuring device is recommended for all liquid medication.
Dramamine Chewable Tablets: To prevent motion sickness, the first dose should be taken one-half to one hour before starting the activity. Additional medication depends on travel conditions. *Adults:* 1 to 2 tablets every 4 to 6 hours.

How Supplied: *Tablets* —scored, white tablets containing 50 mg of dimenhydrinate. Available in packets of 12 and 36 and bottles of 100 (OTC); *Liquid* —12.5 mg dimenhydrinate per 4 ml, ethyl alcohol 5%, bottles of 3 fl oz (OTC).
Shown in Product Identification Section, page 421

ICY HOT® Balm
[*ī'see hot*]
(topical analgesic balm)
ICY HOT® Cream
(topical analgesic cream)
ICY HOT® Stick
(topical analgesic stick)

Active Ingredients: Icy Hot Balm contains methyl salicylate 29%, menthol 7.6%. Icy Hot Cream contains methyl salicylate 30%, menthol 10%. Icy Hot Stick contains methyl salicylate 15%, menthol 8%.
Inactive ingredients of Icy Hot Balm include paraffin and white petrolatum. Inactive ingredients of Icy Hot Cream include carbomer, cetyl esters wax, emulsifying wax, oleth-3 phosphate, stearic acid, trolamine, and water. Inactive ingredients of Icy Hot Stick include ceresin, cyclomethicone, hydrogenated castor oil, microcrystalline wax, paraffin, PEG-150 distearate, propylene glycol, stearic acid, and stearyl alcohol.

Description: Icy Hot Balm, Icy Hot Cream, and Icy Hot Stick are topically applied analgesics containing two active ingredients, methyl salicylate and menthol. It is the particular concentration of these ingredients, in combination with inert ingredients, that results in the distinct, combined heating/cooling sensation of Icy Hot.

Actions: Icy Hot is classified as a counterirritant which, when rubbed into the intact skin, provides relief of deep-seated pain through a counterirritant action rather than through a direct analgesic effect. In acting as a counterirritant, Icy Hot replaces the perception of pain with another sensation that blocks deep pain temporarily by its action on or near the skin surface.

Indications: Icy Hot helps bring temporary relief from minor arthritis pain and its stiffness, helps temporarily block minor pain from simple backache, and helps soothe sore muscles.

Warnings: For external use only as directed. Keep away from children to avoid accidental poisoning. If swallowed, induce vomiting and call a physician immediately. For children under 12, consult a physician before use. Avoid contact with eyes, mouth, genitalia, and mucous membranes. Do not apply to wounds or to damaged, irritated or very sensitive skin. Diabetics and people with impaired circulation should use Icy Hot only upon the advice of a physician. Do not wrap, bandage or apply external heat or hot water. If condition worsens, or if symptoms persist for more than 7 days or clear up and occur again within a few days, discontinue use of this product and consult a physician.

Adverse Reactions: The most common adverse reactions that may occur with Icy Hot use are skin irritation and blistering. The most serious adverse reaction is severe toxicity that occurs if the product is ingested.

Dosage and Administration: Apply Icy Hot to the painful area; massage until Icy Hot is completely absorbed. Repeat as necessary up to four times daily.

How Supplied: Icy Hot Balm is available in jars in two sizes, 3½ oz and 7 oz. Icy Hot Cream is available in tubes in two sizes, 1¼ oz and 3 oz. Icy Hot Stick is available as a 1¾ oz stick.
Shown in Product Identification Section, page 422

PERCOGESIC®
[*pĕrkō-gē'zĭk*]
Analgesic Tablets

Description: Each tablet contains:
Acetaminophen ....325 mg
Phenyltoloxamine citrate ....30 mg

Inactive Ingredients: Cellulose, Flavor, FD&C Yellow No. 6, Hydroxypropyl Methylcellulose, Magnesium Stearate, Polyethylene Glycol, Povidone, Silica Gel, Starch, Stearic Acid, Sucrose.

Indications: For relief of pain and discomfort due to headache, for temporary relief of pain associated with muscle and joint soreness, neuralgia, sinusitis, mi-

Continued on next page

Richardson-Vicks—Cont.

nor menstrual cramps, the common cold, toothache, and minor aches and pains of rheumatism and arthritis.

Warning: May cause excitability especially in children. Do not take this product if you have asthma, glaucoma, emphysema, chronic pulmonary disease, shortness of breath, difficulty in breathing, or difficulty in urination due to enlargement of the prostate gland unless directed by a doctor. May cause drowsiness; alcohol, sedatives, and tranquilizers may increase the drowsiness effect. Avoid alcoholic beverages while taking this product. Do not take this product if you are taking sedatives or tranquilizers without first consulting your doctor. Use caution when driving a motor vehicle or operating machinery. Do not take this product for more than 10 days (adults), 5 days (children under 12). If symptoms persist, or new ones occur, consult your physician. Do not exceed recommended dosage because severe liver damage may occur. If pain persists for more than 10 days or redness is present, or in conditions affecting children under 12 years of age, consult a physician immediately. As with any drug, if you are pregnant or nursing a baby, seek the advice of a health professional before using this preparation.
KEEP OUT OF REACH OF CHILDREN.

Overdosage: In case of overdosage, seek professional assistance or contact a poison control center immediately.

Dosage and Administration:
ADULTS (12 years and over)—1 or 2 tablets every four hours. Maximum daily dose—8 tablets
CHILDREN (6–12 years)—one tablet every 4 hours. Maximum daily dose—4 tablets

How Supplied: Child-resistant bottles of 24 and 90 tablets and bottles of 50 tablets.

Shown in Product Identification Section, page 422

VICKS® CHILDREN'S COUGH SYRUP
Expectorant, Antitussive Cough Syrup

Active Ingredients per tsp. (5 ml.): Dextromethorphan Hydrobromide 3.5 mg., Guaifenesin 50 mg., in a red, cherry-flavored, syrup base. This product contains no alcohol.

Inactive Ingredients: Citric Acid, FD&C Green #3, FD&C Red #40, Flavor, Methylparaben, Propylene Glycol, Purified Water, Sodium Citrate, Sodium Saccharin, Sucrose.

Indications: Provides temporary relief of coughs due to colds, helps loosen phlegm and mucus in the upper chest and promote drainage of bronchial tubes so breathing is made easier. Coats and soothes a cough-irritated throat.

Actions: VICKS COUGH SYRUP is an antitussive, expectorant and demulcent. It calms, quiets coughs of colds, flu and bronchitis; loosens phlegm, promotes drainage of bronchial tubes; and coats and soothes a cough irritated throat.

Warning: Do not use for persistent cough, such as with asthma, emphysema, smoking, or cough with excessive phlegm, unless directed by a doctor. Persistent cough may indicate a serious condition. If cough persists past one week, recurs, or is accompanied by fever, rash or persistent headache, consult a doctor. In case of accidental overdose, seek professional assistance or contact a poison control center immediately. If you are pregnant or nursing a baby, seek the advice of a health professional before using this product.
As with all medicines, keep out of children's reach.

Overdosage: In case of accidental overdose seek professional assistance or contact a Poison Control Center immediately.

Dosage:
12 years and over: 4 teaspoonfuls
6–12 years: 2 teaspoonfuls
2–6 years: 1 teaspoonful
Repeat every 4 hours as needed.

How Supplied: Available in 4 fl. oz. bottles.

VICKS® COUGH SILENCERS
Cough Drops

Active Ingredients per drop: Dextromethorphan (expressed as Dextromethorphan Hydrobromide) 2.5 mg., Benzocaine 1 mg.

Inactive Ingredients: Corn Syrup, FD&C Blue #1, Silicon Dioxide, Sodium Chloride, Sucrose. Special Vicks Medication (menthol, anethole, peppermint oil) 0.35%. Contains FD&C Yellow No. 5 (tartrazine).

Indications: Temporarily relieves coughs due to colds, excessive smoking, dry or irritated throat.

Actions: VICKS COUGH SILENCERS are antitussive, local anesthetic and demulcent throat lozenges.

Warning: Do not take this product for persistent or chronic cough such as occurs with smoking, asthma, or emphysema, or if cough is accompanied by excessive phlegm (mucus) unless directed by a doctor. A persistent cough may be a sign of a serious condition. If cough persists for more than 2 days, tends to recur, or is accompanied by fever, rash or persistent headaches, consult a doctor. Do not use more than 2 days or administer to children under 3 years of age unless directed by a physician. As with any drug, if you are pregnant or nursing a baby, seek the advice of a health professional before using this product.

Overdosage: In case of accidental overdose, seek professional assistance or contact a Poison Control Center immediately.

Directions For Use: Age 12 and over: 4 drops every four hours. Dissolve in mouth one at a time. Do not exceed 48 in 24 hours or as directed by doctor. Ages 6 to under 12: 2 to 4 drops every four hours. Dissolve in mouth one at a time. Do not exceed 24 in 24 hours or as directed by doctor. Ages 2 to under 6: 1 or 2 drops every four hours. Dissolve in mouth one at a time. Do not exceed 12 in 24 hours or as directed by doctor. Children under 2, consult doctor.

How Supplied: Available in boxes of 14's.

VICKS DAYCARE® LIQUID
VICKS DAYCARE® CAPLETS
Multi-Symptom Colds Medicine

Active Ingredients: LIQUID — per fluid ounce (2 tbs.) or **CAPLET** — per **two** caplets, contains Acetaminophen 650 mg., Dextromethorphan HBr 20 mg., Pseudoephedrine Hydrochloride 60 mg., Guaifenesin 200 mg. DAYCARE LIQUID also contains Alcohol 10%.

Inactive Ingredients:
Liquid: Citric Acid, FD&C Yellow #6, Flavor, Glycerin, Propylene Glycol, Purified Water, Saccharin, Sodium Benzoate, Sodium Citrate, Sucrose.
Caplets: Cellulose, Croscarmellose Sodium, FD&C Yellow #6, Magnesium Stearate, Povidone, Starch, Stearic acid.

Indications: For temporary relief of major colds symptoms as follows:
Nasal and sinus congestion, coughing, aches and pains, fever, and cough irritated throat of a cold or flu without drowsy side effects. Loosens upper chest congestion; restores freer breathing.

Actions: VICKS DAYCARE is a decongestant, antitussive, expectorant, analgesic and antipyretic. It helps clear stuffy nose, congested sinus openings. Calms, quiets coughing. Eases headache pain and the ache-all-over feeling. Reduces fever due to colds and flu. It relieves these symptoms without drowsiness. DAYCARE LIQUID is also a demulcent and soothes a cough irritated throat.

Warning: Do not exceed recommended dosage because at higher doses nervousness, dizziness, or sleeplessness may occur. Do not take this product for more than 7 days. If symptoms do not improve or are accompanied by fever, consult a doctor. Do not take this product if you have heart disease, diabetes, high blood pressure, thyroid disease, or difficulty in urination due to enlargement of the prostate gland unless directed by a doctor. Do not take this product for persistent or chronic cough such as occurs with smoking, asthma, or emphysema, or if cough is accompanied by excessive phlegm (mucus) unless directed by a doctor. A persistent cough may be a sign of a serious condition. If cough persists for more than 1 week, tends to recur, or is accompanied by fever, rash, or persistent headaches,

consult a doctor. Do not give this product to children under 3 years of age unless directed by a doctor. Do not take this product for more than 10 days (adults) or 5 days (under age 12). If symptoms persist or new ones occur, consult your physician. Do not exceed recommended dosage because severe liver damage may occur. If fever persists for more than 3 days, consult physician. Severe or persistent sore throat or sore throat accompanied by high fever, headache, nausea, and vomiting may be serious. Consult physician promptly. Do not use more than 2 days or administer to children under 3 years of age unless directed by physician. In case of accidental overdose, seek professional assistance or contact a poison control center immediately. If pregnant or nursing a baby, consult a health professional before using this product.

Drug Interaction Precaution: Do not take this product if you are presently taking a prescription antihypertensive or antidepressant drug containing MAO inhibitor except under the advice and supervision of a physician.

Overdosage: In case of accidental overdose, seek professional assistance or contact a Poison Control Center immediately.

Dosage:
ADULTS one fluid ounce (2 tbs.) LIQUID, or 2 CAPLETS.
CHILDREN (6 to 12 years) One-half ounce (1 tbs.) LIQUID, or 1 CAPLET.
CHILDREN (2 to 6 years) 1½ tsp LIQUID. May be repeated every 4–6 hours as needed. Maximum 4 doses per day.

How Supplied: Available in: **LIQUID** with child resistant cap—6 and 10 fl. oz. plastic bottles; **CAPLET** in child resistant packages—20.
Shown in Product Identification Section, pages 421 & 422

VICKS FORMULA 44® COUGH CONTROL DISCS

Active Ingredients per disc: Dextromethorphan (expressed as Dextromethorphan Hydrobromide) 5 mg., Benzocaine 1.25 mg.

Inactive Ingredients: Caramel, Corn Syrup, Flavor, Silicon Dioxide, Sodium Chloride, Sucrose. Special Vicks Medication (menthol, anethole, peppermint oil) 0.35%.

Indications: Provides temporary relief from coughs and relieves throat irritation caused by colds, flu, bronchitis.

Actions: VICKS FORMULA 44 COUGH CONTROL DISCS are antitussive, local anesthetic and demulcent cough drops. They calm, quiet coughs and help coat and soothe irritated throats.

Warnings: A persistent cough may be a sign of a serious condition. If cough persists for more than 1 week, tends to recur, or is accompanied by fever, rash, or persistent headache, consult a doctor. Do not take this product for persistent or chronic cough such as occurs with smoking, asthma, emphysema, or if cough is accompanied by excessive phlegm (mucus) unless directed by a doctor. As with any drug, if you are pregnant or nursing a baby, seek the advice of a health professional before using this product.

KEEP OUT OF THE REACH OF CHILDREN.

Overdosage: In case of accidental overdose, seek professional assistance or contact a Poison Control Center immediately.

Dosage:
Adults 12 years and over:
Dissolve two discs in mouth, one at a time. Repeat every 4 hours not to exceed 12 discs in 24 hours or as directed by doctor.
Children 2 to under 12 years:
Dissolve one disc in mouth. Repeat every 4 hours not to exceed 6 discs in 24 hours or as directed by doctor.
Under 2 years, consult a doctor.

How Supplied: Available as individual foil wrapped portable packets in boxes of 24.

VICKS FORMULA 44® COUGH MIXTURE

Active Ingredients per 2 tsp. (10 ml.): Dextromethorphan Hydrobromide 30 mg., Chlorpheniramine Maleate 4 mg. in a pleasant tasting, dark brown syrup base. Also contains Alcohol 10%.

Inactive Ingredients: Caramel, Flavor, Propylene Glycol, Purified Water, Sodium Benzoate, Sodium Citrate, Invert Sugar.

Indications: For the temporary relief of coughs and runny nose due to colds, flu, bronchitis.

Actions: VICKS FORMULA 44 COUGH MIXTURE is a cough suppressant, antihistamine and demulcent. Calms and quiets coughs. Reduces sneezing and sniffling. Coats, soothes irritated throat.

Warning: May cause excitability especially in children. Do not take this product if you have asthma, glaucoma, emphysema, chronic pulmonary disease, shortness of breath, difficulty in breathing, or difficulty in urination due to enlargement of the prostate gland unless directed by a doctor. May cause drowsiness; alcohol may increase the drowsiness effect. Avoid alcoholic beverages while taking this product. Use caution when driving a motor vehicle or operating machinery. Do not take this product for persistent or chronic cough such as occurs with smoking, asthma, or emphysema, or if cough is accompanied by excessive phlegm (mucus) unless directed by a doctor. A persistent cough may be a sign of a serious condition. If cough persists for more than one week, tends to recur, or is accompanied by high fever, rash, or persistent headaches, consult a doctor. As with any drug, if you are pregnant or nursing a baby, seek the advice of a

health professional before using this preparation.

Overdosage: In case of accidental overdose, seek professional assistance or contact a Poison Control Center immediately.

Dosage:
Adults: 12 years and over—2 teaspoonfuls
Children: 6 to 12 years: 1 teaspoonful
Children under 6 consult a doctor.
Repeat every 6 hours as needed.
No more than 4 doses per day.

How Supplied: Available in 4 fl. oz. and 8 fl. oz. bottles.
Shown in Product Identification Section, page 422

VICKS FORMULA 44D® DECONGESTANT COUGH MIXTURE

Active Ingredients per 3 tsp. (15 ml.): Dextromethorphan Hydrobromide 30 mg., Pseudoephedrine Hydrochloride 60 mg., Guaifenesin (Glyceryl Guaiacolate) 200 mg. in a red, cherry-flavored, cooling syrup. Also contains alcohol 10%.

Inactive Ingredients: Citric Acid, FD&C Red #40, Flavor, Propylene Glycol, Purified Water, Sodium Benzoate, Sodium Citrate, Sodium Saccharin, Sucrose.

Indications: Relieves coughs, decongests nasal passages and loosens upper chest congestion due to colds, flu, bronchitis.

Actions: VICKS FORMULA 44D is an antitussive, nasal decongestant, expectorant and demulcent. It calms, quiets coughs; relieves nasal congestion; loosens phlegm, mucus; and coats, soothes an irritated throat.

Warning: Do not exceed recommended dosage because at higher doses nervousness, dizziness, or sleeplessness may occur. Do not take this product for more than 7 days. If symptoms do not improve or are accompanied by fever, consult a doctor. Do not take this product if you have heart disease, high blood pressure, thyroid disease, diabetes, or difficulty in urination due to enlargement of the prostate gland unless directed by a doctor. Do not take this product for persistent or chronic cough such as occurs with smoking, asthma, or emphysema, or if cough is accompanied by excessive phlegm (mucus) unless directed by a doctor. A persistent cough may be a sign of a serious condition. If cough persists for more than 1 week, tends to recur, or is accompanied by high fever, rash, or persistent headaches, consult a doctor. Do not give this product to children under 2 years of age unless directed by a doctor. In case of accidental overdose, seek professional assistance or contact a poison control center immediately. As with any drug, if you are pregnant, or nursing a baby, seek the

Continued on next page

Richardson-Vicks—Cont.

advice of a health professional before using this product.

Drug Interaction Precaution: Do not take this product if you are presently taking a prescription drug for high blood pressure or depression without first consulting your doctor.

Overdosage: In case of accidental overdose, seek professional assistance or contact a Poison Control Center immediately.

Dosage:
ADULT DOSE   12 years and over—
               3 teaspoonfuls
CHILD DOSE   6–12 years—
               1½ teaspoonfuls
               2–6 years—
               ¾ teaspoonful.
Repeat ever 6 hours as needed, no more than 4 doses per day.

How Supplied: Available in 4 fl. oz. and 8 fl. oz. bottles.
Shown in Product Identification Section, page 422

VICKS FORMULA 44M®
MULTI-SYMPTOM COUGH MIXTURE

Active Ingredients: per 4 tsp. (20 ml.): Dextromethorphan Hydrobromide 30 mg., Pseudoephedrine Hydrochloride 60 mg., Guaifenesin 200 mg., Acetaminophen 500 mg. in a bluish-red fruit flavored syrup. Also contains alcohol 20%.

Inactive Ingredients: Citric Acid, FD&C Blue No. 1, FD&C Red No. 40, Flavor, Glycerin, Purified Water, Sodium Benzoate, Sodium Citrate, Sodium Saccharin, Sucrose.

Indications: Relieves coughs, decongests nasal passages, loosens upper chest congestion, and eases pain of a cough-irritated throat due to cold, bronchitis, or flu-like conditions.

Actions: VICKS FORMULA 44M is a cough suppressant, nasal decongestant, expectorant demulcent and analgesic. It calms, quiets coughs; relieves nasal congestion; loosens phlegm, mucus; and coats, soothes and eases the pain of an irritated throat.

Warning: Do not exceed recommended dosage because at higher doses nervousness, dizziness, or sleeplessness may occur. Do not take this product for more than 7 days. If symptoms do not improve or are accompanied by fever, consult a doctor. Do not take this product if you have heart disease, high blood pressure, thyroid disease, diabetes, or difficulty in urination due to enlargement of the prostate gland unless directed by a doctor. Do not take this product for persistent or chronic cough such as occurs with smoking, asthma, or emphysema, or if cough is accompanied by excessive phlegm (mucus) unless directed by a doctor. A persistent cough may be a sign of a serious condition. If cough persists for more than 1 week, tends to recur, or is accompanied by fever, rash, or persistent headache, consult a doctor. Do not give this product to children under 2 years of age unless directed by a doctor. Do not take this product for more than 10 days (adults), 5 days (children under 12). If symptoms persist, or new ones occur, consult your physician. Do not exceed recommended dosage because severe liver damage may occur. Do not take this product if fever persists for more than 3 days. In case of accidental overdose, seek professional assistance or contact a poison control center immediately. As with any drug, if you are pregnant or nursing a baby, seek the advice of a health professional before using this product.

Drug Interaction Precaution: Do not take this product if you are presently taking a prescription drug for high blood pressure or depression, without first consulting your doctor.

Overdosage: In case of accidental overdose, seek professional assistance or contact a Poison Control Center immediately.

Dosage: 12 years and over—4 teaspoonfuls
6–12 years—2 teaspoonfuls
Repeat every 6 hours as needed. No more than 4 doses per day.

How Supplied: Available in 4 fl. oz. and 8 fl. oz. bottles.
Shown in Product Identification Section, page 422

VICKS® INHALER
with decongestant action

Active Ingredients per inhaler: l-Desoxyephedrine 50 mg., Special Vicks Medication (menthol, camphor, bornyl acetate) 150 mg.

Inactive Ingredient: Fragrance.

Indications: Provides prompt, temporary relief of nasal congestion of colds and hay fever, allergies and sinusitis.

Actions: VICKS INHALER is an intranasal inhaled decongestant. It shrinks swollen membranes and provides fast relief from a stuffy nose.

Warning: Do not exceed recommended dosage because burning, stinging, sneezing, or increase of nasal discharge may occur. The use of this container by more than one person may spread infection. Do not use this product for more than 7 days. If symptoms persist, consult a doctor.

Overdosage: In case of accidental overdose, seek professional assistance or contact a Poison Control Center immediately.

Directions For Use: Adults (over 12 years): Inhale medicated vapors twice through each nostril while blocking off other nostril. Use every 2 hours as needed. Children (6–12): Inhale once through each nostril every two hours as needed. Children (under 6): Consult a physician.
VICKS INHALER is medically effective for 3 months after first use.

How Supplied: Available as a cylindrical plastic nasal inhaler (net wt. 0.007 oz.).

VICKS CHILDREN'S NYQUIL®

Children's NyQuil was specially formulated with the maximum allowable non-prescription levels of three effective ingredients to relieve nighttime cough, nasal congestion, and runny nose so children can rest. Children's NyQuil is alcohol-free and analgesic free, and has a pleasant cherry flavor.

Active Ingredients: Each ½ oz dose (1 tbs) Chlorpheniramine Maleate 2 mg, Pseudoephedrine HCl 30 mg, Dextromethorphan Hydrobromide 15 mg.

Inactive Ingredients: Citric Acid, Flavor, FD&C Red #40, Grape Juice, Potassium Sorbate, Propylene Glycol, Purified Water, Sodium Citrate, Sucrose.

Indications: Specifically formulated for nighttime relief of nasal congestion, runny nose, sneezing and cough to help children rest.

Administration and Dosage:
[See table left].
Note: Since Children's NyQuil is available without a prescription, the following information appears on the label.

Warning: Do not exceed recommended dosage because at higher doses nervousness, dizziness or sleeplessness may occur. Do not give this product to children

DOSAGE INSTRUCTIONS	Take at bedtime as directed. Use medicine cup provided.	
AGE	WEIGHT	DOSE
Under 2	Under 24 lbs	Physicians Discretion.
2–5	24–47 lbs	¼ oz (½ tbs.)*
6–11	48–95 lbs	½ oz (1 tbs)
12 and over	Over 95 lbs	Use NyQuil Nighttime Cold Medicine Adult Formula as directed.

If cold symptoms keep child confined to bed or at home a total of 4 doses may be taken per day each 6–8 hours apart.
*Administer to children under 6 only on the advice of a physician.

for more than 7 days. If symptoms do not improve or are accompanied by fever, consult a physician. Do not give this product to children who have heart disease, high blood pressure, diabetes or thyroid disease, unless directed by a physician. May cause excitability especially in children. Do not give this product to children who have asthma or glaucoma unless directed by a physician. May cause drowsiness. Do not give this product to children under 6 years except on advice and supervision of a physician. Do not give this product for persistent or chronic cough such as occurs with asthma or if cough is accompanied by excessive mucus unless directed by a physician. A persistent cough may be a sign of a serious condition. If cough persists for more than 1 week, tends to recur, or is accompanied by fever, rash, or persistent headache, consult a physician. In case of accidental overdose, seek professional assistance or contact a poison control center immediately.

Drug Interaction Precaution: Do not give this product to a child who is taking a prescription drug for high blood pressure or depression, without first consulting the child's physician.
TAKE ONLY AS DIRECTED. KEEP OUT OF REACH OF CHILDREN.
Store at room temperature.

How Supplied: 4 fl. oz bottles with dosage cup.
Shown in Product Identification Section, page 422

VICKS NYQUIL®
[nĭ'quĭl]
Nighttime Colds Medicine in oral liquid form.
Regular and Cherry Flavor

Active Ingredients per fluid oz. (2 tbs.): Acetaminophen 1000 mg., Doxylamine Succinate 7.5 mg., Pseudoephedrine HCl 60 mg, and Dextromethorphan Hydrobromide 30 mg. Also contains Alcohol 25%.

Inactive Ingredients: Regular Flavor: Citric Acid, FD&C Blue No. 1, Flavor, Glycerin, Purified Water, Sodium Benzoate, Sodium Citrate, Sucrose.
Contains FD&C Yellow #5 (tartrazine) as a color additive.
Cherry Flavor: Citric Acid, FD&C Blue No. 1, FD&C Red No. 40, Flavor, Glycerin, Purified Water, Sodium Citrate, Sodium Saccharin, Sucrose.

Indications: For the temporary relief of major cold and flu-like symptoms, as follows: nasal & sinus congestion, coughing, sneezing, minor sore throat pain, aches and pains, runny nose, headache, fever.

Actions: Decongestant, antipyretic, antihistaminic, antitussive, analgesic. Helps decongest nasal passages and sinus openings, relieves sniffles and sneezing, eases aches and pains, reduces fever, soothes headache, minor sore throat pain, and quiets coughing due to a cold. By relieving these symptoms, also helps patient to sleep and get the rest he needs.

Warning: Do not exceed recommended dosage because at higher doses nervousness, dizziness or sleeplessness may occur. Do not take this product for more than 7 days. If symptoms do not improve or are accompanied by fever, consult a doctor. Do not take this product if you have heart disease, high blood pressure, thyroid disease, diabetes, or difficulty in urination due to enlargment of the prostate gland unless directed by a doctor. Do not take this product for persistent or chronic cough such as occurs with smoking, asthma, or emphysema, or if cough is accompanied by excessive phlegm (mucus) unless directed by a doctor. A persistent cough may be a sign of a serious condition. If cough persists for more than 1 week, tends to recur, or is accompanied by high fever, rash, or persistent headaches, consult a doctor. May cause marked drowsiness. May cause excitability especially in children. Do not take this product if you have asthma or glaucoma, except under the advice and supervision of a physician. Avoid driving a motor vehicle or operating heavy machinery. If fever persists for more than 3 days, or recurs, consult your physician. Avoid alcoholic beverages while taking this product. In case of accidental overdose, seek professional assistance or contact a poison control center immediately. As with any drug, if you are pregnant or nursing a baby, seek the advice of a health professional before using this product.

Drug Interaction Precaution: Do not take this product if you are presently taking a prescription drug for high blood pressure or depression without first consulting your doctor.
KEEP OUT OF REACH OF CHILDREN

Overdosage: In case of accidental overdose, seek professional assistance or contact a Poison Control Center immediately.

Dosage and Dosage Form: A plastic measuring cup with 2 tablespoonful gradation is supplied.
ADULTS (12 and over): One fluid ounce in medicine cup (2 tablespoonfuls) at bedtime.
Not recommended for children.
If confined to bed or at home, a total of 4 doses may be taken per day, each 6 hours apart.

How Supplied: Available in 6, 10, and 14 fl. oz. plastic bottles.
Shown in Product Identification Section, page 422

VICKS SINEX™
[sĭ'nĕx]
Decongestant Nasal Spray and Ultra Fine Mist

Active Ingredients: Phenylephrine Hydrochloride 0.5%, Cetylpyridinium Chloride 0.04%.

Inactive Ingredients: Aromatic Vapors (Camphor, Eucalyptol, Menthol), Potassium Phosphate, Purified Water, Sodium Chloride, Sodium Phosphate,

Tyloxapol. Preservative: Thimerosal 0.001%.

Indications: For prompt, temporary relief of nasal congestion due to colds, hay fever, allergies, and sinusitis.

Actions: VICKS SINEX is a decongestant nasal spray. The product shrinks swollen membranes to restore freer breathing; gives fast relief of nasal stuffiness and congested sinus openings; allows congested sinuses to drain; and instantly cools irritated nasal passages.

Warning: Do not exceed recommended dosage because burning, stinging, sneezing or increase of nasal discharge may occur. Do not use this product for more than 3 days. If symptoms persist, consult a physician. Do not take this product if you have heart disease, high blood pressure, thyroid disease, diabetes, or difficulty in urination due to enlargement of the prostate gland unless directed by a doctor. The use of this dispenser by more than one person may spread infection. KEEP THIS AND ALL MEDICINES OUT OF THE REACH OF CHILDREN.

Overdosage: In case of accidental ingestion, seek professional assistance or contact a Poison Control Center immediately.

Dosage and Administration: Keep head and dispenser upright. May be used every 4 hours as needed.
Ultra Fine Mist: Remove protective cap. Hold atomizer with thumb at base and nozzle between first and second fingers. Without tilting head, insert nozzle into nostril. Fully depress rim with a firm even stroke and sniff deeply. Adults spray twice up each nostril; children age 6 to 12 years spray once up each nostril.
Squeeze Bottle: Adults spray quickly, firmly, 2 times up each nostril, sniffing the spray upward. Children ages 6 to 12, spray one time up each nostril.

How Supplied: Available in ½ fl. oz. and 1 fl. oz. plastic squeeze bottles and ½ fl. oz. measured dose atomizer.
Shown in Product Identification Section, page 422

VICKS SINEX™ LONG-ACTING
[sĭ'nĕx]
12-hour Formula Decongestant Nasal Spray and Ultra Fine Mist

Active Ingredient: Oxymetazoline Hydrochloride 0.05%.

Inactive Ingredients: Aromatic Vapors (Camphor, Eucalyptol, Menthol), Potassium Phosphate, Purified Water, Sodium Chloride, Sodium Phosphate, Tyloxapol. Preservative: Thimerosal 0.001%.

Indications: For prompt, temporary relief of nasal congestion due to colds, hay fever, allergies, and sinusitis.

Actions: Oxymetazoline constricts the arterioles of the nasal passages—resulting in a nasal decongestant effect which lasts up to twelve hours, restoring freer

Continued on next page

Richardson-Vicks—Cont.

breathing through the nose. SINEX LONG-ACTING helps decongest sinus openings and sinus passages thus promoting sinus drainage.

Warning: Do not exceed recommended dosage because burning, stinging, sneezing or increase of nasal discharge may occur. Do not use this product for more than 3 days. If symptoms persist, consult a physician. Do not take this product if you have heart disease, high blood pressure, thyroid disease, diabetes, or difficulty in urination due to enlargement of the prostate gland unless directed by a doctor. The use of this dispenser by more than one person may spread infection. KEEP THIS AND ALL MEDICINES OUT OF THE REACH OF CHILDREN.

Overdosage: In case of accidental ingestion, seek professional assistance or contact a Poison Control Center immediately.

Dosage and Administration: Keep head and dispenser upright. May be used twice daily (morning and evening) or as directed by a physician.
Ultra Fine Mist: Remove protective cap. Hold atomizer with thumb at base and nozzle between first and second fingers. Without tilting head, insert nozzle into nostril. Fully depress rim with a firm even stroke and sniff deeply. Adults spray twice up each nostril; children age 6 to 12 years spray once up each nostril. Squeeze Bottle: Adults spray quickly, firmly, 2 times up each nostril, sniffing the spray upward. Children ages 6 to 12, spray one time up each nostril.

How Supplied: Available in ½ fl. oz. and 1 fl. oz. plastic squeeze bottles and ½ fl. oz. measured dose atomizer.
Shown in Product Identification Section, page 422

VICKS® THROAT LOZENGES

Active Ingredients per lozenge: Benzocaine 5 mg., Cetylpyridinium Chloride 1.66 mg.

Inactive Ingedients: D&C Red No. 27, D&C Red No. 30, Flavor, Polyethylene Glycol, Sodium Citrate, Sucrose, Talc. Special Vicks Medication (menthol, camphor, eucalyptus oil).

Indications: For fast-acting temporary relief of minor sore throat pain, and minor coughs due to colds.

Actions: VICKS THROAT LOZENGES are local anesthetic and demulcent cough drops. They temporarily soothe minor sore throat irritations—ease pain —and relieve irritation and dryness of mouth and throat.

Warning: Do not exceed recommended dosage. Severe or persistent cough, sore throat, or sore throat accompanied by high fever, headache, nausea, and vomiting may be serious. Consult physician promptly. Do not use more than 2 days or administer to children under 3 years of age unless directed by physician. As with

any drug, if you are pregnant or nursing a baby, seek the advice of a health professional before using this product. As with all medication, keep out of reach of children.

Overdosage: In case of accidental overdosage, seek professional assistance or contact a Poison Control Center immediately.

Dosage: ADULTS AND CHILDREN 3 years and over: allow one lozenge to dissolve slowly in mouth. Repeat hourly as needed.

How Supplied: Box of 12's.

VICKS® VAPORUB®
[vā 'pō-rub]
Decongestant Vaporizing Ointment

For use as a rub or in steam.

Active Ingredients: Special Vicks Medication (menthol 2.6%, camphor 4.73%, eucalyptus oil 1.2%) in a petrolatum base.

Inactive Ingredients: Cedarleaf Oil, Mineral Oil, Nutmeg Oil, Petrolatum, Thymol, Spirits of Turpentine.

Indications: For the symptomatic relief of nasal congestion, bronchial mucous congestion, coughs, and muscular aches and pains due to colds.

Actions: The inhaled vapors of VICKS VAPORUB have a decongestant and antitussive effect.

Warning: For external application and use in steam only. Do not swallow or place in nostrils. If fever is present or cough or other symptoms persist, see your doctor. In case of illness in very young children, it is wise to consult your physician. Never expose VAPORUB to flame or place VAPORUB in boiling water. Do not direct steam from vaporizer toward face. Recommended for infants over six months of age.
KEEP OUT OF CHILDREN'S REACH.

Overdosage: In case of accidental overdosage, seek professional assistance or contact a Poison Control Center immediately.

Dosage:
AS A RUB: For relief of head and chest cold symptoms and coughs due to colds. Rub on throat, chest and back. Cover with a dry warm cloth if desired. Repeat as needed, especially at bedtime for continuous breathing relief.
For relief of muscle tightness, apply hot moist towel to affected area. Remove towel, then massage well with VAPORUB. Cover with a dry, warm cloth if desired.
For chapped hands and skin, apply liberally as a dressing.
IN STEAM: Fill medicine cup of vaporizer with VICKS VAPORUB and follow directions of vaporizer manufacturer. VAPORUB may also be used in a steam bowl. Fill a bowl ¾ full with steaming water (be sure to remove bowl from heat and wait a few seconds until boiling stops) then add 2 teaspoonfuls of Vapo-

rub. Inhale steaming vapors. Do not reheat water after adding Vaporub.

How Supplied: Available in 1.5 oz., 3.0 oz. and 6.0 oz. plastic jars and 2.0 oz. tubes.
Shown in Product Identification Section, page 422

VICKS VAPOSTEAM®
[vā 'pō "stēm]
Liquid Medication for Hot Steam Vaporizers.

Active Ingredients: Menthol 3.2%, Camphor 6.2%, Eucalyptus Oil 1.5%, Alcohol 74%.

Inactive Ingredients: Cedarleaf Oil, Nutmeg Oil, Poloxamer 124, Polyoxyethylene Dodecanol, Silicone.

Indications: For the symptomatic relief of colds, coughs, chest congestion.

Actions: VAPOSTEAM increases the action of steam to help relieve colds symptoms in the following ways: relieves coughs of colds, eases nasal and chest congestion, loosens phlegm, and moistens dry, irritated breathing passages.

Warning: For hot steam medication only. Do not use in cold steam vaporizers/humidifiers. Not to be taken by mouth. Persistent coughing may indicate the presence of a serious condition. If symptoms persist, discontinue use and consult physician. Persons with high fever or persistent cough should not use this preparation except as directed by a physician. Keep away from open flame or extreme heat. Do not direct steam from vaporizer towards face.
KEEP OUT OF REACH OF CHILDREN.

Overdosage: In case of accidental overdose, seek professional assistance or contact a Poison Control Center immediately.

Directions:
In Hot Steam Vaporizers: VAPOSTEAM is formulated for use in HOT STEAM VAPORIZERS. Follow directions for use carefully. Add VAPOSTEAM directly to the water in your electric vaporizer. Add one tablespoonful VAPOSTEAM with each quart of water added to the vaporizer. For best performance, vaporizer should be thoroughly cleaned after each use according to manufacturer's instructions. In soft water areas, it may be necessary to add salt or other steaming aid to promote boiling. Follow directions of vaporizer manufacturer for best results.
In Bowl or Washbasin: Pour boiling water in bowl or washbasin. Then add 1½ teaspoonfuls for each pint of water used. Breathe in vapors.

How Supplied: Available in 4 fl. oz. and 6 fl. oz. bottles.

VICKS VATRONOL®
[vātrōnŏl]
Nose Drops

Active Ingredients: Ephedrine Sulfate 0.5% in an aqueous base.

Inactive Ingredients: Camphor, Cedarleaf Oil, Eucalyptol, Menthol, Nutmeg Oil, Potassium Phosphate, Purified Water, Sodium Chloride, Sodium Phosphate, Tyloxapol.
Preservative: Thimerosal 0.001%.

Indications: Relieves nasal congestion caused by colds and hay fever.

Actions: VICKS VATRONOL is a decongestant nose drop. It helps restore freer breathing by relieving nasal stuffiness and congested sinus openings. VATRONOL also cools irritated nasal passages.

Warning: Do not exceed recommended dosage because burning, stinging, sneezing, or increase of nasal discharge may occur. The use of this container by more than one person may spread infection. Do not use this product for more than 3 days. If symptoms persist, consult a doctor. Do not use this product if you have heart disease, high blood pressure, thyroid disease, diabetes, or difficulty in urination due to enlargement of the prostate gland unless directed by a doctor. **KEEP OUT OF REACH OF CHILDREN.**

Overdosage: In case of accidental overdose, seek professional assistance or contact a Poison Control Center immediately.

Dosage:
  ADULTS: Fill dropper to upper mark.
  CHILDREN (6–12 years): Fill dropper to lower mark.
Apply up one nostril, repeat in other nostril.
Repeat every 4 hours as needed.

How Supplied: Available in ½ fl. oz. and 1 fl. oz. dropper bottles.

Richardson-Vicks USA
**PERSONAL CARE PRODUCTS DIVISION
TEN WESTPORT ROAD
WILTON, CT 06897**

CLEARASIL® Adult Care— Medicated Blemish Cream

Active Ingredient: Sulfur, resorcinol (alcohol 10%) in a cream base which contains water, bentonite, glyceryl stearate SE, propylene glycol, isopropyl myristate, sodium bisulfite, dimethicone, methylparaben, propylparaben, fragrance, iron oxides.

Indications: For the topical treatment of acne vulgaris in adults or persons demonstrating sensitivity to benzoyl peroxide.

Actions: CLEARASIL Adult Care— Medicated Blemish Cream is a blemish medication specially suited for adult usage since it dries acne lesions without overdrying or irritating the skin the way many benzoyl peroxide-containing products do. The product contains sulfur and resorcinol to help heal acne pimples, and bentonite to absorb excess sebum.

Warnings: For external use only. Other topical acne medications should not be used at the same time as this medication. Apply to affected areas only. Do not use on broken skin or apply to large areas of the body. Do not get into eyes. Some people with sensitive skin may experience slight irritation after use of this product. If this occurs, discontinue use of this product. If condition persists, consult a doctor or pharmacist. Keep this and all medicine out of reach of children.

Symptoms and Treatment of Oral Overdosage: These symptoms are based upon medical judgement, not on actual experience. Theoretically, ingestion of very large amounts may cause nausea, vomiting, abdominal discomfort and diarrhea. Treatment is symptomatic, with bedrest and observation.

Dosage and Administration: Cleanse skin thoroughly before applying medication. To clear up the blemishes you have now, apply Clearasil Adult Care directly on and around the affected area two or three times daily. If excessive drying occurs, decrease usage to one or two applications per day.

How Supplied: Available in a .6 oz. tube.
Shown in Product Identification Section, page 422

CLEARASIL® Maximum Strength Medicated Anti-Acne Cream Vanishing and Tinted

Active Ingredient: Benzoyl peroxide 10% in an odorless, greaseless cream base, containing water, propylene glycol, aluminum hydroxide, bentonite, glyceryl stearate SE, isopropyl myristate, dimethicone, PEG-12, potassium carbomer-940, methylparaben, and propylparaben. The tinted formula also contains titanium dioxide and iron oxides.

Indications: For the topical treatment of acne vulgaris.

Actions: CLEARASIL Maximum Strength Medicated Anti-Acne Cream contains benzoyl peroxide, an antibacterial and keratolytic agent as well as bentonite and aluminum hydroxide as oil absorbants. The product 1) helps heal and prevent acne pimples, 2) helps absorb excess skin oil often associated with acne blemishes, 3) helps your skin look fresh. The Vanishing formula works invisibly. The Tinted formula hides pimples while it works.

Warnings: Persons with a known sensitivity to benzoyl peroxide should not use this medication. Excessive dryness or peeling may occur especially in persons with unusually dry, sensitive, or maturing skin. If itching, redness, burning, swelling or undue dryness occurs, reduce dosage or discontinue use. If symptoms persist, consult a physician promptly. For external use only. Keep from eyes, lips, mouth and sensitive areas of the neck. Avoid contact with hair, fabrics and clothing which may be bleached by the benzoyl peroxide in this product. Keep this and all medicine out of the reach of children.

Symptoms and Treatment of Ingestion: These symptoms are based upon medical judgement, not on actual experience. Theoretically, ingestion of very large amounts may cause nausea, vomiting, abdominal discomfort and diarrhea. Treatment is symptomatic, with bedrest and observation.

Directions For Use: 1. Wash thoroughly. (Clearasil® Antibacterial Soap and Clearasil® Medicated Astringent are excellent products to use in your cleansing regimen.) **2.** Try this sensitivity test. Apply cream sparingly with fingertips to one or two small affected areas during the first three days. If no discomfort or reaction occurs, apply up to two times daily, wherever pimples and oil are a problem. **3.** If bothersome dryness or peeling occurs, reduce dosage to one application per day or every other day.

How Supplied: Available in both Vanishing and Tinted formulas in 1 oz. and .65 oz. squeeze tubes.
Shown in Product Identification Section, page 422

CLEARASIL®
10% Benzoyl Peroxide Medicated Anti-Acne Lotion

Active Ingredient: Benzoyl Peroxide 10% in a colorless, greaseless lotion which contains water, aluminum hydroxide, isopropyl stearate, PEG-100 stearate, glyceryl stearate, cetyl alcohol, glycereth-26, isocetyl stearate, glycerin, dimethicone copolyol, sodium citrate, citric acid, methylparaben, propylparaben, fragrance.

Indications: For the topical treatment of acne vulgaris.

Actions: CLEARASIL 10% Benzoyl Peroxide Lotion contains benzoyl peroxide, an antibacterial and keratolytic agent. The product **1. Helps heal and prevent acne pimples.** Benzoyl peroxide dries up existing pimples and kills acne causing bacteria to help prevent new ones.
2. Helps absorb excess skin oil often associated with acne blemishes. Contains aluminum hydroxide which is a special oil absorbing ingredient that allows Clearasil Lotion to absorb **more** excess skin oil than 10% benzoyl peroxide alone.
3. Helps your skin look fresh. Extra oil absorption helps your skin look less oily, more natural.

Warnings: Persons with a known sensitivity to benzoyl peroxide should not use this medication. Excessive dryness or peeling may occur especially in persons

Continued on next page

Richardson-Vicks—Cont.

with unusually dry, sensitive, or maturing skin. If itching, redness, burning, swelling or undue dryness occurs, reduce dosage or discontinue use. If symptoms persist, consult a physician promptly. For external use only. Keep from eyes, lips, mouth and sensitive areas of the neck. Avoid contact with hair, fabrics and clothing which may be bleached by the benzoyl peroxide in this product. of this product. Keep this and all medicine out of the reach of children.

Symptoms and Treatment of Ingestion: These symptoms are based upon medical judgement, not on actual experience. Theoretically, ingestion of very large amounts may cause nausea, vomiting, abdominal discomfort and diarrhea. Treatment is symptomatic, with bedrest and observation.

Directions For Use:
SHAKE WELL BEFORE USING.
1. Wash thoroughly. (Clearasil® Antibacterial Soap and Clearasil® Medicated Astringent are excellent products to use in your cleansing regimen) **2.** Try this sensitivity test. Apply lotion sparingly with fingertips to one or two small affected areas during the first three days. If no discomfort or reaction occurs, apply up to two times daily, wherever pimples and oil are a problem **3.** If bothersome dryness or peeling occurs, reduce dosage to one application per day or every other day.

How Supplied: Available in a 1 fl. oz. squeeze bottle.

CLEARASIL®
Medicated Astringent

Active Ingredient: Salicylic Acid (0.5%), also contains ethyl alcohol (43%).

Indications: Topical Skin Cleanser for treatment of acne vulgaris.

Actions: Clearasil® Medicated Astringent contains a comedolytic agent that penetrates deep into pores to clean out oil and dead skin cells that can clog pores and cause pimples.

Warnings: For external use only. May be irritating to the eyes. If contact occurs, flush thoroughly with water. Keep away from extreme heat or open flame.

Drug Interaction: None known.

Symptoms and Treatment of Ingestion: Product contains ethyl alcohol. If large amounts are ingested, nausea, vomiting, gastrointestinal irritation may develop. Bed rest and observation are indicated if ingested.

Directions for Use: Use up to three times daily as part of your regular cleansing routine. Saturate cotton pad and clean face and neck thoroughly. Repeat with fresh cotton pads until no trace of dirt remains. Do not rinse after use.

How Supplied: 4 oz. plastic bottles.
Shown in Product Identification Section, page 422

A. H. Robins Company, Inc.
CONSUMER PRODUCTS DIVISION
3800 CUTSHAW AVENUE
RICHMOND, VIRGINIA 23230

ALLBEE® C–800 TABLETS
[all-be ']
ALLBEE® C–800
plus IRON TABLETS

Allbee C-800

One tablet daily provides:	Percentage of U.S. Recommended Daily Allowances (U.S. RDA)	
Vitamin E	150	45 I.U.
Vitamin C	1333	800 mg
Thiamine (Vitamin B$_1$)	1000	15 mg
Riboflavin (Vitamin B$_2$)	1000	17 mg
Niacin	500	100 mg
Vitamin B$_6$	1250	25 mg
Vitamin B$_{12}$	200	12 mcg
Pantothenic Acid	250	25 mg

Ingredients: Ascorbic Acid, Niacinamide Ascorbate, Starch, Vitamin E Acetate, Hydrolyzed Protein, Calcium Pantothenate, Hydroxypropyl Methylcellulose, Pyridoxine Hydrochloride, Riboflavin, Stearic Acid, Thiamine Mononitrate, Artificial Color, Silicon Dioxide, Lactose, Magnesium Stearate, Povidone, Polyethylene Glycol 400, Vanillin, Gelatin, Polysorbate 80, Sorbic Acid, Sodium Benzoate, Cyanocobalamin.

Allbee C-800 plus Iron

One tablet daily provides: Vitamin Composition	Percentage of U.S. Recommended Daily Allowances (U.S. RDA)	
Vitamin E	150	45.0 I.U.
Vitamin C	1333	800.0 mg
Folic Acid	100	0.4 mg
Thiamine (Vitamin B$_1$)	1000	15.0 mg
Riboflavin (Vitamin B$_2$)	1000	17.0 mg
Niacin	500	100.0 mg
Vitamin B$_6$	1250	25.0 mg
Vitamin B$_{12}$	200	12.0 mcg
Pantothenic Acid	250	25.0 mg
Mineral Composition		
Iron	150	27.0 mg

Ingredients: Ascorbic Acid, Niacinamide Ascorbate, Ferrous Fumarate, Starch, Vitamin E Acetate, Hydrolyzed Protein, Calcium Pantothenate, Hydroxypropyl Methylcellulose, Pyridoxine Hydrochloride, Riboflavin, Stearic Acid, Thiamine Mononitrate, Povidone, Silicon Dioxide, Artificial Color, Lactose, Magnesium Stearate, Polyethylene Glycol 400, Vanillin, Gelatin, Folic Acid, Polysorbate 80, Sorbic Acid, Sodium Benzoate, Cyanocobalamin.

Actions and Uses: The components of Allbee C-800 have important roles in general nutrition, healing of wounds, and prevention of hemorrhage. Allbee C-800 is recommended for nutritional supplementation of these components in

conditions such as febrile diseases, chronic or acute infections, burns, fractures, surgery, physiologic stress, alcoholism, prolonged exposure to high temperature, geriatrics, gastritis, peptic ulcer, and colitis; and in weight-reduction and other special diets.

In dentistry, Allbee C-800 is recommended for nutritional supplementation of its components in conditions such as herpetic stomatitis, aphthous stomatitis, cheilosis, herpangina and gingivitis.

In addition, Allbee C-800 Plus Iron is recommended as a nutritional source of iron. The iron is present as ferrous fumarate, a well-tolerated salt. The ascorbic acid in the formulation enhances the absorption of iron.

Precautions: Do not take Allbee C-800 Plus Iron within two hours of oral tetracycline antibiotics, since oral iron products interfere with absorption of tetracycline. Not intended for treatment of iron-deficiency anemia.

Adverse Reactions: Iron-containing medications may occasionally cause gastrointestinal discomfort, nausea, constipation or diarrhea.

Dosage: The recommended OTC dosage for adults and children twelve or more years of age is one tablet daily. Under the direction and supervision of a physician, the dose and frequency of administration may be increased in accordance with the patient's requirements.

How Supplied: Allbee C-800—orange, film-coated, elliptically-shaped tablets in bottles of 60 (NDC 0031-0677-62). Allbee C-800 Plus Iron—red, film-coated, elliptically-shaped tablets in bottles of 60 (NDC 0031-0678-62).
Shown in Product Identification Section, page 422

ALLBEE® WITH C CAPLETS
[all-be ']

One caplet daily provides:	Percentage of U.S. Recommended Daily Allowance (U.S. RDA)	
Vitamin C	500	300.0 mg
Thiamine (Vitamin B$_1$)	1000	15.0 mg
Riboflavin (Vitamin B$_2$)	600	10.2 mg
Niacin	250	50.0 mg
Vitamin B$_6$	250	5.0 mg
Pantothenic Acid	100	10.0 mg

Ingredients: Niacinamide Ascorbate; Ascorbic Acid; Microcrystalline Cellulose; Corn Starch; Thiamine Mononitrate; Calcium Pantothenate; Riboflavin; Hydroxypropyl Methylcellulose; Pyridoxine Hydrochloride; Magnesium Stearate; Silicon Dioxide; Propylene Glycol; Lactose; Methacrylic Acid Copolymer; Triethyl Citrate; Titanium Dioxide; Polysorbate 20; Artificial Flavor; Saccharin Sodium; Sodium Sorbate.

Action and Uses: Allbee with C is a high potency formulation of B and C vitamins. Its components have important roles in general nutrition, healing of wounds, and prevention of hemorrhage.

It is recommended for deficiencies of B-vitamins and ascorbic acid in conditions such as febrile diseases, chronic or acute infections, burns, fractures, surgery, toxic conditions, physiologic stress, alcoholism, prolonged exposure to high temperature, geriatrics, gastritis, peptic ulcer, and colitis; and in conditions involving special diets and weight-reduction diets.

In dentistry, Allbee with C is recommended for deficiencies of B-vitamins and ascorbic acid in conditions such as herpetic stomatitis, aphthous stomatitis, cheilosis, herpangina, gingivitis.

Dosage: The recommended OTC dosage for adults and children twelve or more years of age, is one caplet daily. Under the direction and supervision of a physician, the dose and frequency of administration may be increased in accordance with the patient's requirements.

How Supplied: Yellow caplets, monogrammed AHR and Allbee C in bottles of 130 (NDC 0031-0673-66), 1,000 caplets (NDC 0031-0673-74), and in Dis-Co® Unit Dose Packs of 100 (NDC 0031-0673-64).

Shown in Product Identification Section, page 423

CHAP STICK® Lip Balm

Active Ingredients: 44% Petrolatums, 1.5% Padimate O (2-ethyl-hexyl p-dimethylaminobenzoate, 1% Lanolin, 1% Isopropyl Myristate, .5% Cetyl Alcohol.

Inactive Ingredients:
Regular: Arachadyl Propionate, Camphor, Carnauba Wax, D&C Red 6 Barium Lake, FD&C Yellow 5 Aluminum Lake, Fragrance, Isopropyl Lanolate, Methylparaben, Mineral Oil, 2-Octyl Dodecanol, Oleyl Alcohol, Polyphenylmethyl-siloxane 556, Propylparaben, Titanium Dioxide, Wax Paraffin, White Wax.
Cherry: Arachadyl Propionate, Camphor, Carnauba Wax, D&C Red 6 Barium Lake, Flavors, Isopropyl Lanolate, Methylparaben, Mineral Oil, 2-Octyl Dodecanol, Polyphenylmethylsiloxane 556, Propylparaben, Saccharin, Wax Paraffin, White Wax.
Mint: Arachadyl Propionate, Carnauba Wax, FD&C Blue 1 Aluminum Lake, FD&C Yellow 5 Lake, Flavors, Isopropyl Lanolate, Methylparaben, Mineral Oil, 2-Octyl Dodecanol, Polyphenylmethylsiloxane 556, Propylparaben, Saccharin, Wax Paraffin, White Wax.
Orange: Arachadyl Propionate, Carnauba Wax, FD&C Yellow 6 Aluminum Lake, Flavors, Isopropyl Lanolate, Methylparaben, Mineral Oil, 2-Octyl Dodecanol, Polyphenylmethylsiloxane 556, Propylparaben, Saccharin, Wax Paraffin, White Wax.
Strawberry: Arachadyl Propionate, Camphor, Carnauba Wax, D&C Red 6 Barium Lake, Flavors, Isopropyl Lanolate, Methylparaben, Mineral Oil, 2-Octyl Dodecanol, Polyphenylmethylsiloxane 556, Propylparaben, Saccharin, Wax Paraffin, White Wax.

Indications: Helps prevention and healing of dry, chapped, sun and windburned lips.

Actions: A specially designed lipid complex hydrophobic base containing Padimate O which forms a barrier to prevent moisture loss and protect lips from the drying effects of cold weather, wind and sun which cause chapping. The special emollients soften the skin by forming an occlusive film thus inducing hydration, restoring suppleness to the lips, and preventing drying from evaporation of water that diffuses to the surface from the underlying layers of tissue. Chap Stick also protects the skin from the external environment and its sunscreen offers protection from exposure to the sun.

Warning: Discontinue use if signs of irritation appear.

Symptoms and Treatment of Oral Ingestion: The oral LD_{50} in rats is greater than 5 gm/kg. There have been no reported overdoses in humans. There are no known symptoms of overdosage.

Dosage and Treatment: For dry, chapped lips apply as needed. To help prevent dry, chapped sun or windburned lips, apply to lips as needed before, during and following exposure to sun, wind, water and cold weather.

Professional Labeling: None.

How Supplied: Available in 4.25 gm tubes in Regular, Mint, Cherry, Orange, and Strawberry flavors.

Shown in Product Identification Section, page 423

CHAP STICK® SUNBLOCK 15 Lip Balm

Active Ingredients: 44% Petrolatums, 7% Padimate O, 3% Oxybenzone, 0.5% Lanolin, 0.5% Isopropyl Myristate, 0.5% Cetyl Alcohol.

Inactive Ingredients: Camphor, Carnauba Wax, D&C Red 6 Barium Lake, FD&C Yellow 5 Aluminum Lake, Fragrance, Isopropyl Lanolate, Methylparaben, Mineral Oil, Propylparaben, Titanium Dioxide, Wax Paraffin, White Wax.

Indications: Ultra Sunscreen Protection (SPF-15). Helps prevention and healing of dry, chapped, sun and windburned lips. Overexposure to sun may lead to premature aging of skin and lip cancer. Liberal and regular use may help reduce the sun's harmful effects.

Actions: Ultra sunscreen protection for the lips, plus the attributes of Chap Stick® Lip Balm. The emollients in the specially-designed lipid complex hydrophobic base soften the lips by forming an occlusive film while the two sunscreens have specific ultraviolet absorption ranges which overlap to offer ultra sunscreen protection (SPF-15).

Warning: Discontinue use if signs of irritation appear.

Symptoms and Treatment of Oral Ingestion: Toxicity studies indicate this product to be extremely safe. The oral LD_{50} in rats is greater than 5 gm./kg. There are no known symptoms of overdosage.

Dosage and Treatment: For ultra sunscreen protection, apply evenly and liberally to lips before exposure to sun. Reapply as needed. For dry, chapped lips, apply as needed. To help prevent dry, chapped, sun, and windburned lips, apply to lips as needed before, during, and following exposure to sun, wind, water, and cold weather.

How Supplied: 4.25 gm. tube.
Shown in Product Identification Section, page 423

CHAP STICK® PETROLEUM JELLY PLUS

REGULAR:
Active Ingredients: 99% White Petrolatum, USP
Other Ingredients: Aloe, Butylated Hydroxytoluene, Flavor, Lanolin, Phenonip.
CHERRY:
Active Ingredients: 98.85% White Petrolatum, USP.
Other Ingredients: Aloe, Butylated Hydroxytoluene, D&C Red 6 Barium Lake, Flavors, Lanolin, Phenonip, and Saccharin.

Indications: Helps prevent and protect against dry, chapped, sun and windburned lips.

Actions: White Petrolatum, USP forms a barrier to prevent moisture loss and protect lips from the drying effects of cold weather, wind and sun which cause chapping. White Petrolatum, USP helps soften the skin by forming an occlusive film for inducing hydration and restoring suppleness to the lips and preventing drying from evaporation of water that diffuses to the surface from the underlying layers of tissue.

Warning: If condition worsens or does not improve within 7 days, consult a doctor.

Dosage and Treatment: To help prevent dry, chapped, sun or wind-burned lips, apply to lips as needed before, during and following exposure to sun, wind, water and cold weather.

How Supplied: Regular and Cherry flavored available in 0.35 oz. (10 grams) polyethylene tube.
Shown in Product Identification Section page 423

Continued on next page

Robins—Cont.

CHAP STICK® PETROLEUM JELLY PLUS WITH SUNBLOCK 15

Active Ingredients: 89% White Petrolatum, USP, 7% Padimate O, 3% Oxybenzone.

Other Ingredients: Aloe, Butylated Hydroxytoluene, Flavor, Lanolin, Phenonip.

Indications: Ultra Sunscreen Protection (SPF-15). Helps prevent and protect against dry, chapped, sun and windburned lips. Over-exposure to sun may lead to premature aging of skin and skin cancer. Liberal and regular use may help reduce the sun's harmful effects.

Actions: Ultra sunscreen protection for the lips, plus the attributes of Chap Stick® Petroleum Jelly Plus. White Petrolatum, USP forms a barrier to prevent moisture loss and protect lips from the drying effects of wind and sun while two sunscreens, which have specific ultra violet absorption ranges, overlap to provide ultra sunscreen protection (SPF-15).

Warning: For external use only. Avoid contact with eyes. Discontinue use if signs of irritation or rash occur.

Dosage and Treatment: For ultra sunscreen protection, apply evenly and liberally to lips before exposure to sun. Reapply as needed. For dry chapped lips, apply as needed. To help prevent dry, chapped, sun and windburned lips, apply to lips as needed before, during and following exposure to sun, wind, water and cold weather.

How Supplied: Available in 0.35 oz (10 grams) polyethylene tube.
Shown in Product Identification Section, page 423

DIMACOL® Caplets
[di 'mă-col]

Description: Each caplet contains:
Guaifenesin, USP .... 100 mg
Pseudoephedrine
  Hydrochloride, USP .... 30 mg
Dextromethorphan
  Hydrobromide, USP .... 10 mg

Inactive Ingredients: Caplets: D&C Yellow 10 Aluminum Lake, FD&C Yellow 6 Aluminum Lake, Flavor, Hydroxypropyl Methylcellulose, Magnesium Stearate, Methacrylic Acid Copolymer, Methylparaben, Microcrystalline Cellulose, Polysorbate 20, Potassium Sorbate, Povidone, Propylene Glycol, Propylparaben, Saccharin Sodium, Silicon Dioxide, Titanium Dioxide, Triethyl Citrate, Xanthan Gum.

Indications: Temporarily relieves cough due to minor throat and bronchial irritation and nasal congestion as may occur with a cold. Expectorant action to help loosen phlegm and bronchial secretions.

Warnings: A persistent cough may be a sign of a serious condition. If cough persists for more than 1 week, tends to recur, or is accompanied by fever, rash, or persistent headache, consult a doctor. Do not take this product for persistent or chronic cough such as occurs with smoking, asthma, emphysema, or if cough is accompanied by excessive phlegm (mucus) unless directed by a doctor. Persons with high blood pressure, heart disease, diabetes, or thyroid disease should use only as directed by a doctor. As with any drug, if you are pregnant or nursing a baby, seek the advice of a health professional before using this product.

Contraindications: Hypersensitivity to guaifenesin, sympathomimetic amines, or dextromethorphan; marked hypertension, hyperthyroidism or in patients who are receiving monoamine oxidase inhibitors (MAOIs).

Adverse Reactions: The following adverse reactions may possibly occur: nausea, vomiting, dry mouth, nervousness, insomnia and rash (including urticaria).
NOTE: Guaifenesin has been shown to produce a color interference with certain clinical laboratory determinations of 5-hydroxyindoleacetic acid (5-HIAA) and vanillylmandelic acid (VMA).

Drug Interaction Precautions: Concomitant administration of pseudoephedrine with other sympathomimetic agents may produce additive effects and increased toxicity; with MAOIs may produce a hypertensive crisis; with certain antihypertensive agents may diminish their antihypertensive effect. Serious toxicity may result if dextromethorphan is used with MAOIs.

Directions: Adults and children 12 years and over, 2 caplets every 4 hours; children 6 to under 12 years of age, 1 caplet every 4 hours; children under 6 years—consult a doctor. DO NOT EXCEED 4 DOSES IN A 24-HOUR PERIOD.

How Supplied: Orange caplets in bottles of 100 (NDC 0031-1653-63), and 500 (NDC 0031-1653-70) and consumer packages of 12 (NDC 0031-1653-46), and 24 (NDC 0031-1653-54) (individually packaged).
Store at Controlled Room Temperature, Between 15°C and 30°C (59°F and 86°F).
Shown in Product Identification Section, page 423

DIMETANE®
[di 'mĕ-tāne]
brand of Brompheniramine Maleate, USP
Tablets—4 mg
Elixir—2 mg/5 mL (Alcohol, 3%)
Extentabs®—8 mg and 12 mg

Family Description: Dimetane® is Robins brand name for Brompheniramine Maleate, USP, an antihistamine. It comes in several oral dosage forms (tablets, elixir and Extentabs®) and can be used when an antihistamine is indicated.

Inactive Ingredients:
Tablets: Corn Starch, D&C Yellow 10 Aluminum Lake, Dibasic Calcium Phosphate, FD&C Yellow 6 Aluminum Lake, Lactose, Magnesium Stearate, Polyethylene Glycol.
Elixir: Citric Acid, FD&C Yellow 6, Flavors, Glucose, Saccharin Sodium, Sodium Benzoate, Water.
Extentabs® 8 mg: Acacia, Acetylated Monoglycerides, Calcium Carbonate, Calcium Sulfate, Carnauba Wax, Cellulose Acetate Phthalate, Corn Starch, Diethyl Phthalate, Edible Ink, FD&C Blue 2 Aluminum Lake, FD&C Red 3, Gelatin, Guar Gum, Magnesium Stearate, Pharmaceutical Glaze, Polysorbates, Stearic Acid, Sucrose, Titanium Dioxide, Wheat Flour, White Wax and other ingredients, one of which is a corn derivative. May contain FD&C Red 40 and FD&C Yellow 6 Aluminum Lakes.
Extentabs® 12 mg: Acacia, Acetylated Monoglycerides, Calcium Carbonate, Calcium Sulfate, Carnauba Wax, Cellulose Acetate Phthalate, Corn Starch, Diethyl Phthalate, Edible Ink, FD&C Blue 2 Aluminum Lake, FD&C Red 3, FD&C Yellow 6, Gelatin, Guar Gum, Magnesium Stearate, Pharmaceutical Glaze, Polysorbates, Stearic Acid, Sucrose, Titanium Dioxide, Wheat Flour, White Wax and other ingredients, one of which is a corn derivative. May contain FD&C Red 40 and FD&C Yellow 6 Aluminum Lakes.

Indications: For temporary relief of hay fever symptoms: itching of the nose or throat; itchy, watery eyes; sneezing; running nose.

Warnings: May cause drowsiness. May cause excitability, especially in children. This product should not be taken by patients who have asthma, glaucoma or difficulty in urination due to enlargement of the prostate gland. The tablets and liquid should not be given to children under six years, except under the advice and supervision of a physician. The Extentabs should not be given to children under 12 years, except under the advice and supervision of a physician. As with any drug, women who are pregnant or nursing a baby should seek the advice of a health professional before using these products.

Cautions: Driving a motor vehicle, operating heavy machinery and drinking alcoholic beverages should be avoided while this drug is being taken.
THIS AND ALL DRUGS SHOULD BE KEPT OUT OF THE REACH OF CHILDREN. IN CASE OF ACCIDENTAL OVERDOSE, PROFESSIONAL ASSISTANCE SHOULD BE OBTAINED OR A POISON CONTROL CENTER SHOULD BE CONTACTED IMMEDIATELY.

Directions For Use: Tablets and Liquid—The recommended OTC dosage is:
Adults and children 12 years of age and over: 1 tablet or 2 teaspoonfuls every four to six hours, not to exceed 6 tablets or 12 teaspoonfuls in 24 hours.
Children 6 to under 12 years: ½ tablet or 1 teaspoonful every four to six hours, not to exceed 3 whole tablets or 6 teaspoonfuls in 24 hours.
Children under 6 years: Use only as directed by a physician.

Extentabs®—The recommended OTC dosage is: **Adults and children 12 years of age and over:**

8 mg Extentab: One tablet every eight to twelve hours, NOT TO EXCEED 1 TABLET EVERY 8 HOURS OR 3 TABLETS IN A 24-HOUR PERIOD.

12 mg Extentab: One tablet every twelve hours, NOT TO EXCEED 1 TABLET EVERY 12 HOURS OR 2 TABLETS IN A 24-HOUR PERIOD.

Children under 12 years of age should use only as directed by a physician.

How Supplied:
[See table right]

Store at Controlled Room Temperature, Between 15°C and 30°C (59°F and 86°F).

Shown in Product Identification Section, page 423

Product Name	NDC 0031-	Form	Strength	Package Size	Package Type
Dimetane Tablets	1857-54 1857-63	Peach-colored, compressed scored tablets	4 mg tablet	24 100	Blister Unit Bottles
Dimetane Elixir	1807-12 1807-25	Peach-colored liquid	2 mg/5 ml	4 fl. oz. 1 Pint	Bottles Bottles
Dimetane Extentabs 8 mg	1868-46 1868-63	Persian rose-colored, tablets	8 mg tablet	12 100	Blister Unit Bottles
Dimetane Extentabs 12 mg	1843-46 1843-63	Peach-colored, coated tablets	12 mg tablets	12 100	Blister Unit Bottles

DIMETANE® DECONGESTANT ELIXIR
[di'mĕ-tāne]
DIMETANE® DECONGESTANT CAPLETS

Elixir:
Each 5 mL (1 teaspoonful) contains:
Phenylephrine
    Hydrochloride, USP ....5 mg
Brompheniramine
    Maleate, USP ....2 mg
Alcohol 2.3 percent

Inactive Ingredients: Citric Acid, FD&C Blue 1, FD&C Red 40, Flavors, Sodium Benzoate, Sorbitol, Water.
Caplets:
Each caplet contains:
Phenylephrine
    Hydrochloride, USP ....10 mg
Brompheniramine
    Maleate, USP ....4 mg

Inactive Ingredients: Corn Starch, FD&C Blue 1 Aluminum Lake, Magnesium Stearate, Microcrystalline Cellulose.

Indications: For temporary relief of nasal congestion due to the common cold, sinusitis, hay fever or other upper respiratory allergies; runny nose, sneezing, itching of the nose or throat and itchy and watery eyes as may occur in allergic rhinitis (such as hay fever). Temporarily restores freer breathing through the nose.

Warnings: May cause excitability, especially in children. Use with caution in children under 6 years. This product should not be taken by patients with asthma, glaucoma, difficulty in urination due to enlargement of the prostate gland, high blood pressure, heart disease, diabetes or thyroid disease. May cause drowsiness. Doses in excess of the recommended dosage may cause nervousness, dizziness or sleeplessness. As with any drug, if you are pregnant or nursing a baby, seek the advice of a health professional before using this product.

Drug Interaction Precaution: This product should be taken by patients who are taking a prescription antihypertensive drug or antidepressant drug containing an MAO inhibitor only under the advice and supervision of a doctor.

Cautions: Patients should be warned about driving a motor vehicle, operating heavy machinery, or consuming alcoholic beverages while taking this product.

Recommended OTC Dosage: *Elixir:* Adults and children 12 years of age and over: 2 teaspoonfuls every 4 hours, not to exceed 12 teaspoonfuls in a 24-hour period; children 6 to under 12 years: 1 teaspoonful every 4 hours, not to exceed 6 teaspoonfuls in a 24-hour period. *Caplets:* Adults and children 12 years of age and over: 1 caplet every 4 hours, not to exceed 6 caplets in a 24-hour period; children 6 to under 12 years: ½ caplet every 4 hours, not to exceed 3 caplets in a 24-hour period.

How Supplied: *Caplets*—light blue, capsule shaped caplets in cartons of 24 (NDC 0031-2117-54) and 48 (NDC 0031-2117-59) individually packaged blister units.
Elixir—red colored, grape flavored liquid in 4 fl. oz. bottle (NDC 0031-2127-12). Store at Controlled Room Temperature, Between 15°C and 30°C (59°F and 86°F).

Shown in Product Identification Section, page 423

DIMETAPP® Elixir
[di'mĕ-tap]

Description: Each 5 mL (1 teaspoonful) contains:
Brompheniramine
    Maleate, USP ....2 mg
Phenylpropanolamine
    Hydrochloride, USP ....12.5 mg
Alcohol 2.3%
Inactive Ingredients: Citric Acid, FD&C Blue 1, FD&C Red 40, Flavor, Saccharin Sodium, Sodium Benzoate, Sorbitol, Water.

Indications: For temporary relief of nasal congestion due to the common cold, hay fever or other upper respiratory allergies and associated with sinusitis; temporarily relieves running nose, sneezing, and itchy and watery eyes as may occur in allergic rhinitis (such as hay fever). Temporarily restores freer breathing through the nose.

Warnings: This product may cause excitability, especially in children. Do not take this product if you have high blood pressure, heart disease, diabetes, thyroid disease, asthma, glaucoma or difficulty in urination due to enlargement of the prostate gland, except under the advice and supervision of a physician. Do not give this product to children under 6 years except under the advice and supervision of a physician. May cause drowsiness. Do not exceed recommended dosage because at higher doses nervousness, dizziness, or sleeplessness may occur. If symptoms do not improve within 7 days or are accompanied by high fever, consult a physician before continuing use. Do not take if hypersensitive to any of the ingredients. As with any drug, if you are pregnant or nursing a baby, seek the advice of a health professional before using this product.

Caution: Avoid driving a motor vehicle or operating heavy machinery and avoid alcoholic beverages while taking this product.

Drug Interaction Precaution: Do not take this product if you are presently taking a prescription antihypertensive or antidepressant drug containing a monoamine oxidase inhibitor, except under the advice and supervision of a physician.

Dosage and Administration: Adults and children 12 years of age and over: 2 teaspoonfuls every 4 hours, children 6 to under 12 years: 1 teaspoonful every 4 hours. DO NOT EXCEED 6 DOSES IN A 24-HOUR PERIOD. Children under 6 years: consult physician.
Professional Labeling: The suggested dosage for children age 2 to under 6 years, only when the child is under the care of a physician, is ½ teaspoonful every 4 hours, not to exceed 6 doses in a 24-hour period. The dosage for children un-

Continued on next page

Prescribing information on A.H. Robins products listed here is based on official labeling in effect November 1, 1988 with Indications, Contraindications, Warnings, Precautions, Adverse Reactions, and Dosage stated in full.

Robins—Cont.

der 2 years should be determined by the physician on the basis of the patients' weight, physical condition or other appropriate consideration. Dimetapp Elixir is contraindicated in neonates (children under the age of one month).

How Supplied: Purple, grape flavored liquid in bottles of 4 fl. oz. (NDC 0031-2230-12), 8 fl. oz. (NDC 0031-2230-18), 12 fl. oz. (NDC 0031-2230-22), pints (NDC 0031-2230-25), gallons (NDC 0031-2230-29), and 5 mL Dis-Co® Unit Dose Packs (10 × 10s) (NDC 0031-2230-23).
Store at Controlled Room Temperature, Between 15°C and 30°C (59°F and 86°F).
Shown in Product Identification Section, page 423

DIMETAPP® Extentabs®
[di 'mĕ-tap]

Description: Each **Dimetapp Extentabs®** Tablet contains:
Brompheniramine Maleate, USP...................................12 mg
Phenylpropanolamine Hydrochloride, USP ....75 mg
Inactive Ingredients: Acacia, Acetylated Monoglycerides, Calcium Sulfate, Carnauba Wax, Castor Wax or Oil, Citric Acid, Edible Ink, FD&C Blue 1 and FD&C Blue 2 Aluminum Lake, Gelatin, Magnesium Stearate, Magnesium Trisilicate, Pharmaceutical Glaze, Polysorbates, Povidone, Silicon Dioxide, Stearyl Alcohol, Sucrose, Titanium Dioxide, Wheat Flour, White Wax. May contain FD&C Red 40 and FD&C Yellow 6 Aluminum Lakes.

Indications: For temporary relief of nasal congestion due to the common cold, hay fever or other upper respiratory allergies and associated with sinusitis; temporarily relieves running nose, sneezing, and itchy and watery eyes as may occur in allergic rhinitis (such as hay fever). Temporarily restores freer breathing through the nose.

Warnings: This product may cause excitability, especially in children. Do not take this product if you have high blood pressure, heart disease, diabetes, thyroid disease, asthma, glaucoma or difficulty in urination due to enlargement of the prostate gland, except under the advice and supervision of a physician. Do not give to children under 12 years, except under the advice and supervision of a physician. May cause drowsiness. Do not exceed recommended dosage because at higher doses nervousness, dizziness, or sleeplessness may occur. If symptoms do not improve within 7 days or are accompanied by high fever, consult a physician before continuing use. Do not take if hypersensitive to any of the ingredients. As with any drug, if you are pregnant or nursing a baby, seek the advice of a health professional before using this product.

Caution: Avoid driving a motor vehicle or operating heavy machinery and avoid alcoholic beverages while taking this product.

Drug Interaction Precaution: Do not take this product if you are presently taking a prescription antihypertensive or antidepressant drug containing a monoamine oxidase inhibitor, except under the advice and supervision of a physician.

Directions: Adults and children 12 years of age and over: one tablet every 12 hours. **Do not exceed 1 tablet every 12 hours or 2 tablets in a 24-hour period.**

How Supplied: Pale blue sugar-coated tablets monogrammed DIMETAPP AHR in bottles of 100 (NDC 0031-2277-63), 500 (NDC 0031-2277-70); Dis-Co® Unit Dose Packs of 100 (NDC 0031-2277-64); and consumer packages of 12 tablets (NDC 0031-2277-46), and 24 tablets (NDC 0031-2277-54) and 48 tablets (NDC 0031-2277-59) (individually packaged).
Store at Controlled Room Temperature, Between 15°C and 30°C (59°F and 86°F).
Dimetapp Extentabs® Tablets are the A. H. Robins Company's uniquely constructed extended action tablets.
Shown in Product Identification Section, page 423

DIMETAPP® Tablets
[di 'mĕ-tap]

Description: Each **Dimetapp** Tablet contains:
Brompheniramine Maleate, USP.................................4 mg
Phenylpropanolamine Hydrochloride, USP ....25 mg
Inactive Ingredients: Corn starch, FD&C Blue 1 Aluminum Lake, Magnesium Stearate, Microcrystalline Cellulose.

Indications: For temporary relief of nasal congestion due to the common cold, hay fever or other upper respiratory allergies and associated with sinusitis; temporarily relieves running nose, sneezing, and itchy and watery eyes as may occur in allergic rhinitis (such as hay fever). Temporarily restores freer breathing through the nose.

Warnings: This product may cause excitability, especially in children. Do not take this product if you have high blood pressure, heart disease, diabetes, thyroid disease, asthma, glaucoma or difficulty in urination due to enlargement of the prostate gland, except under the advice and supervision of a physician. Do not give this product to children under 6 years except under the advice and supervision of a physician. May cause drowsiness. Do not exceed recommended dosage because at higher doses nervousness, dizziness, or sleeplessness may occur. If symptoms do not improve within 7 days or are accompanied by high fever, consult a physician before continuing use. Do not take if hypersensitive to any of the ingredients. As with any drug, if you are pregnant or nursing a baby, seek the advice of a health professional before using this product.

Caution: Avoid driving a motor vehicle or operating heavy machinery and avoid alcoholic beverages while taking this product.

Drug Interaction Precaution: Do not take this product if you are presently taking a prescription antihypertensive or antidepressant drug containing a monoamine oxidase inhibitor, except under the advice and supervision of a physician.

Directions: Adults and children 12 years of age and over: one tablet every 4 hours. Children 6 to under 12 years: one-half tablet every 4 hours. Do not exceed 6 doses in a 24-hour period.

How Supplied: Blue, scored compressed tablets engraved AHR and 2254 in consumer packages of 24 (NDC 0031-2254-54).
Store at Controlled Room Temperature, Between 15°C and 30°C (59°F and 86°F).
Shown in Product Identification Section, page 423

DIMETAPP® PLUS CAPLETS
[di 'me-tap]

Description: Each **Dimetapp® PLUS Caplet** contains:
Acetaminophen, USP.....................500 mg
Phenylpropanolamine Hydrochloride, USP ....12.5 mg
Brompheniramine Maleate, USP ...2 mg
Inactive Ingredients: Corn starch, FD&C Blue 2 Aluminum Lake, Hydroxypropyl Methylcellulose, Magnesium Stearate, Microcrystalline Cellulose, Polysorbate 20, Povidone, Propylene Glycol, Stearic Acid, Titanium Dioxide. May also contain Calcium Phosphate, Hydroxypropyl Cellulose, Methylparaben, Propylparaben.

Actions: Dimetapp PLUS contains three active ingredients:
a *non-aspirin analgesic* for the temporary relief of aches and pains, headaches and fever.
an *antihistamine* for the temporary relief of runny nose, sneezing, itchy eyes, nose and throat.
a *nasal decongestant* for the temporary relief of stuffy, swollen nasal passages to help restore freer breathing through the nose.

Indications: For the temporary relief of minor aches, pains, and headache; for the reduction of fever; for the relief of nasal congestion due to the common cold or associated with sinusitis; and for the relief of runny nose, sneezing, itching of the nose or throat and itchy and watery eyes as may occur in allergic rhinitis (such as hay fever). Temporarily restores freer breathing through the nose.

Warnings: May cause drowsiness. Avoid alcoholic beverages while taking this product; alcohol may increase the drowsiness effect. Use caution when driving a motor vehicle or operating machinery. May cause excitability, especially in children. Do not give to children under 12 years of age unless under the advice and supervision of a physician. Do not

take this product for more than 7 days. If symptoms do not improve or are accompanied by fever, consult a physician. Do not take this product if you have asthma, glaucoma, heart disease, high blood pressure, thyroid disease, diabetes, emphysema, chronic pulmonary disease, shortness of breath, difficulty in urination due to enlargement of the prostate gland unless directed by a physician. Do not exceed recommended dosage because at higher dosages severe liver damage, nervousness, dizziness, or sleeplessness may occur. As with any drug, if you are pregnant or nursing a baby, seek the advice of a health professional before using this product.

Drug Interaction Precaution: Do not take this product if you are presently taking a prescription drug for high blood pressure or depression without first consulting your physician.

Directions: Adults (12 years and over): Two caplets every 6 hours, NOT TO EXCEED 8 CAPLETS IN A 24-HOUR PERIOD.
Not recommended for children under 12 years of age.

How Supplied: Dimetapp® PLUS Caplets are supplied as blue capsule-shaped film-coated tablets engraved AHR on one side and 2278 on the other in consumer packages of 24 (NDC 0031-2278-54), and 48 (NDC 0031-2278-59) (individually packaged).
Store at Controlled Room Temperature, Between 15°C and 30°C (59°F and 86°F).
Shown in Product Identification Section, page 423

DONNAGEL®
[don 'nă-gel]

Each 30 mL (1 fl. oz.) contains:

Kaolin, USP (90 gr)	6.0 g
Pectin, USP (2 gr)	142.8 mg
Hyoscyamine Sulfate, USP	0.1037 mg
Atropine Sulfate, USP	0.0194 mg
Scopolamine Hydrobromide, USP	0.0065 mg
Sodium Benzoate, N.F. (preservative)	60 mg

Alcohol 3.8 percent

Inactive Ingredients: Citric Acid, D&C Yellow 10, FD&C Blue 1, Flavors, Sodium Carboxymethylcellulose, Sodium Chloride, Sorbitol, Water.

Indications: Donnagel is indicated in the treatment of diarrhea and associated cramping.

Description: Donnagel combines the adsorbent and detoxifying effects of Kaolin and Pectin with the antispasmodic efficacy of the natural Belladonna alkaloids. The latter, present in a specific, fixed ratio, help control hypermotility and hypersecretion in the gastrointestinal tract.

Warnings: As with any drug, if you are pregnant or nursing a baby, seek the advice of a health professional before taking this product.

Contraindications: Glaucoma or increased ocular pressure, advanced renal or hepatic disease or hypersensitivity to any of the ingredients.

Precautions: As with all preparations containing Belladonna alkaloids, Donnagel must be administered cautiously to patients with incipient glaucoma or urinary bladder neck obstruction as in prostatic hypertrophy. Use with caution in elderly patients (where undiagnosed glaucoma or excessive pressure occurs most frequently).

Adverse Reactions: Blurred vision, dry mouth, difficult urination, flushing and dryness of the skin, dizziness or tachycardia may occur at higher dosage levels, rarely at the usual dose.

Dosage and Administration:
[See table above].
Do not take more than 4 doses in any 24-hour period.

How Supplied: Donnagel (light green, aromatic suspension) in 4 fl. oz. (NDC 0031-3016-12), 8 fl. oz. (NDC 0031-3016-18), and pint (NDC 0031-3016-25).
Store at Controlled Room Temperature, Between 15°C and 30°C (59°F and 86°F).
Shown in Product Identification Section, page 423

ROBITUSSIN®
(Guaifenesin Syrup, USP)
[ro "bĭ-tuss 'ĭn]

Ingredients per teaspoonful (5 mL)
Guaifenesin, USP 100 mg in pleasant tasting syrup with alcohol 3.5 percent.
Inactive Ingredients: Caramel, Citric Acid, FD&C Red 40, Flavors, Glucose, Glycerin, High Fructose Corn Syrup, Saccharin Sodium, Sodium Benzoate, Water.

Indications: Expectorant action to help loosen phlegm and bronchial secretions.

Warnings: A persistent cough may be a sign of a serious condition. If cough persists for more than 1 week, tends to recur, or is accompanied by fever, rash, or persistent headache, consult a doctor. Do not take this product for persistent or chronic cough such as occurs with smoking, asthma, emphysema, or if cough is accompanied by excessive phlegm (mucus) unless directed by a doctor. As with any drug, if you are pregnant or nursing a baby, seek the advice of a health professional before using this product.

Contraindications: Hypersensitivity to guaifenesin.

Adverse Reactions: Guaifenesin is well tolerated and has a wide margin of safety. Nausea and vomiting are the side effects that occur most commonly, and other reported adverse reactions have included dizziness, headache, and rash (including urticaria).

	Initial	Every 3 Hours
Adults:	2 Tablespoonfuls (1 Fl. Oz.)	1 Tablespoonful
Children:		
Over 12 Years:	2 Tablespoonfuls	1 Tablespoonful
6–12 Years:	2 Teaspoonfuls	1–2 Teaspoonfuls

Note: Guaifenesin has been shown to produce a color interference with certain clinical laboratory determinations of 5-hydroxyindoleacetic acid (5-HIAA) and vanillylmandelic acid (VMA).

Directions: Adults and children 12 years and over: 2–4 teaspoonfuls every 4 hours; children 6 years to under 12 years: 1–2 teaspoonfuls every 4 hours. Children 2 years to under 6 years: ½–1 teaspoonful every 4 hours; children under 2 years—consult your doctor. DO NOT EXCEED RECOMMENDED DOSAGE.

How Supplied: Robitussin (wine-colored) in bottles of 4 fl. oz. (NDC 0031-8624-12) 8 fl. oz. (NDC 0031-8624-18), pint (NDC 0031-8624-25) and gallon (NDC 0031-8624-29).
Robitussin also available in 1 fl. oz. bottles (4 × 25's NDC 0031-8624-02) and Dis-Co® Unit Dose Packs of 10 × 10's in 5 mL (NDC 0031-8624-23), 10 mL (NDC 0031-8624-26 and 15 mL (NDC 0031-8624-28).
Store at Controlled Room Temperature, Between 15°C and 30°C (59°F and 86°F).
Shown in Product Identification Section, page 424

ROBITUSSIN–CF®
[ro "bĭ-tuss 'ĭn]

Ingredients per teaspoonful (5 mL)
Guaifenesin, USP 100 mg and Phenylpropanolamine Hydrochloride, USP 12.5 mg and Dextromethorphan Hydrobromide, USP 10 mg in pleasant tasting syrup with alcohol 4.75 percent.

Inactive Ingredients: Citric Acid, FD&C Red 40, Flavors, Glycerin, Propylene Glycol, Saccharin Sodium, Sodium Benzoate, Sorbitol, Water.

Indications: Temporarily relieves coughs due to minor throat and bronchial irritation and nasal congestion as may occur with a cold. Expectorant action to help loosen phlegm and bronchial secretions.

Warnings: A persistent cough may be a sign of a serious condition. If cough persists for more than 1 week, tends to recur, or is accompanied by fever, rash, or persistent headache, consult a doctor. Do not take this product for persistent or chronic cough such as occurs with smoking, asthma, emphysema, or if cough is accompanied by excessive phlegm (mu-

Continued on next page

Prescribing information on A.H. Robins products listed here is based on official labeling in effect November 1, 1988 with Indications, Contraindications, Warnings, Precautions, Adverse Reactions, and Dosage stated in full.

Robins—Cont.

cus) unless directed by a doctor. Persons with high blood pressure, heart disease, diabetes, or thyroid disease should use only as directed by a doctor. As with any drug, if you are pregnant or nursing a baby, seek the advice of a health professional before using this product.

Contraindications: Hypersensitivity to guaifenesin, dextromethorphan or sympathomimetic amines; marked hypertension; hyperthyroidism; patients who are receiving monoamine oxidase inhibitors (MAOIs).

Adverse Reactions: The following adverse reactions may occur: nausea, vomiting, dizziness, dry mouth, nervousness, insomnia, restlessness, headache, or rash (including urticaria).
Note: Guaifenesin has been shown to produce a color interference with certain clinical laboratory determinations of 5-hydroxyindoleacetic acid (5-HIAA) and vanillylmandelic acid (VMA).

Drug Interaction Precautions: Concomitant administration of phenylpropanolamine with other sympathomimetic agents may produce additive effects and increased toxicity; with MAOIs may produce a hypertensive crisis; with certain antihypertensive agents may diminish their antihypertensive effect. Serious toxicity may result if dextromethorphan is used with MAOIs.

Directions: Adults and children 12 years and over, 2 teaspoonfuls every 4 hours; children 6 years to under 12 years, 1 teaspoonful every 4 hours; children 2 years to under 6 years, ½ teaspoonful every 4 hours; children under 2 years—consult your doctor. DO NOT EXCEED 6 DOSES IN A 24-HOUR PERIOD.

How Supplied: Robitussin-CF (red-colored) in bottles of 4 fl. oz. (NDC 0031-8677-12), 8 fl. oz. (NDC 0031-8677-18), and one pint (NDC 0031-8677-25).
Store at Controlled Room Temperature, Between 15°C and 30°C (59°F and 86°F).
Shown in Product Identification Section, page 424

ROBITUSSIN-DM®
[ro "bĭ-tuss 'ĭn]

Ingredients per teaspoonful (5 mL)
Guaifenesin, USP 100 mg and Dextromethorphan Hydrobromide, USP 15 mg in pleasant tasting syrup with alcohol 1.4 percent.

Inactive Ingredients: Citric Acid, FD&C Red 40, Flavors, Glucose, Glycerin, High Fructose Corn Syrup, Saccharin Sodium, Sodium Benzoate, Water.

Indications: Temporarily relieves coughs due to minor throat and bronchial irritation as may occur with a cold. Expectorant action to help loosen phlegm and bronchial secretions.

Warnings: A persistent cough may be a sign of a serious condition. If cough persists for more than 1 week, tends to recur, or is accompanied by fever, rash, or

persistent headache, consult a doctor. Do not take this product for persistent or chronic cough such as occurs with smoking, asthma, emphysema, or if cough is accompanied by excessive phlegm (mucus) unless directed by a doctor. As with any drug, if you are pregnant or nursing a baby, seek the advice of a health professional before using this product.

Contraindications: Hypersensitivity to guaifenesin or dextromethorphan, or in patients who are receiving monoamine oxidase inhibitors (MAOIs).

Adverse Reactions: The incidence of side effects is low. Reported side effects include nausea and vomiting, as well as diarrhea, drowsiness, and rash (including urticaria).
Overdose symptoms may include ataxia, respiratory depression and convulsions in children, whereas adults may exhibit altered sensory perception, ataxia, slurred speech and dysphoria.
Note: Guaifenesin has been shown to produce a color interference with certain clinical laboratory determinations of 5-hydroxyindoleacetic acid (5-HIAA) and vanillylmandelic acid (VMA).

Drug Interaction Precautions: Serious toxicity may result if dextromethorphan is used with MAOIs.

Directions: Adults and children 12 years and over, 2 teaspoonfuls every 6 to 8 hours; children 6 years to under 12 years, 1 teaspoonful every 6 to 8 hours; children 2 years to under 6 years, ½ teaspoonful every 6 to 8 hours; children under 2 years—consult your doctor. DO NOT EXCEED 4 DOSES IN A 24-HOUR PERIOD.

How Supplied: Robitussin-DM (cherry-colored) in bottles of 4 fl. oz. (NDC 0031-8684-12), 8 fl. oz. (NDC 0031-8684-18), 12 fl. oz. (NDC 0031-8684-22), pint (NDC 0031-8684-25), and gallon (NDC 0031-8684-29).
Robitussin-DM also available in Dis-Co® Unit Dose Packs of 10 × 10's in 5 mL (NDC 0031-8684-23) and 10 mL (NDC 0031-8684-26).
Store at Controlled Room Temperature, Between 15°C and 30°C (59°F and 86°F).
Shown in Product Identification Section, page 424

ROBITUSSIN-PE®
[ro "bĭ-tuss 'ĭn]

Ingredients per teaspoonful (5 mL)
Guaifenesin, USP 100 mg and Pseudoephedrine Hydrochloride, USP 30 mg in pleasant tasting syrup with alcohol 1.4 percent.

Inactive Ingredients: Citric Acid, FD&C Red 40, Flavors, Glucose, Glycerin, High Fructose Corn Syrup, Saccharin Sodium, Sodium Benzoate, Water.

Indications: Temporarily relieves nasal congestion as may occur with a cold. Expectorant action to help loosen phlegm and bronchial secretions.

Warnings: A persistent cough may be a sign of a serious condition. If cough per-

sists for more than 1 week, tends to recur, or is accompanied by fever, rash, or persistent headache, consult a doctor. Do not take this product for persistent or chronic cough such as occurs with smoking, asthma, emphysema, or if cough is accompanied by excessive phlegm (mucus) unless directed by a doctor. Persons with high blood pressure, heart disease, diabetes, or thyroid disease should use only as directed by a doctor. As with any drug, if you are pregnant or nursing a baby, seek the advice of a health professional before using this product.

Contraindications: Hypersensitivity to guaifenesin or sympathomimetic amines; marked hypertension; hyperthyroidism; or in patients who are receiving monoamine oxidase inhibitors (MAOIs).

Adverse Reactions: Possible side effects include nausea, vomiting, nervousness, restlessness, rash (including urticaria), headache, or dry mouth.
Note: Guaifenesin has been shown to produce a color interference with certain clinical laboratory determinations of 5-hydroxyindoleacetic acid (5-HIAA) and vanillylmandelic acid (VMA).

Drug Interaction Precautions: Concomitant administration of pseudoephedrine with other sympathomimetic agents may produce additive effects and increased toxicity; with MAOIs may produce a hypertensive crisis; with certain antihypertensive agents may diminish their antihypertensive effect.

Directions: Adults and children 12 years and over, 2 teaspoonfuls every 4 hours; children 6 years to under 12 years, 1 teaspoonful every 4 hours; children 2 years to under 6 years, ½ teaspoonful every 4 hours; children under 2 years—consult your doctor. DO NOT EXCEED 4 DOSES IN A 24-HOUR PERIOD.

How Supplied: Robitussin-PE (orange-red) in bottles of 4 fl. oz. (NDC 0031-8695-12), 8 fl. oz. (NDC 0031-8695-18) and pint (NDC 0031-8695-25).
Store at Controlled Room Temperature, Between 15°C and 30°C (59°F and 86°F).
Shown in Product Identification Section, page 424

ROBITUSSIN NIGHT RELIEF®
[ro "bĭ-tuss 'ĭn]
COLDS FORMULA

Composition:
Each fluid ounce contains:
Acetaminophen, USP ....1,000 mg
Phenylephrine HCl, USP ....10 mg
Pyrilamine Maleate, USP ....50 mg
Dextromethorphan
    Hydrobromide, USP ....30 mg
Alcohol 25%

Inactive Ingredients: Citric Acid, FD&C Blue 1, FD&C Red 40, Flavors, Glycerin, Propylene Glycol, Saccharin Sodium, Sodium Benzoate, Sorbitol, Water.

Indications: Temporarily relieves cough, runny nose, sneezing and nasal congestion as may occur with a cold. Also relieves fever, headache, minor sore

throat pain, and body aches and pains as may occur with a cold.

Warnings: This preparation may cause drowsiness. Do not drive or operate machinery while taking this medication. Do not give to children under 12 years of age, unless directed by a doctor. Do not use for more than 10 days. Persons with asthma, glaucoma, high blood pressure, diabetes, heart or thyroid disease or difficulty in urination due to enlargement of the prostate gland should use only as directed by a doctor. Reduce dosage if nervousness, restlessness or sleeplessness occurs. Avoid alcoholic beverages while taking this product. A persistent cough may be a sign of a serious condition. If cough persists for more than 1 week, tends to recur, or is accompanied by fever, rash or persistent headache, consult a doctor. Do not take this product for persistent or chronic cough such as occurs with smoking, asthma, emphysema, or if cough is accompanied by excessive phlegm (mucus) unless directed by a doctor. As with any drug, if you are pregnant or nursing a baby, seek the advice of a health professional before using this product.

Contraindications: Hypersensitivity to any of the ingredients; marked by hypertension, hyperthyroidism or in patients who are receiving monoamine oxidase inhibitors. (MAOIs).

Adverse Effects: The following adverse reactions may possibly occur: nausea, vomiting, dizziness, diarrhea, nervousness, insomnia and drowsiness.

Drug Interaction Precautions: Concomitant administration with other CNS depressants may produce additive sedation; with other sympathomimetic agents may produce additive effects and increased toxicity; with certain antihypertensive agents may diminish their antihypertensive effect; with MAOIs may produce hypertensive crisis, enhanced antimuscarinic effects and other serious toxicity.

Dosage: Adults (12 years and over): one fluid ounce (2 tablespoonfuls) at bedtime. If your cold keeps you confined to bed or at home, take one dose every 6 hours not to exceed 4 doses per 24-hour period.
NOT RECOMMENDED FOR CHILDREN UNDER 12 YEARS.

How Supplied: Bottles of 4 fl. oz. (NDC 0031-8640-12) and 8 fl. oz. (NDC 0031-8640-18).
Store at Controlled Room Temperature, Between 15°C and 30°C (59°F and 86°F).
Shown in Product Identification Section, page 424

Z–BEC® Tablets
[zē'bĕk]

One tablet daily provides:

Vitamin Composition	Percentage of U.S. Recommended Daily Allowance (U.S. RDA)	
Vitamin E	150	45.0 I.U.
Vitamin C	1000	600.0 mg
Thiamine (Vitamin B$_1$)	1000	15.0 mg
Riboflavin (Vitamin B$_2$)	600	10.2 mg
Niacin	500	100.0 mg
Vitamin B$_6$	500	10.0 mg
Vitamin B$_{12}$	100	6.0 mcg
Pantothenic Acid	250	25.0 mg
Mineral Composition		
Zinc	150	22.5 mg*

*22.5 mg zinc (equivalent to zinc content in 100 mg Zinc Sulfate, USP)

Ingredients: Niacinamide Ascorbate; Ascorbic Acid; Microcrystalline Cellulose; Zinc Sulfate; Vitamin E Acetate; Hydrolyzed Protein; Calcium Pantothenate; Modified Starch; Hydroxypropyl Methylcellulose; Thiamine Mononitrate; Stearic Acid; Pyridoxine Hydrochloride; Riboflavin; Silicon Dioxide; Polysorbate 20; Magnesium Stearate; Lactose; Povidone; Propylene Glycol; Artificial Color; Vanillin; Hydroxypropyl Cellulose; Gelatin; Sorbic Acid; Sodium Benzoate; Cyanocobalamin.

Actions and Uses: Z-BEC is a high potency formulation. Its components have important roles in general nutrition, healing of wounds, and prevention of hemorrhage. It is recommended for deficiencies of these components in conditions such as febrile diseases, chronic or acute infections, burns, fractures, surgery, leg ulcers, toxic conditions, physiologic stress, alcoholism, prolonged exposure to high temperature, geriatrics, gastritis, peptic ulcer, and colitis; and in conditions involving special diets and weight-reduction diets.
In dentistry, Z-BEC is recommended for deficiencies of its components in conditions such as herpetic stomatitis, aphthous stomatitis, cheilosis herpangina and gingivitis.

Precaution: Not intended for the treatment of pernicious anemia.

Dosage: The recommended OTC dosage for adults and children twelve or more years of age, is one tablet daily with food or after meals. Under the direction and supervision of a physician, the dose and frequency of administration may be increased in accordance with the patient's requirements.

How Supplied: Green film-coated, capsule shaped tablets in bottles of 60 (NDC 0031-0689-62), 500 (NDC 0031-0689-70), and Dis-Co® Unit Dose Packs of 100 (NDC 0031-0689-64).
Shown in Product Identification Section, page 424

Products are cross-indexed by product classifications in the **BLUE SECTION**

Rorer Consumer Pharmaceuticals
a division of
Rorer Pharmaceutical Corporation
500 VIRGINIA DRIVE
FORT WASHINGTON, PA 19034

Regular Strength
ASCRIPTIN®
[ă"skrĭp'tin]
Analgesic
Aspirin plus Maalox®

Active Ingredients: Each coated tablet contains Aspirin (325 mg) and Maalox (Magnesium Hydroxide 50 mg, Dried Aluminum Hydroxide Gel 50 mg), buffered with Calcium Carbonate.

Inactive Ingredients: Hydroxypropyl Methylcellulose, Magnesium Stearate, Microcrystalline Cellulose, Starch, Talc, Titanium Dioxide, and other ingredients.

Description: Ascriptin is an excellent analgesic, antipyretic, and anti-inflammatory agent for general use, particularly where there is concern over aspirin-induced gastric distress. When large doses are used, as in arthritis and rheumatic disorders, gastric discomfort is rare. Coated tablets make swallowing easy.

Indications: As an analgesic for the relief of pain in such conditions as headache, neuralgia, minor injuries, and dysmenorrhea. As an analgesic and antipyretic in colds and influenza. As an analgesic and anti-inflammatory agent in arthritis and other rheumatic diseases. As an inhibitor of platelet aggregation, see MI's and TIA's indications (page 4).

Usual Adult Dose: Two or three tablets four times daily. For children under 12, at the discretion of the physician. Caution in arthritis and rheumatism, if pain persists for more than 10 days, or redness is present, consult a physician immediately. As an inhibitor of platelet aggregation, see MI's and TIA's dosage information [See next page].

Drug Interaction Precaution: Do not use if you are taking a prescription antibiotic drug containing tetracycline.
WARNINGS: Children and teenagers should not use this medicine for chicken pox or flu symptoms before a doctor is consulted about Reye syndrome, a rare but serious illness reported to be associated with aspirin. Keep this and all medicines out of children's reach. In case of accidental overdose, contact a physician immediately. As with any drug, if you are pregnant or nursing a baby, seek the advice of a health professional before using this product. If you are under medical care or have a history of stomach, kidney, or bleeding disorders, asthma or aspirin sensitivity, or if ringing in the ears occurs, consult a physician before use. Do not use if you are taking a prescription antibiotic drug containing tetracycline.

Continued on next page

Rorer Consumer—Cont.

Professional Labeling:
Aspirin for Myocardial Infarction

Indication: Aspirin is indicated to reduce the risk of death and/or non-fatal myocardial infarction in patients with a previous infarction or unstable angina pectoris.

Dosage and Administration: Although most of the studies used dosages exceeding 300 mg. two trials used only 300 mg. and pharmacologic data indicate that this dose inhibits platelet function fully. Therefore, 300 mg or a conventional 325-mg aspirin dose is a reasonable, routine dose that would minimize gastrointestinal adverse reactions. This use of aspirin applies to both solid, oral dosage forms (buffered and plain aspirin), and buffered aspirin in solution. Note: Complete information and references available.

RECURRENT TIA'S IN MEN

Indications: For reducing the risk of recurrent transient ischemic attacks (TIA's) or stroke in men who have had transient ischemia of the brain due to fibrin platelet emboli. There is inadequate evidence that aspirin or buffered aspirin is effective in reducing TIA's in women at the recommended dosage. There is no evidence that aspirin or buffered aspirin is of benefit in the treatment of completed strokes in men or women.

Precautions: (1) Patients presenting with signs and symptoms of TIA's should have a complete medical and neurologic evaluation. Consideration should be given to other disorders which resemble TIA's. (2) Attention should be given to risk factors; It is important to evaluate and treat, if appropriate, other diseases associated with TIA's and stroke such as hypertension and diabetes. (3) Concurrent administration of absorbable antacids at therapeutic doses may increase the clearance of salicylates in some individuals. The concurrent administration of nonabsorbable antacids may alter the rate of absorption of aspirin, thereby resulting in a decreased acetylsalicylic acid/salicylate ratio in plasma. The clinical significance on TIA's of these decreases in available aspirin is unknown.

Dosage: 1300 mg a day, in divided doses of 650 mg twice a day or 325 mg four times a day.

Supplied: Bottles of 50 tablets (NDC 0067-0145-50), 100 tablets (NDC 0067-0145-68), and 225 tablets (NDC 0067-0145-77) with child-resistant caps. Bottles of 500 tablets (NDC 0067-0145-74) without child-resistant closures (for arthritic patients). Military Stock #NSN 6505-00-135-2783 V.A. Stock #6505-00-890-1979 (bottles of 500).

Shown in Product Identification Section, page 424

ASCRIPTIN® A/D for arthritis pain
Analgesic
Aspirin plus 50% more Maalox® for arthritis
pain relief with extra stomach comfort

Aspirin for arthritis pain relief plus contains 50% more Maalox than does Regular Strength Ascriptin.

Active Ingredients: Each coated caplet contains Aspirin (325 mg) and Maalox (Magnesium Hydroxide 75 mg. Dried Aluminum Hydroxide Gel 75 mg), buffered with Calcium Carbonate.

Inactive Ingredients: Hydroxypropyl Methylcellulose, Magnesium Stearate, Microcrystalline Cellulose, Starch, Talc, Titanium Dioxide, and other ingredients.

Description: Ascriptin A/D is a highly buffered analgesic, anti-inflammatory, and antipyretic agent for use in the treatment of rheumatoid arthritis, osteoarthritis, and other arthritic conditions. It is formulated with added Maalox to provide increased neutralization of gastric acid thus improving the likelihood of GI tolerance when large antiarthritic doses of aspirin are used. Coated caplets make swallowing easy.

Indications: As an analgesic, anti-inflammatory, and antipyretic agent in rheumatoid arthritis, osteoarthritis, and other arthritic conditions.

Usual Adult Dose: Two or three caplets, four times daily, or as directed by the physician for arthritis therapy. For children under twelve, at the discretion of the physician. Caution in arthritis and rheumatism, if pain persists for more than 10 days, or redness is present, consult a physician immediately.

Drug Interaction Precaution: Do not use if you are taking a prescription antibiotic drug containing tetracycline.
WARNINGS: Children and teenagers should not use this medicine for chicken pox or flu symptoms before a doctor is consulted about Reye syndrome, a rare but serious illness reported to be associated with aspirin. Keep this and all medicines out of children's reach. In case of accidental overdose, contact a physician immediately. As with any drug, if you are pregnant or nursing a baby, seek the advice of a health professional before using this product. If you are under medical care or have a history of stomach, kidney, or bleeding disorders, asthma or aspirin sensitivity, or if ringing in the ears occurs, consult a physician. Do not use if you are taking a prescription antibiotic drug containing tetracycline.

Supplied: Available in bottles of 100 caplets (NDC 0067-0147-68), and 225 caplets (NDC 0067-0147-77) with child-resistant caps and in special bottles of 500 caplets (without child-resistant closures) for arthritic patients (NDC 0067-0147-74).

Shown in Product Identification Section, page 424

Extra Strength
ASCRIPTIN®
Analgesic
50% more Aspirin plus Maalox®

Active Ingredients: Each coated caplet contains Aspirin (500 mg) and Maalox (Magnesium Hydroxide 80 mg, Dried Aluminum Hydroxide Gel 80 mg), buffered with Calcium Carbonate.

Inactive Ingredients: Hydroxypropyl Methylcellulose, Magnesium Stearate, Microcrystalline Cellulose, Starch, Talc, Titanium Dioxide, and other ingredients.

Description: Extra Strength Ascriptin contains 50% more aspirin for fast, effective pain relief and Maalox for protection against aspirin-induced gastric distress. Coated caplets make swallowing easy.

Indications: For maximum relief of pain in headache, neuralgia, minor injuries, dysmenorrhea, discomfort and fever of ordinary colds. As an analgesic and anti-inflammatory agent in arthritis and other rheumatic diseases.

Usual Adult Dose: 2 caplets, three or four times daily. Not to exceed a total of 8 tablets in a 24-hour period, or as directed by a physician. Take this product with a full glass of water. For children under 12 at the discretion of physician. Caution: In arthritis and rheumatism, if pain persists for more than 10 days, or redness is present, consult a physician immediately.

Drug Interaction Precaution: Do not use if you are taking a prescription antibiotic drug containing tetracycline.
WARNINGS: Children and teenagers should not use this medicine for chicken pox or flu symptoms before a doctor is consulted about Reye syndrome, a rare but serious illness reported to be associated with aspirin.
Keep this and all medicines out of children's reach. In case of accidental overdose, contact a physician immediately. As with any drug, if your are pregnant or nursing a baby, seek the advice of a health professional before using this product. If you are under medical care or have a history of stomach, kidney, or bleeding disorders, asthma or aspirin sensitivity, or if ringing in the ears occurs, consult a physician. Do not use if you are taking a prescription antibiotic drug containing tetracycline.

Supplied: Bottles of 36 caplets (NDC 0067-0146-63) and 74 caplets (NDC 0067-0146-75) with child-resistant caps.

Shown in Product Identification Section, page 424

CAMALOX®
[kăm 'ă-lŏx "]
Magnesium and Aluminum Hydroxides with Calcium Carbonate Oral Suspension and Tablets, Rorer High-potency antacid

Description: Camalox® Suspension is a carefully balanced formulation of 200 mg magnesium hydroxide, 225 mg aluminum hydroxide and 250 mg calcium carbonate per teaspoonful (5 mL).

This combination of ingredients produces an antacid capability that exceeds that of other leading ethical products in terms of quantity of acid neutralized as well as the speed and duration of antacid activity as measured by laboratory tests. The formulation also minimizes the possibilities of both constipation and diarrhea. Camalox is prepared by a process which enhances its texture and vanilla-mint flavor, making it especially palatable even for patients who must take antacids for extended periods.

Inactive Ingredients: Citric acid, flavors, guar gum, methylparaben, propylparaben, silica, saccharin sodium, sorbitol solution, purified water.

Camalox® Tablets contain 200 mg magnesium hydroxide, 225 mg aluminum hydroxide and 250 mg calcium carbonate per tablet and have a delicate vanilla-mint flavor. They compare favorably with Camalox Suspension in terms of potency, as well as speed and duration of antacid activity, thus, Camalox Tablets overcome the usual deficiencies of antacid tablets. As measured by the *in vitro* test for acid neutralizing capacity, Camalox Tablets exceed the antacid capabilities of the leading ethical antacid suspensions as well as tablets. In addition, the manufacturing process contributes importantly to the flavor and to the texture of the tablets. Patients can take Camalox Tablets in full dosage day after day without tiring of the taste.

Inactive Ingredients: Citric acid, colloidal silicon dioxide, flavors, light mineral oil, magnesium stearate, mannitol, microcrystalline cellulose, silica, saccharin sodium, sorbitol solution, starch.

Acid Neutralizing Capacity
Camalox Suspension—36.9 mEq/10 mL
Camalox Tablets—36.7 mEq/2 tablets
Sodium Content
Camalox Suspension—1.2 mg (0.05 mEq)/5 mL
Camalox Tablets—1.0 mg (0.04 mEq)/tablet

Indications: A high potency antacid for the symptomatic relief of hyperacidity associated with the diagnosis of peptic ulcer, gastritis, peptic esophagitis, gastric hyperacidity, heartburn, or hiatal hernia.

Directions for Use: Camalox Suspension—two to four teaspoonfuls, four times a day, taken one-half hour after meals and at bedtime, or as directed by a physician.
Camalox Tablets—each Camalox Tablet is equivalent to one teaspoonful of Camalox Suspension. Two to four tablets, well-chewed, one-half to one hour after meals and at bedtime, or as directed by a physician.

Patient Warnings: Do not take more than 16 teaspoonfuls or tablets in a 24-hour period or use the maximum dosage for more than two weeks or use if you have kidney disease except under the advice and supervision of a physician. Keep this and all drugs out of the reach of children.

Drug Interaction Precaution: Do not use with patients taking a prescription antibiotic drug containing any form of tetracycline. As with all aluminum-containing antacids, Camalox may prevent the proper absorption of tetracycline.

How Supplied: Camalox Suspension—white liquid in convenient 12 fluid ounce (355 mL) plastic bottles (NDC 0067-0180-71).
Camalox Tablets—Bottles of 50 tablets (NDC 0067-0185-50).

Rationale: Studies reveal that clinical symptoms of gastroesophageal reflux correlate with lower esophageal sphincter (LES) incompetency. Although the mechanism of action is unknown, gastric alkalinization has been shown to increase LES pressure.
Camalox is an ideal antacid for the treatment of reflux esophagitis. The balanced formulation of Camalox exerts its neutralizing effect faster and longer than the leading ethical antacids providing prompt symptomatic relief.
Camalox has been shown to produce significant increases in LES pressure providing a physiological barrier against reflux.*
Because Camalox is a high potency antacid with excellent acid neutralizing capacity, fewer and smaller doses are possible.
The refreshing vanilla-mint flavor and smooth texture of Camalox have earned a high level of patient acceptance and wearability. Available in equally effective dosage forms . . . physician-preferred suspension and convenient tablets.

---

*Higgs, R.H., Smyth, R.D., and Castell, D.O., Gastric Alkalinization—Effect on Lower-Esophageal-Sphincter Pressure and Serum Gastrin, N. Engl. J. Med. 291:486-490, 1974.
Shown in Product Identification Section, page 424

FERMALOX®
[fĕr 'mă-lŏx "]
Hematinic

Formula: Each *uncoated* tablet contains: Ferrous Sulfate 200 mg; Maalox® (magnesium-aluminum hydroxide) 200 mg.

Inactive Ingredients: Confectioners' sugar, ethylcellulose, flavors, iron oxides, magnesium stearate, starch, talc.

Advantages: "A less irritating, more easily tolerated medicinal iron compound (Fermalox) fills an important need in the treatment of iron-deficiency states. The demonstration of effective absorption by means of the radioactive iron tracer, plus thousands of clinical cases showing satisfactory rise of hemoglobin level, fully establishes the efficacy of this medicament. In addition, the almost complete absence of the common adverse reactions to ordinary iron medicaments enables the physician to continue use of the drug until a satisfactory therapeutic result is obtained."[1]

Indications: For use as a hematinic in iron-deficiency conditions as may occur with: rapid growth, pregnancy, blood loss, menorrhagia, post-surgical convalescence, pathologic bleeding.

Usual Adult Dose: Two tablets daily; in mild cases dosage may be reduced to one tablet daily.

Warning: As with any drug, if you are pregnant or nursing a baby, seek the advice of a health professional before using this product. Keep this and all drugs out of the reach of children. In case of accidental overdose, seek professional assistance or contact a poison control center immediately.

Supplied: Bottles of 100 tablets (NDC 0067-0260-68) with child-resistant caps.
1. Price, A.H., Erf, L., and Bierly, J.: J.A.M.A. 167:1612 (July 26), 1958.

MAALOX®
[mă 'lŏx "]
Magnesia and Alumina Oral Suspension and Tablets, Rorer Antacid
A Balanced Formulation of Magnesium and Aluminum Hydroxides

Description: Maalox® Suspension is a balanced combination of magnesium and aluminum hydroxides. . . first in order of preference for all routine purposes of antacid medication. The high neutralizing power of magnesium hydroxide and the established acid binding capacity of aluminum hydroxide support the reputation of Maalox® for reliable antacid action.
Maalox® Suspension: 225 mg Aluminum Hydroxide Equivalent to Dried Gel, USP, and 200 mg Magnesium Hydroxide per 5 mL.

Inactive Ingredients: Citric acid, methylparaben, natural flavor, propylparaben, saccharin sodium, sorbitol, purified water, and other ingredients.
Maalox® Tablets: (200 mg Magnesium Hydroxide, 200 mg Dried Aluminum Hydroxide Gel) per tablet

Inactive Ingredients: Citric acid, flavors, magnesium stearate, mannitol, microcrystalline cellulose, saccharin sodium, sorbitol solution, starch.
Extra Strength Maalox® Tablets: (400 mg Magnesium Hydroxide, 400 mg Dried Aluminum Hydroxide Gel) per tablet

Inactive Ingredients: Confectioner's sugar, flavors, glycerin, magnesium stearate, mannitol, saccharin sodium, sorbitol sucrose, talc.
Acid Neutralizing Capacity
Maalox® Suspension—26.6 mEq/10 ml
Maalox® Tablets—19.4 mEq/2 tablets
Extra Strength Maalox® Tablets—23.4 mEq/tablet
Sodium Content
Maalox® Suspension and Tablets are dietetically sodium-free*. Each teaspoonful (5 mL) of Maalox® Suspension con-

Continued on next page

Rorer Consumer—Cont.

tains approximately 0.06 mEq sodium (1.4 mg) and Maalox® and Extra Strength Maalox® Tablets contain approximately 0.03 mEq (0.7 mg) and 0.06 mEq (1.4 mg) sodium respectively per tablet.

*dietetically insignificant

Indications: As an antacid for symptomatic relief of hyperacidity associated with the diagnosis of peptic ulcer, gastritis, peptic esophagitis, gastric hyperacidity, heartburn or hiatal hernia.

Advantages: Many patients prefer Maalox® whether they are taking it for occasional heartburn or routinely on an ulcer therapy regimen. Once started on Maalox®, patients tend to stay on Maalox® because of effectiveness, taste, and non-constipating characteristics... three important reasons for Maalox® when prolonged therapy is necessary. In addition, Maalox® Suspension and Tablets are sodium-free.

Directions for use:
Maalox® Suspension: Two to four teaspoonfuls, four times a day, taken twenty minutes to one hour after meals and at bedtime, or as directed by a physician.
Maalox® Tablets: Two to four tablets, well chewed, twenty minutes to one hour after meals and at bedtime, or as directed by a physician.
Extra Strength Maalox® Tablets: One or two tablets, well chewed, four times a day, taken twenty minutes to one hour after meals and at bedtime, or as directed by a physician. May be followed with milk or water.
Patient Warnings: Do not take more than 16 teaspoonfuls of Maalox® Suspension, 16 Maalox® Tablets, or 8 Extra Strength Maalox® Tablets in a 24-hour period or use the maximum dosage for more than 2 weeks or use if you have kidney disease, except under the supervision of a physician.

Drug Interaction Precaution: Do not use with patients taking a prescription antibiotic drug containing any form of tetracycline. As with all aluminum-containing antacids, Maalox® may prevent the proper absorption of the tetracycline. Keep this and all drugs out of the reach of children.

Supplied:
Maalox® Suspension is available in plastic bottles of 12 fluid ounces (355 mL) (NDC 0067-0330-71), 5 fluid ounces (148 mL) (NDC 0067-0330-62), and 26 fluid ounces (769 mL) (NDC 0067-0330-44).
Maalox® Tablets (400 mg) available in bottles of 100 tablets (NDC 0067-0335-68).
Extra Strength Maalox® Tablets (800 mg) available in bottles of 50 (NDC 0067-0340-50). Also available in boxes of 24 (NDC 0067-0340-24) and 100 tablets (NDC 0067-0340-67) in easy-to-carry strips.
V.A. Stock #6505-00-993-3507A [boxes of 100 tablets (in cellophane strips)].

Shown in Product Identification Section, page 424

Extra Strength MAALOX® PLUS (Reformulated Maalox Plus)

Alumina, Magnesia and Simethicone Oral Suspension and Tablets, Rorer Antacid/Anti-Gas

☐ **Lemon swiss-creme flavor... the taste preferred by physician and patient.**
☐ **Physician-proven Maalox® formula for antacid effectiveness.**
☐ **Simethicone, at a recognized clinical dose, for antiflatulent action.**

Description: Maalox® Plus, a balanced combination of magnesium and aluminum hydroxides plus simethicone, is a non-constipating, lemon swiss-creme flavored, antacid/anti-gas.

Composition: To provide symptomatic relief of hyperacidity plus alleviation of gas symptoms, each teaspoonful/tablet contains:

Active Ingredients	Extra Strength Maalox® Plus Per Tsp. (5 mL)	Maalox® Plus Per Tablet
Magnesium Hydroxide	450 mg	200 mg
Aluminum Hydroxide	500 mg	200 mg
Simethicone	40 mg	25 mg

Inactive Ingredients: Extra Strength Maalox® Plus Suspension: Citric acid, flavors, methylparaben, propylparaben, saccharin sodium, sorbitol, purified water and other ingredients.
Maalox® Plus Tablets: Citric acid, confectioners' sugar, D&C red No. 30, D&C yellow No. 10, dextrose, flavors, magnesium stearate, mannitol, saccharin sodium, sorbitol solution, starch, talc.
To aid in establishing proper dosage schedules, the following information is provided:

Minimum Recommended Dosage:	Per 2 Tsp. (10 mL)	Per Tablet
Acid neutralizing capacity	58.1 mEq	11.4 mEq
Sodium content*	2.4 mg	0.8 mg
Sugar content	None	0.55 g
Lactose content	None	None

Indications: As an antacid for symptomatic relief of hyperacidity associated with the diagnosis of peptic ulcer, gastri-

tis, peptic esophagitis, gastric hyperacidity, heartburn, or hiatal hernia. As an antiflatulent to alleviate the symptoms of gas, including postoperative gas pain.

Advantages: Among antacids, Maalox® Plus is uniquely palatable—an important feature which encourages patients to follow your dosage directions. Maalox® Plus has the time proven, non-constipating, sodium-free* Maalox® formula—useful for those patients suffering from the problems associated with hyperacidity. Additionally, Maalox® Plus contains simethicone to alleviate discomfort associated with entrapped gas.
*Dietetically insignificant. Contains approximately 0.05 mEq sodium per teaspoonful of Suspension. Each Maalox® Plus Tablet contains approximately 0.03 mEq sodium per Tablet.

Directions for Use:
Extra Strength Maalox® Plus Suspension: Two to four teaspoonfuls, four times a day, taken twenty minutes to one hour after meals and at bedtime, or as directed by a physician.
Maalox® Plus Tablets: One to four tablets, well chewed, four times a day, taken twenty minutes to one hour after meals and at bedtime, or as directed by a physician.

Patient Warnings: Do not take more than 16 teaspoonfuls or 16 tablets in a 24-hour period or use the maximum dosage for more than two weeks or use if you have kidney disease except under the advice and supervision of a physician.

Drug Interaction Precaution: Do not use with patients taking a prescription antibiotic containing any form of tetracycline. As with all aluminum-containing antacids, Maalox® Plus may prevent the proper absorption of the tetracycline. Keep this and all drugs out of the reach of children.

Supplied:
Extra Strength Maalox® Plus Suspension is available in a plastic 12 fluid ounce (355 mL) bottle (NDC 0067-0333-71) and 5 fluid ounce (148 ml) bottle (NDC 0067-0333-62).
Maalox® Plus Tablets are available in bottles of 50 tablets (NDC 0067-0339-50) and 100 tablets (NDC 0067-0339-67), convenience packs of 12 tablets (NDC 0067-0339-19), Roll Packs of 12 tablets (NDC 0067-0339-23), and 36 tablets (NDC 0067-0339-33).

Shown in Product Identification Section, page 424

MAALOX® TC Suspension and Tablets
Therapeutic Concentrate (Magnesium & Aluminum Hydroxides Oral Suspension and Tablets, Rorer)

Description: Maalox® TC Suspension is a potent, concentrated, balanced formulation of 300 mg magnesium hydroxide and 600 mg aluminum hydroxide per teaspoonful (5 mL). This formulation produces a therapeutically concentrated antacid that exceeds standard antacids

in acid neutralizing capacity. Maalox® TC Suspension is formulated to reduce the need to alter therapy due to treatment-induced changes in bowel habits. Palatability is enhanced by a pleasant-tasting peppermint flavor.

Inactive Ingredients: Citric acid, flavor, guar gum, methylparaben, propylparaben, sorbitol solution, purified water.

Maalox® TC Tablets contain 300 mg magnesium hydroxide and 600 mg aluminum hydroxide per tablet, with a pleasant-tasting peppermint-lemon-creme flavor. *In vivo* testing demonstrates a longer duration of action for the tablets when compared with equivalent doses of suspension. Maalox® TC tablets thus overcome the usual deficiencies of antacid tablets.

Inactive Ingredients: Confectioners' sugar, flavors, glycerin, magnesium stearate, mannitol, sorbitol solution, sucrose, talc.

Acid Neutralizing Capacity
Maalox® TC Suspension—27.2 mEq/5 mL
Maalox® TC Tablets—28.0 mEq/tablet

Sodium Content:
Maalox® TC Suspension—0.8 mg/5 mL (0.03 mEq)
Maalox® TC Tablets—0.5 mg/tablet (0.02 mEq)

Indications: Maalox® TC Suspension and Tablets are indicated for the symptomatic relief of hyperacidity associated with the diagnosis of peptic ulcer and other gastrointestinal conditions where a high degree of acid neutralization is desired.

Directions for Use: Maalox® TC Suspension—one or two teaspoonfuls 20 minutes to one hour after meals and at bedtime. Higher dosage regimens may be employed under the direct supervision of a physician in the treatment of active peptic ulcer disease.
Maalox® TC Tablets—each Maalox® tablet is equivalent to one teaspoon of Maalox® TC Suspension. One or two Maalox® TC tablets, well chewed one hour after meals and at bedtime. Higher dosage regimens may be employed under the direct supervision of a physician in the treatment of active peptic ulcer disease.

Patient Warning: Do not take more than 7 teaspoonfuls of the suspension or 8 tablets in a 24-hour period, or use the maximum dosage of this product for more than two weeks except under the advice and supervision of a physician. Also, if you have kidney disease, do not use except under the advice and supervision of a physician.

Drug Interaction Precaution: Do not use with patients taking a prescription antibiotic drug containing any form of tetracycline. As with all aluminum-containing antacids, Maalox® TC may prevent the proper absorption of the tetracycline. Keep this and all drugs out of the reach of children.

Indications: Maalox® TC is indicated for the prevention of stress-induced upper gastrointestinal hemorrhage. As an antacid, for the symptomatic relief of hyperacidity associated with the diagnosis of peptic ulcer and other gastrointestinal conditions where a high degree of acid neutralization is desired.

Directions for Use: PREVENTION OF STRESS-INDUCED UPPER GASTROINTESTINAL HEMORRHAGE: 1) Aspirate stomach via nasogastric tube* and record pH. 2) Instill 10 ml of Maalox® TC followed by 30 ml of water via nasogastric tube. Clamp tube. 3) Wait one hour. Aspirate stomach and record pH. 4a) If pH equals or exceeds 4.0, apply drainage or intermittent suction for one hour, then repeat the cycle. 4b) If pH is less than 4.0, instill double (20 ml) Maalox® TC followed by 30 ml of water. Clamp tube. 5) Wait one hour. If pH equals or exceeds 4.0, see number 7. If pH is still less than 4.0, instill double (40 ml) Maalox® TC followed by 30 ml of water. Clamp tube. 6) Wait one hour. If pH equals or exceeds 4.0, see number 7. If pH is still less than 4.0, instill double (80 ml)** Maalox® TC followed by 30 ml of water. 7) Drain for one hour and repeat cycle with the effective dosage of Maalox® TC. IN HYPERACID STATES FOR SYMPTOMATIC RELIEF: One or two teaspoonfuls as needed between meals and at bedtime or as directed by a physician. Higher dosage regimens may be employed under the direct supervision of a physician in the treatment of active peptic ulcer disease.

*If nasogastric tube is not in place, administer 20 ml of Maalox® TC orally q2h.

**In a recent clinical study[1], 20 ml of Maalox® TC, q2h, was sufficient in more than 85 percent of the patients. No patient studied required more than 80 ml of Maalox® TC q2h.

Precaution: Aluminum-magnesium hydroxide containing antacids should be used with caution in patients with renal impairment.

Adverse Effects: Occasional regurgitation and mild diarrhea have been reported with the dosage recommended for the prevention of stress-induced upper gastrointestinal hemorrhage.

References: 1. Zinner MJ, Zuidema GD, Smith PL, Mignosa M: The prevention of upper gastrointestinal tract bleeding in patients in an intensive care unit. *Surg Gynec & Obstet* 153:214–220, 1981. 2. Lucas CE, Sugawa C, Riddle J et al.: Natural history and surgical dilemma of "stress" gastric bleeding. *Arch Surg* 102:266–273, 1971. 3. Hastings PR, Skillman JJ, Bushnell LS, Silen W: Antacid titration in the prevention of acute gastrointestinal bleeding: a controlled, randomized trial in 100 critically ill patients. *New England J Med* 298:1042–1045, 1978. 4. Day SB, MacMillan BG, Altemeier WA: Curling's Ulcer, An Experiment of Nature. Springfield, IL, Charles C. Thomas Co., 1972, p 205. 5. Skillman JJ, Bushnell LS, Goldman H, Silen W: Respiratory failure, hypotension, sepsis, and jaundice. A clinical syndrome associated with lethal hemorrhage from acute stress ulceration of the stomach. *Am J Surg* 117:523–530, 1969. 6. Priebe HJ, Skillman JJ, Bushnell LS et al.: Antacid versus cimetidine in preventing acute gastrointestinal bleeding. *New England J Med* 302:426–430, 1980. 7. Silen W: The prevention and management of stress ulcers. *Hospital Practice* 15:93–97, 1980. 8. Herrmann V, Kaminski DL: Evaluation of intragastric pH in acutely ill patients. *Arch Surg* 114:511–514, 1979. 9. Martin LF, Staloch DK, Simonowitz DA et al.: Failure of cimetidine prophylaxis in the critically ill. *Arch Surg* 114:492–496, 1979. 10. Zinner MJ, Turtinen L, Gurll N, Reynolds DG: The effect of metiamide on gastric mucosal injury in rat restraint. *Clin Res* 23:484A, 1975. 11. Zinner M, Turtinen BA, Gurll NJ: The role of acid and ischemia in production of stress ulcers during canine hemorrhagic shock. *Surgery* 77:807–816, 1975. 12. Winans CS: Prevention and treatment of stress ulcer bleeding: Antacids or cimetidine? *Drug Therapy* (hospital) 12:37–45, 1981.

How Supplied: Maalox® TC Suspension is available in a 12-fluid ounce (355 mL) plastic bottle (NDC 0067-0334-71). Maalox® TC Tablets are available in plastic bottles of 48 tablets (NDC 0067-0344-48).
* dietetically insignificant
Shown in Product Identification Section, page 424

**Extra Strength
MAALOX WHIP®
Antacid
(Magnesium and Aluminum Hydroxides Oral Suspension, Rorer)**

Indications: For relief of heartburn, acid indigestion, sour stomach and upset stomach associated with these symptoms.

Ingredients: Each 4 gram heaping teaspoonful contains 525 mg of dried aluminum hydroxide gel and 480 mg of magnesium hydroxide. Inactive ingredients: colloidal silicon dioxide, confectioners' sugar, flavors, partially hydrogenated soy bean oil with BHA, propane (propellant), and other ingredients.

Directions for use: one to two heaping teaspoonfuls, four times a day, taken 20 minutes to 1 hour after meals and at bedtime, or as directed by a physician. Hold can upright to dispense. Fill teaspoon to heaping level pictured on front.

Warnings: Do not take more than 8 teaspoonfuls in a 24-hour period or use the maximum dosage for more than 2 weeks or use if you have kidney disease except under the advice and supervision of a physician. Contents under pressure. Do not puncture or incinerate. Do not store at temperatures above 120°F. Keep

Continued on next page

Rorer Consumer—Cont.

this and all drugs out of the reach of children.

Drug Interaction Precaution: Do not use if you are taking a prescription antibiotic drug containing any form of tetracycline.

Acid Neutralizing Capacity: 29.3 mEq/4 gram tsp.

Dietetically sodium free: Less than 0.2 mEq sodium per heaping teaspoonful.

How Supplied: Maalox Whip is available in an 8 ounce aerosol can (NDC 0067-0370-66).

*Shown in Product Identification
Section, page 424*

MYOFLEX® CREME
[mī'ō-flex]
(Trolamine Salicylate)

Description: Trolamine (formerly Triethanolamine) salicylate 10% in a nongreasy base is a nonirritating, nonburning, odorless, stainless, readily absorbed cream. Trolamine salicylate is a topical analgesic. The empirical formula of trolamine salicylate is $C_6H_{15}NO_3 \cdot C_7H_6O_3$, molecular weight 287.31. Its chemical structure is:

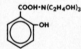

Trolamine salicylate is a light reddish viscous liquid with a faint odor. It is miscible in all proportions with water, glycerin, propylene glycol, and ethyl alcohol.

Clinical Pharmacology: Salicylic acid is the active moiety of MYOFLEX. Salicylic acid is enzymatically biotransformed to salicyluric acid and salicylphenolic glucuronide and eliminated in the urine. Salicylic acid is rapidly distributed throughout all body tissues, mainly by pH-dependent passive processes. It can be detected in synovial, spinal and peritoneal fluids, in saliva and in milk. It readily crosses the placental barrier. About 50% to 90% of salicylic acid is bound to plasma proteins, mainly to albumin.
The urinary excretion of salicylic acid equivalents was studied in 12 normal, healthy male subjects after MYOFLEX application. Salicylic acid was absorbed from MYOFLEX in 11 of 12 normal subjects over the 24-hour period post-application with a mean salicylic acid excretion of 13.5%.
Trolamine salicylate does not block neuronal membranes as do topical anesthetics. Some degree of percutaneous absorption occurs through the skin and blood levels have been demonstrated following topical application in animals and humans. Trolamine salicylate is not a counterirritant analgesic.

Indications: MYOFLEX is indicated as a topical analgesic for the temporary relief of minor aches and pains of mus-

cles and joints due to backache, muscle strains, sprains and bruises or overexertion. It is a useful topical adjunct in arthritis and rheumatism as a cream for patients with minor rheumatic stiffness or sore hands and feet.

Contraindications: MYOFLEX is contraindicated in patients sensitive to its ingredients and patients with advanced chronic renal insufficiency.

Warnings: For external use only. Avoid contact with eyes or mucous membranes. Keep out of the reach of children. If condition worsens, or if symptoms persist for more than 7 days, or clear up and occur again within a few days, discontinue use and consult a doctor.
As with any drug, if you are pregnant or nursing a baby, seek the advice of a health professional before using this product.
As with all salicylates, MYOFLEX should be avoided or used with caution in patients with liver damage, pre-existing hypoprothrombinemia, vitamin K deficiency and before surgery.

Precautions: General—Apply to affected parts only. Do not apply to broken or irritated skin.
Appropriate precautions should be taken by persons known to be sensitive to salicylates or with impairment of renal function. If a reaction develops, the drug should be discontinued.
Drug Interactions—There are no known drug interactions with MYOFLEX. However, salicylates may counteract the effects of uricosuric agents such as probenecid and enhance the effects of oral anticoagulants such as coumadin. Therefore, they must be used with caution in patients on anticoagulants that affect the prothrombin time. Caution should also be exercised in patients concurrently treated with a sulfonylurea hypoglycemic agent, methotrexate, barbiturates and diphenylhydantoin, because these drugs may be displaced from plasma protein binding sites by salicylate resulting in an enhanced effect. Diphenylhydantoin intoxication has been precipitated by concomitant use of aspirin. The diuretic action of spironolactone is inhibited by salicylates.
Usage in Pregnancy (Category C)—Studies have not been performed in animals or humans to determine whether this drug affects fertility in males or females, has mutagenic, carcinogenic or teratogenic potential or other adverse effects on the fetus. Aspirin causes testicular atrophy and inhibition of spermatogenesis in animals and has been shown to be teratogenic in animals and to increase the incidence of still births and neonatal deaths in pregnant women. As with other salicylates, MYOFLEX should be used during pregnancy only if the potential benefit justifies the potential risk to the fetus.
Chronic, high dose salicylate therapy of pregnant women increases the length of gestation and the frequency of post-maturity and prolongs spontaneous labor. It is, therefore, recommended that MYOFLEX be taken during the last three

months of pregnancy only under the close supervision of a physician.
Nursing Mothers—Salicylates are excreted in the breast milk of nursing mothers. Caution should be therefore exercised when MYOFLEX is administered to a nursing woman.
Pediatric Use—Safety and effectiveness of MYOFLEX in children have not been established.

Adverse Reactions: If applied to large skin areas, the absorbed salicylate may cause typical salicylate side effects such as tinnitus, nausea, or vomiting.

Overdosage: Acute overdosage with MYOFLEX is unlikely. A 2 oz. MYOFLEX tube contains the salicylate equivalent of about 56 grains of aspirin. Early signs and symptoms from repeated large doses consist of headache, dizziness, tinnitus (which may be absent in children or the elderly), difficulty in hearing, dimness of vision, mental confusion, lassitude, drowsiness, sweating, thirst, hyperventilation, nausea, vomiting and occasionally diarrhea. Treatment of acute salicylate poisoning is a medical emergency and should be undertaken in a hospital.

Dosage and Administration: Adults —Rub into painful or sore area two or three times daily. Wrists, elbows, knees or ankles may be wrapped loosely with 2″ or 3″ elastic bandage after application.

How Supplied:
NDC 0067-1170-02 Tubes, 2 oz.
NDC 0067-1170-04 Tubes, 4 oz.
NDC 0067-1170-30 Pump Dispenser, 3 oz.
NDC 0067-1170-08 Jars, 8 oz.
NDC 0067-1170-16 Jars, 1 lb.
Store at controlled room temperature (15–30°C, 59–86°F) (jars).
Protect from freezing or excessive heat (tubes and pump).
*Shown in Product Identification
Section, page 425*

PERDIEM®
[pĕr"dē'ŭm]

Actions: Perdiem®, with its gentle action provides comfortable relief from constipation. The vegetable mucilages of Perdiem® soften the stool and provide pain-free evacuation of the bowel. Perdiem® is effective as an aid to elimination for the hemorrhoid or fissure patient prior to and following surgery.

Composition: Perdiem® contains as its active ingredients, 82% psyllium (Plantago Hydrocolloid) and 18% senna (Cassia Pod Concentrate) which are natural vegetable derivatives. Each rounded teaspoonful (6.0 g) contains 3.25 g psyllium, 0.74 g senna, 1.8 mg of sodium, 35.5 mg of potassium, and 4 calories. Perdiem® is "Dye-Free".

Inactive Ingredients: Acacia, iron oxides, natural flavors, paraffin, sucrose, talc.

Indication: For relief of constipation.

Patient Warning: Should not be used in the presence of undiagnosed abdomi-

nal pain. Frequent or prolonged use without the direction of a physician is not recommended, as it may lead to laxative dependence. Do not use in patients with a history of psyllium allergy. Psyllium allergy is rare but can be severe. If an allergic reaction occurs, discontinue use.

Bulk forming agents have the potential to obstruct the esophagus, particularly in the presence of esophageal narrowing or when consumed with insufficient fluid. Patients should be made aware of the symptoms of esophageal obstruction, including chest pain/pressure, regurgitation, and difficulty swallowing. Patients experiencing these symptoms should seek immediate medical attention. Patients with esophageal narrowing or dysphagia should not use Perdiem®.

As with any drug, if you are pregnant or nursing a baby, seek the advice of a health professional before using this product. Keep this and all drugs out of the reach of children. In case of accidental overdose, seek professional assistance or contact a poison control center immediately.

Directions For Use—Adults: In the evening and/or before breakfast, 1–2 rounded teaspoonfuls of Perdiem® granules (in single or partial teaspoon doses) should be placed in the mouth and swallowed with at least 8 fl oz of cool beverage after the dose. Additional liquid would be helpful. Perdiem® granules should not be chewed.

After Perdiem® takes effect (usually after 24 hours, but possibly not before 36–48 hours): reduce the morning and evening doses to one rounded teaspoonful. Subsequent doses should be adjusted after adequate laxation is obtained.

Note: It is extremely important that Perdiem® be taken with at least 8 fl oz of cool liquid.

In Obstinate Cases: Perdiem® may be taken more frequently, up to two rounded teaspoonfuls every six hours.

For Patients Habituated to Strong Purgatives: Two rounded teaspoonfuls of Perdiem® in the morning and evening may be required along with half the usual dose of the purgative being used. The purgative should be discontinued as soon as possible and the dosage of Perdiem® granules reduced when and if bowel tone shows lessened laxative dependence.

For Colostomy Patients: To ensure formed stools, give one to two rounded teaspoonfuls of Perdiem® in the evening.

For Clinical Regulation: For patients confined to bed, for those of inactive habits, and in the presence of cardiovascular disease where straining must be avoided, one rounded teaspoonful of Perdiem® taken once or twice daily will provide regular bowel habits.

For Children: From age 7–11 years, give one rounded teaspoonful one to two times daily. From age 12 and older, give adult dosage.

How Supplied: Granules: 100-gram (3.5 oz) (NDC 0067-0690-68) and 250-gram (8.8 oz) (NDC 0067-0690-70) canisters, Hospital Unit Dose 50 6-gram packets in a gravity feed dispenser.

Shown in Product Identification Section, page 425

PERDIEM® FIBER
[pĕr"dē'ŭm]

100% Bulk Forming Action: Perdiem® Fiber is a light brown, minty tasting, granular, non-irritating bulk fiber which gently softens the stool and promotes regularity through normal elimination of the bowels. Perdiem® Fiber is effective in the treatment of constipation, contains no irritants, and when used under the direction of a physician, can safely be taken for prolonged periods as an aid to regularity.

Composition: Perdiem® Fiber contains as its active ingredient 100% psyllium (Plantago Hydrocolloid), a natural vegetable derivative. Each rounded teaspoonful (6.0 g) contains 4.03 g of psyllium, 1.8 mg of sodium, 36.1 mg of potassium and 4 calories. Perdiem® Fiber is "Dye-Free".

Inactive Ingredients: Acacia, iron oxides, natural flavors, paraffin, sucrose, talc, titanium dioxide.

Indications: Perdiem® Fiber provides gentle relief from simple, chronic, and spastic constipation. In addition, it relieves constipation associated with convalescence, pregnancy, and advanced age. Perdiem® Fiber is also indicated for use in special diets lacking in residue fiber to aid regularity and in the management of constipation associated with irritable bowel syndrome, diverticular disease, hemorrhoids, and anal fissures.

Patient Warning: Should not be used in the presence of undiagnosed abdominal pain. Frequent or prolonged use without the direction of a physician is not recommended.

Do not use in patients with a history of psyllium allergy. Psyllium allergy is rare but can be severe. If an allergic reaction occurs, discontinue use.

Bulk forming agents have the potential to obstruct the esophagus, particularly in the presence of esophageal narrowing or when consumed with insufficient fluid. Patients should be made aware of the symptoms of esophageal obstruction, including chest pain/pressure, regurgitation, and difficulty swallowing. Patients experiencing these symptoms should seek immediate medical attention. Patients with esophageal narrowing or dysphagia should not use Perdiem® Fiber. Keep this and all drugs out of the reach of children. In case of accidental overdose, seek professional assistance or contact a poison control center immediately.

Directions For Use—Adults: In the evening and/or before breakfast, 1 to 2 rounded teaspoonfuls (6.0 to 12.0 g) of Perdiem® Fiber granules (in full or partial teaspoon doses) should be placed in the mouth and swallowed with at least 8 fl oz of cool beverage after the dose. Additional liquid would be helpful. Perdiem® Fiber granules should not be chewed. Children: For children age 7–11, give 1 rounded teaspoonful 1–2 times daily. Age 12 and older, give adult dosage.

Note: It is extremely important that Perdiem® Fiber be taken with at least 8 fl oz of cool liquid.

In Obstinate Cases: Perdiem® Fiber may be taken more frequently, up to 2 rounded teaspoonfuls every 6 hours depending upon need and response. Perdiem® Fiber generally takes effect after 24 hours; however, in obstinate cases, 48 to 72 hours may be required to provide optimal benefit.

After Rectal Surgery: The vegetable mucilages of Perdiem® Fiber soften the stool and ensure pain-free evacuation of the bowel. Perdiem® Fiber is effective as an aid to elimination for the hemorrhoid or fissure patient prior to and following surgery.

For Clinical Regulation: For patients confined to bed—after an operation for example—and for those of inactive habits, 1 rounded teaspoonful of Perdiem® Fiber taken 1–2 times daily will ensure regular bowel habits.

During Pregnancy: Because of its natural ingredient and bulking action, Perdiem® Fiber is effective for expectant mothers when used under a physician's care. In most cases 1–2 rounded teaspoonfuls taken each evening is sufficient.

How Supplied: Granules: 100-gram (3.5 oz) (NDC 0067-0695-68) and 250-gram (8.8 oz) (NDC 0067-0695-70) canisters, Hospital Unit Dose 50 6-gram packets in a gravity feed dispenser.

Shown in Product Identification Section, page 425

Ross Laboratories
COLUMBUS, OH 43216

ADVANCE®
[ad-vans']
Nutritional Beverage With Iron

Usage: As a fortified milk/soy-based feeding more appropriate than 2% lowfat milk for older babies and toddlers.

Features:
- A more appropriate distribution of calories from protein, fat and carbohydrate than in 2% lowfat milk.
- Recommended levels of vitamins and minerals to complement the solid-food diet of older infants.
- 1.8 mg of iron (as ferrous sulfate) per 100 Calories to help avoid iron deficiency.

Continued on next page

Ross—Cont.

- A combination of heat-treated soy and cow's-milk proteins to help reduce the risk of cow's-milk-induced enteric blood loss.
- 16 Calories per fluid ounce.

Availability:
Concentrated Liquid: 13-fl-oz cans; 12 per case; No. 3313.
Ready To Feed: (Prediluted, 16 Cal/fl oz) 32-fl-oz cans; 6 per case; No. 3301.

Preparation:
Concentrated Liquid: Standard dilution (16 Cal/fl oz) is one part Concentrated Liquid to one part water.
Ready To Feed: Do not dilute. For hospital use, Ready To Feed ADVANCE in disposable nursing bottles is available in the Ross Hospital Formula System.

Composition: Ready To Feed (Concentrated Liquid at standard dilution has similar composition and nutrient values. For specific information, refer to product label.)

Ingredients: Ⓤ-D Water, corn syrup, nonfat milk, soy oil, soy protein isolate, corn oil, mono- and diglycerides, soy lecithin, minerals (calcium phosphate tribasic, potassium citrate, magnesium chloride, ferrous sulfate, zinc sulfate, cupric sulfate, manganese sulfate), vitamins (ascorbic acid, choline chloride, m-inositol, alpha-tocopheryl acetate, niacinamide, calcium pantothenate, vitamin A palmitate, thiamine chloride hydrochloride, riboflavin, pyridoxine hydrochloride, folic acid, phylloquinone, biotin, vitamin D_3, cyanocobalamin), carrageenan and taurine.
6.3 fl oz provides 100 Cal; 1 liter provides 540 Cal.

Nutrients:	Per 100 Cal	
Protein	3.7	g
Fat	5.0	g
Carbohydrate	10.2	g
Water	170	g
Linoleic Acid	2300	mg
Vitamins:		
Vitamin A	370	IU
Vitamin D	75	IU
Vitamin E	3.7	IU
Vitamin K	10	mcg
Thiamine (Vit. B_1)	120	mcg
Riboflavin (Vit. B_2)	170	mcg
Vitamin B_6	75	mcg
Vitamin B_{12}	0.3	mcg
Niacin	1300	mcg
Folic Acid (Folacin)	19	mcg
Pantothenic Acid	560	mcg
Biotin	4.4	mcg
Vitamin C		
(Ascorbic Acid)	10	mg
Choline	16	mg
Inositol	4.7	mg
Minerals:		
Calcium	94	mg
Phosphorus	72	mg
Magnesium	7.6	mg
Iron	1.8	mg*
Zinc	0.9	mg
Manganese	6	mcg
Copper	110	mcg
Iodine	18	mcg
Sodium	35	mg
Potassium	146	mg
Chloride	88	mg

*The addition of iron to this beverage conforms to the recommendation of the Committee on Nutrition of the American Academy of Pediatrics.
(FAN 503-03)

CLEAR® EYES
[klēr īz]
Lubricating Eye Redness Reliever

Description: Clear Eyes is a sterile isotonic buffered solution containing the active ingredients naphazoline hydrochloride 0.012% and glycerin 0.2%, as well as boric acid, purified water and sodium borate. Edetate disodium 0.1% and benzalkonium chloride 0.01% are added as preservatives. (Contains vasoconstrictor.)
Clear Eyes contains laboratory tested and scientifically blended ingredients, including an effective vasoconstrictor that narrows swollen blood vessels and rapidly whitens reddened eyes in a formulation that produces a refreshing, soothing effect. Clear Eyes is a sterile solution compatible with the natural fluids of the eye.

Indications: Clear Eyes is a decongestant ophthalmic solution specially designed for temporary relief of redness due to minor eye irritation and to protect against further irritation or dryness of the eye.

Warnings: To avoid contamination, do not touch tip of container to any surface. Replace cap after using. If you experience eye pain, changes in vision, continued redness or irritation of the eye, or if the condition worsens or persists for more than 72 hours, discontinue use and consult a physician. If you have glaucoma, do not use this product except under the advice and supervision of a physician. Overuse of this product may produce increased redness of the eye. If solution changes color or becomes cloudy, do not use. KEEP THIS AND ALL MEDICINES OUT OF THE REACH OF CHILDREN. REMOVE CONTACT LENSES BEFORE USING.

Directions: Instill one or two drops in the affected eye(s), up to four times daily.

How Supplied: In 0.2-fl-oz, 0.5-fl-oz and 1.0-fl-oz plastic dropper bottles.
Shown in Product Identification Section, page 425
(FAN 2202-03)

EAR DROPS BY MURINE®
[myūr'ēn]
See Murine Ear Wax Removal System/Murine Ear Drops
Shown in Product Identification Section, page 425

ISOMIL®
[ī'sō-mil]
Soy Protein Formula With Iron

Usage: As a beverage for infants, children and adults with an allergy or sensitivity to cow's milk. A feeding following diarrhea. A feeding for patients with disorders for which lactose should be avoided: lactase deficiency, lactose intolerance and galactosemia.

Availability:
Powder: 14-oz cans, measuring scoop enclosed; 6 per case; No. 00107.
Concentrated Liquid: 13-fl-oz cans; 24 per case; No. 02110.
Ready To Feed: (Prediluted, 20 Cal/fl oz)
32-fl-oz cans; 6 per case; No. 00230.
8-fl-oz cans; 4 six-packs per case; No. 00173.
For hospital use, Ready To Feed Isomil in disposable nursing bottles is available in the Ross Hospital Formula System.

Preparation:
Powder: Standard dilution (20 Cal/fl oz) is one level, unpacked scoop of Powder (8.7g) for each 2 fl oz of warm water.
Concentrated Liquid: Standard dilution (20 Cal/fl oz) is one part Concentrated Liquid to one part water.
Ready To Feed: Do not dilute.
Note: All forms of Isomil should be shaken well before opening and before feeding.

Composition: Ready To Feed (Concentrated Liquid and Powder at standard dilution have similar composition and nutrient values. For specific information, refer to product labels.)

Ingredients: (Pareve, Ⓤ) 86.4% water, 4.1% corn syrup, 3.2% sucrose, 2.1% soy oil, 2.0% soy protein isolate, 1.4% coconut oil, minerals (calcium citrate, calcium phosphate tribasic, potassium phosphate monobasic, potassium chloride, potassium citrate, magnesium chloride, potassium phosphate dibasic, sodium chloride, ferrous sulfate, zinc sulfate, cupric sulfate, manganese sulfate, potassium iodide), mono- and diglycerides, soy lecithin, vitamins (ascorbic acid, choline chloride, m-inositol, alpha-tocopheryl acetate, niacinamide, calcium pantothenate, vitamin A palmitate, thiamine chloride hydrochloride, riboflavin, pyridoxine hydrochloride, folic acid, phylloquinone, biotin, vitamin D_3, cyanocobalamin), carrageenan, L-methionine, taurine and L-carnitine.
5 fl oz provides 100 Cal; 1 liter provides 676 Cal.

Nutrients:	Per 100 Cal	
Protein	2.66	g
Fat	5.46	g
Carbohydrate	10.1	g
Water	133	g
Linoleic Acid	1300	mg
Vitamins:		
Vitamin A	300	IU
Vitamin D	60	IU
Vitamin E	3.0	IU
Vitamin K	15	mcg
Thiamine (Vit. B_1)	60	mcg
Riboflavin (Vit. B_2)	90	mcg
Vitamin B_6	60	mcg
Vitamin B_{12}	0.45	mcg
Niacin	1350	mcg
Folic Acid (Folacin)	15	mcg
Pantothenic Acid	750	mcg
Biotin	4.5	mcg

Vitamin C		
(Ascorbic Acid)	9	mg
Choline	8	mg
Inositol	5	mg
Minerals:		
Calcium	105	mg
Phosphorus	75	mg
Magnesium	7.5	mg
Iron	1.8	mg*
Zinc	0.75	mg
Manganese	30	mcg
Copper	75	mcg
Iodine	15	mcg
Sodium	44	mg
Potassium	108	mg
Chloride	62	mg

*The addition of iron to this formula conforms to the recommendation of the Committee on Nutrition of the American Academy of Pediatrics.
(FAN 503-04)

ISOMIL® SF
[ī'sō-mil]
Sucrose–Free Soy Protein Formula With Iron

Usage: As a beverage for infants, children and adults with an allergy or sensitivity to cow's-milk protein or an intolerance to sucrose. A feeding following acute diarrhea. A feeding for patients with disorders for which lactose and sucrose should be avoided.

Availability:
Concentrated Liquid: 13-fl-oz cans; 12 per case; No. 00119.
Ready To Feed: (Prediluted, 20 Cal/fl oz) 32-fl-oz cans; 6 per case; No. 00128. For hospital use, Ready To Feed Isomil SF in disposable nursing bottles is available in the Ross Hospital Formula System.

Preparation:
Concentrated Liquid: Standard dilution (20 Cal/fl oz) is one part Concentrated Liquid to one part water.
Ready To Feed: Do not dilute.
Note: All forms of Isomil SF should be shaken well before opening and before feeding.

Composition: Ready To Feed (Concentrated Liquid at standard dilution has similar composition and nutrient values. For specific information, refer to product label.)

Ingredients: (Pareve, Ⓤ) 87.4% water, 6.4% hydrolyzed cornstarch, 2.1% soy oil, 2.0% soy protein isolate, 1.4% coconut oil, minerals (calcium citrate, calcium phosphate tribasic, potassium citrate, potassium phosphate monobasic, potassium chloride, magnesium chloride, potassium phosphate dibasic, sodium chloride, ferrous sulfate, zinc sulfate, cupric sulfate, manganese sulfate, potassium iodide), mono- and diglycerides, soy lecithin, vitamins (ascorbic acid, choline chloride, m-inositol, alpha-tocopheryl acetate, niacinamide, calcium pantothenate, vitamin A palmitate, thiamine chloride hydrochloride, riboflavin, pyridoxine hydrochloride, folic acid, phylloquinone, biotin, vitamin D_3, cyanocobala-

min), carrageenan, L-methionine, taurine and L-carnitine.
5 fl oz provides 100 Cal; 1 liter provides 676 Cal.

Nutrients:	**Per 100 Cal**	
Protein	2.66	g
Fat	5.46	g
Carbohydrate	10.1	g
Water	133	g
Linoleic Acid	1300	mg
Vitamins:		
Vitamin A	300	IU
Vitamin D	60	IU
Vitamin E	3.0	IU
Vitamin K	15	mcg
Thiamine (Vit. B_1)	60	mcg
Riboflavin (Vit. B_2)	90	mcg
Vitamin B_6	60	mcg
Vitamin B_{12}	0.45	mcg
Niacin	1350	mcg
Folic Acid (Folacin)	15	mcg
Pantothenic Acid	750	mcg
Biotin	4.5	mcg
Vitamin C		
(Ascorbic Acid)	9	mg
Choline	8	mg
Inositol	5	mg
Minerals:		
Calcium	105	mg
Phosphorus	75	mg
Magnesium	7.5	mg
Iron	1.8	mg*
Zinc	0.75	mg
Manganese	30	mcg
Copper	75	mcg
Iodine	15	mcg
Sodium	44	mg
Potassium	108	mg
Chloride	62	mg

*The addition of iron to this formula conforms to the recommendation of the Committee on Nutrition of the American Academy of Pediatrics.
(FAN 503-03)

MURINE® EAR WAX REMOVAL SYSTEM/MURINE® EAR DROPS
[myūr'ēn]
Carbamide Peroxide
Ear Wax Removal Aid

Description: MURINE EAR DROPS contains the active ingredient carbamide peroxide, 6.5%. It also contains alcohol (6.3%), glycerin, polysorbate 20 and other ingredients. The MURINE EAR WAX REMOVAL SYSTEM includes a 1.0-fl-oz soft bulb ear washer. This system is the only complete medically approved system to safely remove ear wax. Application of carbamide peroxide drops followed by warm-water irrigation is an effective, medically recommended way to help loosen excessive and/or hardened ear wax.

Actions: The carbamide peroxide formula in MURINE EAR DROPS is an aid in the removal of wax from the ear canal. Anhydrous glycerin penetrates and softens wax while the release of oxygen from carbamide peroxide provides a mechanical action resulting in the loosening of the softened wax accumulation. It is usually necessary to remove the loosened wax by gently flushing the ear with

warm water using the soft bulb ear washer provided.

Indications: The MURINE EAR WAX REMOVAL SYSTEM is indicated for occasional use as an aid to soften, loosen and remove excessive ear wax.

Warning: DO NOT USE if you have ear drainage or discharge, ear pain, irritation, or rash in the ear or are dizzy; consult a doctor. DO NOT USE if you have an injury or perforation (hole) of the eardrum or after ear surgery, unless directed by a doctor.
Do not use for more than 4 days; if excessive ear wax remains after use of this product, consult a doctor. Avoid contact with the eyes. KEEP THIS AND ALL MEDICINES OUT OF THE REACH OF CHILDREN.

Directions: FOR USE IN THE EAR ONLY. Adults and children over 12 years, tilt head sideways and place 5 to 10 drops in ear. Tip of applicator should not enter ear canal. Keep drops in ear for several minutes by keeping head tilted or placing cotton in ear. Use twice daily for up to 4 days if needed, or as directed by a doctor. Any wax remaining after treatment may be removed by gently flushing the ear with warm water, using a soft bulb ear washer. Children under 12 years, consult a doctor.
Used regularly, the Murine Ear Wax Removal System helps keep the ear canal free from blockage due to accumulated ear wax.

Note: When the ear canal is irrigated, the tip of the ear washer should not obstruct the flow of water leaving the ear canal.

How Supplied: The MURINE EAR WAX REMOVAL SYSTEM contains 0.5-fl-oz drops and a 1.0-fl-oz soft bulb ear washer.
Also available in 0.5-fl-oz drops only, MURINE EAR DROPS.
Shown in Product Identification Section, page 425
(FAN 2180-02)

MURINE®
[myūr'ēn]
Eye Lubricant

Description: Murine eye lubricant is a sterile isotonic buffered solution containing the active ingredients 1.4% polyvinyl alcohol and 0.6% povidone. Also contains benzalkonium chloride, dextrose, disodium edetate, potassium chloride, purified water, sodium bicarbonate, sodium chloride, sodium citrate and sodium phosphate (mono- and dibasic). (No vasoconstrictor.)
Murine is a clear solution formulated to more closely match the natural tear fluid of the eye for gentle, soothing relief from minor eye irritation while moisturizing and preventing dryness. Use as desired

Continued on next page

If desired, additional information on any Ross Product will be provided upon request to Ross Laboratories.

Ross—Cont.

to temporarily relieve minor eye irritation, dryness and burning due to conditions such as dust, smoke, smog, sun glare, wearing contact lenses, colds, allergies, swimming, reading, driving, TV or close work.

Indications: For the temporary relief or prevention of further discomfort due to minor eye irritations and symptoms related to dry eyes.

Warning: To avoid contamination, do not touch tip of container to any other surface. Replace cap after using. If you experience eye pain, changes in vision, continued redness or irritation of the eye, or if the condition worsens or persists for more than 72 hours, discontinue use and consult a physician. If solution changes color or becomes cloudy, do not use. KEEP THIS AND ALL MEDICINES OUT OF THE REACH OF CHILDREN. REMOVE CONTACT LENSES BEFORE USING.

Directions: Instill one or two drops in the affected eye(s) as needed.

How Supplied: In 0.2-fl-oz, 0.5-fl-oz and 1.0-fl-oz plastic dropper bottles.
Shown in Product Identification Section, page 425
(FAN 2202-04)

MURINE® PLUS
[*myūr 'ēn*]
Lubricating Eye Redness Reliever

Description: Murine Plus is a sterile, non-staining buffered solution containing the active ingredients 1.4% polyvinyl alcohol, 0.6% povidone and 0.05% tetrahydrozoline hydrochloride. Also contains benzalkonium chloride, dextrose, disodium edetate, potassium chloride, purified water, sodium bicarbonate, sodium chloride, sodium citrate and sodium phosphate (mono- and dibasic).
Murine Plus is an isotonic, sterile ophthalmic solution, formulated to more closely match the natural tear fluid of the eye. Its contains demulcents for gentle, soothing relief from minor eye irritation as well as the sympathomimetic agent, tetrahydrozoline hydrochloride, which produces local vasoconstriction in the eye. Thus, the drug effectively narrows swollen blood vessels locally and provides symptomatic relief of edema and hyperemia of conjunctival tissues due to eye allergies, minor local irritations and conjunctivitis. Use up to 4 times daily, to remove redness due to minor eye irritation caused by conditions such as dust, smoke, smog, sun glare, wearing contact lenses, colds, allergies, swimming, reading, driving, TV or close work. The effect of Murine Plus is prompt (apparent within minutes) and sustained.

Indications: For the temporary relief or prevention of further discomfort due to minor eye irritations and symptoms related to dry eyes plus removal of redness.

Warning: To avoid contamination, do not touch tip of container to any surface. Replace cap after using. If you experience eye pain, changes in vision, continued redness or irritation of the eye, or if the condition worsens or persists for more than 72 hours, discontinue use and consult a physician. If you have glaucoma, do not use this product except under the advice and supervision of a physician. Overuse of this product may produce increased redness of the eye. If solution changes color or becomes cloudy, do not use. KEEP THIS AND ALL MEDICINES OUT OF THE REACH OF CHILDREN. REMOVE CONTACT LENSES BEFORE USING.

Directions: Instill one or two drops in the affected eye(s), up to four times daily.

How Supplied: In 0.5-fl-oz and 1.0-fl-oz plastic dropper bottle.
Shown in Product Identification Section, page 425
(FAN 2202-04)

PEDIALYTE®
[*pē 'dē-ah-līt " *]
Oral Electrolyte Maintenance Solution

Usage: For maintenance of water and electrolytes during mild or moderate diarrhea in infants and children; for maintenance of water and electrolytes following corrective parenteral therapy for severe diarrhea.

Features:
- Ready To Use—no mixing or dilution necessary.
- Balanced electrolytes to replace stool losses and provide maintenance requirements.
- Provides glucose to promote sodium and water absorption.
- Fruit-flavored form available to enhance compliance in older infants and children.
- Plastic quart bottles are resealable, easy to pour and easy to measure.
- No coloring added.
- Widely available in grocery, drug and convenience stores.

Availability:
32-fl-oz plastic bottles; 8 per case; Unflavored, No. 336—NDC 0074-6470-32; Fruit-flavored, No. 365—NDC 0074-6471-32.
8-fl-oz bottles; 4 six-packs per case; Unflavored, No. 160—NDC 0074-6470-08. For hospital use, Pedialyte is available in the Ross Hospital Formula System.

Dosage: See Administration Guide for maintenance of body water and electrolytes in mild or moderate diarrhea (Pedialyte Unflavored or Fruit-Flavored) and management of mild to moderate to severe diarrhea (Rehydralyte® Oral Electrolyte Rehydration Solution).
Pedialyte (Unflavored or Fruit-Flavored) or Rehydralyte should be offered frequently in amounts tolerated. Total daily intake should be adjusted to meet individual needs, based on thirst and response to therapy. The suggested intakes

for maintenance are based on water requirements for ordinary energy expenditure.[1] The suggested intakes for replacement are based on fluid losses of 5% or 10% of body weight, including maintenance requirement.
[See table on next page].

Composition: Unflavored Pedialyte (Fruit-Flavored Pedialyte has similar composition and nutrient value. For specific information, see product label.)

Ingredients: (Pareve, Ⓤ) Water, dextrose, potassium citrate, sodium chloride and sodium citrate.

Provides:	Per 8 Fl Oz	Per Liter	Per 32 Fl Oz
Sodium (mEq)	10.6	45	42.4
Potassium (mEq)	4.7	20	18.8
Chloride (mEq)	8.3	35	33.2
Citrate (mEq)	7.1	30	28.4
Dextrose (g)	5.9	25	23.6
Calories	24	100	96

(FAN 387-01)

RCF®
Ross Carbohydrate Free
Low-Iron Soy Protein Formula Base

Usage: For use in the dietary management of persons unable to tolerate the type or amount of carbohydrate in milk or conventional infant formulas; many of these patients have intractable diarrhea and are not able to tolerate other formulas. This product has been formulated to contain no carbohydrate, which must be added before feeding.

Availability:
Concentrated Liquid only: 13-fl-oz cans; 12 per case; No. 108.

Preparation:
RCF is for use only under the supervision of a physician. Physician's instructions must include the type and amount of carbohydrate and the amount of water to be added to RCF. Standard dilution is one part Formula Base to one part prescribed carbohydrate and water solution. If a physician specifies other types or amounts of carbohydrate, or other amounts of water, to be added to RCF, those instructions should be followed completely.
A full-strength formula, 20 Calories per fluid ounce, may be prepared with one of the following typical carbohydrates:
[See table bottom left next page]

Composition: Concentrated Liquid

Ingredients: (Pareve, Ⓤ) 87% water, 4.4% soy protein isolate, 4.2% soy oil, 2.8% coconut oil, minerals (calcium phosphates [mono- and tribasic], potassium citrate, potassium chloride, magnesium chloride, calcium carbonate, sodium chloride, zinc sulfate, ferrous sulfate, cupric sulfate, manganese sulfate, potassium iodide), carrageenan, mono- and diglycerides, soy lecithin, vitamins (ascorbic acid, choline chloride, m-inositol, alpha-tocopheryl acetate, niacinamide, calcium pantothenate, vitamin A palmitate, thiamine chloride hydrochloride, riboflavin, pyridoxine hydrochloride, folic acid, phylloquinone, biotin,

vitamin D_3, cyanocobalamin), L-methionine, taurine and L-carnitine. 4.2 fl oz of RCF, without added carbohydrate or water, provides 100 Cal (81 Cal/100 mL). 5 fl oz of 20 Cal/fl oz formula provides 100 Cal; see directions. [See table on next page]. (FAN 523-04)

REHYDRALYTE®
[rē-hī′drə-līt″]
Oral Electrolyte Rehydration Solution

Usage: For replacement of water and electrolytes lost during moderate to severe diarrhea.

Features:
- Ready To Use—no mixing or dilution necessary.
- Safe, economical alternative to IV therapy.
- 75 mEq of sodium per liter for effective replacement of fluid deficits.
- 2½% glucose solution to promote sodium and water absorption and provide energy.
- Widely available in pharmacies.

Availability: 8-fl-oz bottles; 4 six-packs per case; No. 162; NDC 0074-0162-01.

Dosage: (See Administration Guide under Pedialyte).

Ingredients: (Pareve, Ⓤ) Water, dextrose, sodium chloride, potassium citrate and sodium citrate.

Provides:	Per 8 Fl Oz	Per Liter
Sodium (mEq)	17.7	75
Potassium (mEq)	4.7	20
Chloride (mEq)	15.4	65
Citrate (mEq)	7.1	30
Dextrose (g)	5.9	25
Calories	24	100

(FAN 437-01)

SELSUN BLUE®
[sel′sən blü]
Dandruff Shampoo
(selenium sulfide lotion, 1%)

Selsun Blue is a non-prescription anti-dandruff shampoo containing the active ingredient selenium sulfide, 1%, in a freshly scented, pH balanced formula to leave hair clean and manageable. Available in Dry, Oily, Normal, Extra Conditioning and Extra Medicated formulas (also contains 0.5% menthol).

Inactive ingredients:
Dry formula—Acetylated lanolin alcohol, ammonium laureth sulfate, ammonium lauryl sulfate, cetyl acetate, citric acid, cocamide DEA, cocamidopropyl betaine, DMDM hydantoin, FD&C blue No. 1, fragrance, hydroxypropyl methylcellu-

Pedialyte, Rehydralyte Administration Guide
For Infants and Young Children

Age	2 Weeks	3 Months	6 Months	9 Months	1 Years	1½ Years	2 Years	2½ Years	3 Years	3½ Years	4 Years
Approximate Weight[2]											
(lb)	7	13	17	20	23	25	28	30	32	35	38
(kg)	3.2	6.0	7.8	9.2	10.2	11.4	12.6	13.6	14.6	16.0	17.0
PEDIALYTE UNFLAVORED or FRUIT-FLAVORED fl oz/day for maintenance*	13 to 16	28 to 32	34 to 40	38 to 44	41 to 46	45 to 50	48 to 53	51 to 56	54 to 58	56 to 60	57 to 62
REHYDRALYTE fl oz/day for Replacement for 5% Dehydration (including maintenance)*	18 to 21	38 to 42	47 to 53	53 to 59	58 to 63	64 to 69	69 to 74	74 to 79	78 to 82	83 to 87	85 to 90
REHYDRALYTE fl oz/day for Replacement for 10% Dehydration (including maintenance)*	23 to 26	48 to 52	60 to 66	68 to 74	75 to 80	83 to 88	90 to 95	97 to 102	102 to 106	110 to 114	113 to 118

Administration Guide does not apply to infants less than 1 week of age. For children over 4 years, maintenance intakes may exceed 2 qt daily.

1. Extrapolated from Barness L: Nutrition and nutritional disorders, in Behrman RE, Vaughan VC III: *Nelson Textbook of Pediatrics*, ed 12. Philadelphia, WB Saunders Co, 1983, pp 136-138.
2. Weight based on the 50th percentile of weight for age of the National Center for Health Statistics (NCHS) reference data. Hamill PVV, Drizd TA, Johnson CL, et al: Physical growth: National Center for Health Statistics percentiles. *Am J Clin Nutr* 1979; 32:607-629.
* Fluid intakes do not take into account ongoing stool losses. Fluid loss in the stool should be replaced by consumption of an extra amount of Pedialyte or Rehydralyte equal to stool losses in addition to the amounts given in this Administration Guide.

lose, magnesium aluminum silicate, polysorbate 80, sodium chloride, titanium dioxide, water and other ingredients.
Normal formula—Ammonium laureth sulfate, ammonium lauryl sulfate, citric acid, cocamide DEA, cocamidopropyl betaine, DMDM hydantoin, FD&C blue No. 1, fragrance, hydroxypropyl methylcellulose, magnesium aluminum silicate, sodium chloride, titanium dioxide, water and other ingredients.
Oily formula—Ammonium laureth sulfate, ammonium lauryl sulfate, citric acid, cocamide DEA, cocamidopropyl betaine, DMDM hydantoin, FD&C blue No. 1, fragrance, hydroxypropyl methylcellulose, magnesium aluminum silicate, so-

dium chloride, titanium dioxide, water and other ingredients.
Extra Conditioning formula—Acetylated lanolin alcohol, aloe, ammonium laureth sulfate, ammonium lauryl sulfate, cetyl acetate, citric acid, cocamide DEA, cocamidopropyl betaine, DMDM hydantoin, FD&C blue No. 1, fragrance, glycol distearate, hydroxypropyl methylcellulose, magnesium aluminum silicate, polysorbate 80, propylene glycol, sodium chloride, TEA-lauryl sulfate, titanium dioxide, water and other ingredients.
Extra Medicated formula—Ammonium laureth sulfate, ammonium lauryl sulfate, citric acid, cocamide DEA, cocamidopropyl betaine, DMDM hydantoin, D&C red No. 33, FD&C blue No. 1, fragrance, hydroxypropyl methylcellulose, magnesium aluminum silicate, sodium chloride, TEA-lauryl sulfate, water and other ingredients.

Continued on next page

If desired, additional information on any Ross Product will be provided upon request to Ross Laboratories.

Type of Carbohydrate	Amount of Carbohydrate*	Water	RCF Formula Base
Table Sugar (sucrose)	4 level tablespoonfuls	12 fl oz	13 fl oz
Dextrose Powder (hydrous)	6 level tablespoonfuls	12 fl oz	13 fl oz
Polycose® Glucose Polymers Powder	9 level tablespoonfuls	12 fl oz	13 fl oz

* Approximately 52 grams needed for 20 Cal/fl oz formula.

Ross—Cont.

Clinical testing has shown Selsun Blue to be as safe and effective as other leading shampoos in helping control dandruff symptoms with regular use.
Directions: Shake well before using. Lather, rinse thoroughly and repeat. For best results, use at least twice a week for effective dandruff control.

Warnings: For external use only. Keep out of eyes—if this happens, rinse thoroughly with water. If used just before or after bleaching, tinting or permanent waving, rinse hair for at least five minutes in cool running water. If irritation occurs, discontinue use. Keep out of the reach of children.

How Supplied: 4-, 7- and 11-fl-oz plastic bottles.

Shown in Product Identification Section, page 425

(FAN 2137-02)

SIMILAC®
[sim 'ə-lak]
Low-Iron Infant Formula

Usage: When an infant formula is needed: if the decision is made to discontinue breastfeeding before age 1 year, if a supplement to breastfeeding is needed, or as a routine feeding if breastfeeding is not adopted.

Availability:
Powder: 1-lb cans, measuring scoop enclosed; 6 per case; No. 03139.
Concentrated Liquid: 13-fl-oz cans; 24 per case; No. 00264.
Ready To Feed: (Prediluted, 20 Cal/fl oz)
32-fl-oz cans; 6 per case; No. 00232.
8-fl-oz cans; 4 six-packs per case; No. 00177.
4-fl-oz nursing bottles; 6 per carry-home carton, 8 cartons per case; No. 00480.
8-fl-oz nursing bottles; 6 per carry-home carton, 4 cartons per case; No. 00880.
For hospital use, Ready To Feed Similac in disposable nursing bottles is available in the Ross Hospital Formula System.

Preparation:
Powder: Standard dilution (20 Cal/fl oz) is one level, unpacked scoop Powder (8.7 g) for each 2 fl oz of warm water.
Concentrated Liquid: Standard dilution (20 Cal/fl oz) is one part Concentrated Liquid to one part water.
Ready To Feed: Do not dilute.

Composition: Ready To Feed (Concentrated Liquid and Powder at standard dilution have similar composition and nutrient values. For specific information, refer to product labels.)

Ingredients: Ⓤ-D Water, nonfat milk, lactose, soy oil, coconut oil, mono- and diglycerides, soy lecithin, vitamins (ascorbic acid, choline chloride, m-inositol, alpha-tocopheryl acetate, niacinamide, calcium pantothenate, vitamin A palmitate, thiamine chloride hydrochloride, riboflavin, pyridoxine hydrochloride, folic acid, phylloquinone, biotin, vitamin D_3, cyanocobalamin), carrageenan, minerals (zinc sulfate, ferrous sulfate, cupric sulfate, manganese sulfate) and taurine. 5 fl oz provides 100 Cal; 1 liter provides 676 Cal.

Nutrients:	Per 100 Cal	
Protein	2.22	g
Fat	5.37	g
Carbohydrate	10.7	g
Water	133	g
Linoleic Acid	1300	mg
Vitamins:		
Vitamin A	300	IU
Vitamin D	60	IU
Vitamin E	3.0	IU
Vitamin K	8	mcg
Thiamine (Vit. B_1)	100	mcg
Riboflavin (Vit. B_2)	150	mcg
Vitamin B_6	60	mcg
Vitamin B_{12}	0.25	mcg
Niacin	1050	mcg
Folic Acid (Folacin)	15	mcg
Pantothenic Acid	450	mcg
Biotin	4.4	mcg
Vitamin C (Ascorbic Acid)	9	mg
Choline	16	mg
Inositol	4.7	mg
Minerals:		
Calcium	75	mg
Phosphorus	58	mg
Magnesium	6	mg
Iron	0.22	mg*
Zinc	0.75	mg
Manganese	5	mcg
Copper	90	mcg
Iodine	15	mcg
Sodium	28	mg
Potassium	108	mg
Chloride	66	mg

*This product, like milk, is deficient in iron; additional iron should be supplied from other sources.

(FAN 503-02)

SIMILAC® PM 60/40
[sim 'ə-lak]
Low-Iron Infant Formula

Usage: For infants who are predisposed to hypocalcemia, or those whose renal, digestive or cardiovascular functions would benefit from lowered mineral levels. Similac PM 60/40 should be used as directed by a physician.

Availability: Powder only: 1-lb cans, measuring scoop enclosed; 6 per case; No. 00850. For hospital use, Ready To Feed Similac PM 60/40 in disposable nursing bottles is available in the Ross Hospital Formula System. (Ready To Feed has composition and nutrient values similar

RCF Nutrients:	Without Carbohydrate Per 100 Cal		With Carbohydrate + Water Per 100 Cal*	
Protein	4.95	g	2.96	g
Fat	8.91	g	5.33	g
Carbohydrate	0.01	g	10.1	g
Water	110	g	133	g
Linoleic Acid	2170	mg	1300	mg
Vitamins:				
Vitamin A	500	IU	300	IU
Vitamin D	100	IU	60	IU
Vitamin E	5	IU	3.0	IU
Vitamin K	25	mcg	15	mcg
Thiamine (Vit. B_1)	100	mcg	60	mcg
Riboflavin (Vit. B_2)	150	mcg	90	mcg
Vitamin B_6	100	mcg	60	mcg
Vitamin B_{12}	0.75	mcg	0.45	mcg
Niacin	2230	mcg	1350	mcg
Folic Acid (Folacin)	25	mcg	15	mcg
Pantothenic Acid	1240	mcg	750	mcg
Biotin	7.5	mcg	4.5	mcg
Vitamin C (Ascorbic Acid)	13.6	mg	9	mg
Choline	13	mg	8	mg
Inositol	8	mg	5	mg
Minerals:				
Calcium	173	mg	105	mg
Phosphorus	124	mg	75	mg
Magnesium	12.4	mg	7.5	mg
Iron	0.37	mg†	0.22	mg†
Zinc	1.24	mg	0.75	mg
Manganese	50	mcg	30	mcg
Copper	124	mcg	75	mcg
Iodine	25	mcg	15	mcg
Sodium	73	mg	44	mg
Potassium	180	mg	108	mg
Chloride	103	mg	62	mg

* When 52 g of carbohydrate and 12 fl oz of water are mixed with 13 fl oz of RCF. Composition will vary depending on quantity of carbohydrate and water used. If carbohydrate is not added to this product, a 1:1 dilution with water provides approximately 12 Cal/fl oz (40.6 Cal/100 mL).

† This product is deficient in iron; additional iron should be supplied from other sources.

to Powder. For specific information see bottle tray.)

Preparation: Standard dilution (20 Cal/fl oz) is one level, unpacked scoop (8.6 g) of Powder for each 2 fl oz of warm water.

Higher caloric feedings are prepared by adding 8.6 g (one level, unpacked scoop) of Similac PM 60/40 to the following amounts of water:

For:	Water:	Yields:	
24 Cal/fl oz	48 mL	55 mL	(1.8 fl oz)
27 Cal/fl oz	42 mL	49 mL	(1.6 fl oz)
30 Cal/fl oz	37 mL	44 mL	(1.5 fl oz)

Composition: Powder (For most current product information, refer to product labels.)

Ingredients: Ⓤ-D Lactose, corn oil, coconut oil, whey protein concentrate, sodium caseinate, minerals (calcium phosphate tribasic, potassium citrate, potassium chloride, magnesium chloride, sodium chloride, calcium carbonate, zinc sulfate, ferrous sulfate, cupric sulfate, manganese sulfate, potassium iodide), vitamins (m-inositol, ascorbic acid, choline chloride, alpha-tocopheryl acetate, niacinamide, calcium pantothenate, vitamin A palmitate, thiamine chloride hydrochloride, riboflavin, pyridoxine hydrochloride, folic acid, phylloquinone, vitamin D_3, biotin, cyanocobalamin), taurine and L-carnitine.

5 fl oz provides 100 Cal when prepared as directed.

1 liter of prepared formula provides 676 Cal.

Nutrients:	Per 100 Cal	
Protein	2.22	g
Fat	5.59	g
Carbohydrate	10.2	g
Water	134	g
Linoleic Acid	1300	mg
Vitamins:		
Vitamin A	300	IU
Vitamin D	60	IU
Vitamin E	2.5	IU
Vitamin K	8	mcg
Thiamine (Vit. B_1)	100	mcg
Riboflavin (Vit. B_2)	150	mcg
Vitamin B_6	60	mcg
Vitamin B_{12}	0.25	mcg
Niacin	1050	mcg
Folic Acid (Folacin)	15	mcg
Pantothenic Acid	450	mcg
Biotin	4.5	mcg
Vitamin C		
(Ascorbic Acid)	9	mg
Choline	12	mg
Inositol	24	mg
Minerals:		
Calcium	56	mg
Phosphorus	28	mg
Magnesium	6	mg
Iron	0.22	mg*
Zinc	0.75	mg
Manganese	5	mcg
Copper	90	mcg
Iodine	6	mcg
Sodium	24	mg
Potassium	86	mg
Chloride	59	mg

*This product, like milk, is deficient in iron; additional iron should be supplied from other sources.

Standard dilution is one level, unpacked scoop of Similac PM 60/40 Powder for each 2 fl oz of water, or 131.7 g of Powder diluted to 1 liter.

Precautions: In conditions where the infant is losing abnormal quantities of one or more electrolytes, it may be necessary to supply electrolytes from sources other than the formula. It may be necessary to supply low-birth-weight infants weighing less than 1500 g at birth additional calcium, phosphorus and sodium during periods of rapid growth.
(FAN 475-03)

SIMILAC® WITH IRON
[sim 'ə-lak]
Infant Formula

Usage: When an iron-fortified infant formula is needed: if the decision is made to discontinue breastfeeding before age 1 year, if a supplement to breastfeeding is needed, or as a routine feeding if breastfeeding is not adopted.

Availability:
Powder: 1-lb cans, measuring scoop enclosed; 6 per case; No. 03360.
Concentrated Liquid: 13-fl-oz cans; 24 cans per case; No. 00414.
Ready To Feed: (Prediluted, 20 Cal/fl oz) 32-fl-oz cans; 6 per case; No. 00241.
8-fl-oz cans; 4 six-packs per case; No. 00179.
4-fl-oz nursing bottles; 6 per carry-home carton, 8 cartons per case; No. 06201.
8-fl-oz nursing bottles; 6 per carry-home carton, 4 cartons per case; No. 06202.
For hospital use, Ready To Feed Similac With Iron in disposable nursing bottles is available in the Ross Hospital Formula System.

Preparation:
Powder: Standard dilution (20 Cal/fl oz) is one level, unpacked scoop Powder (8.7 g) for each 2 fl oz of warm water.
Concentrated Liquid: Standard dilution (20 Cal/fl oz) is one part Concentrated Liquid to one part water.
Ready To Feed: Do not dilute.
Composition: Ready To Feed (Concentrated Liquid and Powder at standard dilution have similar composition and nutrient values. For specific information, refer to product labels.)

Ingredients: Ⓤ-D Water, nonfat milk, lactose, soy oil, coconut oil, mono- and diglycerides, soy lecithin, vitamins (ascorbic acid, choline chloride, m-inositol, alpha-tocopheryl acetate, niacinamide, calcium pantothenate, vitamin A palmitate, thiamine chloride hydrochloride, riboflavin, pyridoxine hydrochloride, folic acid, phylloquinone, biotin, vitamin D_3, cyanocobalamin), carrageenan, minerals (ferrous sulfate, zinc sulfate, cupric sulfate, manganese sulfate) and taurine.
5 fl oz provides 100 Cal; 1 liter provides 676 Cal.

Nutrients:	Per 100 Cal	
Protein	2.22	g
Fat	5.37	g
Carbohydrate	10.7	g
Water	133	g
Linoleic Acid	1300	mg
Vitamins:		
Vitamin A	300	IU
Vitamin D	60	IU
Vitamin E	3.0	IU
Vitamin K	8	mcg
Thiamine (Vit. B_1)	100	mcg
Riboflavin (Vit. B_2)	150	mcg
Vitamin B_6	60	mcg
Vitamin B_{12}	0.25	mcg
Niacin	1050	mcg
Folic Acid (Folacin)	15	mcg
Pantothenic Acid	450	mcg
Biotin	4.4	mcg
Vitamin C		
(Ascorbic Acid)	9	mg
Choline	16	mg
Inositol	4.7	mg
Minerals:		
Calcium	75	mg
Phosphorus	58	mg
Magnesium	6	mg
Iron	1.8	mg*
Zinc	0.75	mg
Manganese	5	mcg
Copper	90	mcg
Iodine	15	mcg
Sodium	28	mg
Potassium	108	mg
Chloride	66	mg

*The addition of iron to this formula conforms to the recommendation of the Committee on Nutrition of the American Academy of Pediatrics.
(FAN 503-02)

TRONOLANE®
[tron 'ə-lān]
Anesthetic Cream for Hemorrhoids
Anesthetic Suppositories for Hemorrhoids

Description: The active ingredient in Tronolane is a topical anesthetic agent (Cream: pramoxine hydrochloride 1%; Suppositories: pramoxine 1% as pramoxine and pramoxine HCl), chemically unrelated to the benzoate esters of the "caine" type, which is chemically designated as a 4-n-butoxyphenyl gammamorpholinopropyl-ether hydrochloride. The cream contains the following inactive ingredients: A nongreasy zinc oxide cream base containing beeswax, cetyl alcohol, cetyl esters wax, glycerin, methylparaben, propylparaben, sodium lauryl sulfate, water and zinc oxide. The suppository contains the following inactive ingredients: A base containing hydrogenated cocoa glycerides and zinc oxide.

Indications: Tronolane is a topical anesthetic indicated for the temporary relief of the pain, burning, itching and dis-

Continued on next page

Ross—Cont.

comfort that accompany hemorrhoids. It has a soothing, lubricating action on mucous membranes.

Tronolane contains a rapidly acting topical anesthetic producing analgesia that lasts up to 5 hours. Because the drug is chemically unrelated to other anesthetics, cross-sensitization is unlikely. Patients who are already sensitized to the "caine" anesthetics can generally use Tronolane.

The emollient/emulsion base of Tronolane cream provides soothing lubrication, making bowel movements more comfortable. Tronolane cream is in a nondrying base that is nongreasy and nonstaining to undergarments.

Warnings: If bleeding is present, consult physician. Certain persons can develop allergic reactions to ingredients in this product. During treatment, if condition worsens or persists 7 days, consult physician. For children under 12 years, use only as directed by physician. Keep out of the reach of children. As with any drug, if you are pregnant or nursing a baby, we recommend that you seek the advice of a health care professional before using this product.

Dosage and Administration: CREAM: Apply up to five times daily, especially morning, night, and after bowel movements, or as directed by physician. *External*—Apply liberally to affected area. *Intrarectal*—Remove cap from tube and attach clean applicator. Remove protective cover from clean applicator. Squeeze tube to fill applicator and lubricate tip with cream. Gently insert applicator into rectum and squeeze tube again. Thoroughly cleanse applicator after use.

Dosage and Administration: SUPPOSITORIES: Use up to five times daily, especially morning, night, and after bowel movements, or as directed by physician. Detach one suppository from pack. Separate foil at rounded end and peel apart until suppository is exposed. Insert suppository into the rectum, pointed end first.

How Supplied: Tronolane is available in 1-oz and 2-oz cream tubes and 10- and 20-count suppository boxes.

*Shown in Product Identification
Section, page 425*

(FAN 2093-03)

Products are cross-indexed by
generic and chemical names
in the
YELLOW SECTION

Rydelle Laboratories, Inc.

Subsidiary of S. C. Johnson & Son, Inc.
**1525 HOWE STREET
RACINE, WI 53403**

AVEENO® BATH TREATMENTS
[ah-ve´no]
REGULAR FORMULA AND OILATED FOR DRY SKIN

AVEENO® BATH TREATMENTS contain colloidal oatmeal, a natural oat derivative developed especially for soothing and cleaning itchy, sore, sensitive skin.

AVEENO® BATH TREATMENTS contain no soaps or synthetic detergents that may be harmful to the skin. They cleanse naturally because of their unique adsorptive properties.

AVEENO BATH TREATMENTS can be used in the care of itch due to dry skin, rashes, psoriasis, hemorrhoidal and genital irritations, poison ivy/oak, and sunburn. They are safe for use on children and can be used in the treatment of chicken pox, diaper rash, prickly heat and hives.

Ingredients: Aveeno Bath Regular: 100% colloidal oatmeal; Aveeno Bath Oilated: 43% colloidal oatmeal, mineral oil, and a specially selected emollient.

*Shown in Product Identification
Section, page 425*

AVEENO® CLEANSING BAR
[ah-ve´no]
FOR NORMAL TO OILY SKIN

AVEENO® Cleansing Bar For Normal To Oily Skin is made especially for itchy, sensitive skin that is irritated by ordinary soaps.

More than 50% of this mild skin cleanser is colloidal oatmeal, noted for its soothing and protective qualities.

Aveeno® Cleansing Bar is completely soap-free. It leaves no harsh alkaline film to irritate delicate skin, and it leaves skin feeling soft and comfortable.

Ingredients: Aveeno® Colloidal Oatmeal, 51%; in a sudsing soap-free base containing a mild surfactant.

*Shown in Product Identification
Section, page 425*

AVEENO® CLEANSING BAR
[ah-ve´no]
FOR ACNE

AVEENO® Cleansing Bar For Acne is a unique soap-free cleanser. It combines colloidal oatmeal, a long recognized, natural anti-itch treatment and gentle adsorbing cleanser, with special medication to eliminate most blackheads or acne pimples.

Ingredients: Aveeno® Colloidal Oatmeal, 51%; salicylic acid 2%; in a sudsing soap-free base containing a mild surfactant.

*Shown in Product Identification
Section, page 425*

AVEENO® CLEANSING BAR
[ah-ve´no]
FOR DRY SKIN

AVEENO® Cleansing Bar For Dry Skin is a unique, soap-free cleanser for itchy, dry, sensitive skin that is irritated by ordinary soaps. It contains over 15% skin-softening emollients to help replace natural skin oils and 51% colloidal oatmeal, recommended for its soothing and protective qualities.

Ingredients: Aveeno® Colloidal Oatmeal, 51%, in a sudsing soap-free base containing vegetable oils, glycerine, and a mild surfactant.

*Shown in Product Identification
Section, page 425*

AVEENO® LOTION
[ah-ve´no]
FOR RELIEF OF DRY, ITCHY SKIN

AVEENO® Lotion has been clinically proven to relieve dry skin. It contains natural colloidal oatmeal to relieve the itch often associated with dry skin. It is noncomedogenic and contains no fragrance, parabens, or lanolin which can cause allergic reactions.

Active Ingredients: Colloidal oatmeal 1%, allantoin 0.5%.

Also Contains: Water, glycerin, distearyldimonium chloride, petrolatum, isopropyl palmitate, cetyl alcohol, dimethicone, sodium chloride, benzyl alcohol.

*Shown in Product Identification
Section, page 425*

AVEENO® SHOWER AND BATH OIL
[ah-ve´no]
FOR RELIEF OF DRY ITCHY SKIN

AVEENO® Shower and Bath Oil combines the lubricating properties of mineral oil with the natural anti-itch benefits of colloidal oatmeal for the relief of dry, itchy skin. It contains no fragrance, parabens or lanolin which can cause allergic reactions.

Active Ingredient: Colloidal oatmeal 5%

Also contains: Mineral oil, glyceryl stearate and PEG 100 stearate, laureth-4, benzyl alcohol, silica, benzaldehyde.

*Shown in Product Identification
Section, page 425*

RHULIGEL®
(External analgesic)

Rhuligel® is uniquely formulated to provide penetrating cooling relief of itching and pain associated with many common skin irritations. Rhuligel® provides fast, soothing itch-relief in a cool, clear medicated gel. Rhuligel® is especially effective in relieving the annoying itch of poison ivy/oak/sumac, insect bites and sunburn.

Rhuligel® contains no hydrocortisone and is suitable for use on children age 2 years and older.

Indications: For temporary relief of pain and itching associated with minor

burns, sunburn, insect bites, or minor skin irritations.

Active Ingredients: Benzyl Alcohol 2% w/w, Menthol 0.3% w/w, Camphor 0.3% w/w, SD 23A Alcohol 32% w/w.

Also Contains: Benzophenone-4, Carbomer 940, EDTA, Propylene Glycol, Purified Water, Triethanolamine.

Directions: Adults and children 2 years of age and older: Apply liberally to affected area no more than 3 to 4 times daily. Children under 2 years of age: Consult a physician.

Warnings: For external use only. Avoid contact with eyes. If condition worsens or if symptoms persist for more than seven days, or clear up and occur again within a few days, discontinue use and consult a physician. Keep this and all medications out of the reach of children.

How Supplied: 2 oz. tube.

Shown in Product Identification Section, page 425

RHULISPRAY®
(External analgesic)

Soothing Rhulispray® with Calamine and Benzocaine works on contact to provide fast, cooling relief of the itching and pain of poison ivy/oak/sumac, insect bites, sunburn, and minor skin irritations.

Spray action provides immediate itch relief on contact without touching delicate, inflamed skin.

Rhulispray® contains no hydrocortisone and is suitable for use on children age 2 years and older.

Active Ingredients: Phenylcarbinol 1.9% w/w, Menthol 0.07%, Camphor 0.7%, Calamine 13.9%, Benzocaine 3.4%, Isopropyl Alcohol 71.92% (in concentrate).

Also Contains: Hydrated Silica, Oleyl Alcohol, Isobutane, Sorbitan Trioleate.

Directions: Adults and children 2 years of age and older: Apply liberally to affected area no more than 3 to 4 times daily for the relief of itching and pain. Children under 2 years of age: Consult a physician.

Warnings: For external use only. Avoid contact with eyes. If condition worsens or if symptoms persist for more than seven days, or clear up and occur again within a few days, discontinue use and consult a physician. Keep this and all medication out of the reach of children.

Caution: Flammable. Contents under pressure. Do not puncture or incinerate. Do not store at temperatures above 120°F (49°C). Intentional misuse by deliberately concentrating and inhaling the contents can be harmful or fatal. Store at room temperature 59–86°F (15–30°C).

How Supplied: 4 oz. aerosol.

Shown in Product Identification Section, page 425

Sandoz Consumer
59 ROUTE 10
EAST HANOVER, NJ 07936

ACID MANTLE® CREME
[ă'sĭd-mănt'l]

Description: A greaseless, water-miscible preparation containing buffered aluminum acetate. Other ingredients: aluminum sulfate, calcium acetate, cetearyl alcohol, glycerin, light mineral oil, methylparaben, purified water, sodium lauryl sulfate, synthetic beeswax, white petrolatum, white potato dextrin. May also contain: ammonium hydroxide, citric acid.

Indications: A vehicle for compatible topical drugs. Restores and maintains protective acidity of the skin. Provides relief of mildly irritated skin due to exposure to soaps, detergents, chemicals, alkalis. Aids in the treatment of diaper rash, bath dermatitis, athlete's foot, anogenital pruritis, acne, winter eczema and dry, rough, scaly skin of varied causes.

Caution: Limited compatibility and stability with Vitamin A, neomycin and other water-sensitive antibiotics. For external use only. Not for ophthalmic use.

Warnings: Keep this and all drugs out of the reach of children. In case of accidental ingestion, seek professional assistance or contact a Poison Control Center immediately.

Directions: Apply several times daily, especially after wet work.

How Supplied: 1 oz tubes; 4 oz and 1 lb jars.

BiCOZENE® Creme External Analgesic
[bī-cō-zēn]

Active Ingredients: Benzocaine 6%, resorcinol 1.67% in a specially prepared cream base.

Inactive Ingredients: Castor Oil, Chlorothymol, Ethanolamine Stearates, Glycerin, Glyceryl Borate, Glyceryl Stearates, Parachlorometaxylenol, Polysorbate 80, Sodium Stearate, Triglycerol Diisostearate, Perfume.

Indications: For the temporary relief of minor skin irritation and minor burns, sunburn, minor cuts, abrasions, and insect bites. For all kinds of external itching skin conditions; vaginal, rectal, poison ivy, heat rash, chafing, eczema, and common itching of the skin.

Actions: Benzocaine is a topical anesthetic and resorcinol is a topical antipruritic, at the concentrations used in BiCozene Creme. Both exert their actions by depressing cutaneous sensory receptors.

Warnings: Caution: Use only as directed. Keep away from the eyes. Not for prolonged use. If the condition for which this preparation is used persists, or if a rash or irritation develops, discontinue use and consult a physician. For external

use only. KEEP ALL MEDICINES OUT OF THE REACH OF CHILDREN.

Drug Interaction Precautions: No known drug interaction.

Dosage and Administration: Apply liberally to affected area as needed, several times a day.

How Supplied: BiCozene Creme is available in 1-ounce tubes.

Shown in Product Identification Section, page 425

CAMA® ARTHRITIS PAIN RELIEVER
[kă'măh]

Description: Each CAMA Inlay-Tab® contains: Active ingredients: aspirin, USP, 500 mg (7.7 grains); magnesium oxide, USP, 150 mg; dried aluminum hydroxide gel, USP, 150 mg. Other ingredients: colloidal silicon dioxide, croscarmellose sodium, hydrogenated vegetable oil, methylcellulose, methylparaben, microcrystalline cellulose, polyethylene glycol, povidone, pregelatinized starch, starch, Yellow 6, Yellow 10.

Indications: For the temporary relief of minor arthritic pain.

Warnings: Children and teenagers should not use this medicine for chicken pox or flu symptoms before a doctor is consulted about Reye syndrome, a rare but serious illness reported to be associated with aspirin. If pain persists for more than 10 days, consult a physician immediately. As with any drug, if you are pregnant or nursing a baby, seek the advice of a health professional before using this product. Stop taking this product if ringing in the ears or dizziness occurs. Do not take this product if you are presently taking a prescription drug for anticoagulation (thinning the blood), gout or if you have an aspirin allergy. **Keep this and all medicines out of the reach of children. In case of accidental overdose, contact a physician immediately.**

Directions For Use: Adults—2 tablets with a full glass of water every 6 hours. Not to exceed 8 tablets in 24 hours unless directed by a physician. Do not use in children under 12 years of age except under the advice and supervision of a physician.

How Supplied: CAMA Arthritis Pain Reliever Tablets (white with salmon inlay), imprinted "Cama 500" on one side, "Dorsey" on the other, in bottles of 100.

CHEXIT® TABLETS
[chex'it]

Description: Each CHEXIT Timed Release Tablet contains: phenylpropanolamine hydrochloride 25 mg, pheniramine maleate 12.5 mg, pyrilamine maleate 12.5 mg, dextromethorphan hydrobromide 30 mg, terpin hydrate 180 mg and acetaminophen 325 mg. Other ingredients: alginic acid, calcium

Continued on next page

stearate, colloidal silicon dioxide, magnesium stearate, methylcellulose, methylparaben, pharmaceutical glaze, polyethylene glycol, polysorbate 20, povidone, Red 30, starch, stearic acid, sucrose, titanium dioxide.

Indications: For relief of flu-like symptoms due to the common cold, such as cough, nasal congestion, simple headache and minor muscular aches and pains.

Warnings: Do not exceed recommended dosage because at higher doses, nervousness, dizziness or sleeplessness may occur. Do not take this product if you have heart disease, high blood pressure, thyroid disease, diabetes, asthma, glaucoma, emphysema, chronic pulmonary disease, shortness of breath, difficulty in breathing or difficulty in urination due to enlargement of the prostate gland unless directed by a doctor. May cause marked drowsiness; alcohol may increase the drowsiness effect. Avoid alcoholic beverages while taking this product. Use caution when driving a motor vehicle or operating machinery. May cause excitability especially in children. If symptoms do not improve within seven days or new ones occur or if fever persists for more than three days (72 hours) or recurs, consult a doctor. Do not take this product for persistent or chronic cough such as occurs with smoking, asthma or emphysema or if cough is accompanied by excessive phlegm (mucus) unless directed by a doctor. A persistent cough may be a sign of a serious condition. If cough persists for more than one week, tends to recur or is accompanied by high fever, rash or persistent headaches, consult a doctor. As with any drug, if you are pregnant or nursing a baby, seek the advice of a health professional before using this product. Keep this and all drugs out of the reach of children. In case of accidental overdose, seek professional assistance or contact a Poison Control Center immediately. *Drug Interaction Precaution:* Do not take this product if you are presently taking a prescription drug for high blood pressure or depression without first consulting your doctor.

Dosage: Adults—1 tablet morning, midafternoon and before retiring, swallowed whole to preserve the timed-release feature.

How Supplied: CHEXIT Tablets (pink), in blister packs of 12.

DENCLENZ® DENTURE CLEANSER
[děn-clěnz]

Indications: For daily cleaning of removable dentures.

Actions: Denclenz liquid works in combination with the mechanical action of the brush-applicator bottle. The combined action breaks up mineral deposits, plaque, and stain which adhere to dentures, and are responsible for denture odor and discoloration.

Caution: Not for use in mouth. Use with care. Keep away from eyes and out of children's reach. Contains dilute solution of hydrochloric acid. If spilled on eyes, skin, clothing, chrome or Formica® surfaces, rinse immediately with cold water.

Directions for use: Hold bottle upside down over sink. Squeeze bottle gently and brush Denclenz on dentures inside and out. Rinse thoroughly in running water (at least 30 seconds) to remove all of the Denclenz liquid. (Rinse brush too).

How Supplied: In bottles of 2 and 3.5 fluid ounce.

DORCOL® CHILDREN'S COUGH SYRUP
[door 'call]

Description: Each teaspoonful (5 ml) of DORCOL Children's Cough Syrup contains pseudoephedrine hydrochloride 15 mg, guaifenesin 50 mg, dextromethorphan hydrobromide 5 mg. Other ingredients: benzoic acid, Blue 1, edetate disodium, flavors, glycerin, propylene glycol, purified water, Red 40, sodium hydroxide, sucrose, tartaric acid.

Indications: Temporarily relieves your child's cough due to minor throat and bronchial irritation as may occur with the common cold. Helps loosen phlegm (mucus) and bronchial secretions to rid the bronchial passageways of bothersome mucus. Relieves irritated membranes in the respiratory passageways by preventing dryness through increased mucus flow. Temporarily relieves nasal stuffiness due to the common cold and promotes nasal and/or sinus drainage.

Warnings: EXCEPT UNDER THE ADVICE AND SUPERVISION OF A PHYSICIAN: DO NOT give your child more than the recommended dosage because at higher doses nervousness, dizziness or sleeplessness may occur. DO NOT give this preparation if your child has high blood pressure, heart disease, diabetes or thyroid disease. DO NOT give this product for persistent or chronic cough such as occurs with asthma or where cough is accompanied by excessive secretions. Keep this and all drugs out of the reach of children. In case of accidental overdose, seek professional assistance or contact a Poison Control Center immediately. A persistent cough may be a sign of a serious condition. If cough or other symptoms persist for more than one week, tend to recur or are accompanied by high fever, rash or persistent headache, consult a physician before continuing use. *Drug Interaction Precaution:* Do not give this product if your child is presently taking a prescription antihypertensive or antidepressant drug containing a monoamine oxidase inhibitor except under the advice and supervision of a physician.

Directions For Use: Children under 2 years—consult physician.

By age:
Children 2 to under 6 years: 1 teaspoonful every 4 hours.
Children 6 to under 12 years: 2 teaspoonfuls every 4 hours.
By weight:
Children 25 to 45 pounds: 1 teaspoonful every 4 hours.
Children 46 to 85 pounds: 2 teaspoonfuls every 4 hours.
Unless directed by a physician, do not exceed 4 doses in 24 hours.

Professional Labeling: The suggested dosage for pediatric patients is:

3–12 months	3 drops/Kg of body weight every 4 hours	
12–24 months	7 drops (0.2 ml)/Kg of body weight every 4 hours	

Maximum 4 doses in 24 hours.

How Supplied: DORCOL Children's Cough Syrup (grape colored), in 4 fl oz and 8 fl oz plastic bottles with tamper-evident band around child-resistant cap.
Shown in Product Identification Section, page 425

DORCOL® CHILDREN'S DECONGESTANT LIQUID
[door 'call]

Description: Each teaspoonful (5 ml) of DORCOL Children's Decongestant Liquid contains pseudoephedrine hydrochloride 15 mg. Other ingredients: benzoic acid, edetate disodium, flavors, purified water, sodium hydroxide, sorbitol, sucrose, Yellow 6, Yellow 10.

Indications: Provides temporary relief of nasal congestion due to the common cold, hay fever or other upper respiratory allergies, or associated with sinusitis. Reduces swelling of nasal passages; to restore freer breathing through the nose. Promotes nasal and sinus drainage; relieves sinus pressure.

Directions For Use: Children under 2 years—consult physician.
By age:
Children 2 to under 6 years: 1 teaspoonful every 4 to 6 hours.
Children 6 years: 2 teaspoonfuls every 4 to 6 hours.
By weight:
Children 25 to 45 pounds: 1 teaspoonful every 4 to 6 hours.
Children 46 to 85 pounds: 2 teaspoonfuls every 4 to 6 hours.
Unless directed by a physician, do not exceed 4 doses in 24 hours.

Professional Labeling: The suggested dosage for pediatric patients is:

3–12 months	3 drops/Kg of body weight every 4–6 hours	
12–24 months	7 drops (0.2 ml)/Kg of body weight every 4–6 hours	

Maximum of 4 doses in 24 hours.

Warnings: Do not give your child more than the recommended dosage because at higher doses nervousness, dizziness, or sleeplessness may occur. If symptoms do not improve within seven days or are accompanied by high fever, consult a physi-

cian before continuing use. Do not give this preparation if your child has high blood pressure, heart disease, diabetes, or thyroid disease except under the advice and supervision of a physician. Keep this and all drugs out of the reach of children. In case of accidental overdose, seek professional assistance or contact a Poison Control Center immediately. *Drug Interaction Precaution:* Do not give this product if your child is presently taking a prescription antihypertensive or antidepressant drug containing a monoamine oxidase inhibitor except under the advice and supervision of a physician.

How Supplied: DORCOL Children's Decongestant Liquid (pale orange), in 4 fl oz bottles with tamper-evident band around child-resistant cap.

Shown in Product Identification Section, page 425

DORCOL® CHILDREN'S FEVER & PAIN REDUCER
[door 'call]

Description: Each teaspoonful (5 ml) of DORCOL Children's Fever & Pain Reducer contains acetaminophen 160 mg. Other ingredients: benzoic acid, edetate disodium, flavors, glycerin, polyethylene glycol, purified water, Red 40, sodium chloride, sucrose.

Indications: For temporary relief of your child's fever and occasional minor aches, pains and headache.

Directions For Use: Children under 2 years—consult physician.
By age:
Children 2 to under 4 years: 1 teaspoonful
Children 4 to under 6 years: 1½ teaspoonfuls
Children 6 years of age: 2 teaspoonfuls
By weight:
Children 25 to 35 pounds: 1 teaspoonful
Children 36 to 45 pounds: 1½ teaspoonfuls
Children 46 to 60 pounds: 2 teaspoonfuls
Give every 4 hours while symptoms persist or as directed by a physician. Unless directed by a physician do not exceed 5 doses in 24 hours.

Professional Labeling: The suggested dosage for pediatric patients is:

3–12 months	3 drops/Kg of body weight every 4 hours	
12–24 months	7 drops (0.2 ml)/Kg of body weight every 4 hours	

Maximum of 5 doses in 24 hours.

Warnings: Do not give this product to your child for more than 5 days. Consult your physician if symptoms persist, new ones occur, or if fever persists for more than 3 days (72 hours) or recurs. DO NOT exceed recommended dosage. Keep this and all drugs out of the reach of children. In case of accidental overdose, seek professional assistance or contact a Poison Control Center immediately.

How Supplied: DORCOL Children's Fever & Pain Reducer (red), in 4 fl oz bottles with tamper-evident band around child-resistant cap.

Shown in Product Identification Section, page 425

DORCOL® CHILDREN'S LIQUID COLD FORMULA
[door 'call]

Description: Each teaspoonful (5 ml) of DORCOL Children's Liquid Cold Formula contains: pseudoephedrine hydrochloride 15 mg and chlorpheniramine maleate 1 mg. Other ingredients: benzoic acid, Blue 1, flavors, purified water, Red 40, sorbitol, sucrose, Yellow 10. May also contain sodium hydroxide.

Indications: Provides temporary relief of nasal congestion, sneezing and rhinorrhea due to the common cold, hay fever or other upper respiratory allergies or associated with sinusitis. Reduces swelling of nasal passages and restores freer breathing. Promotes nasal and sinus drainage; relieves sinus pressure.

Directions For Use: Children under 6 years—consult physician.
By age:
Children 6 to under 12 years: 2 teaspoonfuls every 4 to 6 hours.
By weight:
Children 45 to 85 pounds: 2 teaspoonfuls every 4 to 6 hours.
Unless directed by a physician, do not exceed 4 doses in 24 hours.

Professional Labeling: The suggested dosage for pediatric patients is:

3–12 months	2 drops/Kg of body weight every 4–6 hours	
12–24 months	5 drops (0.2 ml)/Kg of body weight every 4–6 hours	
2–6 years	1 teaspoonful every 4–6 hours	

Maximum of 4 doses in 24 hours.

Warnings: Do not give your child more than the recommended dosage because at higher doses nervousness, dizziness, or sleeplessness may occur. Do not give this preparation if your child has high blood pressure, heart disease, diabetes, thyroid disease, asthma, glaucoma, or difficulty in urination due to enlargement of the prostate gland except under the advice and supervision of a physician. If symptoms do not improve within 7 days or are accompanied by high fever, consult a physician before continuing use. May cause drowsiness. May cause excitability especially in children. Keep this and all drugs out of the reach of children. In case of accidental overdose, seek professional assistance or contact a Poison Control Center immediately. *Drug Interaction Precaution:* Do not give this product if your child is presently taking a prescription antihypertensive or antidepressant drug containing a monoamine oxidase inhibitor except under the advice and supervision of a physician.

Caution: Avoid alcoholic beverages or operating a motor vehicle or heavy machinery while taking this product.

How Supplied: DORCOL Children's Liquid Cold Formula (light brown), in 4 fl oz bottles with tamper-evident band around child-resistant cap.

Shown in Product Identification Section, page 425

EX–LAX® Chocolated Laxative

Active Ingredient: Yellow phenolphthalein, 90 mg phenolphthalein per tablet.

Inactive Ingredients: Cocoa, Confectioners' Sugar, Hydrogenated Palm Kernel Oil, Lecithin, Nonfat Dry Milk, Vanillin.

Indication: For relief of occasional constipation (irregularity).

Caution: Do not take any laxative when abdominal pain, nausea, or vomiting are present. Frequent or prolonged use of this or any other laxative may result in dependence on laxatives. If skin rash appears, do not use this or any other preparation containing phenolphthalein.

Warnings: Keep this and all drugs out of the reach of children. In case of accidental overdose, seek professional assistance or contact a poison control center immediately. As with any drug, if you are pregnant or nursing a baby, seek the advice of a health care professional before using this product.

Drug Interaction Precautions: No known drug interaction.

Dosage and Administration: Adults: Chew 1 to 2 tablets, preferably at bedtime. Children over 6 years: Chew ½ to 1 tablet.

How Supplied: Available in boxes of 6, 18, 48, and 72 chewable chocolate-flavored tablets.

Shown in Product Identification Section, page 426

EX–LAX® Unflavored Laxative Pills

Active Ingredient: Yellow phenolphthalein, 90 mg phenolphthalein per pill.

Inactive Ingredients: Acacia, Alginic Acid, Carnauba Wax, Colloidal Silicon Dioxide, Dibasic Calcium Phosphate, Iron Oxides, Magnesium Stearate, Microcrystalline Cellulose, Sodium Benzoate, Sodium Lauryl Sulfate, Starch, Stearic Acid, Sucrose, Talc, Titanium Dioxide.

Indication: For relief of occasional constipation (irregularity).

Caution: Do not take any laxative when abdominal pain, nausea, or vomiting are present. Frequent or prolonged use of this or any other laxative may result in dependence on laxatives. If skin rash appears, do not use this or any other preparation containing phenolphthalein.

Warnings: Keep this and all drugs out of the reach of children. In case of accidental overdose, seek professional assistance or contact a poison control center

Continued on next page

Sandoz Consumer—Cont.

immediately. As with any drug, if you are pregnant or nursing a baby, seek the advice of a health care professional before using this product.

Drug Interaction Precautions: No known drug interaction.

Dosage and Administration: Adults take 1 to 2 pills with a glass of water, preferably at bed time. Children over 6 years: 1 pill.

How Supplied: Available in boxes of 8, 30, and 60 unflavored pills.
Shown in Product Identification Section, page 426

EXTRA GENTLE EX-LAX®

Active Ingredients: Docusate Sodium, 75 mg. and Yellow Phenolphthalein 65 mg. per tablet.

Inactive Ingredients: Acacia, Croscarmellose Sodium, Dibasic Calcium Phosphate, Colloidal Silicon Dioxide, Magnesium Stearate, Microcrystalline Cellulose, Red 7, Stearic Acid, Sucrose, Talc, Titanium Dioxide.

Indication: For relief of occasional constipation (irregularity).

Caution: Do not take any laxative when abdominal pain, nausea or vomiting are present. Frequent or prolonged use of this or any other laxative may result in dependence on laxatives. If skin rash appears, do not use this or any other preparation containing phenolphthalein.

Warnings: Keep this and all drugs out of the reach of children. In case of accidental overdose, seek professional assistance or contact a poison control center immediately. As with any drug, if you are pregnant or nursing a baby, seek the advise of a health care professional before using this product.

Drug Interaction Precautions: No known drug interaction.

Dosage and Administration: Adults take 1 or 2 pills with water, preferably at bedtime, or as directed by physician. Children over 6 years: 1 pill, as needed.

How Supplied: Available in boxes of 24 pills.
Shown in Product Identification Section, page 426

GAS-X® AND EXTRA STRENGTH GAS-X®
High–Capacity Antiflatulent

Active Ingredients: GAS-X®—Each tablet contains 80 mg. simethicone. EXTRA STRENGTH GAS-X®—Each tablet contains 125 mg. simethicone.

Inactive Ingredients: calcium phosphates dibasic and tribasic, colloidal silicon dioxide, calcium silicate, microcrystalline cellulose, flavors, compressible sugar and talc. Extra strength Gas-X also contains Red 30 and Yellow 10.

Indications: For relief of the pain and pressure symptoms of excess gas in the digestive tract, which is often accompanied by complaints of bloating, distention, fullness, pressure, pain, cramps or excess anal flatus.

Actions: GAS-X acts in the stomach and intestines to disperse and reduce the formation of mucus-trapped gas bubbles. The GAS-X defoaming action reduces the surface tension of gas bubbles so that they are more easily eliminated.

Warning: Keep this and all medicines out of the reach of children.

Drug Interaction Precautions: No known drug interaction.

Dosage and Administration: Adults: Chew thoroughly and swallow one or two tablets as needed after meals and at bedtime. Do not exceed six GAS-X tablets or four EXTRA STRENGTH GAS-X tablets in 24 hours, except under the advice and supervision of a physician.

Professional Labeling: GAS-X may be useful in the alleviation of postoperative gas pain, and for use in endoscopic examination.

How Supplied: GAS-X is available in white, chewable, scored tablets in boxes of 36 tablets and convenience packages of 12 tablets.
EXTRA STRENGTH GAS-X is available in yellow, chewable, scored tablets in boxes of 18 tablets.
Shown in Product Identification Section, page 426

GENTLE NATURE®
NATURAL VEGETABLE LAXATIVE

Active Ingredients: 20 mg. Sennosides per tablet.

Inactive Ingredients: Alginic Acid, Calcium Phosphate Dibasic, Magnesium stearate, Microcrystalline Cellulose, Silicon Dioxide, Sodium Lauryl Sulfate, Starch, Stearic Acid.

Indications: For short-term relief of constipation.

Actions: Sennosides is a highly purified form of senna. The purification process removes components found in senna concentrate which may cause griping and cramps.
Sennosides has no laxative effect until they are carried to the lower part of the alimentary system by the regular working of the digestive process. In the bowel, the active glycosides are freed by the natural bowel micro-organisms. The freed laxative agent then gently encourages the muscle wave action of elimination. The gentle, predictable working of the laxative in the bowel, usually in 8–10 hours, or overnight if taken at bedtime, is apt to produce a well-formed stool in a natural-feeling way.

Caution: Not to be used when abdominal pain, nausea, or vomiting are present. Take only as needed. Frequent or prolonged use may result in dependence on laxatives. Keep this and all medications out of reach of children.

Drug Interaction Precautions: No known drug interaction.

Dosage and Administration: Adults— Take 1 or 2 tablets daily with water, preferably at bedtime, or as directed by your physician. Children over 6 years—1 tablet daily as required.

How Supplied: Available in boxes of 16 blister packed uncoated pills.
Shown in Product Identification Section, page 426

TRIAMINIC® ALLERGY TABLETS
[trī″ah-mĭn′ĭc]

Description: Each TRIAMINIC Allergy Tablet contains: phenylpropanolamine hydrochloride 25 mg, chlorpheniramine maleate 4.0 mg. Other ingredients: calcium stearate, calcium sulfate, colloidal silicon dioxide, methylcellulose, methylparaben, microcrystalline cellulose, polyethylene glycol, povidone, pregelatinized starch, titanium dioxide, Yellow 10.

Indications: For the temporary relief of runny nose, nasal congestion, sneezing, itching of the eyes, nose or throat and watery eyes as may occur in hay fever or other upper respiratory allergies (allergic rhinitis).

Warnings: Do not exceed the recommended dosage because at higher doses nervousness, dizziness or sleeplessness may occur. This preparation may cause drowsiness; this preparation may cause excitability especially in children. Do not take this preparation if you have high blood pressure, heart disease, diabetes, thyroid disease or are presently taking a prescription antihypertensive or antidepressant drug containing a monoamine oxidase inhibitor except under the advice and supervision of a physician. Do not give this preparation to children under 6 years except under the advice and supervision of a physician. Do not take this preparation if you have asthma, glaucoma or difficulty in urination due to enlargement of the prostate gland except under the advice and supervision of a physician. If symptoms do not improve within 7 days or are accompanied by high fever, consult a physician before continuing use. As with any drug, if you are pregnant or nursing a baby, seek the advice of a health professional before using this product. Keep this and all drugs out of the reach of children. In case of accidental overdose, seek professional assistance or contact a Poison Control Center immediately.

Caution: Avoid alcoholic beverages, operating a motor vehicle or heavy machinery while taking this product.

Dosage: Adults and children 12 and over—1 tablet every 4 hours. Children 6 to under 12 years—½ tablet every 4 hours. Unless directed by physician, do not exceed 6 doses in 24 hours or give to children under 6 years.

How Supplied: TRIAMINIC Allergy Tablets (yellow), scored, in blister packs of 24.

Shown in Product Identification Section, page 426

TRIAMINIC® CHEWABLES
[trī"ah-mĭn'ĭc]

Description: Each TRIAMINIC Chewable contains: phenylpropanolamine hydrochloride 6.25 mg, chlorpheniramine maleate 0.5 mg. Other ingredients: calcium stearate, citric acid, flavors, magnesium trisilicate, mannitol, microcrystalline cellulose, saccharin sodium, sucrose, Yellow 6, Yellow 10.

Indications: For the temporary relief of children's nasal congestion, runny nose, and sneezing due to the common cold or hay fever.

Warnings: Do not exceed recommended dosage because at higher doses nervousness, dizziness, or sleeplessness may occur. Do not give this product to children for more than 7 days. If symptoms do not improve or are accompanied by fever, consult a doctor. Do not give this product to children who have heart disease, high blood pressure, thyroid disease, diabetes, asthma or glaucoma unless directed by a doctor. May cause drowsiness. May cause excitability. *Drug Interaction Precaution:* Do not give this product to a child who is taking a prescription drug for high blood pressure or depression, without first consulting the child's doctor. Keep this and all drugs out of the reach of children. In case of accidental overdose, seek professional assistance or contact a Poison Control Center immediately.

Dosage: Children 6 to 12 years—2 tablets every 4 hours. Children under 6, consult your physician.

Professional Labeling: The suggested dosage for children 2 to 6 years is 1 tablet every 4 hours.

How Supplied: TRIAMINIC Chewables (hexagonal, yellow), in blister packs of 24.

TRIAMINIC® COLD SYRUP
[trī"ah-mĭn'ĭc]

Description: Each teaspoonful (5 ml) of TRIAMINIC Cold Syrup contains: phenylpropanolamine hydrochloride 12.5 mg and chlorpheniramine maleate 2 mg in a nonalcoholic vehicle. Other ingredients: benzoic acid, edetate disodium, flavors, purified water, sodium hydroxide, sorbitol, sucrose, Yellow 6.

Indications: Provides temporary relief of nasal congestion, runny nose and sneezing that may occur with the common cold or with hay fever or other upper respiratory allergies. Relieves itching of the nose or throat and itchy, watery eyes.

Warnings: Unless directed by a doctor, do not take this product if you have heart disease, high blood pressure, thyroid disease, diabetes, asthma, glaucoma, difficulty in breathing, enlargement of the prostate gland or are taking a prescription drug for high blood pressure or depression. Do not exceed recommended dosage or take for more than 7 days. If symptoms persist or are accompanied by fever, consult a doctor. May cause excitability especially in children. May cause drowsiness. Avoid drinking alcohol, driving or operating machinery while taking this product. As with any drug, if you are pregnant or nursing a baby, seek the advice of a health professional before using this product. Keep this and all drugs out of the reach of children. In case of accidental overdose, seek professional assistance or contact a Poison Control Center immediately.

Dosage and Administration: Adults and children 12 and over—2 teaspoonfuls every 4 hours. Children 6 to under 12 years—1 teaspoonful every 4 hours. Unless directed by physician, do not exceed 6 doses in 24 hours. Consult physician for dosage under 6 years of age.

Professional Labeling: The suggested dosage for pediatric patients is:

3–12 months	1 drop/Kg of body weight every 4 hours
12–24 months	3 drops/Kg of body weight every 4 hours
2–6 years	½ teaspoonful every 4 hours

How Supplied: TRIAMINIC Cold Syrup (orange), in 4 fl oz and 8 fl oz plastic bottles with tamper-evident band around child-resistant cap.

Shown in Product Identification Section, page 426

TRIAMINIC® COLD TABLETS
[trī"ah-mĭn'ĭc]

Description: Each TRIAMINIC Cold Tablet contains: phenylpropanolamine hydrochloride 12.5 mg and chlorpheniramine maleate 2 mg. Other ingredients: calcium stearate, colloidal silicon dioxide, flavor, lactose, methylcellulose, methylparaben, microcrystalline cellulose, polyethylene glycol, povidone, pregelatinized starch, Red 40, saccharin sodium, titanium dioxide, Yellow 6.

Indications: Temporarily relieves runny nose, nasal congestion and sneezing due to colds and allergies. Also relieves itching nose or throat and itchy, watery eyes associated with allergies.

Warnings: Unless directed by a doctor, do not take this product if you have heart disease, high blood pressure, thyroid disease, diabetes, asthma, glaucoma, difficulty in breathing, enlargement of the prostate gland or are taking a prescription drug for high blood pressure or depression. Do not exceed recommended dosage or take for more than 7 days. If symptoms persist or are accompanied by fever, consult a doctor. May cause excitability especially in children. May cause drowsiness. Avoid drinking alcohol, driving or operating machinery while taking this product. As with any drug, if you are pregnant or nursing a baby, seek the advice of a health professional before using this product. Keep this and all drugs out of the reach of children. In case of accidental overdose, seek professional assistance or contact a Poison Control Center immediately.

Caution: Avoid alcoholic beverages, operating a motor vehicle or heavy machinery while taking this product.

Dosage and Administration: Adults and children 12 and over—2 tablets every 4 hours. Children 6 to under 12 years—1 tablet every 4 hours. Unless directed by physician, do not exceed 6 doses in 24 hours.

How Supplied: TRIAMINIC Cold Tablets (orange), imprinted "DORSEY" on one side, "TRIAMINIC" on the other, in blister packs of 24.

Shown in Product Identification Section, page 426

TRIAMINIC® EXPECTORANT
[trī"ah-mĭn'ĭc]

Description: Each teaspoonful (5 ml) of TRIAMINIC Expectorant contains: phenylpropanolamine hydrochloride 12.5 mg and guaifenesin 100 mg. Other ingredients: alcohol (5%), benzoic acid, edetate disodium, flavors, purified water, saccharin, saccharin sodium, sodium hydroxide, sorbitol, sucrose, Yellow 6, Yellow 10.

Indications: Provides prompt relief of cough and nasal congestion due to the common cold. The expectorant component helps loosen bronchial secretions and rid the bronchial passageways of bothersome mucus. The decongestant and expectorant are provided in an antihistamine-free formula.

Warnings: Unless directed by a doctor, do not take this product if you have heart disease, high blood pressure, thyroid disease, diabetes, enlargement of the prostate gland or are taking a prescription drug for high blood pressure or depression. Do not exceed recommended dosage or take for more than 7 days. If symptoms persist, are accompanied by fever, rash or persistent headache or if cough recurs, consult a doctor. As with any drug, if you are pregnant or nursing a baby, seek advice from a health professional before using this product. Keep this and all drugs out of the reach of children. In case of accidental overdose, seek professional assistance or contact a Poison Control Center immediately.

Dosage and Administration: Adults and children 12 and over—2 teaspoonfuls every 4 hours. Children 6 to under 12 years—1 teaspoonful every 4 hours. Children 2–6 years—½ teaspoonful every 4 hours. Unless directed by physician, do not exceed 6 doses in 24 hours or give to children under 2 years of age.

Professional Labeling: The suggested dosage for pediatric patients is:

3–12 months	2 drops/Kg of body weight every 4 hours

Continued on next page

Sandoz Consumer—Cont.

12–24 months   3   drops/Kg of body weight every 4 hours

How Supplied: TRIAMINIC Expectorant (yellow), in 4 fl oz and 8 fl oz plastic bottles with tamper-evident band around child-resistant cap.

Shown in Product Identification Section, page 426

TRIAMINIC–DM® COUGH FORMULA
[trī″ah-mĭn′ĭc]

Description: Each teaspoonful (5 ml) of TRIAMINIC-DM Cough Formula contains: phenylpropanolamine hydrochloride 12.5 mg and dextromethorphan hydrobromide 10 mg in a nonalcoholic vehicle. Other ingredients: benzoic acid, Blue 1, flavors, propylene glycol, purified water, Red 40, sodium chloride, sorbitol, sucrose.

Indications: Provides relief of cough due to minor throat and bronchial irritation as may occur with the common cold or inhaled irritants. Promotes nasal and sinus drainage. The decongestant and antitussive are provided in an antihistamine-free formula.

Warnings: Unless directed by a doctor, **DO NOT** take this product: **1)** if cough is accompanied by excessive secretions, **2)** for persistent cough such as occurs with smoking, asthma or emphysema, or **3)** if you have heart disease, high blood pressure, thyroid disease, diabetes, enlargement of the prostate gland or are taking a prescription drug for high blood pressure or depression. Do not exceed recommended dosage or take for more than 7 days. If symtoms persist, are accompanied by fever, rash or persistent headache or if cough recurs, consult a doctor. As with any drug, if you are pregnant or nursing a baby, seek advice from a health professional before using this product. Keep this and all drugs out of the reach of children. In case of accidental overdose, seek professional assistance or contact a Poison Control Center immediately.

Dosage and Administration: Adults and children 12 and over—2 teaspoonfuls every 4 hours. Children 6 to under 12 years—1 teaspoonful every 4 hours. Children 2–6 years—½ teaspoonful every 4 hours. Unless directed by physician, do not exceed 6 doses in 24 hours or give to children under 2 years of age.

Professional Labeling: The suggested dosage for pediatric patients is:
3–12 months   1 drop/Kg of body weight every 4 hours
12–24 months   3   drops/Kg of body weight every 4 hours

How Supplied: TRIAMINIC-DM Cough Formula (dark red), in 4 fl oz and 8 fl oz plastic bottles with tamper-evident band around child-resistant cap.

Shown in Product Identification Section, page 426

TRIAMINIC–12® TABLETS
[trī″ah-mĭn′ĭc]

Description: Each TRIAMINIC - 12 Tablet contains: phenylpropanolamine hydrochloride 75 mg and chlorpheniramine maleate 12 mg. Other ingredients: carnauba wax, colloidal silicon dioxide, lactose, methylcellulose, polyethylene glycol, povidone, Red 30, stearic acid, titanium dioxide, Yellow 6.
TRIAMINIC-12 Tablets contain the nasal decongestant phenylpropanolamine, and the antihistamine chlorpheniramine, in a formulation providing 12 hours of symptomatic relief.

Indications: For the temporary relief of nasal congestion due to the common cold, hay fever or other upper respiratory allergies and associated with sinusitis. Helps decongest sinus openings, sinus passages; promotes nasal and/or sinus drainage; temporarily restores freer breathing through the nose. For temporary relief of running nose, sneezing, itching of the nose or throat and itchy and watery eyes as may occur in allergic rhinitis (such as hay fever).

Warnings: Do not give this product to children under 12 years except under the advice and supervision of a physician. Do not take this preparation if you have high blood pressure, heart disease, diabetes, thyroid disease, asthma, glaucoma or difficulty in urination due to enlargement of the prostate gland except under the advice and supervision of a physician. Do not exceed the recommended dosage because at higher doses nervousness, dizziness, or sleeplessness may occur. This preparation may cause drowsiness; this preparation may cause excitability, especially in children. If symptoms do not improve within seven days or are accompanied by high fever, consult a physician before continuing use. As with any drug, if you are pregnant or nursing a baby, seek the advice of a health professional before using this product.
Keep this and all drugs out of the reach of children. In case of accidental overdose, seek professional assistance or contact a Poison Control Center immediately.

Caution: Avoid driving a motor vehicle or operating heavy machinery. Avoid alcoholic beverages while taking this product.

Drug Interaction Precaution: Do not take this product if you are presently taking a prescription antihypertensive or antidepressant drug containing a monoamine oxidase inhibitor except under the advice and supervision of a physician.

Directions: Adults and children over 12 years of age—1 tablet swallowed whole every 12 hours. Unless directed by physician, do not exceed 2 tablets in 24 hours.

Note: The nonactive portion of the tablet that supplies the active ingredients may occasionally appear in your stool as a soft mass.

How Supplied: TRIAMINIC-12 Tablets (orange), imprinted "DORSEY" on one side, "TRIAMINIC 12" on the other, in blister packs of 10 and 20.

Shown in Product Identification Section, page 426

TRIAMINICIN® TABLETS
[trī″ah-mĭn′ĭ-sĭn]

Description: Each TRIAMINICIN Tablet contains: phenylpropanolamine hydrochloride 25 mg, chlorpheniramine maleate 4 mg and acetaminophen 650 mg. Other ingredients: calcium stearate, colloidal silicon dioxide, croscarmellose sodium, lactose, methylcellulose, methylparaben, polyethylene glycol, povidone, pregelatinized starch, Red 40, titanium dioxide, Yellow 10.

Indications: Temporarily relieves runny nose, sneezing, itching of the nose or throat, and itchy, watery eyes due to hay fever (allergic rhinitis) or other upper respiratory allergies. For the temporary relief of nasal congestion due to hay fever or other upper respiratory allergies or associated with sinusitis. Temporarily relieves nasal congestion, runny nose and sneezing associated with the common cold. For the temporary relief of occasional minor aches, pains and headache.

Warnings: Do not take this product if you have heart disease, high blood pressure, thyroid disease, diabetes, asthma, glaucoma, emphysema, chronic pulmonary disease, shortness of breath, difficulty in breathing, or difficulty in urination due to enlargement of the prostate gland unless directed by a doctor. Do not exceed recommended dosage because at higher doses nervousness, dizziness, or sleeplessness may occur. Do not take this product for more than 7 days. If symptoms do not improve, new ones occur, or if fever persists for more than three days (72 hours) or recurs, consult a doctor. May cause drowsiness; alcohol may increase the drowsiness effect. Avoid alcoholic beverages while taking this product. Use caution when driving a motor vehicle or operating machinery. May cause excitability especially in children. As with any drug, if you are pregnant or nursing a baby, seek the advice of a health professional before using this product. *Drug Interaction Precaution:* Do not take this product if you are presently taking a prescription drug for high blood pressure or depression, without first consulting your doctor. Keep this and all drugs out of the reach of children. In case of accidental overdose, seek professional assistance or contact a Poison Control Center immediately.

Dosage and Administration: Adults and children 12 years and older: Take 1 tablet every 4 hours while symptoms persist or as directed by a physician. Unless directed by a physician, do not exceed 6 doses in 24 hours or give to children under 12 years.

How Supplied: TRIAMINICIN Tablets (yellow), imprinted "DORSEY" on

one side, "TRIAMINICIN" on the other, in blister packs of 12, 24 and 48, and bottles of 100 tablets.

Shown in Product Identification Section, page 426

TRIAMINICOL® MULTI-SYMPTOM COLD SYRUP
[trī"ah-mĭn'ĭ-call]

Description: Each teaspoonful (5 ml) of TRIAMINICOL Multi-Symptom Cold Syrup contains: phenylpropanolamine hydrochloride 12.5 mg, chlorpheniramine maleate 2 mg, dextromethorphan hydrobromide 10 mg in a palatable nonalcoholic vehicle. Other ingredients: benzoic acid, flavors, propylene glycol, purified water, Red 40, saccharin sodium, sodium chloride, sorbitol, sucrose.

Indications: Provides relief of runny nose, nasal congestion and sneezing that may occur with the common cold. Suppresses cough due to minor throat and bronchial irritation. Promotes nasal and sinus drainage.

Warnings: Unless directed by a doctor, **DO NOT** take this product: **1)** if cough is accompanied by excessive secretions, **2)** for persistent cough such as occurs with smoking, asthma or emphysema, or **3)** if you have heart disease, high blood pressure, thyroid disease, diabetes, asthma, glaucoma, difficulty in breathing, enlargement of the prostate gland or are taking a prescription drug for high blood pressure or depression. Do not exceed recommended dosage or take for more than 7 days. If symtoms persist, are accompanied by fever, rash or persistent headache or if cough recurs, consult a doctor. May cause excitability especially in children. May cause drowsiness. Avoid drinking alcohol, driving or operating machinery while taking this product. As with any drug, if you are pregnant or nursing a baby, seek the advice of a health professional before using this product. Keep this and all drugs out of the reach of children. In case of accidental overdose, seek professional assistance or contact a Poison Control Center immediately.

Dosage and Administration: Adults and children 12 and over—2 teaspoonfuls every 4 hours. Children 6 to under 12 years—1 teaspoonful every 4 hours. Unless directed by physician, do not exceed 6 doses in 24 hours or give to children under 6 years of age.

Professional Labeling: The suggested dosage for pediatric patients is:

3–12 months	1 drop/Kg of body weight every 4 hours
12–24 months	3 drops/Kg of body weight every 4 hours
2–6 years	½ teaspoonful every 4 hours

How Supplied: TRIAMINICOL Multi-Symptom Cold Syrup (red), in 4 fl oz and 8 fl oz plastic bottles with tamper-evident band around child-resistant cap.

Shown in Product Identification Section, page 426

TRIAMINICOL® MULTI-SYMPTOM COLD TABLETS
[trī"ah-mĭn'ĭ-call]

Description: Each TRIAMINICOL Multi-Symptom Cold Tablet contains: phenylpropanolamine hydrochloride 12.5 mg, chlorpheniramine maleate 2 mg, dextromethorphan hydrobromide 10 mg. Other ingredients: calcium stearate, colloidal silicon dioxide, lactose, methylcellulose, methylparaben, microcrystalline cellulose, polyethylene glycol, povidone, pregelatinized starch, Red 40, titanium dioxide.

Indications: Temporarily relieves coughs due to minor throat and bronchial irritation. Temporarily relieves runny nose, nasal congestion and sneezing due to colds and allergies. Also relieves itching nose or throat and itchy, watery eyes associated with allergies.

Warnings: Unless directed by a doctor, **DO NOT** take this product: **1)** if cough is accompanied by excessive secretions, **2)** for persistent cough such as occurs with smoking, asthma or emphysema, or **3)** if you have heart disease, high blood pressure, thyroid disease, diabetes, asthma, glaucoma, difficulty in breathing, enlargement of the prostate gland or are taking a prescription drug for high blood pressure or depression. Do not exceed recommended dosage or take for more than 7 days. If symtoms persist, are accompanied by fever, rash or persistent headache or if cough recurs, consult a doctor. May cause excitability especially in children. May cause drowsiness. Avoid drinking alcohol, driving or operating machinery while taking this product. As with any drug, if you are pregnant or nursing a baby, seek the advice of a health professional before using this product. Keep this and all drugs out of the reach of children. In case of accidental overdose, seek professional assistance or contact a Poison Control Center immediately.

Dosage and Administration: Adults and children 12 and over—2 tablets every 4 hours. Children 6 to under 12 years—1 tablet every 4 hours. For nighttime cough relief, give the last dose at bedtime. Unless directed by physician, do not exceed 6 doses in 24 hours or give to children under 6 years.

How Supplied: TRIAMINICOL Multi-Symptom Cold Tablets (cherry pink), imprinted "DORSEY" on one side, "TRIAMINICOL" on the other, in blister packs of 24.

Shown in Product Identification Section, page 426

TUSSAGESIC® TABLETS
[tuss"a-geez'ĭc]

Description: Each TUSSAGESIC Timed Release Tablet contains: phenylpropanolamine hydrochloride 25 mg, pheniramine maleate 12.5 mg, pyrilamine maleate 12.5 mg, dextromethorphan hydrobromide 30 mg, terpin hydrate 180 mg and acetaminophen 325 mg.

Other ingredients: alginic acid, calcium stearate, colloidal silicon dioxide, magnesium stearate, methylcellulose, methylparaben, pharmaceutical glaze, polyethylene glycol, polysorbate 20, povidone, Red 30, starch, stearic acid, sucrose, titanium dioxide.

Indications: For prompt relief of symptoms associated with the common cold such as cough, nasal congestion, simple headache and minor muscular aches and pains.

Warnings: Do not exceed recommended dosage because at higher doses, nervousness, dizziness or sleeplessness may occur. Do not take this product if you have heart disease, high blood pressure, thyroid disease, diabetes, asthma, glaucoma, emphysema, chronic pulmonary disease, shortness of breath, difficulty in breathing or difficulty in urination due to enlargement of the prostate gland unless directed by a doctor. May cause marked drowsiness; alcohol may increase the drowsiness effect. Avoid alcoholic beverages while taking this product. Use caution when driving a motor vehicle or operating machinery. May cause excitibility especially in children. If symptoms do not improve within seven days or new ones occur or if fever persists for more than three days (72 hours) or recurs, consult a doctor. Do not take this product for persistent or chronic cough such as occurs with smoking, asthma or emphysema or if cough is accompanied by excessive phlegm (mucus) unless directed by a doctor. A persistent cough may be a sign of a serious condition. If cough persists for more than one week, tends to recur or is accompanied by high fever, rash or persistent headaches, consult a doctor. As with any drug, if you are pregnant or nursing a baby, seek the advice of a health professional before using this product. Keep this and all drugs out of the reach of children. In case of accidental overdose, seek professional assistance or contact a Poison Control Center immediately. *Drug Interaction Precaution:* Do not take this product if you are presently taking a prescription drug for high blood pressure or depression without first consulting your doctor.

Dosage: Adults—1 tablet, swallowed whole, in the morning, midafternoon and before retiring.

How Supplied: TUSSAGESIC Tablets (pink), in bottles of 100.

URSINUS® INLAY–TABS®
[yur"sīgn'us]

Description: Each URSINUS INLAY-TAB contains: pseudoephedrine hydrochloride 30 mg and aspirin 325 mg. Other ingredients: calcium stearate, lactose, microcrystalline cellulose, pregelatinized starch, sodium starch glycolate, starch, Yellow 6, Yellow 10.

Indications: For the temporary relief of nasal congestion due to the common cold, hay fever or associated with sinusi-

Continued on next page

Sandoz Consumer—Cont.

tis. For the temporary relief of occasional minor aches, pains and headache.

Warnings: Children and teenagers should not use this medicine for chicken pox or flu symptoms before a doctor is consulted about Reye syndrome, a rare but serious illness reported to be associated with aspirin. Unless directed by a doctor: 1) Do not take this product if you are allergic to aspirin or if you have asthma; 2) Do not take this product if you have heart disease, high blood pressure, thyroid disease, diabetes, or difficulty in urination due to enlargement of the prostate gland, and 3) Do not take this product during the last 3 months of pregnancy. Do not exceed recommended dosage because at higher doses nervousness, dizziness, or sleeplessness may occur. Do not take this product for more than 7 days. If symptoms do not improve, are accompanied by fever, or new symptoms occur, consult a doctor. Stop taking this product if ringing in the ears or other symptoms occur. Drink a full glass of water with each dose. Caution: Do not take this product if you are presently taking a prescription drug for anticoagulation (thinning the blood), diabetes, gout or arthritis or if you have stomach distress, ulcers or bleeding problems except under the advice and supervision of a physician. *Drug Interaction Precaution:* Do not take this product if you are presently taking a prescription drug for high blood pressure or depression, without first consulting your doctor. As with any drug, if you are pregnant or nursing a baby, seek the advice of a health professional before using this product.
Keep this and all medicines out of the reach of children. In case of accidental overdose, contact a physician immediately.

Directions: Adults and children 12 years and older: 2 tablets every 4 hours while symptoms persist or as directed by a physician. Do not take more than 4 doses in 24 hours. For chicken pox or flu see Warnings.

How Supplied: URSINUS INLAY-TABS (white with yellow inlay), in bottles of 24 and 100.

IDENTIFICATION PROBLEM?
Consult the
Product Identification Section
where you'll find
products pictured
in full color.

Schering Corporation
GALLOPING HILL ROAD
KENILWORTH, NJ 07033

A and D Ointment
REG. T.M.

Description: An ointment containing the emollients, anhydrous lanolin and petrolatum. Also contains: Fragrance, Mineral Oil, Fish Liver Oil and Cholecalciferol.

Indications: *Diaper rash*—**A and D Ointment** provides prompt, soothing relief for diaper rash and helps heal baby's tender skin; forms a moisture-proof shield that helps protect against urine and detergent irritants; comforts baby's skin and helps prevent chafing.
Chafed Skin—**A and D Ointment** helps skin retain its vital natural moisture; quickly soothes chafed skin in adults and children and helps prevent abnormal dryness.
Abrasions and Minor Burns—**A and D Ointment** soothes and helps relieve the smarting and pain of abrasions and minor burns, encourages healing and prevents dressings from sticking to the injured area.

Warning: Keep this and all drugs out of the reach of children.

Overdosage: In case of accidental ingestion, seek professional assistance or contact a poison control center immediately.

Dosage and Administration: *Diaper Rash*—Simply apply a thin coating of **A and D Ointment** at each diaper change. A modest amount is all that is needed to provide protective and healing action.
Chafed Skin—Gently smooth a small quantity of **A and D Ointment** over the area to be treated.
Abrasions, Minor Burns—Wash with lukewarm water and mild soap. When dry, apply **A and D Ointment** liberally. When a sterile dressing is used, change the dressing daily and apply fresh **A and D Ointment.** If no improvement occurs after 48 to 72 hours or if condition worsens, consult your physician.

How Supplied: A and D Ointment is available in 1½-ounce (42.5 g) and 4-ounce (113 g) tubes and 1-pound (454 g) jars.
Store away from heat.
Copyright© 1973, 1977, Schering Corporation. All rights reserved.
Shown in Product Identification Section, page 426

AFRIN®
[a'frin]
Nasal Spray 0.05%
Nasal Spray Pump 0.05%
Menthol Nasal Spray 0.05%
Nose Drops 0.05%
Children's Strength Nose Drops 0.025%

Description: AFRIN products contain oxymetazoline hydrochloride, the longest acting topical nasal decongestant

available. Each ml of AFRIN Nasal Spray, Nasal Spray Pump, and Nose Drops contains Oxymetazoline Hydrochloride, USP 0.5 mg (0.05%); Benzalkonium Chloride, Glycine, Phenylmercuric Acetate (0.02 mg/ml), Sorbitol, and Water.
Each ml of AFRIN Children's Strength Nose Drops contains Oxymetazoline Hydrochloride, USP 0.25 mg (0.025%); Benzalkonium Chloride, Glycine, Phenylmercuric Acetate (0.02 mg/ml), Sorbitol, and Water.
AFRIN Menthol Nasal Spray contains cooling aromatic vapors of menthol, eucalyptol and camphor and polysorbate, in addition to the ingredients of AFRIN Nasal Spray.

Indications: For temporary relief of nasal congestion "associated with" colds, hay fever and sinusitis.

Actions: The sympathomimetic action of AFRIN products constrict the smaller arterioles of the nasal passages, producing a prolonged, gentle and predictable decongesting effect. In just a few minutes a single dose, as directed, provides prompt, temporary relief of nasal congestion that lasts up to 12 hours. AFRIN products last up to 3 or 4 times longer than most ordinary nasal sprays. AFRIN products used at bedtime help restore freer nasal breathing through the night.

Warnings: Do not exceed recommended dosage because burning, stinging, sneezing or increase of nasal discharge may occur. Do not use these products for more than 3 days. If nasal congestion persists, consult a physician. The use of the dispensers by more than one person may spread infection. Keep these and all medicines out of the reach of children.

Overdosage: In case of accidental ingestion, seek professional assistance or contact a Poison Control Center immediately.

Dosage and Administration: Because AFRIN has a long duration of action, twice-a-day administration—in the morning and at bedtime—is usually adequate.
AFRIN Nasal Spray and Menthol Nasal Spray, 0.05%—For adults and children 6 years of age and over: With head upright, spray 2 or 3 times into each nostril twice daily—morning and evening. To spray, squeeze bottle quickly and firmly. Do not tilt head backward while spraying. Wipe nozzle clean after use. Not recommended for children under six.
Afrin Nasal Spray Pump, 0.05%—For adults and children 6 years of age and over: Two or three sprays in each nostril twice daily—morning and bedtime. Remove protective cap. Hold bottle with thumb at base and nozzle between first and second fingers. With head upright, insert metered pump spray nozzle in nostril. Depress pump 2 or 3 times, all the way down, with a firm even stroke and sniff deeply. Repeat in other nostril. Do not tilt head backward while spraying. Wipe tip clean after each use. Before us-

ing the first time, remove the protective cap from the tip and prime the metered pump by depressing pump firmly several times.

AFRIN Nose Drops—For adults and children 6 years of age and over: Tilt head back, apply 2 or 3 drops into each nostril twice daily—morning and evening. Immediately bend head forward toward knees. Hold a few seconds, then return to upright position. Wipe dropper clean after each use. Not recommended for children under six.

AFRIN Children's Strength Nose Drops—Children 2 through 5 years of age: Tilt head back, apply 2 or 3 drops into each nostril twice daily—morning and evening. Promptly move head forward toward knees. Hold a few seconds, then return child to upright position. Wipe dropper clean after each use. For children under 2 years, use only as directed by a physician.

How Supplied: AFRIN Nasal Spray 0.05% (1:2000), 15 ml and 30 ml plastic squeeze bottles.
AFRIN Nasal Spray Pump 0.05% (1:2000), 15 ml spray pump bottles.
AFRIN Menthol Nasal Spray 0.05% (1:2000), 15 ml plastic squeeze bottle.
AFRIN Nose Drops, 0.05% (1:2000), 20 ml dropper bottle.
AFRIN Children's Strength Nose Drops, 0.025% (1:4000), 20 ml dropper bottle.
Store all nasal sprays and nose drops between 2° and 30°C (36° and 86°F).

Shown in Product Identification Section, page 426

AFRINOL®
[a 'frin-ol]
Repetabs® Tablets
Long-Acting Nasal Decongestant

Active Ingredients: Each Repetabs Tablet contains: 120 mg pseudoephedrine sulfate. Each Repetab also contains: Acacia, Butylparaben, Calcium Sulfate, Carnauba Wax, Corn Starch, FD&C Blue No. 1, FD&C Yellow No. 6, Gelatin, Lactose, Magnesium Stearate, Neutral Soap, Oleic Acid, Povidone, Rosin, Sugar, Talc, White Wax, Zein. Half the dose (60 mg) is released after the tablet is swallowed and the other half is released hours later; continuous relief is provided for up to 12 hours . . . without drowsiness.

Indications: For temporary relief of nasal congestion due to the common cold, hay fever or other upper respiratory allergies, and nasal congestion associated with sinusitis.

Actions: Promotes nasal and/or sinus drainage, helps decongest sinus openings, sinus passages.

Warnings: Do not exceed recommended dosage because at higher doses nervousness, dizziness or sleeplessness may occur. Do not take this preparation if you have high blood pressure, heart disease, diabetes, or thyroid disease, except under the advice and supervision of a physician. If symptoms do not improve within 7 days or are accompanied by fever, consult a physician before continuing use.

Keep this and all drugs out of the reach of children.
As with any drug, if you are pregnant or nursing a baby, seek the advice of a health professional before using this product.

Drug Interactions: Do not take this product if you are presently taking a prescription drug for high blood pressure or depression, without first consulting your physician.

Overdosage: In case of accidental overdose, seek professional assistance or contact a poison control center immediately.

Dosage and Administration: Adults and children 12 years and over—One tablet every 12 hours. AFRINOL is not recommended for children under 12 years of age.

How Supplied: AFRINOL Repetabs Tablets—Boxes of 12 and bottles of 100. Store between 2° and 30°C (36° and 86° F) Protect from excessive moisture.
Shown in Product Identification Section, page 426

CHLOR–TRIMETON®
[klor-tri 'mĕ-ton]
Allergy Syrup
Allergy Tablets 4 mg
Long Acting Allergy REPETABS®
  Tablets 8 mg and 12 mg.

Active Ingredients: Each Allergy Tablet contains: 4 mg CHLOR-TRIMETON (brand of chlorpheniramine maleate, USP); also contains: Corn Starch, D&C Yellow No. 10 Al Lake, Lactose, Magnesium Stearate. Each REPETABS® Tablet contains: 8 mg or 12 mg CHLOR-TRIMETON (brand of chlorpheniramine maleate); 8 mg Repetabs also contains: Acacia, Butylparaben, Calcium Phosphate, Calcium Sulfate, Carnauba Wax, Corn Starch, D&C Yellow No. 10 Al Lake, FD&C Yellow No.6 Al Lake, Lactose, Magnesium Stearate, Neutral Soap, Oleic Acid, Povidone, Rosin, Sugar, Talc, White Wax, Zein. 12 mg Repetabs also contains: Acacia, Butylparaben, Calcium Phosphate, Calcium Sulfate, Carnauba Wax, Corn Starch, D&C Yellow No. 10 Al Lake, FD&C Blue No. 2 Al Lake, FD&C Yellow No. 6, FD&C Yellow No. 6 Al Lake, Lactose, Magnesium Stearate, Neutral Soap, Oleic Acid, Potato Starch, Rosin, Sugar, Talc, White Wax, Zein. Half the dose is released after the tablet is swallowed, and the other half is released hours later; continuous relief is provided for up to 12 hours.
Each teaspoonful (5 ml) of Allergy Syrup contains: 2 mg CHLOR-TRIMETON (brand of chlorpheniramine maleate) in a pleasant-tasting syrup containing approximately 7% alcohol. Also contains: Benzaldehyde, FD&C Green No. 3, FD&C Yellow No. 6, Flavor, Glycerin, Menthol, Methylparaben, Propylene Glycol, Propylparaben, Sugar, Vanillin, Water.

Indications: For temporary relief of hay fever symptoms: sneezing; runny nose; watery, itchy eyes, itching of the nose or throat.

Actions: The active ingredient in CHLOR-TRIMETON is an antihistamine with anticholinergic (drying) and sedative side effects. Antihistamines appear to compete with histamine for cell receptor sites on effector cells.

Warnings: May cause drowsiness. May cause excitability especially in children. Do not take these products if you have asthma, glaucoma or difficulty in urination due to enlargement of the prostate gland, or give the REPETABS Tablets to children under 12 years, or the Allergy Syrup and Tablets to children under 6 years, except under the advice and supervision of a physician. Keep these and all drugs out of the reach of children.
As with any drug, if you are pregnant or nursing a baby, seek the advice of a health professional before using this product.

Precautions: Avoid driving a motor vehicle or operating heavy machinery. Avoid alcoholic beverages while taking these products.

Overdosage: In case of accidental overdose, seek professional assistance or contact a Poison Control Center immediately.

Dosage and Administration: Allergy Syrup—Adults and Children 12 years and over: Two teaspoonfuls (4 mg) every 4 to 6 hours, not to exceed 12 teaspoonfuls in 24 hours; Children 6 through 11 years: one teaspoonful (2 mg) every 4 to 6 hours, not to exceed 6 teaspoonfuls in 24 hours; For children under 6 years, consult a physician.
Allergy Tablets—Adults and Children 12 years and over: One tablet (4 mg) every 4 to 6 hours, not to exceed 6 tablets in 24 hours. Children 6 through 11 years: One half the adult dose (break tablet in half) every 4 to 6 hours, not to exceed 3 whole tablets in 24 hours. For children under 6 years, consult a physician.
Allergy REPETABS Tablets—Adults and Children 12 years and over: One tablet in the morning and one tablet in the evening, not to exceed 24 mg (3 tablets of 8 mg; 2 tablets of 12 mg.) in 24 hours. For children under 12 years, consult a physician.

Professional Labeling: Dosage—Allergy Syrup: Children 2 through 5 years: ½ teaspoonful (1 mg) every 4 to 6 hours; Allergy Tablets: Children 2 through 5 years: one-quarter tablet (1 mg) every 4 to 6 hours.
Allergy REPETABS Tablets—Children 6 to 12 years: One tablet (8 mg) at bedtime or during the day, as indicated.

How Supplied: CHLOR-TRIMETON Allergy Tablets, 4 mg, yellow compressed, scored tablets impressed with the Schering trademark and product

Continued on next page

Schering—Cont.

identification letters, TW or numbers, 080; box of 24, bottles of 100.
CHLOR-TRIMETON Allergy Syrup: 2 mg per 5 ml, blue-green-colored liquid; 4-fluid ounce (118 ml). Protect from light; however, if color fades potency will not be affected.
CHLOR-TRIMETON Allergy REPETABS Tablets, 8 mg, sugar-coated, yellow tablets branded in red with the Schering trademark and product identification letters, CC or numbers, 374; boxes of 24, 48, bottles of 100.
CHLOR-TRIMETON REPETABS Tablets, 12 mg, sugar coated orange tablets branded in black with Schering trademark and product identification letters AAE or numbers 009; boxes of 12 and 24, bottles of 100.
Store the tablets and syrup between 2° and 30°C (36° and 86°F).

*Shown in Product Identification
Section, page 427*

CHLOR-TRIMETON®
[*klor 'tri 'mĕ-ton*]
Decongestant Tablets
Long Acting CHLOR-TRIMETON®
Decongestant REPETABS® Tablets

Active Ingredients: Each tablet contains: 4 mg CHLOR-TRIMETON (brand of chlorpheniramine maleate, USP) and 60 mg pseudoephedrine sulfate. Each tablet also contains: Corn Starch, FD&C Blue No. 1, Lactose, Magnesium Stearate, Povidone.
Each REPETABS Tablet contains: 8 mg CHLOR-TRIMETON (brand of chlorpheniramine maleate) and 120 mg pseudoephedrine sulfate. Each repetab also contains: Acacia, Butylparaben, Calcium Sulfate, Carnauba Wax, Corn Starch, D&C Yellow No. 10 Al Lake, FD&C Blue No. 1 Al Lake, FD&C Yellow No. 6 Al Lake, Gelatin, Lactose, Magnesium Stearate, Neutral Soap, Oleic Acid, Povidone, Rosin, Sugar, Talc, White Wax, Zein. Half the dose of each ingredient is released after the tablet is swallowed and the other half is released hours later providing continuous long-lasting relief up to 12 hours.

Indications: For temporary relief of hay fever symptoms (sneezing; running nose; watery, itchy eyes, itching of the nose or throat) and nasal congestion due to hay fever and associated with sinusitis.

Actions: The antihistamine, chlorpheniramine maleate, provides temporary relief of running nose, sneezing, itching of the nose or throat, and itchy and watery eyes as may occur in allergic rhinitis (such as hayfever). The decongestant, pseudoephedrine sulfate reduces swelling of nasal passages; shrinks swollen membranes; and temporarily restores freer breathing through the nose.

Warnings: If symptoms do not improve within seven days or are accompanied by high fever, consult your physician before continuing use. May cause drowsiness. May cause excitability especially in children. Do not exceed recommended dosage because at higher doses nervousness, dizziness or sleeplessness may occur. Do not give the Decongestant Tablets to children under 6 years or the REPETABS Tablets to children under 12 years except under the advice and supervision of a physician. Do not take these products if you have asthma, glaucoma, difficulty in urination due to enlargement of the prostate gland, high blood pressure, heart disease, diabetes or thyroid disease, except under the advice and supervision of a physician.
As with any drug, if you are pregnant or nursing a baby, seek the advice of a health professional before using this product.

Drug Interaction: Do not take this product if you are presently taking a prescription antihypertensive or antidepressant medication containing a monoamine oxidase inhibitor, except under the advice and supervision of a physician.

Precautions: Avoid driving a motor vehicle or operating heavy machinery. Avoid alcoholic beverages while taking this product. Keep these and all drugs out of the reach of children.

Overdosage: In case of accidental overdose, seek professional assistance or contact a Poison Control Center immediately.

Dosage and Administration: Tablets —ADULTS AND CHILDREN 12 YEARS AND OVER: One tablet every 4 to 6 hours, not to exceed 4 tablets in 24 hours. CHILDREN 6 THROUGH 11 YEARS —One half the adult dose (break tablet in half) every 4 to 6 hours not to exceed 2 whole tablets in 24 hours. For children under 6 years, consult a physician. REPETABS Tablets—ADULTS AND CHILDREN 12 YEARS AND OVER: one tablet every 12 hours.

Professional Labeling: Tablets— Children 2-5 years—one quarter the adult dose every 4 hours, not to exceed 1 tablet in 24 hours.

How Supplied: CHLOR-TRIMETON Decongestant Tablets—boxes of 24 and 48. Long Acting CHLOR-TRIMETON Decongestant REPETABS Tablets boxes of 12 and 36.
Store these CHLOR-TRIMETON Products between 2° and 30°C (36°& 86°F); and protect from excessive moisture.

*Shown in Product Identification
Section, page 427*

COD LIVER OIL CONCENTRATE
[*kod liv 'er oyl kon-sen-trāt*]
Tablets
Capsules
Tablets with Vitamin C

Active Ingredients: Tablets—A pleasantly flavored concentrate of cod liver oil with Vitamins A & D added. Each tasty, chewable tablet provides: 4000 IU of vitamin A and 200 IU of cholecalciferol (vitamin D).
Capsules—A concentrate of cod liver oil with Vitamins A and D added. Each capsule provides: 10,000 IU of vitamin A and 400 IU of cholecalciferol (vitamin D).
Tablets with Vitamin C—A pleasantly-flavored concentrate of cod liver oil with Vitamins A, D and C added. Each tablet provides, 4000 IU of Vitamin A, 200 IU of cholecalciferol (vitamin D) and 50 mg of Vitamin C.
Tablets may be chewed or swallowed.

Inactive Ingredients: Capsules—Corn oil, gelatin, glycerin, vitamin E.
Tablets with Vitamin C—Acacia, Butylparaben, Carnauba Wax, Confectioners Glaze, FD&C Yellow No. 5 Aluminum Lake, FD&C Yellow No. 6 Aluminum Lake, Flavor, Gelatin, Magnesium Stearate, Sugar, Wheat Flour, White Wax.

Indications: Cod Liver Oil Concentrate Tablets and Capsules are recommended for prevention and treatment of diseases due to deficiencies in Vitamins A and D. The tablets with Vitamin C are recommended for prevention and treatment of diseases due to deficiencies of Vitamins A, D and C.

Warnings: Keep these and all drugs out of the reach of children.
As with any drug, if you are pregnant or nursing a baby, seek the advice of a health professional before using these products.

Precautions: Cod Liver Oil Concentrate Tablets and Tablets with Vitamin C contain FD&C Yellow No. 5 (tartrazine) as a color additive.
Persons sensitive to tartrazine or aspirin should consult a physician.

Overdosage: In case of accidental overdose, seek professional assistance or contact a Poison Control Center immediately.

Dosage and Administration: Tablets: Two tablets daily, or as prescribed by a physician, taken preferably before meals.
Capsules: One capsule daily, or as prescribed by a physician, taken preferably before meals.
Tablets with Vitamin C: Two tablets daily, taken preferably before meals.

How Supplied: Cod Liver Oil Concentrate Tablets: bottles of 100. Cod Liver Oil Concentrate Capsules: bottles of 40 and 100. Cod Liver Oil Concentrate Tablets with Vitamin C: bottles of 100 tablets.

*Shown in Product Identification
Section, page 427*

COMPLEX 15®
Phospholipid Hand & Body
Moisturizing Cream
Formulated For Mild To Severe Dry Skin

Ingredients: Water, Mineral Oil, Glycerin, Squalane, Caprylic/Capric Triglyceride, Dimethicone, Glyceryl Stearate, Glycol Stearate, PEG-50 Stearate, Stearic Acid, Cetyl Alcohol, Myristyl Myris-

tate, Lecithin, Diazolidinyl Urea, Carbomer 934, Magnesium Aluminum Silicate, C10–30 Carboxylic Acid Sterol Ester, Sodium Hydroxide, Tetrasodium EDTA, BHT

COMPLEX 15® Hand and Body Cream is formulated for mild to severe dry skin with a system modeled from nature. It contains lecithin, a phospholipid water-binding agent found naturally in the skin. Each phospholipid molecule holds 15 molecules of water, restoring the natural moisture balance. COMPLEX 15 Hand and Body Cream is nongreasy and absorbs quickly into the skin. COMPLEX 15 Hand and Body Cream is unscented, contains no parabens or lanolin. COMPLEX 15 Hand and Body Cream is proven to be hypoallergenic and noncomedogenic.

Directions: Apply to the hands and body as needed or as directed by a physician. Avoid contact with eyes.

FOR EXTERNAL USE ONLY

How Supplied: COMPLEX 15® Hand & Body Moisturizing Cream is available in 4 ounce jars (0085-4151-04).

Manufactured for:
Schering Corporation
Kenilworth, NJ 07033 USA

COMPLEX 15®
Phospholipid Hand & Body
Moisturizing Lotion
Formulated For Mild To Severe Dry Skin

Ingredients: Water, Caprylic/Capric Triglyceride, Glycerin, Glyceryl Stearate, Dimethicone, PEG-50 Stearate, Squalane, Cetyl Alcohol, Glycol Stearate, Myristyl Myristate, Stearic Acid, Lecithin, C10–30 Carboxylic Acid Sterol Ester, Diazolidinyl Urea, Carbomer 934, Magnesium Aluminum Silicate, Sodium Hydroxide, BHT, Tetrasodium EDTA

COMPLEX 15® Hand and Body Lotion is formulated for mild to severe dry skin with a system modeled from nature. It contains lecithin, a phospholipid water-binding agent found naturally in the skin. Each phospholipid molecule holds 15 molecules of water, restoring the natural moisture balance. COMPLEX 15 Hand and Body Lotion is nongreasy and absorbs quickly into the skin. COMPLEX 15 Hand and Body Lotion is unscented, contains no parabens, lanolin, or mineral oil. COMPLEX 15 Hand and Body Lotion is proven to be hypoallergenic and noncomedogenic.

Directions: Apply to the hands and body as needed, or as directed by a physician. Avoid contact with eyes.

FOR EXTERNAL USE ONLY

How Supplied: COMPLEX 15® Hand and Body Moisturizing Lotion is available in 8 fluid ounce bottles (0085-4115-08).

Manufactured for:
Schering Corporation
Kenilworth, NJ 07033

COMPLEX 15®
Phospholipid Moisturizing Face Cream

Ingredients: Water, Caprylic/Capric Triglyceride, Glycerin, Squalane, Glyceryl Stearate, Propylene Glycol, PEG-50 Stearate, Cetyl Alcohol, Dimethicone, Glycol Stearate, Myristyl Myristate, Stearic Acid, Carbomer 934, Magnesium Aluminum Silicate, Diazolidinyl Urea, Lecithin, Sodium Hydroxide, C10–30 Carboxylic Acid Sterol Ester, BHT, Tetrasodium EDTA

COMPLEX 15® Face Cream is formulated for mild to severe dry skin with a system modeled from nature. It contains lecithin, a phospholipid water-binding agent found naturally in the skin. Each phospholipid molecule holds 15 molecules of water, restoring the natural moisture balance. COMPLEX 15 Face Cream is nongreasy and absorbs quickly into the skin. COMPLEX 15 Face Cream is unscented, contains no parabens, lanolin or mineral oil. COMPLEX 15 Face Cream is proven to be hypoallergenic and noncomedogenic.

Directions: Apply to the face as needed or as directed by a physician. Avoid contact with eyes.

FOR EXTERNAL USE ONLY.

How Supplied: COMPLEX 15® Moisturizing Face Cream is available in 2.5 oz. tubes (0085-4100-25).

Manufactured for:
Schering Corporation
Kenilworth, NJ 07033

CORICIDIN® Tablets
[kor-a-see 'din]
CORICIDIN 'D'® Decongestant Tablets
CORICIDIN® Nasal Mist

Active Ingredients: CORICIDIN Tablets—2 mg CHLOR-TRIMETON® (brand of chlorpheniramine maleate, USP); 325 mg (5gr) acetaminophen. CORICIDIN 'D' Decongestant Tablets—2 mg chlorpheniramine maleate, USP; 12.5 mg phenylpropanolamine hydrochloride, USP; 325 mg (5 gr) acetaminophen. CORICIDIN Nasal Mist—.05% oxymetazoline hydrochloride.

Inactive Ingredients: CORICIDIN Tablets—Acacia, Butylparaben, Calcium Sulfate, Carnauba Wax, Cellulose, Corn Starch, FD&C Red No. 40, FD&C Yellow No. 6 Aluminum Lake, Lactose, Magnesium Stearate, Povidone, Sugar, Titanium Dioxide, and White Wax. May also contain Talc.
CORICIDIN 'D' Decongestant Tablets —Acacia, Butylparaben, Calcium Sulfate, Carnauba Wax, Cellulose, Corn Starch, Magnesium Stearate, Povidone, Sugar, Titanium Dioxide, and White Wax. May also contain Talc.
CORICIDIN Nasal Mist—Benzalkonium Chloride, Glycine, Phenylmercuric Acetate (0.02 mg/ml), Sorbitol, and Water.

Indications: CORICIDIN Tablets—For effective, temporary relief of cold and flu symptoms.
CORICIDIN 'D' Decongestant Tablets— For effective, temporary relief of congested cold, flu and sinus symptoms.
CORICIDIN Nasal Mist— For temporary relief of nasal congestion associated with the common cold, hay fever or sinusitis.

Actions: CORICIDIN Tablets relieve annoying cold and flu symptoms such as minor aches and pains, fever, sneezing, running nose and watery/itchy eyes.
CORICIDIN 'D' Tablets relieve the same annoying cold and flu symptoms as well as stuffy nose, nasal membrane swelling and sinus headache.
CORICIDIN Nasal Mist is "symptom specific" and designed to shrink swollen nasal membranes promptly and help restore freer breathing through the nose.

Warnings: CORICIDIN Tablets: Adults should not take this product for more than 10 days; children 6 through 11 not more than 5 days. If fever persists or recurs, neither adults nor children should use for more than 3 days. If symptoms persist or new ones occur, consult your physician. May cause drowsiness. May cause excitability, especially in children. Do not take this product if you have asthma, glaucoma, difficulty in urination due to enlargement of the prostate gland, or give this product to children under 6 years, except under the advice and supervision of a physician. Keep this and all drugs out of the reach of children. As with any drug, if you are pregnant or nursing a baby, seek the advice of a health professional before using this product.
CORICIDIN 'D' Decongestant Tablets: Adults should not take this product for more than 7 days; children 6 through 11 not more than 5 days. If fever persists or recurs, neither adults nor children should use for more than 3 days. If symptoms persist or new ones occur, consult your physician. May cause drowsiness. May cause excitability, especially in children. Do not exceed recommended dosage because at higher doses nervousness, dizziness, elevation of blood pressure, or sleeplessness may occur. Do not take this product you have asthma, glaucoma, difficulty in urination due to enlargement of the prostate gland, high blood pressure, heart disease, diabetes or thyroid disease, or give this product to children under 6 years, except under the advice and supervision of a physician. Keep this and all drugs out of the reach of children. As with any drug, if you are pregnant or nursing a baby, seek the advice of a health professional before using this product.
CORICIDIN Nasal Mist—Do not exceed recommended dosage because burning, stinging, sneezing, or increase of nasal

Continued on next page

Information on Schering products appearing on these pages is effective as of November 1, 1988.

Schering—Cont.

discharge may occur. Do not use this product for more than 3 days. If nasal congestion persists, consult a physician. The use of this dispenser by more than one person may spread infection. For adult use only. Keep this and all medicines out of the reach of children.

Drug Interactions: CORICIDIN Tablets: Avoid alcoholic beverages while taking this product. Also avoid driving a motor vehicle or operating heavy machinery.
CORICIDIN 'D' Decongestant Tablets: Do not take this product if you are presently taking a prescription antihypertensive or antidepressant medication containing a monoamine oxidase inhibitor or an appetite controlling medication containing phenylpropanolamine except under the advice and supervision of a physician. Avoid alcoholic beverages while taking this product. Also avoid driving a motor vehicle or operating heavy machinery.

Overdosage: In case of accidental overdose of the tablets or syrup or accidental ingestion of the nasal mist, seek professional assistance or contact a Poison Control Center immediately.

Dosage and Administration: CORICIDIN Tablets—Adults and children 12 years and over—2 tablets every 4 hours not to exceed 12 tablets in 24 hours. Children 6 through 11 years: 1 tablet every 4 hours not to exceed 5 tablets in 24 hours. CORICIDIN 'D' Decongestant Tablets —Adults and children 12 years and over: 2 tablets every 4 hours not to exceed 12 tablets in 24 hours. Children 6 through 11 years: 1 tablet every 4 hours not to exceed 5 tablets in 24 hours. CORICIDIN Nasal Mist— For adults and children 6 years of age and over: With head upright spray two or three times in each nostril twice daily—morning and evening, to spray squeeze bottle quickly and firmly. Do not tilt head backward while spraying. Wipe nozzle clean after use. Not recommended for children under six.

How Supplied: CORICIDIN Tablets— bottles of 12, 24, 48 , and 100.
CORICIDIN 'D' Decongestant Tablets— bottles of 12, 24, 48, and 100.
CORICIDIN Decongestant Nasal Mist— Plastic squeeze bottles of ½ fl. oz. (15 ml.)
Store the tablets, nasal mist, and syrup between 2° and 30°C (36° and 86°F).
Shown in Product Identification Section, page 427

CORICIDIN® DEMILETS®
[kor-a-see 'din dem 'ē-lets]
Tablets for Children

CORICIDIN DEMILETS Tablets—1.0 mg chlorpheniramine maleate, USP; 80 mg acetaminophen, USP; 6.25 mg phenylpropanolamine hydrochloride, USP.

Inactive Ingredients: Corn Starch, D&C Yellow No. 10 Al Lake, FD&C Yellow No. 6 Al Lake, Flavor, Lactose, Mag-

nesium Stearate, Mannitol, Saccharin, Stearic Acid.

Indications: CORICIDIN DEMILETS Tablets—For temporary relief of children's congested cold, flu and sinus symptoms.

Actions: CORICIDIN DEMILETS Tablets provide relief of annoying cold, flu and sinus symptoms: running nose, stuffy nose, sneezing, watery/itchy eyes, minor aches, pains and fever.

Warnings: CORICIDIN DEMILETS Tablets—Give water with each dose. Do not give this product for more than 5 days, but if fever is present, persists or recurs, limit dosage to 3 days; if symptoms persist or new ones occur, consult a physician. This product may cause drowsiness, therefore, driving a motor vehicle or operating heavy machinery must be avoided while taking it. Alcoholic beverages must also be avoided while taking this product. It may cause excitability, especially in children. Do not exceed recommended dosage because at higher doses severe liver damage, nervousness, dizziness, elevation of blood pressure or sleeplessness are more likely to occur. Do not administer this product to persons who have asthma, glaucoma, difficulty in urination due to enlargement of the prostate gland, high blood pressure, heart disease, diabetes or thyroid disease, or give this product to children less than 6 years old, except under the advice and supervision of a physician. Keep this and all drugs out of the reach of children. As with any drug, if you are pregnant or nursing a baby, seek the advice of a health professional before using this product.

Drug Interactions: CORICIDIN DEMILETS Tablets—Do not give this product to persons who are presently taking a prescription antihypertensive or antidepressant medication containing a monoamine oxidase inhibitor or an appetite-controlling medication containing phenylpropanolamine except under the advice and supervision of a physician.

Overdosage: In case of accidental overdose, seek professional assistance or contact a Poison Control Center immediately.

Dosage and Administration: CORICIDIN DEMILETS Tablets—Under 6 years: As directed by a physician. 6 through 11 years: Two DEMILETS Tablets every 4 hours not to exceed 12 tablets in a 24-hour period, or as directed by a physician.

How Supplied: CORICIDIN DEMILETS Tablets—boxes of 36, individually wrapped in a child's protective pack. Store the tablets between 2° and 30°C (36° and 86°F). Protect from excessive moisture.
Shown in Product Identification Section, page 427

CORICIDIN® Maximum Strength Sinus Headache Caplets
[kor-a-see 'din]

Active Ingredients: Each caplet contains: acetaminophen 500 mg (500 mg is a non-standard extra strength dosage of acetaminophen, as compared to the standard of 325 mg); CHLOR-TRIMETON® (brand of chlorpheniramine maleate) 2 mg; phenylpropanolamine hydrochloride 12.5 mg.

Inactive Ingredients: Each caplet also contains Carnauba Wax, Cellulose, FD&C Yellow No. 6 Al Lake, Hydroxypropyl Methylcellulose, Magnesium Stearate, Povidone.

Indications: For temporary relief of sinus headache and congestion.

Actions: CORICIDIN Sinus Headache Caplets have been formulated with an antihistamine for temporary relief of the running nose that often accompanies upper respiratory allergies and sinusitis; a non-aspirin pain reliever for temporary relief of sinus headache pain and a decongestant for temporary relief of nasal membrane swelling, thus promoting freer breathing.

Warnings: Consult your physician: if symptoms persist, do not improve within 7 days, if new symptoms occur, or if fever persists for more than 3 days (72 hours) or recurs. May cause drowsiness. May cause excitability, especially in children. Do not exceed recommended dosage because severe liver damage may occur and at higher doses nervousness, dizziness, elevation of blood pressure, or sleeplessness are more likely to occur. Except under the advice and supervision of a physician, this product should not be used in children less than 12 years old or by persons with high blood pressure, heart disease, diabetes or thyroid disease, asthma, glaucoma or difficulty in urination due to enlargement of the prostate gland. Keep this and all drugs out of the reach of children. As with any drug, if you are pregnant or nursing a baby, seek the advice of a health professional before using this product.

Drug Interactions: Do not take this product if you are presently taking a prescription antihypertensive or antidepressant medication containing a monoamine oxidase inhibitor or an appetite controlling medication containing phenylpropanolamine, except under the advice and supervision of a physician.

Precautions: Avoid alcoholic beverages while taking this product. Also, avoid driving a motor vehicle or operating heavy machinery.

Overdosage: In case of accidental overdose, seek professional assistance or contact a poison control center immediately.

Dosage and Administration: Adults and children 12 years and older: 2 caplets every 6 hours not to exceed 8 caplets in a 24-hour period, or as directed by a physician. Swallow one caplet at a time. Store between 2° and 30°C (36° and 86°F). Protect from excessive moisture.

How Supplied: Box of 24 coated caplets.
Shown in Product Identification Section, page 427

DEMAZIN®
[dem'a-zin]
Nasal Decongestant/Antihistamine
TIMED-RELEASE Tablets
Syrup

Description: Each **TIMED-RELEASE Tablet** contains: 25 mg phenylpropanolamine hydrochloride and 4 mg CHLOR-TRIMETON® (brand of chlorpheniramine maleate, USP). Half the dose is released after the tablet is swallowed and the other half is released hours later; continuous relief is provided for up to 8 hours.
Each **TIMED-RELEASE Tablet** also contains: Acacia, Butylparaben, Calcium Phosphate, Calcium Sulfate, Carnauba Wax, Corn Starch, Diatomaceous Earth, FD&C Blue No. 1, FD&C Blue No. 2 Al Lake, Kaolin, Lactose, Magnesium Stearate, Neutral Soap, Oleic Acid, Stearic Acid, Sugar, Talc, White Wax, and Zein.
Each teaspoonful (5 ml) of **Syrup** contains 12.5 mg phenylpropanolamine hydrochloride, USP and 2 mg CHLOR-TRIMETON® (brand of chlorpheniramine maleate, USP) in a pleasant-tasting syrup containing approximately 7.5% alcohol.
Each teaspoonful of **Syrup** also contains: Benzaldehyde, FD&C Blue No. 1, FD&C Green No. 3, FD&C Yellow No. 6, Flavor, Glycerin, Menthol, Methylparaben, Propylene Glycol, Propylparaben, Sugar, Vanillin, and Water.

Indications: For temporary relief of running nose, sneezing, itching of the nose or throat, and itchy and watery eyes as may occur in allergic rhinitis (such as hay fever); nasal congestion due to the common cold (cold), hay fever or other upper respiratory allergies, or associated with sinusitis.

Actions: Phenylpropanolamine hydrochloride is a sympathomimetic agent which acts as an upper respiratory and pulmonary decongestant and mild bronchodilator. It exerts desirable sympathomimetic action with relatively little central nervous system excitation, so that wakefulness and nervousness are reduced to a minimum. Chlorpheniramine maleate antagonizes many of the characteristic effects of histamine. It is of value clinically in the prevention and relief of many allergic manifestations.
The oral administration of phenylpropanolamine hydrochloride with chlorpheniramine maleate produces a complementary action on congestive conditions of the upper respiratory tract, thus often obviating the need for topical nasal therapy.

Warnings: If symptoms do not improve within 7 days or are accompanied by high fever, consult a physician before continuing use. May cause drowsiness. May cause excitability especially in children. Do not exceed recommended dosage because at higher doses nervousness, dizziness, elevation of blood pressure or sleeplessness may occur. Except under the advice and supervision of a physician, these products should not be used in children under 6 years of age or by persons with high blood pressure, heart disease, diabetes, thyroid disease, asthma, glaucoma or difficulty in urination due to enlargement of the prostate gland.
Keep these and all drugs out of the reach of children.
As with any drug, if you are pregnant or nursing a baby, seek the advice of a health professional before using this product.

Drug Interaction: Do not take this product if you are presently taking a prescription antihypertensive or antidepressant drug containing a monoamine oxidase inhibitor or an appetite-controlling medication containing phenylpropanolamine except under the advice and supervision of a physician.

Precautions: Avoid alcoholic beverages while taking these products. Also avoid driving a motor vehicle or operating heavy machinery.

Overdosage: In case of accidental overdose, seek professional assistance or contact a Poison Control Center immediately.

Dosage and Administration: TIMED-RELEASE Tablets—Adults and children 12 years and older: 2 tablets every 8 hours not to exceed 6 tablets in 24 hours. **Children 6 through 11 years:** 1 tablet every 8 hours not to exceed 3 tablets in 24 hours. For children under 6 years, consult a physician. **Syrup—Adults and children 12 years and older:** Two teaspoonfuls every 4–6 hours not to exceed 12 teaspoonfuls in 24 hours, or as directed by a physician. **Children 6 through 11 years:** One teaspoonful every 4 hours not to exceed 6 teaspoonfuls in 24 hours or as directed by a physician. For children under 6 years, consult a physician.

How Supplied: DEMAZIN TIMED-RELEASE Tablets, blue, sugar-coated tablets branded in red with the Schering trademark and product identification number 751; box of 24 and bottle of 100. DEMAZIN Syrup, blue-colored liquid, bottles of 4 fluid ounces (118 ml).
Store DEMAZIN TIMED-RELEASE Tablets and Syrup between 2° and 30°C (36° and 86°F).
Copyright © 1983, 1985 Schering Corporation.
All rights reserved.
Shown in Product Identification Section, page 427

DERMOLATE® Anti-Itch Cream
[dur'mō-lāt]

Active Ingredients: DERMOLATE Anti-Itch Cream contains hydrocortisone 0.5% in a greaseless, vanishing cream. It also contains: Ceteareth-30, Cetearyl Alcohol, Mineral Oil, Petrolatum, Propylene Glycol, Sodium Phosphate, Water.

Indications: For the temporary relief of minor skin irritations, itching and rashes due to eczema, dermatitis, insect bites, poison ivy, poison oak, poison sumac, soaps, detergents, cosmetics and jewelry.

Actions: DERMOLATE Anti-Itch Cream provides temporary relief of itching and minor skin irritation.

Warnings: DERMOLATE Anti-Itch Cream is for external use only. Avoid contact with the eyes. Discontinue use and consult a physician if condition worsens or if symptoms persist for more than seven days.
Do not use on children under 2 years of age except under the advice and supervision of physician. Keep these and all drugs out of the reach of children.

Overdosage: In case of accidental ingestion, seek professional assistance or contact a Poison Control Center immediately.

Dosage and Administration: *For adults and children 2 years of age and older:* Gently massage into affected skin area not more than 3 or 4 times daily. *For children under 2 years of age,* there is no recommended dosage except under the advice and supervision of a physician.

How Supplied: DERMOLATE Anti-Itch Cream—30 g (1.0 oz.) tube, and 15 g (½ oz) tubes.
Store between 2° and 30°C (36° and 86°F).

DIASORB®
[dī'ah-zorb]
Antidiarrheal
Liquid and Tablets

Description: Each tablet or teaspoonful of Diasorb contains 750 mg activated nonfibrous attapulgite.

Inactive Ingredients: DIASORB Liquid—Benzoic Acid, Citric Acid, Flavor, Glycerin, Magnesium Aluminum Silicate, Methylparaben, Polysorbate, Propylene Glycol, Propylparaben, Saccharin, Sodium Hypochlorite Solution, Sorbitol, Xanthan Gum, Water.
DIASORB Tablets—D&C Red No. 30 Al Lake, Distilled Acetylated Monoglycerides, Ethylcellulose, Gelatin, Hydroxypropyl Methylcellulose, Magnesium Stearate, Mannitol, Titanium Dioxide, Water. Diasorb does not contain aspirin, salicyclates, alcohol, caffeine, or sugar.

Indications: Diasorb is indicated for fast effective relief of diarrhea. DIASORB relieves cramps and pain associated with diarrhea.

Precautions: Do not use for more than 2 days or in the presence of fever; or in infants and children under 3 years of age unless directed by a physician.

Continued on next page

Information on Schering products appearing on these pages is effective as of November 1, 1988.

Schering—Cont.

Overdosage: In case of accidental overdosage, seek professional assistance or contact a Poison Control Center immediately.

Dosage and Administration: Take the full recommended starting dose at the first sign of diarrhea and repeat after each subsequent bowel movement. DO NOT EXCEED MAXIMUM RECOMMENDED DOSE PER DAY. DO NOT CHEW TABLETS—THEY SHOULD BE SWALLOWED WITH WATER.

Recommended Dose for Acute Diarrhea
[See table below].

How Supplied: Diasorb is available as a beige-colored, pleasant tasting cola flavored liquid; bottles of 4 fl. oz. (118 ml). SHAKE WELL BEFORE USING. Diasorb is also available in tablet form. Each pink tablet is individually foil wrapped in boxes of 24.

Store products at room temperature.

DISOPHROL® Chronotab®
[dĭ'sō-frŏl]
Sustained–Action Tablets

Description: EACH DISOPHROL® Chronotab® SUSTAINED-ACTION TABLET CONTAINS: 120 mg of pseudoephedrine sulfate and 6 mg of dexbrompheniramine maleate. Half of the medication is released after the tablet is swallowed and the remaining amount of medication is released hours later providing continuous long-lasting relief for 12 hours. Also contains: Acacia, Butylparaben, Calcium Sulfate, Carnauba Wax, Corn Starch, FD&C Yellow No. 6 Al Lake, FD&C Red No. 40 Al Lake, Gelatin, Lactose, Magnesium Stearate, Neutral Soap, Oleic Acid, Povidone, Rosin, Sugar, Talc, White Wax, Zein.

Indications: For temporary relief of nasal congestion due to the common cold, hay fever, or other upper respiratory allergies, and associated with sinusitis. Helps decongest sinus openings, sinus passages. Reduces swelling of nasal passages; shrinks swollen membranes; and temporarily restores freer breathing through the nose. Alleviates running nose, sneezing, itching of the nose or throat, and itchy and watery eyes as may occur in allergic rhinitis (such as hay fever).

Warnings: If symptoms do not improve within 7 days or are accompanied by high fever, consult a physician before continuing use. May cause drowsiness. May cause excitability especially in children. Do not exceed recommended dosage because at higher doses nervousness, dizziness, or sleeplessness may occur. Do not give this product to children under 12 years except under the advice and supervision of a physician. Do not take this product if you have asthma, glaucoma, difficulty in urination due to enlargement of the prostate gland, high blood pressure, heart disease, diabetes, or thyroid disease except under the advice and supervision of a physician.

As with any drug, if you are pregnant or nursing a baby, seek the advice of a health professional before using this product.

Drug Interaction: Do not take this product if you are presently taking a prescription antihypertensive or antidepressant drug containing a monoamine oxidase inhibitor except under the advice and supervision of a physician.

Precaution: Avoid driving a motor vehicle or operating heavy machinery. Avoid alcoholic beverages while taking this product.
Keep this and all drugs out of the reach of children.

Overdosage: In case of accidental overdose, seek professional assistance or contact a Poison Control Center immediately.

Dosage and Administration: ADULTS AND CHILDREN 12 YEARS AND OVER—one tablet every 12 hours. Do not exceed two tablets in 24 hours.

How Supplied: DISOPHROL Chronotab Sustained-Action Tablets, sugar-coated, cherry-red tablets branded in black with either the product identification code 85-WMH or one of the Schering trademarks and the numbers, 231; bottle of 100.

Store between 2° and 30°C (36° and 86°F).

© 1982, 1985, Schering Corporation.

DRIXORAL®
[dricks-or'al]
Antihistamine/Nasal Decongestant Syrup

Description: Each 5 ml (1 teaspoonful) of DRIXORAL Syrup contains 2 mg brompheniramine maleate and 30 mg pseudoephedrine sulfate; also contains Citric Acid, D&C Red No. 33, FD&C Yellow No. 6, Flavor, Propylene Glycol, Sodium Benzoate, Sodium Citrate, Sorbitol, Sugar, Water. Drixoral Syrup is alcohol-free.

Indications: DRIXORAL Syrup contains a nasal decongestant with an antihistamine in a pleasant-tasting wild cherry flavor to provide temporary relief of nasal congestion due to the common cold, hay fever or other upper respiratory allergies. Helps decongest sinus openings, sinus passages. Alleviates running nose, sneezing, itching of the nose or throat, and itchy and watery eyes due to hay fever. DRIXORAL Syrup is ideal for adults and children who prefer a syrup instead of tablets or capsules.

Warnings: If symptoms do not improve within 7 days or are accompanied by high fever, consult a physician before continuing use. May cause drowsiness. May cause excitability especially in children. Do not exceed recommended dosage because at higher doses nervousness, dizziness, or sleeplessness may occur. Do not give this product to children under 6 years except under the advice and supervision of a physician. Do not take this product if you have asthma, glaucoma, difficulty in urination due to enlargement of the prostate gland, high blood pressure, heart disease, diabetes, or thyroid disease except under the advice and supervision of a physician. As with any drug, if you are pregnant or nursing a baby, seek the advice of a health professional before using this product.

Caution: Avoid driving a motor vehicle or operating heavy machinery. Avoid alcoholic beverages while taking this product. Keep this and all drugs out of the reach of children.

Drug Interaction Precaution: Do not take this product if you are presently taking a prescription antihypertensive or antidepressant drug containing a monoamine oxidase inhibitor except under the advice and supervision of a physician.

Directions: Adults and children 12 years of age and over: two teaspoonfuls every 4–6 hours. Children 6 to under 12 years of age: 1 teaspoonful every 4–6 hours. Do not exceed 4 doses in 24 hours. Children under 6 years of age, consult a physician.

Store between 2° and 30°C (36° and 86°F).

Overdosage: In case of accidental overdose, seek professional assistance or contact a Poison Control Center immediately.

How Supplied: DRIXORAL Syrup is available in 4 fl. oz. (118 ml) bottles. Copyright © 1984, 1985, Schering Corporation, Kenilworth, NJ, USA 07033. All rights reserved.

Shown in Product Identification Section, page 427

DRIXORAL®
[dricks-or'al]
Sustained-Action Tablets

Description: EACH DRIXORAL SUSTAINED-ACTION TABLET CONTAINS: 120 mg of pseudoephedrine sulfate and 6 mg of dexbrompheniramine maleate. Half of the medication is released after the tablet is swallowed and the remaining amount of medication is

Age	Initial Dose		Maximum dose per 24 hours
	Liquid	Tablets	
Adults and children over 12 years	4 tsps.	4 tablets	12 tsps./12 tablets
Children 6–12 years	2 tsps.	2 tablets	6 tsps./6 tablets
Children 3–6 years	1 tsps.	1 tablet	3 tsps./3 tablets
Infants and children under 3 years	ONLY AS DIRECTED BY A PHYSICIAN		

released hours later providing continuous long-lasting relief for 12 hours. Also contains: Acacia, Butylparaben, Calcium Sulfate, Carnauba Wax, Corn Starch, D&C Yellow No. 10 Al Lake, FD&C Blue No. 1 Al Lake, FD&C Yellow No. 6 Al Lake, Gelatin, Lactose, Magnesium Stearate, Neutral Soap, Oleic Acid, Povidone, Rosin, Sugar, Talc, White Wax, Zein.

Indications: For temporary relief of nasal congestion due to the common cold, hay fever, or other upper respiratory allergies, and associated with sinusitis. Helps decongest sinus openings, sinus passages. Reduces swelling of nasal passages; shrinks swollen membranes; and temporarily restores freer breathing through the nose. Alleviates running nose, sneezing, itching of the nose or throat, and itchy and watery eyes as may occur in allergic rhinitis (such as hay fever).

Actions: The antihistamine, dexbrompheniramine maleate, provides temporary relief of sneezing; watery, itchy eyes; running nose due to hay fever and other upper respiratory allergies. The decongestant, pseudoephedrine sulfate, temporarily restores freer breathing through the nose and promotes sinus drainage.

Warnings: If symptoms do not improve within 7 days or are accompanied by high fever, consult a physician before continuing use. May cause drowsiness. May cause excitability especially in children. Do not exceed recommended dosage because at higher doses nervousness, dizziness, or sleeplessness may occur. Do not give this product to children under 12 years except under the advice and supervision of a physician. Do not take this product if you have asthma, glaucoma, difficulty in urination due to enlargement of the prostate gland, high blood pressure, heart disease, diabetes, or thyroid disease except under the advice and supervision of a physician.
As with any drug, if you are pregnant or nursing a baby, seek the advice of a health professional before using this product.

Drug Interaction: Do not take this product if you are presently taking a prescription antihypertensive or antidepressant drug containing a monoamine oxidase inhibitor except under the advice and supervision of a physician.

Precaution: Avoid driving a motor vehicle or operting heavy machinery. Avoid alcoholic beverages while taking this product.
Keep this and all drugs out of the reach of children.

Overdosage: In case of accidental overdose, seek professional assistance or contact a Poison Control Center immediately.

Dosage and Administration: ADULTS AND CHILDREN 12 YEARS AND OVER—one tablet every 12 hours. Do not exceed two tablets in 24 hours.

How Supplied: DRIXORAL Sustained-Action Tablets, green, sugar-coated tablets branded in black with the product name, boxes of 10, 20, and 40, bottle of 100.
Store between 2° and 30°C (36° and 86°F).
© 1982, 1985, Schering Corporation.
Shown in Product Identification Section, page 427

DRIXORAL® PLUS
[*dricks-or 'al*]
Extended-Release Tablets

Active Ingredients: Acetaminophen, Dexbrompheniramine Maleate, Pseudoephedrine Sulfate.

Also Contains: Calcium Phosphate, Carnauba Wax, D&C Yellow No. 10 Al Lake, FD&C Blue No. 1 Al Lake, FD&C Yellow No. 6 Al Lake, Hydroxypropyl Methylcellulose, Magnesium Stearate, Methylparaben, PEG, Propylparaben, Stearic Acid.
DRIXORAL® *PLUS* Extended-Release Tablets combine a nasal decongestant, and an antihistamine with a nonaspirin analgesic in a special 12 hour continuous-acting timed-release tablet.

Indications: The *decongestant* temporarily relieves nasal congestion due to the common cold, hay fever or other upper respiratory allergies, and associated with sinusitis. Reduces swelling of nasal passages; shrinks swollen membranes; and temporarily restores freer breathing through the nose. Also helps decongest sinus openings, sinus passages. The *nonaspirin analgesic* temporarily relieves occasional minor aches, pains, and headache and reduces fever due to the common cold. The *antihistamine* alleviates running nose, sneezing, itching of the nose or throat, and itchy and watery eyes as may occur in allergic rhinitis (such as hay fever).

EACH DRIXORAL PLUS EXTENDED-RELEASE TABLET CONTAINS: 60 mg of pseudoephedrine sulfate, 3 mg of dexbrompheniramine maleate and 500 mg of acetaminophen. These ingredients are released continuously, providing long-lasting relief for 12 hours.

Directions: ADULTS AND CHILDREN 12 YEARS AND OVER—two tablets every 12 hours. Do not exceed four tablets in 24 hours. Children under 12 years of age: consult a doctor.

Warnings: Do not take this product for more than 7 days. If symptoms do not improve, or are accompanied by fever that lasts for more than three days (72 hours) or recurs, or if new symptoms occur, consult a physician before continuing use. May cause drowsiness. May cause excitability especially in children. Do not exceed recommended dosage because at higher doses nervousness, dizziness or sleeplessness may occur. Do not take this product if you have asthma, glaucoma, difficulty in urination due to enlargement of the prostate gland, high blood pressure, heart disease,

diabetes, or thyroid disease except under the advice and supervision of a physician. As with any drug, if you are pregnant or nursing a baby, seek the advice of a health professional before using this product. CAUTION: Avoid driving a motor vehicle or operating heavy machinery. Avoid alcoholic beverages while taking this product. Keep this and all drugs out of the reach of children. In case of accidental overdose, seek professional assistance or contact a Poison Control Center immediately.

Drug Interaction Precaution: Do not take this product if you are presently taking a prescription antihypertensive or antidepressant drug containing a monoamine oxidase inhibitor except under the advice and supervision of a physician.

How Supplied: DRIXORAL PLUS Extended-Release Tablets are available in boxes of 12's and 24's and bottles of 48.
Store between 2° and 30°C (36° and 86°F).
Protect from excessive moisture.
Shown in Product Identification Section, page 427

EMKO® BECAUSE®
[*em 'ko bē-koz '*]
Vaginal Contraceptive Foam

Description: A non-hormonal, non-scented aerosol foam contraceptive in a portable applicator/foam unit containing six applications of an 8.0% concentration of the spermicide nonoxynol-9. Also contains: Benzethonium Chloride, Glyceryl Monostearate, PEG, Pluronic F-68 (Poloxamer 188), Quaternium-15, Stearic Acid, Triethanolamine, and Water.

Indications: Vaginal contraceptive intended for the prevention of pregnancy. BECAUSE Foam provides effective protection alone or it may be used instead of spermicidal jelly or cream to give added protection with a diaphragm.
BECAUSE Foam also may be used to give added protection to other methods of contraception: with a condom; as a backup to the IUD or oral contraceptives during the first month of use; in the event more than one oral contraceptive pill is forgotten and extra protection is needed during that menstrual cycle.

Actions: Each applicatorful of BECAUSE Foam provides the correct amount of nonoxynol-9, the most widely used spermicide, to prevent pregnancy effectively. The foam covers the inside of the vagina and forms a layer of spermicidal material between the sperm and the cervix. The powerful spermicide prevents pregnancy by killing sperm after contact. BECAUSE Foam is effective immediately upon insertion. No waiting

Continued on next page

Schering—Cont.

period is needed for effervescing or melting to take place since BECAUSE is introduced into the vagina as a foam.

Warnings: If vaginal or penile irritation occurs and continues, a physician should be consulted. Not effective orally. Where pregnancy is contraindicated, further individualization of the contraceptive program may be needed. Do not burn, incinerate or puncture container. Keep this and all drugs out of the reach of children and in case of accidental ingestion, call a Poison Control Center, emergency medical facility, or a doctor.

Dosage and Administration: Although no contraceptive can guarantee 100% effectiveness, for reliable protection against pregnancy follow directions. One applicatorful of BECAUSE Contraceptive Foam must be inserted before each act of sexual intercourse. BECAUSE Foam can be inserted immediately or up to one hour before intercourse. If more than one hour has passed before intercourse or if intercourse is repeated, another applicatorful of BECAUSE Foam must be inserted.

Directions for Use: The BECAUSE CONTRACEPTOR has a foam container attached to an applicator barrel.
With the container pushed all the way into the barrel, shake well. Pull the container upward until it stops. Tilt container to side to release foam into barrel. Allow foam to fill barrel to about one inch from end and return container to straight position. Foam will expand to fill remainder of barrel.
Hold contraceptor at top of the barrel part and gently insert applicator barrel deep into the vagina (close to the cervix). For ease of insertion, lie on your back with knees bent. With applicator barrel in place, push container all the way into the barrel. This deposits the foam properly. Remove the Contraceptor with the container still pushed all the way in the applicator barrel to avoid withdrawing any of the foam. No waiting period is needed before intercourse. BECAUSE Contraceptive Foam is effective immediately after proper insertion.
As with other vaginal contraceptive foam, cream and jelly products, douching is *not* recommended after using BECAUSE Foam. However, if douching is desired for cleansing purposes, you *must* wait at least six hours following your last act of sexual intercourse to allow BECAUSE Foam's full spermicidal activity to take place. Refer to package insert directions and diagrams for further details and applicator cleansing instructions.
How to Use the BECAUSE CONTRACEPTOR with a Diaphragm.
Insert one applicatorful of BECAUSE Foam directly into the vagina according to above directions and then insert diaphragm. After insertion, BECAUSE Foam is effective immediately and remains effective up to one hour before intercourse. If more than one hour has passed or you are going to repeat inter-

course, insert another applicatorful of BECAUSE Foam *without removing your diaphragm.*

Storage: Contents under pressure. Do not burn, incinerate, or puncture the applicator. Store at normal room temperature. Do not expose to extreme heat or open flame or store at temperatures above 120°F. If stored at temperatures below 60°F, warm to room temperature before using.

How Supplied: Disposable 10 gm CONTRACEPTOR containing six applications of BECAUSE Contraceptive Foam. This foam is also available in the original form of EMKO® Foam with the regular applicator.
Copyright © 1985, Schering Corporation
Shown in Product Identification Section, page 428

EMKO®
[em′kō]
Vaginal Contraceptive Foam

Description: A non-hormonal, non-scented aerosol foam contraceptive containing an 8.0% concentration of the spermicide nonoxynol-9. Also contains: Benzethonium Chloride, Glyceryl Monostearate, PEG, Pluronic F-68 (Poloxamer 188), Quaternium-15, Stearic Acid, Triethanolamine, and Water.

Indications: Vaginal contraceptive intended for the prevention of pregnancy. EMKO Foam provides effective protection alone or it may be used instead of spermicidal jelly or cream to give added protection with a diaphragm.
EMKO Foam also may be used to give added protection to other methods of contraception: with a condom; as a backup to the IUD or oral contraceptives during the first month of use; in the event more than one oral contraceptive pill is forgotten and extra protection is needed during that menstrual cycle.

Actions: Each applicatorful of EMKO Foam provides the correct amount of nonoxynol-9, the most widely used spermicide, to prevent pregnancy effectively. The foam covers the inside of the vagina and forms a layer of spermicidal material between the sperm and the cervix. The powerful spermicide prevents pregnancy by killing sperm after contact. EMKO Foam is effective immediately upon insertion. No waiting period is needed for effervescing or melting to take place since EMKO is introduced into the vagina as a foam.

Warnings: If vaginal or penile irritation occurs and continues, a physician should be consulted. Where pregnancy is contraindicated, further individualization of the contraceptive program may be needed. Do not burn, incinerate or puncture can. Keep this and all drugs out of the reach of children and in case of accidental ingestion, call a Poison Control Center, emergency medical facility, or a doctor.

Dosage and Administration: Although no contraceptive can guarantee

100% effectiveness, for reliable protection against pregnancy read and follow directions carefully. One applicatorful of EMKO Contraceptive Foam must be inserted before each act of sexual intercourse. EMKO Foam can be inserted immediately or up to one hour before intercourse. If more than one hour has passed before intercourse or if intercourse is repeated, another applicatorful of EMKO Foam must be inserted.

Directions for Use:
Check Foam Supply with Weigh Cap.
With the cap on the can, hold the can in midair by the white button. As long as the black is showing, a full dose of foam is available. When the black begins to disappear, purchase a new can of EMKO Foam. USE *only if black is showing* to assure a full application. SHAKE CAN WELL before filling applicator. *Remove cap and place the can in an upright position on a level surface.* Place the EMKO regular applicator in an upright position over valve on top of can. Press down on the applicator gently. Allow foam to fill to the ridge in applicator barrel. The plunger will rise up as the foam fills the applicator. Remove the filled applicator from the can to stop flow. Hold the filled applicator by the barrel and gently insert deep into the vagina (close to the cervix). For ease of insertion, lie on your back with knees bent. With the applicator in place, push plunger into applicator until it stops. This deposits the foam properly. Remove the applicator with the plunger still pushed all the way in to avoid withdrawing any of the foam. No waiting period is needed before intercourse. EMKO Contraceptive Foam is effective immediately after proper insertion. As with other vaginal contraceptive foam, cream, and jelly products, douching is *not* recommended after using EMKO Foam. However, if douching is desired for cleansing purposes, you *must* wait at least six hours following your last act of sexual intercourse to allow EMKO Foam's full spermicidal activity to take place. Refer to package insert directions and diagrams for further details and applicator cleansing instructions.
How to Use EMKO with a Diaphragm.
Insert one applicatorful of EMKO Foam directly into the vagina according to above directions and then insert your diaphragm. After insertion, EMKO Foam is effective immediately and remains effective up to one hour before intercourse. If more than one hour has passed or you are going to repeat intercourse, insert another applicatorful of EMKO Foam *without removing your diaphragm.*

Storage: Contents under pressure. Do not burn, incinerate or puncture can. Store at normal room temperature. Do not expose to extreme heat or open flame or store at temperatures above 120°F. If stored at temperatures below 60°F, warm to room temperature before using.

How Supplied: EMKO Contraceptive Foam, 40 gm can with applicator and storage purse. Refill cans without applicator and purse available in 40 gm and 90

gm sizes. All sizes feature a unique weighing cap that indicates when a new foam supply is needed. EMKO Foam also comes in the convenient BECAUSE® CONTRACEPTOR®, a portable six-use, combination foam/applicator unit.

Copyright © 1985, Schering Corporation

Shown in Product Identification Section, page 428

MOL-IRON®
[mōl-i'ern]
Tablets
Tablets with Vitamin C

Active Ingredients: MOL-IRON products are highly effective and unusually well tolerated even by children and pregnant women.
Tablets: Each tablet contains 195 mg ferrous sulfate, USP (39 mg elemental iron).
Tablets with Vitamin C: Each tablet contains 195 mg ferrous sulfate (39 mg elemental iron) and 75 mg ascorbic acid.

Inactive Ingredients: Each MOL-IRON Tablet contains Acacia, Butylparaben, Calcium Sulfate, Carnauba Wax, FD&C Blue No. 1 Aluminum Lake, FD&C Red No. 40 Aluminum Lake, Magnesium Stearate, Povidone, Stearic Acid, Sugar, Talc, Titanium Dioxide, White Wax.

In addition to the above ingredients, MOL-IRON Tablets with Vitamin C contain confectioners glaze.

Indications: For the prevention and treatment of iron-deficiency anemias.

Warnings: Keep these and all drugs out of the reach of children. In case of accidental overdose, seek professional assistance or contact a Poison Control Center immediately. As with any drug, if you are pregnant or nursing a baby, seek the advice of a health professional before using this product.

Dosage and Administration: Tablets—(Taken preferably after meals): Adults and Children 12 years and older—1 or 2 tablets 3 times daily; Children 6 through 11 years—1 tablet 3 times daily; or as prescribed by a physician. Tablets with Vitamin C—(Taken preferably after meals): Adults and Children 12 years and older—1 or 2 tablets 3 times daily; Children 6 through 11 years—1 tablet 3 times daily; or as prescribed by a physician.

How Supplied: MOL-IRON Tablets—brownish colored tablets, bottles of 100; MOL-IRON Tablets with Vitamin C—bottles of 100.
Store between 2° and 30°C (36° and 86°F).

Shown in Product Identification Section, page 428

TINACTIN® Antifungal
[tin-ak'tin]
Cream 1%
Solution 1%
Powder 1%
Powder (1%) Aerosol
Liquid (1%) Aerosol
Jock Itch Cream 1%
Jock Itch Spray Powder 1%

Description: TINACTIN Cream 1% is a white homogeneous, nonaqueous preparation containing the highly active synthetic fungicidal agent, tolnaftate. Each gram contains 10 mg tolnaftate solubilized in BHT, Carbomer 934 P, Monoamylamine, PEG, Propylene Glycol, and Titanium Dioxide.
TINACTIN Jock Itch Cream 1% is a smooth white homogeneous cream containing the highly active synthetic fungicidal agent, tolnaftate. Each gram contains 10 mg tolnaftate finely dispersed in a water-washable emulsion containing: Cetearyl Alcohol, Ceteareth-30, Chlorocresol, Mineral Oil, Petrolatum, Propylene Glycol, Sodium Phosphate and Water. Phosphoric acid and sodium hydroxide used to adjust pH .
TINACTIN Solution 1% contains in each ml tolnaftate 10 mg, BHT, and PEG. The solution solidifies at low temperatures but liquefies readily when warmed, retaining its potency.
TINACTIN Liquid Aerosol contains 91 mg tolnaftate in a vehicle of Alcohol SD-40-2 (36% w/w), BHT and PPG-12 Buteth-16. The spray deposits solution containing a concentration of 1% tolnaftate.
Each gram of **TINACTIN Powder 1%** contains tolnaftate 10 mg in a vehicle of corn starch and talc.
TINACTIN Powder Aerosol contains 91 mg tolnaftate in a vehicle of Alcohol SD-40-2 (14% w/w), BHT, Hydrocarbon Propellant, PPG-12 Buteth-16 and Talc. The spray deposits a white clinging powder containing a concentration of 1% tolnaftate.
TINACTIN Jock Itch Spray Powder contains 91 mg tolnaftate in a vehicle of Alcohol SD-40-2 (14% w/w), BHT, Hydrocarbon Propellant, PPG-12 Buteth-16, Talc. The spray deposits a white clinging powder containing a concentration of 1% tolnaftate.

Indications: TINACTIN Cream, Solution, Liquid Aerosol and **TINACTIN Jock Itch Cream** are highly active antifungal agents that are effective in killing superficial fungi of the skin which cause tinea pedis (athlete's foot), tinea cruris (jock itch) and tinea corporis (body ringworm).
TINACTIN Powder, Powder Aerosol and **TINACTIN Jock Itch Spray Powder** are effective in killing superficial fungi of the skin which cause tinea cruris (jock itch) and tinea pedis (athlete's foot). All forms begin to relieve burning, itching and soreness within 24 hours. The powder and powder aerosol forms aid the drying of naturally moist areas.

Actions: The active ingredient in TINACTIN, tolnaftate, is a highly active

synthetic fungicidal agent that is effective in the treatment of superficial fungous infections of the skin. It is inactive systemically, virtually nonsensitizing, and does not ordinarily sting or irritate intact or broken skin, even in the presence of acute inflammatory reactions. TINACTIN products are odorless, greaseless, and do not stain or discolor the skin, hair, or nails.

Warnings: Keep these and all drugs out of the reach of children. Do not use in children under 2 years of age except under the advice and supervision of a physician.
TINACTIN Powder Aerosol and **Liquid Aerosol:** Avoid spraying in eyes. Contents under pressure. Do not puncture or incinerate. Flammable mixture, do not use or store near heat or open flame. Exposure to temperatures above 120°F may cause bursting. Never throw container into fire or incinerator. Use only as directed. Intentional misuse by deliberately concentrating and inhaling the contents can be harmful or fatal.

Precautions: If irritation occurs or symptoms do not improve within 10 days, discontinue use and consult your physician or podiatrist.
TINACTIN products are for external use only. Keep out of eyes.
TINACTIN is not effective on nail or scalp infections.

Overdosage: In case of accidental ingestion, seek professional assistance or contact a Poison Control Center immediately.

Dosage and Administration: Children under 12 years of age should be supervised in the use of TINACTIN.
TINACTIN Cream and **TINACTIN Jock Itch Cream**—Wash and dry infected area. Then apply one-half inch ribbon of cream and rub gently on infected area morning and evening or as directed by a doctor. Spread evenly. Best results in athlete's foot and body ringworm are usually obtained with 4 weeks' use of this product and in jock itch, with 2 weeks' use. To help prevent recurrence of athlete's foot, continue treatment for two weeks after disappearance of all symptoms.
TINACTIN Solution—Wash and dry infected area. Then apply two or three drops morning and evening or as directed by a doctor, and massage gently to cover the infected area. Best results in athlete's foot and body ringworm are usually obtained with 4 weeks' use of this product and in jock itch, with 2 weeks' use. To help prevent recurrence of athlete's foot, continue treatment for two weeks after disappearance of all symptoms.
TINACTIN Liquid Aerosol—Wash and dry infected area. Spray from a distance of 6 to 10 inches morning and evening or

Continued on next page

Information on Schering products appearing on these pages is effective as of November 1, 1988.

Schering—Cont.

as directed by a doctor. For athlete's foot, spray between toes and on feet. For jock itch, spray infected area. Best results in athlete's foot are usually obtained with 4 weeks' use of this product and in jock itch, with 2 weeks' use. Continue treatment for two weeks after symptoms disappear. To help prevent reinfection of athlete's foot, bathe daily, dry carefully and apply **TINACTIN Powder** daily.

TINACTIN Powder—Wash and dry infected area. Sprinkle powder liberally on all areas of infection and in shoes or socks morning and evening or as directed by a doctor. Best results in athlete's foot are usually obtained with 4 weeks' use of this product and in jock itch, with 2 weeks' use. Continue treatment for two weeks after symptoms disappear. To prevent recurrence of athlete's foot, bathe daily, dry carefully and apply **TINAC-TIN Powder.**

TINACTIN Powder Aerosol and **TINACTIN Jock Itch Spray Powder**—Wash and dry infected area. Shake container well before using. Spray liberally from a distance of 6 to 10 inches onto affected area morning and night or as directed by a doctor. Best results in athlete's foot are usually obtained with 4 weeks' use of this product and in jock itch, with 2 weeks' use. To help prevent recurrence of athlete's foot, bathe daily, dry carefully and apply **TINACTIN Powder Aerosol.**

How Supplied: TINACTIN Antifungal Cream 1%, 15 g (½ oz) and 30 g (1 oz) collapsible tube with dispensing tip. **TINACTIN Antifungal Solution 1%,** 10 ml (⅓ oz) plastic squeeze bottle. **TINACTIN Antifungal Liquid (1%) Aerosol,** 113 g (4 oz) spray can. **TINACTIN Antifungal Powder 1%,** 45 g (1.5 oz) and 90 g (3.0 oz) plastic containers. **TINACTIN Antifungal Powder (1%) Aerosol,** 100 g (3.5 oz) and 150 g (5.0 oz) spray containers. **TINACTIN Antifungal Jock Itch Cream 1%,** 15 g (½ oz) collapsible tube with dispensing tip. **TINACTIN Antifungal Jock Itch Spray Powder (1%),** 100 g (3.5 oz) spray can.

Store TINACTIN products between 36° and 86°F (2° and 30°C).
© 1984, 1985, 1987 Schering Corporation, Kenilworth NJ 07033
Shown in Product Identification Section, page 428

IDENTIFICATION PROBLEM?
Consult the
Product Identification Section
where you'll find
products pictured
in full color.

Schwarz Pharma
Kremers Urban Company
P.O. BOX 2038
5600 W. COUNTY LINE ROAD
MILWAUKEE, WI 53201

FEDAHIST® Decongestant Syrup
FEDAHIST® Tablets
[fed 'a-hist "]

Description: Decongestant Syrup: Each 5 mL (teaspoonful) of FEDAHIST® Decongestant Syrup contains 30 mg of pseudoephedrine hydrochloride USP and 2 mg of chlorpheniramine maleate USP. **Tablets:** Each FEDAHIST® Tablet contains 60 mg of pseudoephedrine hydrochloride USP and 4 mg of chlorpheniramine maleate USP.

Inactive Ingredients: Decongestant Syrup: citric acid, FD&C blue No. 1, FD&C red No. 40, flavors, glycerin, methylparaben, purified water, saccharin sodium, sodium benzoate, sorbitol solution, sucrose and other ingredients. **Tablets:** colloidal silicon dioxide, lactose, magnesium stearate, microcrystalline cellulose, stearic acid, and talc.

Indications: For the temporary relief of nasal congestion, runny nose, sneezing, itching of the nose or throat, and itchy, watery eyes due to the common cold, hay fever, sinusitis, or other upper respiratory allergies.

Warnings: May cause excitability, especially in children. May cause drowsiness; alcohol, sedatives, and tranquilizers may increase the drowsiness effect. Avoid alcoholic beverages while taking this product. Do not take this product if you are taking sedatives or tranquilizers without first consulting your doctor. Use caution when driving a motor vehicle or operating machinery. Do not exceed recommended dosage because at higher doses nervousness, dizziness or sleeplessness may occur. If symptoms do not improve within 7 days, or are accompanied by high fever, consult a doctor before continuing use. Do not take this product if you have high blood pressure, heart disease, diabetes, thyroid disease, asthma, glaucoma, emphysema, chronic pulmonary disease, shortness of breath, difficulty in breathing or difficulty in urination due to enlargement of the prostate gland unless directed by a doctor. As with any drug, if you are pregnant or nursing a baby, seek the advice of a health professional before using this product.
Keep this and all medications out of children's reach. In case of accidental overdose contact a doctor or poison control center immediately.
Drug Interaction Precaution: Do not take this product if you are presently taking a prescription drug for high blood pressure or depression without first consulting your doctor.

Directions: Decongestant Syrup: *Adults and children 12 years of age and older:* 2 teaspoonfuls every 4 to 6 hours not to exceed 8 teaspoonfuls in 24 hours.

Children 6 to under 12 years of age: 1 teaspoonful every 4 to 6 hours not to exceed 4 teaspoonfuls in 24 hours.
Children under 6 years of age: consult a doctor.
Professional Labeling: *Children 2 to under 6 years of age:* ½ teaspoonful every 4 to 6 hours not to exceed 2 teaspoonfuls in 24 hours.
Tablets: *Adults and children 12 years of age and older:* 1 tablet every 4 to 6 hours not to exceed 4 tablets in 24 hours.
Children 6 to under 12 years of age: ½ tablet every 4 to 6 hours not to exceed 2 tablets in 24 hours.
Children under 6 years of age: consult a doctor.

How Supplied: FEDAHIST Decongestant Syrup is a grape colored and flavored syrup in 4 oz bottles (NDC 0091-0052-04).
FEDAHIST Tablets are white, scored and imprinted with "KU" on one side and "050" on the other. Bottles of 100 tablets (NDC 0091-0050-01) and blister packs of 24 tablets (NDC 0091-0050-24). Store at controlled room temperature 15–30° C (59–86° F).
Shown in Product Identification Section, page 428

FEDAHIST® Expectorant Syrup
FEDAHIST® Expectorant Pediatric Drops
[fed 'a-hist "]

Description: Expectorant Syrup: Each 5 mL (teaspoonful) of FEDAHIST® Expectorant Syrup contains 30 mg of pseudoephedrine hydrochloride USP and 200 mg of guaifenesin USP.
Expectorant Pediatric Drops: Each mL of FEDAHIST® Expectorant Pediatric Drops contains 7.5 mg of pseudoephedrine hydrochloride USP and 40 mg of guaifenesin USP.
Inactive Ingredients: Expectorant Syrup: benzoic acid, citric acid, FD&C red No. 40, flavors, glycerin, polyethylene glycol, povidone, purified water, saccharin sodium, sodium citrate, sorbitol solution, and other ingredients.
Expectorant Pediatric Drops: benzoic acid, citric acid, FD&C yellow No. 6, flavors, glycerin, polyethylene glycol, povidone, purified water, saccharin sodium, sodium citrate, sorbitol solution, and other ingredients.

Indications: Helps loosen phlegm and bronchial secretions and rids the bronchial passageways of bothersome mucus making coughs more productive. For the temporary relief of nasal and bronchial congestion due to the common cold, bronchitis, sinusitis, or croup.

Warnings: Do not take this product for persistent or chronic cough such as occurs with smoking, asthma, emphysema, or where cough is accompanied by excessive secretions unless directed by a doctor. A persistent cough may be a sign of a serious condition. If cough persists for more than 1 week, tends to recur, or is accompanied by fever, rash, or persistent headache, consult a doctor.

Do not exceed recommended dosage because at higher doses nervousness, dizziness, or sleeplessness may occur. Do not take this product for more than 7 days. If symptoms do not improve or are accompanied by fever, consult a doctor. Do not take this product if you have heart disease, high blood pressure, thyroid disease, diabetes, or difficulty in urination due to enlargement of the prostate gland unless directed by a doctor.

As with any drug, if you are pregnant or nursing a baby, seek the advice of a health professional before using this product.

Keep this and all medications out of children's reach. In case of accidental overdose, contact a doctor or poison control center immediately.

Drug Interaction Precaution: Do not take this product if you are presently taking a prescription drug for high blood pressure or depression without first consulting your doctor.

Directions: Expectorant Syrup: *Adults and children 12 years of age and older:* 2 teaspoonfuls every 4 to 6 hours not to exceed 8 teaspoonfuls in 24 hours.

Children 6 to under 12 years of age: 1 teaspoonful every 4 to 6 hours not to exceed 4 teaspoonfuls in 24 hours.

Children 2 to under 6 years of age: ½ teaspoonful every 4 to 6 hours not to exceed 2 teaspoonfuls in 24 hours.

Children under 2 years of age: consult a doctor.

Expectorant Pediatric Drops: Take by mouth only.

Children 6 to under 12 years of age: 4 mL every 4 to 6 hours not to exceed 4 doses (16 mL) in 24 hours.

Children 2 to under 6 years of age: 2 mL every 4 to 6 hours not to exceed 4 doses (8 mL) in 24 hours.

Professional Labeling: *Children under 2 years of age:* The dose should be adjusted to age or weight and be given every 4 to 6 hours not to exceed 4 doses in 24 hours.

Age or Weight	Starting Dose
1–3 months (8–12 lbs)	¼ mL
4–6 months (13–17 lbs)	½ mL
7–9 months (18–20 lbs)	¾ mL
10–23 months (21–30 lbs)	1 mL

How Supplied: FEDAHIST Expectorant Syrup is a red colored and fruit flavored syrup in 4 oz bottles (NDC 0091-0057-04).

FEDAHIST Expectorant Pediatric Drops is an orange colored and fruit flavored solution in 1 oz bottles (NDC 0091-0051-30).

Store at controlled room temperature 15°–30°C (59°–86°F).

Shown in Product Identification Section, page 428

LACTRASE® Capsules
[lăk 'trās]
(lactase)

Description: Each LACTRASE® Capsule contains 250 mg of standardized enzyme dispersed in a lactose-free base.

Inactive Ingredients: gelatin, magnesium stearate, maltodextrin, red iron oxide, titanium dioxide, yellow iron oxide, and other ingredients.

Indications: LACTRASE is indicated for individuals exhibiting symptoms of lactose intolerance or lactase insufficiency as identified by a lactose tolerance test or by exhibiting gastrointestinal disturbances after consumption of milk or dairy products.

Action: Though lactase is normally present in adequate quantities in infants, in many populations its concentration naturally declines starting at about 4–5 years of age and is low in a substantial number of individuals by their teens or early 20's. Within certain geographic and ethnic groups, especially in adult Blacks, Orientals, American Indians, and Eastern European Jews, the lactase activity may be low even earlier. Although many of them can easily digest smaller quantities of lactose in milk, after consumption of an excessive volume of milk or dairy products, they may exhibit symptoms of lactose intolerance.

Lactose is a non-absorbable disaccharide found as a common constituent in most dairy products. Under normal conditions, dietary lactose is hydrolyzed in the jejunum and proximal ileum by beta-D-galactosidase or lactase. Lactase is produced in the brush border of the columnar epithelial cells of the intestinal villi. Lactase hydrolyzes lactose into two monosaccharides, glucose and galactose, that are readily absorbed by the intestine.

When available lactase is insufficient to split the lactose, the unabsorbable sugar remains in the small intestine for an extended period, presenting an osmotic load that increases and retains intraluminal fluid and intensifies intestinal motility; thus the individual reports a bloated feeling and cramps. The undigested lactose is decomposed by the intestinal flora in the lower intestine and excessive carbon dioxide and hydrogen is produced. These gases contribute to flatulence and increased abdominal discomfort. The lactic acid and other short-chain acids raise the osmolality, hinder fluid reabsorption and decrease transit time of the contents of the colon, leading to diarrhea. Often hydrogen is noticed in the expired breath of a lactase-deficient patient.

Precautions: It should be noted that in diabetic persons who use LACTRASE, the milk sugar will be metabolically available and may result in increased blood glucose levels. Individuals with galactosemia may not have milk in any form, lactose enzyme modified or not.

Directions: Generally, one or two LACTRASE Capsules swallowed with milk or dairy products is all that is necessary to digest the milk sugar contained in a normal serving. If the individual is severely intolerant to lactose, additional capsules may be taken until a satisfactory response is achieved as recognized by resolution of the symptoms. LACTRASE Capsules are safe to take and higher quantities in severe cases will be well-tolerated.

If the individual cannot swallow capsules, the contents of the capsules may be sprinkled onto dairy products before consuming. LACTRASE will not alter the taste of the dairy product when used in this manner.

Milk may also be pretreated with LACTRASE; simply add the contents from one or two capsules to each quart of milk, shake gently, and store the milk in the refrigerator for 24 hours. LACTRASE will break down milk sugars to digestible simple sugars. LACTRASE powder will not alter the appearance of milk, however the taste may be slightly sweeter than untreated milk.

How Supplied: LACTRASE Capsules are opaque orange and opaque white and are imprinted "KREMERS URBAN" and "505". They are supplied in blister packs containing 10 capsules (NDC 0091-3505-10) or 30 capsules (NDC 0091-3505-03) and in bottles containing 100 capsules (NDC 0091-3505-01).

Store at controlled room temperature 15°–30°C (59°–86°F).

Shown in Product Identification Section, page 428

EDUCATIONAL MATERIAL

Good News For People Who Can't Digest Milk.

For people who cannot digest dairy products because they lack the enzyme necessary for the digestion of milk sugar, this pamphlet explains how the problem comes about, its symptoms and how it can be treated with Lactrase®, an enzyme supplement. A table addressing the lactose content of food is included.

Scot-Tussin Pharmacal Co., Inc.
**50 CLEMENCE STREET
CRANSTON, RI 02920-0217**

**SCOT–TUSSIN® DM
No Sugar, Alcohol or Decongestant
COUGH & COLD MEDICINE**

Composition: Each 5 ml (1 teaspoonful) contains:
Dextromethorphan
  HBr., USP .... 15 mg.
Chlorpheniramine
  Maleate, USP .... 2 mg.
Recommended for use by diabetics and others on sugar restricted diets.

How Supplied: Bottles of 4 fl. oz. (NDC 0372-0036-04)

Continued on next page

Scot-Tussin—Cont.

SCOT–TUSSIN® Sugar-Free Expectorant
No Sugar, Sodium, Dye

Composition: Each 5 ml (1 teaspoonful) contains:
Guaifenesin, USP........................ 100 mg
Alcohol 3.5 per cent
Recommended for use by diabetics and others on sugar restricted diets.

How Supplied: Bottles of 4 fl. oz. (NDC 0372-0006-04).

SmithKline Consumer Products
A SmithKline Beckman Company
ONE FRANKLIN PLAZA
P. O. BOX 8082
PHILADELPHIA, PA 19101

A.R.M.® Allergy Relief Medicine
Maximum Strength Caplets

Product Information: A.R.M. combines two important medicines in one safe, fast-acting caplet:
- The highest level of antihistamine available without prescription—for better relief of sneezing, runny nose and itchy, weepy eyes.
- A clinically proven sinus decongestant to help ease breathing and drain sinus congestion for hours.

Directions: One caplet every 4 hours, not to exceed 6 caplets daily.
Children (6–12 years): one-half the adult dose. Children under 6 years use only as directed by physician.
TAMPER-RESISTANT PACKAGE FEATURES FOR YOUR PROTECTION:
- The carton has been sealed at the factory with a clear overwrap printed with "safety sealed."
- Each caplet is encased in a clear plastic cell with a foil back.
- The name A.R.M. appears on each caplet (see product illustration on front of carton).
- DO NOT USE THIS PRODUCT IF ANY OF THESE TAMPER-RESISTANT FEATURES ARE MISSING OR BROKEN. IF YOU HAVE ANY QUESTIONS, PLEASE CALL 1-800-543-3434 TOLL FREE.

Warning: Do not exceed recommended dosage. If symptoms do not improve within 7 days, or are accompanied by high fever, consult a physician before continuing use. Stop use if dizziness, sleeplessness or nervousness occurs. If you have or are being treated for depression, high blood pressure, glaucoma, diabetes, asthma, difficulty in urination due to enlarged prostate, heart disease or thyroid disease, use only as directed by physician. Do not take this product if you are taking another medication containing phenylpropanolamine.
Avoid alcoholic beverages while taking this product. Do not drive or operate heavy machinery. May cause drowsiness. May cause excitability, especially in children. Keep this and all drugs out of reach of children. In case of accidental overdose, seek professional assistance or contact a poison control center immediately. As with any drug, if you are pregnant or nursing a baby, seek the advice of a health professional before using this product. Store at controlled room temperature (59°–86°F.).

Formula: Active Ingredients: Each caplet contains Chlorpheniramine Maleate, 4 mg., Phenylpropanolamine Hydrochloride, 25 mg. **Inactive Ingredients (listed for individuals with specific allergies:** Carnauba Wax, D&C Yellow 10, FD&C Yellow 6 (Sunset Yellow) as a color additive, Gelatin, Hydroxypropyl Methylcellulose, Lactose, Magnesium Stearate, Polyethylene Glycol, Sodium Starch Glycolate, Starch.

How Supplied: Consumer packages of 20 and 40 caplets.
Shown in Product Identification Section, page 428

ACNOMEL® CREAM
acne therapy

Description: Cream—sulfur, 8%; resorcinol, 2%; alcohol, 11% (w/w); nongreasy, dries oily skin, easy to apply.

Indications: Acnomel Cream is highly effective in the treatment of pimples and blemishes due to acne.

Directions: Wash and dry affected areas thoroughly. Apply a thin coating of Acnomel Cream once or twice daily, making sure it does not get into the eyes or on eyelids. Do not rub in. If a marked chapping effect occurs, discontinue use temporarily.

Warning: Acnomel should not be applied to acutely inflamed area. If undue skin irritation develops or increases, discontinue use and consult physician. Keep this and all drugs out of reach of children. In case of accidental ingestion, seek professional assistance or contact a poison control center immediately. Keep tube tightly closed to prevent drying. Store at controlled room temperature (59°–86°F.).

Inactive Ingredients: Bentonite, Fragrance, Iron Oxides, Potassium Hydroxide, Propylene Glycol, Titanium Dioxide, Purified Water.

How Supplied: Cream—in specially lined 1 oz. tubes.
Shown in Product Identification Section, page 428

AQUA CARE® CREAM
Effective Medication for Dry Skin Relief

Product Information: AQUA CARE, with 10% urea, is a topical cream formulated to restore nature's moisture balance to rough, dry skin. The special urea ingredient penetrates the surface of the skin to both restore lost moisture and soften dry, rough skin.

Directions: Apply two or three times daily to affected area or as your physician directs.

Warning: Discontinue use if irritation occurs.
Store at controlled room temperature (59°–86°F.).
FOR EXTERNAL USE ONLY

Formula: Purified water, urea 10%, cetyl esters wax, DEA-oleth-3 phosphate, petrolatum, trolamine, glycerin, carbomer 934, mineral oil and lanolin alcohol, lanolin oil, benzyl alcohol, and fragrance.

How Supplied: Available in 2.5 oz. cream.
Shown in Product Identification Section, page 428

AQUA CARE® LOTION
Effective Medication for Dry Skin Relief

Product Information: AQUA CARE, with 10% urea, is a topical lotion formulated to restore nature's moisture balance to rough, dry skin. The special urea ingredient penetrates the surface of the skin to both restore lost moisture and soften dry, rough skin.

Directions: Apply two or three times daily to affected area or as your physician directs.

Warning: Discontinue use if irritation occurs.
Store at controlled room temperature (59°–86°F.).
FOR EXTERNAL USE ONLY

Formula: 10% urea with purified water, mineral oil, petrolatum, propylene glycol stearate, sorbitan stearate, cetyl alcohol, lactic acid, magnesium aluminum silicate, sodium lauryl sulfate, methylparaben and propylparaben.

How Supplied: Available in 8 oz. lotion.
Shown in Product Identification Section, page 428

BENZEDREX® INHALER
Nasal Decongestant

Description: Each inhaler packed with propylhexedrine, 250 mg. Inactive ingredients: Lavender Oil, Menthol.

Indications: For temporary relief of nasal congestion in colds and hay fever; also for ear block and pressure pain during air travel.

Directions: Insert in nostril. Close other nostril. Inhale twice. Treat other nostril the same way. Avoid excessive use.
Inhaler loses potency after 2 or 3 months' use but some aroma may linger.

Warning: Ill effects may result if taken internally. In the case of accidental overdose or ingestion of contents, seek professional assistance or contact a poison control center immediately. Keep this and all drugs out of reach of children.

TAMPER-RESISTANT PACKAGE FEATURES FOR YOUR PROTECTION:

- The carton has been sealed at the factory with a clear overwrap printed with "safety sealed."
- Inhaler sealed with imprinted cellophane.
- DO NOT USE THIS PRODUCT IF ANY OF THESE TAMPER-RESISTANT FEATURES ARE MISSING OR BROKEN. IF YOU HAVE ANY QUESTIONS, PLEASE CALL 1-800-543-3434 TOLL FREE.

How Supplied: In single plastic tubes.
Shown in Product Identification Section, page 429

CLEAR BY DESIGN®
Medicated Acne Gel for Sensitive Skin

Product Information: CLEAR BY DESIGN contains benzoyl peroxide, an effective anti-acne agent available without a prescription in a lower 2.5% strength. CLEAR BY DESIGN is as effective as 10% benzoyl peroxide but with less of the irritation and redness that you may get with the higher strengths. Greaseless, colorless CLEAR BY DESIGN is invisible while it works fast. Helps prevent new acne pimples and blackheads from forming.

Directions: Wash problem areas thoroughly but gently and dry well. Using fingertip, apply CLEAR BY DESIGN to all affected and surrounding areas of face, neck, and body. Apply one or two times a day as directed by a physician.

Warning: Persons with a known allergy to benzoyl peroxide should not use this medication. To test for an allergy, apply CLEAR BY DESIGN on a small affected area once a day for two days. If discomforting irritation or undue dryness occurs during treatment, reduce frequency of use or amount. If excessive itching, redness, burning, swelling, irritation or dryness occurs, discontinue use and consult a physician. Avoid contact with eyes, lips and mouth. May bleach hair or dyed fabrics. Keep tightly closed. Keep this and all drugs out of reach of children. Store at controlled room temperature (59°–86°F.); avoid excessive heat.
FOR EXTERNAL USE ONLY

Formula: Benzoyl Peroxide, 2.5% in a gel base. Also contains: Purified water, carbomer 940, dioctyl sodium sulfosuccinate, sodium hydroxide, and edetate disodium.

How Supplied: Available in 1.5 oz. gel.
Shown in Product Identification Section, page 429

CONGESTAC®
Congestion Relief Medicine Decongestant/Expectorant Caplets

Product Information: Helps you breathe easier by temporarily relieving nasal congestion associated with the common cold, sinusitis, hay fever and allergies. Also helps relieve chest congestion by loosening phlegm and clearing bronchial passages of excess mucus. Contains no antihistamines which may overdry or make you drowsy.

Directions: One caplet every 4 hours not to exceed 4 caplets in 24 hours. Children (6 to 12 years): one-half the adult dose (break caplet in half). Children under 6 years use only as directed by physician.

TAMPER-RESISTANT PACKAGE FEATURES FOR YOUR PROTECTION:

- The carton has been sealed at the factory with a clear overwrap printed with "safety sealed."
- Each caplet is encased in a clear plastic cell with a foil back.
- The letter "C" appears on each caplet (see product illustration on front of carton).
- DO NOT USE THIS PRODUCT IF ANY OF THESE TAMPER-RESISTANT FEATURES ARE MISSING OR BROKEN. IF YOU HAVE ANY QUESTIONS, PLEASE CALL 1-800-543-3434 TOLL FREE.

Warning: Do not exceed recommended dosage. If symptoms do not improve within 7 days or are accompanied by high fever, rash, shortness of breath or persistent headache, consult a physician before continuing use. Do not use if you have high blood pressure, heart disease, diabetes, thyroid disease or a persistent or chronic cough, except under the advice and supervision of a physician. Keep this and all drugs out of reach of children. In case of accidental overdose, seek professional assistance or contact a poison control center immediately. As with any drug, if you are pregnant or nursing a baby, seek the advice of a health professional before using this product.

Drug Interaction Precaution: Do not take this product if you are presently taking a prescription antihypertensive or antidepressant drug containing a monoamine oxidase inhibitor except under the advice and supervision of a physician.

Formula: Active Ingredients: Each caplet contains Pseudoephedrine Hydrochloride 60 mg., Guaifenesin 400 mg. **Inactive Ingredients (listed for individuals with specific allergies):** Cellulose, Croscarmellose Sodium, Hydroxypropyl Methylcellulose, Magnesium Stearate, Polyethylene Glycol, Povidone, Silica Gel, Starch.

Store at controlled room temperature (59°–86°F.).
The Congestac horizontal color bar is a trademark.

How Supplied: In consumer packages of 12 and 24 caplets.
Shown in Product Identification Section, page 429

CONTAC®
**MAXIMUM STRENGTH
Continuous Action Nasal Decongestant/Antihistamine Caplets**

Composition:
[See table next page] .

Product Information: Each CONTAC Maximum Strength continuous action caplet provides up to 12 hours of relief. Part of the caplet goes to work right away for fast relief; the rest is released gradually to provide up to 12 hours of prolonged relief. With just *one* caplet in the morning and *one* at bedtime, you feel better all day, sleep better at night, breathing freely without congestion. CONTAC Maximum Strength provides:

- A NASAL DECONGESTANT which helps clear nasal passages, shrinks swollen membranes and helps decongest sinus openings.
- AN ANTIHISTAMINE at the maximum level to help relieve itchy, watery eyes, sneezing, and runny nose.

Indications: For temporary relief of nasal congestion due to the common cold, hay fever or other upper respiratory allergies, and nasal congestion associated with sinusitis.

Directions: One caplet every 12 hours. Do not exceed 2 caplets in 24 hours.

NOTE: The nonactive portion of the caplet that supplies the active ingredients may occasionally appear in your stool as a soft mass.

TAMPER-RESISTANT PACKAGING FEATURES FOR YOUR PROTECTION:

- The carton is protected by a clear overwrap printed with "safety sealed"; do not use if overwrap is missing or broken.
- Each caplet is encased in a plastic cell with a foil back; do not use if cell or foil is broken.
- The name CONTAC appears on each caplet; do not use this product if the CONTAC name is missing.
- A package insert is provided for information on tamper-resistant packaging.

Warnings: Do not give this product to children under 12 years except under the advice and supervision of a physician. Do not exceed recommended dosage because at higher doses nervousness, dizziness, or sleeplessness may occur. Do not take this product if you have high blood pressure, heart disease, diabetes or thyroid disease except under the advice and supervision of a physician. If symptoms do not improve within 7 days or are accompanied by high fever, consult a physician before continuing use. Do not take this product if you have asthma, glaucoma or difficulty in urination due to enlargement of the prostate gland except under the advice and supervision of a physician. Do not take this product if you are taking another medication containing phenylpropanolamine. Avoid alcoholic beverages while taking this product. Do not drive or operate heavy machinery. May

Continued on next page

SmithKline Consumer—Cont.

cause drowsiness. May cause excitability, especially in children. Keep this and all drugs out of reach of children. In case of accidental overdose, seek professional assistance or contact a poison control center immediately. As with any drug, if you are pregnant or nursing a baby, seek the advice of a health professional before using this product. Store at controlled room temperature (59°–86°F.).

Drug Interaction Precaution: Do not take this product if you are presently taking a prescription antihypertensive or antidepressant drug containing monoamine oxidase inhibitor except under the advice and supervision of a physician.

Formula: Active Ingredients: Each Maximum Strength caplet contains Phenylpropanolamine Hydrochloride 75 mg.; Chlorpheniramine Maleate 12 mg. (which is a higher dose of antihistamine than CONTAC capsules). **Inactive Ingredients (listed for individuals with specific allergies):** Acetylated Monoglycerides, Carnauba Wax, Colloidal Silicon Dioxide, Ethylcellulose, Hydroxypropyl Methylcellulose, Lactose, Stearic Acid, Titanium Dioxide.

How Supplied: Consumer packages of 10, 20 and 40 caplets.
Note: There are other CONTAC products. Make sure this is the one you are interested in.
Shown in Product Identification Section, page 429

CONTAC®
Continuous Action Nasal Decongestant/Antihistamine Capsules

Composition:
[See table below].

Product Information: Each CONTAC continuous action capsule contains over 600 "tiny time pills." Some go to work right away. The rest are scientifically timed to dissolve slowly to give up to 12 hours of relief. With just *one* capsule in the morning and *one* at bedtime, you feel better all day, sleep better at night, breathing freely without congestion. CONTAC provides:

- A NASAL DECONGESTANT which helps clear nasal passages, shrinks swollen membranes and helps decongest sinus openings.

- AN ANTIHISTAMINE to help relieve itchy, watery eyes, sneezing, and runny nose.

Indications: For temporary relief of nasal congestion due to the common cold, hay fever or other upper respiratory allergies, and nasal congestion associated with sinusitis.

Directions: One capsule every 12 hours. Do not exceed 2 capsules in 24 hours.

TAMPER-RESISTANT PACKAGING FEATURES FOR YOUR PROTECTION:
- The carton is protected by a clear overwrap printed with "safety sealed"; do not use if overwrap is missing or broken.
- Each capsule is encased in a plastic cell with a foil back; do not use if cell or foil is broken.
- Each CONTAC capsule is protected by a red Perma-Seal™ band which bonds the two capsule halves together; do not use if capsule or band is broken.
- A package insert is provided for information on tamper-resistant packaging.

Warnings: Do not give this product to children under 12 years except under the advice and supervision of a physician. Do not exceed recommended dosage because at higher doses nervousness, dizziness, or sleeplessness may occur. Do not take this product if you have high blood pressure, heart disease, diabetes or thyroid disease except under the advice and supervision of a physician. If symptoms do not improve within 7 days or are accompanied by a high fever, consult a physician before continuing use. Do not take this product if you have asthma, glaucoma or difficulty in urination due to enlargement of the prostate gland except under the advice and supervision of a physician. Do not take this product if you are taking another medication containing phenylpropanolamine. Avoid alcoholic beverages while taking this product. Do not drive or operate heavy machinery. May cause drowsiness. May cause excitability, especially in children. Keep this and all drugs out of reach of children. In case of accidental overdose, seek professional assistance or contact a poison control center immediately. As with any drug, if you are pregnant or nursing a baby, seek the advice of a health professional before using this product. Store at controlled room temperature (59°–86°F.).

Drug Interaction Precaution: Do not take this product if you are presently taking a prescription antihypertensive or antidepressant drug containing mono-

amine oxidase inhibitor except under the advice and supervision of a physician.

Formula: Active Ingredients: Each capsule contains Phenylpropanolamine Hydrochloride 75 mg.; Chlorpheniramine Maleate 8 mg. **Inactive Ingredients (listed for individuals with specific allergies):** Benzyl Alcohol, Cetylpyridinium Chloride, D&C Red 33, Yellow 10, FD&C Red 3, Yellow 6 (Sunset Yellow) as a color additive, Gelatin, Glyceryl Distearate, Microcrystalline Wax, Silicon Dioxide, Sodium Lauryl Sulfate, Starch, Sucrose, and trace amounts of other inactive ingredients.

How Supplied: Consumer packages of 10, 20 and 40 capsules.
Note: There are other CONTAC products. Make sure this is the one you are interested in.
Shown in Product Identification Section, page 429

CONTAC®
Severe Cold Formula Caplets
Analgesic • Decongestant
Antihistamine • Cough Suppressant

Composition:
[See table below].

Product Information: Two caplets every 6 hours to help relieve the discomforts of severe colds with flu-like symptoms.

Product Benefits: CONTAC Severe Cold Formula contains a non-aspirin analgesic, a decongestant, an antihistamine and a cough suppressant. These safe and effective ingredients provide temporary relief from these major cold symptoms: fever, body aches and pains, minor sore throat pain, headache, runny nose, postnasal drip, sneezing, itchy, watery eyes, nasal and sinus congestion, and temporarily relieves cough due to the common cold.

Directions: Two caplets every 6 hours, not to exceed 8 caplets in any 24 hour period. Children under 12 should use only as directed by physician.

TAMPER-RESISTANT PACKAGING FEATURES FOR YOUR PROTECTION:
- The carton is protected by a clear overwrap printed with "safety sealed"; do not use if overwrap is missing or broken.
- Each caplet is encased in a plastic cell with a foil back; do not use if cell or foil is broken.
- The letters SCF appear on each caplet; do not use this product if these letters are missing.
- A package insert is provided for information on tamper-resistant packaging.

Warnings: Do not exceed recommended dosage. If symptoms do not improve within 7 days, or worsen, consult a physician before continuing use. Individuals being treated for depression, high blood pressure, asthma, heart disease, diabetes, thyroid disease, glaucoma or difficulty in urinating due to an enlarged prostate should use only as directed by a

CONTAC	CONTAC Maximum Strength Continuous Action Decongestant Caplets	CONTAC Continuous Action Decongestant Capsules	CONTAC Severe Cold Formula Caplets (each 2 caplet dose)
Phenylpropanolamine HCl	75.0 mg	75.0 mg	25.0 mg
Chlorpheniramine Maleate	12.0 mg	8.0 mg	4.0 mg
Acetaminophen	—	—	1000.0 mg
Dextromethorphan Hydrobromide	—	—	30.0 mg

CONTAC Liquid	CONTAC Cough Formula (each adult dose)	CONTAC Cough & Sore Throat Formula (each adult dose)	CONTAC JR. (each 5cc)	CONTAC Nighttime Cold Medicine (each fluid ounce)
Pseudoephedrine Hydrochloride	—	—	15.0 mg	60.0 mg
Acetaminophen	—	650.0 mg	160.0 mg	1000.0 mg
Dextromethorphan Hydrobromide	30.0 mg	20.0 mg	5.0 mg	30.0 mg
Doxylamine Succinate	—	—	—	7.5 mg
Guaifenesin	200.0 mg	200.0 mg	—	—
Alcohol	—	—	—	25%

physician. Do not take this product if you are taking another medication containing phenylpropanolamine. Avoid alcoholic beverages while taking this product. Do not drive or operate heavy machinery. May cause drowsiness. Stop use if dizziness, sleeplessness or nervousness occurs. A persistent cough may be a sign of a serious condition. If cough persists for more than 1 week, tends to recur, or is accompanied by fever, rash or persistent headache, consult a doctor. Do not take this product for persistent or chronic cough such as occurs with smoking, asthma, emphysema, or if cough is accompanied by excessive phlegm (Mucus), unless directed by a doctor. May cause excitability, especially in children. Keep this and all drugs out of reach of children. In case of accidental overdose, seek professional assistance or contact a poison control center immediately. As with any drug, if you are pregnant or nursing a baby, seek the advice of a health professional before using this product.

Store at controlled room temperature (59°–86°F.).

Drug Interaction Precaution: Do not take if you are presently taking a prescription antihypertensive or antidepressant drug containing monoamine oxidase inhibitor except under the advice and supervision of a physician.

Formula: Active Ingredients: Each caplet contains Acetaminophen, 500 mg. *(500 mg. is a non-standard dose of acetaminophen, as compared to the standard of 325 mg.);* Dextromethorphan Hydrobromide, 15 mg.; Phenylpropanolamine Hydrochloride, 12.5 mg.; Chlorpheniramine Maleate, 2 mg. **Inactive Ingredients (listed for individuals with specific allergies):** Cellulose, FD&C Blue 1, Hydroxypropyl Methylcellulose, Polyethylene Glycol, Polysorbate 80, Povidone, Sodium Starch Glycolate, Starch, Stearic Acid, Titanium Dioxide.

How Supplied: Consumer packages of 10 and 20 caplets.
Note: There are other CONTAC products. Make sure this is the one you are interested in.
Shown in Product Identification Section, page 429

CONTAC® Cough Formula
Cough Suppressant and Expectorant With 6–8 Hour Cough Control

Composition:
[See table above].

Product Information: ALCOHOL-FREE, cherry flavored CONTAC Cough Formula provides temporary relief of coughs due to the common cold and chest congestion. It contains:
● A non-narcotic cough suppressant **to temporarily relieve your cough for 6–8 hours.**
● An expectorant to **break up phlegm and mucus** that cause upper chest congestion.

Directions: Take every 6–8 hours. ADULTS: Fill medicine cup provided to "ADULT DOSE" line (3 teaspoons). Do not exceed 4 doses (12 teaspoons) in 24 hours. CHILDREN 6–12: Fill medicine cup provided to "CHILDREN 6–12 DOSE" line (1½ teaspoons). Do not exceed 4 doses (6 teaspoons) in 24 hours.
TAMPER-RESISTANT PACKAGING FEATURES FOR YOUR PROTECTION:
● The carton has been sealed at the factory with a clear overwrap printed with "Safety Sealed."
● Imprinted seal around bottle cap. Seal is printed with "SKCP."
● DO NOT USE THIS PRODUCT IF ANY OF THESE TAMPER-RESISTANT FEATURES ARE MISSING OR BROKEN. IF YOU HAVE ANY QUESTIONS ABOUT CONTAC COUGH FORMULA OR OUR PACKAGING, PLEASE CALL TOLL FREE 1-800-543-3434.

Warnings: Do not take this product for persistent or chronic cough such as occurs with smoking, asthma, or emphysema, or if cough is accompanied by excessive phlegm (mucus), unless directed by a doctor. A persistent cough may be a sign of a serious condition. If cough persists for more than 1 week, tends to recur, or is accompanied by fever, rash or persistent headache, consult a doctor. Do not give this product to children under 6 years of age unless directed by a doctor. As with any drug, if you are pregnant or nursing a baby, seek the advice of a health professional before using this product. Keep this and all drugs out of the reach of children. In case of accidental overdose, seek professional assistance or contact a poison control center immediately.

Formula: Active Ingredients: Each Adult Dose Contains Dextromethorphan Hydrobromide 30 mg. (Cough Suppressant), Guaifenesin 200 mg. (Expectorant). **Inactive Ingredients (listed for individuals with specific allergies):** Citric Acid, FD&C Red 40, Natural & Artificial Flavors, Menthol, Methylparaben, Polyethylene Glycol, Propylene Glycol, Propylparaben, Sodium Benzoate, Sodium Citrate, Sodium Saccharin, Sugar and Water.

Store at controlled room temperature (59°–86°F.).

How Supplied: In 4 fl. oz. bottles.
Note: There are other CONTAC products. Make sure this is the one you are interested in.
Shown in Product Identification Section, page 429

CONTAC® Cough & Sore Throat Formula
Cough Suppressant ● Expectorant and Non-Aspirin Analgesic

Composition:
[See table above].

Product Information: ALCOHOL-FREE, cherry flavored CONTAC Cough & Sore Throat Formula provides temporary relief of coughs due to the common cold, and chest congestion and minor sore throat pain and irritation. It contains:
● A non-narcotic cough suppressant to **temporarily relieve your cough,**
● An expectorant to **break up phlegm and mucus** that cause upper chest congestion,
● A non-aspirin analgesic to **relieve minor sore throat pain and irritation,** and
● A soothing liquid formulation to **coat a raw and irritated throat.**

Directions: Take every 4 hours as needed. ADULTS: Fill medicine cup provided to "ADULT DOSE" line (3 teaspoons). Do not exceed 6 doses (18 teaspoons) in 24 hours. CHILDREN 6–12: Fill medicine cup provided to "CHILDREN 6–12 DOSE" line (1½ teaspoons). Do not exceed 6 doses (9 teaspoons) in 24 hours.
TAMPER-RESISTANT PACKAGING FEATURES FOR YOUR PROTECTION:
● The carton has been sealed at the factory with a clear overwrap printed with "Safety Sealed."
● Imprinted seal around bottle cap. Seal is printed with "SKCP."
● DO NOT USE THIS PRODUCT IF ANY OF THESE TAMPER-RESISTANT FEATURES ARE MISSING OR BROKEN. IF YOU HAVE ANY QUESTIONS ABOUT CONTAC COUGH & SORE THROAT FORMULA OR OUR PACKAGING, PLEASE CALL TOLL FREE 1-800-543-3434.

Continued on next page

SmithKline Consumer—Cont.

Warnings: Do not take this product for persistent or chronic cough such as occurs with smoking, asthma, or emphysema, or if cough is accompanied by excessive phlegm (mucus), unless directed by a doctor. A persistent cough may be a sign of a serious condition. If cough persists for more than 1 week, tends to recur, or is accompanied by fever, rash or persistent headache, consult a doctor. Do not give this product to children under 6 years of age unless directed by a doctor. Adults: do not take this product for more than 10 days. Children under 12 years: do not take this product for more than 5 days. Do not exceed recommended dosage because severe liver damage may occur. Do not take additional pain relievers/fever reducers while using this product. As with any drug, if you are pregnant or nursing a baby, seek the advice of a health professional before using this product. Keep this and all drugs out of the reach of children. In case of accidental overdose, seek professional assistance or contact a poison control center immediately.

Formula: Active Ingredients: Each Adult Dose Contains Acetaminophen 650 mg. (Analgesic/Fever Reducer), Dextromethorphan Hydrobromide 20 mg. (Cough Suppressant), Guaifenesin 200 mg. (Expectorant). **Inactive Ingredients (listed for individuals with specific allergies):** Citric Acid, D&C Red 33, FD&C Red 40, Menthol, Methylparaben, Natural & Artificial Flavors, Polyethylene Glycol, Propylene Glycol, Propylparaben, Sodium Benzoate, Sodium Citrate, Sodium Saccharin, Sugar and Water.

Store at controlled room temperature (59°–86°F.).

How Supplied: In 4 fl. oz. bottles.
Note: There are other CONTAC products. Make sure this is the one you are interested in.

Shown in Product Identification Section, page 429

CONTAC JR.®
Non-Drowsy Cold Liquid
Analgesic • Decongestant
Cough Suppressant

Composition:
[See table on preceding page].

Product Information: For nasal and sinus congestion, coughing and body aches and pains due to colds. Relieves symptoms with these reliable medicines. A gentle decongestant. For temporary relief of nasal and sinus congestion. Helps your child breathe more freely. A safe, sensible, non-narcotic cough quieter. Calms worrisome coughs due to colds.
A trusted, aspirin-free pain reliever and fever reducer. Provides temporary relief of muscular aches and pains, headaches and discomforts of fever due to colds and "flu."

Product Benefits: The good medicines in CONTAC Jr. were specially chosen to help gently relieve your child's nasal and sinus congestion, coughing, body aches and pains due to colds. DOES NOT CONTAIN ANTIHISTAMINES WHICH MAY CAUSE DROWSINESS.
Medical authorities know that for children, dose by weight—not age—means the dose you give is right for consistent, controlled relief. Use the CONTAC Jr. Accu-Measure Cup to select the right dose for your child's body weight.

Directions: Shake well before using. One dose every 4 to 6 hours, not to exceed 4 times daily. Use the CONTAC Jr. Accu-Measure Cup to measure the right dose for your child. For dose by teaspoon see bottle label.

TAMPER-RESISTANT PACKAGING FEATURES FOR YOUR PROTECTION:
- The carton has been sealed at the factory with a clear overwrap printed with "Safety Sealed."
- Imprinted seal around bottle-cap. Seal is printed with "SKCP."
- DO NOT USE THIS PRODUCT IF ANY OF THESE TAMPER-RESISTANT FEATURES ARE MISSING OR BROKEN. IF YOU HAVE ANY QUESTIONS ABOUT CONTAC JR. OR OUR PACKAGING, PLEASE CALL TOLL FREE 1-800-543-3434.

Warning: Do not exceed recommended dosage for your child's body weight. For children under 31 lbs. or under 3 years of age, consult a physician. If symptoms persist for 7 days or are accompanied by high fever, severe or recurrent pain, or if child is being treated for depression, high blood pressure, diabetes, heart disease or thyroid disease, consult a physician. Stop use if dizziness, sleeplessness or nervousness occurs. Do not give this product for persistent or chronic cough such as occurs with asthma or if cough is accompanied by excessive phlegm (mucus) unless directed by a doctor. Keep this and all drugs out of reach of children. In case of accidental overdose, seek professional assistance or contact a poison control center immediately.

Formula: Active Ingredients: Each 5 cc. (average teaspoon) contains Pseudoephedrine Hydrochloride 15.0 mg. (nasal decongestant); Acetaminophen 160.0 mg. (analgesic/antipyretic); Dextromethorphan Hydrobromide 5.0 mg. (anti-tussive). **Inactive Ingredients (listed for individuals with specific allergies):** Citric Acid, D&C Red 33, FD&C Yellow 6 (Sunset Yellow) as a color additive, Flavors, Methyl and Propyl Paraben, Polyethylene Glycol, Propylene Glycol, Saccharin Sodium, Sodium Benzoate, Sodium Citrate, Sorbitol, Purified Water.

Store at controlled room temperature (59°–86°F.).

How Supplied: A clear red liquid in 4 oz. size bottle.
Note: There are other CONTAC products. Make sure this is the one you are interested in.

Shown in Product Identification Section, page 429

CONTAC®
Nighttime Cold Medicine
Antihistamine • Analgesic
Cough Suppressant • Nasal Decongestant

Composition:
[See table on preceding page].

Product Information: CONTAC Nighttime Cold Medicine:

- Provides temporary relief from nasal and sinus congestion, runny nose, coughing due to the common cold, postnasal drip, headache, body aches and pains, minor sore throat pain, sneezing, fever, and itchy, watery eyes, so you can get the rest you need.

- Contains a non-aspirin analgesic and fever reducer, a cough suppressant, a nasal decongestant and an antihistamine.

In consumer testing, the soothing mint taste of CONTAC Nighttime Cold Medicine was preferred over the taste of original NYQUIL* Nighttime Colds Medicine.

Directions: ADULTS—Take 1 fluid ounce at bedtime in dosage cup provided. May be repeated every 6 hours as needed, not to exceed 4 fluid ounces in 24 hours. Children under 12 should use only as directed by physician.

TAMPER-RESISTANT FEATURES FOR YOUR PROTECTION:
- The carton has been sealed at the factory with a clear overwrap printed with "safety sealed."
- Imprinted seal around bottle cap. Seal is printed with "SKCP."
- DO NOT USE THIS PRODUCT IF ANY OF THESE TAMPER-RESISTANT FEATURES ARE MISSING OR BROKEN. IF YOU HAVE ANY QUESTIONS ABOUT CONTAC NIGHTTIME COLD MEDICINE OR PACKAGING, PLEASE CALL 1-800-543-3434 TOLL FREE.

Warnings: Do not exceed recommended dosage. If symptoms do not improve or worsen within 7 days, or are accompanied by high fever, or difficulty in breathing, consult a physician before continuing use. A persistent cough may be a sign of a serious condition. If cough persists for more than one week, tends to recur or is accompanied by a high fever, a fever lasting more than 3 days, a rash, a persistent headache, shortness of breath or chest pain when breathing, consult a physician. Do not take this product for persistent or chronic cough such as occurs with smoking, asthma, emphysema, or if cough is accompanied by excessive phlegm (mucus) unless directed by a doctor. Stop use if dizziness, sleeplessness, or nervousness occurs. Individuals who have been or are being treated for depression, high blood pressure, glaucoma, diabetes, asthma, difficulty in urination due to enlarged prostate, heart disease or thyroid disease should use only as directed by a physician. Avoid alcoholic beverages while taking this product. Do

not drive or operate heavy machinery. May cause marked drowsiness. May cause excitability, especially in children. **This package is child-safe;** however, keep this and all drugs out of reach of children. In case of accidental overdose, seek professional assistance or contact a poison control center immediately. As with any drug, if you are pregnant or nursing a baby, seek the advice of a health professional before using this product.

Formula: Active Ingredients: Each 1 oz. Dose Contains: Acetaminophen 1000 mg. (Analgesic/Fever Reducer), Dextromethorphan Hydrobromide 30 mg. (Cough Suppressant), Pseudoephedrine Hydrochloride 60 mg. (Nasal Decongestant), Doxylamine Succinate 7.5 mg. (Antihistamine), Alcohol 25%. **Inactive Ingredients (listed for individuals with specific allergies):** Citric Acid, FD&C Green 3, Yellow 6 (Sunset Yellow) as a color additive, Flavor, Polyethylene Glycol, Sodium Benzoate, Sodium Citrate, Sodium Saccharin, Sorbitol, Sugar and Water.

Store at controlled room temperature (59°–86°F.).

How Supplied: In 6 fl. oz. bottles.
Note: There are other CONTAC products. Make sure this is the one you are interested in.
*NYQUIL is a registered trademark of Richardson-Vicks Inc.

Shown in Product Identification Section, page 429

ECOTRIN®
Enteric-Coated Aspirin
Antiarthritic, Antiplatelet

Description: 'Ecotrin' is enteric-coated aspirin (acetylsalicylic acid, ASA) available in tablet and caplet forms in 325 mg. and 500 mg. dosage units. *(500 mg. is a non-standard, maximum strength dosage of aspirin, as compared to the standard of 325 mg.)*
The enteric coating covers a core of aspirin and is designed to resist disintegration in the stomach, dissolving in the more neutral-to-alkaline environment of the duodenum. Such action tends to protect the stomach from injury that may result from ingestion of plain, i.e., non-enteric-coated, aspirin (see SAFETY).

Indications: 'Ecotrin' is indicated for:
- conditions requiring chronic or long-term aspirin therapy for pain and/or inflammation, e.g., rheumatoid or osteoarthritis,
- antiplatelet indications of aspirin (see the ANTIPLATELET-EFFECT section) and
- situations in which compliance with aspirin therapy may be affected because of the gastrointestinal side effects of plain, i.e., non-enteric-coated, or buffered aspirin.

Dosage: For analgesic or anti-inflammatory indications, the OTC maximum dosage for aspirin is 4000 mg. per day in divided doses, i.e., 2,325 mg. tablets or caplets q4h or 3,325 mg. tablets or caplets or 2,500 mg. tablets or caplets q6h.
For antiplatelet effect dosage: see the ANTIPLATELET EFFECT section.
Under a physician's direction, the dosage can be increased or otherwise modified as appropriate to the clinical situation. When 'Ecotrin' is used for anti-inflammatory effect, the physician should be attentive to plasma salicylate levels, and may also caution the patient to be alert to the development of tinnitus as an indicator of elevated salicylate levels. It should be noted that patients with a high frequency hearing loss (such as may occur in older individuals) may have difficulty perceiving the tinnitus. Tinnitus would then not be a reliable indicator in such individuals.

Inactive Ingredients: Inactive ingredients (listed for individuals with specific allergies): Cellulose, Cellulose Acetate Phthalate, D&C Yellow 10, Diethyl Phthalate, FD&C Yellow 6 (Sunset Yellow) as a color additive, Silicon Dioxide, Sodium Starch Glycolate, Starch, Stearic Acid, Titanium Dioxide, and trace amounts of other inactive ingredients.

Bioavailability: The bioavailability of aspirin from 'Ecotrin' has been demonstrated in a number of salicylate excretion studies. The studies show levels of salicylate (and metabolites) in urine excreted over 48 hours for 'Ecotrin' do not differ statistically from plain, i.e., non-enteric-coated, aspirin.
Plasma studies, in which tablet form of 'Ecotrin' has been compared with plain aspirin in steady-state studies over eight days, also demonstrate that 'Ecotrin' provides plasma salicylate levels not statistically different from plain aspirin.
Information regarding salicylate levels over a range of doses was generated in a study in which 24 healthy volunteers (12 male and 12 female) took daily (divided) doses of either 2600 mg., 3900 mg., or 5200 mg. of 'Ecotrin'. Plasma salicylate levels generally acknowledged to be anti-inflammatory (15 mg./dL.) were attained at daily doses of 5200 mg., on Day 2 by females and Day 3 by males. At 3900 mg., anti-inflammatory levels were attained at Day 3 by females and Day 4 by males. Dissolution of the enteric coating occurs at a neutral-to-basic pH and is therefore dependent on gastric emptying into the duodenum. With continued dosing, appropriate plasma levels are maintained.

Safety: The safety of 'Ecotrin' has been demonstrated in a number of endoscopic studies comparing 'Ecotrin', plain aspirin, as well as plain buffered and "arthritis-strength" buffered preparations. In these studies, all forms of aspirin were dosed to the OTC maximum (3900–4000 mg. per day) for up to 14 days. The normal healthy volunteers participating in these studies were gastroscoped before and after the courses of treatment, and 14-day drug-free periods followed active drug. Compared to all the other preparations, there was statistically significantly less gastric damage during the 'Ecotrin' courses. There was also statistically less duodenal damage when compared with the plain, i.e., non-enteric-coated, aspirin.
Details of studies demonstrating the safety and bioavailability of 'Ecotrin' are available to health care professionals. Write: Medical Affairs Department, SmithKline Consumer Products, P.O. Box 8082, Philadelphia, PA 19101.

Warning:
Consumer Warning: Children and teenagers should not use this medicine for chicken pox or flu symptoms before a doctor is consulted about Reye syndrome, a rare but serious illness reported to be associated with aspirin. If pain persists for more than 10 days, or if redness is present, or in arthritic or rheumatic conditions affecting children under 12, consult a physician immediately. Discontinue use if dizziness, ringing in ears, or impaired hearing occurs. If you experience persistent or unexplained stomach upset, consult a physician. Keep this and all drugs out of children's reach. In case of accidental overdose, seek professional assistance or contact a poison control center immediately. As with any medicine, if you are pregnant or nursing a baby, seek the advice of a health professional before using this product. Store at controlled room temperature (59°–86°F.).
Professional Warning: There have been occasional reports in the literature concerning individuals with impaired gastric emptying in whom there may be retention of one or more 'Ecotrin' tablets over time. This phenomenon may occur as a result of outlet obstruction from ulcer disease alone or combined with hypotonic gastric peristalsis. Because of the integrity of the enteric coating in an acidic environment, these tablets may accumulate and form a bezoar in the stomach. Individuals with this condition may present with complaints of early satiety or of vague upper abdominal distress. Diagnosis may be made by endoscopy or by abdominal films which show opacities suggestive of a mass of small tablets *(Ref.: Bogacz, K. and Caldron, P.: Enteric-coated Aspirin Bezoar: Elevation of Serum Salicylate Level by Barium Study. Amer. J. Med. 1987:83, 783–6.).* Management may vary according to the condition of the patient. Options include: gastrotomy and alternating slightly basic and neutral lavage *(Ref.: Baum, J.: Enteric-Coated Aspirin and the Problem of Gastric Retention. J. Rheum., 1984:11, 250–1.).* While there have been no clinical reports, it has been suggested that such individuals may also be treated with parenteral cimetidine (to reduce acid secretion) and then given sips of slightly basic liquids to effect gradual dissolution of the enteric coating. Progress may be followed with plasma salicylate levels or via recognition of tinnitus by the patient. It should be kept in mind that individuals with a history of partial or complete gastrectomy may produce reduced amounts of acid and therefore have less acidic gastric pH. Under these circumstances, the benefits offered by the acid-resistant enteric coating may not exist.

Continued on next page

SmithKline Consumer—Cont.

Antiplatelet Effect: FDA has approved the professional labeling of aspirin to reduce the risk of death and/or nonfatal myocardial infarction (MI) in patients with a previous infarction or unstable angina pectoris. Previously, wording was added to the professional labeling of aspirin approving its use in reducing the risk of transient ischemic attacks in men.

Labeling for both indications follows:

Aspirin for Myocardial Infarction

Indication: Aspirin is indicated to reduce the risk of death and/or nonfatal myocardial infarction in patients with a previous infarction or unstable angina pectoris.

Clinical Trials: The indication is supported by the results of six, large, randomized multicenter, placebo-controlled studies involving 10,816 predominantly male, post-myocardial infarction (MI) patients and one randomized placebo-controlled study of 1,266 men with unstable angina.[1-7] Therapy with aspirin was begun at intervals after the onset of acute MI varying from less than three days to more than five years and continued for periods of from less than one year to four years. In the unstable angina study, treatment was started within one month after the onset of unstable angina and continued for 12 weeks, and patients with complicating conditions such as congestive heart failure were not included in the study.

Aspirin therapy in MI patients was associated with about a 20 percent reduction in the risk of subsequent death and/or nonfatal reinfarction, a median absolute decrease of 3 percent from the 12 to 22 percent event rates in the placebo groups. In aspirin-treated unstable angina patients, the reduction in risk was about 50 percent, a reduction in event rate in the placebo group over the 12 weeks of the study.

Daily dosage of aspirin in the post-myocardial infarction studies was 300 mg. in one study and 900 to 1500 mg. in five studies. A dose of 325 mg. was used in the study of unstable angina.

Adverse Reactions

Gastrointestinal Reactions: Doses of 1000 mg. per day of aspirin caused gastrointestinal symptoms and bleeding that in some cases were clinically significant. In the largest postinfarction study (the Aspirin Myocardial Infarction Study [AMIS] with 4,500 people), the percentage incidences of gastrointestinal symptoms of a standard, solid-tablet formulation) and placebo-treated subjects, respectively, were: stomach pain (14.5%; 4.4%); heartburn (11.9%; 4.8%); nausea and/or vomiting (7.6%; 2.1%); hospitalization for gastrointestinal disorder (4.9%; 3.5%). In the AMIS and other trials, aspirin-treated patients had increased rates of gross gastrointestinal bleeding. Symptoms and signs of gastrointestinal irritation were not significantly increased in subjects treated for

unstable angina with buffered aspirin in solution.

Cardiovascular and Biochemical: In the AMIS trial, the dosage of 1000 mg. per day of aspirin was associated with small increases in systolic blood pressure (BP) (average 1.5 to 2.1 mmHg) and diastolic BP (0.5 to 0.6 mmHg), depending upon whether maximal or last available readings were used. Blood urea nitrogen and uric acid levels were also increased, but by less than 1.0 mg.%. Subjects with marked hypertension or renal insufficiency had been excluded from the trial so that the clinical importance of these observations for such subjects or for any subjects treated over more prolonged periods is not known. It is recommended that patients placed on long-term aspirin treatment, even at doses of 300 mg. per day, be seen at regular intervals to assess changes in these measurements.

Sodium in Buffered Aspirin for Solution Formulations: One tablet daily of buffered aspirin in solution adds 553 mg. of sodium to that in the diet and may not be tolerated by patients with active sodium-retaining states such as congestive heart or renal failure. This amount of sodium adds about 30 percent to the 70 to 90 meq. intake suggested as appropriate for dietary hypertension in the 1984 Report of the Joint National Committee on Detection, Evaluation, and Treatment of High Blood Pressure.[8]

Dosage and Administration: Although most of the studies used dosages exceeding 300 mg. daily, two trials used only 300 mg. and pharmacologic data indicate that this dose inhibits platelet function fully. Therefore, 300 mg. or a conventional 325 mg. aspirin dose daily is a reasonable, routine dose that would minimize gastrointestinal adverse reactions for both solid, oral dosage forms (buffered and plain aspirin) and buffered aspirin in solution.

References:

1. Elwood, P.C., et al.: A Randomized Controlled Trial of Acetylsalicylic Acid in the Secondary Prevention of Mortality from Myocardial Infarction, *Br. Med. J.* 1:436–440, 1974.
2. The Coronary Drug Project Research Group: Aspirin in Coronary Heart Disease, *J. Chronic Dis.* 29:625–642, 1976.
3. Breddin, K., et al.: Secondary Prevention of Myocardial Infarction: A Comparison of Acetylsalicylic Acid, Phenprocoumon or Placebo, *Homeostasis* 470:263–268, 1979.
4. Aspirin Myocardial Infarction Study Research Group: A Randomized Controlled Trial of Aspirin in Persons Recovered from Myocardial Infarction, *J.A.M.A.* 243:661–669, 1980.
5. Elwood, P.C., and Sweetnam, P.M.: Aspirin and Secondary Mortality After Myocardial Infarction, *Lancet* pp. 1313–1315, Dec. 22–29, 1979.
6. The Persantine-Aspirin Reinfarction Study Research Group, Persantine and Aspirin in Coronary Heart Disease, *Circulation* 62: 449–469, 1980.
7. Lewis, H.D., et al.: Protective Effects of Aspirin Against Acute Myocardial In-

farction and Death in Men with Unstable Angina, Results of a Veterans Administration Cooperative Study, *N. Engl. J. Med.* 309:396–403, 1983.
8. 1984 Report of the Joint National Committee on Detection, Evaluation, and Treatment of High Blood Pressure, U.S. Department of Health and Human Services and U.S. Public Health Service, National Institutes of Health. NIH Pub. No. 84–1088.

For Recurrent TIAs in Men

There is evidence that aspirin is safe and effective for reducing the risk of recurrent transient ischemic attacks (TIAs) or stroke in men who have transient ischemia of the brain due to fibrin emboli. There is no evidence that aspirin is effective in reducing TIAs in women, or is of benefit in the treatment of completed strokes in men or women.

Patients presenting with signs and/or symptoms of TIAs should have a complete medical and neurologic evaluation. Consideration should be given to other disorders which may resemble TIAs. It is important to evaluate and treat, if appropriate, diseases associated with TIAs and stroke, such as hypertension and diabetes.

Dosage: The recommended dosage for this new indication is 1300 mg./day (650 mg. b.i.d. or 325 mg. q.i.d.).

Store at controlled room temperature (59°–86°F.).

Supplied:
'Ecotrin' Tablets
　　325 mg. in bottles of 100, 250 and 1000.
　　500 mg. in bottles of 60 and 150.
'Ecotrin' Caplets
　　325 mg. in bottles of 75.
　　500 mg. in bottles of 50.

TAMPER-RESISTANT PACKAGE FEATURES:

- The carton has been sealed at the factory with a clear overwrap printed with "safety sealed."
- Bottle has imprinted "SKCP" seal under cap.
- The words ECOTRIN REG or ECOTRIN MAX appear on each tablet or caplet (see product illustration printed on carton).
- **DO NOT USE THIS PRODUCT IF ANY OF THESE TAMPER-RESISTANT FEATURES ARE MISSING OR BROKEN. IF YOU HAVE ANY QUESTIONS, PLEASE CALL 1-800-543-3434 TOLL FREE.**

Shown in Product Identification Section, page 429

FEOSOL® CAPSULES
Hematinic

Product Information: FEOSOL capsules provide the body with ferrous sulfate, iron in its most efficient form, for simple iron deficiency and iron-deficiency anemia.

The special targeted-release capsule is formulated to reduce stomach upset, a common problem with iron.

Directions: *Adults:* 1 or 2 capsules daily or as directed by a physician. *Children:* As directed by a physician.

TAMPER-RESISTANT PACKAGING FEATURES FOR YOUR PROTECTION:

- The carton is protected by a clear overwrap printed with "safety sealed"; do not use if overwrap is missing or broken.
- Each capsule is encased in a plastic cell with a foil back; do not use if cell or foil is broken.
- Each FEOSOL capsule is protected by a red Perma-Seal™ band which bonds the two capsule halves together; do not use if capsule is broken or band is missing or broken.
- A package insert is provided for information on tamper-resistant packaging.

Warnings: Do not exceed recommended dosage. The treatment of any anemic condition should be under the advice and supervision of a physician. Iron-containing medication may occasionally cause constipation or diarrhea. Since oral iron products interfere with absorption of oral tetracycline antibiotics, these products should not be taken within two hours of each other. This package is child-safe; however, keep this and all drugs out of reach of children. In case of accidental overdose, seek professional assistance or contact a poison control center immediately. As with any drug, if you are pregnant or nursing a baby, seek the advice of a health professional before using this product. Store at controlled room temperature (59°–86°F.).

Formula: Active Ingredients: Each capsule contains 159 mg. of dried ferrous sulfate USP (50 mg. of elemental iron), equivalent to 250 mg. of ferrous sulfate USP. **Inactive Ingredients (listed for individuals with specific allergies):** Benzyl Alcohol, Cetylpyridinium Chloride, D&C Red 33, Yellow 10, FD&C Blue 1, Red 3, Red 40, Gelatin, Glyceryl Stearates, Iron Oxide, Polyethylene Glycol, Povidone, Sodium Lauryl Sulfate, Starch, Sucrose, White Wax and trace amounts of other inactive ingredients.

How Supplied: Packages of 30 and 60 capsules; in Single Unit Packages of 100 capsules (intended for institutional use only).
Also available in Tablets and Elixir.
Note: There are other FEOSOL products. Make sure this is the one you are interested in.
Shown in Product Identification Section, page 429

FEOSOL® ELIXIR
Hematinic

Product Information: FEOSOL Elixir, an unusually palatable iron elixir, provides the body with ferrous sulfate—iron in its most efficient form. The standard elixir for simple iron deficiency and iron-deficiency anemia when the need for such therapy has been determined by a physician.

Directions: Adults: 1 to 2 teaspoonfuls three times daily. Children: ½ to 1 teaspoonful three times daily preferably between meals. Infants: as directed by physician. Mix with water or fruit juice to avoid temporary staining of teeth; do not mix with milk or wine-based vehicles.

TAMPER-RESISTANT PACKAGE FEATURE: Imprinted seal around top of bottle; do not use if seal is missing.

Warning: The treatment of any anemic condition should be under the advice and supervision of a physician. Since oral iron products interfere with absorption of oral tetracycline antibiotics, these products should not be taken within two hours of each other. Occasional gastrointestinal discomfort (such as nausea) may be minimized by taking with meals and by beginning with one teaspoonful the first day, two the second, etc. until the recommended dosage is reached. Iron-containing medication may occasionally cause constipation or diarrhea, and liquids may cause temporary staining of the teeth (this is less likely when diluted). Keep this and all drugs out of reach of children. In case of accidental overdose, seek professional assistance or contact a poison control center immediately.
As with any drug, if you are pregnant or nursing a baby, seek the advice of a health professional before using this product. Store at controlled room temperature (59°–86°F.).

Formula: Each 5 ml. (1 teaspoonful) contains ferrous sulfate USP, 220 mg. (44 mg. of elemental iron); alcohol, 5%. **Inactive Ingredients (listed for individuals with specific allergies):** Citric Acid, FD&C Yellow 6 (Sunset Yellow) as a color additive, Flavors, Glucose, Saccharin Sodium, Sucrose, Purified Water.

How Supplied: A clear orange liquid in 16 fl. oz. bottles.
Also available in Tablets and Capsules.
Note: There are other FEOSOL products. Make sure this is the one you are interested in.
Shown in Product Identification Section, page 429

FEOSOL® TABLETS
Hematinic

Product Information: FEOSOL Tablets provide the body with ferrous sulfate, iron in its most efficient form, for iron deficiency and iron-deficiency anemia when the need for such therapy has been determined by a physician. The distinctive triangular-shaped tablet has a coating to prevent oxidation and improve palatability.

Directions: *Adults* —one tablet 3 to 4 times daily after meals and upon retiring or as directed by a physician. *Children 6 to 12 years* —one tablet three times a day after meals. *Children under 6 and infants* —use Feosol® Elixir.

TAMPER-RESISTANT PACKAGE FEATURES FOR YOUR PROTECTION:

- The carton has been sealed at the factory with a clear overwrap printed with "safety sealed."
- Bottle has imprinted "SKCP" seal under cap.
- FEOSOL Tablets are triangular shaped (see product illustration printed on carton).
- **DO NOT USE THIS PRODUCT IF ANY OF THESE TAMPER-RESISTANT FEATURES ARE MISSING OR BROKEN. IF YOU HAVE ANY QUESTIONS, PLEASE CALL 1-800-543-3434 TOLL FREE.**

Warning: Do not exceed recommended dosage. The treatment of any anemic condition should be under the advice and supervision of a physician. Since oral iron products interfere with absorption of oral tetracycline antibiotics, these products should not be taken within two hours of each other.
Occasional gastrointestinal discomfort (such as nausea) may be minimized by taking with meals and by beginning with one tablet the first day, two the second, etc. until the recommended dosage is reached. Iron-containing medication may occasionally cause constipation or diarrhea.
Keep this and all drugs out of reach of children. In case of accidental overdose, seek professional assistance or contact a poison control center immediately.
As with any drug, if you are pregnant or nursing a baby, seek the advice of a health professional before using this product. Store at controlled room temperature (59°–86°F.).

Formula: Active Ingredients: Each tablet contains 200 mg. of dried ferrous sulfate USP (65 mg. of elemental iron), equivalent to 325 mg. (5 grains) of ferrous sulfate USP. **Inactive Ingredients (listed for individuals with specific allergies):** Calcium Sulfate, D&C Yellow 10, FD&C Blue 2, Glucose, Hydroxypropyl Methylcellulose, Mineral Oil, Polyethylene Glycol, Sodium Lauryl Sulfate, Starch, Stearic Acid, Talc, Titanium Dioxide, and trace amounts of other inactive ingredients.

How Supplied: Bottles of 100 and 1000 tablets; in Single Unit Packages of 100 tablets (intended for institutional use only).
Also available in Capsules and Elixir.
Note: There are other FEOSOL products. Make sure this is the one you are interested in.
Shown in Product Identification Section, page 430

ORNEX®
decongestant/analgesic
Caplets

Product Information: For temporary relief of nasal congestion, headache, aches, pains and fever due to colds, sinusitis and flu.
NO ANTIHISTAMINE DROWSINESS

Directions: Adults—TWO CAPLETS every 4 hours, not to exceed 8 caplets in any 24-hour period. Children (6 to 12

Continued on next page

SmithKline Consumer—Cont.

years)—ONE CAPLET every 4 hours, not to exceed 4 caplets in 24 hours.

TAMPER-RESISTANT PACKAGE FEATURES FOR YOUR PROTECTION:

- The carton has been sealed at the factory with a clear overwrap printed with "safety sealed."
- Each caplet is encased in a clear plastic cell with a foil back.
- The name ORNEX appears on each caplet (see product illustration on front of carton).
- DO NOT USE THIS PRODUCT IF ANY OF THESE TAMPER-RESISTANT FEATURES ARE MISSING OR BROKEN. IF YOU HAVE ANY QUESTIONS, PLEASE CALL 1-800-543-3434 TOLL FREE.

Warnings: Do not exceed recommended dosage. Do not give to children under 6 or use for more than 10 days, unless directed by physician. If you have or are being treated for depression, high blood pressure, diabetes, heart disease or thyroid disease, use only as directed by physician. Stop use if dizziness, sleeplessness or nervousness occurs. This package is for households without young children. Keep this and all medicines out of reach of children. In case of accidental overdose, seek professional assistance or contact a poison control center immediately. As with any drug, if you are pregnant or nursing a baby, seek the advice of a health professional before using this product.
Store at controlled room temperature (59°–86°F.).

Formula: Active Ingredients: Each caplet contains Pseudoephedrine Hydrochloride 30 mg., Acetaminophen 325 mg. **Inactive Ingredients (listed for individuals with specific allergies):** Cellulose, Crospovidone, FD&C Blue 1, Hydroxypropyl Methylcellulose, Magnesium Stearate, Polyethylene Glycol, Polysorbate 80, Povidone, Starch, Titanium Dioxide, and trace amounts of other inactive ingredients.

How Supplied: In consumer packages of 24 and 48 caplets. Also, Dispensary Packages of 792 caplets for industrial dispensaries and student health clinics only.
Shown in Product Identification Section, page 430

SINE–OFF® Maximum Strength Allergy/Sinus Formula Caplets

Composition:
[See table below].

Product Information: SINE-OFF Maximum Strength Allergy/Sinus Formula provides maximum strength relief from upper respiratory allergy, hay fever and sinusitis symptoms. This formula contains acetaminophen, a non-aspirin pain reliever.

Product Benefits: Relieves itchy, watery eyes, sneezing, runny nose and post nasal drip • Eases headache pain and pressure • promotes sinus drainage • shrinks swollen membranes to relieve congestion.

Directions: Adults and children over 12 years of age: 2 caplets every 6 hours, not to exceed 8 caplets in any 24-hour period. Children under 12 should use only as directed by a physician.

TAMPER-RESISTANT PACKAGE FEATURES FOR YOUR PROTECTION:

- The carton has been sealed at the factory with a clear overwrap printed with "safety sealed."
- Each caplet is encased in a clear plastic cell with a foil back.
- The name SINE-OFF appears on each caplet (see product illustration on front of carton).
- DO NOT USE THIS PRODUCT IF ANY OF THESE TAMPER-RESISTANT FEATURES ARE MISSING OR BROKEN. IF YOU HAVE ANY QUESTIONS, PLEASE CALL 1-800-543-3434 TOLL FREE.

Warnings: Do not exceed recommended dosage. If symptoms do not improve within 7 days, consult a physician before continuing use. Individuals being treated for depression, high blood pressure, asthma, heart disease, diabetes, thyroid disease, glaucoma or difficulty urinating due to an enlarged prostate gland should use only as directed by a physician. Do not take this product if you are taking sedatives or tranquilizers. Avoid alcoholic beverages while taking this product. Do not drive or operate heavy machinery. May cause drowsiness. Stop use if dizziness, sleeplessness or nervousness occurs. May cause excitability, especially in children. **This package is child-safe**; however, keep this and all drugs out of reach of children. In case of accidental overdose, seek professional assistance or contact a poison control center immediately. As with any drug, if you are pregnant or nursing a baby, seek

the advice of a health professional before using this product.
Store at controlled room temperature (59°–86°F.).

Formula: Active Ingredients: Each caplet contains Chlorpheniramine Maleate 2 mg., Pseudoephedrine Hydrochloride 30 mg., Acetaminophen 500 mg. *(500 mg. is a non-standard dosage of acetaminophen as compared to the standard of 325 mg.).* **Inactive Ingredients (listed for individuals with specific allergies):** Cellulose, Crospovidone, D&C Red 30, D&C Yellow 10, FD&C Blue 2, Hydroxypropyl Methylcellulose, Magnesium Stearate, Polyethylene Glycol, Povidone, Starch, Titanium Dioxide, and trace amounts of other inactive ingredients.

How Supplied: Consumer packages of 24 caplets.
Note: There are other SINE-OFF products. Make sure this is the one you are interested in.

Also Available: SINE-OFF® Sinus Medicine Tablets with Aspirin in 24's, 48's, 100's. SINE-OFF® Maximum Strength No Drowsiness Formula Caplets 24's.
Shown in Product Identification Section, page 430

SINE–OFF® Maximum Strength No Drowsiness Formula Caplets

Composition:
[See table below].

Product Information: SINE-OFF Maximum Strength No Drowsiness Formula provides maximum strength relief from headache and sinus pain. Relieves pressure and congestion due to sinusitis, allergic sinusitis or the common cold. This formula contains acetaminophen, a non-aspirin pain reliever.

NO ANTIHISTAMINE DROWSINESS

Product Benefits: Eases headache, pain and pressure. Promotes sinus drainage • shrinks swollen membranes to relieve congestion.

Directions: Adults and children over 12 years of age: 2 caplets every 6 hours, not to exceed 8 caplets in any 24-hour period. Children under 12 should use only as directed by physician.

TAMPER-RESISTANT PACKAGE FEATURES FOR YOUR PROTECTION:

- The carton has been sealed at the factory with a clear overwrap printed with "safety sealed."
- Each caplet is encased in a clear plastic cell with a foil back.

Each tablet/ caplet contains:	SINE-OFF Tablets-Aspirin Formula	SINE-OFF Maximum Strength Allergy/Sinus Formula Caplets	SINE-OFF Maximum Strength No Drowsiness Formula Caplets
Chlorpheniramine maleate	2.0 mg	2.0 mg	—
Phenylpropanolamine HCl	12.5 mg	—	—
Aspirin	325.0 mg	—	—
Acetaminophen	—	500.0 mg	500.0 mg
Pseudoephedrine HCl	—	30.0 mg	30.0 mg

- The name SINE-OFF appears on each caplet (see product illustration on front of carton).
- **DO NOT USE THIS PRODUCT IF ANY OF THESE TAMPER-RESIST-ANT FEATURES ARE MISSING OR BROKEN. IF YOU HAVE ANY QUESTIONS, PLEASE CALL 1-800-543-3434 TOLL FREE.**

Warnings: Do not exceed recommended dosage. If symptoms do not improve within 7 days, consult a physician before continuing use. Individuals being treated for depression, high blood pressure, heart disease, diabetes, thyroid disease, or difficulty in urination due to enlargement of the prostate gland should use only as directed by a physician. Stop use if dizziness, sleeplessness or nervousness occurs. This package is child-safe; however, keep this and all drugs out of reach of children. In case of accidental overdose, seek professional assistance or contact a poison control center immediately. As with any drug, if you are pregnant or nursing a baby, seek the advice of a health professional before using this product.
Store at controlled room temperature (59°–86°F.).

Formula: Active Ingredients: Each caplet contains: 30 mg. Pseudoephedrine Hydrochloride, 500 mg. Acetaminophen *(500 mg. is a non-standard dosage of acetaminophen, as compared to the standard of 325 mg.).* **Inactive Ingredients (listed for individuals with specific allergies):** Cellulose, Crospovidone, FD&C Red 3, FD&C Yellow 6 (Sunset Yellow) as a color additive, Hydroxypropyl Methylcellulose, Magnesium Stearate, Polyethylene Glycol, Polysorbate 80, Povidone, Starch, Titanium Dioxide, and trace amounts of other inactive ingredients.

How Supplied: Consumer packages of 24 caplets.

Note: There are other SINE-OFF products. Make sure this is the one you are interested in.

Also Available:
SINE-OFF® Tablets with Aspirin
SINE-OFF® Maximum Strength Allergy/Sinus Formula Caplets
Shown in Product Identification Section, page 430

SINE-OFF® Sinus Medicine Tablets–Aspirin Formula
Relieves sinus headache and congestion.

Composition:
[See table on preceding page].

Product Information: SINE-OFF relieves headache, pain, pressure and congestion due to sinusitis, allergic sinusitis, or the common cold.

Product Benefits: Eases headache, pain and pressure; promotes sinus drainage; shrinks swollen membranes to relieve congestion; relieves postnasal drip.

Directions: Adults: 2 tablets every 4 hours, not to exceed 8 tablets in any 24-hour period. Children (6–12) one-half the adult dosage. Children under 6 years should use only as directed by a physician.

TAMPER-RESISTANT PACKAGE FEATURES FOR YOUR PROTECTION:
- The carton has been sealed at the factory with a clear overwrap printed with "safety sealed."
- Each tablet is encased in a clear plastic cell with a foil back.
- The name SINE-OFF appears on each tablet (see product illustration on front of carton).
- **DO NOT USE THIS PRODUCT IF ANY OF THESE TAMPER-RESIST-ANT FEATURES ARE MISSING OR BROKEN. IF YOU HAVE ANY QUESTIONS, PLEASE CALL 1-800-543-3434 TOLL FREE.**

Warning: Children and teenagers should not use this medicine for chicken pox or flu symptoms before a doctor is consulted about Reye syndrome, a rare but serious illness reported to be associated with aspirin. Do not exceed recommended dosage. If symptoms do not improve within 7 days, consult a physician before continuing use. Individuals being treated for depression, high blood pressure, asthma, heart disease, diabetes, thyroid disease, glaucoma or enlarged prostate should use only as directed by a physician. Do not take this product if you are taking another medication containing phenylpropanolamine. □ Avoid alcoholic beverages while taking this product. Do not drive or operate heavy machinery as this preparation may cause drowsiness. □ Stop use if dizziness, sleeplessness or nervousness occurs. □ May cause excitability, especially in children. Keep this and all drugs out of reach of children. In case of accidental overdose, seek professional assistance or contact a poison control center immediately. As with any drug, if you are pregnant or nursing a baby, seek the advice of a health professional before using this product.
Store at controlled room temperature (59°–86°F.).

Formula: Active Ingredients: Chlorpheniramine Maleate 2 mg.; Phenylpropanolamine Hydrochloride 12.5 mg. Aspirin 325 mg. **Inactive Ingredients (listed for individuals with specific allergies):** Acacia, Calcium Sulfate, D&C Yellow 10, Ethylcellulose, FD&C Yellow 6 (Sunset Yellow) as a color additive, Gelatin, Guar Gum, Polysorbate 80, Silicon Dioxide, Starch, Sucrose, Titanium Dioxide, and trace amounts of other inactive ingredients.

How Supplied: Consumer packages of 24, 48 and 100 tablets.

Note: There are other SINE-OFF products. Make sure this is the one you are interested in.

Also Available: SINE-OFF® Maximum Strength Allergy/Sinus Formula Caplets 24's. SINE-OFF® Maximum Strength No Drowsiness Formula Caplets 24's.
Shown in Product Identification Section, page 430

TELDRIN®
Chlorpheniramine Maleate
Timed-Release Allergy Capsules
Maximum Strength 12 mg.

Product Information: Hay fever and allergies are caused by grass and tree pollen, dust and pollution. TELDRIN provides up to 12 hours of relief from hay fever/upper respiratory allergy symptoms: sneezing, runny nose, itchy, watery eyes. TELDRIN is formulated to release some medication initially and the rest gradually over a prolonged period.

Directions: Adults and children over 12: Just one capsule in the morning, and one in the evening. Do not give to children under 12 without the advice and consent of a physician. Not to exceed 24 mg. (2 capsules) in 24 hours.

TAMPER-RESISTANT PACKAGING FEATURES FOR YOUR PROTECTION:
- The carton is protected by a clear overwrap printed with "safety sealed"; do not use if overwrap is missing or broken.
- Each capsule is encased in a plastic cell with a foil back; do not use if the cell or foil is broken.
- Each TELDRIN capsule is protected by a green PERMA-SEAL™ band which bonds the two capsule halves together; do not use if capsule or band is broken.
- A package insert is provided for information on tamper-resistant packaging.

Warning: Do not take this product if you have asthma, glaucoma, or difficulty in urination due to enlargement of the prostate gland, except under the advice and supervision of a physician. Do not drive or operate heavy machinery. May cause drowsiness. Avoid alcoholic beverages while taking this product. May cause excitability, especially in children. Keep this and all drugs out of the reach of children. In case of accidental overdose, seek professional assistance or contact a poison control center immediately. As with any drug, if you are pregnant or nursing a baby, seek the advice of a health professional before using this product.

Formula: Active Ingredient: Each capsule contains Chlorpheniramine Maleate, 12 mg. **Inactive Ingredients (listed for individuals with specific allergies):** Benzyl Alcohol, Cetylpyridinium Chloride, D&C Red 33, Ethylcellulose, FD&C Green 3, Red 3, Red 40, Yellow 6 (Sunset Yellow) as a color additive, Gelatin, Hydrogenated Castor Oil, Silicon Dioxide, Sodium Lauryl Sulfate, Starch, Sucrose, and trace amounts of other inactive ingredients.

Store at controlled room temperature (59°–86°F.).

How Supplied: Maximum Strength 12 mg. Timed-Release capsules in packages of 12, 24 and 48 capsules.
Shown in Product Identification Section, page 430

Continued on next page

SmithKline Consumer—Cont.

TROPH–IRON®
Vitamins B₁, B₁₂ and Iron

Indications: For deficiencies of vitamins B₁, B₁₂ and iron.

Directions: Liquid—One teaspoonful daily, or as directed by physician. While its effectiveness is in no way affected, TROPH-IRON Liquid may darken as it ages.

TAMPER-RESISTANT PACKAGE FEATURE: Sealed, imprinted bottle cap; do not use if broken.

Warning: The treatment of any anemic condition should be under the advice and supervision of a physician. Since oral iron products interfere with absorption of oral tetracycline antibiotics, these products should not be taken within two hours of each other.
Iron-containing medications may occasionally cause gastrointestinal discomfort, such as nausea, constipation or diarrhea.
Keep this and all drugs out of reach of children. In case of accidental overdose, seek professional assistance or contact a poison control center immediately.
As with any drug, if you are pregnant or nursing a baby, seek the advice of a health professional before using this product.
Store at room temperature (59°–86°F).

Formula: Each 5 ml. (1 teaspoonful) contains Thiamine Hydrochloride (vitamin B₁), 10 mg.; Cyanocobalamin (vitamin B₁₂), 25 mcg.; Iron, 20 mg., present as soluble ferric pyrophosphate. **Inactive Ingredients (listed for individuals with specific allergies):** Citric Acid, FD&C Red 40, Flavor, Glucose, Glycerin, Methyl and Propyl Paraben, Saccharin Sodium, Sodium Citrate, Purified Water.

How Supplied: Liquid—in 4 fl. oz. (118 ml) bottles.
Shown in Product Identification Section, page 430

TROPHITE®
Vitamins B₁ and B₁₂

Indications: For deficiencies of vitamins B₁ and B₁₂.

Directions: One 5 ml. teaspoonful or one tablet daily—or as directed by physician.

Important: Dispense liquid only in original bottle or an amber bottle. This product is light-sensitive. Never dispense in a flint, green, or blue bottle.
Trophite Liquid may be mixed with water, milk, or fruit or vegetable juices immediately before taking.
Store at controlled room temperature (59°–86°F).

TAMPER-RESISTANT PACKAGE FEATURE: Liquid—Sealed, imprinted bottle cap; do not use if broken.
Tablets—Bottle has imprinted seal under cap; do not use if broken.

Warning: Keep this and all drugs out of reach of children. In case of accidental overdose, seek professional assistance or contact a poison control center immediately.
As with any drug, if you are pregnant or nursing a baby, seek the advice of a health professional before using this product.

Formula: Each 5 ml. (1 teaspoonful) and each tablet contains Thiamine Hydrochloride (vitamin B₁), 10 mg.; and Cyanocobalamin (vitamin B₁₂), 25 mcg. **Inactive Ingredients (listed for individuals with specific allergies):** LIQUID—D&C Red 33, Yellow 10, Dextrose, FD&C Blue 1, Flavor, Glycerin, Methyl and Propyl Paraben, Sodium Tartrate, Tartaric Acid, Purified Water. TABLETS—Calcium Sulfate, FD&C Red 3, Yellow 6 (Sunset Yellow) as a color additive, Gelatin, Magnesium Stearate, Mannitol, Mineral Oil, Starch, Tartaric Acid.

How Supplied: Liquid—4 fl. oz. (118 ml.) bottles. Tablets—bottles of 50.
Shown in Product Identification Section, page 430

E. R. Squibb & Sons, Inc.
GENERAL OFFICES
P.O. BOX 4000
PRINCETON, NJ 08540

PROTO–CHOL®
Natural Fish Oil Gelcaps (1000 mg)

PROTO-CHOL gelcaps are one-piece hermetically sealed soft elastic capsules.
Each PROTO-CHOL gelcap contains 1 gram triglyceride marine lipid concentrate, a dietary source of omega-3 fatty acids [180 mg eicosapentaenoic acid (EPA) and 120 mg docosahexaenoic acid (DHA)].

NUTRITIONAL INFORMATION PER SERVING:

Serving Size	2 gelcaps
Servings per container	30 or 45
Calories	20
Protein	less than 1 gram
Carbohydrates	less than 1 gram
Fat*	2 grams
(90% of calories from fat)	
Polyunsaturated	1 gram
Saturated	less than 1 gram
Cholesterol-Free*	less than 2 mg
Sodium	0

Percentage of US Recommended Daily Allowances:
Contains less than 2% of the US RDA of protein, vitamin A, vitamin C, thiamine, riboflavin, niacin, calcium and iron.
*Information on fat and cholesterol content is provided for individuals who, on the advice of their physicians, are modifying their total dietary intake of fat and cholesterol.

Ingredients: Fish oils, gelatin, glycerin, and d-alpha tocopherol (Vitamin E) as an antioxidant.
SUGGESTED USE: As a convenient dietary source of EPA and DHA, 1 or 2 gelcaps with each meal.

The materials in this product are derived from all natural sources.
Gelcaps contain no sugar, starch, wax, artificial colors or flavors, or preservatives. Natural color of product can range from light gold to amber.

How Supplied: Bottles of 60 and 90.

Storage: Store at room temperature; avoid excessive heat. Keep tightly closed. (C0744)
Shown in Product Identification Section, page 430

PROTO–CHOL® Mini-Caps™
Natural Fish Oil Gelcaps (500 mg)

PROTO-CHOL **Mini-Caps** are one-piece hermetically sealed soft elastic capsules. Each PROTO-CHOL **Mini-Cap** contains 500 mg triglyceride marine lipid concentrate, a dietary source of omega-3 fatty acids [90 mg eicosapentaenoic acid (EPA) and 60 mg docosahexaenoic acid (DHA)].

NUTRITIONAL INFORMATION PER SERVING:

Serving Size	4 **Mini-Caps**
Servings per container	18
Calories	20
Protein	less than 1 gram
Carbohydrates	less than 1 gram
Fat*	2 grams
(90% of calories from fat)	
Polyunsaturated	1 gram
Saturated	less than 1 gram
Cholesterol-Free*	less than 2 mg
Sodium	0

Percentage of US Recommended Daily Allowances:
Contains less than 2% of the US RDA of protein, vitamin A, vitamin C, thiamine, riboflavin, niacin, calcium and iron.
*Information on fat and cholesterol content is provided for individuals who, on the advice of their physicians, are modifying their total dietary intake of fat and cholesterol. **PROTO-CHOL is cholesterol free (less than 0.5 mg per mini-cap).**

Ingredients: Fish oils, gelatin, glycerin, and d-alpha tocopherol (Vitamin E) as an antioxidant.
SUGGESTED USE: As a convenient dietary source of EPA and DHA, 2 to 4 **Mini-Caps** with each meal.
The materials in this product are derived from all natural sources.
Gelcaps contain no sugar, starch, wax, artificial colors or flavors, or preservatives. Natural color of product can range from light gold to amber.

How Supplied: Bottles of 75.

Storage: Store at room temperature; avoid excessive heat. Keep tightly closed. (C0733)
Shown in Product Identification Section, page 430

THERAGRAN JR.®
Children's Chewable Sugar Free* Vitamin Formula

	Percent US RDA** Ages 4–12	
Vitamin A (as Palmitate)	5,000 IU	100
Vitamin D (Ergocalciferol)	400 IU	100

Vitamin E	30 IU	100
(dl-α-Tocopheryl Acetate)		
Vitamin C	60 mg	100
(as Sodium Ascorbate and Ascorbic Acid)		
Folic Acid	0.4 mg	100
Vitamin B₁	1.5 mg	100
(Thiamine Mononitrate)		
Vitamin B₂	1.7 mg	100
(Riboflavin)		
Niacin	20 mg	100
(as Niacinamide)		
Vitamin B₆	2 mg	100
(Pyridoxine Hydrochloride)		
Vitamin B₁₂	6 mcg	100
(Cyanocobalamin)		

*Does not promote tooth decay
**US Recommended Daily Allowance

Usage: Chew one tablet daily

How Supplied: Bottle of 75 tablets.

Storage: Store at room temperature; avoid excessive heat; keep tightly closed. (C0578)

Shown in Product Identification Section, page 430

THERAGRAN JR.®
Children's Chewable Sugar Free*
Vitamin Formula
with Extra Vitamin C

		Percent US RDA** Ages 4–12
Vitamin A	5,000 IU	100
(as Palmitate)		
Vitamin D	400 IU	100
(Ergocalciferol)		
Vitamin E	30 IU	100
(dl-α- Tocopheryl Acetate)		
Vitamin C	250 mg	417
(as Sodium Ascorbate and Ascorbic Acid)		
Folic Acid	0.4 mg	100
Vitamin B₁	1.5 mg	100
(Thiamine Mononitrate)		
Vitamin B₂	1.7 mg	100
(Riboflavin)		
Niacin	20 mg	100
(as Niacinamide)		
Vitamin B₆	2 mg	100
(as Pyridoxine Hydrochloride)		
Vitamin B₁₂	6 mcg	100
(Cyanocobalamin)		

*Does not promote tooth decay
**US Recommended Daily Allowance

Usage: Chew one tablet daily

How Supplied: Bottle of 75 tablets.
Storage: Store at room temperature; avoid excessive heat; keep tightly closed. (C0579)

Shown in Product Identification Section, page 430

THERAGRAN JR.®
Children's Chewable Sugar Free*
Vitamin Formula
With Iron

		Percent US RDA** Ages 4–12
Vitamin A	5,000 IU	100
(as Palmitate)		
Vitamin D	400 IU	100
(Ergocalciferol)		
Vitamin E	30 IU	100
(dl-α-Tocopheryl Acetate)		

Vitamin C	60 mg	100
(as Sodium Ascorbate and Ascorbic Acid)		
Folic Acid	0.4 mg	100
Vitamin B₁	1.5 mg	100
(Thiamine Mononitrate)		
Vitamin B₂	1.7 mg	100
(Riboflavin)		
Niacin	20 mg	100
(as Niacinamide)		
Vitamin B₆	2 mg	100
(Pyridoxine Hydrochloride)		
Vitamin B₁₂	6 mcg	100
(Cyanocobalamin)		
Iron	18 mg	100
(as Ferrous Fumarate)		

* Does not promote tooth decay
**US Recommended Daily Allowance

Usage: Chew one tablet daily

How Supplied: Bottle of 75 tablets.

Storage: Store at room temperature; avoid excessive heat; keep tightly closed. (C0580)

Shown in Product Identification Section, page 430

THERAGRAN® LIQUID
High Potency Vitamin Supplement

Each 5 ml. teaspoonful contains:

		Percent US RDA*
Vitamin A	10,000 IU	200
Vitamin D	400 IU	100
Vitamin C	200 mg	333
Thiamine	10 mg	667
Riboflavin	10 mg	588
Niacin	100 mg	500
Vitamin B₆	4.1 mg	205
Vitamin B₁₂	5 mcg	83
Pantothenic Acid	21.4 mg	214

*US Recommended Daily Allowance

Ingredients: water, sugar, glycerin, propylene glycol, sodium ascorbate, niacinamide, polysorbate 80, ascorbic acid, carboxymethylcellulose sodium, d-panthenol, riboflavin-5-phosphate sodium, thiamine hydrochloride, vitamin A palmitate, pyridoxine hydrochloride, (sodium benzoate and methylparaben as preservatives), ferric ammonium citrate, artificial and natural flavors, cholecalciferol, cyanocobalamin

Usage: For 12 year olds and older—1 teaspoonful daily.

How Supplied: In bottles of 4 fl. oz.

Storage: Store at room temperature; avoid excessive heat. (C0262D)

Shown in Product Identification Section, page 430

ADVANCED FORMULA
THERAGRAN® TABLETS
(High Potency Multivitamin Formula)

Each FILMLOK® tablet contains:		Percent US RDA*
Vitamin A	5,000 IU	100
Beta Carotene	2500 IU	**
Vitamin C	120 mg	200
Vitamin D	400 IU	100
Vitamin B₁	3 mg	200
(Thiamine)		

Vitamin B₂	3.4 mg	200
(Riboflavin)		
Niacin	30 mg	150
Vitamin B₆	3 mg	150
Vitamin B₁₂	9 mcg	150
Vitamin E	30 IU	100
Folic Acid	0.4 mg	100
Pantothenic Acid	10 mg	100
Biotin	15 mcg	5

*US Recommended Daily Allowance (age 12 and older)
**US RDA not established

Ingredients: Ascorbic Acid, Lactose, Gelatin, Sucrose, Microcrystalline Cellulose, dl-alpha Tocopheryl Acetate, Niacinamide, Starch, Sodium Caseinate, Calcium Pantothenate, Hydroxypropyl Methylcellulose, Hydrogenated Coconut Oil, Vitamin A Palmitate, Pyridoxine Hydrochloride, Silicon Dioxide, Riboflavin, Magnesium Stearate, Thiamine Mononitrate, Povidone, Polyethylene Glycol, Triacetin, Beta Carotene, Stearic Acid, Titanium Dioxide, Annatto Powder, Red 40, Folic Acid, Biotin, Ergocalciferol, Cyanocobalamin.

Usage: 1 tablet daily.

How Supplied: Bottles of 1000; Packs of 30, 100, and 180; and Unimatic® cartons of 100.

Storage: Store at room temperature; avoid excessive heat; keep tightly closed. FILMLOK® is an E.R. Squibb & Sons, Inc. trademark for veneer-coated tablets. UNIMATIC® is a trademark of E.R. Squibb & Sons, Inc.

Shown in Product Identification Section, page 430

ADVANCED FORMULA
THERAGRAN-M® TABLETS
(High Potency Multivitamin Formula with Minerals)

Each FILMLOK® tablet contains:

VITAMINS		Percent US RDA*
Vitamin A	5000 IU	100
Beta Carotene	2500 IU	**
Vitamin C	120 mg	200
Vitamin D	400 IU	100
Vitamin B₁	3 mg	200
(Thiamine)		
Vitamin B₂	3.4 mg	200
(Riboflavin)		
Niacin	30 mg	150
Vitamin B₆	3 mg	150
Vitamin B₁₂	9 mcg	150
Vitamin E	30 IU	100
Folic Acid	0.4 mg	100
Pantothenic Acid	10 mg	100
Biotin	15 mcg	5
MINERALS		
Iodine	150 mcg	100
Iron	27 mg	150
Magnesium	100 mg	25
Copper	2 mg	100
Zinc	15 mg	100
Manganese	5 mg	**
Calcium	40 mg	4
Selenium	10 mcg	**
Chromium	15 mcg	**
Molybdenum	15 mcg	**
Phosphorus	31 mg	3

Continued on next page

Squibb—Cont.

ELECTROLYTES

Potassium	7.5 mg	**
Chloride	7.5 mg	**

*US Recommended Daily Allowance (age 12 and older)
**US RDA not established

Ingredients: Dibasic Calcium Phosphate, Magnesium Oxide, Lactose, Ascorbic Acid, Ferrous Fumarate, Gelatin, Sucrose, dl-alpha Tocopheryl Acetate, Crospovidone, Niacinamide, Starch, Zinc Oxide, Povidone, Manganese Sulfate, Hydroxypropyl Methylcellulose, Potassium Chloride, Sodium Caseinate, Calcium Pantothenate, Hydrogenated Coconut Oil, Silicon Dioxide, Cupric Sulfate, Magnesium Stearate, Vitamin A Palmitate, Pyridoxine Hydrochloride, Stearic Acid, Riboflavin, Thiamine Mononitrate, Polyethylene Glycol, Triacetin, Beta Carotene, Red 40, Titanium Dioxide, Potassium Citrate, Folic Acid, Potassium Iodide, Blue 2, Chromic Chloride, Sodium Molybdate, Sodium Selenate, Biotin, Erogocalciferol, Cyanocobalamin.

Usage: 1 tablet daily.

How Supplied: Bottles of 1000; Packs of 30, 60, 100, and 180; and Unimatic® cartons of 100.
Storage: Store at room temperature; avoid excessive heat; keep tightly closed.
FILMLOK® is an E.R. Squibb & Sons, Inc. trademark for veneer-coated tablets.
UNIMATIC® is a trademark of E.R. Squibb & Sons, Inc.

Shown in Product Identification Section, page 430

THERAGRAN® STRESS FORMULA
High Potency Multivitamin Formula with Iron and Biotin

Each FILMLOK® tablet contains:		Percent US RDA*
Vitamin E (dl-α- Tocopheryl Acetate)	30 IU	100
Vitamin C (Ascorbic Acid)	600 mg	1000
B VITAMINS		
Folic Acid	400 mcg	100
Vitamin B$_1$ (as Thiamine Mononitrate)	15 mg	1000
Vitamin B$_2$ (Riboflavin)	15 mg	882
Niacin (as Niacinamide)	100 mg	500
Vitamin B$_6$ (as Pyridoxine Hydrochloride)	25 mg	1250
Vitamin B$_{12}$ (Cyanocobalamin)	12 mcg	200
Biotin	45 mcg	15
Pantothenic Acid (as Calcium Pantothenate)	20 mg	200
Iron (as Ferrous Fumarate)	27 mg	150

*US Recommended Daily Allowance for Adults

Usage: For adults—1 tablet daily or as directed by physician.

How Supplied: Bottles of 75.
Storage: Store at room temperature; avoid excessive heat.

FILMLOK® is a Squibb trademark for veneer-coated tablets.
(C0584)

Shown in Product Identification Section, page 430

Stellar Pharmacal Corp.
**Div./Star Pharmaceuticals, Inc.
1990 N.W. 44TH STREET
POMPANO BEACH, FL
33064-1278**

STAR-OTIC®
**Antibacterial, Antifungal, Nonaqueous Ear Solution
For Prevention of "Swimmer's Ear"**

Active Ingredients: Acetic acid nonaqueous, Burow's solution, Boric acid, in a propylene glycol vehicle, with an acid pH and a low surface tension.

Indications: For the prevention of otitis externa, commonly called "Swimmer's Ear".

Actions: Star-Otic is antibacterial, antifungal, hydrophilic, has an acid pH and a low surface tension. Acetic acid and boric acid inhibit the rapid multiplication of microorganisms and help maintain the lining mantle of the ear canal in its normal acid state. Burow's solution (aluminum acetate) is a mild astringent. Propylene glycol reduces moisture in the ear canal.

Warning: Do not use in ear if tympanic membrane (ear drum) is perforated or punctured.

Symptoms and Treatment of Overdosage: Discontinue use if undue irritation or sensitivity occurs.

Dosage and Administration: Adults and Children: For the prevention of otitis externa (Swimmer's Ear). In susceptible persons, instill 2–3 drops of Star-Otic in each ear before and after swimming or bathing, or as directed by physician.

Professional Labeling: Same as those outlined under Indications.

How Supplied: Available in ½ oz measured drop, safety tip, plastic bottle.
Shown in Product Identification Section, page 431

EDUCATIONAL MATERIAL

First Aid Prevention for Swimmer's Ear
Public health information on cause and care of preventing swimmer's ear.
Star-Otic Patient Instruction Pads
Instructions for patients on use of Star-Otic to prevent swimmer's ear.

Products are cross-indexed by generic and chemical names in the
YELLOW SECTION

Stuart Pharmaceuticals
**Div. of ICI Americas Inc.
WILMINGTON, DE 19897**

ALternaGEL®
[al-tern 'a-jel]
**Liquid
High-Potency Aluminum Hydroxide Antacid**

Description: ALternaGEL is available as a white, pleasant-tasting, high-potency aluminum hydroxide liquid antacid.

Ingredients: Each 5 mL teaspoonful contains: Active: 600 mg aluminum hydroxide (equivalent to dried gel, USP) providing 16 milliequivalents (mEq) of acid-neutralizing capacity (ANC), and less than 2.5 mg (0.109 mEq) of sodium and no sugar. Inactive: butylparaben, flavors, propylparaben, purified water, simethicone, and other ingredients.

Indications: ALternaGEL is indicated for the symptomatic relief of hyperacidity associated with peptic ulcer, gastritis, peptic esophagitis, gastric hyperacidity, hiatal hernia, and heartburn.
ALternaGEL will be of special value to those patients for whom magnesium-containing antacids are undesirable, such as patients with renal insufficiency, patients requiring control of attendant G.I. complications resulting from steroid or other drug therapy, and patients experiencing the laxation which may result from magnesium or combination antacid regimens.

Directions: One to two teaspoonfuls, as needed, between meals and at bedtime, or as directed by a physician: May be followed by a sip of water if desired. Concentrated product. Shake well before using. Keep tightly closed.

Warnings: As with all medications, ALternaGEL should be kept out of the reach of children. ALternaGEL may cause constipation.
Except under the advice and supervision of a physician: do not take more than 18 teaspoonfuls in a 24-hour period, or use the maximum dose of ALternaGEL for more than two weeks.

Drug Interaction Precaution: ALternaGEL should not be taken concurrently with an antibiotic containing any form of tetracycline.

How Supplied: ALternaGEL is available in bottles of 12 fluid ounces and 5 fluid ounces, and 1 fluid ounce hospital unit doses. NDC 0038-0860.
Shown in Product Identification Section, page 431

DIALOSE® Capsules
[di 'a-lose]
Stool Softener Laxative

Description: DIALOSE is a sodium-free, nonhabit forming, stool softener containing docusate potassium in capsules of 100 mg.
The docusate in DIALOSE is a highly efficient surfactant which facilitates ab-

sorption of water by the stool to form a soft, easily evacuated mass. Unlike stimulant laxatives, DIALOSE does not interfere with normal peristalsis, neither does it cause griping nor sensations of urgency.

Ingredients: Each capsule contains: Active: docusate potassium. Inactive: Blue 1, gelatin, lactose, magnesium stearate, Red 28, Red 40, silicon dioxide, titanium dioxide.

Indications: DIALOSE is an effective aid to soften or prevent formation of hard stools in a wide range of conditions that may lead to constipation. DIALOSE helps to eliminate straining associated with obstetric, geriatric, cardiac, surgical, anorectal, or proctologic conditions. In cases of mild constipation, the fecal softening action of DIALOSE can prevent constipation from progressing and relieve painful defecation.

Directions: *Adults:* Adjust dosage as needed, one capsule one to three times daily. *Children:* 6 years and over—One capsule at bedtime, or as directed by physician. *Children:* under 6 years—As directed by physician. It is helpful to increase the daily intake of fluids by taking a glass of water with each dose.

Warnings: As with any drug, if you are pregnant or nursing a baby, seek the advice of a health professional before using this product. Keep out of the reach of children.

How Supplied: Bottles of 36 and 100 pink capsules, identified "STUART 470". Also available in 100 capsule unit dose boxes (10 strips of 10 capsules each). NDC 0038-0470
Shown in Product Identification Section, page 431

DIALOSE® PLUS Capsules
[di 'a-lose Plus]
Stool Softener/Stimulant Laxative

Description: DIALOSE PLUS provides a sodium-free formulation of docusate potassium in capsules of 100 mg and casanthranol, 30 mg.

Ingredients: Each capsule contains: Active: docusate potassium, casanthranol. Inactive: gelatin, lactose, magnesium stearate, Red 33, silicon dioxide, titanium dioxide, Yellow 10.

Indications: DIALOSE PLUS is indicated for the treatment of constipation characterized by lack of moisture in the intestinal contents, resulting in hardness of stool and decreased intestinal motility. DIALOSE PLUS combines the advantages of the stool softener, docusate potassium, with the peristaltic activating effect of casanthranol.

Directions: *Adults:* Initially, one capsule two times a day. *Children:* As directed by physician. When adequate bowel function is restored, the dose may be adjusted to meet individual needs. It is helpful to increase the daily intake of fluids by taking a glass of water with each dose.

Warnings: As with any drug, if you are pregnant or nursing a baby, seek the advice of a health professional before using this product. And, as with any laxative, DIALOSE PLUS should not be used when abdominal pain, nausea, or vomiting are present. Frequent or prolonged use may result in dependence on laxatives. Keep out of the reach of children.

How Supplied: Bottles of 36, 100, and 500 yellow capsules, identified "STUART 475". Also available in 100 capsule unit dose boxes (10 strips of 10 capsules each). NDC 0038-0475
Shown in Product Identification Section, page 431

EFFER-SYLLIUM®
[ef 'fer-sil 'lium]
Natural Fiber Bulking Agent

Description: EFFER-SYLLIUM is a tan, granular powder. Each rounded teaspoonful, or individual packet (7 g) contains psyllium hydrocolloid, 3 g.

Ingredients: Active: psyllium hydrocolloid. Inactive: citric acid, ethyl vanillin, lemon and lime flavors, potassium bicarbonate, potassium citrate, saccharin calcium, starch, sucrose. EFFER-SYLLIUM contains less than 5 mg sodium per rounded teaspoonful and is considered dietetically sodium free.

Indications: EFFER-SYLLIUM is indicated to restore normal bowel habits in chronic constipation, to promote normal elimination in irritable bowel syndrome, and to ease passage of stools in presence of anorectal disorders. EFFER-SYLLIUM produces a soft, lubricating bulk which promotes natural elimination.
EFFER-SYLLIUM is not a one-dose, fast-acting bowel regulator. Administration for several days may be needed to establish regularity.

Directions:
Adults: One rounded teaspoonful, or one packet, in a glass of water one to three times a day, or as directed by physician. *Children, 6 years and over:* One level teaspoonful, or one-half packet (3.5 g) in one-half glass of water at bedtime, or as directed by physician. *Children, under 6 years:* As directed by physician.

Instructions: Pour EFFER-SYLLIUM into a *dry* glass, add water and stir briskly. Drink immediately. To avoid caking, always use a *dry* spoon to remove EFFER-SYLLIUM from its container. Replace cap tightly. Keep in a dry place.

Caution: People sensitive to psyllium powder should avoid inhalation as it may cause an allergic reaction such as wheezing.

Warning: As with all medications, keep out of the reach of children.

How Supplied: Bottles of 9 oz and 16 oz, and individual convenience packets (7 g each) packaged in boxes of 12 and 24. NDC 0038-0440
Shown in Product Identification Section, page 431

FERANCEE®
[fer 'an-see]
Chewable Hematinic

Two Tablets Daily Provide:

	US RDA*	
Iron	744%	134 mg
Vitamin C	500%	300 mg

*Percentage of US Recommended Daily Allowances for adults and children 4 or more years of age.

Ingredients: Active: ferrous fumarate, sodium ascorbate, ascorbic acid. Inactive: confectioner's sugar, flavors, magnesium stearate, mannitol, povidone, saccharin calcium, starch, Yellow 5 (tartrazine), Yellow 6.

Indications: A pleasant-tasting hematinic for iron deficiency anemias, well-tolerated FERANCEE is particularly useful when chronic blood loss, onset of menses, or pregnancy create additional demands for iron supplementation. Available information indicates a low incidence of staining of the teeth by ferrous fumarate, alone or in combination with ascorbic acid. The peach-cherry flavored chewable tablets dissolve quickly in the mouth and may be either chewed or swallowed.

Directions:
Adults: Two tablets daily, or as directed by physician.
Chidren over 6 years of age: One tablet daily, or as directed by physician.
Children under 6 years of age: As directed by physician.

Warnings: As with any drug, if you are pregnant or nursing a baby, seek the advice of a health professional before using this product. Keep out of the reach of children. In case of accidental overdose, seek professional assistance or contact a Poison Control Center immediately.

How Supplied: Bottles of 100 brown and yellow, two-layer tablets identified "STUART 650" on brown layer. A child-resistant cap is standard on each bottle as a safeguard against accidental ingestion by children. Keep in a dry place. Replace cap tightly. NDC 0038-0650.

FERANCEE®–HP Tablets
[fer-an-see hp]
High Potency Hematinic

One Tablet Daily Provides:

	US RDA*	
Iron	611%	110 mg
Vitamin C	1000%	600 mg

*Percentage of US Recommended Daily Allowances for adults and children 4 or more years of age.

Ingredients: Active: ferrous fumarate, sodium ascorbate, ascorbic acid. Inactive: flavor, hydrogenated vegetable oil, microcrystalline cellulose, povidone, Red 40, and other ingredients.

Indications: FERANCEE-HP is a high potency formulation of iron and vitamin C and is intended for use as either:

Continued on next page

Stuart—Cont.

(1) a maintenance hematinic for those patients needing a daily iron supplement to maintain normal hemoglobin levels, or

(2) intensive therapy for the acute and/or severe iron deficiency anemia where a high intake of elemental iron is required.

The use of well-tolerated ferrous fumarate provides high levels of elemental iron with a low incidence of gastric distress. The inclusion of 600 mg of vitamin C per tablet serves to maintain more of the iron in the absorbable ferrous state.

Precautions: Because FERANCEE-HP contains 110 mg of elemental iron per tablet, it is recommended that its use be limited to adults, ie over 12 years of age.

Directions: One tablet per day after a meal or as directed by a physician. Should be sufficient to maintain normal hemoglobin levels in most patients with a history of recurring iron deficiency anemia. Not recommended for children under 12 years of age.

For acute and/or severe iron deficiency anemia, two or three tablets per day taken one tablet per dose after meals. (Each tablet provides 110 mg elemental iron).

Warnings: As with all medications, keep out of the reach of children. In case of accidental overdose, seek professional assistance or contact a Poison Control Center immediately.

How Supplied: FERANCEE-HP is supplied in bottles of 60 red, film coated, oval shaped tablets.
NDC 0038-0863.
Note: A child-resistant safety cap is standard on each bottle of 60 tablets as a safeguard against accidental ingestion by children.

Shown in Product Identification Section, page 431

HIBICLENS® Antiseptic Antimicrobial
[*hibi-klenz*]
Skin Cleanser
(chlorhexidine gluconate)

Description: HIBICLENS is an antiseptic antimicrobial skin cleanser possessing bactericidal activities. HIBICLENS contains 4% w/v HIBITANE® (chlorhexidine gluconate), a chemically unique hexamethylenebis biguanide with inactive ingredients: fragrance, isopropyl alcohol 4%, purified water, Red 40, and other ingredients, in a mild, sudsing base adjusted to pH 5.0–6.5 for optimal activity and stability as well as compatability with the normal pH of the skin.

Action: HIBICLENS is bactericidal on contact. It has antiseptic activity and a persistent antimicrobial effect with rapid bactericidal activity against a wide range of microorganisms, including gram-positive bacteria, and gram-negative bacteria such as *Pseudomonas aeruginosa.* The effectiveness of HIBICLENS is not significantly reduced by the presence of organic matter, such as blood.[1]

In a study[2] simulating surgical use, the immediate bactericidal effect of HIBICLENS after a single six-minute scrub resulted in a 99.9% reduction in resident bacterial flora, with a reduction of 99.98% after the eleventh scrub. Reductions on surgically gloved hands were maintained over the six-hour test period.

HIBICLENS displays persistent antimicrobial action. In one study[2], 93% of a radiolabeled formulation of HIBICLENS remained present on uncovered skin after five hours.

HIBICLENS prevents skin infection thereby reducing the risk of cross-infection.

Indications: HIBICLENS is indicated for use as a surgical scrub, as a health-care personnel handwash, for patient preoperative showering and bathing, as a patient preoperative skin preparation, and as a skin wound cleanser and general skin cleanser.

Safety: The extensive use of chlorhexidine gluconate for over 20 years outside the United States has produced no evidence of absorption of the compound through intact skin. The potential for producing skin reactions is extremely low. HIBICLENS can be used many times a day without causing irritation, dryness, or discomfort. Experimental studies indicate that when used for cleaning superficial wounds, HIBICLENS will neither cause additional tissue injury nor delay healing.

Warnings: FOR EXTERNAL USE ONLY. KEEP OUT OF EYES, EARS AND MOUTH. HIBICLENS SHOULD NOT BE USED AS A PREOPERATIVE SKIN PREPARATION OF THE FACE OR HEAD. MISUSE OF HIBICLENS HAS BEEN REPORTED TO CAUSE SERIOUS AND PERMANENT EYE INJURY WHEN IT HAS BEEN PERMITTED TO ENTER AND REMAIN IN THE EYE DURING SURGICAL PROCEDURES. IF HIBICLENS SHOULD CONTACT THESE AREAS, RINSE OUT PROMPTLY AND THOROUGHLY WITH WATER. Avoid contact with meninges. HIBICLENS should not be used by persons who have a sensitivity to it or its components. Chlorhexidine gluconate has been reported to cause deafness when instilled in the middle ear through perforated ear drums. Irritation, sensitization and generalized allergic reactions have been reported with chlorhexidine-containing products, especially in the genital areas. If adverse reactions occur, discontinue use immediately and if severe, contact a physician. Keep this and all drugs out of the reach of children. In case of accidental ingestion, seek professional assistance or contact a Poison Control Center immediately.

Accidental ingestion: Chlorhexidine gluconate taken orally is poorly absorbed. Treat with gastric lavage using milk, egg white, gelatin or mild soap. Employ supportive measures as appropriate. Avoid excessive heat (above 104°F).

Directions for Use:
Patient preoperative skin preparation
Apply HIBICLENS liberally to surgical site and swab for at least two minutes. Dry with a sterile towel. Repeat procedure for an additional two minutes and dry with a sterile towel.

Preoperative showering and whole-body bathing
The patient should be instructed to wash the entire body, including the scalp, on two consecutive occasions immediately prior to surgery. Each procedure should consist of two consecutive thorough applications of HIBICLENS followed by thorough rinsing. If the patient's condition allows, showering is recommended for whole-body bathing. The recommended procedure is: Wet the body, including hair. Wash the hair using 25 mL of HIBICLENS and the body with another 25 mL of HIBICLENS. Rinse. Repeat. Rinse thoroughly after second application.

Skin wound and general skin cleansing
Wounds which involve more than the superficial layers of the skin should not be routinely treated with HIBICLENS. HIBICLENS should not be used for repeated general skin cleansing of large body areas except in those patients whose underlying condition makes it necessary to reduce the bacterial population of the skin. To use, thoroughly rinse the area to be cleansed with water. Apply the minimum amount of HIBICLENS necessary to cover the skin or wound area and wash gently. Rinse again thoroughly.

Health-care personnel use
SURGICAL HAND SCRUB
Directions for use of HIBICLENS Liquid: Wet hands and forearms to the elbows with warm water. (Avoid using very cold or very hot water.) Dispense about 5 mL of HIBICLENS into cupped hands. Spread over both hands. Scrub hands and forearms for 3 minutes without adding water, using a brush or sponge. (Avoid using extremely hard-bristled brushes.) While scrubbing, pay particular attention to fingernails, cuticles, and interdigital spaces. (Do not use excessive pressure to produce additional lather.) Rinse thoroughly with warm water. Dispense about 5 mL of HIBICLENS into cupped hands. Wash for an additional 3 minutes. (No need to use brush or sponge.) Then rinse thoroughly. Dry thoroughly.

HAND WASH
Wet hands with water. (Avoid using very cold or very hot water.) Dispense about 5 mL of HIBICLENS into cupped hands. Wash for 15 seconds. (Do not use excessive pressure to produce additional lather.) Rinse thoroughly with warm water. Dry thoroughly.

Directions for use of HIBICLENS® Sponge/Brush: Open package and remove nail cleaner. Wet hands. Use nail cleaner under fingernails and to clean cuticles. Wet hands and forearms to the elbow with warm water. (Avoid using very cold or very hot water.) Wet sponge side of sponge/brush. Squeeze and pump

immediately to work up adequate lather. Apply lather to hands and forearms using *sponge* side of the product. *Start 3 minute scrub* by using the brush side of the product to scrub *only* nails, cuticles, and interdigital areas. Use sponge side for scrubbing hands and forearms. (Avoid using brush on these more sensitive areas.) Rinse thoroughly with warm water. Scrub for an additional 3 minutes *using sponge side* only. To produce additional lather, add a small amount of water and pump the sponge. (While scrubbing, do not use excessive pressure to produce lather—a small amount of lather is all that is required to adequately cleanse skin with HIBICLENS.) Rinse and dry thoroughly, blotting hands and forearms with a soft sterile towel.

Operation	Water Level	Temperature	Time (Min)	Supplies/ 100 lb
Break	Low	180°F	20	1.5 lb oxalic acid
Flush	High	Cold	1	—
Emulsify	Low	160°F	5	18 oz emulsifier
Flush	High	Cold	1	—
Bleach	Low	180°F	20	2 lb alkali builder and 1 lb organic bleach
Rinse	High	Cold	1	—
Antichlor	High	Cold	2	4 oz antichlor
Rinse	High	Cold	1	—
Rinse	High	Cold	1	—
Sour	Low	Cold	4	2 oz rust removing sour

IMPORTANT LAUNDERING ADVICE FOR HOSPITAL STAFF AND OTHER USERS OF ANTISEPTIC PATIENT SKIN PREPARATIONS CONTAINING CHLORHEXIDINE GLUCONATE

Chlorhexidine gluconate is a unique agent that most closely fits the definition of an ideal antimicrobial agent, having (among others) one of the most important characteristics of persistent activity. This persistence is due to chlorhexidine gluconate binding to the protein of the skin and, thus, being available for residual activity over a relatively long period of time.

Chlorhexidine gluconate, however, binds not only to protein of the skin, but also to many fabrics, particularly cotton. Thus, special laundering procedures should be considered when such products contact these fabrics. As a result of such contact, chlorhexidine gluconate may become adsorbed onto the fabric and not be removed by washing. If sufficient available chlorine is present during the washing procedure, a fast brown stain may develop due to a chemical reaction between chlorhexidine gluconate and chlorine.

SUGGESTED LAUNDERING PROCEDURES TO LIMIT STAINING

1. **Not Aging.** Avoid allowing the product to age (set) on unwashed linens.
2. **Flushing and Washing.** A flush operation as the initial step in the wash process is helpful in the laundering of linen exposed to chlorhexidine gluconate. Such flushing is also important in the laundering of linen which contains organic materials such as blood or pus. For best results, warm water flushes (90°–100°F) are recommended. After a number of initial flushings followed by a washing with a low alkaline/nonchlorine detergent, most articles which come in contact with chlorhexidine gluconate should have an acceptable level of whiteness. If a rewash process using bleach is necessary to achieve a greater degree of whiteness, the bleach used should be a nonchlorine bleach.
3. **Not Using Chlorine Bleach.** Modern laundering methods often make the use of chlorine bleach unnecessary. It is worthwhile trying to wash without chlorine to ascertain if the resulting degree of whiteness is acceptable. Omission of chlorine from the laundering process can extend the useful life of cotton articles since oxidizing bleaches such as chlorine may cause some damage to cellulose even when used in low concentration.
4. **Changing to a Peroxide-Type Bleach, Such as Sodium Perborate, Sodium Percarbonate or Hydrogen Peroxide.** This should eliminate the reaction which could occur with the use of chlorine bleaches. If a chlorine bleach must be used, a concentration of less than 7 ppm available chlorine ($1/10$ the normal bleach level) is suggested to minimize possible staining.

A NOTE ON LAUNDERING OF PERSONAL CLOTHING

The laundering procedures set forth above using low alkaline, nonchlorinated laundry detergents are also applicable to laundering of uniforms and lab coats. Commercially available laundry detergents which do not contain chlorine include Borax, Borateem, Dreft, Oxydol, and Ivory Snow. These products, however, will not remove stains previously set into the fabric.

RECLAMATION OF STAINED LINENS

For those linens which previously have been stained due to the chemical reaction between chlorhexidine gluconate and chlorine, the following laundering procedure may be helpful in reducing the visible stain:

[See table above].

How Supplied: *For general handwashing locations:* pocket-size, 15 mL foil Packettes; plastic disposable bottles of 4 oz and 8 oz with dispenser caps; and 16 oz filled globes. *For surgical scrub areas:* disposable, unit-of-use 22 mL impregnated Sponge/Brushes with nail cleaner; plastic disposable bottles of 32 oz and 1 gal. The 32-oz bottle is designed for a special foot-operated wall dispenser. A hand-operated wall dispenser is available for the 16-oz globe. Hand pumps are available for 16 oz, 32 oz, and 1 gal sizes.
NDC 0038-0575 (liquid).
NDC 0038-0577 (sponge/brush).

References:
1. Lowbury EJL, and Lilly HA: The effect of blood on disinfection of surgeons' hands, Brit. J. Surg. 61:19–21 (Jan.) 1974.
2. Peterson AF, Rosenberg A, Alatary SD: Comparative evaluation of surgical scrub preparations, Surg. Gynecol. Obstet. 146:63–65 (Jan.) 1978.

Shown in Product Identification Section, page 431

HIBISTAT®
Germicidal Hand Rinse
HIBISTAT® TOWELETTE
Germicidal Hand Wipe
[hi-bi-stat]
(chlorhexidine gluconate)

Description: HIBISTAT is a germicidal hand rinse which provides rapid bactericidal action and has a persistent antimicrobial effect against a wide range of microorganisms. HIBISTAT is a clear, colorless liquid containing 0.5% w/w HIBITANE® (chlorhexidine gluconate) with inactive ingredients: emollients, isopropyl alcohol 70%, purified water.

Indications: HIBISTAT is indicated for health-care personnel use as a germicidal hand rinse. HIBISTAT is for hand hygiene on physically clean hands. It is used in those situations where hands are physically clean, but in need of degerming, when routine handwashing is not convenient or desirable. HIBISTAT provides rapid germicidal action and has a persistent effect.

HIBISTAT should be used in-between patients and procedures where there are no sinks available or continued return to the sink area is inconvenient. HIBISTAT can be used as an alternative to detergent-based products when hands are physically clean. Also, HIBISTAT is an effective germicidal hand rinse following a soap and water handwash.

Warnings: Flammable. This product is alcohol based. Alcohol is extremely flammable. It should be kept away from flame or devices which may generate an electrical spark.

FOR EXTERNAL USE ONLY. KEEP OUT OF EYES, EARS AND MOUTH. HIBISTAT SHOULD NOT BE USED AS A PREOPERATIVE SKIN PREPARATION OF THE FACE OR HEAD. MISUSE OF CHLORHEXIDINE-CONTAINING PRODUCTS HAS BEEN REPORTED TO CAUSE SERIOUS AND PERMANENT EYE INJURY WHEN IT HAS BEEN PERMITTED TO ENTER AND REMAIN IN THE EYE DURING SURGICAL PROCEDURES. IF HIBISTAT SHOULD CONTACT THESE

Continued on next page

Stuart—Cont.

AREAS, RINSE OUT PROMPTLY AND THOROUGHLY WITH WATER. Avoid contact with meninges. HIBISTAT should not be used by persons who have a sensitivity to it or its components. Chlorhexidine gluconate has been reported to cause deafness when instilled in the middle ear through perforated ear drums. Irritation, sensitization and generalized allergic reactions have been reported with chlorhexidine-containing products, especially in the genital areas. If adverse reactions occur, discontinue use immediately and if severe, contact a physician. Keep this and all drugs out of the reach of children. In case of accidental ingestion, seek professional assistance or contact a Poison Control Center immediately.

Avoid excessive heat (above 104°F).

Accidental ingestion: Chlorhexidine gluconate taken orally is poorly absorbed. Treat with gastric lavage using milk, egg white, gelatin or mild soap avoiding pulmonary aspiration. Do not use apomorphine. Assist respiration if necessary and keep patient warm. Intravenous levulose can accelerate alcohol metabolism. In severe cases, hemodialysis or peritoneal dialysis may be appropriate.

Directions for Use: HIBISTAT Towelette: Rub hands vigorously with the HIBISTAT Towelette for approximately 15 seconds, paying particular attention to nails and interdigital spaces. HIBISTAT dries rapidly in use. No water or towel drying are necessary. The emollients contained in the HIBISTAT Towelette protect the hands from the potential drying effect of alcohol.

HIBISTAT Liquid: Dispense about 5 mL of HIBISTAT into cupped hands and rub vigorously until dry (about 15 seconds), paying particular attention to nails and interdigital spaces. HIBISTAT dries rapidly in use. No water or toweling are necessary. The emollients contained in HIBISTAT protect the hands from the potential drying effect of alcohol.

Laundering: Chlorhexidine gluconate chemically reacts with chlorine to form a brown stain on fabric. Fabric which has come in contact with chlorhexidine gluconate should be rinsed well and washed without the addition of chlorine products. If bleach is desired, only nonchlorine bleach should be used. Full laundering instructions are packed with each case of HIBISTAT. (Please see HIBICLENS for full laundering instructions.)

How Supplied: In plastic disposable bottles of 4 oz and 8 oz with flip-top cap, and in disposable towelettes containing 5 mL, packaged 50 towelettes to a carton.
NDC 0038-0585 (bottles)
NDC 0038-0587 (towelettes)

KASOF® Capsules
[kay 'sof]
High Strength Stool Softener Laxative

Ingredients: Each capsule contains: Active: docusate potassium, 240 mg. Inactive: Blue 1, gelatin, glycerin, methylparaben, polyethylene glycol, propylparaben, purified water, Red 40, sorbitol, Yellow 10.

Indications: KASOF provides a highly efficient wetting action to restore moisture to the bowel, thus softening the stool to prevent straining. The action of KASOF does not interfere with normal peristalsis and generally does not cause griping or extreme sensation of urgency. KASOF is sodium-free, containing a unique potassium formulation, without the problems associated with sodium intake. KASOF is especially valuable for the severely constipated, as well as patients with anorectal disorders, such as hemorrhoids and anal fissures. KASOF is ideal for patients with any condition that can be complicated by straining at stool, for example, cardiac patients. The simple, one-a-day dosage helps assure patient compliance in maintaining normal bowel function.

Directions: Adults: One KASOF capsule daily for several days, or until bowel movements are normal and gentle. It is helpful to increase the daily intake of fluids by drinking a glass of water with each dose.

Store in a closed container, protect from freezing and avoid excessive heat (104°F).

Warnings: As with any drug, if you are pregnant or nursing a baby, seek the advice of a health professional before using this product. Keep out of the reach of children.

How Supplied: KASOF is available in bottles of 30 and 60 brown, gelatin capsules, identified "Stuart 380".
NDC 0038-0380.

Shown in Product Identification Section, page 431

MYLANTA®
[my-lan 'ta]
Liquid and Tablets
Antacid/Anti-Gas

Ingredients: Each chewable tablet or each 5 mL (one teaspoonful) of liquid contains: Active: Aluminum hydroxide (Dried Gel, USP in tablet and equiv. to Dried Gel, USP in liquid) 200 mg, Magnesium hydroxide 200 mg, Simethicone 20 mg. Inactive: Tablets: dextrates, flavors, magnesium stearate, mannitol, sorbitol, starch, Yellow 10. Liquid: butylparaben, carboxymethylcellulose sodium, flavors, hydroxypropyl methylcellulose, microcrystalline cellulose, propylparaben, purified water, sorbitol solution with no added sugar.

Sodium Content: MYLANTA contains an insignificant amount of sodium per daily dose and is considered dietetically sodium free. Typical values are 0.68 mg (0.03 mEq) sodium per 5 mL teaspoonful of liquid and 0.77 mg (0.03 mEq) per tablet.

Acid Neutralizing Capacity: Two teaspoonfuls of MYLANTA liquid will neutralize 25.4 mEq of acid. Two MYLANTA tablets will neutralize 23.0 mEq.

Indications: MYLANTA, a well-balanced combination of two antacids and simethicone, provides consistently dependable relief of symptoms associated with gastric hyperacidity, and mucus-entrapped air or "gas". These indications include:

    Common heartburn (pyrosis)
    Hiatal hernia
    Peptic esophagitis
    Gastritis
    Peptic ulcer

The exceptionally pleasant tasting liquid and soft, easy-to-chew tablets encourage patients' acceptance, thereby minimizing the skipping of prescribed doses. MYLANTA is appropriate whenever there is a need for effective relief of temporary gastric hyperacidity and mucus-entrapped gas.

Directions: *Liquid:* Shake well, 2–4 teaspoonfuls between meals and at bedtime or as directed by a physician. *Tablets:* 2–4 tablets, well chewed, between meals and at bedtime or as directed by a physician.

Warnings: Keep this and all drugs out of the reach of children.

Except under the advice and supervision of a physician: Do not take more than 24 teaspoonfuls or 24 tablets in a 24 hour period or use the maximum dose for more than two weeks. Do not use this product if you have kidney disease. Magnesium hydroxide and other magnesium salts, in the presence of renal insufficiency, may cause central nervous system depression and other symptoms of hypermagnesemia.

Drug Interaction Precaution: Do not use this product for any patient receiving a prescription antibiotic containing any form of tetracycline.

How Supplied: MYLANTA is available as a white, pleasant tasting liquid suspension, and as a two-layer yellow and white chewable tablet, identified on yellow layer "STUART 620". Liquid supplied in 5 oz, 12 oz and 24 oz bottles. Tablets supplied in boxes of individually wrapped 40's and 100's, economy size bottles of 180, consumer convenience pocket packs of 48 and roll packs of 12 tablets each. Also available for hospital use in liquid unit doses of 1 oz, and bottles of 5 oz.
NDC 0038-0610 (liquid). NDC 0038-0620 (tablets).

Shown in Product Identification Section, page 431

MYLANTA®-II
[my-lan 'ta]
Liquid and Tablets
Double Strength Antacid/Anti-Gas

Ingredients: Each chewable tablet or each 5 mL (one teaspoonful) of liquid contains: Active: Aluminum hydroxide

(Dried Gel, USP in tablet and equiv. to Dried Gel, USP in liquid) 400 mg
Magnesium hydroxide 400 mg
Simethicone 40 mg
Tablets: Blue 1, cereal solids, confectioner's sugar, flavors, glycerin, lactose, mannitol, starch, Yellow 10. Liquid: butylparaben, carboxymethylcellulose sodium, flavors, hydroxypropyl methylcellulose, microcrystalline cellulose, potassium citrate, propylparaben, purified water, sorbitol solution with no added sugar.

Sodium Content: MYLANTA-II contains an insignificant amount of sodium per daily dose. Typical values are 1.14 mg (0.05 mEq) sodium per 5 mL teaspoonful of liquid and 1.3 mg (0.06 mEq) per tablet.

Acid Neutralizing Capacity: Two teaspoonfuls of MYLANTA-II liquid will neutralize 50.8 mEq of acid. Two MYLANTA-II tablets will neutralize 46.0 mEq.

Indications: MYLANTA-II is a double strength antacid with an anti-gas ingredient for the relief of heartburn, acid indigestion, sour stomach and accompanying gas. The exceptionally pleasant tasting liquid and soft, easy-to-chew tablets encourage patient acceptance, thereby minimizing the skipping of prescribed doses. MYLANTA-II provides consistently dependable relief of the symptoms of peptic ulcer and other problems related to acid hypersecretion. The high potency of MYLANTA-II is achieved through its concentration of noncalcium antacid ingredients. Thus MYLANTA-II can produce both rapid and long lasting neutralization without the acid rebound associated with calcium carbonate. The balanced formula of aluminum and magnesium hydroxides minimizes undesirable bowel effects. Simethicone is effective for the relief of concomitant distress caused by mucus-entrapped gas and swallowed air.

Directions: Liquid: Shake well, 2–4 teaspoonfuls between meals and at bedtime, or as directed by a physician. Tablets: 2–4 tablets, well-chewed, between meals and at bedtime, or as directed by a physician.
Because patients with peptic ulcer vary greatly in both acid output and gastric emptying time, the amount and schedule of dosages should be varied accordingly.

Warnings: Keep this and all drugs out of the reach of children.
Except under the advice and supervision of a physician: Do not take more than 12 teaspoonfuls or 12 tablets in a 24 hour period or use the maximum dose for more than two weeks. Do not use this product if you have kidney disease. Magnesium hydroxide and other magnesium salts, in the presence of renal insufficiency, may cause central nervous system depression and other symptoms of hypermagnesemia.

Drug Interaction Precaution: Do not use this product for any patient receiving a prescription antibiotic containing any form of tetracycline.

How Supplied: MYLANTA-II is available as a white, pleasant tasting liquid suspension, and a two-layer green and white chewable tablet, identified on green layer "STUART 651". Liquid supplied in 5 oz, 12 oz and 24 oz bottles. Tablets supplied in boxes of 60 individually wrapped chewable tablets and consumer convenience pocket packs of 24. Also available for hospital use in liquid unit dose bottles of 1 oz, and bottles of 5 oz. NDC 0038-0652 (liquid). NDC 0038-0651 (tablets).
Shown in Product Identification Section, page 431

MYLICON® Tablets and Drops
[my'li-con]
Antiflatulent

Ingredients: Each tablet or 0.6 mL of drops contains: Active: simethicone, 40 mg. Inactive: Tablets: calcium silicate, lactose, povidone, saccharin calcium. Drops: carbomer 934P, citric acid, flavors, hydroxypropyl methylcellulose, purified water, Red 3, saccharin calcium, sodium benzoate, sodium citrate.

Indications: For relief of the painful symptoms of excess gas in the digestive tract. Such gas is frequently caused by excessive swallowing of air or by eating foods that disagree. If condition persists consult your physician. MYLICON is a valuable adjunct in the treatment of many conditions in which the retention of gas may be a problem, such as: postoperative gaseous distention, air swallowing, functional dyspepsia, peptic ulcer, spastic or irritable colon, diverticulosis. The defoaming action of MYLICON relieves flatulence by dispersing and preventing the formation of mucus-surrounded gas pockets in the gastrointestinal tract. MYLICON acts in the stomach and intestines to change the surface tension of gas bubbles enabling them to coalesce; thus the gas is freed and is eliminated more easily by belching or passing flatus.
Infants: MYLICON drops are also useful for relief of the painful symptoms of excess gas associated with such conditions as colic, lactose intolerance, or air swallowing.

Directions:
Tablets—One or two tablets four times daily after meals and at bedtime. May also be taken as needed up to 12 tablets daily or as directed by a physician. TABLETS SHOULD BE CHEWED THOROUGHLY.
Drops—Adults and Children 0.6 mL four times daily after meals and at bedtime or as directed by a physician. Shake well before using.
Infants (under 2 years): Initially, 0.3 mL four times daily, after meals and at bedtime, or as directed by a physician. The dosage can also be mixed with 1 oz of cool water, infant formula, or other suitable liquids to ease administration. Dosage should not exceed 12 doses per day.

Warnings: Keep this and all drugs out of the reach of children.

How Supplied: Bottles of 100 and 500 white, scored, chewable tablets, identified front "STUART", reverse "450," and dropper bottles of 30 mL (1 fl oz) pink, pleasant tasting liquid. Also available in 100 tablet unit dose boxes (10 strips of 10 tablets each).
NDC 0038-0450 (tablets).
NDC 0038-0630 (drops).
Shown in Product Identification Section, page 431

MYLICON®-80 Tablets
[my'li-con]
High-Capacity Antiflatulent

Ingredients: Each tablet contains: Active: simethicone, 80 mg. Inactive: flavor, cereal solids, lactose, mannitol, povidone, Red 3, talc.

Indications: For relief of the painful symptoms of excess gas in the digestive tract. Such gas is frequently caused by excessive swallowing of air or by eating foods that disagree. If condition persists, consult your physician. MYLICON-80 is a high capacity antiflatulent for adjunctive treatment of many conditions in which the retention of gas may be a problem, such as the following: air swallowing, functional dyspepsia, postoperative gaseous distention, peptic ulcer, spastic or irritable colon, diverticulosis.
MYLICON-80 has a defoaming action that relieves flatulence by dispersing and preventing the formation of mucus-surrounded gas pockets in the gastrointestinal tract. MYLICON-80 acts in the stomach and intestines to change the surface tension of gas bubbles enabling them to coalesce; thus, the gas is freed and is eliminated more easily by belching or passing flatus.

Directions: One tablet four times daily after meals and at bedtime. May also be taken as needed up to 6 tablets daily or as directed by a physician. TABLETS SHOULD BE CHEWED THOROUGHLY.

Warnings: Keep this and all drugs out of the reach of children.

How Supplied: Economical bottles of 100 and convenience packages of individually wrapped 12 and 48 pink, scored, chewable tablets identified "STUART 858". Also available in 100 tablet unit dose boxes (10 strips of 10 tablets each).
NDC 0038-0858.
Shown in Product Identification Section, page 431

MYLICON®-125 Tablets
[my'li-con]
Maximum Strength Antiflatulent

Ingredients: Each tablet contains: Active: simethicone, 125 mg. Inactive: cereal solids, flavor, lactose, mannitol, povidone, Red 3, talc.

Continued on next page

Stuart—Cont.

Indications: MYLICON-125 is useful for relief of the painful symptoms of excess gas in the digestive tract. Such gas is frequently caused by excessive swallowing of air or by eating foods that disagree. If condition persists, consult your physician. MYLICON-125 is the strongest possible antiflatulent for adjunctive treatment of many conditions in which the retention of gas may be a problem, such as the following: air swallowing, functional dyspepsia, postoperative gaseous distention, peptic ulcer, spastic or irritable colon, diverticulosis. MYLICON-125 has a defoaming action that relieves flatulence by dispersing and preventing the formation of mucus-surrounded gas pockets in the gastrointestinal tract. MYLICON-125 acts in the stomach and intestines to change the surface tension of gas bubbles enabling them to coalesce; thus, the gas is freed and is eliminated more easily by belching or passing flatus.

Directions: One tablet four times daily after meals and at bedtime or as directed by physician. TABLETS SHOULD BE CHEWED THOROUGHLY.

Warnings: Keep this and all drugs out of the reach of children.

How Supplied: Convenience packages of individually wrapped 12 and 60 dark pink, scored chewable tablets identified "STUART 455". Also available in 100 tablet unit dose boxes (10 strips of 10 tablets each). NDC 0038-0455.
Shown in Product Identification Section, page 431

OREXIN® SOFTAB® Tablets
[*or 'ex-in*]
High Potency Vitamin Supplement

One Tablet Daily Provides:

VITAMINS:	US RDA*	
B$_1$	540%	8.1 mg
(thiamin)		
B$_6$	205%	4.1 mg
(pyridoxine hydrochloride)		
B$_{12}$	417%	25 mcg
(cyanocobalamin)		

*Percentage of US Recommended Daily Allowances for adults and children 4 or more years of age.

Ingredients: Active: thiamin mononitrate, pyridoxine hydrochloride, cyanocobalamin. Inactive: flavor, mannitol, saccharin calcium, sodium chloride, starch.

Indications: OREXIN is a high-potency vitamin supplement providing vitamins B$_1$, B$_6$, and B$_{12}$.
OREXIN SOFTAB tablets are specially formulated to dissolve quickly in the mouth. They may be chewed or swallowed. Dissolve tablet in a teaspoonful of water or fruit juice if liquid is preferred.

Directions: One tablet daily or as directed by a physician.

Warnings: Keep this and all drugs out of the reach of children.

How Supplied: Bottles of 100 pale pink SOFTAB tablets, identified "STUART".
NDC 0038-0280.
Shown in Product Identification Section, page 431

PROBEC®–T Tablets
[*pro 'bec-t*]
Vitamin B Complex Supplement
One Tablet Daily Provides:

VITAMINS:	US RDA*	
C	1000%	600 mg
B$_1$	813%	12.2 mg
(thiamin)		
B$_2$	588%	10 mg
(riboflavin)		
Niacin	500%	100 mg
B$_6$	205%	4.1 mg
(pyridoxine hydrochloride)		
B$_{12}$	83%	5 mcg
(cyanocobalamin)		
Pantothenic Acid	184%	18.4 mg

*Percentage of US Recommended Daily Allowances for adults and children 4 or more years of age.

DOSAGE: One tablet a day with a meal or as directed by physician.

Ingredients: Active: sodium ascorbate, niacinamide, calcium pantothenate, ascorbic acid, thiamin mononitrate, riboflavin, pyridoxine hydrochloride, cyanocobalamin. Inactive: calcium sulfate, carnauba wax, magnesium oxide, pharmaceutical glaze, povidone, Red 30, sucrose, titanium dioxide, white wax, Yellow 10.

Indications: PROBEC-T is a high-potency B complex supplement with 600 mg of vitamin C in easy to swallow odorless tablets.

Directions: One tablet a day with a meal or as directed by physician.

Warnings: As with all medications, keep out of the reach of children.

How Supplied: Bottles of 60, peach colored, capsule-shaped tablets. NDC 0038-0840.
Shown in Product Identification Section, page 431

THE STUART FORMULA® Tablets
Multivitamin/Multimineral Supplement
One Tablet Daily Provides:

VITAMINS:	US RDA*	
A	100%	5,000 IU
D	100%	400 IU
E	50%	15 IU
C	100%	60 mg
Folic Acid	100%	0.4 mg
B$_1$	80%	1.2 mg
(thiamin)		
B$_2$	100%	1.7 mg
(riboflavin)		
Niacin	100%	20 mg
B$_6$	100%	2 mg
(pyridoxine hydrochloride)		
B$_{12}$	100%	6 mcg
(cyanocobalamin)		

MINERALS:	US RDA	
Calcium	16%	160 mg
Phosphorus	12%	125 mg
Iodine	100%	150 mcg
Iron	100%	18 mg
Magnesium	25%	100 mg

*Percentage of US Recommended Daily Allowances for adults and children 4 or more years of age.

Ingredients: Each tablet contains: Active: dibasic calcium phosphate, magnesium oxide, ascorbic acid, ferrous fumarate, dl-alpha tocopheryl acetate, folic acid, niacinamide, vitamin A palmitate, cyanocobalamin, pyridoxine hydrochloride, riboflavin, thiamin mononitrate, ergocalciferol, potassium iodide. Inactive: calcium sulfate, carnauba wax, pharmaceutical glaze, povidone, sodium starch glycolate, starch, sucrose, titanium dioxide, white wax.

Indications: The STUART FORMULA tablet provides a well-balanced multivitamin/multimineral formula intended for use as a daily dietary supplement for adults and children over age four.

Directions: One tablet daily or as directed by physician.

Warnings: Keep this and all drugs out of the reach of children. In case of accidental overdose, seek professional assistance or contact a Poison Control Center immediately.

How Supplied: Bottles of 100 and 250 white round tablets. Child-resistant safety caps are standard on both bottles as a safeguard against accidental ingestion by children.
NDC 0038-0866.
Shown in Product Identification Section, page 431

STUART PRENATAL® Tablets
Multivitamin/Multimineral Supplement
One Tablet Daily Provides:

VITAMINS:	RDA*	
A	100%	4,000 IU
D	100%	400 IU
E	100%	11 mg
C	100%	100 mg
Folic Acid	100%	0.8 mg
B$_1$	100%	1.5 mg
(thiamin)		
B$_2$	100%	1.7 mg
(riboflavin)		
Niacin	100%	18 mg
B$_6$	100%	2.6 mg
(pyridoxine hydrochloride)		
B$_{12}$	100%	4 mcg
(cyanocobalamin)		

MINERALS:	RDA*	
Calcium	17%	200 mg
Iron	330%**	60 mg
Zinc	100%	25 mg

*Recommended Dietary Allowances (Food and Nutrition Board, NAS/NRC-1980) for pregnant and lactating women.
**Recommended Dietary Allowances (Food and Nutrition Board, NAS/NRC-1980) for adults, not pregnant and lactating women.

Ingredients: Each tablet contains:
Active: calcium sulfate, ferrous fumarate, ascorbic acid, dl-alpha tocopheryl acetate, zinc oxide, niacinamide, Vitamin A acetate, pyridoxine hydrochloride, riboflavin, thiamin mononitrate, folic acid, cholecalciferol, cyanocobalamin. Inactive: croscarmellose sodium, hydroxypropyl methylcellulose, microcrystalline cellulose, pregelatinized starch, red iron oxide, titanium dioxide.

Indications: STUART PRENATAL is a nonprescription multivitamin/multimineral supplement for use before, during, and after pregnancy. It provides vitamins equal to 100% or more of the RDA for pregnant and lactating women, plus essential minerals, including 60 mg of elemental iron as well-tolerated ferrous fumarate, and 200 mg of elemental calcium (nonalkalizing and phosphorus-free), and 25 mg zinc. Stuart Prenatal also contains 0.8 mg folic acid.

Directions: Before, during and after pregnancy, one tablet daily, or as directed by a physician.

Warning: In case of accidental overdose, seek professional assistance or contact a Poison Control Center immediately.

How Supplied: Bottles of 100 light pink tablets imprinted "STUART 071". A child-resistant safety cap is standard on 100 tablet bottles as a safeguard against accidental ingestion by children. NDC 0038-0071.
Shown in Product Identification Section, page 432

STUARTINIC® Tablets
[stu "are-tin 'ic]
Hematinic

One Tablet Daily Provides:

	US RDA*	
Iron	556%	100 mg
VITAMINS:		
C	833%	500 mg
B₁	327%	4.9 mg
(thiamin)		
B₂	353%	6 mg
(riboflavin)		
Niacin	100%	20 mg
B₆	40%	0.8 mg
(pyridoxine hydrochloride)		
B₁₂	417%	25 mcg
(cyanocobalamin)		
Pantothenic		
Acid	92%	9.2 mg

*Percentage of US Recommended Daily Allowances for adults and children 4 or more years of age.

Ingredients: Active: ferrous fumarate, ascorbic acid, sodium ascorbate, niacinamide, calcium pantothenate, thiamin mononitrate, riboflavin, pyridoxine hydrochloride, cyanocobalamin. Inactive: flavor, hydrogenated vegetable oil, microcrystalline cellulose, povidone, Yellow 6, Yellow 10, and other ingredients.

Indications: STUARTINIC is a complete hematinic for patients with history of iron deficiency anemia who also lack proper amounts of vitamin C and B-complex vitamins due to inadequate diet. The use of well-tolerated ferrous fumarate in STUARTINIC provides a high level of elemental iron with a low incidence of gastric distress. The inclusion of 500 mg of Vitamin C per tablet serves to maintain more of the iron in the absorbable ferrous state. The B-complex vitamins improve nutrition where B-complex deficient diets contribute to the anemia.

Warnings: As with any drug, if you are pregnant or nursing a baby, seek the advice of a health professional before using this product. Keep out of the reach of children. In case of accidental overdose, seek professional assistance or contact a Poison Control Center immediately.

Dosage: One tablet daily taken after a meal or as directed by physician. Because of the high amount of iron per tablet, STUARTINIC is not recommended for children under 12 years of age.

How Supplied: STUARTINIC is supplied in bottles of 60 yellow, film coated, oval shaped tablets. NDC 0038-0862.
Note: A child-resistant safety cap is standard on each 60 tablet bottle as a safeguard against accidental ingestion by children.
Shown in Product Identification Section, page 432

Syntex Laboratories, Inc
**3401 HILLVIEW AVENUE
PALO ALTO, CA 94304**

CARMOL® 10
**10% urea lotion
for total body
dry skin care.**

Active Ingredient: Urea 10% in a scented lotion of purified water, carbomer 940, cetyl alcohol, isopropyl palmitate, PEG-8 dioleate, PEG-8 distearate, propylene glycol, propylene glycol dipelargonate, stearic acid, sodium laureth sulfate, trolamine, and xanthan gum.

Indications: For total body dry skin care.

Actions: Keratolytic CARMOL 10 is non-occlusive, contains no mineral oil or petrolatum. CARMOL 10 is hypoallergenic; contains no lanolin, parabens or other preservatives.

Precautions: For external use only. Discontinue use if irritation occurs. Keep out of the reach of children. In case of accidental ingestion, seek professional assistance or contact a poison control center immediately.

Dosage and Administration: Rub in gently on hands, face or body. Repeat as necessary.

How Supplied: 6 fl. oz. bottle.

CARMOL® 20
**20% Urea Cream
Extra strength for
rough, dry skin**

Active Ingredients: Urea 20% in a non-lipid vanishing cream containing carbomer 940, hypoallergenic fragrance, isopropyl myristate, isopropyl palmitate, propylene glycol, purified water, sodium laureth sulfate, stearic acid, trolamine, xanthan gum.

Indications: Especially useful on rough, dry skin of hands, elbows, knees and feet.

Actions: Keratolytic. Contains no parabens, lanolin or mineral oil.

Precautions: For external use only. Keep away from eyes. Use with caution on face or broken or inflamed skin; transient stinging may occur. Discontinue use if irritation occurs. Keep out of the reach of children. In case of accidental ingestion, seek professional assistance or contact a poison control center immediately.

Dosage and Administration: Apply once or twice daily or as directed. Rub in well.

How Supplied: 3 oz. tubes, 1 lb. jars.

Thompson Medical Company, Inc.
**919 THIRD AVENUE
NEW YORK, NY 10022**

ASPERCREME®
[ăs-per-crēme]
External Analgesic Rub

Description: ASPERCREME® is available as an odor-free creme and lotion for use as a topical massage rub that temporarily relieves minor muscle aches and pains without stomach upset. Aspercreme does not contain aspirin.

Active Ingredients: Salycin® 10% (Thompson Medical's brand of Trolamine Salicylate).

Other Ingredients:
Cream: Cetyl Alcohol, Glycerin, Methylparaben, Mineral Oil, Potassium Phosphate, Propylparaben, Stearic Acid, Triethanolamine, Water.
Lotion: Cetyl Alcohol, Fragrance, Glyceryl Stearate, Isopropyl Palmitate, Lanolin, Methylparaben, Potassium Phosphate, Propylene Glycol, Propylparaben, Sodium Lauryl Sulfate, Stearic Acid, Water.

Actions: External analgesic rub.

Indications: Analgesic rub for temporary relief of minor aches and pains of muscles associated with simple backaches, strains and sprains. Aspercreme is aspirin free.

Warnings: Use only as directed. If prone to allergic reaction from aspirin or salicylate, consult your doctor before using. If redness is present or condition

Continued on next page

Thompson—Cont.

worsens, or if pain persists for more than 7 days or clears up and occurs again within a few days, discontinue use and consult a doctor. Do not use on children under 10 years of age. Do not apply if skin is irritated or if irritation develops. As with any drug, if you are pregnant or nursing a baby, seek the advice of a health professional before using this product. For external use only. Avoid contact with eyes. Keep this and all medicines out of the reach of children. In case of accidental ingestion seek professional assistance or contact a Poison Control Center immediately.

Dosage and Administration: Apply generously directly to affected area. Massage into painful area until thoroughly absorbed into skin, repeat as necessary, especially before retiring but not more than 4 times daily.

How to Store: Protect from freezing and temperatures above 100°F. Close cap tightly after use.

How Supplied: Cream: 1¼ oz., 3 oz. and 5 oz. tubes. Lotion: 6 oz. bottle.
Shown in Product Identification Section, page 432

CORTIZONE–5
Creme and Ointment
Antipruritic
(hydrocortisone)

Description: CORTIZONE-5 creme and ointment are topical anti-itch preparations

Active Ingredient: Hydrocortisone 0.5%

Other Ingredients:
Cream: Aluminum Sulfate, Calcium Acetate, Glycerin, Light Mineral Oil, Methylparaben, Potato Dextrin, Purified Water, Sodium Lauryl Sulfate, White Petroleum. May Also Contain: Cetearyl Alcohol, Propylparaben, Sodium C12–15 Alcohols Sulfate, Synthetic Beeswax, White Wax.
Ointment: White Petrolatum

Indications: CORTIZONE-5 is recommended for the temporary relief of itching associated with minor skin irritations, inflammations and rashes due to: eczema, dermatitis, psoriasis, insect bites, poison ivy, oak, sumac, detergents, soaps, cosmetics, jewelry, external anal and genital itching.

Warnings: For external use only. Avoid contact with the eyes. In case of accidental ingestion get professional assistance or contact a poison control center immediately. Do not use on children under two years of age unless under the advice and supervision of a doctor. If condition worsens, or symptoms persist for more than seven days, discontinue use and consult a doctor. Do not use for external genital itching if vaginal discharge is present.
KEEP THIS AND ALL MEDICINES OUT OF THE REACH OF CHILDREN.

Dosage and Administration: For use by adults and children 2 years of age and older. Apply to affected area, not more than three or four times daily.

How to Store: Store at room temperature

How Supplied: CORTIZONE-5 creme: ½oz., 1oz, and 2oz. tubes. CORTIZONE-5 ointment: 1oz tube
Shown in Product Identification Section, page 432

DEXATRIM® Capsules
[dĕx-a-trĭm]
**Prolonged action anorectic for weight control contains
phenylpropanolamine HCl   50mg
(time release)**

**DEXATRIM® Maximum Strength Plus Vitamin C/Caffeine-Free Capsules
phenylpropanolamine HCl   75mg
(time release)
Vitamin C   180mg
(immediate release)**

**DEXATRIM® Maximum Strength Caffeine-Free Capsules
phenylpropanolamine HCl   75mg
(time release)**

**DEXATRIM® Maximum Strength Plus Vitamin C/Caffeine-Free Caplets
phenylpropanolamine HCl   75mg
(time release)
Vitamin C   180mg
(immediate release)**

**DEXATRIM® Maximum Strength Caffeine-Free Caplets
phenylpropanolamine HCl   75mg
(time release)**

**DEXATRIM® Maximum Strength Pre-Meal Caplets
phenylpropanolamine HCl   25mg
(immediate release)**

Indication: DEXATRIM® is an appetite suppressant for use in conjunction with a calorie restricted diet for fast weight loss. It is available in time release and immediate release dosage forms.

Caution: READ BEFORE USING. For adult use only. Do not give this product to children under 12 years of age. Persons between the ages of 12 and 18 or over 60 are advised to consult their doctor or pharmacist before using this or any drug. If nervousness, dizziness, headaches, rapid pulse, palpitations, sleeplessness, or other symptoms occur, stop using and consult your physician.

Warning: DO NOT EXCEED RECOMMENDED DOSAGE. Taking more of this or any drug than is recommended can cause untoward health complications. It is sensible to check your blood pressure regularly. Do not use if you have high blood pressure, diabetes, heart, thyroid, kidney, or other disease or are being treated for high blood pressure or depression except under the advice and supervision of a doctor. As with any drug if you are pregnant or nursing a baby, seek the advice of a health professional before using this product. Do not

use continuously for more than 3 months. When you have reached your desired weight or are able to control your appetite by yourself, use DEXATRIM only as needed.

Drug Interaction Precaution: Do not take if you are presently taking another medication containing phenylpropanolamine, or any type of nasal decongestant, or a prescription drug for high blood pressure or depression, or any other type of prescription medication except under the advice and supervision of a doctor.
KEEP THIS AND ALL MEDICATION OUT OF THE REACH OF CHILDREN. In case of accidental overdose seek professional assistance or contact a Poison Control Center immediately.

Dosage and Administration:
Capsule Dosage Forms: DEXATRIM®, DEXATRIM® Maximum Strength Plus Vitamin C, DEXATRIM® Maximum Strength/Caffeine-Free.
Caplet Dosage Forms: DEXATRIM® Maximum Strength Plus Vitamin C, DEXATRIM® Maximum Strength/Caffeine-Free.
Administration: One capsule or caplet at mid-morning (10am) with a full glass of water.
Immediate Release Caplet Dosage Form: DEXATRIM® Maximum Strength Pre-Meal Caplets:
Administration: One caplet 30 minutes before each meal with one or two full glasses of water. Do not exceed 3 caplets in 24 hours.

How Supplied: All Dexatrim products are supplied in tamper evident blister packages. Do not use if individual seals are broken.
DEXATRIM® Capsules: Packages of 28 with 1250 calorie DEXATRIM Diet Plan.
DEXATRIM® Maximum Strength Plus Vitamin C/Caffeine-Free Capsules: Packages of 10, 20 and 40 with 1250 calorie DEXATRIM Diet Plan.
DEXATRIM® Maximum Strength Capsules/Caffeine-Free: Packages of 10, 20 and 40 with 1250 calorie DEXATRIM Diet Plan.
DEXATRIM® Maximum Strength Plus Vitamin C/Caffeine-Free Caplets: Packages of 10, 20 and 40 with 1250 calorie DEXATRIM Diet Plan.
DEXATRIM® Maximum Strength Caplets/Caffeine-Free: Packages of 10, 20 and 40 with 1250 calorie DEXATRIM Diet Plan.
DEXATRIM® Maximum Strength Pre-Meal Caplets: Packages of 30 and 60 with 1250 calorie DEXATRIM Diet Plan.

References: Altschuler, S. and Frazer, D.L., Double-Blind Clinical Evaluation of the Anorectic Activity of Phenylpropanolamine Hydrochloride Drops and Placebo Drops in the Treatment of Exogenous Obesity. Current Therapeutic Research, 40(1), 211–217, July 1986.
Sebok, M., A Double-Blinded, Placebo-Controlled Clincial Study of the Efficacy of a Phenylpropanolamine/Caffeine Combination Product as an Aid to Weight Loss in Adults. Current Thera-

peutic Research, 37(4), 701–708, April 1985.

Lasagna, L., *Phenylpropanolamine—A Review*, New York, John Wiley and Sons, 1988.

All referenced materials available on request.

Shown in Product Identification Section, page 432

NP-27®
Cream, Solution, Spray Powder and Powder
Antifungal
(Tolnaftate)

Description: NP-27 contains the maximum strength available without a prescription of tolnaftate, a clinically proven ingredient which kills athlete's foot fungus and jock itch fungus on contact. It is available as a cream, solution, spray powder and powder.

Active Ingredients:
Cream, Solution and Powder: Tolnaftate 1%
Aerosol: Tolnaftate 1%, Contains: SD Alcohol 40 14.9%

Other Ingredients:
Cream: BHT, Polyethylene Glycol 400, Propylene Glycol, Titanium Dioxide. May also Contain: n-Amylamine, Carbomer 934P, Carbomer 940, Diisopropanolamine.
Solution: BHT, Polyethylene Glycol 400. May also contain: Propylene Glycol.
Aerosol: Isobutane, Isopropyl Myristate, Talc.
Powder: Corn Starch, Talc.

Indications: An effective antifungal agent that kills athlete's foot fungus and jock itch fungus on contact and helps prevent reinfection. Provides quick relief of the itching, burning, scaling and discomfort that can accompany these conditions.

Warnings: For external use only. Do not use on children under 2 years of age except under the advice and supervision of a doctor. Children under 12 years of age should be supervised in the use of the product. If irritation occurs or if there is no improvement within 2 weeks, discontinue use and consult a doctor or pharmacist. Keep this and all medications out of the reach of children. In case of accidental ingestion, seek professional assistance or contact a Poison Control Center immediately. Avoid eye contact. Not effective on scalp or nails.

Dosage and Administration: Cleanse skin with soap and water and dry thoroughly. Apply a thin layer over affected area morning and night or as directed by a doctor. To help prevent recurrence, continue treatment for 2 weeks after disappearance of all symptoms. For athlete's foot pay special attention to the spaces between the toes.

How Supplied: Available in ½oz. and 1oz. cream; ½oz. solution; ⅗oz. spray powder; 1.5oz powder.

How to Store: Store at room temperature.

Shown in Product Identification Section, page 432

SLEEPINAL®
Night-time Sleep Aid Capsules
(Diphenhydramine HCl)

Description: SLEEPINAL is a nighttime sleep aid. When taken prior to bedtime, it helps to increase drowsiness and aids in falling asleep.

Active Ingredient: Diphenhydramine HCl 50 mg

Other Ingredients: FD&C Blue No. 1, Gelatin, Lactose, Magnesium Stearate, Povidone, Talc

Indications: Aids in relieving sleeplessness

Action: SLEEPINAL is an antihistamine with anticholinergic and sedative action

Warnings: Read before using. Do not exceed recommended dosage. Do not give to children under 12 years of age. Do not use if you are taking any other type of medication without first consulting a doctor or pharmacist. Take this product with caution if alcohol is being consumed. If sleeplessness perists continuously for more than 2 weeks, consult a doctor since insomnia may be a sign of serious underlying medical illness. As with any drug, if you are pregnant or nursing a baby, seek the advice of a health professional before using this product. DO NOT TAKE THIS PRODUCT IF YOU HAVE ASTHMA, GLAUCOMA OR ENLARGEMENT OF THE PROSTATE GLAND EXCEPT UNDER THE ADVICE AND SUPERVISION OF A DOCTOR.
KEEP THIS AND ALL MEDICATIONS OUT OF THE REACH OF CHILDREN. In the case of accidental overdose, contact a doctor immediately.

Dosage and Administration: Take 1 capsule 20 minutes before going to bed, or as directed by a doctor.

How to Store: Store in a dry place at controlled room temperature 15° C–30° C (59° F–86° F)

How Supplied: Sleepinal is supplied in tamper evident blister packages. Do not use if individual seals are broken. Packages of 16 and 32 capsules.

Shown in Product Identification Section, page 432

ULTRA SLIM·FAST
Nutritional Meal Replacement Drink—Part of the Ultra SlimFast Program

Description: A precisely portioned, nutritionally complete liquid meal replacement to be used in conjunction with real-food meals for weight loss or weight-loss maintenance. Unlike "fasting" diets, the ULTRA Slim·Fast program provides a combination of convenient, palatable meal replacements and whole-food meals in an integrated program that makes it pleasant to lose weight and keep it off.

The delicious, thick ULTRA Slim·Fast "milkshake" provides a nutritious, low-calorie answer to cravings for "sweet" or "forbidden" food, while the high fiber content promotes feelings of satiety. The ULTRA Slim·Fast Program, scientifically developed with the help of physicians and dietitians, includes diet suggestions for the whole-food dinners or other meals that accompany the "shakes". The Program promotes behavior modification to aid in the eating-pattern and lifestyle changes that can make weight reduction succeed permanently.

Uses: The ULTRA Slim·Fast program is recommended to help the moderately obese patient (up to 50 pounds or more overweight) to achieve safe, rapid weight loss. It is also indicated for the patient who wishes to maintain weight loss, or to control or reverse modest weight gains.

Professional Supplementary Materials: Physicians and dietitians may also send for patient samples and free support materials, including physicians' weight-loss manuals, prepared diet sheets, "wallet cards" with patient dieting tips. Write to Ultra SlimFast Medical Program, Thompson Medical Company, 919 Third Ave., New York, NY 10022, for details.

Nutritional Information: ULTRA Slim·Fast provides an exceptionally safe, nutritious weight-loss regimen. One ULTRA Slim·Fast "shake" made with 1% low-fat milk includes 33% of the U.S. RDA of 19 essential nutrients. It is an excellent source of dietary fiber (5 grams in chocolate flavor; 4.2 grams in vanilla or strawberry), calcium (50% of adult RDA), and protein (13 grams, largely from casein, providing 24% of total calories). And it is low in fat (just 4 grams—16% of calories).
[See table on next page].

Ingredients: Sucrose, Whey powder, Dutch processed cocoa (in Chocolate Royale only); Calcium caseinate, Bran fiber, Purified cellulose; Soy protein, Nonfat dry milk, Fructose, Carrageenan, Natural and artificial flavors, Malto-dextrins, Lecithin, Guar gum, DL-methionine, Aspartame, and the following vitamins and mineral: magnesium carbonate, calcium phosphate, sodium phosphate, potassium chloride, calcium carbonate, ferric orthophosphate, vitamin E acetate, ascorbic acid, niacinamide, zinc oxide, vitamin A palmitate, manganese sulfate, calcium pantothenate, copper sulfate, pyridoxine hydrochloride, thiamine mononitrate, vitamin D_3, riboflavin, biotin, folic acid, potassium iodide, vitamine B_{12}.

Directions: The ULTRA Slim·Fast Program for weight loss consists of "shakes" to replace two of three regular meals (and another for a snack, if needed) PLUS one well-balanced whole-food meal as specified in the enclosed diet booklet. (This plan provides for approximately 1200 calories per day).

Continued on next page

Thompson—Cont.

IMPORTANT: USE A SHAKER OR BLENDER. Simply add 1 rounded measuring scoopful of ULTRA Slim·Fast powder to 8 oz. of 1% low fat milk. SHAKE OR BLEND for about 20 seconds. For best results, use very cold milk and wait about one minute as the shake thickens into a rich, creamy drink. If 1% low fat milk is not available, use 2% low fat milk (nutritional information will change slightly).

FOR FAST, SAFE WEIGHT LOSS: Enjoy ULTRA Slim·Fast twice daily in place of breakfast and lunch. (Enjoy a third serving, as needed, in place of snacks). For dinner, eat a well-balanced meal as specified in enclosed diet booklet.

FOR WEIGHT MAINTENANCE AND GOOD HEALTH: Enjoy ULTRA Slim·Fast daily in place of EITHER breakfast OR lunch (and a second time, as needed,

The Ultra Slim·Fast™ Medical Program . . .

. . . is NOT . . .

- **A fasting program** requiring abstinence from solid foods.
- **A fad diet** with questionable nutritioinal balance.
- **An inconvenient diet** requiring complex preparation.
- **An unappealing diet** with unappetizing ingredients.
- **A "miracle" diet** promising unhealthy, overly rapid weight loss, with no follow-through.
- **Expensive** (as some clinic- or hospital-based programs are)

. . . IS . . .

- **A combination** of meal replacements and "real" foods.
- **A precisely proportioned, highly nutritious food** low in calories and fat.
- **Convenient and readily available** (without prescription).
- **Palatable, delicious** "milkshake" meals plus tasty solid-food meals.
- **An aid to behavior modification** vital for achieving and maintaining weight loss.
- **Economical** (usually less costly than the meal or snack it replaces).

Starter kit includes 7 oz. (6 servings) can with patient instruction. [See table above].

Shown in Product Identification Section, page 432

Serving Size: 1.16 oz (12 servings per 14 oz can)

Each Serving Provides:	One Serving	One Serving with 8 Fl. Oz. Vitamin A&D Protein Fortified 1% Low Fat Milk
Calories	100	220
Protein	5 grams	15 grams
Carbohydrate	19 grams	33 grams
Fat	1 gram	4 grams
Sodium	110 mg.	250 mg.
Potassium	240 mg.	680 mg.
Fiber (Dietary)	5 grams	5 grams
Percentage of Adult U.S. Recommended Daily Allowance (U.S. RDA):		
Protein	10%	35%
Vitamin A	25%	35%
Vitamin C (Ascorbic Acid)	30%	35%
Thiamine (Vitamin B_1)	30%	35%
Riboflavin (Vitamin B_2)	10%	35%
Niacin	35%	35%
Calcium	15%	50%
Iron	35%	35%
Vitamin D	10%	35%
Vitamin E	35%	35%
Vitamin B_6	30%	35%
Folic Acid	25%	30%
Vitamin B_{12}	20%	35%
Phosphorous	15%	40%
Iodine	10%	35%
Magnesium	25%	35%
Zinc	30%	35%
Copper	35%	35%
Biotin	35%	35%
Pantothenic Acid	25%	35%
Manganese	1 mg.*	1 mg.*

*No U.S. RDA established

Nutritional information may vary slightly in Strawberry Supreme and French Vanilla flavors.

in place of snacks). For the other two regular meals, follow a nutritionally balanced eating program.

Warnings: Phenylketonurics—Contains phenylalanine. Anyone who is pregnant or nursing, is under 18 years of age, or has a health problem should consult a physician before starting any weight-loss program.

How Supplied: Flavors: Chocolate Royale, French Vanilla, Strawberry Supreme. Available in 14-oz. cans (397 grams, 12 servings)—including measuring scoop and diet plan suggestions. Professional starter kit available on request to physicians and registered dietitians.

IDENTIFICATION PROBLEM?
Consult the
Product Identification Section
where you'll find
products pictured
in full color.

Triton Consumer Products, Inc.
5105 TOLLVIEW DRIVE
SUITE 190
ROLLING MEADOWS, IL 60008

MG 217® Psoriasis Ointment

Active Ingredients: Sulfur 1.5%, salicylic acid 1.5% and coal tar solution USP in Guy-Base™, a specially formulated ointment base designed to retain the skin's natural moisture and enhance the therapeutic effectivess of the three active ingredients.

Action and Uses: Specially formulated to control the discomfort, itching, flaking and scaling of Psoriasis.

Caution: For external use only. Keep out of the reach of children. Keep away from eyes and other mucous membranes. Do not use on scalp. If undue skin irritation develops or increases, discontinue use.

Administration: Wash affected areas with warm water and a mild soap. Dry well, then rub MG 217 in with finger tips. Apply twice daily.

How Supplied: MG 217 Psoriasis Ointment in 4 oz. and 16 oz. plastic jars.

MG 217® Psoriasis Shampoo

Active Ingredients: Coal tar solution USP 5%, colloidal sulfur 2% and salicylic acid 2% in a base of surface active cleansers, wetting agents and lanolin.

Action and Uses: Specially formulated for long-term control of scalp psoriasis, dandruff and other seborrheic conditions. Reduces scaling and flaking and relieves itching.

Caution: For external use only. Keep out of the reach of children. In isolated cases temporary discoloration of blond, bleached or tinted hair may occur. Avoid contact with eyes. If undue skin irritation occurs, discontinue use.

Administration: Shake well before using. Massage in a liberal amount of shampoo and leave on the scalp 5–10 minutes. Rinse thoroughly and repeat.

How Supplied: MG 217 Psoriasis Shampoo in 8 oz. and 16 oz. plastic bottles.

UAS Laboratories
9201 PENN AVENUE SOUTH
#10
MINNEAPOLIS, MN 55431

DDS–ACIDOPHILUS
Capsule, Tablet & Powder free of dairy products, corn, soy, and preservatives

Description: DDS-Acidophilus is the source of a special strain of Lactobacillus acidophilus free of dairy products, corn, soy and preservatives. Each capsule or tablet contain one billion viable DDS-1 L.acidophilus at the time of manufacturing. One gram of powder contains two billion viable DDS-1 L.acidophilus.

Indications and Usages: An aid in implanting the gut with beneficial Lactobacillus acidophilus under conditions of digestive disorders, acne, yeast infections, and following antibiotic therapy.

Administration: One to two capsules or tablets twice daily before meals. One-fourth teaspoon powder can be substituted for two capsules or tablets.

How Supplied: Bottles of 100 capsules or tablets. 12 bottles per case. Powder is available in 2 oz. bottle; 12 bottles per case.

Storage: Keep refrigerated under 40°F.

EDUCATIONAL MATERIAL

DDS-Acidophilus
Booklet describing superior-strain Acidophilus without dairy products, corn, soy, or preservatives. Two billion viable DDS-L. acidophilus per gram.

UltraBalance Products
3215 56TH STREET NW
GIG HARBOR, WA 98335

ULTRABALANCE WEIGHT MANAGEMENT PRODUCT
ULTRABALANCE PROTEIN FORMULA

Description: UltraBalance Protein Formula is a partially predigested, lactalbumin-based formula that is vitamin/mineral enriched and contains no common allergen-derived materials. Contains no corn, wheat, soy, egg, milk casein, lactose, yeast, sweetener, artificial flavoring/coloring or stimulants.

Composition: Hydrolyzed lactalbumin, rice protein concentrate, potassium citrate, tricalcium phosphate, natural vanilla flavors, magnesium oxide, beta carotene, high oleic safflower oil, potassium chloride, calcium carbonate, ascorbic acid, iron amino acid chelate, zinc amino acid chelate, dl alpha tocopheryl acetate, ChromeMate-GTF™, molybdenum amino acid chelate, selenium amino acid chelate, manganese amino acid chelate, copper amino acid chelate, niacinamide, pyridoxine hydrochloride, calcium pantothenate, riboflavin, thiamine hydrochloride, folic acid, potassium iodide, vitamin D3 (cholecalciferol), biotin and cyanocobalamin.

Actions/Uses: Used for weight management as well as food allergy testing/treatment. Provides 100% RDA for all vitamins and minerals except calcium.

Preparation: 1 level scoop of Protein mixed with 8 oz diluted fruit juice either 2 or 3 times per day depending on patient's needs.

ULTRABALANCE HERBULK

Description: Used as a part of the UltraBalance Program for weight management or separately as a soluble fiber supplement. Completely natural, contains no narcotics or stimulants.

Composition: Psyllium seed powder, rice flour, guar gum, Mezotrace™ (dolomite-limestone), prune fiber concentrate, cellulose gum, ascorbic acid.

Actions/Uses: Provides fiber for the digestive system without contributing excessive calories.

Preparation: 1 level scoop of Herbulk mixed with 8 oz diluted juice either 2 or 3 times per day depending on patient's needs.

How Supplied: UltraBalance Weight Management "Kit" consists of one can Protein, one can Herbulk, Program Description Booklet. Also available are Patient Workbook, Recipe Book/Menu Planner, Lifestyle Modification Tapes. Available through licensed health practitioners.

United Medical
Division of Pfizer Hospital Products Group, Inc.
11775 STARKEY ROAD
LARGO, FL 34643-4799

ONE–PIECE SYSTEM WITH SOFT GUARD SHEER PLUS™

Description: System consisting of skin barrier wafer attached directly to colostomy or wound management pouch. The special thin barrier wafer provides greater flexibility for patient comfort and ease of application.

Ingredients (pouches): Vinyl or MF film with oxygen barrier (coextruded three layer EVA/PVDC/EVA).

Ingredients (skin barrier): Polyisobutylene, polyvinylpyrrolidone, pectin, 2-propenamide-co-2-propenic acid, mixed sodium and aluminum salt, regenerated cellulose fibers, mineral oil, substituted hydroxy toluene, triclosan.

Indications and Use: The one-piece system is used in ostomy, wound management (post-op), fistula care and incontinence.

Contraindications: Hypersensitivity to any ingredient of the skin barrier and/or to the material of the pouch.

Precautions and Adverse Reaction: For external use only. Discontinue use if itching or irritation occurs.

Dosage and Administration: Use as needed. Pouches may be left in place as long as they perform efficiently. Remove release paper and attach to skin.

How Supplied:
1818-04 One-Piece Drainable Pouch with Soft Guard Sheer Plus™ (Clear)
1821-04 One-Piece Pouch with Soft Guard Sheer Plus™ (Opaque)
1835-04 One-Piece Pouch, Closed-End with Filter (Opaque)

SOFT GUARD XL™ SKIN BARRIER

Description: Synthetic, soft and pliable skin barrier for use in ostomy and wound management applications. Formulation designed to inhibit growth of odor producing microorganisms.

Ingredients: Polyisobutylene, sodium carboxy methyl cellulose, pectin, acrylamide based polymer, mineral oil and 2,4,4' tricholoro 2' hydroxy diphenyl ether.

Indications and Usage: Long lasting skin barrier resisting bacterial growth and odor. Forms a soft protective seal that substantially reduces stoma cuts and peristomal skin irritation from effluent. For use around stomas, wound drainage, fistula care and incontinence.

Contraindications: Hypersensitivity to any ingredient of the formulation.

Precautions and Adverse Reactions: For external use only. Discontinue use if itching or irritation appears.

Dosage and Administration: Use as needed. Remove barrier wafer from package, cut to fit the desired stoma or wound size, peel off white paper backing, and apply to clean, dry skin.

How Supplied:
4600 4" × 4" wafer, 5/box
4610 8" × 8" wafer, 3/box

ONE-PIECE SYSTEM WITH SOFT GUARD XL™

Description: System consisting of skin barrier wafer attached directly to colostomy, ileostomy, urinary diversion or wound management pouch. The urinary pouches contain anti-reflux valves to keep fluid from returning to site.

Ingredients (pouches): Vinyl or MF film with oxygen barrier (coextruded three layer EVA/PVDC/EVA).

Ingredients (skin barrier): Polyisobutylene, polyvinylpyrrolidone, pectin, 2-propenamide-co-2-propenic acid, mixed sodium and aluminum salt, regenerated cellulose fibers, mineral oil, substituted hydroxy toluene, acrylic polymer, triclosan.

Indications and Use: The one-piece system is used in ostomy, wound manage-

Continued on next page

United Medical—Cont.

ment (post-op), fistula care and incontinence.

Contraindications: Hypersensitivity to any ingredient of the skin barrier and/or to the material of the skin pouch.

Precautions and Adverse Reaction: For external use only. Discontinue use if itching or irritation occurs.

Dosage and Administration: Use as needed. Pouches may be left in place as long as they perform efficiently. Remove release paper and attach to skin.

How Supplied:
4675-04 One-Piece Urinary Pouch with Soft Guard XL™ (580 ml)
4676-04 One-Piece Urinary Pouch with Soft Guard XL™ (800 ml)
4620-04 One-Piece Drainable Pouch with Soft Guard XL™

TWO-PIECE SYSTEM WITH SOFT GUARD XL™

Description: System consisting of skin barrier wafer with male flange attached, and colostomy, ileostomy, urinary diversion or wound management pouch with female flange. The urinary pouches contain anti-reflux valves to keep fluid from returning to site.

Ingredients (pouches): Vinyl or MF film with oxygen barrier (coextruded three layer EVA/PVDC/EVA).

Ingredients (skin barrier w/flange): Polyisobutylene, polyvinylpyrrolidone, pectin, 2-propenamide-co-2-propenic acid, mixed sodium and aluminum salt, regenerated cellulose fibers, mineral oil, substituted hydroxy toluene, acrylic polymer, triclosan.

Indications and Use: The two-piece system is used in ostomy, wound management, fistula care and incontinence. The pouch is secured to the barrier which is attached to the skin around stoma or wound.

Contraindications: Hypersensitivity to any ingredient of the skin barrier and/or to the material of the pouch.

Precautions and Adverse Reactions: For external use. Discontinue use if itching or irritation occurs.

Dosage and Administration: Use as needed. Attach pouch to barrier flange by aligning rim of pouch flange with rim of barrier flange. Press pouch securely around entire ring - walking your fingers around the ring until it locks in place. Pouch may be left in place on barrier flange until barrier is removed, or changed on a daily or every other day basis, according to performance.

How Supplied:
4700 4″ × 4″ wafer with male flanges 1½″, 1¾″, 2¼″ and 2¾″ to fit the fol-

lowing pouches/sleeves:
1095 Urinary Pouch (550 ml)
1096 Urinary Pouch (850 ml)
1840 Drainable Opaque Pouch
1844 Drainable Clear Pouch
1849 Closed-End Pouch with Gas Filter
1850 Closed-End Pouch
2800 Irrigation Sleeve

UNIFLEX™ TRANSPARENT DRESSINGS AND DRAPES

Description: UniFlex is a bacteria proof, moisture vapor permeable, elastic, transparent dressing or drape. A low allergy polyurethane film is coated with a medical grade adhesive.

Ingredients: Collagen filled polyurethane film and vinyl acetate-acrylate multipolymer adhesive.

Indications and Uses: The UniFlex dressings can be used in a wide variety of applications, including primary IV sites (peripheral and central line), preventive skin care, for pressure related dermal ulcers, and in wound care. The UniFlex drapes can be used in hospitals as incise sheets. The UniFlex Incision Dressing is for use as a post surgical dressing.

Contraindication: Hypersensitivity to any ingredients of the dressing or drape.

Precautions and Adverse Reactions: Discontinue use if irritation occurs.

Dosage and Administration: Per instructions on box and on individual dressing.

How Supplied:

5610-00 5cm × 7.5 cm	IV
5620-00 6cm × 8.5	IV
5630-00 10cm × 14cm	IV
5640-00 10cm × 25cm Wound	
5645-00 6.4cm × 35.6cm Post Surgical	
5650-00 14cm × 25cm Wound	
5660-00 30cm × 28cm Surgical Drape	
5670-00 45cm × 28cm Surgical Drape	
5680-00 45cm × 55cm Surgical Drape	
5690-00 56cm × 84cm Surgical Drape	

The Upjohn Company
KALAMAZOO, MI 49001

BACIGUENT® Antibiotic Ointment

Active Ingredient: Each gram contains 500 units of bacitracin. Also contains anhydrous lanolin, mineral oil, and white petrolatum.

Indications: *Baciguent* is a first aid ointment to help prevent infection and aid in the healing of minor cuts, burns and abrasions.

How Supplied: Available in ½ oz and 1 oz tubes.

CHERACOL D® Cough Formula

Active Ingredients: Each teaspoonful (5 ml) contains dextromethorphan hydrobromide, 10 mg; guaifenesin, 100 mg; alcohol, 4.75%. Also contains benzoic acid, FD & C Red #40, flavors, fragrances,

fructose, glycerin, propylene glycol, sodium chloride, sucrose, and purified water.

Indications: *Cheracol D* Cough Formula helps quiet dry, hacking coughs, and helps loosen phlegm and mucus. Recommended for adults and children 2 years of age and older.

Dosage and Administration: Adults: 2 teaspoonfuls. Children 6 to 12 years: 1 teaspoonful. Children 2 to 6 years: ½ teaspoonful. These doses may be repeated every four hours if necessary.

How Supplied: Available in 2 oz, 4 oz and 6 oz bottles.
Shown in Product Identification Section, page 432

CHERACOL PLUS®
Head Cold/Cough Formula

Active Ingredients: Each tablespoonful (15 ml) contains phenylpropanolamine hydrochloride, 25 mg; dextromethorphan hydrobromide, 20 mg; chlorpheniramine maleate, 4 mg, and alcohol, 8%. Also contains flavors, glycerin, methylparaben, propylene glycol, propylparaben, FD&C Red #40, sodium chloride, sorbitol solution, and purified water.

Indications: *Cheracol Plus* syrup is an effective 3-ingredient, maximum strength formula for the temporary relief of head cold symptoms and cough (without narcotic side effects).

Dosage and Administration: Adults and children over 12 years of age: 1 tablespoonful every 4 hours or as directed by a physician. Do not take more than 6 tablespoonfuls in a 24-hour period. Do not administer to children under 12 years of age.

How Supplied: Available in 4 oz and 6 oz bottles.
Shown in Product Identification Section, page 432

CITROCARBONATE® Antacid

Active Ingredients: When dissolved, each 3.9 grams (1 teaspoonful) contains approximately: sodium bicarbonate, 0.78 gram and sodium citrate, 1.82 grams. **As derived from: (per teaspoonful):** Sodium bicarbonate 2.34 gram; citric acid anhydrous, 1.19 gram; sodium citrate hydrous, 254 mg; calcium lactate pentahydrate, 151 mg; sodium chloride, 79 mg; monobasic sodium phosphate anhydrous, 44 mg; and, magnesium sulfate dried, 42 mg. Each teaspoonful contains 30.46 mEq (700.6 mg) of sodium.

Indications: For the relief of heartburn, acid indigestion, and sour stomach; and upset stomach associated with these symptoms.

Dosage and Administration: Adults: 1 to 2 teaspoonfuls (not to exceed 5 level teaspoonfuls per day) in a glass of cold water after meals. Children 6 to 12 years: ¼ to ½ adult dose. For children under 6 years: Consult physician. Persons 60

years or older: ½ to 1 teaspoonful after meals.

How Supplied: Available in 4 oz and 8 oz bottles.

CORTAID® Cream with Aloe
CORTAID® Ointment with Aloe
CORTAID® Lotion
(hydrocortisone acetate)
CORTAID® Spray
(hydrocortisone)

Antipruritic

Description: *Cortaid* Cream with Aloe contains hydrocortisone acetate (equivalent to 0.5% hydrocortisone) in a greaseless, odorless, vanishing cream that leaves no residue. Also contains aloe vera, butylparaben, cetyl palmitate, glyceryl stearate, methylparaben, polyethylene glycol, stearamidoethyl diethylamine, and purified water.
Cortaid Ointment with Aloe contains hydrocortisone acetate (equivalent to 0.5% hydrocortisone) in a soothing, lubricated ointment. Also contains aloe vera, butylparaben, cholesterol, methylparaben, mineral oil, white petrolatum, and microcrystaline wax.
Cortaid Lotion contains hydrocortisone acetate (equivalent to 0.5% hydrocortisone) in a greaseless, odorless, vanishing lotion. Also contains butylparaben, cetyl palmitate, glyceryl monostearate, methylparaben, polysorbate 80, propylene glycol, stearamidoethyl diethylamine, and purified water.
Cortaid Spray contains 0.5% hydrocortisone in a quick drying, non-staining, non-aerosol, vanishing liquid spray. Also contains alcohol (46%), glycerin, methylparaben, and purified water.

Indications: All *Cortaid* forms are indicated for the temporary relief of minor itchy skin irritations, inflammation, and rashes due to eczema, dermatitis, insect bites, poison ivy, poison oak, poison sumac, soaps, detergents, cosmetics, and jewelry, and with the exception of *Cortaid* Spray, for external genital and anal itching.

Uses: The vanishing action of *Cortaid* Cream with Aloe makes it cosmetically acceptable when the skin rash treated is on an exposed part of the body such as the hands or arms. *Cortaid* Ointment with Aloe is best used where protection, lubrication and soothing of dry and scaly lesions is required; the ointment is also preferred for treating itchy genital and anal areas. *Cortaid* Lotion is thinner than the cream and is especially suitable for hairy body areas such as the scalp or arms. *Cortaid* Spray is a quick drying, non-staining formulation suitable for covering large areas of the skin.

Warnings: All *Cortaid* formulations are for external use only. Avoid contact with the eyes. If condition worsens or if symptoms persist for more than 7 days, discontinue use of this product and consult a physician. Do not use on children under 2 years of age except under the advice and supervision of a physician. Keep this and all drugs out of the reach of chil-

dren. In case of accidental ingestion, seek professional assistance or contact a poison control center immediately.

Dosage and Administration: For adults and children 2 years of age and older, apply as follows: *Cortaid* Cream with Aloe, *Cortaid* Ointment with Aloe or *Cortaid* Lotion: gently massage into the affected area not more than 3 to 4 times daily. *Cortaid* Spray: spray on affected area not more than 3 to 4 times daily.

How Supplied: *Cortaid* formulations (hydrocortisone acetate) are available in: Cream with Aloe ½ oz and 1 oz tubes; Ointment with Aloe ½ oz and 1 oz tubes; Lotion 1 oz bottle. *Cortaid* Spray (hydrocortisone) is available in 1.5 fluid oz pump spray bottles.

Shown in Product Identification Section, page 432

CORTEF® Feminine Itch Cream
(hydrocortisone acetate)
Antipruritic

Description: *Cortef* Feminine Itch Cream contains hydrocortisone acetate (equivalent to hydrocortisone 0.5%) in an odorless, vanishing cream base that quickly disappears into the skin to avoid staining of clothing. Also contains butylparaben, cetyl palmitate, glyceryl monostearate, methylparaben, polyethylene glycol, stearamidoethyl diethylamine, and purified water.

Indications: For effective temporary relief of minor skin irritations and external genital itching. It relieves the itch and takes the redness out of the skin to break the annoying itch/scratch cycle.

Warnings: For external use only. Avoid contact with the eyes. If condition worsens, or if symptoms persist for more than 7 days, discontinue use of this product and consult a physician. Do not use on children under 2 years of age except under the advice and supervision of a physician. Keep this and all drugs out of the reach of children. In case of accidental ingestion, seek professional assistance or contact a poison control center immediately.

Dosage and Administration: Apply to affected area not more than 3 to 4 times daily.

How Supplied: *Cortef* Feminine Itch Cream (hydrocortisone acetate) is available in ½ oz tubes.

HALTRAN® Tablets
Ibuprofen/Analgesic
MENSTRUAL CRAMP RELIEVER
WARNING: ASPIRIN SENSITIVE PATIENTS. Do not take this product if you have had a severe allergic reaction to aspirin, eg—asthma, swelling, shock or hives, because even though this product contains no aspirin or salicylates cross-reactions may occur in patients allergic to aspirin.

Indications: For the pain of menstrual cramps and also the temporary relief of

minor aches and pains associated with the common cold, headache, toothache, muscular aches, backache, for the minor pain of arthritis and for reduction of fever.

Directions: *Adults:* Take 1 tablet every 4 to 6 hours while symptoms persist. If pain or fever does not respond to 1 tablet, 2 tablets may be used, but do not exceed 6 tablets in 24 hours, unless directed by a doctor. The smallest effective dose should be used. Take with food or milk if occasional and mild heartburn, upset stomach, or stomach pain occurs with use. Consult a doctor if these symptoms are more than mild or if they persist. *Children:* Do not give this product to children under 12 except under the advice and supervision of a doctor.

Warnings: Do not take for pain for more than 10 days or for fever for more than 3 days unless directed by a doctor. If pain or fever persists or gets worse, if new symptoms occur, or if the painful area is red or swollen, consult a doctor. These could be signs of serious illness. If you are under a doctor's care for any serious condition, consult a doctor before taking this product. As with aspirin and acetaminophen, if you have any condition which requires you to take prescription drugs or if you have had any problems or serious side effects from taking any non-prescription pain reliever, do not take HALTRAN Tablets (ibuprofen) without first discussing it with your doctor. If you experience any symptoms which are unusual or seem unrelated to the condition for which you took ibuprofen, consult a doctor before taking any more of it. Although ibuprofen is indicated for the same conditions as aspirin and acetaminophen, it should not be taken with them except under a doctor's direction. Before using any drug, including HALTRAN, you should seek the advice of a health professional if you are pregnant or nursing a baby. IT IS ESPECIALLY IMPORTANT NOT TO USE IBUPROFEN DURING THE LAST 3 MONTHS OF PREGNANCY UNLESS SPECIFICALLY DIRECTED TO DO SO BY A DOCTOR BECAUSE IT MAY CAUSE PROBLEMS IN THE UNBORN CHILD OR COMPLICATIONS DURING DELIVERY. Keep this and all drugs out of the reach of children. In case of accidental overdose, seek professional assistance or contact a poison control center immediately.

Active Ingredient: Each tablet contains ibuprofen USP 200 mg.

Other Ingredients: Carnauba wax, cornstarch, hydroxypropylmethylcellulose, propylene glycol, silicon dioxide, pregelatinized starch, stearic acid, and titanium dioxide.
Store at room temperature. Avoid excessive heat 40°C (104°F).

How Supplied: Blister package of 12; bottles of 30 and 50.
Shown in Product Identification Section, page 432

Continued on next page

Upjohn—Cont.

Advanced Formula
KAOPECTATE®
Concentrated Anti-Diarrheal

Active Ingredient: Each tablespoon contains 600 mg attapulgite.

Inactive Ingredients: Flavors, gucono-delta-lactone, magnesium aluminum silicate, methylparaben, sorbic acid, sucrose, titanium dioxide, xanthan gum and purified water; Peppermint flavor contains FD&C Red #40.

Indications: For the relief of diarrhea and cramps. Relieves diarrhea within 24 hours.

Dosage and Administration: For best results, take full recommended dose at first sign of diarrhea and after each subsequent bowel movement. (Maximum 7 times in 24 hours): Adults and children 12 years of age and over: 2 tablespoons. Children 6 to under 12 years of age: 1 tablespoon. Children 3 to under 6 years of age: $\frac{1}{2}$ tablespoon.

How Supplied: Regular flavor available in 3 oz, 8 oz, 12 oz and 16 oz bottles. Peppermint flavor available in 3 oz, 8 oz and 12 oz bottles.
Shown in Product Identification Section, page 432

Maximum Strength
KAOPECTATE® Tablets
Anti-Diarrhea Medicine

Active Ingredient: Each tablet contains 750 mg attapulgite.

Inactive Ingredients: Croscarmellose Sodium, Pectin, Sucrose and Zinc Stearate.

Indications: For the relief of diarrhea and cramps. Relieves diarrhea within 24 hours.

Dosage and Administration: Swallow whole tablets with water; do not chew. For best results, take full recommended dose.
Adults: Take 2 tablets after the initial bowel movement and 2 tablets after each subsequent bowel movement, not to exceed 12 tablets in 24 hours. Children 6 to 12 years of age: Take 1 tablet after the initial bowel movement and 1 tablet after each subsequent bowel movement, not to exceed 6 tablets in 24 hours. Children 3 to under 6 years of age: Use liquid *Kaopectate* Anti-Diarrheal.

How Supplied: Available in 12 tablet and 20 tablet packages.
Shown in Product Identification Section, page 432

MYCIGUENT® Antibiotic Ointment

Active Ingredient: Each gram contains 5 mg of neomycin sulfate (equivalent to 3.5 mg neomycin). Also contains anhydrous lanolin, mineral oil, and white petrolatum.

Indications: *Myciguent* is a first aid ointment to help prevent infection and aid in the healing of minor cuts, burns and abrasions.

How Supplied: Available in $\frac{1}{2}$ oz, 1 oz and 4 oz tubes.

MYCITRACIN® Triple Antibiotic Ointment

Active Ingredients: Each gram contains 500 units of bacitracin, 5 mg of neomycin sulfate (equivalent to 3.5 mg neomycin) and 5000 units of polymyxin B sulfate. Also contains butylparaben, cholesterol, methylparaben, microcrystalline wax, mineral oil, and white petrolatum.

Indications: *Mycitracin* is a first aid ointment to help prevent infection and aid in the healing of minor cuts, burns and abrasions.

How Supplied: Available in $\frac{1}{32}$ oz unit-dose, $\frac{1}{2}$ oz and 1 oz tubes.
Shown in Product Identification Section, page 432

PYRROXATE® Capsules
Extra Strength
Decongestant/Antihistamine/
Analgesic Capsules

Description: *Pyrroxate* provides single-capsule, multisymptom relief for colds, allergies, nasal/sinus congestion, runny nose, sneezing, and watery eyes. Because it contains the non-aspirin analgesic **acetaminophen,** *Pyrroxate* gives temporary relief of occasional minor aches, pains, headache, and helps in the reduction of fever. *Pyrroxate* is caffeine and aspirin-free.

Ingredients: Each *Pyrroxate* Capsule contains: chlorpheniramine maleate, 4 mg; phenylpropanolamine HCl, 25 mg; acetaminophen, 500 mg. The 500 mg (7.69 gr) strength of acetaminophen per capsule is non-standard, as compared to the established standard of 325 mg (5 gr) acetaminophen per capsule. Also contains benzyl alcohol, butylparaben, D & C yellow No. 10, erythrosine sodium, FD & C blue No. 1, FD & C yellow No. 6 (sunset yellow) as a color additive, gelatin, glycerin, magnesium stearate, methylparaben, propylparaben, sodium lauryl sulfate, sodium propionate, starch, and talc.

Indications: *Pyrroxate* Capsules are for the temporary relief of runny nose, sneezing, itching of the nose or throat; for the temporary relief of nasal congestion due to the common cold, allergies (hay fever), and sinus congestion; for the temporary relief of occasional minor aches, pains, headache, and for the reduction of fever.

Actions: Chlorpheniramine maleate is an antihistamine effective in controlling runny nose, sneezing, watery eyes, and itching of the nose and throat. Phenylpropanolamine HCl is an oral nasal decongestant effective in relieving nasal/sinus congestion due to the common cold or allergies (hay fever). Acetaminophen is a clinically effective analgesic and antipyretic without aspirin side effects.

Warnings: Do not take this product for more than 7 days. If symptoms persist, do not improve, or new ones occur, or if fever persists for more than 3 days, discontinue use and consult your physician. Do not take this product if you have asthma, glaucoma, difficulty in urination due to the enlargement of the prostate gland, high blood pressure, diabetes, thyroid disease, or if you are presently taking a prescription antihypertensive or antidepressant drug containing a monamine oxidase inhibitor, except under the advice and supervision of a physician. As with any drug, if you are pregnant or nursing a baby, seek the advice of a health professional before using this product. Do not exceed recommended dosage because severe liver damage may occur and at higher doses, nervousness, dizziness or sleeplessness may occur. Do not take this product for the treatment of arthritis except under the advice and supervision of a physician.

Cautions: Avoid alcoholic beverages, driving a motor vehicle, or operating heavy machinery while taking this product. This product may cause drowsiness or excitability, especially in children. Keep this and all drugs out of the reach of children. In case of accidental overdose, seek professional assistance or contact a poison control center immediately.

Dosage and Administration: Take 1 capsule every 4 hours or as directed by a physician. Do not take more than 6 capsules in a 24-hour period. Do not administer to children under 12 years of age.

How Supplied: Black/yellow capsules available in blister packages of 24 and bottles of 500.
Shown in Product Identification Section, page 432

SIGTAB® Tablets
High Potency Vitamin Supplement

Each tablet contains:		% U.S. RDA*
Vitamin A	5000 IU	100
Vitamin D	400 IU	100
Vitamin E	15 IU	50
Vitamin C	333 mg	555
Folic Acid	0.4 mg	100
Thiamine	10.3 mg	686
Riboflavin	10 mg	588
Niacin	100 mg	500
Vitamin B_6	6 mg	300
Vitamin B_{12}	18 mcg	300
Pantothenic Acid	20 mg	200

*Percentage of U.S. Recommended Daily Allowances

Recommended dosage: 1 tablet daily

Ingredient List: Sucrose, Sodium Ascorbate (Vit. C), Calcium Sulfate, Niacinamide, Vitamin E Acetate, Calcium Pantothenate, Vitamin A Acetate. Thiamine Mononitrate (B-1), Riboflavin (B-2), Gelatin, Pyridoxine HCl (B-6), Povidone, Lacca, Magnesium Stearate, Silica, Artificial Color, Sodium Benzoate, Folic Acid, Polyethylene Glycol, Cholecalciferol

(Vit. D), Carnauba Wax, Cyanocobalamin (B-12), Medical Antifoam.

How Supplied: Available in bottles of 90 and 500 tablets.

UNICAP® Capsules/Tablets
Multivitamin Supplement in Original Capsule Form
Sugar and Sodium Free Tablet

Indications: Dietary multivitamin supplement of ten essential vitamins in easy to swallow capsule or tablet form for adults and children 4 or more years of age.
Each capsule (or tablet) contains:

		% U.S. RDA*
Vitamin A	5000 Int. Units	100
Vitamin D	400 Int. Units	100
Vitamin E	15 Int. Units	50
Vitamin C	60 mg	100
Folic Acid	400 mcg	100
Thiamine	1.5 mg	100
Riboflavin	1.7 mg	100
Niacin	20 mg	100
Vitamin B_6	2 mg	100
Vitamin B_{12}	6 mcg	100

*Percentage of U.S. Recommended Daily Allowances

Ingredient List:
Capsules: Corn Oil, Gelatin, Ascorbic Acid (Vit. C), Glycerin, Niacinamide, Vitamin E Acetate, Cellulose, Pyridoxine HCl (B-6), Thiamine HCl (B-1), Riboflavin (B-2), Vitamin A Palmitate, Folic Acid, Methylparaben, Lecithin, Ethyl Vanillin, F D & C Yellow No. 5, Vanilla Enhancer, Cholecalciferol (Vit. D), Cyanocobalamin (B-12).
Tablets: Calcium Phosphate, Ascorbic Acid (Vit. C), Vitamin E Acetate, Hydroxypropyl Methylcellulose, Niacinamide Ascorbate, Artifical Color, Vitamin A Acetate, Magnesium Stearate, Pyridoxine Hydrochloride (B-6), Riboflavin (B-2), Silica Gel, Thiamine Mononitrate (B-1), F D & C Yellow No. 5, Folic Acid, Artificial Flavor, Cholecalciferol (Vit. D), Carnauba Wax, Cyanocobalamin (B-12).

Recommended Dosage: 1 capsule or tablet daily

How Supplied: Available in bottles of 120 and 240 capsules; bottles of 120 tablets.

UNICAP JR™ Chewable Tablets

Indications: Dietary multivitamin supplement with essential vitamins in an orange-flavored tablet. For **children** 4 or more years of age.

Each tablet contains:

		% U.S. RDA*
Vitamin A	5000 Int. Units	100
Vitamin D	400 Int. Units	100
Vitamin E	15 Int. Units	50
Vitamin C	60 mg	100
Folic Acid	400 mcg	100
Thiamine	1.5 mg	100
Riboflavin	1.7 mg	100
Niacin	20 mg	100
Vitamin B_6	2 mg	100
Vitamin B_{12}	6 mcg	100

* Percentage of U.S. Recommended Daily Allowances

Ingredient List: Sucrose, Mannitol, Sodium Ascorbate (Vit C), Lactose, Cornstarch, Niacinamide, Citric Acid, Vitamin E Acetate, Povidone, Artificial Flavor, Dextrins, Silica, Calcium Stearate, Pyridoxine HCl (B-6), Artificial Color, Vitamin A Acetate, Thiamine Mononitrate (B-1), Riboflavin (B-2), Folic Acid, Cyanocobalamin (B-12), Cholecalciferol (Vit D).

Recommended Dosage: 1 tablet daily

How Supplied: Available in bottles of 120 tablets.

UNICAP M® Tablets
Multivitamins and Minerals
Sugar Free and Sodium Free

Indications: Dietary supplement of essential vitamins and minerals including iron and calcium for persons 12 or more years of age.

Each tablet contains:

		% U.S. RDA
Vitamin A	5000 Int. Units	100
Vitamin D	400 Int. Units	100
Vitamin E	30 Int. Units	100
Vitamin C	60 mg	100
Folic Acid	400 mcg	100
Thiamine	1.5 mg	100
Riboflavin	1.7 mg	100
Niacin	20 mg	100
Vitamin B_6	2 mg	100
Vitamin B_{12}	6 mcg	100
Pantothenic Acid	10 mg	100
Iodine	150 mcg	100
Iron	18 mg	100
Copper	2 mg	100
Zinc	15 mg	100
Calcium	60 mg	6
Phosphorus	45 mg	5
Manganese	1 mg	+
Potassium	5 mg	+

\+ Recognized as essential in human nutrition, but no U.S. Recommended Daily Allowance (U.S. RDA) has been established.

Ingredient List: Calcium Phosphate, Ascorbic Acid (Vit C) Vitamin E Acetate, Ferrous Fumarate, Cellulose, Niacinamide Ascorbate, Artificial Color, Zinc Oxide, Calcium Pantothenate, Vitamin A Acetate, Potassium Sulfate, Magnesium Stearate, Cupric Sulfate, Silica Gel, Manganese Sulfate, Pyridoxine Hydrochloride, Riboflavin (B-2), Thiamine Mononitrate (B-1), F D & C Yellow No. 5, Folic Acid, Artificial Flavor, Cholecalciferol (Vit D), Potassium Iodide, Carnauba Wax, Cyanocobalamin (B-12).

Recommended Dosage: 1 tablet daily

How Supplied: Available in bottles of 120 and 180 tablets.

Shown in Product Identification Section, page 433

UNICAP® Plus Iron Tablets
Multivitamin Supplement with 100% of the U.S. RDA for Iron
Low in Sodium

Indications: Dietary multivitamin supplement with essential vitamins plus iron for persons 12 or more years of age.

Each tablet contains:

		% U.S. RDA*
Vitamin A	5000 Int. Units	100
Vitamin D	400 Int. Units	100
Vitamin E	15 Int. Units	50
Vitamin C	60 mg	100
Folic Acid	400 mcg	100
Thiamine	1.5 mg	100
Riboflavin	1.7 mg	100
Niacin	20 mg	100
Vitamin B_6	2 mg	100
Vitamin B_{12}	6 mcg	100
Pantothenic Acid	10 mg	100
Iron	18 mg	100

* Percentage of U.S. Recommended Daily Allowances.

Ingredient List: Sucrose, Calcium Sulfate, Sodium Ascorbate (Vit C) Calcium Carbonate, Ferrous Sulfate, Cellulose, Tocopheryl Acetate (Vit E), Niacinamide, Calcium Pantothenate, Vitamin A Acetate, Gelatin, Lacca, Pyridoxine HCl (B-6), Magnesium Stearate, Silica, Riboflavin (B-2), Thiamine Mononitrate (B-1), Povidone, Artificial Color, Folic Acid, Cholecalciferol (Vit D), Polyethylene Glycol, Sodium Benzoate, Carnauba Wax, Cyanocobalamin (B-12), Sesame Oil, Medical Antifoam.

Recommended Dosage: 1 tablet daily

How Supplied: Available in bottles of 120 tablets.

UNICAP® Senior Tablets
Multivitamins and Minerals including Calcium
Sugar Free and Sodium Free

Indications: Dietary supplement of essential vitamins and minerals especially formulated for people 50 years and over to reflect the recommendations of the National Academy of Sciences—National Research Council.

Each tablet contains:

		% U.S. RDA
Vitamin A (includes 200 IU Beta-Carotene)	5000 Int. Units	100
Vitamin D	200 Int. Units	50
Vitamin E	15 Int. Units	50
Vitamin C	60 mg	100
Folic Acid	400 mcg	100
Thiamine	1.2 mg	80
Riboflavin	1.4 mg	70
Niacin	16 mg	80
Vitamin B_6	2.2 mg	110
Vitamin B_{12}	3 mcg	50
Pantothenic Acid	10 mg	100
Iodine	150 mcg	100
Iron	10 mg	56
Copper	2 mg	100
Zinc	15 mg	100
Calcium	100 mg	10

Continued on next page

Upjohn—Cont.

Phosphorus	77 mg	8
Magnesium	30 mg	8
Manganese	1 mg	+
Potassium	5 mg	+

+ Recognized as essential in human nutrition, but no U.S. Recommended Daily Allowance (U.S. RDA) has been established.

Ingredient List: Calcium Phosphate, Cellulose, Ascorbic Acid (Vit C), Magnesium Oxide, Vitamin E Acetate, Ferrous Fumarate, Artificial Color, Zinc Oxide, Niacinamide, Calcium Pantothenate, Vitamin A Acetate, Magnesium Stearate, Potassium Sulfate, Cupric Sulfate, Silica Gel, Beta Carotene, Manganese Sulfate, Pyridoxine Hydrochloride (B-6), Riboflavin (B-2), Thiamine Mononitrate (B-1), Folic Acid, Artificial Flavor, Cholecalciferol (Vit D), Potassium Iodide, Carnauba Wax, Cyanocobalamin (B-12).

Recommended Dosage: 1 tablet daily

How Supplied: Available in bottles of 120 tablets.
Shown in Product Identification Section, page 433

UNICAP T® Tablets
Stress Formula
High Potency
Vitamin-Mineral Supplement with Zinc and Selenium
Sugar Free and Sodium Free

Indications: High potency dietary supplement of essential vitamins and minerals for persons 12 or more years of age.

Each tablet contains:		% U.S. RDA
Vitamin A	5000 Int. Units	100
Vitamin D	400 Int. Units	100
Vitamin E	30 Int. Units	100
Vitamin C	500 mg	833
Folic Acid	400 mcg	100
Thiamine	10 mg	667
Riboflavin	10 mg	588
Niacin	100 mg	500
Vitamin B$_6$	6 mg	300
Vitamin B$_{12}$	18 mcg	300
Pantothenic Acid	25 mg	250
Iodine	150 mcg	100
Iron	18 mg	100
Copper	2 mg	100
Zinc	15 mg	100
Manganese	1 mg	+
Potassium	5 mg	+
Selenium	10 mcg	+

+ Recognized as essential in human nutrition, but no U.S. Recommended Daily Allowance (U.S. RDA) has been established.

Ingredient List: Ascorbic Acid (Vit C), Niacinamide Ascorbate, Cellulose, Hydroxypropyl Methylcellulose, Vitamin E Acetate, Ferrous Fumarate, Artificial Color, Calcium Pantothenate, Calcium Phosphate, Zinc Oxide, Vitamin A Acetate, Magnesium Stearate, Potassium Sulfate, Thiamine Mononitrate (B-1), Riboflavin (B-2), Selenium Yeast, Pyridoxine Hydrochloride (B-6), Cupric Sulfate, Silica Gel, Manganese Sulfate, F D & C Yellow No. 5, Folic Acid, Artificial Flavor, Cholecalciferol (Vit D), Potassium Iodide, Carnauba Wax, Cyanocobalamin (B-12).

Recommended Dosage: 1 tablet daily

How Supplied: Available in bottles of 60 tablets.
Shown in Product Identification Section, page 433

Wakunaga of America Co., Ltd.
Subsidiary of Wakunaga Pharmaceutical Co., Ltd.
23501 MADERO
MISSION VIEJO, CA 92691

KYOLIC®
Odor Modified Garlic

Active Ingredient: Aged Garlic Extract.

Indications: Dietary Supplement.

Suggested Use: Average serving, four capsules or tablets a day during or after meals.

How Supplied: Liquid—Kyolic-Aged Garlic Extract Flavor and Odor Modified Enriched with Vitamin B$_1$ and B$_{12}$ (and empty gelatine capsules) 2 fl oz (62 capsules) and 4 fl oz (124 capsules). Kyolic-Aged Garlic Extract Flavor and Odor Modified Plain (and empty gelatine capsules) 2 fl oz (62 capsules) and 4 fl oz (124 capsules).
Tablets and Capsules—Kyolic-Formula 101 Tablets: Aged Garlic Extract Powder (270 mg) blended with Brewers Yeast (27 mg), Kelp (9 mg) and Algin (9 mg) bottles of 100 and 200 tablets. Kyolic-Formula 101 Capsules: Aged Garlic Extract Powder (270 mg) blended with Brewers Yeast (27 mg), Kelp (9 mg) and Algin (9 mg) bottles of 100 and 200 capsules. Kyolic-Formula 103 Capsules: Aged Garlic Extract Powder (220 mg) blended with Calcium Lactate (200 mg), and Vitamin C (100 mg) bottles of 100 capsules. Kyolic-Super Formula 100 Tablets: Aged Garlic Extract Powder (270 mg) blended with natural vegetable sources: Cellulose and Algin, bottles of 100 and 200 tablets. Kyolic Super Formula 104 Capsules: Aged Garlic Extract Powder (300 mg) with Lecithin (200 mg), bottles of 100 capsules. Formula 105 capsules: Ingredients (per capsule): Kyolic aged garlic extract (200mg) blended with alfalfa leaf (100mg), parsley leaf (50mg) and beta carotene (7.5mg equivalent to 1,250 IU of vitamin A).
Formula 106 capsules: Ingredients (per capsule): Kyolic aged garlic extract powder (300mg), vitamin E (d-alpha tocopheryl succinate) 100 IU blended with; hawthorne berry (50mg) and cayenne pepper (10mg).
Shown in Product Identification Section, page 433

From Soil to Shelf
Brochure describing our company, garlic fields, aging tanks and factory, plus our product line.

Walker, Corp & Co., Inc.
P.O. BOX 1320
EASTHAMPTON PL. &
N. COLLINGWOOD AVE.
SYRACUSE, NY 13201

EVAC–U–GEN®

Description: Evac-U-Gen® is available as purple scored tablets, each containing 97.2 mg of yellow phenolphthalein. Also contains anise oil, corn syrup solids, D&C red 7, FD&C blue 1, lactose, magnesium stearate, saccharin sodium and sugar.

Action and Uses: For temporary relief of occasional constipation and to help restore a normal pattern of evacuation. A mild, non-griping, stimulant laxative in chewable, anise-flavored form, Evac-U-Gen provides gentle, overnight relief by softening of the feces through selective action on the intramural nerve plexus of intestinal smooth muscle, and increases the propulsive peristaltic activity of the colon. It is frequently helpful in preparing the bowel for diagnostic procedures.

Indications: Because of its gentle and non-toxic nature, Evac-U-Gen is suitable in pregnancy, in the presence of hemorrhoids, for children and the elderly. Safe for nursing mothers, it does not affect the infant. It may be especially useful when straining at the stool is a hazard, as in hernia, cardiac or hypertensive patients.

Contraindications: Contraindicated in patients with a history of sensitivity to phenolphthalein. Evac-U-Gen should not be used when abdominal pain, nausea, vomiting, or other symptoms of appendicitis are present.

Side Effects: If skin rash appears, use of Evac-U-Gen or other preparations containing phenolphthalein should be discontinued. May cause coloration of feces or urine if such are sufficiently alkaline.

Warning: Frequent or prolonged use may result in dependence on laxatives. Keep this and all medication out of reach of children.

Administration and Dosage: Adults: chew one or two tablets night or morning. **Children:** Over 6, chew ½ tablet daily. Intensity of action is proportional to dosage, but individually effective doses vary. Evac-U-Gen is usually active 6 to 8 hours after administration, but residual action may last 3 to 4 days.

How Supplied: Evac-U-Gen is available in bottles of 35, 100, 500, 1000 and 6000 tablets.
Shown in Product Identification Section, page 433

Walker Pharmacal Company
4200 LACLEDE AVENUE
ST. LOUIS, MO 63108

PRID SALVE
(Smile's PRID Salve)
Drawing Salve and Anti-infectant

Active Ingredients: Ichthammol (Ammonium Ichthosulfonate) Phenol (Carbolic Acid) Lead Oleate, Rosin, Bees Wax, Lard.

Description: PRID has a very stiff consistency and is almost black in color.

Indication: PRID is an anti-infective salve, which also serves as a skin protective ointment. As a drawing salve, PRID softens the skin around the foreign body, and assists the natural rejection. PRID also helps to prevent the spread of infection. PRID aids in relieving the discomfort of minor skin irritations, superficial cuts, scratches and wounds. PRID is also helpful in the treatment of boils and carbuncles. PRID has been used with some success in the treatment of acne and furunculosis as well as other skin disorders.

Warning: When applied to fingers or toes, do not use a bandage; use loose gauze so as to not interfere with circulation. Apply according to directions for use and in no case to large areas of the body without a physician's direction. Keep out of eyes.

Caution: If PRID salve is not effective in 10 days, see your physician.

Directions For Use: Wash affected parts thoroughly with hot water; dry and apply PRID at least twice daily on a clean bandage or gauze. After irritation subsides, repeat application once a day for several days. DO NOT irritate by squeezing or pressing skin area.

How Supplied: PRID is packaged in a telescoping orange metal can containing 20 grams of PRID salve.

Wallace Laboratories
HALF ACRE ROAD
CRANBURY, NJ 08512

MALTSUPEX®
(malt soup extract)
Powder, Liquid, Tablets

Composition: 'Maltsupex' is a nondiastatic extract from barley malt, which is available in powder, liquid, and tablet form. 'Maltsupex' has a gentle laxative action and promotes soft, easily passed stools. Each **Tablet** contains 750 mg of 'Maltsupex' and approximately 0.15 to 0.25 mEq of potassium. Tablet Ingredients: acetylated monoglycerides, FD&C Yellow #5, FD&C Yellow #6, flavor (artificial), hydroxypropyl methylcellulose, polyethylene glycol, povidone, stearic acid, talc, titanium dioxide. Each tablespoonful (½ fl oz) of **Liquid** and each heaping tablespoonful of **Powder** contains the equivalent of 16 g of Malt Soup Extract Powder and 3.1 to 5.5 mEq of potassium. Other Ingredients: none.

Indications: 'Maltsupex' is indicated for the dietary management and treatment of functional constipation in infants and children. It is also useful in treating constipation in adults, including those with laxative dependence.

Warnings: Do not use when abdominal pain, nausea or vomiting are present. If constipation persists, consult a physician. Keep this and all medications out of the reach of children.
'Maltsupex' Powder and Liquid only—Do not use these products except under the advice and supervision of a physician if you have kidney disease.
As with any drug, if you are pregnant or nursing a baby, seek the advice of a health professional before using this product.

Precautions: In patients with diabetes, allow for carbohydrate content of approximately 14 grams per tablespoonful of **Liquid** (56 calories), 13 grams per tablespoonful of **Powder** (52 calories), and 0.6 grams per Tablet (3 calories). **Tablets only:** This product contains FD&C Yellow No. 5 (tartrazine) which may cause allergic-type reactions (including bronchial asthma) in certain susceptible individuals. Although the overall incidence of FD&C Yellow No. 5 (tartrazine) sensitivity in the general population is low, it is frequently seen in patients who also have aspirin hypersensitivity.

Dosage and Administration: General—The recommended daily dosage of 'Maltsupex' may vary from 6 to 32 grams for infants (2 years or less) and 12 to 64 grams for children and adults, accompanied by adequate fluid intake with each dose. Use the smallest dose that is effective and lower dosage as improvement occurs. Use heaping measures of the **Powder.** 'Maltsupex' **Liquid** mixes more easily if stirred first in one or two ounces of warm water.
Powder and Liquid (Usual Dosage)—
Adults: 2 tablespoonfuls (32 g) twice daily for 3 or 4 days, or until relief is noted, then 1 to 2 tablespoonfuls at bedtime for maintenance, as needed. Drink a full glass (8 oz) of liquid with each dose.
Children: 1 or 2 tablespoonfuls in 8 ounces of liquid once or twice daily (with cereal, milk or preferred beverage). **Bottle-Fed Infants (over 1 month):** ½ to 2 tablespoonfuls in the day's total formula, or 1 to 2 teaspoonfuls in a single feeding to correct constipation. To prevent constipation (as when switching to whole milk) add 1 to 2 teaspoonfuls to the day's formula or 1 teaspoonful to every second feeding. **Breast-Fed Infants (over one month):** 1 to 2 teaspoonfuls in 2 to 4 ounces of water or fruit juice once or twice daily.
Tablets—**Adults:** Start with 4 tablets (3 g) four times daily (with meals and bedtime) and adjust dosage according to response. Drink a full glass (8 oz) of liquid with each dose.

How Supplied: 'Maltsupex' is supplied in 8 ounce (NDC 0037-9101-12) and 16 ounce (NDC 0037-9101-08) jars of 'Maltsupex' Powder; 8 fluid ounce (NDC 0037-9001-12) and 1 pint (NDC 0037-9001-08) bottles of 'Maltsupex' Liquid; and in bottles of 100 'Maltsupex' Tablets (NDC 0037-9201-01).
'Maltsupex' **Powder** and **Liquid** are Distributed by
WALLACE LABORATORIES
Division of
CARTER-WALLACE, INC.
Cranbury, New Jersey 08512
'Maltsupex' **Tablets** are Manufactured by
WALLACE LABORATORIES
Division of
CARTER-WALLACE, INC.
Cranbury, New Jersey 08512
Rev. 10/85
Shown in Product Identification Section, page 433

RYNA™
(Liquid)
RYNA–C®
(Liquid)
RYNA–CX®
(Liquid)

Description:
RYNA Liquid—Each 5 mL (one teaspoonful) contains:
Chlorpheniramine maleate..............2 mg
Pseudoephedrine hydrochloride....30 mg
Other ingredients: flavor (artificial), glycerin, malic acid, sodium benzoate, sorbitol, purified water, in a clear, slightly yellow colored, lemon-vanilla flavored demulcent base containing no sugar, dyes, or alcohol.
RYNA-C Liquid—Each 5 mL (one teaspoonful) contains, in addition:
Codeine phosphate..........................10 mg
(WARNING: May be habit-forming)
Other ingredients: flavor (artificial), glycerin, malic acid, purified water, saccharin sodium, sodium benzoate, sorbitol, in a clear, colorless to slightly yellow, cinnamon-flavored, demulcent base containing no sugar, dyes, or alcohol.
RYNA-CX Liquid—Each 5 mL (one teaspoonful) contains:
Codeine phosphate..........................10 mg
(WARNING: May be habit-forming)
Pseudoephedrine hydrochloride....30 mg
Guaifenesin.....................................100 mg
Other ingredients: flavors (artificial), glycerin, glycine, malic acid, povidone, propylene glycol, purified water, saccharin sodium, sorbitol, in a clear, colorless, cherry-vanilla-menthol flavored demulcent base containing no sugar, dyes, or alcohol.

Actions:
Chlorpheniramine maleate in RYNA and RYNA-C is an antihistamine that antagonizes the effects of histamine.
Codeine phosphate in RYNA-C and RYNA-CX is a centrally-acting antitussive that relieves cough.
Pseudoephedrine hydrochloride in RYNA, RYNA-C and RYNA-CX is a sym-

Continued on next page

Wallace—Cont.

pathomimetic nasal decongestant that acts to shrink swollen mucosa of the respiratory tract.

Guaifenesin in RYNA-CX is an expectorant that increases mucus flow to help prevent dryness and relieve irritated respiratory tract membranes.

Indications:

RYNA: For the temporary relief of the concurrent symptoms of nasal congestion, sneezing, itchy and watery eyes, and running nose as occur with the common cold or allergic rhinitis.

RYNA-C: Temporarily relieves cough, nasal congestion, runny nose and sneezing as may occur with the common cold.

RYNA-CX: Temporarily relieves cough and nasal congestion as may occur with the common cold. Relieves irritated membranes in the respiratory passageways by preventing dryness through increased mucus flow.

Warnings:

For RYNA:

Do not give this product to children taking other medication or to children under 6 years except under the advice and supervision of a physician. Do not exceed recommended dosage unless directed by a physician because nervousness, dizziness, or sleeplessness may occur at higher doses. If symptoms do not improve within 3 days or are accompanied by high fever, discontinue use and consult a physician. Do not take this product except under the advice and supervision of a physician if you have any of the following symptoms or conditions: high blood pressure; heart disease; thyroid disease; diabetes; asthma; glaucoma; or difficulty in urination due to enlargement of the prostate.

For RYNA-C and RYNA-CX:

Adults and children who have a chronic pulmonary disease or shortness of breath, or children who are taking other drugs, should not take these products unless directed by a physician. Do not give these products to children under 6 years of age except under the advice and supervision of a physician. A persistent cough may be a sign of a serious condition. If cough persists for more than one week, tends to recur, or is accompanied by fever, rash or persistent headache, consult a physician. Do not take these products for persistent or chronic cough such as occurs with smoking, asthma, emphysema, or if cough is accompanied by excessive phlegm (mucus) unless directed by a physician. Do not take these products if you have glaucoma, asthma, emphysema, difficulty in breathing, difficulty in urination due to enlargement of the prostate gland, heart disease, high blood pressure, thyroid disease, or diabetes unless directed by a physician. May cause or aggravate constipation.

Do not take these products or give to children for more than 7 days. If symptoms do not improve or are accompanied by fever, consult a physician. Unless directed by a physician, do not exceed recommended dosage because nervous-

ness, dizziness or sleeplessness may occur at higher doses.

For RYNA and RYNA-C:

These products contain an antihistamine which may cause excitability, especially in children, or drowsiness or may impair mental alertness. Combined use with alcohol, sedatives, or other depressants may have an additive effect. Do not drive motor vehicles, operate machinery, or drink alcoholic beverages while taking these products.

As with any drug, if you are pregnant or nursing a baby, seek the advice of a health professional before using these products.

Drug Interaction Precaution: Persons who are presently taking a prescription drug for high blood pressure or depression should not use these products without consulting a physician.

Dosage and Administration:

Adults: 2 teaspoonfuls every 6 hours.
Children 6 to under 12 years: 1 teaspoonful every 6 hours.
Children under 6 years: consult a physician.
DO NOT EXCEED 4 DOSES IN 24 HOURS.

Ryna-C and Ryna-CX:

A special measuring device should be used to give an accurate dose of these products to children under 6 years of age. Giving a higher dose than recommended by a physician could result in serious side effects for the child.

How Supplied:

RYNA: bottles of 4 fl oz (NDC 0037-0638-66) and one pint (NDC 0037-0638-68).

RYNA-C: bottles of 4 fl oz (NDC 0037-0522-66) and one pint (NDC 0037-0522-68).

RYNA-CX: bottles of 4 fl oz (NDC 0037-0801-66) and one pint (NDC 0037-0801-68).

TAMPER-RESISTANT BAND ON CAP, PRINTED "WALLACE LABORATORIES". DO NOT USE IF BAND IS MISSING OR BROKEN.

Storage:

RYNA: Store below 30° (86°F).

RYNA-C and RYNA-CX: Store at controlled room temperature. Protect from excessive heat and freezing.

KEEP THESE AND ALL DRUGS OUT OF THE REACH OF CHILDREN. IN CASE OF ACCIDENTAL OVERDOSE, SEEK PROFESSIONAL ASSISTANCE OR CONTACT A POISON CONTROL CENTER IMMEDIATELY.

WALLACE LABORATORIES
Division of
CARTER-WALLACE, Inc.
Cranbury, New Jersey 08512
Rev. 8/88

Shown in Product Identification Section, page 433

SYLLACT®
(Powdered Psyllium Seed Husks)

Description: Each rounded teaspoonful of fruit-flavored **'Syllact'** contains approximately 3.3 g of powdered psyl-

lium seed husks and an equal amount of dextrose as a dispersing agent, and provides about 14 calories. Potassium sorbate, methyl and propylparaben are added as preservatives. Other ingredients: citric acid, dextrose, FD&C Red #40, flavor (artificial), and saccharin sodium.

Actions: The active ingredient in 'Syllact' is hydrophilic mucilloid, non-absorbable dietary fiber derived from the powdered husks of natural psyllium seed, which acts by increasing the water content and bulk volume of stools. It gives 'Syllact' a bland, non-irritating, laxative action and promotes physiologic evacuation of the bowel.

Indications: 'Syllact' is indicated for the treatment of constipation and, when recommended by a physician, in other disorders where the effect of additional bulk and fiber is desired.

Warnings: Do not swallow dry. Drink a full glass (8 oz) of water or other liquid with each dose. If constipation persists, consult a physician. Do not use if fecal impaction, intestinal obstruction, or abdominal pain, nausea or vomiting are present. Keep this and all medications out of the reach of children.

As with any drug, if you are pregnant or nursing a baby, seek the advice of a health professional before using this product.

Dosage and Administration: The actual daily dosage depends on the need and response of the patient. Adults may take up to 9 teaspoonfuls daily, in divided doses, for several days to provide optimum benefit when constipation is chronic or severe. Lower the dosage as improvement occurs. Use a dry spoon to measure powder. Tighten lid to keep out moisture.

Usual Adult Dosage—One rounded teaspoonful of 'Syllact' in a full glass (8 oz) of cool water or other beverage taken orally one to three times daily. If desired, an additional glass of liquid may be taken after each dose.

Children's Dosage—6 years and older—Half the adult dosage with the same fluid intake requirement.

How Supplied: 'Syllact' Powder—in 10 oz jars (NDC 0037-9501-13).

Rev. 10/85
WALLACE LABORATORIES
Division of
CARTER-WALLACE, INC.
Cranbury, New Jersey 08512
Shown in Product Identification Section, page 433

Products are
indexed alphabetically
in the
PINK SECTION

Warner-Lambert Company
Consumer Health Products Group
201 TABOR ROAD
MORRIS PLAINS, NJ 07950

PROFESSIONAL STRENGTH EFFEREDENT
Denture Cleanser

Active Ingredients: Potassium monopersulfate, sodium perborate, sodium carbonate, sodium tripolyphoshate and surfactants.

Inactive Ingredients: Sodium bicarbonate, citric acid, colors and flavors.

Indications: For effective and convenient daily denture cleaning to remove plaque and stains and to inhibit bacterial growth on dentures and removable orthodontic appliances.

Actions: Efferdent's effervescent cleansing action removes stubborn stains between teeth, whitens and brightens, flights plaque and leaves dentures and orthodontic appliances fresh tasting and odor free.

Warnings: Keep out of the reach of children. DO NOT PUT TABLETS IN MOUTH

Dosage and Administration: For best results, use at least once daily. Dentures may be soaked safely in Efferdent overnight.

How Supplied: Available in boxes of 20, 40, 60 and 96 tablets
Shown in Product Identification Section, page, 433

HALLS® MENTHO–LYPTUS®
Cough Suppressant Tablets

Active Ingredients: Each tablet contains eucalyptus oil and menthol.

Inactive Ingredients: Corn Syrup, Flavoring, Sugar and Artificial Colors.

Indications: For temporary relief of minor throat irritation and coughs due to colds or inhaled irritants. Makes nasal passages feel clearer.

Warning: A persistent cough or sore throat may be a sign of a serious condition. If cough persists for more than 1 week, tends to recur, or is accompanied by fever, rash or persistent headache, or if sore throat is severe, persistent or accompanied by high fever, headache, nausea, and vomiting, consult a doctor. Do not take this product for sore throat lasting more than 2 days or persistent or chronic cough such as occurs with smoking, asthma, emphysema, or if cough is accompanied by excessive phlegm (mucus) unless directed by a doctor. Keep this and all drugs out of the reach of children.

Dosage and Administration: Adults and children 3 years and over dissolve one tablet slowly in mouth. Repeat every hour as needed or as directed by a doctor. Children under 3 years: consult a doctor.

How Supplied: Halls Mentho-Lyptus Cough Suppressant Tablets are available in single sticks of 9 tablets each, in 3-stick packs, and in bags of 30 tablets. They are available in five flavors: Regular, Cherry, Honey-Lemon, Ice Blue, and Spearmint.
Shown in Product Identification Section, page 433

HALLS® Vitamin C Drops

Description: Halls Vitamin C Drops are a delicious way to get 100% of the U.S. Recommended Daily Allowance of Vitamin C. Each drop provides 60 mg. of Vitamin C (100% U.S. RDA)

Ingredients: Sugar, Glucose Syrup, Sodium Ascorbate, Citric Acid, Ascorbic Acid, Natural Flavoring and Artificial Color (Including Yellow 5 and Yellow 6).

Indication: Dietary Supplementation.

How Supplied: Halls Vitamin C Drops are available in single sticks of 9 drops each and in bags of 30 drops. They are available in 5 great tasting all-natural citrus flavors: tangerine, lemon, sweet grapefruit, lime and orange.

LISTERINE® Antiseptic

Active Ingredients: Thymol .06%, Eucalyptol .09%, Methyl Salicylate .06% and Menthol .04%. Also contains: Water, Alcohol 26.9%, Benzoic Acid, Poloxamer 407 and Caramel.

Indications: To help prevent and reduce supragingival plaque and gingivitis; for general oral hygiene and bad breath.

Actions: Listerine Antiseptic has been shown to help prevent and reduce supragingival plaque and gingivitis when used in a conscientiously applied program of daily oral hygiene and regular professional care. Its effect on periodontitis has not been demonstrated. Listerine is the only non-prescription mouthrinse that has received the American Dental Association's Council on Dental Therapeutics Seal of Acceptance for helping to prevent and reduce plaque above the gumline and gingivitis.

Directions: Rinse full strength for 30 seconds with ⅔ ounce (4 teaspoonfuls) morning and night. If bad breath persists, see your dentist.

How Supplied: Listerine Antiseptic is supplied in 3, 6, 12, 18, 24, 32 and 48 fl. oz. bottles.
Shown in Product Identification Section, page 433

LISTERINE ANTISEPTIC THROAT LOZENGES

Active Ingredients: Each lozenge contains: Hexylresorcinol.

Inactive Ingredients: Caramel, Corn Syrup, Flavoring, Glycerin and Sugar.

Indications: For fast temporary relief of minor sore throat pain.

Actions: When allowed to dissolve slowly in the mouth Listerine Lozenges bathes the throat with the soothing pain relieving action of Hexylresorcinol a safe and effective topical anesthetic. Listerine Lozenges provide fast temporary relief from minor sore throat pain of colds, smoking and mouth irritations.

Warnings: Severe or persistent sore throat, or sore throat accompanied by high fever, headache, nausea and vomiting, may be serious. Consult physician promptly. Do not use more than 2 days or administer to children under 3 years of age unless directed by a physician. Keep this and all drugs out of the reach of children.

Dosage: 1 lozenge every 2 hours as needed.

Storage: Store at room temperature.

How Supplied: 24 count packages

Available In: Regular Strength (Hexylresorcinol 2.4 mg.) in Cherry, Lemon-Mint and Regular flavors and Maximum Strength (Hexylresorcinol 4.0 mg.).
Shown in Product Identification Section, page 433

LISTERMINT®
Mouthwash with Fluoride

Active Ingredient: Sodium Fluoride (0.02%). Also contains: Water, SD alcohol 38-B (6.65%), glycerin, poloxamer 407, sodium lauryl sulfate, sodium citrate, flavoring, sodium saccharin, zinc chloride, citric acid, D&C Yellow No. 10, FD&C Green No. 3.

Indications: Aids in prevention of dental cavities and freshens breath.

Directions: Adults and children 6 years of age and older: Use twice a day after brushing teeth with toothpaste. Vigorously swish 10 ml. (2 teaspoonfuls) of rinse between teeth for 1 minute and spit out. Do not swallow the rinse. Do not eat or drink for 30 minutes after rinsing.

Warnings: Children under 12 years of age should be supervised in the use of this product. Consult a dentist or physician for use in children under 6 years of age. Developing teeth of children under 6 years of age may become permanently discolored if excessive amounts of fluoride are repeatedly swallowed. This is not a dentifrice and should not be used as a substitute for regular toothbrushing. Keep this and all drugs out of reach of children.

How Supplied: Listermint with Fluoride is supplied to consumers in 6, 12, 18, 24 and 32 fl. oz. bottles.
Shown in Product Identification Section, page 433

LUBRIDERM® CREAM
Skin Lubricant Moisturizer

Composition:
Scented—Contains Water, Mineral Oil, Petrolatum, Glycerin, Glyceryl Stearate,

Continued on next page

Warner-Lambert—Cont.

PEG 100 Stearate, Hydrogenated Polyisobutene, Lanolin, Lanolin Alcohol, Lanolin Oil, Cetyl Alcohol, Sorbitan Laurate, Fragrance, Methylparaben, Butylparaben, Propylparaben, Quaternium-15.

Fragrance Free—Contains Water, Mineral Oil, Petrolatum, Glycerin, Glyceryl Stearate, PEG 100 Stearate, Hydrogenated Polyisobutene, Lanolin, Lanolin Alcohol, Lanolin Oil, Cetyl Alcohol, Sorbitan Laurate, Methylparaben, Butylparaben, Propylparaben, Quaternium-15.

Actions and Uses: Lubriderm Cream is an emollient-rich formula designed for extremely dry skin. Lubriderm cream relieves the roughness, dryness, and discomfort associated with dry or chapped skin and helps protect the skin from drying.

Lubriderm Cream is ideal for overnight treatment of extra dry skin. It smooths on easily and penetrates to help smooth, soften, and moisturize.

Administration and Dosage: Apply as often as needed to extra dry skin areas.

Precautions: For external use only.

How Supplied:
Scented: Available in 2.7 oz. pump container.
Fragrance Free: Available in a 2.7 oz. pump container.
Shown in Product Identification Section, page 434

LUBRIDERM® LOTION
Skin Lubricant Moisturizer

Composition:
Scented—Contains Water, Mineral Oil, Petrolatum, Sorbitol, Lanolin, Lanolin Alcohol, Stearic Acid, Triethanolamine, Cetyl Alcohol, Fragrance, Butylparaben, Methylparaben, Propylparaben, Sodium Chloride.
Fragrance Free—Contains Water, Mineral Oil, Petrolatum, Sorbitol, Lanolin, Lanolin Alcohol, Stearic Acid, Triethanolamine, Cetyl Alcohol, Butylparaben, Methylparaben, Propylparaben, Sodium Chloride.

Actions and Uses: Lubriderm Lotion is an oil-in-water emulsion indicated for use in softening, soothing and moisturizing dry chapped skin. Lubriderm relieves the roughness, tightness and discomfort associated with dry or chapped skin and helps protect the skin from further drying.

Lubriderm's extra rich formula smoothes easily into skin without leaving a sticky film.

Administration and Dosage: Apply as often as needed to hands, face and body for skin protection.

Precautions: For external use only.

How Supplied:
Scented: Available in 1, 4, 8 and 16 fl. oz. plastic bottles.

Fragrance Free: Available in 8 and 16 fl. oz. plastic bottles.
Shown in Product Identification Section, page 434

LUBRIDERM LUBATH®
Skin Conditioning Oil

Composition: Contains Mineral Oil, PPG-15 Stearyl Ether, Oleth-2, Nonoxynol-5, Fragrance, D&C Green No. 6.

Actions and Uses: Lubriderm Skin Conditioning Oil is a lanolin-free, mineral oil based, bath oil designed for softening and soothing dry skin during the bath. The formula disperses into countless droplets of oil that coat the skin and help lubricate and soften. It is equally effective in hard or soft water and provides an excellent way to moisturize the skin, and help counterbalance the drying effects of harsh soaps and hot water.

Administration and Dosage: One to two capfuls (16 oz. size) or two to four capfuls (8 oz. size) in bath, or apply with moistened cloth in shower and rinse. For use as a skin cleanser, rub into wet skin and rinse.

Precautions: Avoid getting in eyes, if this occurs, flush with clear water. When using any bath oil, take precautions against slipping. For external use only.

How Supplied: Available in 8 and 16 fl. oz. plastic bottles.
Shown in Product Identification Section, page 434

REMEGEL

Active Ingredients: Each piece contains: Aluminum hydroxide-magnesium carbonate codried gel 476.4 mg.

Inactive Ingredients: Corn syrup, D&C Yellow No. 10, egg white, flavoring, FD&C Green No. 3, glyceryl monostearate, modified food starch, partially hydrogenated palm kernel oil, preservative (BHA), sugar and titanium dioxide. Contains 25 mg. sodium per piece. Store at room temperature.

Indications: For the relief of heartburn, sour stomach or acid indigestion and upset stomach associated with these symptoms.

Action: Remegel is a fast-acting, highly effective antacid in a pleasant-tasting, soft, chewable form. Each square has an acid-neutralizing capacity of 132 ml of 0.1 N hydrochloric acid which is comparable to the leading liquid antacids. It has been clinically proven to relieve the symptoms of acid indigestion, heartburn and sour stomach and associated upset stomach. The superior palatability of Remegel has been demonstrated in consumer tests and the soft, chewable, mint-flavored dosage form encourages patient compliance with recommended and antacid regimens.

Warnings: Do not take more than 12 pieces in a 24-hour period, nor use the maximum dosage for more than two weeks, nor use this product if you are on

a sodium restricted diet, except under the advice and supervision of a physician. Keep this and all drugs out of the reach of children.

Drug Interaction Precaution: Do not take this product if you are presently taking a prescription antibiotic drug containing any form of tetracycline.

Directions: Chew one or two pieces as symptoms occur. Repeat hourly if symptoms return or as directed by a physician.

How Supplied: Single sticks with 8 pieces. 3-Packed Single Sticks with a total of 24 pieces.
Shown in Product Identification Section, page 434

ROLAIDS®

Active Ingredient: Dihydroxyaluminum Sodium Carbonate. 334 mg. contains 53 mg. sodium per tablet.

Inactive Ingredients: Corn Starch, Corn Syrup, Flavoring, Magnesium Stearate and Sugar.

Indications: For the relief of heartburn, sour stomach or acid indigestion and upset stomach associated with these symptoms.

Actions: Rolaids® provides rapid neutralization of stomach acid. Each tablet has acid neutralizing capacity of 75–80 ml. of 0.1N hydrochloric acid and the ability to maintain the pH of the stomach contents close to 3.5 for a significant period of time—the pH never reaching into the alkaline region.

Due to the relatively low solubility and other physical and chemical properties of dihydroxyaluminum sodium carbonate (DASC), it is for the most part nonabsorbed.

Although sodium is present in DASC, the sodium is available for absorption only when the antacid reacts with stomach acid. When Rolaids are consumed in excess of the amount of acid present in the stomach, this sodium is unavailable for absorption and the active ingredient is passed through the digestive system unchanged, with no sodium released.

Warnings: Keep this and all drugs out of the reach of children. Do not take more than 24 tablets in a 24 hour period, nor use the maximum dosage of this product for more than two weeks, nor use this product if you are on a sodium restricted diet, except under the advice and supervision of a physician.

Drug Interaction Precaution: Do not take this product if you are presently taking a prescription antibiotic drug containing any form of tetracycline.

Dosage and Administration: Chew 1 or 2 tablets as symptoms occur. Repeat hourly if symptoms return or as directed by a physician.

How Supplied: Rolaids is available in Regular (Peppermint), Spearmint and Wintergreen Flavors. One roll contains 12 tablets; 3-Pack contains three 12-tab-

let rolls; One bottle contains 75 tablets; one bottle contains 150 tablets.

Shown in Product Identification Section, page 434

CALCIUM RICH ROLAIDS®

Active Ingredient: Calcium Carbonate 550 mg. per tablet.

Inactive Ingredients:
Cherry Flavor: Corn Starch, FD&C Red No. 3, Flavoring, Magnesium Stearate, Mannitol, Polyethylene Glycol, Sugar and Titanium Dioxide.
Assorted Fruit Flavors: Colors (FD&C Blue No. 1, Red 3, Red 40, Yellow 5 [Tartrazine] and Yellow 6), Corn Starch, Flavoring, Magnesium Stearate, Mannitol, Pregelatinized Starch and Sugar.

Indications: For the relief of heartburn, sour stomach or acid indigestion and upset stomach associated with these symptoms.

Actions: Calcium Rich Rolaids provides rapid neutralization of stomach acid. Each tablet has an acid neutralizing capacity of 110 ml of 0.1N hydrochloric acid and the ability to maintain the pH of the stomach contents at 3.5 or greater for a significant period of time—the pH never reaches into the alkaline region. Each tablet provides 22% of the Adult U.S. RDA for calcium.

Warnings: Do not take more than 14 tablets in a 24 hour period or use the maximum dosage of this product for more than 2 weeks except under the advice and supervision of a physician. Keep this and all drugs out of the reach of children.

Drug Interaction Precaution: None.

Dosage and Administration: Chew 1 or 2 tablets as symptoms occur. Repeat hourly if symptoms return or as directed by a physician.

How Supplied: Calcium Rich Rolaids is available in Cherry and Assorted Fruit Flavors. One roll contains 12 tablets: 3-pack contains three 12-tablet rolls; one bottle contains 75 tablets; one bottle contains 150 tablets.

Shown in Product Identification Section, page 434

SODIUM FREE ROLAIDS®

Active Ingredients: Calcium Carbonate 317 mg. and magnesium hydroxide 64 mg. per tablet.

Inactive Ingredients: Corn starch, corn syrup, flavoring, magnesium stearate, mannitol and sugar.

Indications: For the relief of heartburn, sour stomach or acid indigestion and upset stomach associated with these symptoms.

Actions: Rolaids Sodium Free provides rapid neutralization of stomach acid. Each tablet has an acid neutralizing capacity of 85 ml of 0.1N hydrochloric acid

and the ability to maintain the pH of the stomach contents close to 3.5 for a significant period of time—the pH never reaching into the alkaline region.

Warnings: Do not take more than 18 tablets in a 24 hour period or use the maximum dosage of this product for more than 2 weeks except under the advice and supervision of a physician. Keep this and all drugs out of the reach of children.

Drug Interaction Precaution: None.

Dosage and Administration: Chew 1 or 2 tablets as symptoms occur. Repeat hourly if symptoms return, or as directed by a physician.

How Supplied: One roll contains 12 tablets: 3-pack contains three 12-tablet rolls; one bottle contains 75 tablets; one bottle contains 150 tablets.

Shown in Product Identification Section, page 434

Westwood Pharmaceuticals Inc.
**100 FOREST AVENUE
BUFFALO, NY 14213**

ALPHA KERI®
Moisture Rich Body Oil

Composition: Contains mineral oil, Hydroloc™ brand of Westwood's PEG-4 dilaurate, lanolin oil, fragrance, benzophenone-3, D&C green 6.

Action and Uses: ALPHA KERI is a water-dispersible, antipruritic oil for the care of dry skin. ALPHA KERI effectively deposits a thin, uniform, emulsified film of oil over the skin. This film helps relieve itching, lubricates and softens the skin. ALPHA KERI Moisture Rich Body Oil is an all-over skin moisturizer. Only Alpha Keri contains Hydroloc™—the unique emulsifier that provides a more uniform distribution of the therapeutic oils to moisturize dry skin. ALPHA KERI is valuable as an aid in the treatment of dry, pruritic skin and mild skin irritations such as chronic atopic dermatitis; pruritus senilis and hiemalis; contact dermatitis; "bath-itch"; xerosis or asteatosis; ichthyosis; soap dermatitis; psoriasis.

Adminstration and Dosage: ALPHA KERI *should always be used with water, either added to water or rubbed on to wet skin.* Because of its inherent cleansing properties it is not necessary to use soap when ALPHA KERI is being used.
For exact dosage, label directions should be followed.
BATH: Added as directed to bathtub of water. For optimum relief: 10 to 20 minute soak.
SHOWER: Dispense a small amount into hand and rub onto wet skin. Rinse as desired and pat dry.
SPONGE BATH: Added as directed to a basin of warm water then rubbed over entire body with washcloth.

SITZ BATH: Added as directed to tub water. Soak should last for 10 to 20 minutes.
INFANT BATH: Added as directed to basin or bathinette of water.
SKIN CLEANSING OTHER THAN BATH OR SHOWER: A small amount is rubbed onto wet skin. Rinse. Pat dry.

Precaution: The patient should be warned to guard against slipping in tub or shower.

How Supplied: 4 fl. oz. (NDC 0072-3600-04) 8 fl. oz. (NDC 0072-3600-08), 12 fl. oz. (NDC 0072-3600-12) and 16 fl. oz. (NDC 0072-3600-16) plastic bottles. Also available in non-aerosol pump spray, 3.5 oz. (NDC 0072-3601-35)

Shown in Product Identification Section, page 434

ALPHA KERI®
Moisture Rich Cleansing Bar
Non-detergent Soap

Composition: Sodium tallowate, sodium cocoate, water, mineral oil, fragrance, PEG-75, glycerin, titanium dioxide, lanolin oil, sodium chloride, BHT, trisodium HEDTA, D&C Green 5, D&C Yellow 10.

Action and Uses: ALPHA KERI Moisture Rich Cleansing Bar, rich in emollient oils, thoroughly cleanses as it soothes and softens the skin.

Indications: Adjunctive use in dry skin care.

Administration and Dosage: To be used as any other soap.

How Supplied: 4 oz. (NDC 0072-3500-04) bar.

BALNETAR®
Water-dispersible Emollient Tar

Composition: Contains WESTWOOD® TAR (equivalent to 2.5% Coal Tar USP) in mineral oil, laureth-4, lanolin oil, PEG-4 dilaurate, fragrance, and sodium dioctyl sulfosuccinate.

Action and Uses: For temporary relief of itching and scaling due to psoriasis, eczema, and other tar-responsive dermatoses. Tar ingredient is chemically and biologically standardized to insure uniform therapeutic activity. BALNETAR exerts keratoplastic, antieczematous, antipruritic, and emollient actions. It deposits microfine particles of tar over the skin in a lubricant-moisturizing film that helps soften and remove scales and crusts, making the skin smoother and more supple. BALNETAR is an important adjunct in a wide range of dermatoses, including: atopic dermatitis; chronic eczematoid dermatitis; seborrheic dermatitis.

Contraindications: Not indicated when acute inflammation is present.

Administration and Dosage: BALNETAR *should always be used with water... either added to water or rubbed onto wet*

Continued on next page

Westwood—Cont.

skin. For exact dosage label directions are to be followed.

IN THE TUB—Add as directed to a bathtub of water. Soap is not used. The patient soaks for 10 to 20 minutes and then pats dry.

FOR DIRECT APPLICATION—A small amount is rubbed onto the wet skin. Excess is wiped off with tissue to help prevent staining of clothes or linens.

FOR SCALP APPLICATION—A small amount is rubbed onto the wet scalp with fingertips.

Caution: If irritation persists, discontinue use. May temporarily discolor blond, bleached or tinted hair. In rare cases BALNETAR may cause allergic sensitization attributable to coal tar. For external use only. Keep this and all drugs out of reach of children.

Precaution: After use of BALNETAR, patient should avoid exposure to direct sunlight unless sunlight is being used therapeutically in a supervised, modified Goeckerman regimen. Contact with the eyes should be avoided. Patient should be cautioned against slipping when BALNETAR is used in bathtub. Also advise patient that use in a plastic or fiberglass tub may cause staining of the tub.

How Supplied: 8 fl. oz. (NDC 0072-4200-08) plastic shatterproof bottle.

ESTAR®
Therapeutic Tar Gel

Active Ingredient: Westwood tar (biologically equivalent to 5% coal tar USP). Also contains: B-alanine, benzyl alcohol, carbomer 940, glycereth-7 coconate, polysorbate 80, 15.6% SD alcohol 40, simethicone, sorbitol and water.

Actions and Uses: A therapeutic aid in the treatment of eczema, psoriasis, and other tar-responsive dermatoses such as atopic dermatitis, lichen simplex chronicus, and nummular eczema. ESTAR exerts keratoplastic, antieczematous, and antipruritic actions. It is equivalent in its photodynamic activity to 5% crude coal tar in either hydrophilic ointment or petrolatum. ESTAR provides the characteristic benefits of tar therapy in a form that is readily accepted by patients and nursing staff, due to its negligible tar odor and staining potential, and the superior cosmetic qualities of its gel base. ESTAR is suitable for use in a modified Goeckerman regimen, either in the hospital or on an outpatient basis; it also can be used in followup treatment to help maintain remissions. Substantivity to the skin can be demonstrated by examination with a Wood's light, which shows residual microfine particles of tar on the skin several days after application.

Contraindications: ESTAR should not be applied to acutely inflamed skin or used by individuals who are known to be sensitive to coal tar.

Administration and Dosage: *Psoriasis:* ESTAR can be applied at bedtime in

the following manner: the patient should massage ESTAR into affected areas, allowing the gel to remain for five minutes, and then remove excess by patting with tissues. This procedure minimizes staining of skin and clothing, leaving behind an almost invisible layer of the active tar. If any staining of fabric should occur, it can be removed easily by standard laundry procedures.

The same technique of application may be used the following morning. If dryness occurs, an emollient may be applied one hour after ESTAR.

Because of ESTAR's superior substantivity and cosmetic qualities, patients who might otherwise be hospitalized for tar/UV therapy can now be treated as outpatients. The patient can easily apply ESTAR at bedtime and the following morning, then report for UV treatment that day. Laboratory tests and clinical experience to date suggest that it may be advisable to carefully regulate the length of UV exposure.

Chronic atopic dermatitis, lichen simplex chronicus, nummular eczema, and seborrheic dermatitis: One or two applications per day as described above, are suggested. If dryness occurs, an emollient may be applied one hour after ESTAR and between applications as needed.

Caution: PROTECT TREATED AREAS FROM DIRECT SUNLIGHT, FOR AT LEAST 24 HOURS AFTER APPLICATION, UNLESS DIRECTED BY A PHYSICIAN. AVOID USE ON INFECTED, HIGHLY INFLAMED OR BROKEN SKIN. DO NOT APPLY TO GENITAL AREA. If used on the scalp, temporary discoloration of blond, bleached, or tinted hair may occur. If undue irritation develops or increases, the usage schedule should be changed or ESTAR discontinued. Contact with the eyes should be avoided. In case of contact, flush eyes with water.

Slight staining of clothing may occur. Standard laundry procedures will usually remove stains. For external use only.

How Supplied: 3 oz. (NDC 0072-7603-03) plastic tube.

FOSTEX® MEDICATED CLEANSING BAR
Acne Skin Cleanser

Active Ingredients: Sulfur 2%, salicylic acid 2%. Also Contains: Boric acid, cellulose gum, dextrin, disodium EDTA, docusate sodium, fragrance, lactic acid, ochre, sodium lauryl sulfoacetate (or sodium dodecyl benzene sulfonate and trisodium sulfosuccinate), sodium octoxynol-2 ethane sulfonate, sorbitol, urea and water.

Action and Uses: FOSTEX MEDICATED CLEANSING BAR is a surface-active, penetrating anti-seborrheic cleanser for therapeutic washing of the skin in the local treatment of acne and other skin conditions characterized by excessive oiliness. Degreases, dries and mildly desquamates.

Administration and Dosage: Use FOSTEX MEDICATED CLEANSING BAR instead of soap. Wash entire affected area 2 or 3 times daily, or as physician directs. Rinse well. The desired degree of dryness and peeling may be obtained by regulating frequency of use.

Caution: Avoid contact with eyes. In case of contact, flush with water. If undue skin irritation develops or increases, discontinue use and consult physician. For external use only. Keep this and all drugs out of the reach of children.

How Supplied: 3¾ oz. (NDC 0072-3000-01) bar.

Shown in Product Identification Section, page 434

FOSTEX® MEDICATED CLEANSING CREAM
Acne Skin Cleanser and Dandruff Shampoo

Active Ingredients: Sulfur 2% and salicylic acid 2%. Also contains: Ceteareth-20, D&C yellow #10, docusate sodium, EDTA, food starch, fragrance, methylcellulose, poloxamer 188, sodium chloride, sodium dodecyl benzene sulfonate, sodium octoxynol-2 ethane sulfonate, stearyl alcohol and water.

Action and Uses: A penetrating antiseborrheic cleanser for the local treatment of acne, dandruff and other seborrheic skin conditions, characterized by excessive oiliness. Degreases, dries and mildly desquamates.

Administration and Dosage: AS A WASH: Wet skin; wash entire affected area with FOSTEX MEDICATED CLEANSING CREAM instead of soap. Rinse thoroughly. Use 2 or 3 times daily or as physician directs. The desired degree of dryness and peeling may be obtained by regulating frequency of use.

AS A SHAMPOO: Use liberal amount on wet scalp and hair. Shampoo thoroughly, rinse, and repeat shampoo. Rinse thoroughly. No other shampoos are required. To help keep scalp free from excessive oiliness or scaling, use FOSTEX MEDICATED CLEANSING CREAM as often as necessary or as physician directs.

Caution: Avoid contact with eyes. In case of contact, flush with water. If undue skin irritation develops or increases, discontinue use and consult physician. For external use only.

How Supplied: FOSTEX MEDICATED CLEANSING CREAM in 4 oz. (NDC 0072-3200-01) tube.

FOSTEX® 5% BENZOYL PEROXIDE GEL
Antibacterial Acne Gel

Active Ingredient: Benzoyl peroxide 5%. Also contains: Carbomer 940, diisopropanolamine, disodium EDTA, laureth-4 and water.

Action and Uses: FOSTEX 5% BENZOYL PEROXIDE GEL is a penetrating,

disappearing gel which helps kill bacteria that cause acne. Helps prevent new pimples before they appear. Drying action promotes gentle peeling to help clear acne skin.

Indications: A topical aid for the control of acne vulgaris.

Administration and Dosage: After washing, rub FOSTEX 5% BENZOYL PEROXIDE GEL into entire affected area twice daily, or as physician directs. In fair-skinned individuals or in excessively dry climates start with only one application daily. The desired degree of dryness and peeling may be obtained by regulating frequency of use.

Caution: Avoid contact with eyes, lips and mucous membranes. In case of contact, flush with water. Persons with very sensitive skin or a known allergy to benzoyl peroxide should not use this medication. If itching, redness, burning or swelling occurs, discontinue use. For external use only. May bleach dyed fabrics. Keep this and all drugs out of the reach of children. Store at controlled room temperature (59°–86°F).

How Supplied: 1.5 oz (NDC 0072-3300-02) plastic tube.

FOSTEX 10% BENZOYL PEROXIDE CLEANSING BAR
Antibacterial Acne Cleanser

Active Ingredient: Benzoyl peroxide 10%. Also contains: Boric acid, cellulose gum, dextrin (may contain wheat starch), disodium EDTA, docusate sodium, lactic acid, sodium lauryl sulfoacetate (or sodium dodecyl benzene sulfonate and trisodium sulfosuccinate), sodium octoxynol-2 ethane sulfonate, sorbitol, urea and water.

Action and Uses: FOSTEX 10% BENZOYL PEROXIDE CLEANSING BAR helps kill bacteria that can cause acne. Helps prevent new pimples before they appear. Drying action promotes gentle peeling to help clear your skin.

Indications: A topical aid for the control of acne vulgaris.

Administration and Dosage: Use FOSTEX 10% BENZOYL PEROXIDE CLEANSING BAR instead of soap. For best results, wash entire affected area gently with fingertips for 1 to 2 minutes, 2 to 3 times daily, or as physician directs. Rinse well. The desired degree of dryness and peeling may be obtained by regulating frequency of use.

Caution: Avoid contact with eyes, lips and mucous membranes. In case of contact, flush with water. Persons with very sensitive skin or a known allergy to benzoyl peroxide should not use this medication. If itching, redness, burning or swelling occurs, discontinue use. If symptoms persist, consult a physician. For external use only. May bleach dyed fabrics. Keep this and all drugs out of the reach of children. Store at controlled room temperature (59°–86°F).

How Supplied: 3¾ oz. (NDC 0072-2900-03) bar.

Shown in Product Identification Section, page 434

FOSTEX® 10% BENZOYL PEROXIDE GEL
Antibacterial Acne Gel

Active Ingredient: 10% benzoyl peroxide. Also contains: Carbomer 940, diisopropanolamine, disodium EDTA, laureth-4, and water.

Action and Uses: FOSTEX 10% BENZOYL PEROXIDE GEL provides super strong protection against acne with 10% benzoyl peroxide... the strongest concentration of the most effective acne fighter you can buy without a prescription. Penetrates to kill bacteria that can cause acne. Helps prevent new pimples before they appear. Drying action promotes peeling to help clear skin. Wear day and night for invisible acne treatment.

Administration and Dosage: Before applying FOSTEX 10% BENZOYL PEROXIDE GEL, start fresh with a Fostex cleanser—to clean skin effectively. After washing, rub Fostex 10% Benzoyl Peroxide Gel into entire affected area twice daily, or as physician directs. In fair-skinned individuals or in excessively dry climates, start with only one application daily. The desired degree of dryness and peeling may be obtained by regulating frequency of use.

Caution: Avoid contact with eyes, lips and mucous membranes. In case of contact, flush with water. Persons with very sensitive skin or a known allergy to benzoyl peroxide should not use this medication. If itching, redness, burning or swelling occurs, discontinue use. If symptoms persist, consult a physician. For external use only. May bleach dyed fabrics. Keep this and all drugs out of the reach of children.

How Supplied: 1.5 oz. (NDC 0072-4300-01) plastic tube.

Shown in Product Identification Section, page 434

FOSTEX 10% BENZOYL PEROXIDE TINTED CREAM
Antibacterial Acne Cream

Active Ingredient: Benzoyl peroxide 10%. Also contains: Citric acid, disodium EDTA, glyceryl stearate, hydroxypropyl methylcellulose, isopropyl palmitate, magnesium aluminum silicate, ochre, POE-21 stearyl ether, propylene glycol, red oxide, simethicone, steareth-2, talc, titanium dioxide, umber and water.

Action and Uses: FOSTEX 10% BENZOYL PEROXIDE TINTED CREAM provides super-strong protection against acne with 10% benzoyl peroxide... the strongest concentration of the most effective acne fighter you can buy without a prescription. Conceals as it helps heal. Helps prevent new pimples. Drying action promotes peeling to help clear skin.

Wear this skin-tone acne medication day and night.

Administration and Dosage: Start fresh with a Fostex cleanser to clean skin effectively. After washing, rub FOSTEX 10% BENZOYL PEROXIDE TINTED CREAM into entire affected area twice daily, or as physician directs. In fair-skinned individuals or in excessively dry climates, start with only one application daily. The desired degree of dryness and peeling may be obtained by regulating frequency of use.

Caution: Avoid contact with eyes, lips and mucous membranes. In case of contact, flush with water. Persons with very sensitive skin or a known allergy to benzoyl peroxide should not use this medication. If itching, redness, burning or swelling occurs, discontinue use. If symptoms persist consult a physician. For external use only. May bleach dyed fabrics. Keep this and all drugs out of reach of children. Store at controlled room temperature (59°–86°F).

How Supplied: 1½ oz. (NDC 0072-4002-01).

FOSTEX 10% BENZOYL PEROXIDE WASH
Antibacterial Acne Wash

Active Ingredient: Benzoyl peroxide 10%. Also contains: Citric acid, disodium EDTA, docusate sodium, magnesium aluminum silicate, methylcellulose, sodium chloride, sodium laureth sulfate and water.

Action and Uses: FOSTEX 10% BENZOYL PEROXIDE WASH helps kill bacteria that can cause acne. Helps prevent new pimples before they appear. Drying action promotes gentle peeling to help clear your acne.

Indications: A topical aid for the control of acne vulgaris.

Administration and Dosage: Shake well. Wet skin; wash entire affected area with FOSTEX 10% BENZOYL PEROXIDE WASH instead of soap. Wash gently for 1 to 2 minutes, 2 to 3 times daily, or as physician directs. The desired degree of dryness and peeling may be obtained by regulating frequency of use.

Caution: Avoid contact with eyes, lips and mucous membranes. In case of contact, flush with water. Persons with very sensitive skin or a known allergy to benzoyl peroxide should not use this medication. If itching, redness, burning or swelling occurs, discontinue use. If symptoms persist, consult a physician. For external use only. May bleach dyed fabrics. Keep this and all drugs out of reach of children. Store at controlled room temperature (59°–86°F).

How Supplied: 5 oz. (NDC 0072-3100-05) plastic bottles.

Continued on next page

Westwood—Cont.

FOSTRIL®
Drying Lotion for Acne

Active Ingredient: Sulfur 2%. Also contains: Bentonite, citric acid, EDTA, fragrance, hydroxypropyl methylcellulose, laureth-4, magnesium aluminium silicate, methylparaben, ochre, PEG-8 stearate, PEG-40 stearate, propylparaben, quaternium-15, red oxide, simethicone, talc, umber, water and zinc oxide.

Action and Uses: Promotes drying and peeling of the skin in the treatment of acne. Daily use of FOSTRIL should result in a desirable degree of dryness and peeling in about 7 days. FOSTRIL removes excess oil and follicular obstruction, helping to remove comedones. It also helps prevent epithelial closure of pores and formation of new lesions.

Administration and Dosage: A thin film is applied to affected areas once or twice daily, or as directed.

Caution: If undue skin irritation develops or increases, adjust usage schedule or discontinue use. Anti-inflammatory measures may be used if necessary. For external use only. Contact with eyes should be avoided. In case of contact, flush eyes thoroughly with water.

How Supplied: 1 oz. (NDC 0072-3800-01) tube.

KERI® CREME
Concentrated Moisturizer— Non-greasy Emollient

Composition: Contains water, mineral oil, talc, sorbitol, ceresin, lanolin alcohol/mineral oil, magnesium stearate, glyceryl oleate/propylene glycol, isopropyl myristate, methylparaben, propylparaben, fragrance, quaternium-15.

Actions and Uses: KERI CREME is a concentrated moisturizer and non-greasy emollient for problem dry skin— hands, face, elbows, feet, legs. KERI CREME helps retain moisture that makes skin feel soft, smooth, supple. Helps resist the drying effects of soaps, detergents and chemicals.

Administration and Dosage: A small amount is rubbed into dry skin areas as needed.

How Supplied: 2.25 oz. (NDC 0072-5800-01) tube.

KERI® FACIAL SOAP
Non-detergent Facial Soap

Composition: KERI LOTION® concentrate in a gentle, non-detergent soap containing: sodium tallowate, sodium cocoate, water, mineral oil, octyl hydroxystearate, fragrance, glycerin, titanium dioxide, PEG-75, lanolin oil, dioctyl sodium sulfosuccinate, PEG-4 dilaurate, propylparaben, PEG-40 stearate, glyceryl monostearate, PEG-100 stearate, sodium chloride, BHT, trisodium HEDTA.

Action and Uses: KERI FACIAL SOAP helps keep skin soft while thoroughly cleansing.

Administration and Dosage: To be used as facial soap.

How Supplied: 3.25 oz. (NDC 0072-4900-03) bar.

KERI LOTION
Skin Lubricant—Moisturizer

Available in two formulations:
KERI Original—recommended for extremely dry skin.

Composition: Contains mineral oil in water, propylene glycol, PEG-40 stearate, glyceryl stearate, PEG-100 stearate, PEG-4 dilaurate, laureth-4, lanolin oil, methylparaben, propylparaben, carbomer-934, triethanolamine, fragrance, dioctyl sodium sulfosuccinate, quaternium-15. Freshly-scented: FD&C blue 1, D&C yellow 10.

KERI-Silky Smooth—recommended for daily use on dry skin.

Composition: Water, petrolatum, glycerin, dimethicone, steareth-2, cetyl alcohol, benzyl alcohol, laureth-23, carbomer-934, MgAl silicate, fragrance, quaternium-15, sodium hydroxide.

Action and Uses: KERI Lotion lubricates and helps hydrate the skin, making it soft and smooth. It relieves itching, helps maintain a normal moisture balance and supplements the protective action of skin lipids. Indicated for generalized dryness and itching; detergent hands; chapped or chafed skin; sunburn; "winter-itch", aging, dry skin; diaper rash; heat rash.

Administration and Dosage: Apply as often as needed. Use particularly after bathing and exposure to sun, water, soaps and detergents.

How Supplied: KERI Lotion Original 6½ oz. (NDC 0072-4600-56), 13 oz. (NDC 0072-4600-63) and 20 oz. (NDC 0072-4600-70) plastic bottles. KERI Lotion Fresh Herbal Scent 6½ oz. (NDC 0072-4500-56), 13 oz. (NDC 0072-4500-63), and 20 oz. (NDC 0072-4500-70) plastic bottles. KERI Silky Smooth 6½ oz. (NDC 0072-4400-65), 13 oz. (NDC 0072-4400-13) and 20 oz. (NDC 0072-4400-20) plastic bottle.

Shown in Product Identification Section, page 434

LOWILA® CAKE
Soap-free Skin Cleanser

Composition: Contains dextrin, sodium lauryl sulfoacetate, water, boric acid, urea, sorbitol, mineral oil, PEG-14 M, lactic acid, dioctyl sodium sulfosuccinate, cellulose gum, fragrance.

Action and Uses: LOWILA CAKE is indicated when soap should not be used, for cleansing skin that is sensitive or irritated, or in dermatitic and eczematous conditions. Used for general bathing, infant bathing, routine washing of hands

and face and shampooing. The pH of LOWILA CAKE helps protect the skin's normal acid mantle and create an environment favorable to therapy and healing.

Administration and Dosage: LOWILA CAKE is used in place of soap. Lathers well in both hard and soft water.

How Supplied: 3¾ oz. (NDC 0072-2300-01) bar.

MOISTUREL® CREAM
Skin Lubricant—Moisturizer

Composition: Water, petrolatum, glycerin, PG dioctanoate, cetyl alcohol, steareth-2, dimethicone, PVP/hexadecene copolymer, laureth-23, Mg Al silicate, diazolidinyl urea, carbomer-934, sodium hydroxide, methylchloroisothiazolinone and methylisothiazolinone.

Actions and Uses: A highly effective concentrated formula clinically proven to relieve dry skin. Free of lanolins, fragrances, and parabens that can sensitize or irritate skin. Indicated for generalized dry skin, chapped or chafed skin, diaper rash, sunburn, windburn, heat rash, itching and dryness associated with eczema.

Administration and Dosage: Apply a small amount as often as needed.

How Supplied: 4 oz. (NDC 0072-9500-04) and 16 oz. (NDC 0072-9500-16) plastic jars.
Shown in Product Identification Section, page 434

MOISTUREL® LOTION
Skin Lubricant—Moisturizer

Composition: Water, petrolatum, glycerin, dimethicone, steareth-2, cetyl alcohol, benzyl alcohol, laureth-23, Mg Al silicate, carbomer-934, sodium hydroxide, quaternium-15.

Action and Uses: MOISTUREL is a non-greasy formula that leaves the skin feeling smooth and soft. Clinically proven to relieve dry skin. Free of parabens and fragrances that can sensitize or irritate skin. Indicated for generalized dry skin, chapped or chafed skin, diaper rash, sunburn, heat rash, itching and dryness associated with eczema.

Administration and Dosage: Apply liberally as often as needed.

How Supplied: 8 oz. (NDC 0072-9100-08) and 12 oz. (NDC 0072-9100-12) plastic bottles.
Shown in Product Identification Section, page 434

MOISTUREL®
SENSITIVE SKIN CLEANSER
Pure, Clear and Soap-Free

Composition: Sodium laureth sulfate and laureth 6 carboxylic acid and disodium laureth sulfosuccinate, methyl gluceth-20, cocamidopropyl betaine, water, diazolidinyl urea, and methylchloroisothiazolinone and methylisothiazolinone.

Actions and Uses: Moisturel Sensitive Skin Cleanser is a crystal clear, lathering, soap-free cleanser. It cleans thoroughly without stinging, irritating, or drying. Unlike soaps, Moisturel Sensitive Skin Cleanser rinses refreshingly clean without leaving a film or residue. Its pure and gentle formula makes it ideal for facial use. Its non-drying, noncomedogenic, and fragrance-free formula makes it ideal for cleansing:
• Sensitive skin—even a baby's
• Dry, itchy skin caused by cold and wind, or overexposure to sun
• Skin robbed of moisture by use and removal of cosmetics
• Irritated, allergic skin
• Skin that breaks out
• Skin dried by harsh acne medications

Administration and Dosage: With skin wet, gently work Moisturel Sensitive Skin Cleanser into a rich lather by massaging in a circular motion. Rinse thoroughly and pat dry with a soft cloth.

Caution: Avoid contact with eyes. For external use only.

How Supplied: 8.75 oz. (NDC 0072-6420-08) plastic bottle with pump.
Shown in Product Identification Section, page 434

PERNOX® LOTION
Lathering Scrub Cleanser for Acne

Active Ingredients: Sulfur 2% and salicylic acid 2%. Also contains: Docusate sodium, EDTA, fragrance, magnesium aluminum silicate, methylcellulose, modified starch, polyethylene, sodium dodecyl benzene sulfonate, sodium octoxynol-2 ethane sulfonate and water.

Actions and Uses: PERNOX LOTION is a therapeutic scrub cleanser in lotion form that is to be used routinely instead of soap. It gently desquamates or peels acne or oily skin. PERNOX LOTION also removes excessive oil from the skin surface and will produce mild drying of the affected skin areas when used regularly. It helps skin feel fresher and smoother with each wash.

Contraindications: Not indicated when acute inflammation is present or in nodular or cystic acne.

Administration and Dosage: To be shaken well before using. PERNOX may be used instead of soap one or two times daily or as directed. The skin should be wet first and PERNOX applied with the fingertips. The lather should be massaged into skin for one-half to one minute. The patient then rinses thoroughly and pats dry.

Caution: If undue skin irritation develops or increases, adjust usage schedule or discontinue use. For external use only. Contact with eyes should be avoided. In case of contact, flush eyes with water.

How Supplied: 5 oz. (NDC 0072-7900-05) plastic bottle.

PERNOX®
Medicated Scrub Cleanser for Acne

Active Ingredients: Sulfur 2% and salicylic acid 1.5%. Also contains: D&C yellow #10, docusate sodium, EDTA, FD&C Blue #1, food starch, fragrance, methylcellulose, poloxamer 184, polyethylene, sodium dodecyl benzene sulfonate, sodium octoxynol-2-ethane sulfonate and water. Lemon formulation does not contain FD&C Blue #1.

Actions and Uses: A lathering scrub cleanser for acne, oily skin. PERNOX provides microfine, uniform-size scrub particles with a rounded surface area to enable patients to achieve effective and gentle desquamation as they wash their skin. PERNOX helps loosen and remove comedones, dries, peels and degreases acne skin. It lathers abundantly and leaves the skin feeling smooth.

Contraindications: Not indicated when acute inflammation is present or in nodular or cystic acne.

Administration and Dosage: After wetting the skin, PERNOX is applied with the fingertips and massaged onto the skin for about one-half to one minute. The skin is then thoroughly rinsed. May be used instead of soap one to two times daily, or as directed.

Caution: If undue skin irritation develops or increases, adjust usage schedule or discontinue use. If necessary, anti-inflammatory measures may be used after discontinuance. For external use only. Contact with eyes should be avoided. In case of contact, flush eyes thoroughly with water.

How Supplied: 2 oz. (NDC 0072-5200-02); and 4 oz. (NDC 0072-5200-04) tubes; lemon scented: 2 oz. (NDC 0072-5300-02), and 4 oz. (NDC 0072-5300-04) tubes.

PERNOX® SHAMPOO
For Oily Hair

Composition: A blend of biodegradable cleansers and hair conditioners, containing: sodium laureth sulfate, water, lauramide DEA, quaternium 22, PEG-75 lanolin/hydrolyzed animal protein, sodium chloride, fragrance, lactic acid, sorbic acid, disodium EDTA, FD&C yellow 6, FD&C blue 1.

Actions and Uses: A gentle but thorough shampoo especially formulated to cleanse, control and condition oily hair. Especially suitable for adjunctive use with acne patients. PERNOX SHAMPOO works into a rich, pleasant lather, leaves the hair lustrous and manageable. Its special conditioners help prevent tangles and fly away hair. Gentle enough to be used every day. It contains a refreshing natural scent.

Administration and Dosage: A liberal amount is massaged into wet hair and scalp. A good lather is worked up, massaging thoroughly. This is followed by a rinse and repeat application. A final rinse is used. No other shampoos or hair conditioners are necessary. May be used as needed.

Caution: For external use only. Contact with the eyes should be avoided. In case of contact, flush eyes with water. Keep this and all drugs out of reach of children.

How Supplied: 8 fl. oz. (NDC 0072-5500-08) shatterproof plastic bottle.

PRESUN® FOR KIDS
Children's Sunscreen

Active Ingredients: Octyl methoxycinnamate, oxybenzone, octyl salicylate. Also contains: Carbomer-940, cetyl alcohol, diazolidinyl urea, dimethicone, methylchloroisothiazolinone and methylisothiazolinone, stearic acid, triethanolamine, water and other ingredients.

Actions and Uses: 29 TIMES NATURAL PROTECTION: Used as directed, PRESUN For Kids provides 29 times your child's natural sunburn protection and may help reduce the chance of premature aging and wrinkling of the skin. Clinical research indicates that regular use of a sunscreen (SPF 15) during the first 18 years of life may reduce the risk of developing the two most common forms of skin cancer by as much as 78%.
NON-STINGING: A non-PABA, fragrance-free formula that is designed not to sting sensitive skin. (Avoid contact with eyes since all sunscreens can cause irritation and stinging of the eye.)
HYPOALLERGENIC: PRESUN For Kids is hypoallergenic and, because the known sensitizers common to most sunscreens have been removed, is suitable for your child's sensitive skin.
WATERPROOF 29: PRESUN For Kids maintains its degree of protection (SPF 29) even after 80 minutes in the water.

Warnings: For external use only. Protect from freezing. *As with all sunscreens:* Apply to a small area; check after 24 hours. Discontinue use if irritation or rash appears. Avoid contact with eyes. In case of contact, flush eyes with water. Keep out of the reach of children. Use on children under six months of age only with the advice of a physician.

Administration and Dosage: For maximum protection, smooth evenly and liberally onto dry skin before sun exposure. Massage in gently. Reapplication to dry skin after prolonged swimming, excessive perspiration or towel drying is recommended for all day protection.

How Supplied: 4 oz (NDC 0072-9399-04) plastic bottle.

PRESUN® 8, 15 and 39 CREAMY SUNSCREENS

Active Ingredients: Octyl dimethyl PABA, oxybenzone. Also contains: Carbomer-940, cetyl alcohol, diazolidinyl urea, dimethicone, fragrance, methylchloroisothiazolinone and methyliso-

Continued on next page

Westwood—Cont.

thiazolinone, stearic acid, triethanolamine, water, and other ingredients.

Action and Uses: **8, 15 or 39 TIMES NATURAL PROTECTION:** Used as directed. PRESUN Creamy Sunscreens provide 8, 15 or 39 times your natural *sunscreen* protection and may help reduce the chance of premature aging and wrinkling of the skin as well as skin cancer caused by overexposure to the sun.

UVA/UVB PROTECTION: PRESUN Sunscren is formulated to provide protection from the harmful effects of both UVA and UVB rays.

WATERPROOF PRESUN Creamy Sunscreen maintains its degree of protection even after 80 minutes in the water.

Warnings: For external use only. Protect from freezing. Do not use if sensitive to P-aminobenzoic acid (PABA) or related compounds. *As with all sunscreens:* Apply to a small area; check after 24 hours. Discontinue use if irritation or rash appears. Avoid contact with eyes. In case of contact, flush eyes with water. Keep out of the reach of children. Use on children under six months of age only with the advice of a physician.

Administration and Dosage: Smooth evenly onto dry skin before sun exposure. Massage in gently. Reapply to dry skin after prolonged swimming, excessive perspiration or towel drying. Repeated applications during prolonged sun exposure are recommended.

How Supplied: 8 Creamy: 4 oz. (NDC 0072-8506-04) plastic bottle. 15 Creamy: 4 oz. (NDC 0072-8906-04) plastic bottle. 39 Creamy: 4 oz. (NDC 0072-9600-04) plastic bottle.

PRESUN® 15 FACIAL STICK/LIP PROTECTOR SUNSCREEN

Active Ingredients: 8% Octyl dimethyl PABA, 3% oxybenzone. Also contains: Flavoring, lanolin oil, mineral oil, ozokerite, PEG-4 dilaurate, petrolatum and propylparaben.

Actions and Uses: **15 TIMES NATURAL PROTECTION:** Used as directed, PRESUN 15 Facial Sunscreen Stick and Sunscreen Lip Protector provide 15 times your natural *sunburn* protection and may help reduce the chance of premature aging and wrinkling of the skin as well as skin cancer caused by overexposure to the sun.

UVA/UVB PROTECTION: PRESUN 15 Facial Sunscreen Stick and Sunscreen Lip Protector are formulated to provide protection from the harmful effects of both UVA and UVB rays.

MOISTURIZES: PRESUN 15 Facial Sunscreen Stick helps keep your skin soft and smooth—even after long hours in the sun.

PRESUN 15 Sunscreen Lip Protector helps prevent drying, cracking and chapping from the sun, wind or cold.

Warnings: For external use only. Do not use if sensitive to P-aminobenzoic

acid (PABA) or related compounds. *As with all sunscreens:* Apply to a small area; check after 24 hours. Discontinue use if irritation or rash appears. Avoid contact with eyes. In case of contact, flush eyes with water. Keep out of the reach of children. Use on children under six months of age only with the advice of a physician.

Administration and Dosage: Facial Stick: Apply evenly to dry skin before sun exposure. Reapply to dry skin after swimming, excessive perspiration or towel drying. Repeated applications during prolonged sun exposure are recommended.

Lip Protector: Apply to lips as needed. Repeated applications during prolonged exposure to the sun, wind or cold are recommended.

How Supplied: .42 oz. (NDC 0072-8703-04) plastic facial stick, .15 oz. (NDC 0072-8703-01) plastic lip stick.

PRESUN® 15 FACIAL SUNSCREEN
Ultra Sunscreen Protection

Active Ingredients: 8% Octyl dimethyl PABA, 3% oxybenzone. Also contains: Benzyl alcohol, carbomer 934, cetyl alcohol, dimethicone, glyceryl stearate, laureth-23, magnesium aluminum silicate, petrolatum, propylene glycol dioctanoate, quaternium-15, sodium hydroxide, steareth-2 and water.

Action and Uses: **15 TIMES NATURAL PROTECTION:** Used as directed, PRESUN 15 Facial Sunscreen provides 15 times your natural *sunburn* protection and may help reduce the chance of premature aging and wrinkling of the skin as well as skin cancer caused by overexposure to the sun.

UVA/UVB PROTECTION: PRESUN 15 Facial Sunscreen is formulated to provide protection from the harmful effects of both UVA and UVB rays.

MOISTURIZES: PRESUN 15 Facial Sunscreen was developed especially for use on the face. The special moisturizers soften and smooth your skin while protecting it from the drying effects of the sun.

SUITABLE UNDER MAKE-UP: A non-greasy cream made especially for daily use under facial make-up and designed not to clog pores or cause acne or blemishes.

Administration and Dosage: Gently smooth evenly onto dry skin before sun exposure. Reapply to dry skin after swimming, excessive perspiration or towel drying. Repeated applications during prolonged sun exposure are recommended.

Warnings: For external use only. Do not use if sensitive to p-aminobenzoic acid (PABA) or related compounds. *As with all sunscreens:* Apply to a small area; check after 24 hours. Discontinue use if irritation or rash appears. Avoid contact with eyes. In case of contact, flush eyes with water. Keep out of reach of children. Use on children under six

months of age only with the advice of a physician.

How Supplied: 2 oz. (NDC 0072-9200-02) plastic tube.

PRESUN® 15 and 29 SENSITIVE SKIN SUNSCREENS
PABA-FREE Sunscreen Protection

Active Ingredients: Octyl methoxycinnamate, oxybenzone, octyl salicylate. Also contains: Carbomer-940, cetyl alcohol, diazolidinyl urea, dimethicone, methylchloroisothiazolinone and methylisothiazolinone, stearic acid, triethanolamine, water, and other ingredients.

Actions and Uses:
15 or 29 TIMES NATURAL PROTECTION: Used as directed, PRESUN 15 or 29 Sensitive Skin Sunscreen provides 15 or 29 times your natural *sunburn* protection and may help reduce the chance of premature aging and wrinkling of the skin as well as skin cancer caused by overexposure to the sun.

UVA/UVB PROTECTION: PRESUN 15 or 29 Sensitive Skin Sunscreen is formulated to provide protection from the harmful effects of both UVA and UVB rays.

PABA-FREE FORMULA: A PABA- and fragrance-free formula that provides a very high degree of sunburn protection and, because the known sensitizers common to most sunscreens have been removed, is suitable for sensitive skin.

WATERPROOF: PRESUN Sensitive Skin Sunscreen maintains its degree of protection even after 80 minutes in the water.

Administration and Dosage: For maximum protection, smooth evenly and liberally onto dry skin before sun exposure. Massage in gently. Reapplication to dry skin after prolonged swimming, excessive perspiration or towel drying is recommended for all day protection.

Warnings: For external use only. Protect from freezing. *As with all sunscreens:* Apply to a small area; check after 24 hours. Discontinue use if irritation or rash appears. Avoid contact with eyes. In case of contact, flush eyes with water. Keep out of the reach of children. Use on children under six months of age only with the advice of a physician.

How Supplied: 29 Sensitive Skin: 4 oz. (NDC 0072-9300-04; NSN 6505-01-267-1483) plastic bottle. 15 Sensitive Skin: 4 oz. (NDC 0072-9370-04) plastic bottle.

Shown in Product Identification Section, page 434

SEBUCARE®
Antiseborrheic Scalp Lotion

Contains: 1.8% Salicylic acid, 61% alcohol, water, PPG-40 butyl ether, laureth-4, dihydroabietyl alcohol, fragrance.

Action and Uses: An aid in the treatment of dandruff, seborrhea capitis and other scaling conditions of the scalp.

SEBUCARE helps control scaling, oiliness and itching. The unique base helps soften brittle hair and grooms the hair, thus eliminating the need for hair dressing which often impedes antiseborrheic treatment. SEBUCARE should be used every day in conjunction with a therapeutic shampoo such as SEBULEX®.

Administration and Dosage: SEBUCARE is applied directly to scalp and massaged thoroughly with fingertips. Comb or brush as usual. Grooms as it medicates. Use once or twice daily or as directed.

Precaution: Volatile—Avoid flame. For external use only. Keep this and all drugs out of reach of children. Avoid contact with eyes. In case of contact, flush eyes with water.

How Supplied: 4 fl. oz. (NDC 0072-4800-04) plastic bottle.

SEBULEX®
Antiseborrheic Treatment Shampoo

Active Ingredients: 2% sulfur and 2% salicylic acid. Also contains: D&C yellow #10, docusate sodium, EDTA, FD&C blue #1, fragrance, PEG-6 lauramide, PEG-14M, sodium dodecyl benzene sulfonate, sodium octoxynol-2 ethane sulfonate and water.

Action and Uses: A penetrating therapeutic shampoo for the temporary relief of itchy scalp and the scaling of dandruff. SEBULEX helps to relieve dandruff and itching, and removes excess oil. It penetrates and softens the crusty, matted layers of scales adhering to the scalp, and leaves the hair soft and manageable.

Administration and Dosage: SEBULEX liquid should be shaken before being used. SEBULEX is massaged into wet scalp. Lather should be allowed to remain on scalp for about 5 minutes and then rinsed. Application is repeated, followed by a thorough rinse. Initially, SEBULEX can be used daily, or every other day, or as directed, depending on the condition. Once symptoms are under control, one or two treatments a week usually will maintain control of itching, oiliness and scaling.

Caution: If undue skin irritation develops or increases, discontinue use. For external use only. Contact with eyes should be avoided. In case of contact, flush eyes thoroughly with water. Keep this and all drugs out of reach of children.

How Supplied: SEBULEX in 4 oz. (NDC 0072-2700-04) and 8 oz. (NDC 0072-2700-08) plastic bottles.

Shown in Product Identification Section, page 434

SEBULEX® SHAMPOO WITH CONDITIONERS
Antiseborrheic Treatment and Conditioning Shampoo

Active Ingredients: 2% sulfur, 2% salicylic acid. Also contains: water, sodium octoxynol-3 sulfonate, sodium lauryl sulfate, lauramide DEA, acetamide MEA, amphoteric-2, hydrolyzed animal protein, magnesium aluminum silicate, propylene glycol, methylcellulose, PEG-14 M, fragrance, disodium EDTA, dioctyl sodium sulfosuccinate, FD & C blue 1, D & C yellow 10.

Action and Uses: SEBULEX SHAMPOO WITH CONDITIONERS provides effective temporary control of the scaling and itching of dandruff and seborrheic dermatitis, while adding protein to the hair shaft to increase its manageability.

Administration and Dosage: SEBULEX SHAMPOO WITH CONDITIONERS should be shaken well before use. Shampoo five minutes. For optimum dandruff control and conditioning leave lather on scalp for the full five minutes. Rinse. Repeat. Use daily until control is achieved. Use to to three times weekly to maintain control, although daily use may be continued. Consult physician for severe or unresponsive scalp conditions.

Caution: If undue skin irritation develops or increases, discontinue use and consult physician. Contact with eyes should be avoided. In cases of contact, eyes should be flushed thoroughly with water. For external use only. Keep this and all drugs out of reach of children.

How Supplied: 4 oz. (NDC 0072-2600-04) and 8 oz. (NDC 0072-2600-08) plastic bottles.

SEBULON® DANDRUFF SHAMPOO
Antiseborrheic Treatment and Conditioning Shampoo

Composition: 2% Zinc pyrithione. Also contains: Water, TEA-lauryl sulfate, disodium oleamido PEG-2 sulfosuccinate, cocamide DEA, acetamide MEA, magnesium aluminum silicate, hydroxypropyl guar, benzyl alcohol, fragrance, quaternium-15, FD & C green 3 and D & C green 5.

Action and Uses: SEBULON SHAMPOO—specially formulated to relieve the itching and flaking of dandruff and seborrheic dermatitis. Leaves hair clean and manageable.

Administration and Dosage: Shake well before using. For best results use at least twice a week. Can be used daily, if desired. Wet hair, apply to scalp and massage vigorously. Rinse and repeat.

Caution: For external use only. If condition worsens or does not improve after regular use of this product as directed, consult a physician. Avoid contact with the eyes—if this occurs, rinse thoroughly with water. Do not use on children under 2 years of age except as directed by a physician. Keep this and all drugs out of reach of children.

How Supplied: 4 oz. (NDC 0072-2500-04) and 8 oz. (NDC 0072-2500-08) plastic bottles.

SEBUTONE® and SEBUTONE® CREAM
Antiseborrheic Tar Shampoo

Active Ingredients: Coal tar 0.5%, salicylic acid 2%, sulfur 2%. SEBUTONE also contains: D&C yellow #10, docusate sodium, EDTA, FD&C blue #1, fragrance, lanolin oil, PEG-6 lauramide, PEG-90M, sodium dodecyl benzene sulfonate, sodium octoxynol-2 ethane sulfonate, titanium dioxide, and water. SEBUTONE CREAM also contains: Ceteareth-20, D&C yellow #10, dextrin, docusate sodium, EDTA, FD&C blue #1, fragrance, laureth-4, lanolin oil, magnesium aluminum silicate, PEG-6 lauramide, PEG-14 M, sodium dodecyl benzene sulfonate, sodium octoxynol-2 ethane sulfonate, stearyl alcohol, titanium dioxide and water.

Action and Uses: A surface-active, penetrating therapeutic shampoo for the temporary relief of itchy scalp and the scaling of stubborn dandruff and psoriasis. Provide prompt and prolonged relief of itching, helps control oiliness and rid the scalp of scales and crust. Tar ingredient is chemically and biologically standardized to produce uniform therapeutic activity. Wood's light demonstrates residual microfine particles of tar on the scalp several days after a course of SEBUTONE shampoo. In addition to its antipruritic and antiseborrheic actions, SEBUTONE also helps offset excessive scalp dryness with a special moisturizing emollient.

Administration and Dosage: SEBUTONE liquid should be well shaken before use. A liberal amount of SEBUTONE or SEBUTONE CREAM is massaged into the wet scalp for 5 minutes and the scalp is then rinsed. Application is repeated, followed by a thorough rinse. Use as often as necessary to keep the scalp free from itching and scaling or as directed. No other shampoo or soap washings are required.

Caution: If undue skin irritation develops or increases, discontinue use. In rare instances, temporary discoloration of white, blond, bleached or tinted hair may occur. Contact with the eyes is to be avoided. In case of contact, flush eyes with water. For external use only. Keep this and all drugs out of reach of children.

How Supplied: SEBUTONE in 4 oz. (NDC 0072-5000-04) and 8 oz. (NDC 0072-5000-08) plastic bottles. SEBUTONE CREAM in 4 oz. (NDC 0072-5100-01) tubes.

Shown in Product Identification Section, page 434

Products are cross-indexed by product classifications in the **BLUE SECTION**

Whitehall Laboratories Inc.

Division of American Home
Products Corporation
685 THIRD AVENUE
NEW YORK, NY 10017

ADVIL®

[ad 'vil]
Ibuprofen Tablets, USP
Ibuprofen Caplets
Pain Reliever/Fever Reducer

**Warning: ASPIRIN SENSITIVE PA-
TIENTS.** Do not take this product if
you have had a severe allergic reaction to aspirin, e.g.—asthma, swelling, shock or hives, because even
though this product contains no aspirin or salicylates, cross-reactions may
occur in patients allergic to aspirin.

Active Ingredient: Each tablet contains Ibuprofen 200 mg.

Inactive Ingredients: Acacia, Acetylated Monoglycerides, Beeswax or Carnauba Wax, Calcium Sulfate, Colloidal
Silicon Dioxide, Dimethicone, Iron Oxide, Lecithin, Pharmaceutical Glaze, Povidone, Sodium Benzoate, Sodium Carboxymethylcellulose, Starch, Stearic
Acid, Sucrose, Titanium Dioxide.

Indications: For the temporary relief
of minor aches and pains associated with
the common cold, headache, toothache,
muscular aches, backache, for the minor
pain of arthritis, for the pain of menstrual cramps and for reduction of fever.

Dosage and Administration: Adults:
Take one tablet every 4 to 6 hours while
symptoms persist. If pain or fever does
not respond to one tablet, two tablets
may be used but do not exceed six tablets
in 24 hours unless directed by a doctor.
The smallest effective dose should be
used. Take with food or milk if occasional
and mild heartburn, upset stomach, or
stomach pain occurs with use. Consult a
doctor if these symptoms are more than
mild or if they persist. Children: Do not
give this product to children under 12
except under the advice and supervision
of a doctor.

Warnings: Do not take for pain for
more than 10 days or for fever for more
than 3 days unless directed by a doctor. If
pain or fever persists or gets worse, if
new symptoms occur, or if the painful
area is red or swollen, consult a doctor.
These could be signs of serious illness. If
you are under a doctor's care for any serious condition, consult a doctor before
taking this product. As with aspirin and
acetaminophen, if you have any condition which requires you to take prescription drugs or if you have had any problems or serious side effects from taking
any non-prescription pain reliever, do
not take this product without first discussing it with your doctor. If you experience any symptoms which are unusual or
seem unrelated to the condition for
which you took ibuprofen, consult a doctor before taking any more of it. Although ibuprofen is indicated for the

same conditions as aspirin and acetaminophen, it should not be taken with them
except under a doctor's direction. Do not
combine this product with any other ibuprofen-containing product. As with any
drug, if you are pregnant or nursing a
baby, seek the advice of a health professional before using this product. IT IS
ESPECIALLY IMPORTANT NOT TO
USE IBUPROFEN DURING THE LAST
3 MONTHS OF PREGNANCY UNLESS
SPECIFICALLY DIRECTED TO DO SO
BY A DOCTOR BECAUSE IT MAY
CAUSE PROBLEMS IN THE UNBORN
CHILD OR COMPLICATIONS DURING
DELIVERY. Keep this and all drugs out
of the reach of children. In case of accidental overdose, seek professional assistance or contact a poison control center
immediately.

Professional Labeling: Same as
stated under Indications.

How Supplied: Coated tablets in bottles of 8, 24, 50, 100, 165 and 250. Coated
caplets in bottles of 24, 50, 100 and 165.

Storage: Store at room temperature;
avoid excessive heat 40℃ (104°F).
*Shown in Product Identification
Section, page 434*

ANACIN®

[an 'a-sin]
Analgesic Coated Tablets
Analgesic Coated Caplets

Description: Each tablet or caplet contains: Aspirin 400 mg., Caffeine 32 mg.
Anacin® has a special protective coating
that makes each tablet or caplet easy to
swallow.

Indications and Usage: Anacin provides fast relief from the pain of headaches, neuralgia, neuritis, sprains, muscular aches, sinus pressure... discomforts and fever of colds... pain caused by
tooth extraction and toothache... menstrual discomfort. Anacin also temporarily relieves the minor aches and pains of
arthritis and rheumatism.

Warnings: Children and teenagers
should not use this medicine for chicken
pox or flu symptoms before a doctor is
consulted about Reye's Syndrome, a rare
but serious illness reported to be associated with aspirin. As with any drug, if
you are pregnant or nursing a baby, seek
the advice of a health professional before
using this product. Keep this and all
medicines out of children's reach. In case
of accidental overdose, contact a physician immediately.

Precautions: If pain persists for more
than 10 days, or redness is present, or in
arthritic or rheumatic conditions affecting children under 12 years of age, consult a physician immediately.

Dosage and Administration: Two tablets or caplets with water every 4 hours,
as needed. Do not exceed 10 tablets or 10
caplets daily. For children 6–12, administer half the adult dosage.

Professional Labeling: Same as those
outlined under Indications.

Inactive Ingredients: Tablets contain
Hydroxypropyl Methylcellulose, Micro-
crystalline Cellulose, Polyethylene Gly-
col, Starch, Surfactant.
Caplets contain Hydroxypropyl Methyl-
cellulose, Iron Oxide, Microcrystalline
Cellulose, Polyethylene Glycol, Starch,
Surfactant.

How Supplied: Tablets: In tins of 12's
and bottles of 30's, 50's, 100's, 200's and
300's. Caplets: In bottles of 30's, 50's and
100's. Professional Samples: Available
upon request. Write Whitehall Laboratories, New York, New York 10017.
*Shown in Product Identification
Section, page 434*

MAXIMUM STRENGTH ANACIN®

[an 'a-sin]
Analgesic Coated Tablets

Description: Each tablet contains: Aspirin 500 mg., Caffeine 32 mg. Maximum
Strength Anacin has a special protective
coating that makes each tablet easy to
swallow.

Indications and Actions: See Anacin
Tablets.

Warnings: See Anacin Tablets.

Precautions: See Anacin Tablets.

Dosage and Administration: Adults: 2
Tablets with water 3 or 4 times a day. Do
not exceed 8 tablets in any 24-hour period. Not recommended for children under 12 years of age.

Inactive Ingredients: Hydroxypropyl
Methylcellulose, Microcrystalline Cellulose, Polyethylene Glycol, Starch, Surfactant.

How Supplied: Tablets: Tins of 12's
and bottles of 20's, 40's, 75's, and 150's.

Children's ANACIN-3®

[an 'a-sin thre]
Acetaminophen
Chewable Tablets, Alcohol-Free
Liquid and Drops

Description: Chewable Tablets: Each
Children's ANACIN-3 Chewable Tablet
is cherry flavored and contains 80 mg
acetaminophen.
Liquid: Children's ANACIN-3 Liquid is
stable, cherry flavored, red in color. It
contains no alcohol or saccharin. Each 5
mL contains 160 mg acetaminophen.
Infants' Drops: Infants' Anacin-3 Drops
are stable, fruit flavored, red in color and
contain no alcohol. Each 0.8 mL (one calibrated dropperful) contains 80 mg acetaminophen.

Actions: Children's Anacin-3 Chewable
Tablets, Liquid and Infants' Drops are
safe and effective 100% aspirin free products designed for treatment of infants
and children with conditions requiring
reduction of fever or relief of pain.

Indications: Children's Anacin-3 is used
for the treatment of fever and pain which
may accompany conditions such as mild
upper respiratory infections (tonsillitis,

common cold, "grippe"), headache, myalgia, post-immunization reactions, post-tonsillectomy discomfort and gastroenteritis. Anacin-3 acetaminophen is useful as an analgesic and antipyretic in infections such as bronchitis, pharyngitis, tracheobronchitis, sinusitis, pneumonia, otitis media and cervical adenitis of viral origin or of bacterial origin when used in conjunction with an antibiotic.

Warnings: Keep this and all medicines out of children's reach. In case of accidental overdose contact a physician immediately.

Precautions: If fever persists for more than 3 days or recurs, or if pain continues for more than 5 days, consult your physician immediately.
If a rare sensitivity reaction occurs, the drug should be stopped. It is usually well tolerated by aspirin-sensitive patients. Phenylketonurics: tablets contain Phenylalanine 3.1 mg per tablet.

Dosage and Administration: All dosages may be repeated every 4 hours. Do not exceed 5 dosages in any 24-hour period.

Age	Wt (lb)	Tablet	Liquid
4–11 mo	12–17	—	½ teaspoon
1–2 yr	18–23	1–1½	¾ "
2–3 "	24–35	2	1 "
4–5 "	36–47	3	1½ "
6–8 "	48–59	4	2 "
9–10 "	60–71	5	2½ "
11–12 "	72–95	6	3 "

Infants' Drops: 0–3 months, 6 to 11 lbs: one-half dropperful. 4–11 months, 12 to 17 lbs: one dropperful. 12–23 months, 18 to 23 lbs: one and one-half droppersful. 2–3 years, 24 to 35 lbs: 2 droppersful. 4–5 years, 36 to 47 lbs: 3 droppersful.

Overdosage: Acetaminophen in massive overdosage may cause hepatic toxicity in some patients. In all cases of suspected overdose, immediately call your regional poison center or the Rocky Mountain Poison Center for assistance in diagnosis and for directions in the use of N-acetylcysteine as an antidote. The occurrence of acetaminophen overdose toxicity is uncommon in the pediatric age group. Even with large overdoses, children appear to be less vulnerable than adults to developing hepatotoxicity. This may be due to age-related differences that have been demonstrated in the metabolism of acetaminophen. Despite these differences, the measures outlined below should be immediately initiated in any child suspected of having ingested an overdose of acetaminophen.
Early symptoms following a potentially hepatotoxic overdose may include: nausea, vomiting, diaphoresis and general malaise. Clinical and laboratory evidence of hepatic toxicity may not be apparent until 48 to 72 hours post-ingestion. The stomach should be emptied promptly by lavage or by induction of emesis with syrup of ipecac. If an acute dose of 150 mg/kg body weight or greater was ingested, or if the dose cannot be accurately determined, a serum acetaminophen assay should be obtained as early as possible, but no sooner than four hours

post-ingestion. Liver function studies should be obtained initially and repeated at 24-hour intervals. The antidote N-acetylcysteine should be administered as early as possible and within 16 hours of the overdose ingestion for optimal results. Following recovery there are no residual, structural or functional hepatic abnormalities.

Inactive Ingredients: Chewable Tablets: Aspartame, Cetyl Alcohol, Colloidal Silicon Dioxide, Dibutyl Sebacate, Ethyl Cellulose, FD&C Red No. 40 Lake, Flavor, Hydrogenated Vegetable Oil, Magnesium Stearate, Mannitol, Microcrystalline Cellulose, Simethicone, Sucrose and Surfactant.
Liquid: Citric Acid, D&C Red No. 33, Disodium Edetate, FD&C Red No. 40, Flavor, Glycerin, Methylparaben, Polyethylene Glycol, Propylene Glycol, Sorbitol, Sodium Benzoate, Sucrose and Water.
Infants' Drops: FD&C Red No. 40, FD&C Yellow No. 6, Flavors, Glycerin, Polyethylene Glycol 1450, Propylene Glycol, Saccharin, Sodium Benzoate, Sorbitol and Water.

How Supplied: Chewable Tablets (colored pink, scored, imprinted "Children A–3")—bottles of 30. Liquid (colored red)—bottles of 2 and 4 fl. oz. Drops (colored red)—bottles of ½ oz. (15 mL) with calibrated plastic dropper.
All packages listed above have child-resistant safety caps and tamper resistant packaging.

**Maximum Strength
ANACIN–3®**
[an 'a-sin thre]
**Film Coated Acetaminophen Tablets
Film Coated Acetaminophen Caplets
Regular Strength
ANACIN–3®
Film Coated Acetaminophen Tablets**

Description: Maximum Strength Tablets and Caplets: Each film coated tablet and caplet contains acetaminophen, 500 mg.
Regular Strength: Each film coated tablet contains acetaminophen, 325 mg.

Indications and Actions: Anacin-3 is a safe and effective 100% aspirin-free analgesic and antipyretic that acts fast to provide temporary relief from pain of headache, colds or "flu", sinusitis, muscle aches, bursitis, sprains, overexertion, backache and menstrual discomfort. Also for temporary relief of minor arthritis pain, toothaches and to reduce fever. Anacin-3 is particularly well suited in the presence of aspirin sensitivity, upper gastrointestinal disorders and anticoagulant therapy. It is usually well tolerated by aspirin-sensitive patients.

Warnings: Keep this and all medicines out of children's reach. In case of accidental overdose, contact a physician immediately. As with any drug, if you are pregnant or nursing a baby, seek the advice of a health professional before using this product.

Precautions: If pain persists for more than 10 days or redness is present or in arthritic or rheumatic conditions affecting children under 12, consult a physician immediately.

Dosage and Administration: Maximum Strength—Adults: Two tablets or caplets 3 or 4 times a day. Do not exceed 8 tablets or caplets in any 24-hour period. Regular Strength—Adults: 2 or 3 tablets every 4 hours not to exceed 12 tablets in any 24-hour period. Children (6–12): ½ to 1 tablet 3 to 4 times daily. Consult a physician for use by children under 6 or for use longer than 10 days.

Overdosage: Acetaminophen in massive overdosage may cause hepatic toxicity in some patients. In all cases of suspected overdose, immediately call your regional poison control center or the Rocky Mountain Poison Control Center for assistance in diagnosis and for directions in the use of N-acetylcysteine as an antidote. In adults, hepatic toxicity has rarely been reported with acute overdoses of less than 10 grams and fatalities with less than 15 grams. Importantly, young children seem to be more resistant than adults to the hepatotoxic effect of an acetaminophen overdose. Despite this, the measures outined below should be initiated in any adult or child suspected of having ingested an acetaminophen overdose.
Early symptoms following a potentially hepatotoxic overdose may include: nausea, vomiting, diaphoresis and general malaise. Clinical and laboratory evidence of hepatic toxicity may not be apparent until 48 to 72 hours post-ingestion. The stomach should be emptied promptly by lavage or by induction of emesis with syrup of ipecac. Patients' estimates of the quantity of a drug ingested are notoriously unreliable. Therefore, if an acetaminophen overdose is suspected, a serum acetaminophen assay should be obtained as early as possible, but no sooner than four hours following ingestion. Liver function studies should be obtained initially and at 24-hour intervals. The antidote, N-acetylcysteine, should be administered as early as possible and within 16 hours of the overdose ingestion for optimal results. Following recovery, there is no residual, structural or functional hepatic abnormalities.

Professional Labeling: Same as those outlined under Indications.

Inactive Ingredients: Maximum and Regular Strength Tablets:
Calcium Stearate, Croscarmellose Sodium, FD&C Blue No. 1 Lake, Hydroxypropyl Methylcellulose, Microcrystalline Cellulose, Polyethylene Glycol, Povidone, Propylene Gylcol, Starch, Stearic Acid and Titanium Dioxide.
Maximum Strength Caplets:
Calcium Stearate, Croscarmellose Sodium, D&C Red No. 7 Lake, FD&C Blue No. 1 Lake, Hydroxypropyl Methylcellulose, Microcrystalline Cellulose, Polyethylene Glycol, Povidone, Propylene Gly-

Continued on next page

Whitehall—Cont.

col, Starch, Stearic Acid and Titanium Dioxide.

How Supplied: Maximum Strength Film Coated—Tablets (colored white, imprinted "A-3" and "500")—tins of 12 and bottles of 30, 60, and 100: Caplets (colored white, imprinted "Anacin-3")—bottles of 30's, 60's and 100's. Regular Strength Film Coated—Tablets (colored white, scored, imprinted "A-3") in bottles of 24, 50, and 100.

Shown in Product Identification Section, page 435

ANBESOL® Liquid and Gel
[an ʹba-sol ʺ]
Antiseptic-Anesthetic

Description: Anbesol is an antiseptic-anesthetic which is available in a Maximum Strength and Regular Strength gel and liquid. Baby Anbesol, available in gel, is an anesthetic only and is alcohol-free.

The Maximum Strength formulations contain Benzocaine 20% and Alcohol 60%.

The Regular Strength formulations contain Benzocaine 6.3%, Alcohol 70%, and Phenol 0.5%.

The Baby Anbesol Gel contains Benzocaine 7.5%.

Indications: Maximum Strength and Regular Strength Anbesol are indicated for the fast temporary relief of pain due to toothache, braces, denture and orthodontic irritation, sore gums, cold and canker sores and fever blisters. Regular Strength Anbesol and Baby Anbesol Gel are also indicated for the fast temporary relief of teething pain.

Actions: Temporarily deadens sensations of nerve endings to provide relief of pain and discomfort; reduces oral bacterial flora temporarily as an aid in oral hygiene (Regular and Maximum Stengths only).

Warnings: Flammable. Keep away from fire or flame. Avoid smoking during application and until product has dried. Do not use near eyes. For persistent or excessive teething pain, consult a physician or dentist. Localized allergic reactions may occur after prolonged or repeated use. KEEP THIS AND ALL MEDICINES OUT OF THE REACH OF CHILDREN.

Precautions: Not for prolonged use. If the condition persists or irritation develops, discontinue use and consult your physician or dentist. NOT FOR USE UNDER DENTURES OR OTHER DENTAL WORK.

Dosage and Administration: Apply topically to the affected area on or around the lips, or within the mouth.

For Denture Irritation: Apply thin layer to affected area and do not reinsert dental work until irritation/pain is relieved. Rinse mouth before reinserting. If irritation/pain persists, contact your physician.

Professional Labeling: Same as outlined under Indications.

Inactive Ingredients:
Maximum Strength Gel: Carbomer 934P, D&C Yellow #10, FD&C Red #40, Flavor, Polyethylene Glycol, Saccharin.
Maximum Strength Liquid: D&C Yellow #10, FD&C Red #40, Flavor, Polyethylene Glycol, Saccharin.
Regular Liquid: Camphor, Glycerin, Menthol, Potassium Iodide, Povidone Iodine.
Regular Gel: Carbomer 934P, D&C Red #33 and Yellow #10, FD&C Blue #1 and Yellow #6, Flavor, Glycerin.
Baby Gel: Carbomer 934, D&C Red #33, Disodium Edetate, Flavor, Glycerin, Polyethylene Glycol, Saccharin, Water.

How Supplied: Maximum Strength Gel in .25 oz (7.2 gram) tube, Maximum Strength Liquid in .31 oz (9mL) bottle. Regular Liquid in two sizes— .31 fl. oz. (9 mL) and .74 fl. oz. (22 mL) bottles. Gel and Baby Gel in .25 oz. (7.2 gram) tubes.

Shown in Product Identification Section, page 435

ARTHRITIS PAIN FORMULA™
[är ʹthrīt-is ʹ pān ʹ for-mye-la]
By the Makers of Anacin® Analgesic Tablets and Caplets

Description: Each caplet contains 500 mg. microfined aspirin and two buffers, 27 mg. Aluminum Hydroxide and 100 mg. Magnesium Hydroxide.
Arthritis Pain Formula is a buffered analgesic and antipyretic with microfined aspirin. The buffering agents help provide protection against stomach upset that could be associated with large anti-arthritic doses of aspirin.

Indications and Actions: Arthritis Pain Formula provides hours of relief from minor aches and pain of arthritis and rheumatism and low back pain. Also relieves the pain of headache, neuralgia, neuritis, sprains, muscular aches, discomforts and fever of colds, pain caused by tooth extraction and toothache, and menstrual discomfort.

Warnings: Children and teenagers should not use this medicine for chicken pox or flu symptoms before a doctor is consulted about Reye syndrome, a rare but serious illness reported to be associated with aspirin. Keep this and all medications out of children's reach. In case of accidental overdose, contact a physician immediately. As with any drug, if you are pregnant or nursing a baby, seek the advice of a health professional before using this product.

Precautions: If pain persists for more than 10 days, or redness is present, or in arthritic or rheumatic conditions affecting children under 12, consult a physician immediately.

Dosage and Administration: Adult Dosage: 2 caplets, 3 or 4 times a day. Do not exceed 8 caplets in any 24 hour period. For children under 12, consult a physician.

Professional Labeling: Same as stated under "Indications".

Inactive Ingredients: Hydrogenated Vegetable Oil, Microcrystalline Cellulose, Starch, Surfactant.

How Supplied: In plastic bottles of 40, 100 and 175 caplets.

Shown in Product Identification Section, page 435

BEMINAL® 500
[bē ʹmĭn-awl]
Vitamin B Complex with Vitamin C

Each tablet contains:		% US RDA*
Thiamine mononitrate (vit. B$_1$)...	25.0 mg	1717%
Riboflavin (vit. B$_2$)...	12.5 mg	735%
Niacinamide (vit. B$_3$) as niacinamide ascorbate...	100.0 mg	500%
Pyridoxine hydrochloride (vit. B$_6$)...	10.0 mg	500%
Calcium pantothenate..	20.0 mg	92%
Ascorbic acid (vit. C) as ascorbic acid and niacinamide ascorbate...	500.0 mg	833%
Cyanocobalamin (vit. B$_{12}$)...	5.0 mcg	83%

Does not contain saccharin or other sweeteners.
*US Recommended Daily Allowance

Inactive Ingredients: Calcium Carboxymethylcellulose, ethylcellulose, FD&C Blue #2 Lake, FD&C Red #40 Lake, FD&C Yellow #6 Lake, Flavor, Iron Oxide, Lactose, Magnesium Stearate, Mannitol, Microcrystalline Cellulose, Pharmaceutical Glaze, Polyethylene Glycol, Starch, Talc, Titanium Dioxide.

Indication: Dietary Supplement

Uses: BEMINAL 500 can help replenish the vitamins depleted by the stress of sickness, infections, and surgery. BEMINAL 500 may also be used when the demand on the body's store of vitamins may be increased by dieting, lack of sleep, the use of alcohol or cigarettes, jogging, and other strenuous physical exercise.

Recommended Intake: 12-year-olds and older, one tablet daily.

How Supplied: In bottles of 100 tablets.

COMPOUND W®
[ʹkäm-pound W]
Solution and Gel

Description: Compound W is a Salicylic Acid (17% w/w) preparation available as a solution or gel.

Indication: Compound W is indicated for the removal of common warts.

Actions: Warts are common benign skin lesions which appear mainly on the back of hands and on fingers, but can also

appear on other parts of the body. The common wart exhibits a rough, raised cauliflower-like surface. They are caused by an infectious virus which stimulates mitosis in the basal cell layer resulting in the production of elevated epithelial growths. The keratolytic action of salicylic acid in a flexible collodion vehicle causes the cornified epithelium to swell, soften, macerate and then desquamate.

Warnings: Highly Flammable. Keep away from fire or flame. Avoid smoking during application and until product has dried. Do not use this product if you are a diabetic or have poor blood circulation as serious complications may result. Do not use on moles, birthmarks, warts with hair growing from them, genital warts, or warts on the face or mucous membranes (inside mouth, nose, anus, genitals, or on lips). If pain should develop or if infection is present, consult your physician. Do not use near eyes. If product accidentally comes in contact with eyes flush with water to remove film and continue to flush with water for 15 minutes. Do not inhale. Keep bottle tightly capped. For external use only. In case of accidental ingestion, contact a physician or a Poison Control Center immediately. Keep this and all medicines out of the reach of children.

Precautions: If redness or irritation occurs, discontinue product for 2 days and then reapply. Should stinging or irritation recur, discontinue use. Covering the treated wart with a bandage will increase effectiveness but may also increase the chance of irritation. If a bandage is used, first allow the solution or gel to dry thoroughly.

Dosage and Administration: Use on common warts once daily. 1. Soak affected area in hot water for 5 minutes. If any tissue has loosened, remove by rubbing with a washcloth or soft brush. Do not rub hard enough to cause bleeding. Dry thoroughly. 2. Using the plastic rod provided with the solution or by squeezing the tube to apply, completely cover the wart with solution or gel. To avoid irritating the skin surrounding the wart, confine the solution or gel to the wart only. To help achieve this, circle the wart with a ring of petroleum jelly. Allow the solution or gel to dry, then reapply. The area covered with the medicine will appear white. 3. Follow this procedure daily for the next 6 to 7 days. Most warts should clear within this time period. However, if the wart remains, continue the treatment for up to 12 weeks. If the wart shows no improvement, see your physician.

Professional Labeling: Same as those outlined under Indication.

Inactive Ingredients: Solution: Acetone Collodion, Alcohol 2.2% w/w, Camphor, Castor Oil, Ether 63.5%, Menthol, Polysorbate 80. Gel: Alcohol 67.5% by vol., Camphor, Castor Oil, Collodion, Colloidal Silicon Dioxide, Hydroxypropyl Cellulose, Hypophosphorous Acid, Polysorbate 80.

How Supplied: Compound W is available in .31 fluid oz. clear bottles with plastic applicators. Compound W Gel is available in .25 oz. tubes. Store at room temperature.

DENOREX®
[dĕn 'ō-reks]
Medicated Shampoo
DENOREX®
Mountain Fresh Herbal Scent Medicated Shampoo
DENOREX®
Medicated Shampoo and Conditioner
DENOREX®
Extra Strength Medicated Shampoo

Description: The Shampoo (Regular and Mt. Fresh Herbal) and the Shampoo with Conditioner contain Coal Tar Solution 9.0%, Menthol 1.5%. The Extra Strength Shampoo contains Coal Tar Solution 12.5% and Menthol 1.5%.

Indications: Relieves scaling, itching, flaking of dandruff, seborrhea and psoriasis. Regular use promotes cleaner, healthier hair and scalp.

Actions: Denorex Shampoo is an antiseborrheic and antipruritic which loosens and softens scales and crusts. Coal tar helps correct abnormalities of keratinization by decreasing epidermal proliferation and dermal infiltration. Denorex also contains the antipruritic agent, menthol.

Warnings: For external use only. Discontinue treatment if irritation develops. Avoid contact with eyes. Keep this and all medicines out of children's reach.

Directions: For best results, shampoo every other day. For severe scalp problems use daily. Wet hair thoroughly and briskly massage until you obtain a rich lather. Rinse thoroughly and repeat. Your scalp may tingle slightly during treatment.

Professional Labeling: Same as stated under Indications.

Inactive Ingredients:
Shampoo: Also contains Chloroxylenol, Lauramide DEA, Stearic Acid, TEA-Lauryl Sulfate, Water (plus Hydroxypropyl Methylcellulose in the Mountain Fresh Herbal scent formula), Alcohol 7.5%.
Shampoo and Conditioner: Chloroxylenol, Citric Acid, Fragrance, Hydroxypropyl Methylcellulose, Lauramide DEA, PEG-27 Lanolin, Polyquaternium-11, TEA-Lauryl Sulfate, Water, Alcohol 7.5%.
Extra Strength: Chloroxylenol, FD&C Red #40, Fragrance, Glycol Distearate, Lauramide DEA, Methylcellulose, TEA-Lauryl Sulfate, Water, Alcohol 10.4%.

How Supplied:
Lotion: 4 oz. and 8 oz. and 12 oz. bottles in Regular Scent, Mountain Fresh Herbal Scent, Shampoo and Conditioner, and Extra Strength Shampoo.
Shown in Product Identification Section, page 435

DERMOPLAST®
[der 'mō-plăst]
Anesthetic Pain Relief Lotion

Description: Dermoplast Lotion contains Benzocaine, 8% and Menthol, 0.5%.

Actions: Dermoplast is a topical anesthetic and antipruritic.

Indications: Dermoplast is indicated for the fast, temporary relief of pain and itching from sunburn, insect bites, minor cuts, abrasions, minor burns, and minor skin irritations.

Warnings: FOR EXTERNAL USE ONLY.
In case of accidental ingestion, seek professional assistance or contact a Poison Control Center. Avoid contact with eyes. If symptoms persist, discontinue use and consult physician. Keep this and all drugs out of the reach of children.

Directions: Apply freely over sunburned or irritated skin. Repeat three or four times daily, as needed.

Inactive Ingredients: Aloe Vera Gel, Carbomer 934P, Ceteth-16, Glycerin, Glyceryl Stearate, Laneth-16, Methylparaben, Oleth-16, Propylparaben, Simethicone, Steareth-16, Triethanolamine, Water.

How Supplied: DERMOPLAST Anesthetic Pain Relief Lotion, in Net Wt 3 fl oz.
Shown in Product Identification Section, page 435

DERMOPLAST®
[der 'mō-plăst]
Anesthetic Pain Relief Spray

Description: DERMOPLAST is an aerosol containing Benzocaine, 20% and Menthol, 0.5%.

Indications: DERMOPLAST is indicated for the fast, temporary relief of skin pain and itching, due to sunburn, minor cuts, insect bites, abrasions, minor burns, and minor skin irritations. May be applied without touching sensitive affected areas. Widely used in hospitals for pain and itch of episiotomy, pruritus vulvae, postpartum hemorrhoids.

Warnings: FOR EXTERNAL USE ONLY. Avoid spraying in eyes. Contents under pressure. Do not puncture or incinerate. Do not use near open flame. Use only as directed. Intentional misuse by deliberately concentrating and inhaling the contents can be harmful or fatal. Do not take orally. Not for prolonged use. If the condition for which this preparation is used persists, or if a rash or irritation develops, discontinue use and consult physician.

Directions for Use: Hold can in a comfortable position 6–12 inches away from affected area. Point spray nozzle and press button. To apply to face, spray in palm of hand. May be administered three or four times daily, or as directed by physician.

Continued on next page

Whitehall—Cont.

Inactive Ingredients: Acetylated Lanolin Alcohol, Aloe Vera Oil, Butane, Cetyl Acetate, Hydrofluorocarbon, Methylparaben, PEG-8 Laurate, Polysorbate 85.

How Supplied: DERMOPLAST Anesthetic Pain Relief Spray, in Net Wt 2¾ oz (78 g). Do not expose to heat or temperatures above 120° F.

Shown in Product Identification Section, page 435

DRISTAN®
[drĭs 'tăn]
Decongestant/Antihistamine/Analgesic
Coated Tablets and Coated Caplets

Description: Each Dristan Coated Tablet or Coated Caplet contains: Phenylephrine HCl 5 mg., Chlorpheniramine Maleate 2 mg., Acetaminophen 325 mg.

Actions: Acetaminophen is both an analgesic and an antipyretic. Therapeutic doses of acetaminophen will effectively reduce an elevated body temperature. Also, acetaminophen is effective in reducing the discomfort of pain associated with headache. Phenylephrine HCl is an oral nasal decongestant (sympathomimetic amine), effective as a vasoconstrictor to help reduce nasal/sinus congestion. Phenylephrine produces little or no Central Nervous System stimulation. Chlorpheniramine Maleate is an antihistamine effective in the control of rhinorrhea, sneezing and lacrimation associated with elevated histamine levels in disorders of the respiratory tract.

Indications: Dristan is indicated for effective multi-symptom relief of colds/flu, sinusitis, hay fever, or other upper respiratory allergies: nasal congestion, sneezing, runny nose, fever, headache and minor aches and pains.

Warnings: Avoid alcoholic beverages and driving a motor vehicle or operating heavy machinery while taking this product. May cause drowsiness or excitability, especially in children. Persons with asthma, glaucoma, high blood pressure, diabetes, heart or thyroid disease, difficulty in urination due to enlarged prostate gland, or taking an antidepressant drug, should use only as directed by a physician. Do not exceed recommended dosage because at higher doses nervousness, dizziness, or sleeplessness may occur. If symptoms do not improve within 7 days or are accompanied by high fever, discontinue use and see a physician. As with any drug, if you are pregnant or nursing a baby, seek the advice of a health professional before using this product.
Do not give to children under 6. Keep this and all medication out of children's reach. In case of accidental overdose contact a physician immediately.

Professional Labeling: Same as those outlined under Indications.

Dosage and Administration: Adults: Two tablets or caplets every four hours, not to exceed 12 tablets or caplets in 24 hours. Children 6–12: One tablet or caplet every four hours, not to exceed six tablets or caplets in 24 hours.

Inactive Ingredients: Tablets and Caplets—Calcium Stearate, Croscarmellose Sodium, D&C Yellow #10 Lake, FD&C Yellow #6 Lake, Hydroxypropyl Methylcellulose, Microcrystalline Cellulose, Polyethylene Glycol, Povidone, Starch, Stearic Acid.

How Supplied: Yellow/White coated tablets in tins of 12 and blister packages of 24, 48, and 100. Yellow/White coated caplets in blister packages of 20 and 40.

Shown in Product Identification Section, page 435

DRISTAN®
[drĭs 'tăn]
Nasal Spray
Menthol Nasal Spray

Description: Dristan Nasal Spray contains Phenylephrine HCl 0.5%, Pheniramine Maleate 0.2%.

Actions: Phenylephrine HCl is a sympathomimetic agent that constricts the smaller arterioles of the nasal passages producing a gentle and predictable decongesting effect. Pheniramine Maleate is an antihistamine that controls rhinorrhea, sneezing, and lacrimation associated with elevated histamine levels in disorders of the respiratory tract.

Indications: Dristan Nasal Spray provides prompt temporary relief of nasal congestion due to colds, sinusitis, hay fever or other upper respiratory allergies.

Warnings: Do not exceed recommended dosage because symptoms may occur such as burning, stinging, sneezing, or increase of nasal discharge. Do not use this product for more than 3 days. If symptoms persist, consult a physician. The use of the dispenser by more than one person may spread infection. For adult use only. Do not give this product to children under 12 years except under the advice and supervision of a physician. Keep these and all medicines out of children's reach. In case of accidental ingestion, seek professional assistance or contact a Poison Control Center immediately.

Dosage and Administration: (Squeeze Bottle) With head upright, insert nozzle in nostril. Spray quickly, firmly and sniff deeply.
Metered Dose Pump—Prime the metered dose pump by depressing pump firmly several times. With head upright, insert nozzle in nostril. Depress pump 2 or 3 times, all the way down, with a firm, even stroke and sniff deeply.
Adults: Spray 2 or 3 times into each nostril. Repeat every 4 hours as needed. Children under 12 years: As directed by a physician.

Professional Labeling: Same as those outlined under Indications.

Inactive Ingredients: Dristan Nasal Spray: Alcohol 0.4%, Benzalkonium

---

Chloride 1:5000 in buffered isotonic aqueous solution, Eucalyptol, Hydroxypropyl Methylcellulose, Menthol, Sodium Chloride, Sodium Phosphate, Thimerosal Preservative 0.002%, and Water.
Dristan Menthol Nasal Spray: Benzalkonium Chloride 1:5000 in buffered isotonic aqueous solution, aromatics consisting of Camphor, Eucalyptol, Menthol, Methyl Salicylate; Polysorbate 80, Sodium Chloride, Sodium Phosphate, Thimerosal Preservative 0.002%, and Water.

How Supplied: 15 mL and 30 mL plastic squeeze bottle and 15 mL metered dose pump.

Shown in Product Identification Section, page 435

DRISTAN®
[drĭs 'tăn]
Long Lasting Nasal Spray
Long Lasting Menthol Nasal Spray

Description: Dristan Long Lasting Nasal Spray contains Oxymetazoline HCl 0.05%.

Actions: The sympathomimetic action of Dristan Long Lasting Nasal Spray and Dristen Long Lasting Menthol Nasal Spray constricts the smaller arterioles of the nasal passages, producing a prolonged, up to 12 hours, gentle and predictable decongesting effect.

Indications: Dristan Long Lasting Nasal Spray and Dristan Long Lasting Menthol Nasal Spray provide prompt temporary relief of nasal congestion due to colds, sinusitis, hay fever, or other upper respiratory allergies for up to 12 hours.

Warnings: Do not exceed recommended dosage because symptoms may occur such as burning, stinging, sneezing, or increase of nasal discharge. Do not use this product for more than 3 days. If symptoms persist, consult a physician. The use of the dispenser by more than one person may spread infection. Keep these and all medicines out of the reach of children. In case of accidental ingestion, seek professional assistance or contact a Poison Control Center immediately.

Dosage and Administration: (Squeeze Bottle) With head upright, insert nozzle in nostril. Spray quickly, firmly and sniff deeply.
Metered Dose Pump—Prime the metered dose pump by depressing pump firmly several times. With head upright, insert nozzle in nostril. Depress pump 2 or 3 times, all the way down, with a firm even stroke and sniff deeply.
Adults and children 6 years of age and over, spray 2 or 3 times into each nostril. Repeat twice daily—morning and evening. Not recommended for children under six.

Professional Labeling: Same as those outlined under Indications.

Inactive Ingredients: Dristan Long Lasting Nasal Spray—Benzalkonium Chloride 1:5000 in buffered isotonic aqueous solution, Hydroxypropyl Methylcellulose, Potassium Phosphate, So-

dium Chloride, Sodium Phosphate, Thimerosal Preservative 0.002%, and Water.

Dristan Long Lasting Menthol Nasal Spray—Alcohol 0.04%, Benzalkonium Chloride 1:5000 in buffered isotonic aqueous solution, Aromatics consisting of Camphor, Eucalyptol, Menthol; Potassium Phosphate, Sodium Chloride, Sodium Phosphate, Thimerosal Preservative 0.002%, and Water.

How Supplied: Dristan Long Lasting Nasal Spray: 15 mL and 30 mL plastic squeeze bottle and 15 mL metered dose pump. Dristan Long Lasting Menthol Nasal Spray: 15 mL plastic squeeze bottle.

Shown in Product Identification Section, page 435

Maximum Strength DRISTAN®
[drĭs'tăn]
Decongestant/Analgesic Coated Caplets

Description: Each Maximum Strength Dristan Coated Caplet contains: Acetaminophen 500 mg and Pseudoephedrine HCl 30 mg.

Actions: Acetaminophen is both an analgesic and an antipyretic. This maximum strength non-aspirin pain reliever effectively reduces headache pain and the pain of a sinus cold. Acetaminophen also reduces an elevated body temperature. Pseudoephedrine HCl is an oral nasal decongestant and is effective in reducing nasal/sinus congestion.

Indications: Maximum Strength Dristan is indicated for effective relief without drowsiness from sinus congestion, sinus pressure and sinus pain due to colds and sinusitis.

Warnings: Do not exceed recommended dosage because at higher doses nervousness, dizziness or sleeplessness may occur. Persons with high blood pressure, heart disease, diabetes, thyroid disease, asthma, glaucoma, difficulty in urination due to an enlarged prostate gland, or taking an antidepressant drug should use only as directed by a physician. If symptoms do not improve within 7 days, or are accompanied by high fever, discontinue use and see a physician. Do not give to children under 12. As with any drug, if you are pregnant or nursing a baby, seek the advice of a health professional before using this product. Keep this and all medication out of children's reach. In case of accidental overdose, contact a physician immediately.

Dosage and Administration: Adults and children over 12: Two caplets every 6 hours, not to exceed 8 caplets in any 24-hour period. Children under 12 should use only as directed by a physician.

Professional Labeling: Same as those outlined under Indications.

Inactive Ingredients: Calcium Stearate, Croscarmellose Sodium, D&C Yellow #10 Lake, FD&C Yellow #6 Lake, Hydrogenated Vegetable Oil, Hydroxypropyl Methylcellulose, Microcrystalline Cellulose, Polyethylene Glycol, Povidone, Starch, Stearic Acid, Titanium Dioxide.

How Supplied: Yellow coated caplets in blister packages of 24, 48 and bottles of 100.

Shown in Product Identification Section, page 435

FREEZONE®
['frēz-ōn]
Solution

Description: Freezone is a solution which contains Salicylic Acid 13.6% w/w in a collodion vehicle.

Indications: Freezone is indicated for removal of corns and calluses.

Actions: Freezone penetrates corns and calluses painlessly, layer by layer, loosening and softening the corn or callus so that the whole corn or callus can be lifted off or peeled away in just a few days.

Warnings: DO NOT USE THIS PRODUCT IF YOU ARE A DIABETIC OR HAVE POOR BLOOD CIRCULATION BECAUSE SERIOUS COMPLICATIONS MAY RESULT. DO NOT USE ON IRRITATED SKIN OR ON ANY AREA THAT IS INFECTED OR REDDENED. IF INFECTION OR INFLAMMATION OCCURS OR IF DISCOMFORT PERSISTS, STOP USING THE PRODUCT AND SEE YOUR PODIATRIST OR PHYSICIAN IMMEDIATELY. Care should be used to avoid contact of product with skin surrounding corn and callus. Do not use this product on soft corns (usually occurring between toes). If product gets into the eye, flush with water to remove film and continue to flush with water 15 more minutes. Avoid inhaling vapors. HIGHLY FLAMMABLE, KEEP AWAY FROM FIRE OR FLAME. AVOID SMOKING DURING USE AND UNTIL PRODUCT HAS DRIED. Keep bottle tightly capped. For external use only on the foot or toes. In case of accidental ingestion, contact a physician or call a Poison Control Center immediately. Keep this and all medicine out of children's reach.

Dosage and Administration: Cleanse feet thoroughly with soap. Soak in warm water for 15 to 30 minutes and dry feet thoroughly. Circle corn or callus with a ring of petroleum jelly to protect surrounding skin. Apply product one drop at a time using rod in cap to cover sufficiently each hard corn or callus only; let dry. Repeat this procedure daily until the corn or callus is removed or partially removed to provide comfort. Do not use medication for more than 14 days.

Professional Labeling: Same as outlined under Indications.

Inactive Ingredients: Alcohol (20.5%), Balsam Oregon, Castor Oil, Ether (64.8%), Hypophosphorus Acid and Zinc Chloride.

How Supplied: Available in a .31 fl. oz. glass bottle.

Store at room temperature away from heat.

MEDICATED CLEANSING PADS
[mĕd'i-kāt-ĭd klĕnz-ĭng păds]
By The Makers of Preparation H®
Hemorrhoidal Remedies

Description: Each cleansing pad contains Witch Hazel (50% w/v).

Indications: Medicated Cleansing Pads can be used for hemorrhoidal tissue irritation, anal cleansing wipe; everyday hygiene of the outer vaginal area, final cleansing step at diaper changing time.

Actions: Medicated Cleansing Pads are scientifically developed, soft cloth pads which are impregnated with a solution specially designed to gently soothe, freshen and cleanse the anal or genital area. Medicated Cleansing Pads are superior for a multitude of types of personal hygiene uses and are especially recommended for hemorrhoid sufferers.

Warnings: In case of rectal bleeding, consult physician promptly. In case of continued irritation, discontinue use and consult a physician.

Precaution: Keep this and all medicines out of the reach of children.

Dosage and Administration: As a personal wipe—use as a final cleansing step after regular toilet tissue or instead of tissue, in cases of special sensitivity. As a compress—hemorrhoid sufferers will get additional relief by using Medicated Cleansing Pads as a compress. Fold pad and hold in contact with inflamed anal tissue for 10 to 15 minutes. Repeat several times daily while inflammation lasts.

Inactive Ingredients: Alcohol 7.4%, (glycerin 10% w/v) Methylparaben, Octoxynol-9, Water.

How Supplied: Jars of 40's and 100's.

MOMENTUM®
[mō-mĕn'tum]
Muscular Backache Formula

Description: Momentum contains Aspirin 500 mg., Phenyltoloxamine Citrate 15 mg., per caplet.

Indications: Momentum is indicated for the relief of pain due to stiffness and tight, inflamed muscles.

Actions: The combination of aspirin and phenyltoloxamine citrate act to relieve the pain of tense, knotted muscles. As pain subsides, muscles loosen and become less stiff, more relaxed and mobility is increased.

Warnings: Children and teenagers should not use this medicine for chicken pox or flu symptoms before a doctor is consulted about Reye syndrome, a rare but serious illness reported to be associated with aspirin. Do not drive a car or operate machinery while taking this medication as this preparation may cause drowsiness in some persons. Keep

Continued on next page

Whitehall—Cont.

this and all medicines out of children's reach. In case of accidental overdose, contact a physician immediately.

Precaution: As with any drug, if you are pregnant or nursing a baby, seek the advice of a health professional before using this product.

Dosage and Administration: Adults: Two caplets upon rising, then two caplets as needed at lunch, dinner, and bedtime. Dosage should not exceed 8 caplets in any 24-hour period. Not recommended for children.

Professional Labeling: Same as those outlined under Indications.

Inactive Ingredients: Alginic Acid, Citric Acid, Colloidal Silicon Dioxide, Hydrogenated Vegetable Oil, Microcrystalline Cellulose, Starch and Surfactant.

How Supplied: Bottles of 24 and 48 white, uncoated caplets.

OUTGRO®
[*'aut-grō*]
Solution

Description: Outgro solution contains Tannic Acid 25%, Chlorobutanol 5%.

Indications: Outgro provides fast, temporary pain relief of ingrown toenails.

Actions: Outgro temporarily relieves pain, reduces swelling and eases inflammation accompanying ingrown toenails. Daily use of Outgro toughens tender skin—allowing the nail to be cut and thus preventing further pain and discomfort. Outgro does not affect the growth, shape or position of the nail.

Warnings: For external use only. Do not use Outgro solution for more than 7 days unless directed by a doctor. Consult a doctor if no improvement is seen after 7 days. IF YOU HAVE DIABETES OR POOR CIRCULATION, SEE A DOCTOR FOR TREATMENT OF INGROWN TOENAIL. DO NOT APPLY THIS PRODUCT TO OPEN SORES. IF REDNESS AND SWELLING OF YOUR TOE INCREASE, OR IF A DISCHARGE IS PRESENT AROUND THE NAIL, STOP USING THIS PRODUCT AND SEE YOUR DOCTOR IMMEDIATELY. Flammable. Keep away from fire or flame. Avoid smoking during use and until product has dried. In case of accidental ingestion, contact a physician or call a Poison Control Center immediately. KEEP THIS AND ALL MEDICINES OUT OF CHILDREN'S REACH.

Directions: Cleanse affected toes thoroughly. Using rod in cap, either apply Outgro Solution in the crevice where the nail is growing into the flesh or place a small piece of cotton in the nail groove (the side of the nail where the pain is) and wet cotton thoroughly with Outgro solution several times daily until nail discomfort is relieved. Change cotton at least once daily. Do not use product for more than 7 days unless directed by a

doctor (podiatrist or physician). In some instances, temporary discoloration of the nail and surrounding skin may occur.

Professional Labeling: Same as outlined under Indications.

Inactive Ingredients: Ethylcellulose, Isopropyl Alcohol 83% (by volume).

How Supplied: Available in .31 fl. oz. glass bottles.

OXIPOR VHC®
[*'äk-si-pōr VHC*]
Lotion for Psoriasis

Description: OXIPOR VHC lotion for psoriasis contains Coal Tar Solution 48.5%, Salicylic Acid 1.0%, Benzocaine 2.0%.

Actions: Coal tar solution helps control cell growth and therefore prevents formation of new scales. Salicylic acid has a keratolytic action which helps peel off and dissolve away scales. Benzocaine is a local anesthetic that gives prompt relief from pain and itching. Alcohol is the solvent vehicle.

Indications: OXIPOR VHC has been clinically proven to relieve itching, redness and help dissolve and clear away the scales and crusts of psoriasis.

Warnings: For external use only. Avoid contact with eyes or mucous membranes. Use caution in exposing skin to sunlight after applying product. It may increase your tendency to sunburn for up to 24 hours after application. DO NOT USE in or around rectum or in genital area or groin except on advice of a doctor. Flammable. Keep away from fire or flame. Avoid smoking during application and until product has dried. Do not chill. Not for prolonged use. If condition persists or if rash or irritation develops, discontinue use and consult physician. Keep out of children's reach.

Dosage and Administration: Shake bottle well before each application. <u>SKIN:</u> Wash affected area before applying to remove loose scales. With a small wad of cotton, apply twice daily. Allow to dry before contact with clothing. <u>SCALP:</u> Apply to scalp with fingertips making sure to get down to the skin itself. Leave on for as long as possible, even overnight. Shampoo. Then remove all loose scales with a fine comb. This product may temporarily discolor light-colored hair. Discoloration can be prevented by reducing the time the product is left on the scalp. Also be sure to rinse product out of hair thoroughly.

Professional Labeling: Same as those outlined under Indications.

Inactive Ingredients: Alcohol 81% by volume, water.

How Supplied: Available in 1.9 oz. and 4.0 oz. bottles. Store at room temperature.

POSTURE®
[*pos'tūr*]
600 mg
High Potency Calcium Supplement for Healthy Bones

Description: Each film-coated tablet of POSTURE® contains 600 mg of elemental calcium (as calcium phosphate) specially formulated not to produce gas.

For Adults—

Two tablets contain:	% U.S. RDA*
Elemental Calcium...... 1200 mg ...120% (as calcium phosphate)	

*Percentage of U.S. Recommended Daily Allowance

Indication: POSTURE® Tablets provide a daily source of calcium for healthy bones or, when recommended by a physician, to increase dietary intake of calcium.

Recommended Intake: One or two tablets daily, or as recommended by a physician. Keep Out of Reach of Children.

Inactive Ingredients: Croscarmellose Sodium, Ethylcellulose, Magnesium Stearate, Microcrystalline Cellulose, Polyethylene Glycol, Povidone, Sodium Lauryl Sulfate, Talc.

How Supplied: In bottles of 60 tablets.

Shown in Product Identification Section, page 435

POSTURE®-D
600 mg
High Potency Calcium Supplement with Vitamin D for Healthy Bones

Description: Each film-coated tablet of POSTURE®-D contains 600 mg of elemental calcium (as calcium phosphate) and 125 IU of Vitamin D, specially formulated not to produce gas.

For Adults—

Two tablets contain:	% U.S. RDA*
Elemental Calcium...... 1200 mg ...120% (as calcium phosphate)	
Vitamin D..................... 250 IU 63%	

*Percentage of U.S. Recommended Daily Allowance.

Indication: POSTURE®-D Tablets provide a daily source of calcium for healthy bones or, when recommended by a physician, to increase dietary intake of calcium.

Recommended Intake: One or two tablets daily, or as recommended by a physician. Keep Out of Reach of Children.

Inactive Ingredients: Croscarmellose Sodium, Ethylcellulose, Magnesium Stearate, Microcrystalline Cellulose, Polyethylene Glycol, Povidone, Sodium Lauryl Sulfate, Talc.

How Supplied: In bottles of 60 tablets.

Shown in Product Identification Section, page 435

PREPARATION H®
[prep-e 'rā-shen-āch]
Hemorrhoidal Ointment and Cream
PREPARATION H®
Hemorrhoidal Suppositories

Description: Preparation H is available in ointment, cream and suppository product forms. The **Ointment** contains Live Yeast Cell Derivative supplying 2,000 units Skin Respiratory Factor per ounce of Ointment, and Shark Liver Oil 3.0%; in a specially prepared Rectal Petrolatum Base.

The **Cream** contains Live Yeast Cell Derivative supplying 2,000 units Skin Respiratory Factor per ounce of Cream and Shark Liver Oil 3.0% in a specially prepared Rectal Cream Base containing Petrolatum.

The **Suppositories** contain Live Yeast Cell Derivative, supplying 2,000 units Skin Respiratory Factor per ounce of Cocoa Butter Suppository Base and Shark Liver Oil 3.0%.

Actions: Live Yeast Cell Derivative acts by increasing the oxygen uptake of dermal tissues and facilitating collagen formation. Shark Liver Oil has been incorporated to act as a protectant which softens and soothes the tissues. Preparation H also lubricates inflamed, irritated surfaces to help make bowel movements less painful.

Indications: Preparation H helps shrink swelling of hemorrhoidal tissues caused by inflammation, and to give prompt, temporary relief in many cases from pain and itch in tissues.

Precautions: In case of bleeding, or if your condition persists, a physician should be consulted.

Dosage and Administration: Ointment/Cream: Before applying, remove protective cover from applicator. Lubricate applicator before each application and thoroughly cleanse after use. It is recommended that Preparation H Hemorrhoidal ointment/cream be applied freely to the affected rectal area whenever symptoms occur, from three to five times per day, especially at night, in the morning, and after each bowel movement. Frequent application with Preparation H ointment/cream provides continual therapy which leads to more rapid improvement of rectal conditions. **Suppositories:** Whenever symptoms occur, remove wrapper, insert one suppository rectally from three to five times per day, especially at night, in the morning, and after each bowel movement. Frequent application with Preparation H suppositories provides continual therapy which leads to more rapid improvement of rectal conditions.

Professional Labeling: Same as those outlined under Indications.

Inactive Ingredients: Ointment—Beeswax, Glycerin, Lanolin, Lanolin Alcohol, Mineral Oil, Paraffin, Phenylmercuric Nitrate 1:10,000 (as a preservative), Thyme Oil.
Cream—Beeswax, BHA, Citric Acid, Glycerin, Glyceryl Oleate, Lanolin, Lanolin Alcohol, Magnesium Aluminum Silicate, Mineral Oil, Paraffin, Phenylmercuric Nitrate 1:10,000 (as a preservative), Polysorbate 80, Propyl Gallate, Propylene Glycol, Silica, Water. May also contain Methylparaben and Propylparaben.
Suppositories — Beeswax, Glycerin, Phenylmercuric Nitrate 1:10,000 (as a preservative), Polyethylene Glycol 600 Dilaurate.

How Supplied: Ointment: Net Wt. 1 oz. and 2 oz. **Cream:** Net wt. 0.9 oz. and 1.8 oz. **Suppositories:** 12's, 24's, 36's and 48's. Store at controlled room temperature in cool place but not over 80° F.
Shown in Product Identification Section, page 435

PRIMATENE®
[prĭm 'a-tēn]
Mist
(Epinephrine Inhalation Aerosol Bronchodilator)

Description: Primatene Mist contains Epinephrine 5.5 mg./mL.

Action: Epinephrine is a sympathomimetic agent which eases breathing for asthma patients by reducing spasms of bronchial muscles.

Indications: Primatene Mist is indicated for temporary relief of shortness of breath, tightness of chest, and wheezing due to bronchial asthma.

Dosage and Administration: Inhalation dosage for adults and children 4 years of age and older: Start with one inhalation, then wait at least 1 minute. If not relieved, use once more. Do not use again for at least 3 hours. The use of this product by children should be supervised by an adult. Children under 4 years of age: Consult a physician. Each inhalation delivers 0.22 mg. of epinephrine.

Warnings: Do not use this product unless a diagnosis of asthma has been made by a physician. Do not use this product if you have heart disease, high blood pressure, thyroid disease, diabetes or difficulty in urination due to enlargement of the prostate gland unless directed by a physician. As with any drug, if you are pregnant or nursing a baby, seek the advice of a health professional before using this product. Do not use this product if you have ever been hospitalized for asthma or if you are taking any prescription drug for asthma unless directed by a physician. Keep this and all drugs out of the reach of children. In case of accidental overdose, seek professional assistance or contact a poison control center immediately. DRUG INTERACTION PRECAUTION: Do not use this product if you are presently taking a prescription drug for high blood pressure or depression, without first consulting your physician. DO NOT CONTINUE TO USE THIS PRODUCT, BUT SEEK MEDICAL ASSISTANCE IMMEDIATELY IF SYMPTOMS ARE NOT RELIEVED WITHIN 20 MINUTES OR BECOME WORSE. DO NOT USE THIS PRODUCT MORE FREQUENTLY OR AT HIGHER DOSES THAN RECOMMENDED UNLESS DIRECTED BY A PHYSICIAN. EXCESSIVE USE MAY CAUSE NERVOUSNESS AND RAPID HEART BEAT AND POSSIBLY, ADVERSE EFFECTS ON THE HEART.

Precautions: Contents under pressure. Do not puncture or throw container into incinerator. Using or storing near open flame or heating above 120° F may cause bursting.

Directions For Use of The Mouthpiece:
The Primatene Mist mouthpiece, which is enclosed in the Primatene Mist 15mL size (not the refill size), should be used for inhalation only with Primatene Mist.
1. Take plastic cap off mouthpiece. (For refills, use mouthpiece from previous purchase.)
2. Take plastic mouthpiece off bottle.
3. Place other end of mouthpiece on bottle.
4. Turn bottle upside down. Place thumb on bottom of mouthpiece over circular button and forefinger on top of vial. Empty the lungs as completely as possible by exhaling.
5. Place mouthpiece in mouth with lips closed around opening. Inhale deeply while squeezing mouthpiece and bottle together. Release immediately and remove unit from mouth, then complete taking the deep breath, drawing medication into your lungs, holding breath as long as comfortable.
6. Then exhale slowly keeping lips nearly closed. This distributes the medication in the lungs.
7. Replace plastic cap on mouthpiece.

Inactive Ingredients: Alcohol 34%, Ascorbic Acid, Fluorocarbons (Propellant), Water. Contains No Sulfites.

How Supplied:
½ Fl. oz. (15mL) With Mouthpiece
½ Fl. oz. (15mL) Refill
¾ Fl. oz. (22.5mL) Refill
Shown in Product Identification Section, page 435

PRIMATENE®
[prĭm 'a-tēn]
Mist Suspension
(Epinephrine Bitartrate Inhalation Aerosol Bronchodilator)

Description: Primatene Mist Suspension contains Epinephrine Bitartrate 7.0 mg./mL.

Action: Epinephrine is a sympathomimetic agent which eases breathing for asthma patients by reducing spasms of bronchial muscles.

Indications: Primatene Mist Suspension is indicated for temporary relief of shortness of breath, tightness of chest, and wheezing due to bronchial asthma.

Dosage and Administration: Shake before using. Inhalation dosage for adults and children 4 years of age and older: Start with one inhalation, then wait at least 1 minute. If not relieved, use once more. Do not use again for at least 3

Continued on next page

Whitehall—Cont.

hours. The use of this product by children should be supervised by an adult. Children under 4 years of age: Consult a physician. Each inhalation delivers 0.3 mg. Epinephrine Bitartrate equivalent to 0.16 mg. Epinephrine Base.

Warnings: Do not use this product unless a diagnosis of asthma has been made by a physician. Do not use this product if you have heart disease, high blood pressure, thyroid disease, diabetes or difficulty in urination due to enlargement of the prostate gland unless directed by a physician. As with any drug, if you are pregnant or nursing a baby, seek the advice of a health professional before using this product. Do not use this product if you have ever been hospitalized for asthma or if you are taking any prescription drug for asthma unless directed by a physician. Keep this and all drugs out of the reach of children. In case of accidental overdose, seek professional assistance or contact a poison control center immediately. DRUG INTERACTION PRECAUTION: Do not use this product if you are presently taking a prescription drug for high blood pressure or depression, without first consulting your physician. DO NOT CONTINUE TO USE THIS PRODUCT, BUT SEEK MEDICAL ASSISTANCE IMMEDIATELY IF SYMPTOMS ARE NOT RELIEVED WITHIN 20 MINUTES OR BECOME WORSE. DO NOT USE THIS PRODUCT MORE FREQUENTLY OR AT HIGHER DOSES THAN RECOMMENDED UNLESS DIRECTED BY A PHYSICIAN. EXCESSIVE USE MAY CAUSE NERVOUSNESS AND RAPID HEART BEAT AND POSSIBLY, ADVERSE EFFECTS ON THE HEART.

Precautions: Contents under pressure. Do not puncture or throw container into incinerator. Using or storing near open flame or heating above 120° F may cause bursting.

Directions For Use of The Inhaler:
1. SHAKE BEFORE USING.
2. HOLD INHALER WITH NOZZLE DOWN WHILE USING. Empty the lungs as completely as possible by exhaling.
3. Purse the lips as in saying "O" and hold the nozzle up to the lips keeping the tongue flat. As you start to take a deep breath, squeeze nozzle and can together, releasing one full application. Complete taking deep breath, drawing medication into your lungs.
4. Hold breath for as long as comfortable. Then exhale slowly, keeping the lips nearly closed. This distributes the medication in the lungs.

Inactive Ingredients: Fluorocarbons (Propellant), Sorbitan Trioleate. Contains No Sulfites.

How Supplied: ⅓ Fl. oz. (10mL) pocket-size aerosol inhaler.

Shown in Product Identification Section, page 435

PRIMATENE®
[prĭm'a-tēn]
Tablets

Description: Depending upon the state (see How Supplied), Primatene Tablets are available in 3 formulations:
(regular formula): Theophylline Anhydrous 130 mg., Ephedrine Hydrochloride 24 mg.
P Formula: Theophylline Hydrous 130 mg., Ephedrine Hydrochloride 24 mg., Phenobarbital 8 mg. (¼ gr.) per tablet. (Warning: May be habit forming.)
M Formula: Theophylline Anhydrous 130 mg., Ephedrine Hydrochloride 24 mg., Pyrilamine Maleate 16.6 mg. per tablet.

Actions: Primatene Tablets contain two bronchodilators, theophylline, a methylxanthine, and ephedrine, a sympathomimetic. The pharmacologic action of theophylline may be mediated through inhibition of phosphodiesterase with a resulting increase in intracellular cyclic AMP. The β-adrenergic ephedrine acts by a different mechanism to produce cyclic AMP. Used at the start of an asthma attack, Primatene acts to (1) open bronchial tubes so breathing is natural, (2) relax bronchial muscles, (3) reduce congestion. Primatene helps relieve the asthma spasms, thus permitting sleep at night and freedom from associated anxiety by day.

Indications: Primatene Tablets are indicated for relief and control of attacks of bronchial asthma and associated hay fever.

Warnings: If symptoms persist, consult your physician. Some people are sensitive to ephedrine and, in some cases, temporary sleeplessness and nervousness may occur. These reactions will disappear if the use of the medication is discontinued. Do not exceed recommended dosage.
People who have heart disease, high blood pressure, diabetes or thyroid trouble or difficulty in urination due to enlarged prostate gland should take this preparation only on the advice of a physician. Both "M" and "P" formulae may cause drowsiness. People taking the "M" or "P" formulae should not drive or operate machinery.
As with any drug, if you are pregnant or nursing a baby, seek the advice of a health professional before using this product. Keep all medicines out of reach of children.

Dosage and Administration: Adults: 1 or 2 tablets initially and then one every 4 hours, as needed, not to exceed 6 tablets in 24 hours. Children (6–12): One half adult dose. For children under 6, consult a physician.

Inactive Ingredients:
(regular formula): FD&C Yellow No. 6 Lake, D&C Yellow No. 10 Lake, Hydrogenated Vegetable Oil, Magnesium Stearate, Microcrystalline Cellulose, Sodium Starch Glycolate, Surfactant, Talc.

P Formula (Phenobarbital): Colloidal Silicon Dioxide, D&C Yellow No. 10, FD&C Yellow No. 6, Magnesium Stearate, Sodium Starch Glycolate, Starch, Surfactant.
M Formula (Pyrilamine Maleate): D&C Yellow No. 10 Lake, FD&C Yellow No. 6 Lake, Hydrogenated Vegetable Oil, Magnesium Stearate, Microcrystalline Cellulose, Sodium Starch Glycolate, Surfactant.

Contains No Sulfites.

How Supplied: Available in three forms (regular) Primatene Tablets, "M" Formula, and "P" Formula. In those states where Phenobarbital is Rx only, "M" Formula, containing pyrilamine maleate, is available.
"P" Formula, containing phenobarbital, is available in other states.
(Regular) Primatene Tablets are currently available in the West and Southwest only. Both "M" and "P" formulas are supplied in glass bottles of 24 and 60 tablets. (Regular) Primatene Tablets are supplied in 24 and 60 tablet thermoform blister cartons.

Shown in Product Identification Section, page 435

RIOPAN®
[rī'opan]
magaldrate
Antacid

Description: RIOPAN is a buffer antacid containing the unique chemical entity Magaldrate. Each teaspoonful (5 mL) of suspension contains Magaldrate, 540 mg. Each Chew Tablet or Swallow Tablet contains Magaldrate, 480 mg. RIOPAN is considered dietetically sodium-free (containing not more than 0.004 mEq, 0.1 mg sodium per teaspoonful or tablet).

Actions: The active ingredient in RIOPAN, Magaldrate demonstrates a rapid and uniform buffering action. The acid-neutralizing capacity of RIOPAN is 15.0 mEq/5mL and 13.5 mEq/tablet. RIOPAN does not produce acid rebound or alkalinization.

Indications: Riopan is indicated for the relief of heartburn, sour stomach, and acid indigestion. For symptomatic relief of hyperacidity associated with the diagnosis of peptic ulcer, gastritis, peptic esophagitis, gastric hyperacidity, and hiatal hernia.

Dosage and Administration: RIOPAN (magaldrate) Antacid *Suspension* —Take one or two teaspoonfuls, between meals and at bedtime, or as directed by the physician. RIOPAN Antacid *Chew Tablets* —Chew one or two tablets, between meals and at bedtime, or as directed by the physician. RIOPAN Antacid *Swallow Tablets* —Take one or two tablets, between meals and at bedtime, or as directed by the physician. Take with enough water to swallow promptly.

Warnings: Patients should not take more than 18 teaspoonfuls (or 20 tablets) in a 24-hour period or use the maximum dosage for more than two weeks, or use if they have kidney disease except under

the advice and supervision of a physician.

Drug Interaction Precaution: Do not use in patients taking a prescription antibiotic drug containing any form of tetracycline.

Inactive Ingredients: Chew Tablets: Flavor, Magnesium Stearate, Polyethylene Glycol, Sorbitol, Starch, Sucrose, Titanium Dioxide. Swallow Tablets: Flavor, Magnesium Stearate, Menthol, Microcrystalline Cellulose, Polyethylene Glycol, Starch, Talc, Titanium Dioxide. Suspension: Acacia, Flavor, Hydroxypropyl Methylcellulose, Menthol, Saccharin, Water.

How Supplied: RIOPAN Antacid *Suspension* —in 12 fl oz (355 mL) plastic bottles. Individual Cups, 1 fl oz (30 mL) ea., tray of 10—10 trays per packer. Store at room temperature (approximately 25°C). Avoid freezing. RIOPAN Antacid *Chew Tablets* —in bottles of 60 and 100. Also, single roll-packs of 12 tablets and 3-roll rollpacks of 36 tablets. RIOPAN Antacid *Swallow Tablets* —Boxes of 60 and 100 in individual film strips (6 x 10 and 10 x 10, respectively).
Shown in Product Identification Section, page 435

RIOPAN PLUS®
[rī′opan]
magaldrate and simethicone
Antacid plus Anti-Gas

Description: RIOPAN PLUS is a buffer antacid plus anti-gas combination product containing the unique chemical entity Magaldrate. Each teaspoonful (5mL) of suspension contains Magaldrate, 540 mg and Simethicone, 20 mg. Each Chew Tablet contains Magaldrate, 480 mg and Simethicone, 20 mg. RIOPAN PLUS is considered dietetically sodium-free (containing not more than 0.004 mEq, 0.1 mg sodium per teaspoonful or tablet).

Actions: The active antacid ingredient in RIOPAN PLUS, Magaldrate, demonstrates a rapid and uniform buffering action. The acid-neutralizing capacity of RIOPAN PLUS is 15.0 mEq/5mL and 13.5 mEq/tablet. RIOPAN PLUS does not produce acid rebound or alkalinization.

Indications: RIOPAN PLUS is indicated for the relief of heartburn, sour stomach and acid indigestion, accompanied by the symptoms of gas. For symptomatic relief of hyperacidity associated with the diagnosis of peptic ulcer, gastritis, peptic esophagitis, gastric hyperacidity, and hiatal hernia. For postoperative gas pain.

Dosage and Administration: RIOPAN PLUS (magaldrate and simethicone) Antacid plus Anti-Gas *Suspension* —Take one or two teaspoonfuls between meals and at bedtime, or as directed by the physician.
RIOPAN PLUS Antacid plus Anti-Gas *Chew Tablets* —Chew one or two tablets,

between meals and at bedtime, or as directed by the physician.

Warnings: Patients should not take more than 18 teaspoonfuls (or 20 tablets) in a 24-hour period, or use the maximum dosage for more than two weeks, or use if they have kidney disease, except under the advice and supervision of a physician.

Drug Interaction Precaution: Do not use in patients taking a prescription antibiotic drug containing any form of tetracycline.

Inactive Ingredients: Chew Tablets: Flavor, Magnesium Stearate, Methylcellulose, Polyethylene Glycol, Silica, Sorbitol, Starch, Sucrose, Titanium Dioxide. Suspension: Acacia, Flavor, Hydroxypropyl Methylcellulose, Menthol, PEG-8 Stearate, Saccharin, Sorbitan Stearate, Water.

How Supplied: RIOPAN PLUS Antacid plus Anti-Gas *Suspension* —in 12 fl oz (355 mL) plastic bottles. Individual Cups, 1 fl oz (30 mL) ea., tray of 10—10 trays per packer. Store at room temperature (approximately 25°C). Avoid freezing.
RIOPAN PLUS Antacid plus Anti-Gas *Chew Tablets* —in bottles of 60 and 100. Also, single rollpacks of 12 tablets and 3-roll rollpacks of 36 tablets.
Shown in Product Identification Section, page 435

RIOPAN PLUS® 2
[rī′opan plus 2]
magaldrate and simethicone
Double Strength
Antacid plus Anti-Gas

Description: RIOPAN PLUS 2 is a double strength buffer antacid plus antigas combination product containing the unique chemical entity Magaldrate. Each teaspoonful (5mL) of suspension contains Magaldrate, 1080 mg and Simethicone, 30 mg. Each Chew Tablet contains Magaldrate, 1080 mg and Simethicone, 30 mg. RIOPAN PLUS 2 is considered dietetically sodium-free (containing not more than 0.013 mEq, 0.3 mg per teaspoonful or 0.021 mEq, 0.5 mg per tablet).

Actions: The active antacid ingredient in RIOPAN PLUS 2, Magaldrate, demonstrates a rapid and uniform buffering action. The acid-neutralizing capacity of Double Strength RIOPAN PLUS 2 is 30 mEq/5mL and 30.0 mEq/tablet. RIOPAN PLUS 2 does not produce acid rebound or alkalinization.

Indications: RIOPAN PLUS 2 is indicated for the relief of heartburn, sour stomach and acid indigestion accompanied by the symptoms of gas. For symptomatic relief of hyperacidity associated with the diagnosis of peptic ulcer, gastritis, peptic esophagitis, gastric hyperacidity, and hiatal hernia. For postoperative gas pain.

Dosage and Administration: RIOPAN PLUS 2 (magaldrate and simethicone) *Suspension* —Take one or two tea-

spoonfuls between meals and at bedtime, or as directed by the physician.
RIOPAN PLUS 2 Chew Tablets—Chew one or two tablets, between meals and at bedtime, or as directed by the physician.

Warnings: Patients should not take more than 9 teaspoonfuls (or 9 tablets) in a 24-hour period, or use the maximum dosage for more than two weeks, or use if they have kidney disease, except under the advice and supervision of a physician.

Drug Interaction Precaution: Do not use in patients taking a prescription antibiotic drug containing any form of tetracycline.

Inactive Ingredients: Chew Tablets: Flavor, Magnesium Stearate, Methylcellulose, Polyethylene Glycol, Saccharin, Silica, Sorbitol, Starch, Sucrose, Titanium Dioxide. Supension: Flavor, Glycerin, PEG-8 Stearate, Potassium Citrate, Saccharin, Sorbitan Stearate, Sorbitol, Xanthan Gum, Water.

How Supplied: RIOPAN PLUS 2 *Suspension* —in 12 fl oz (355 mL) plastic bottles. RIOPAN PLUS 2 Chew Tablets—in bottles of 60.
Shown in Product Identification Section, page 436

SEMICID®
[sĕm′ē-sĭd]
Vaginal Contraceptive Inserts

Description: Semicid is a safe and effective, non-systemic, reversible method of birth control. Each vaginal contraceptive insert contains 100 mg of the spermicide nonoxynol-9. It contains no hormones and is odorless and non-messy. When used consistently and according to directions, the effectiveness of Semicid is approximately equal to vaginal foam contraceptives, but less than the pill or diaphragm.

Actions: Semicid dissolves in the vagina and blends with natural vaginal secretions to provide double birth control protection: a physical barrier, plus an effective sperm killing barrier that covers the cervical opening and adjoining vaginal walls.
Semicid requires no applicator and has no unpleasant taste. Unlike foams, creams and jellies, Semicid does not drip or run, and Semicid inserts are easier to use than the diaphragm. Also, Semicid does not effervesce like some inserts, so it is not as likely to cause a burning feeling. Semicid provides effective contraceptive protection when used properly. However, no contraceptive method or product can provide an absolute guarantee against becoming pregnant.

Indication: For the prevention of pregnancy.

Warnings: Do not insert in urinary opening (urethra). Do not take orally. If irritation occurs, discontinue use. If irritation persists, consult your physician.

Continued on next page

Whitehall—Cont.

Keep this and all contraceptives out of the reach of children.

Precautions: If douching is desired, one should wait at least six hours after intercourse before douching. If either partner experiences irritation, discontinue use. If irritation persists, consult a physician.

If your doctor has told you that it is dangerous to become pregnant, ask your doctor if you can use Semicid.

If menstrual period is missed, a physician should be consulted.

Dosage and Administration: To use, unwrap one insert and insert it deeply into the vagina. It is essential that Semicid be inserted at least <u>15 minutes</u> before intercourse, however, Semicid is also effective when inserted up to 1 hour before intercourse. If intercourse is delayed for more than 1 hour after Semicid is inserted, or if intercourse is repeated, then another insert must be inserted. Semicid can be used as frequently as needed.

Inactive Ingredients: Benzethonium Chloride, Citric Acid, D&C Red #21 Lake, D&C Red #33 Lake, Methylparaben, Polyethylene Glycol, Water.

How Supplied: Strip Packaging of 10's and 20's.

Keep Semicid at room temperature (Not over 86°F or 30°C).

Shown in Product Identification Section, page 436

SLEEP–EZE 3®
[slēp-ēz]
Nighttime Sleep Aid Tablets
Diphenhydramine Hydrochloride

Description: Sleep-eze 3 is a nighttime sleep-aid that contains Diphenhydramine Hydrochloride, 25 mg. per tablet.

Indication: Sleep-eze 3 helps to reduce difficulty in falling asleep.

Action: Sleep-eze 3 contains diphenhydramine, an antihistamine with anticholinergic and sedative action.

Warnings: Do not give to children under 12 years of age. Insomnia may be a symptom of serious underlying medical illness. If sleeplessness persists continuously for more than 2 weeks, consult your physician. As with any drug, if you are pregnant or nursing a baby, seek the advice of a health professional before using this product.

Do not take this product if you have asthma, glaucoma, or enlargement of the prostate gland except under the advice and supervision of a physician.

In case of accidental ingestion or overdose, contact a physician or Poison Control Center immediately. Keep this and all medicines out of children's reach.

Drug Interaction: Take this product with caution if alcohol is being consumed.

Precaution: This product contains an antihistamine and will cause drowsiness. It should be used only at bedtime.

Dosage and Administration: Take 2 tablets 20 minutes before going to bed.

Professional Labeling: Same as outlined under Indication.

Inactive Ingredients: Calcium Phosphate, D&C Yellow No. 10, FD&C Yellow No. 6, Magnesium Stearate, Microcrystalline Cellulose and Starch.

How Supplied: Packages of 12's, 24's, and 48's.

TODAY®
[tü-dā]
Vaginal Contraceptive Sponge

Description: Today Vaginal Contraceptive Sponge is a soft polyurethane foam sponge containing nonoxynol-9, a spermicide used by millions of women for over 25 years.

Today Sponge is Effective, Safe, and Convenient. Today Sponge provides 24-hour contraceptive protection without hormones, allowing spontaneity. Today Sponge is easy to use, non-messy and disposable.

Active Ingredient: Each Today Sponge contains nonoxynol-9, one gram.

Inactive Ingredients: Benzoic acid, citric acid, sodium dihydrogen citrate, sodium metabisulfite, sorbic acid, water in a polyurethane foam sponge.

Indication: For the prevention of pregnancy.

Actions: Used as directed, Today Vaginal Contraceptive Sponge prevents pregnancy in three ways: 1) the spermicide nonoxynol-9 kills sperm before they can reach the egg; 2) Today Sponge traps and absorbs sperm; 3) Today Sponge blocks the cervix so that sperm cannot enter. Today Sponge is designed for easy insertion into the vagina. It is positioned against the cervix, and while in place provides protection against pregnancy for 24 hours. The soft polyurethane foam sponge is formulated to feel like normal vaginal tissue and has a specially-designed ribbon loop attached to an interior web for maximum strength.

In clinical trials of Today Sponge in over 1,800 women worldwide who completed over 12,000 cycles of use, the method-effectiveness, i.e., the level of effectiveness seen in women who followed the printed instructions exactly and who used Today Sponge every time that they had intercourse, was 89 to 91%.

Instructions: Remove one Today Sponge from airtight inner pack, wet thoroughly with clean tap water, and squeeze gently until it becomes very sudsy. The water activates the spermicide. Fold the sides of Today Sponge upward until it looks long and narrow and then insert it deeply into the vagina with the string loop dangling below. Protection begins immediately and continues for 24 hours. It is <u>not</u> necessary to add creams, jellies,

foams, or any other additional spermicide as long as Today Sponge is in place, no matter how many acts of intercourse may occur during a 24-hour period. Always wait 6 hours after your last act of intercourse before removing Today Sponge. If you have intercourse when Today Sponge has been in place for 24 hours, it must be left in place an additional 6 hours after intercourse before removing it.

To remove Today Sponge, place a finger in the vagina and reach up and back to find the string loop. Hook a finger around the loop. Slowly and gently pull the Sponge out. Some women, especially first-time users, may have difficulty removing the Sponge. This situation may be due to tension or unusually strong muscular pressure. Simple relaxation of the vaginal muscles and bearing down should make it possible to remove the Sponge without difficulty. See User Instruction Booklet (Section 7) for details on removing Today Sponge or call the Today TalkLine 1-800-223-2329.

Warnings: For best protection against pregnancy, follow instructions exactly. Any delay in your menstrual period may be an early sign of pregnancy. If this happens, consult your physician or clinic as soon as possible. A small number of men and women may be sensitive to the spermicide in this product (nonoxynol-9) or any of its other components and should not use this product if irritation occurs and persists. If genital burning or itching occurs in either partner, stop using Today Sponge and contact your physician. If you have ever had Toxic Shock Syndrome, do not use Today Sponge. If you experience two or more of the warning signs of Toxic Shock Syndrome (TSS), including fever, vomiting, diarrhea, muscular pain, dizziness, and rash similar to sunburn, consult your physician or clinic immediately. Today Sponge should not be used during the menstrual period. After childbirth, miscarriage, other termination of pregnancy, or if you are nursing a baby, it is important to consult your physician or clinic before using this product. Today Sponge should be removed within the specified time limit (maximum wear time is 30 hours). In clinical trials, approximately one-half of all unintended pregnancies occurred during the first three months of Today Sponge use. A back-up contraceptive, such as Today Condom, is recommended for additional contraceptive protection during this time, until the user becomes familiar with Today Sponge.

Keep this and all drugs out of the reach of children. In case of accidental ingestion of Today Sponge, call a poison control center, emergency medical facility or doctor.

How To Store: Store at normal room temperature.

How Supplied: Packages of 3s, 6s, and 12s.

Shown in Product Indentification Section, page 436

TRENDAR®
Ibuprofen Tablets, USP
Menstrual Pain & Cramp Reliever

Warning: ASPIRIN SENSITIVE PATIENTS. Do not take this product if you have had a severe allergic reaction to aspirin, e.g. asthma, swelling, shock or hives, because even though this product contains no aspirin or salicylates cross-reactions may occur in patients allergic to aspirin.

Indications: For the temporary relief of painful menstrual cramps (Dysmenorrhea); also headaches, backaches and muscular aches and pains associated with Premenstrual Syndrome.

Dosage and Administration: Adults: Take 1 tablet every 4 to 6 hours at the onset of menstrual symptoms and while pain persists. If pain does not respond to 1 tablet, 2 tablets may be used but do not exceed 6 tablets in 24 hours, unless directed by a doctor. The smallest effective dose should be used. Take with food or milk if occasional and mild heartburn, upset stomach, or stomach pain occurs with use. Consult a doctor if these symptoms are more than mild or if they persist. Children: Do not give this product to children under 12 except under the advice or supervision of a doctor.

Warnings: Do not take for pain for more than 10 days unless directed by a doctor. If pain persists or gets worse, or if new symptoms occur, consult a doctor. These could be signs of serious illness. If you are under a doctor's care for any serious condition, consult a doctor before taking this product. As with aspirin and acetaminophen, if you have any condition which requires you to take prescription drugs or if you have had any problems or serious side effects from taking any nonprescription pain reliever, do not take this product without first discussing it with your doctor. If you experience any symptoms which are unusual or seem unrelated to the condition for which you took ibuprofen, consult a doctor before taking any more of it. Although ibuprofen is indicated for the same conditions as aspirin and acetaminophen, it should not be taken with them except under a doctor's direction. Do not combine this product with any other ibuprofen-containing product. As with any drug, if you are pregnant or nursing a baby, seek the advice of a health professional before using this product. IT IS ESPECIALLY IMPORTANT NOT TO USE IBUPROFEN DURING THE LAST 3 MONTHS OF PREGNANCY UNLESS SPECIFICALLY DIRECTED TO DO SO BY A DOCTOR BECAUSE IT MAY CAUSE PROBLEMS IN THE UNBORN CHILD OR COMPLICATIONS DURING DELIVERY. Keep this and all drugs out of the reach of children. In case of accidental overdose, seek professional assistance or contact a poison control center immediately.

Active Ingredient: Each tablet contains Ibuprofen 200 mg.

Inactive Ingredients: Acacia, Acetylated Monoglycerides, Beeswax, Calcium Sulfate, Colloidal Silicon Dioxide, Dimethicone, Iron Oxide, Lecithin, Pharmaceutical Glaze, Povidone, Sodium Benzoate, Sodium Carboxymethylcellulose, Starch, Stearic Acid, Sucrose, Titanium Dioxide.

Professional Labeling: Same as stated under Indications.

How Supplied: Coated tablets in bottles of 20's & 40's.

Storage: Store at room temperature; avoid excessive heat 40°C (104°F).

Winthrop Consumer Products
Division of Sterling Drug Inc.
90 PARK AVENUE
NEW YORK, NY 10016

BRONKAID® Mist
(Epinephrine)

Description: BRONKAID Mist, brand of epinephrine inhalation aerosol. Contains: Epinephrine, USP, 0.5% (w/w) (as nitrate and hydrochloric salts). Also contains: Alcohol 33% (w/w), ascorbic acid dichlorodifluoromethane, dichlorotetrafluoroethane, purified water. Each spray delivers 0.25 mg epinephrine. Contains no sulfites.

Indication: For temporary relief of shortness of breath, tightness of chest and wheezing due to Bronchial Asthma.

Warnings: FOR ORAL INHALATION ONLY. Do not use unless a diagnosis of asthma has been established by a doctor. Reduce dosage if nervousness, restlessness, sleeplessness, or bronchial irritation occurs. Do not use if high blood pressure, heart disease, diabetes, thyroid disease is present, difficulty in urination due to enlargement of the prostate gland or if you have ever been hospitalized for asthma or if you are taking any prescription drug for asthma, unless directed by a physician. Do not use this product more frequently or at higher doses than recommended, unless directed by a doctor. If prompt relief is not obtained, consult your physician.
Avoid spraying in eyes. Contents under pressure. Do not break or incinerate. Do not use near open flame or store at temperature above 120°F. Keep this and all drugs out of the reach of children. In case of accidental overdose, seek professioinal assistance or contact a poison control center immediately. If you are pregnant or nursing a baby, seek the advice of a health professional before using this product. Do not use if you are presently taking a prescription drug for high blood pressure or depression, without first consulting your doctor.

Precaution: Children under 4 years of age should use BRONKAID Mist only on the advice of a physician. Avoid indiscriminate use of BRONKAID Mist as many people do with similar medications. Use only when actually needed for relief. Overdose may cause rapid heart beat and nervousness.

Dosage and Administration: For adults and children 4 years of age or older: Start with one inhalation, then wait at least one minute. If not relieved, use BRONKAID Mist once more. Do not repeat treatment for at least 3 hours. If difficulty in breathing persists, consult your physician.

Directions for Use:
1. Remove cap and mouthpiece from bottle.
2. Remove cap from mouthpiece.
3. Turn mouthpiece sideways and fit metal stem of nebulizer into hole in flattened end of mouthpiece.
4. Exhale, as completely as possible. Now, hold bottle upside down between thumb and forefinger and close lips loosely around end of mouthpiece.
5. Inhale deeply while pressing down firmly on bottle, once only.
6. Remove mouthpiece and hold your breath a moment to allow for maximum absorption of medication. Then exhale slowly through nearly closed lips.
After use, remove mouthpiece from bottle and replace cap. Slide mouthpiece over bottle for protection. When possible rinse mouthpiece with tap water immediately after use. Soap and water will not hurt it. A clean mouthpiece always works better.

How Supplied: Bottles of ½ fl oz (15 ml) NDC 0024-4082-15 with actuator. Also available—refills (no mouthpiece) in 15 ml (½ fl oz) NDC 0024-4083-16 and 22.5 ml (¾ fl oz) NDC 0024-4083-22.
Shown in Product Identification Section, page 436

BRONKAID® Mist Suspension
(Epinephrine Bitartrate)

Active Ingredients: Each spray delivers 0.3 mg Epinephrine Bitartrate equivalent to 0.16 mg Epinephrine base. Contains Epinephrine Bitartrate 7.0 mg per cc. Also contains: Cetylpyridinium Chloride, Dichlorodifluoromethane, Dichlorotetrafluoroethane, Sorbitan Trioleate, Trichloromonofluoromethane. Contains no Sulfites.

Indication: Provides temporary relief of shortness of breath, tightness of chest and wheezing due to Bronchial Asthma.

Warnings: For—ORAL INHALATION ONLY. Contents under pressure. Do not puncture or throw container into incinerator. Using or storing near open flame or heating above 120°F may cause burst-

Continued on next page

This product information was effective as of January 1, 1989. Current detailed information may be obtained directly from Winthrop Consumer Products, Division of Sterling Drug Inc., by writing to 90 Park Avenue, New York, NY 10016.

Winthrop Consumer—Cont.

ing. Do not use unless a diagnosis of asthma has been established by a physician. Reduce dosage if bronchial irritation, nervousness, restlessness, or sleeplessness occurs. Overdose may cause nervousness and rapid heartbeat. Use only on the advice of a physician if heart disease, high blood pressure, diabetes, thyroid disease is present, difficulty in urination due to enlargement of the prostate gland, if you have ever been hospitalized for asthma, or if you are taking any prescription drug for asthma. If difficulty in breathing persists, or if relief does not occur within 20 minutes of inhalation, discontinue use and seek medical assistance immediately. Children under 4 years of age should use BRONKAID Mist Suspension only on the advice of a physician. Keep this and all drugs out of the reach of children. In case of accidental overdose, seek professional assistance or contact a poison control center immediately. If you are pregnant or nursing a baby, seek the advice of a health professional before using this product. Do not use this product if you are presently taking a prescription drug for high blood pressure or depression, without first consulting a physician.

Administration: (1) SHAKE WELL. (2) HOLD INHALER WITH NOZZLE DOWN WHILE USING. Empty the lungs as completely as possible by exhaling. (3) Purse the lips as in saying the letter "O" and hold the nozzle up to the lips, keeping the tongue flat. As you start to take a deep breath, squeeze nozzle and can together, releasing one full application. Complete taking deep breath, drawing medication into your lungs. (4) Hold breath for as long as comfortable. This distributes the medication in the lungs. Then exhale slowly keeping the lips nearly closed. (5) Rinse nozzle daily with soap and hot water after removing from vial. Dry with clean cloth. Before each use, remove dust cap and inspect mouthpiece for foreign objects. Replace dust cap after each use.

Dosage: Start with one inhalation—then wait at least one minute; if not relieved, use BRONKAID Mist Suspension once more; do not repeat treatment for at least 3 hours.

Professional Labeling: Same as stated under Indication.

How Supplied: $\frac{1}{3}$ fl oz (10 cc) pocket-size aerosol inhaler (NDC 0024-4082-10) with actuator.

BRONKAID® Tablets

Description: Each tablet contains ephedrine sulfate 24 mg, guaifenesin (glyceryl guaiacolate) 100 mg, and theophylline 100 mg. Also contains: magnesium stearate, magnesium trisilicate, microcrystalline cellulose, starch.

Indication: For symptomatic control of bronchial congestion and bronchial asthma. Clears bronchial passages.

Helps relieve shortness of breath. Plus helps loosen phlegm.

Precautions: Do not use this product unless a diagnosis of asthma has been made by a doctor, if you have heart disease, diabetes, difficulty in urination due to enlargement of the prostate gland, if you have ever been hospitalized for asthma or if you are taking any prescription drug for asthma unless directed by a doctor, do not continue to use this product, but seek medical assistance immediately if symptoms are not relieved within an hour or become worse. Some users of this product may experieence nervousness, tremor, sleeplessness, nausea, and loss of appetite. If these symptoms persist or become worse, consult your doctor. Do not use this product if you are presently taking a prescription drug for high blood pressure or depression. Do not exceed recommended dosage unless directed by a physician.

Warnings: As with any drug, if you are pregnant or nursing a baby, seek the advice of a health professional before using this product. Keep this and all drugs out of the reach of children. In case of accidental overdose, seek professional assistance or contact a poison control center immediately.

Dosage and Administration:
Adult Dosage: 1 tablet every four hours. Do not take more than 5 tablets in a 24-hour period. Swallow tablets whole with water.
Children under 12 years of age: Consult a doctor.
Morning Dose: An early dose of 1 tablet (for adults) can relieve the coughing and wheezing caused by the night's accumulation of mucus, and can help you start the day with better breathing capacity.
Before an Attack: Many persons feel an attack of asthma coming on. One BRONKAID tablet beforehand may stop the attack before it starts.
During the Day: The precise dose of BRONKAID tablets can be varied to meet your individual needs as you gain experience with this product. It is advisable to take 1 tablet before going to bed, for nighttime relief. However, be sure not to exceed recommended daily dosage.

How Supplied:
Boxes of 24 (NDC 0024-4081-02)
Boxes of 60 (NDC 0024-4081-06)
Shown in Product Identification
Section, page 436

CAMPHO–PHENIQUE®
[*kam'fo-finēk*]
COLD SORE GEL

Description: Contains phenol 4.7% (w/w) and camphor 10.8% (w/w). Also contains: Colloidal silicon dioxide, eucalyptus oil, glycerin, light mineral oil.

Actions: Use at the first sign of cold sore, fever blister and sun blister symptoms (tingling, pain, itching).

Indications: For relief of pain and itching due to cold sores, fever blisters

and sun blisters. To combat infection from minor injuries and skin lesions.
Also effective for:
Minor Skin Injuries: abrasions, cuts, scrapes, burns, razor nicks, and chafed or irritated skin.
Insect Bites: Mosquitoes, black flies, sand fleas, chiggers.

Warnings: Not for prolonged use. Not to be used on large areas. In case of deep or puncture wounds, serious burns, or persisting redness, swelling or pain, or if rash or infection develops, discontinue use and consult physician. Do not bandage if applied to fingers or toes.
Avoid using near eyes. If product gets into the eye, flush thoroughly with water and obtain medical attention. Keep this and all drugs out of the reach of children. In case of accidental ingestion, seek professional assistance or contact a poison control center immediately.

Directions for Use: For external use. Apply directly to cold sore, fever blister or injury three or four times a day.

How Supplied: Tubes of .23 oz (6.5 g) NDC 0024-0212-01 and .50 oz (14 g) NDC 0024-0212-02.
Shown in Product Identification
Section, page 436

CAMPHO–PHENIQUE® Liquid
[*kam'fo-finēk*]

Description: Contains phenol 4.7% (w/w) and camphor 10.8% (w/w). Also contains: Eucalyptus oil, light mineral oil.

Actions: Pain-relieving antiseptic for scrapes, cuts, burns, insect bites, fever blisters and cold sores.

Indications: For relief of pain and to combat infection from minor injuries and skin lesions.

Warnings: Not for prolonged use. Not to be used on large areas or in or near the eyes. In case of deep or puncture wounds, serious burns, or persisting redness, swelling or pain, or if rash or infection develops, discontinue use and consult physician. Do not bandage if applied to fingers or toes.
Keep this and all drugs out of the reach of children. In case of accidental ingestion, seek professional assistance or contact a poison control center immediately.

Directions for Use: For external use. Apply with cotton three or four times daily.
4 oz size only:
Do not use more than $\frac{1}{2}$ the contents of the 4 fl oz bottle in any 24-hour period.

How Supplied:
Bottles of $\frac{3}{4}$ fl oz (NDC 0024-5150-05)
        $1\frac{1}{2}$ fl oz (NDC 0024-5150-06)
        4 fl oz (NDC 0024-5150-04)
Shown in Product Identification
Section, page 436

CAMPHO–PHENIQUE®
[kam'fo-finēk]
STING RELIEF FORMULA

Description: Contains: Benzocaine U.S.P. 20% and Menthol 1.0%. Also contains: D&C Green No. 5 and D&C Yellow No. 10, FD&C Blue No. 1, Isopropyl Alcohol 29.3%, Polyethylene Glycol 300, Purified Water.

Actions: External analgesic for fast, effective relief of pain and itching from stings and bites of Bees, Wasps, Hornets, Yellow Jackets and other insects.

Indications: Also effective for the temporary relief of pain and itching associated with stings and bites from Ants, Mosquitos, Deer Flies, Horse Flies and Chiggers.

Warning: For EXTERNAL use only. Avoid contact with eyes. If condition worsens or if symptoms persist for more than 7 days, discontinue use of this product and consult a physician. Keep this and all drugs out of the reach of children. In case of accidental ingestion, seek professional assistance or contact a poison control center immediately.

Directions: For adults and children two years of age and older. Do not use on children under two years of age except under the advice and supervision of a physician. Apply to affected areas not more than three to four times daily.

How Supplied: Cartons of 5 0.5 ml vials (NDC 0024-0300-25).

CAMPHO–PHENIQUE™
[kam'fo-finēk]
TRIPLE ANTIBIOTIC OINTMENT PLUS PAIN RELIEVER

Description: Contains Bacitracin 400 units, Neomycin Sulfate 5mg (equiv. to 3.5 mg Neomycin Base), Polymyxin B Sulfate 5000 units, Diperodon HCl 10mg (Pain Reliever). Also contains mineral oil and white petrolatum.

Actions: Pain-relieving triple antibiotic with anesthetic to help prevent infection in minor cuts, scrapes, burns and other minor wounds.

Indications: Helps prevent infections in minor cuts, burns, and other minor wounds. Provides soothing, non-stinging temporary relief of pain and itching associated with these conditions.

Warnings: For external use only. In case of deep or puncture wounds, animal bites or serious burns, consult physician. If redness, irritation, swelling or pain persists or increases, or if infection occurs, discontinue use and consult physician. Do not use in eyes or over large areas. Keep this and all medicines out of children's reach. In case of accidental ingestion seek professional assistance or contact a poison control center immediately.

Directions: Apply directly to the affected area and cover with a sterile gauze if necessary. May be applied 1 to 3 times daily as the condition indicates.

How Supplied: Tubes of .50 oz. (NDC 0024-2015-05) and 1.0 oz. (NDC 0024-2015-01).

FERGON® CAPSULES
FERGON® TABLETS
[fur-gone]
brand of ferrous gluconate
FERGON® ELIXIR

Description: FERGON (ferrous gluconate, USP) is stabilized to maintain a minimum of ferric ions. It contains not less than 11.5 percent iron. Each FERGON Capsule contains 435 mg of ferrous gluconate, yielding 50 mg of elemental iron. Also contains: Benzyl Alcohol, Calcium Stearate, D&C Red #7, Red #28, Red #36, FD&C Blue #1, Red #40, Gelatin, Glycerin, Hydroxypropyl Cellulose, Parabens, Pharmaceutical Glaze, Povidone, Sodium Propionate, Sucrose, Talc.
Each FERGON tablet contains 320 mg (5 grains) ferrous gluconate equal to approximately 36 mg ferrous iron. Also contains: Acacia, Carnauba Wax, Dextrose Excipient, FD&C Red #40, D & C Yellow #10, FD & C Blue #1, Gelatin, Kaolin, Magnesium Stearate, Parabens, Povidone, Precipitated Calcium Carbonate, Sodium Benzoate, Starch, Sucrose, Talc, Titanium Dioxide, Yellow Wax. Not USP for dissolution.
FERGON Elixir contains: Ferrous Gluconate 6%. Also contains: Alcohol 7%, Flavor, Glycerin, Liquid Glucose, Purified Water, Saccharin Sodium. Each teaspoon (5 ml) contains 300 mg (5 grains) Ferrous Gluconate equivalent to approximately 34 mg Ferrous Iron.

Action and Uses: FERGON preparations produce rapid hemoglobin regeneration in patients with iron deficiency anemias. FERGON is better utilized and better tolerated than other forms of iron because of its low ionization constant and solubility in the entire pH range of the gastrointestinal tract. It does not precipitate proteins or have the astringency of more ionizable forms of iron, does not interfere with proteolytic or diastatic activities of the digestive system, and will not produce nausea, abdominal cramps, constipation or diarrhea in the great majority of patients. The pellets of ferrous gluconate contained in FERGON Capsules are coated to permit maximum availability of iron in the upper small bowel, the site of maximum absorption. FERGON preparations are for use in the prevention and treatment of iron deficiency. They should be taken when the need for iron supplement therapy has been determined by a physician.

Warnings: Since oral iron products interfere with absorption of oral tetracycline antibiotics, these products should not be taken within two hours of each other. Keep this and all drugs out of the reach of children. As with any drug, if you are pregnant or nursing a baby, seek the advise of a health professional before using this product. In case of accidental overdose, seek professional assistance or contact a poison control center immediately.

Dosage and Administration: *Adults* —One to two FERGON capsules or tablets or one to two teaspoonsful of FERGON Elixir daily. *For children and infants,* as prescribed by physician.

How Supplied: FERGON Capsules, bottle of 30 (NDC 0024-1016-03). FERGON, tablets of 320 mg (5 grains), bottle of 100 (NDC 0024-1015-10), bottle of 500 (NDC 0024-1015-50), and bottle of 1,000 (NDC 0024-1015-00). FERGON Elixir 6% (5 grains per teaspoonful) bottle of 1 pint (NDC 0024-1019-16).
Shown in Product Identification Section, page 436

FERGON® IRON PLUS CALCIUM CAPLETS
[fur-gone]

Description: Each Caplet contains Ferrous Fumarate in a time released system (yielding 18 mg of elemental iron), 1500 mg Calcium Carbonate (yielding 600 mg of elemental Calcium) and 125 IU of Vitamin D.
Also contains: Diethyl Phthalate, Ethylcellulose, Hydroxypropyl Methylcellulose, Magnesium Stearate, Microcrystalline Cellulose, Pharmaceutical Glaze, Povidone, FD&C Red 40, Colloidal Silicon Dioxide, Sodium Starch Glycolate, Stearic Acid, Talc, Titanium Dioxide and other ingredients.

Actions and Uses: Fergon Iron Plus Calcium contains pure calcium and time-released iron for diets deficient in both minerals.

Indications: For use in the prevention of iron (calcium) deficiency when the need for such therapy has been determined by a physician.

Warnings: Since oral iron products interfere with absorption of oral tetracycline antibiotics, these products should not be taken within two hours of each other. Keep this and all drugs out of the reach of children. As with any drug, if you are pregnant or nursing a baby, seek the advice of a health professional before using this product. In case of accidental overdose, seek professional assistance or contact a poison control center immediately. The treatment of any anemic condition should be under the advice and supervision of a physician.

Directions: Adults, one to two caplets daily. For children and infants, consult physician.

Continued on next page

This product information was effective as of January 1, 1989. Current detailed information may be obtained directly from Winthrop Consumer Products, Division of Sterling Drug Inc., by writing to 90 Park Avenue, New York, NY 10016.

Winthrop Consumer—Cont.

How Supplied: Fergon® Iron Plus Calcium Caplets (bottle of 60) (NDC 0024-0596-60).

NaSal™
Saline (buffered)
0.65% Sodium chloride
Nasal Spray
Nose Drops

Description: Both the nasal spray and nose drops contain Sodium Chloride 0.65%. Also contains: Benzalkonium Chloride and Thimerosal 0.001% as preservative, Mono- and Dibasic Sodium Phosphates as buffers, Purified Water. **Contains No Alcohol**

Actions: Immediate relief for dry nose. Formulated to match the pH of normal nasal secretions to help prevent stinging or burning.

Indications: Provides soothing relief for clogged nasal passages—without stinging or burning. Provides immediate relief for dry, inflamed nasal membranes due to colds, low humidity, allergies, minor nose bleeds, overuse of topical nasal decongestants, and other nasal irritations. As an ideal nasal moisturizer, it can be used in conjunction with oral decongestants.

Adverse Reactions: No associated side effects.

Warnings: Keep this and all drugs out of the reach of children. In case of accidental ingestion seek professional assistance or contact a poison control center immediately. The use of the dispenser by more than one person may spread infection.

Dosage and Administration: *Spray*— For adults and children six years of age and over: with head upright, spray twice in each nostril as needed or as directed by physician. To spray, squeeze bottle quickly and firmly. *Nose Drops*—For infants and adults: 2 to 6 drops in each nostril as needed or as directed by physician.

How Supplied: Nasal Spray—plastic squeeze bottles of 15 ml (½ fl oz) NDC 0024-1316-01.
Nose Drops—MonoDrop® bottles of 15 ml (½ fl oz) NDC 0024-1315-01.
Shown in Product Identification Section, page 436

NEO-SYNEPHRINE®
phenylephrine hydrochloride

Description: This line of Nasal Spray, Nose Drops and Nasal Spray Pumps contain Phenylephrine Hydrochloride in strengths ranging from .125% (drops only) to 1%. Also contains: Benzalkonium Chloride and Thimerosal 0.001% as preservatives, Citric Acid, Purified Water, Sodium Chloride, Sodium Citrate.

Action: Rapid-acting nasal decongestant.

Indications: For temporary relief of nasal congestion due to common cold, hay fever or other upper respiratory allergies, or associated with sinusitis.

Precautions: Some hypersensitive individuals may experience a mild stinging sensation. This is usually transient and often disappears after a few applications. Do not exceed recommended dosage. Follow directions for use carefully. If symptoms are not relieved after several applications, a physician should be consulted. Frequent and continued usage of the higher concentrations (especially the 1% solution) occasionally may cause a rebound congestion of the nose. Therefore, long-term or frequent use of this solution is not recommended without the advice of a physician.
Prolonged exposure to air or strong light will cause oxidation and some loss of potency. Do not use if brown in color or contains a precipitate.

Adverse Reactions: Generally very well tolerated; systemic side effects such as tremor, insomnia, or palpitation rarely occur.

Warnings: Keep these and all drugs out of the reach of children. In case of accidental ingestion seek professional assistance or contact a poison control center immediately. The use of the dispenser by more than one person may spread infection.

Dosage and Administration: *Topical* —dropper or spray. The *0.25% solution* is adequate in most cases *(0.125% for children 2 to 6 years.).* In resistant cases, or if more powerful decongestion is desired, the *0.5 or 1% solution* should be used. Also used as *0.5% jelly.*

How Supplied: Nasal spray 0.25%—15 ml (for children and for adults who prefer a mild nasal spray)—NDC 0024-1348-03; nasal spray 0.5%—15 ml (for adults)—NDC 0024-1353-01 and 30 ml (1 fl oz) NDC 0024-1353-05; nasal spray 1%—15 ml (extra strength for adults)—NDC 0024-1352-02; nasal spray pump 0.5%—15 ml bottle (½ fl oz) NDC 0024-1353-04; nasal solution 0.125% (for infants and small children), 15 ml bottles—NDC 0024-1345-05; nasal solution 0.25% (for children and adults who prefer a mild solution), 15 ml bottles—NDC 0024-1347-05; nasal solution 0.5% (for adults), 15 ml bottles—NDC 0024-1351-05; nasal solution 1% (extra strength for adults), 15 ml bottles—NDC 0024-1355-05; and 16 fl oz bottles—NDC 0024-1355-06; and water soluble nasal jelly 0.5%, ⅝ oz tubes—NDC 0024-1367-01.
Also available — NEO-SYNEPHRINE Mentholated Nasal Spray 0.5% (for adults), ½ fl oz bottles—NDC 0024-1364-01.
Shown in Product Identification Section, page 436

NEO-SYNEPHRINE® 12 HOUR
oxymetazoline hydrochloride
Nasal Spray 0.05%
Vapor Nasal Spray 0.05%
Nose Drops 0.05%

Description: *Adult Strength Nasal Spray, Nose Drops* and *Nasal Spray Pump* contain: Oxymetazoline Hydrochloride 0.05%. Also contains: Benzalkonium Chloride and Phenylmercuric Acetate 0.002% as preservatives, Glycine, Purified Water, Sorbitol, may also contain Sodium Chloride. *Adult Strength Vapor Nasal Spray* contains Oxymetazoline Hydrochloride 0.05%. Also contains: Benzalkonium Chloride and Thimerosal 0.001% as preservatives, Camphor, Citric Acid, Eucalyptol, Menthol, Methyl Salicylate, Purified Water, Sodium Chloride, Sodium Citrate, Tyloxapol.

Action: 12 HOUR Nasal Decongestant.

Indications: Provides temporary relief, for up to 12 HOURS, of nasal congestion due to colds, hay fever, sinusitis, or allergies. NEO-SYNEPHRINE 12-HOUR Nasal Sprays, Nose Drops and Nasal Spray Pump contain oxymetazoline which provides the longest-lasting relief of nasal congestion available.

Warnings: Do not exceed recommended dosage because symptoms may occur such as burning, stinging, sneezing, or increase of nasal discharge. Nasal Spray 0.05%, Vapor Nasal Spray 0.05%, Nasal Spray Pump 0.05%, Nose Drops 0.05% not recommended for children under 6. Do not use these products for more than 3 days. If symptoms persist, consult a physician. The use of the dispenser by more than one person may spread infection.
Keep this and all drugs out of the reach of children. In case of accidental ingestion, seek professional assistance or contact a poison control center immediately.

Dosage and Administration: *Adult Strength Nasal Spray and Vapor Nasal Spray*—For adults and children 6 years of age and over: With head upright, spray two or three times in each nostril twice daily—morning and evening. To spray, squeeze bottle quickly and firmly.
Nasal Spray Pump—For adults and children 6 to under 12 years of age (with adult supervision): spray 2 or 3 times in each nostril daily—morning and evening. Do not exceed 2 applications in any 24 hour period. Children under 6 years of age: consult a doctor. Hold bottle with thumb at base and nozzle between first and second fingers. With head upright insert spray nozzle in nostril. Depress pump 2 or 3 times, all the way down, with a firm even stroke and sniff deeply. Repeat in other nostril. Do not tilt head backward while spraying.
Adult Strength Nose Drops—For adults and children 6 years of age and over: two or three drops in each nostril twice daily—morning and evening.

How Supplied: *Nasal Spray Adult Strength*—plastic squeeze bottles of 15 ml (½ fl oz) NDC 0024-1390-03 and 30 ml (1 fl oz) NDC 0024-1394-01; Nasal Spray Pump—15 ml bottle (½ fl oz) NDC 0024-1389-01; *Vapor Nasal Spray Adult Strength*—squeeze bottles of 15 ml (½ fl oz) NDC 0024-1391-03; *Nose Drops Adult*

Strength —bottles of 15 ml (½ fl oz) with dropper NDC 0024-1392-01.
Shown in Product Identification Section, page 436

NTZ®
Long Acting
Oxymetazoline hydrochloride
Nasal Spray 0.05%
Nose Drops 0.05%

Description: Both the nasal spray and nose drops contain Oxymetazoline Hydrochloride 0.05%. Also contains: Benzalkonium Chloride and Phenylmercuric Acetate 0.002% as preservatives, Glycine, Purified Water, Sorbitol, and may also contain Sodium Chloride.

Actions: 12 Hour Nasal Decongestant

Indications: Provides temporary relief, for up to 12 hours, of nasal congestion due to colds, hay fever, sinusitis, or allergies. Oxymetazoline hydrochloride provides the longest-lasting relief of nasal congestion available. It decongests nasal passages up to 12 hours, reduces swelling of nasal passages, and temporarily restores freer breathing through the nose.

Warnings: Not recommended for children under six. Do not exceed recommended dosage because symptoms may occur such as burning, stinging, sneezing, or increase of nasal discharge. Do not use these products for more than 3 days. If symptoms persist, consult a physician. The use of the dispenser by more than one person may spread infection. Keep these and all drugs out of the reach of children. In case of accidental ingestion seek professional assistance or contact a poison control center immediately.

Dosage and Administration: Intranasally by spray and dropper. *Nasal Spray* —For adults and children 6 years of age and over: With head upright, spray 2 or 3 times in each nostril twice daily—morning and evening. To spray, squeeze bottle quickly and firmly. *Nose Drops* —For adults and children 6 years of age and over: 2 or 3 drops in each nostril twice daily—morning and evening.

How Supplied:
Nasal Spray —plastic squeeze bottles of 15 ml (½ fl oz) NDC 0024-1312-02
Nose Drops —bottles of 15 ml (½ fl oz) with dropper NDC 0024-1311-03

pHisoDerm®
[*fi 'zo-derm*]
Skin Cleanser and Conditioner

Description: pHisoDerm, a nonsoap emollient skin cleanser, is a unique liquid emulsion containing Sodium Octoxynol-2 Ethane Sulfonate Solution, Water, Petrolatum, Octoxynol-3, Mineral Oil (with Lanolin Alcohol and Oleyl Alcohol), Cocamide MEA, Imidazolidinyl Urea, Sodium Benzoate, Tetrasodium EDTA, and Methylcellulose. Adjusted to normal skin pH with Hydrochloric Acid. Contains no hexachlorophene. pHisoDerm contains no soap, perfumes, or irritating alkali. Its pH value, unlike that of soap, lies within the pH range of normal skin.

Actions: pHisoDerm is well tolerated and can be used frequently by those persons whose skin may be irritated by the use of soap or other alkaline cleansers, or by those who are sensitive to the fatty acids contained in soap. pHisoDerm contains an effective detergent for removing soil and acts as an active emulsifier of all types of oil—animal, vegetable, and mineral.

pHisoDerm produces suds when used with any kind of water—hard or soft, hot or cold (even cold sea water)—at any temperature and under acid, alkaline, or neutral conditions.

pHisoDerm deposits a fine film of lanolin components and petrolatum on the skin during the washing process and, thereby, helps protect against the dryness that soap can cause.

Indications: A sudsing emollient cleanser for use on skin of infants, children, and adults.
Useful for removal of ointments and cosmetics from the skin.

Directions: For external use only.
HANDS. Squeeze a few drops of pHisoDerm into the palm, add a little water, and work up a lather. Rinse thoroughly.
FACE. After washing your hands, squeeze a small amount of pHisoDerm into the palm or onto a small sponge or washcloth, and work up a lather by adding a little water. Massage the suds onto the face for approximately one minute. Rinse thoroughly. Avoid getting suds into the eyes.
BATHING. First wet the body. Work a small amount of pHisoDerm into a lather with hands or a soft wet sponge, gradually adding small amounts of water to make more lather. Rinse thoroughly.

Caution: pHisoDerm suds that get into the eyes accidentally during washing should be rinsed out promptly with a sufficient amount of water.
pHisoDerm is intended for external use only. pHisoDerm should not be poured into measuring cups, medicine bottles, or similar containers since it may be mistaken for baby formula or medications. If swallowed, pHisoDerm may cause gastrointestinal irritation.
pHisoDerm should not be used on persons with sensitivity to any of its components.

How Supplied: pHisoDerm is supplied in two formulations for regular and oily skin. It is packaged in sanitary squeeze bottles of 5 and 16 ounces. The regular formula is also supplied in squeeze bottles of 9 ounces and plastic bottles of 1 gallon.
Shown in Product Identification Section, page 436

pHisoDerm® FOR BABY
[*fi 'zo-derm*]
Skin Cleanser

Description: pHisoDerm FOR BABY, a nonsoap emollient skin cleanser, is a unique liquid emulsion containing Sodium Octoxynol-2 Ethane Sulfonate Solution, Water, Petrolatum, Octoxynol-3, Mineral Oil (with Lanolin Alcohol and Oleyl Alcohol), Cocamide MEA, Fragrance, Imidazolidinyl Urea, Sodium Benzoate, Tetrasodium EDTA, and Methylcellulose. Adjusted to normal skin pH with Hydrochloric Acid. Contains no hexachlorophene or irritating alkali. Its pH value, unlike that of soap, lies within the pH range of normal skin.

Actions: pHisoDerm FOR BABY gently cleans babies' delicate skin without irritating. Petrolatum and lanolin leave skin soft and smooth and protect against dryness.
pHisoDerm FOR BABY rinses easily without leaving a soapy film. The powder fragrance leaves skin smelling fresh and clean.

Precautions: pHisoDerm FOR BABY suds that get into babies' eyes accidentally during washing should be rinsed out promptly with a sufficient amount of water.
pHisoDerm FOR BABY is intended for external use only. It should not be poured into measuring cups, medicine bottles, or similar containers since it may be mistaken for baby formula or medications. If swallowed, pHisoDerm FOR BABY may cause gastrointestinal irritation.
pHisoDerm FOR BABY should not be used on babies with sensitivity to any of its components.

Administration: First wet the baby's body. Work a small amount of pHisoDerm FOR BABY into a lather with hands or a soft wet sponge, gradually adding small amounts of water to make more lather. Spread the lather over all parts of the baby's body, including the head. Avoid getting suds into the baby's eyes. Wash the diaper area last. Be sure to carefully cleanse all folds and creases. Rinse thoroughly. Pat the baby dry with a soft towel.

How Supplied: pHisoDerm FOR BABY is packaged in soft plastic, sanitary, squeeze bottles of 5 and 9 ounces and can be opened and closed with one hand.
Shown in Product Identification Section, page 436

pHisoPUFF®
[*fi-zo-puf*]
Nonmedicated Cleansing Sponge

Description: pHisoPUFF is a nonmedicated cleansing sponge with a special dual layer construction combining a white polyester fiber side and a green sponge side.

Continued on next page

This product information was effective as of January 1, 1989. Current detailed information may be obtained directly from Winthrop Consumer Products, Division of Sterling Drug Inc., by writing to 90 Park Avenue, New York, NY 10016.

Winthrop Consumer—Cont.

Actions: pHisoPUFF cleanses two ways: (1) white fiber side for extra thorough cleansing to gently remove the top layer of dead skin cells, free dirt, debris, and oil trapped in this layer and reveal new, fresh skin cells and (2) green sponge side works to cleanse and rinse skin clean. Using this side will help apply your cleanser or soap more evenly. Also good for removing eye makeup.

Precautions: Do not use pHisoPUFF fiber side on skin that is irritated, sunburned, windburned, damaged, broken, or infected. Do not use on skin which is prone to rashes or itching.

Administration: For the green sponge side: Wet pHisoPUFF with warm water, apply pHisoDerm® or another skin cleanser of your choice, and develop a lather. Glide sponge over your face up and down, back and forth, or in a circle; whatever is the easiest for you. Rinse face and dry.
For the white fiber side: Wet pHisoPUFF with warm water, apply pHisoDerm or another skin cleanser of your choice, and develop a lather. Try pHisoPUFF on the back of your hand before using it on your face. Experiment by changing the pressure and speed with which you move it. Now move pHisoPUFF gently and slowly over your face. Use no more than a few seconds on each area. You can move it in any direction, whichever comes natural to you. Rinse face and dry. As you use this fiber side more often, usage and pressure may be increased to best fit your skin sensitivity. Always rinse your pHisoPUFF thoroughly each time you use it. Hold under running water, let it drain, then give it a few quick shakes.

How Supplied: Box of 1 pHisoPUFF.
Shown in Product Identification Section, page 436

pHisoPUFF® Disposa–PUFFS™
[fi-zo-puf dis-po-za-pufs]
Nonmedicated Cleansing Sponges

Description: pHisoPUFF Disposa-PUFFS are nonmedicated cleansing sponges of white polyester fiber.

Action: For extra thorough cleansing; gently removes the top layer of dead skin cells, frees dirt, debris and oil trapped in this layer frees and reveals new, fresh skin cells.

Precautions: Do not use on skin that is irritated, sunburned, windburned, damaged, broken or infected. Do not use on skin which is prone to rashes or itching.

Administration: Wet a pHisoPUFF Disposa-PUFF with warm water. Apply your favorite cleanser to the sponge and develop a lather. Glide sponge over your face in a slow circular motion. Apply only light pressure for sensitive or dry skin. For oily skin, more pressure may be required for best results. Rinse face thoroughly to remove cleanser. Pat dry. Discard sponge after use.

How Supplied: Box of 36 pHisoPUFF Disposa-PUFFS.
Shown in Product Identification Section, page 436

WinGel®
[win 'jel]
Liquid and Tablets

Description: Each teaspoon (5 ml) of liquid contains a specially processed, short polymer, hexitol stabilized aluminum-magnesium hydroxide equivalent to 180 mg of aluminum hydroxide and 160 mg of magnesium hydroxide. Also contains: Benzoic acid, flavor, methylcellulose, purified water, red ferric oxide, saccharin sodium, sodium hypochlorite solution, sorbitol solution.
Each tablet contains a specially processed, short polymer, hexitol stabilized aluminum-magnesium hydroxide equivalent to 180 mg of aluminum hydroxide and 160 mg of magnesium hydroxide. Also contains: D&C Red #28, FD&C Red #40, flavor, magnesium stearate, mannitol, saccharin sodium, starch. Smooth, easy-to-chew tablets.

Action: Antacid.

Indications: An antacid for the relief of acid indigestion, heartburn, and sour stomach. Nonconstipating. For the symptomatic relief of hyperacidity associated with the diagnosis of peptic ulcer, gastritis, peptic esophagitis, gastric hyperacidity, and hiatal hernia.

WARNINGS: *Adults and children over 6*—Patients should not take more than eight teaspoonfuls or eight tablets in a 24-hour period or use the maximum dosage of the product for more than 2 weeks, except under the advice and supervision of a physician.
Keep this and all drugs out of the reach of children. In case of accidental overdose, seek professional assistance or contact a poison control center immediately.

Drug Interaction Precautions: Antacids may react with certain prescription drugs. Do not take this product if you are presently taking a prescription antibiotic drug containing any form of tetracycline. If the patient is presently taking a prescription drug, this product should not be taken without checking with the physician.

Dosage and Administration: *Adults and children over 6*—1 to 2 teaspoonfuls or 1 to 2 tablets up to four times daily, or as directed by a physician.

Acid Neutralization: The acid neutralizing capacity of WINGEL liquid and tablets is not less than 10 mEq/5 ml.

How Supplied: Liquid—bottles of 6 fl oz (NDC 0024-2247-03) and 12 fl oz (NDC 0024-2247-05).
Tablets—boxes of 50 (NDC 0024-2249-05) and 100 (NDC 0024-2249-06).

Winthrop Pharmaceuticals
**90 PARK AVENUE
NEW YORK, NY 10016**

BREONESIN®
**brand of guaifenesin capsules, USP
Expectorant**

Description: Each red, oval-shaped capsule contains 200 mg of guaifenesin in an easy-to-swallow, soft gelatin capsule. Also contains: FD&C Red #40, Gelatin, Glycerin, Hydrogenated Vegetable Oil and Solids, Lecithin, Parabens, Soybean Oil, Yellow Wax. BREONESIN does not contain any sugar or alcohol.

Indications: BREONESIN is indicated for the temporary relief of coughs. BREONESIN is an expectorant which helps to loosen phlegm (sputum) and bronchial secretions, and acts to thin mucus. Coughs due to minor throat and bronchial irritation that occur with the common cold are temporarily relieved.

Warnings: Persistent cough may indicate a serious condition. Consult your physician if cough persists for more than 1 week, recurs, or is accompanied by high fever, rash, or persistent headache. Do not take this product for persistent coughs due to smoking, asthma, or emphysema, or coughs accompanied by excessive secretions, except under the advice and supervision of your physician. As with any drug, if you are pregnant or nursing a baby, seek the advice of a health professional before using this product.

Dosage: *Adults and Children 12 years of age and over:* 1 or 2 capsules every 4 hours, not to exceed 12 capsules in a 24-hour period. *Children under 12 years:* as directed by your physician.
Store at controlled room temperature, between 15°C and 30°C (59°F and 86°F).

How Supplied: Capsules of 200 mg (red), bottle of 100 (NDC 0024-1050-10)
Distributed by
Winthrop Pharmaceuticals
New York, NY 10016
Mfd. by R.P. Scherer Corp.
Clearwater, Florida 33518

BRONKOLIXIR®
Bronchodilator • Decongestant

Description: Each 5 mL teaspoonful contains:
Ephedrine sulfate, USP..................12 mg
Guaifenesin, USP............................50 mg
Theophylline, USP ....15 mg
Phenobarbital, USP..........................4 mg
(Warning: May be habit forming.)
Also contains: Alcohol 19% (v/v), FD&C Red #40, Flavors, Glycerin, Purified Water, Saccharin Sodium, Sodium Chloride, Sodium Citrate, Sucrose.

Indications: For symptomatic control of bronchial asthma. BRONKOLIXIR is also helpful in overcoming the nonproductive cough often associated with bronchitis or colds.

Warnings: Frequent or prolonged use may cause nervousness, restlessness, or sleeplessness. Phenobarbital may cause drowsiness. Do not use if high blood pressure, heart disease, diabetes, or thyroid disease is present, unless directed by a physician. Ephedrine may cause urinary retention, especially in the presence of partial obstruction, as in prostatism. Keep this and all drugs out of the reach of children. In case of accidental overdose, seek professional assistance or contact a poison control center immediately. As with any drug, if you are pregnant or nursing a baby, seek the advice of a health professional before using this product.

Dosage: *Adults*—2 teaspoons every three or four hours, not to exceed four times daily. *Children*—**over six**—one half the adult dose; **under six**—as directed by physician.

How Supplied: Bottle of 16 fl oz (NDC 0024-1004-16)

BRONKOTABS®
Bronchodilator • Decongestant

Description: Each tablet contains ephedrine sulfate, USP, 24 mg; guaifenesin, USP, 100 mg; theophylline, USP, 100 mg; phenobarbital, USP, 8 mg. (Warning: May be habit forming.)
Also contains: Magnesium Stearate, Magnesium Trisilicate, Microcrystalline Cellulose, Starch.

Indications: For symptomatic control of bronchial asthma.

Warnings: Frequent or prolonged use may cause nervousness, restlessness, or sleeplessness. Phenobarbital may cause drowsiness. Do not use if high blood pressure, heart disease, diabetes, or thyroid disease is present unless directed by a physician. Ephedrine may cause urinary retention, especially in the presence of partial obstruction, as in prostatism. Keep this and all drugs out of the reach of children. In case of accidental overdose, seek professional assistance or contact a poison control center immediately. As with any drug, if you are pregnant or nursing a baby, seek the advice of a health professional before using this product.

Dosage: *Adults*—1 tablet every three or four hours, four to five times daily. *Children:* **over six**—one half the adult dose; **under six**—as directed by physician.

How Supplied: Bottle of 100 (NDC 0024-1006-10)
Bottle of 1000 (NDC 0024-1006-00)

DRISDOL®
brand of ergocalciferol oral solution, USP (in propylene glycol)
Vitamin D Supplement

Description: 200 International Units (5 µg) per drop. The dropper supplied delivers 40 drops per mL.

Indication: For the prevention of vitamin D deficiency in infants, children, and adults.

Warnings: Keep this and all drugs out of the reach of children. In case of accidental overdose, seek professional assistance or contact a poison control center immediately.

Dosage: 2 drops daily. This dose provides the US Recommended Daily Allowance for vitamin D for infants, children, and adults.

How Supplied: Bottles of 2 fl oz (NDC 0024-0391-02)

MEASURIN®
Timed-Released Aspirin

Description: Each caplet contains 10 grains aspirin.
Also contains: Guar Gum, Microcrystalline Cellulose, Starch, and other ingredients.

Indications: For the temporary relief of minor aches and pains associated with rheumatism, or arthritis, bursitis, sprains, or neuralgia. For the temporary relief of minor aches and pains due to overexertion or fatigue, sinusitis, and the common cold or "flu." For simple headache. For the temporary relief of toothache. For the temporary relief of minor cramps associated with the menstrual period.

Caution: If pain persists for more than 10 days, or redness is present, or in conditions affecting children under 12 years of age, consult a physician immediately.

Warnings: Children and teenagers should not use this medicine for chicken pox or flu symptoms before a doctor is consulted about Reye Syndrome, a rare but serious illness reported to be associated with aspirin. Keep this and all drugs out of the reach of children. In case of accidental overdose, seek professional assistance or contact a poison control center immediately. As with any drug, if you are pregnant or nursing a baby, seek the advice of a health professional before using this product.

Dosage—*Adults:* 2 CAPLETS® with water, followed by 1 to 2 CAPLETS every 8 hours, as required. For maximum nighttime and early morning relief, take 2 CAPLETS at bedtime. Do not exceed 6 CAPLETS in 24 hours.

How Supplied: CAPLETS—bottle of 60 (NDC 0024-1025-06)

pHisoDerm
(See Winthrop Consumer Products.)

ZEPHIRAN® CHLORIDE
brand of benzalkonium chloride
ANTISEPTIC
AQUEOUS SOLUTION 1:750
TINTED TINCTURE 1:750
SPRAY—TINTED TINCTURE 1:750

Description: ZEPHIRAN Chloride, brand of benzalkonium chloride, NF, a mixture of alkylbenzyldimethylammonium chlorides, is a cationic quaternary ammonium surface-acting agent. It is very soluble in water, alcohol, and acetone. Aqueous solutions of ZEPHIRAN Chloride are neutral to slightly alkaline, generally colorless, and nonstaining. They have a bitter taste, aromatic odor, and foam when shaken. ZEPHIRAN Chloride Tinted Tincture 1:750 contains alcohol 50 percent and acetone 10 percent by volume. ZEPHIRAN Chloride Spray—Tinted Tincture 1:750 contains alcohol 92 percent. The Tinted Tincture and Spray also contain an orange-red coloring agent.

Clinical Pharmacology: ZEPHIRAN Chloride solutions are rapidly acting anti-infective agents with a moderately long duration of action. They are active against bacteria and some viruses, fungi, and protozoa. Bacterial spores are considered to be resistant. Solutions are bacteriostatic or bactericidal according to their concentration. The exact mechanism of bactericidal action is unknown but is thought to be due to enzyme inactivation. Activity generally increases with increasing temperature and pH. Gram-positive bacteria are more susceptible than gram-negative bacteria (TABLE 1).

TABLE 1
Highest Dilution of ZEPHIRAN Chloride Aqueous Solution Destroying the Organism in 10 but not in 5 Minutes

Organisms	20°C
Streptococcus pyogenes	1:75,000
Staphylococcus aureus	1:52,500
Salmonella typhosa	1:37,500
Escherichia coli	1:10,500

Pseudomonas is the most resistant gram-negative genus. Using the AOAC Use-Dilution Confirmation Method, no growth was obtained when *Staphylococcus aureus, Salmonella choleraesuis,* and *Pseudomonas aeruginosa* (strain PRD-10) were exposed for ten minutes at 20°C to ZEPHIRAN Chloride Aqueous Solution 1:750 and Tinted Tincture 1:750. ZEPHIRAN Chloride Aqueous Solution 1:750 has been shown to retain its bactericidal activity following autoclaving for 30 minutes at 15 lb pressure, freezing, and then thawing.

Continued on next page

This product information was effective as of January 1, 1989. Current detailed information may be obtained directly from Winthrop Pharmaceuticals, Division of Sterling Drug Inc., by writing to 90 Park Avenue, New York NY, 10016.

Winthrop Pharm.—Cont.

The tubercle bacillus may be resistant to aqueous ZEPHIRAN Chloride solutions but is susceptible to the 1:750 tincture (AOAC Method, 10 minutes at 20°C). ZEPHIRAN Chloride solutions also demonstrate deodorant, wetting, detergent, keratolytic, and emulsifying activity.

Indications and Usage: ZEPHIRAN Chloride aqueous solutions in appropriate dilutions (see Recommended Dilutions) are indicated for the antisepsis of skin, mucous membranes, and wounds. They are used for preoperative preparation of the skin, surgeons' hand and arm soaks, treatment of wounds, preservation of ophthalmic solutions, irrigations of the eye, body cavities, bladder, urethra, and vaginal douching. ZEPHIRAN Chloride Tinted Tincture 1:750 and Spray are indicated for preoperative preparation of the skin and for treatment of minor skin wounds and abrasions.

Contraindication: The use of ZEPHIRAN Chloride solutions in occlusive dressings, casts, and anal or vaginal packs is inadvisable, as they may produce irritation or chemical burns.

Warnings: Sterile Water for Injection, USP, should be used as diluent in preparing diluted aqueous solutions intended for use on deep wounds or for irrigation of body cavities. Otherwise, freshly distilled water should be used. Tap water, containing metallic ions and organic matter, may reduce antibacterial potency. Resin deionized water should not be used since it may contain pathogenic bacteria.

Organic, inorganic, and synthetic materials and surfaces may adsorb sufficient quantities of ZEPHIRAN Chloride to significantly reduce its antibacterial potency in solutions. This has resulted in serious contamination of solutions of ZEPHIRAN Chloride with viable pathogenic bacteria. Solutions should not be stored in bottles stoppered with cork closures, but rather in those equipped with appropriate screw-caps. Cotton, wool, rayon, and other materials should not be stored in ZEPHIRAN Chloride solutions. Gauze sponges and fiber pledgets used to apply solutions of ZEPHIRAN Chloride to the skin should be sterilized and stored in separate containers. Only immediately prior to application should they be immersed in ZEPHIRAN Chloride solutions.

Since ZEPHIRAN Chloride solutions are inactivated by soaps and anionic detergents, thorough rinsing is necessary if these agents are employed prior to their use.

Antiseptics such as ZEPHIRAN Chloride solutions must not be relied upon to achieve complete sterilization, because they do not destroy bacterial spores and certain viruses, including the etiologic agent of infectious hepatitis, and may not destroy *Mycobacterium tuberculosis* and other rare bacterial strains.

ZEPHIRAN Chloride Tinted Tincture 1:750 and Spray contain flammable organic solvents and should not be used near an open flame or cautery.

If solutions stronger than 1:3000 enter the eyes, irrigate immediately and repeatedly with water. Prompt medical attention should then be obtained. Concentrations greater than 1:5000 should not be used on mucous membranes, with the exception of the vaginal mucosa (see Recommended Dilutions).

Precautions: In preoperative antisepsis of the skin, ZEPHIRAN Chloride solutions should not be permitted to remain in prolonged contact with the patient's skin. Avoid pooling of the solution on the operating table. ZEPHIRAN Chloride solutions that are used on inflamed or irritated tissues must be more dilute than those used on normal tissues (see Recommended Dilutions). ZEPHIRAN Chloride Tincture 1:750 and Spray, which contain irritating organic solvents, should be kept away from the eyes or other mucous membranes.

Preoperative periorbital skin or head prep should be performed only before the patient, or eye, is anesthetized.

Adverse Reactions: ZEPHIRAN chloride solutions in normally used concentrations have low systemic and local toxicity and are generally well tolerated, although a rare individual may exhibit hypersensitivity.

Directions for Use:

General: For most surgical applications, the recommended concentration of ZEPHIRAN Chloride Aqueous Solution or ZEPHIRAN Chloride Tinted Tincture is 1:750 (0.13 percent). Liberal use of the solution is recommended to compensate for any adsorption of ZEPHIRAN Chloride by cotton or other materials.

To use ZEPHIRAN Chloride Spray—Tinted Tincture 1:750, remove protective cap, hold in an UPRIGHT position several inches away from the surgical field or injured area, and apply by spraying freely.

Preoperative preparation of skin: ZEPHIRAN Chloride solutions 1:750 are recommended as an antiseptic for use on unbroken skin in the preoperative preparation of the surgical field. Detergents and soaps should be thoroughly rinsed from the skin before applying ZEPHIRAN Chloride solutions. The detergent action of ZEPHIRAN Chloride solutions, particularly when used alternately with alcohol, leaves the skin smooth and clean. When ZEPHIRAN Chloride solutions are applied by friction (using several changes of sponges), dirt, skin fats, desquamating epithelium, and superficial bacteria are effectively removed, thus exposing the underlying skin to the antiseptic activity of the solutions.

The following procedure has been found satisfactory for preparation of the surgical field. On the day prior to surgery, the operative site is shaved and then scrubbed thoroughly with ZEPHIRAN Chloride Aqueous Solution 1:750. Immedi-

ately before surgery, ZEPHIRAN Chloride Tinted Tincture 1:750 or Spray is applied to the site in the usual manner (see Precautions). If the red tinted solution turns yellow during the preparation of patient's skin for surgery, it usually indicates the presence of soap (alkali) residue which is incompatible with ZEPHIRAN solutions. Therefore, rinse thoroughly and reapply the antiseptic. Because ZEPHIRAN Chloride Tinted Tincture 1:750 contains alcohol and acetone, its cleansing action on the skin is particularly effective and it dries more rapidly than the aqueous solution. The Tinted Tincture is recommended when it is desirable to outline the operative site.

Recommended Dilutions: For specific directions, see TABLES 2 and 3.

Surgery
Preoperative preparation of skin: Aqueous solution 1:750 and Tinted Tincture 1:750 or Spray
Surgeons' hand and arm soaks: Aqueous solution 1:750
Treatment of minor wounds and lacerations: Tinted Tincture 1:750 or Spray
Irrigation of deep infected wounds: Aqueous solution 1:3000 to 1:20,000
Denuded skin and mucous membranes: Aqueous solution 1:5000 to 1:10,000

Obstetrics and Gynecology
Preoperative preparation of skin: Aqueous solution 1:750 and Tinted Tincture 1:750 or Spray
Vaginal douche and irrigation: Aqueous solution 1:2000 to 1:5000
Postepisiotomy care: Aqueous solution 1:5000 to 1:10,000
Breast and nipple hygiene: Aqueous solution 1:1000 to 1:2000

Urology
Bladder and urethral irrigation: Aqueous solution 1:5000 to 1:20,000
Bladder retention lavage: Aqueous solution 1:20,000 to 1:40,000

Dermatology
Oozing and open infections: Aqueous solution 1:2000 to 1:5000
Wet dressings by irrigation or open dressing (Use in occlusive dressings is inadvisable.): Aqueous solution 1:5000 or less

Ophthalmology
Eye irrigation: Aqueous solution 1:5000 to 1:10,000
Preservation of ophthalmic solutions: Aqueous solution 1:5000 to 1:7500
[See tables on next page].

Accidental Ingestion: If ZEPHIRAN Chloride solution, particularly a concentrated solution, is ingested, marked local irritation of the gastrointestinal tract, manifested by nausea and vomiting, may occur. Signs of systemic toxicity include restlessness, apprehension, weakness, confusion, dyspnea, cyanosis, collapse, convulsions, and coma. Death occurs as a result of paralysis of the respiratory muscles.

Treatment: Immediate administration of several glasses of a mild soap solution, milk, or egg whites beaten in water is

TABLE 2
Correct Use of ZEPHIRAN Chloride

ZEPHIRAN Chloride solutions must be prepared, stored, and used correctly to achieve and maintain their antiseptic action. Serious inactivation and contamination of ZEPHIRAN Chloride solutions may occur with misuse.

CORRECT DILUENTS	INCOMPATIBILITIES	PREFERRED FORM
Sterile Water for Injection is recommended for irrigation of body cavities.	Anionic detergents and soaps should be thoroughly rinsed from the skin or other areas prior to use of ZEPHIRAN Chloride solutions because they reduce the antibacterial activity of the solutions.	ZEPHIRAN Chloride Tinted Tincture 1:750 is recommended for preoperative skin preparation because it contains alcohol and acetone which enhance its cleansing action and promote rapid drying.

Sterile distilled water is recommended for irrigating traumatized tissue and in the eye.

Serum and protein material also decrease the activity of ZEPHIRAN Chloride solutions.

ZEPHIRAN Chloride Tinted Tincture 1:750, containing acetone, is recommended when it is desirable to outline the operative site. (Aqueous solutions of ZEPHIRAN Chloride used in skin preparation have a tendency to "run off" the skin.)

Freshly distilled water is recommended for skin antisepsis.

Resin deionized water should not be used because the deionizing resins can carry pathogens (especially gram-negative bacteria); they also inactivate quaternary ammonium compounds.

Corks should not be used to stopper bottles containing ZEPHIRAN Chloride solutions.

Caution: Because of the flammable organic solvents in ZEPHIRAN Chloride Tinted Tincture 1:750 and Spray, these products should be kept away from open flame or cautery.

Stored water is not recommended since it may contain many organisms.

Fibers of fabrics when stored in ZEPHIRAN Chloride solutions adsorb ZEPHIRAN from the surrounding liquid. Examples are:

Saline should not be used since it may decrease the antibacterial potency of ZEPHIRAN Chloride solutions.

Cotton	Gauze sponges
Wool	Rayon
	Rubber materials

Applicators or sponges, intended for a skin prep, should be stored separately and dipped in ZEPHIRAN Chloride solutions immediately before use.

Under certain circumstances the following commonly encountered substances are incompatible with ZEPHIRAN Chloride solutions:

Iodine	Aluminum
Silver nitrate	Caramel
Fluorescein	Kaolin
Nitrates	Pine oil
Peroxide	Zinc sulfate
Lanolin	Zinc oxide
Potassium permanganate	Yellow oxide of mercury

TABLE 3
Dilutions of ZEPHIRAN Chloride Aqueous Solution 1:750

Final Dilution	ZEPHIRAN Chloride Aqueous Solution 1:750 (parts)	Distilled Water (parts)
1:1000	3	1
1:2000	3	5
1:2500	3	7
1:3000	3	9
1:4000	3	13
1:5000	3	17
1:10,000	3	37
1:20,000	3	77
1:40,000	3	157

recommended. This may be followed by gastric lavage with a mild soap solution. Alcohol should be avoided as it promotes absorption.

To support respiration, the airway should be clear and oxygen should be administered, employing artificial respiration if necessary. If convulsions occur, a short-acting barbiturate may be given parenterally with caution.

How Supplied:
ZEPHIRAN Chloride Aqueous Solution 1:750
    Bottles of 8 fl oz (NDC 0024-2521-04) and 1 gallon (NDC 0024-2521-08)
ZEPHIRAN Chloride Tinted Tincture 1:750 (*flammable*)
    Bottles of 1 gallon (NDC 0024-2523-08)
ZEPHIRAN Chloride Spray—Tinted Tincture 1:750 (*flammable*)
    Bottles of 1 fl oz (NDC 0024-2527-01) and 6 fl oz (NDC 0024-2527-03)
                   ZW-83-H

This product information was effective as of January 1, 1989. Current detailed information may be obtained directly from Winthrop Pharmaceuticals, Division of Sterling Drug Inc., by writing to 90 Park Avenue, New York, NY 10016.

Products are cross-indexed by generic and chemical names in the
YELLOW SECTION

Wyeth-Ayerst Laboratories
Division of American Home Products Corporation
P.O. BOX 8299
PHILADELPHIA, PA 19101

Wyeth-Ayerst
Tamper-Resistant/Evident
Packaging

Statements alerting consumers to the specific type of Tamper-Resistant/Evident Packaging appear on the bottle labels and cartons of all Wyeth-Ayerst over-the-counter products. This includes plastic cap seals on bottles, individually wrapped tablets or suppositories, and sealed cartons. This packaging has been developed to better protect the consumer.

Continued on next page

Wyeth-Ayerst—Cont.

ALUDROX®
[al 'ū-drox]
Antacid
(alumina and magnesia)
ORAL SUSPENSION

Composition: *Suspension* —each 5 ml teaspoonful contains 307 mg aluminum hydroxide [Al(OH)$_3$] as a gel and 103 mg of magnesium hydroxide. The inactive ingredients present are artificial and natural flavors, benzoic acid, butylparaben, glycerin, hydroxypropyl methylcellulose, methylparaben, propylparaben, saccharin, simethicone, sorbitol solution, and water. Sodium content is 0.10 mEq per 5 ml suspension.

Indications: For temporary relief of heartburn, upset stomach, sour stomach, and/or acid indigestion.

Directions: *Suspension* —Two teaspoonfuls (10 ml) every 4 hours or as directed by a physician. Medication may be followed by a sip of water if desired.

Warnings: Do not take more than 12 teaspoonfuls (60 ml) of suspension in a 24-hour period or use maximum dosage for more than two weeks except under the advice and supervision of a physician. As with any drug, if you are pregnant or nursing a baby, seek the advice of a health professional before using this product.

Drug Interaction Precautions: Do not take this product if you are presently taking a prescription antibiotic drug containing any form of tetracycline.
Keep at Room Temperature, Approx. 77°F (25°C)
Suspension should be kept tightly closed and shaken well before use. Avoid freezing.
Keep this and all drugs out of the reach of children.

How Supplied: *Oral Suspension* —bottles of 12 fluidounces.
Shown in Product Identification Section, page 436

Professional Labeling: Consult 1989 Physicians' Desk Reference.

AMPHOJEL®
[am 'fo-jel]
Antacid
(aluminum hydroxide gel)
ORAL SUSPENSION • TABLETS

Composition: *Suspension* —Each 5 ml teaspoonful contains 320 mg aluminum hydroxide [Al(OH)$_3$] as a gel, and not more than 0.10 mEq of sodium. The inactive ingredients present are artificial and natural flavors, butylparaben, calcium benzoate, glycerin, hydroxypropyl methylcellulose, methylparaben, propylparaben, saccharin, simethicone, sorbitol solution, and water. *Tablets* are available in 0.3 and 0.6 g strengths. Each contains, respectively, the equivalent of 300 mg and 600 mg aluminum hydroxide as a dried gel. The 0.3 g (5 grain) tablet is equivalent to about 1 teaspoonful of the

suspension and the 0.6 g (10 grain) tablet is equivalent to about 2 teaspoonfuls. Each 0.3 g tablet contains 0.08 mEq of sodium and each 0.6 g tablet contains 0.13 mEq of sodium.

Indications: For temporary relief of heartburn, upset stomach, sour stomach, and/or acid indigestion.

Directions: *Suspension* —Two teaspoonfuls (10 ml) to be taken five or six times daily, between meals and at bedtime or as directed by a physician. Medication may be followed by a sip of water if desired. *Tablets* —Two tablets of the 0.3 g strength, or one tablet of the 0.6 g strength, five or six times daily, between meals and at bedtime or as directed by a physician. It is unnecessary to chew the 0.3 g tablet before swallowing.

Warnings: Do not take more than 12 teaspoonfuls (60 ml) of suspension, or more than twelve 0.3 g tablets, or more than six 0.6 g tablets in a 24-hour period or use this maximum dosage for more than two weeks except under the advice and supervision of a physician. May cause constipation. As with any drug, if you are pregnant or nursing a baby, seek the advice of a health professional before using this product.

Drug Interaction Precautions: Do not use this product if you are presently taking a prescription antibiotic containing any form of tetracycline.
Keep tightly closed and store at room temperature, Approx. 77°F (25°C)
Suspension should be shaken well before use. Avoid freezing.
Keep this and all drugs out of the reach of children.

How Supplied: *Suspension* —Peppermint flavored; without flavor—bottles of 12 fluidounces. *Tablets* —a convenient auxiliary dosage form—0.3 g (5 grain) bottles of 100; 0.6 g (10 grain), boxes of 100.
Shown in Product Identification Section, page 436

Professional Labeling: Consult 1989 Physicians' Desk Reference.

BASALJEL®
[bā 'sel-jel]
(basic aluminum carbonate gel)
ORAL SUSPENSION •CAPSULES
•TABLETS

Composition: *Suspension* —each 5 ml teaspoonful contains basic aluminum carbonate gel equivalent to 400 mg aluminum hydroxide [Al(OH)$_3$]. The inactive ingredients present are artificial and natural flavors, butylparaben, calcium benzoate, glycerin, hydroxypropyl methylcellulose, methylparaben, mineral oil, propylparaben, saccharin, simethicone, sorbitol solution, and water. *Capsule* contains dried basic aluminum carbonate gel equivalent to 608 mg of dried aluminum hydroxide gel or 500 mg aluminum hydroxide [Al(OH)$_3$]. The inactive ingredients present are D&C Yellow 10, FD&C Blue 1, FD&C Red 40, FD&C Yellow 6, gelatin, polacrilin potas-

sium, polyethylene glycol, talc, and titanium dioxide. *Tablet* contains dried basic aluminum carbonate gel equivalent to 608 mg of dried aluminum hydroxide gel or 500 mg aluminum hydroxide. The inactive ingredients present are cellulose, hydrogenated vegetable oil, magnesium stearate, polacrilin potassium, starch, and talc.

Indications: For the symptomatic relief of hyperacidity, associated with the diagnosis of peptic ulcer, gastritis, peptic esophagitis, gastric hyperacidity, and hiatal hernia.

Warnings: Do not take more than 24 tablets / capsules / teaspoonfuls of BASALJEL in a 24-hour period, or use this maximum dosage for more than two weeks except under the advice and supervision of a physician. Dosage should be carefully supervised since continued overdosage, in conjunction with restriction of dietary phosphorous and calcium, may produce a persistently lowered serum phosphate and a mildly elevated alkaline phosphatase. A usually transient hypercalciuria of mild degree may be associated with the early weeks of therapy. As with any drug, if you are pregnant or nursing a baby, seek the advice of a health professional before using this product.

Dosage and Administration: *Suspension* —two teaspoonfuls (10 ml) in water or fruit juice taken as often as every two hours up to twelve times daily. Two teaspoonfuls have the capacity to neutralize 23 mEq of acid. *Capsules* —two capsules as often as every two hours up to twelve times daily. Two capsules have the capacity to neutralize 24 mEq of acid. *Tablets* —two tablets as often as every two hours up to twelve times daily. Two tablets have the capacity to neutralize 25 mEq of acid. The sodium content of each dosage form is as follows: 0.13 mEq/5 ml for the suspension, 0.12 mEq per capsule, and 0.12 mEq per tablet.

Precautions: May cause constipation. Adequate fluid intake should be maintained in addition to the specific medical or surgical management indicated by the patient's condition.

Drug Interaction Precautions: Alumina-containing antacids should not be used concomitantly with any form of tetracycline therapy.

How Supplied: Suspension—bottles of 12 fluidounces.
Capsules—bottles of 100 and 500.
Tablets (scored)—bottles of 100.
Shown in Product Identification Section, page 436

Professional Labeling: Consult 1989 Physicians' Desk Reference.

CEROSE–DM®
[se-ros 'DM]
Cough/Cold Preparation with
Dextromethorphan
Sugar Free • Non-Narcotic

Description: Each teaspoonful (5 mL) contains 15 mg dextromethorphan hy-

drobromide, 4 mg chlorpheniramine maleate, and 10 mg phenylephrine hydrochloride. Alcohol 2.4%. The inactive ingredients present are artificial flavors, citric acid, edetate disodium, FD&C Yellow 6, glycerin, saccharin sodium, sodium benzoate, sodium citrate, sodium propionate, and water.

Indications: For the symptomatic control of cough due to colds.

Dosage and Administration: Adults, and children 12 years and over, one to two teaspoonfuls 4 times daily. Children over 6 years, one teaspoonful 4 times daily. Children under 6, as directed by a physician only.

Caution: Do not exceed recommended dosage. Individuals with high blood pressure, heart disease, diabetes, or thyroid disease should consult a physician before using. If there is persistent cough or high fever which may indicate a serious condition, consult your physician. Drowsiness may occur; if so, do not drive or operate machinery or do not permit hazardous childhood activities.

Warning: As with any drug, if you are pregnant or nursing a baby, seek the advice of a health professional before using this product.
Keep this and all drugs out of the reach of children. In case of accidental overdose, seek professional assistance or contact a Poison Control Center immediately.
Keep tightly closed below 77° F (25° C).

How Supplied: Cases of 12 bottles of 4 fl. oz.; bottles of 1 pint.
Shown in Product Identification Section, page 437

COLLYRIUM for FRESH EYES
[*ko-lir'e-um*]
a neutral borate solution
EYE WASH

Description: A neutral borate solution that contains boric acid, sodium borate, thimerosal (not more than 0.002% as a preservative) and water.

Indications: For soothing, refreshing, and cleansing tired or irritated eyes and for flushing or irrigating the eye to remove loose foreign material, dust, pollutants, or chlorinated water.

Directions: To open, twist off sealed, tamper resistant top and discard. Rinse eyecup with clean water immediately before and after each use. Avoid contamination of rim and inside surfaces of cup. Fill cup one-half full with Collyrium Eye Wash. Apply cup tightly to the affected eye to prevent the escape of the liquid and tilt head backward. Open eyelids wide and rotate eyeballs to thoroughly wash eye. Rinse cup with clean water after use and recap by twisting threaded eye cup on bottle.

Warnings: To avoid contamination do not touch tip of container to any surface. Replace cap after using. If you experience eye pain, changes in vision, continued redness, irritation of the eye, or if the

condition worsens or persists, consult a doctor. Not for use in open wounds in or near the eyes. Consult a doctor.
This product contains thimerosal as a preservative. Do not use this product if you are sensitive to mercury. Do not use if solution changes color or becomes cloudy, or with a wetting solution for contact lens or other eye care products containing polyvinyl alcohol.
Keep tightly closed at Room Temperature, Approx. 77°F (25°C)
Keep this and all medication out of the reach of children.

How Supplied: Bottles of 6 fl. oz. (177 ml) with eyecup.
Shown in Product Identification Section, page 437

COLLYRIUM FRESH™
[*ko-lir'e-um*]
Eye Drops with Tetrahydrozoline plus glycerin
Eye redness reliever
Eye lubricant

Collyrium Fresh contains tetrahydrozoline hydrochloride (0.05%), and glycerin (1.0%), with benzalkonium chloride (0.01%) and edetate disodium (0.1%) as preservatives, and boric acid, hydrochloric acid and sodium borate as buffering agents.

Indications: For soothing, refreshing, moisturizing and removing redness due to minor eye irritation caused by dust, smoke, smog, sun glare, wearing contact lenses, colds, allergies, swimming, reading, driving, TV or close work.

Directions: Tilt head back, and squeeze 1 to 2 drops into each eye up to four times daily, or as directed by a physician.

Warnings: To avoid contamination, do not touch tip of container to any surface. Replace cap after using. If you experience eye pain, changes in vision, continued redness or irritation of the eye, or if the condition worsens or persists for more than 72 hours, discontinue use and consult a physician. If you have glaucoma, do not use this product except under the advice and supervision of a physician.
Overuse of this product may produce increased redness of the eye. Do not use if solution changes color or becomes cloudy. Remove contact lenses before using.
Keep this and all medication out of the reach of children.
Keep bottle tightly closed at Room Temperature, Approx. 77°F (25°C).

How Supplied: Bottles of ½ fl. oz. (15 ml) with built-in eye dropper.
Shown in Product Identification Section, page 437

NURSOY®
[*nur-soy*]
Soy protein formula
READY–TO–FEED
CONCENTRATED LIQUID
POWDER

Breast milk is preferred feeding for newborns. NURSOY® milk-free formula is intended to meet the nutritional needs of infants and children who are allergic to cow's milk protein or intolerant to lactose. NURSOY Ready-to-Feed and Concentrated Liquid contain sucrose as their carbohydrate. NURSOY Powder contains corn syrup solids as its carbohydrate. Professional advice should be followed.

Ingredients: (in normal dilution supplying 20 calories per fluidounce): 87% water; 6.7% sucrose; 3.4% oleo, coconut, oleic (safflower) and soybean oils; 2.3% soy protein isolate; 0.10% potassium citrate; 0.09% monobasic sodium phosphate; 0.04% calcium carbonate; 0.04% dibasic calcium phosphate; 0.03% magnesium chloride; 0.03% calcium chloride; 0.03% soy lecithin; 0.03% calcium carrageenan; 0.03% calcium hydroxide; 0.03% l-methionine; 0.01% sodium chloride; 0.01% potassium bicarbonate; ferrous, zinc, and cupric sulfates; (68ppb) potassium iodide; ascorbic acid; choline chloride; alpha tocopheryl acetate; niacinamide; calcium pantothenate; riboflavin; vitamin A palmitate; thiamine hydrochloride; pyridoxine hydrochloride; beta-carotene; phytonadione; folic acid; biotin; activated 7-dehydrocholesterol; cyanocobalamin. NURSOY Powder contains corn syrup solids. NURSOY Ready-to-Feed and Concentrated Liquids contain sucrose.
PROXIMATE ANALYSIS
at 20 calories per fluidounce
READY-TO-FEED, CONCENTRATED LIQUID, and POWDER

	(W/V)
Protein	2.1%
Fat	3.6%
Carbohydrate	6.9%
Ash	0.35%
Water	87.0%
Crude fiber	not more than 0.01%
Calories/fl. oz.	20

Vitamins, Minerals: In normal dilution, each quart contains:

A	2,500	IU
D$_3$	400	IU
E	9	IU
K$_1$	0.1	mg
C (ascorbic acid)	55	mg
B$_1$ (thiamine)	0.67	mg
B$_2$ (riboflavin)	1	mg
B$_6$	0.4	mg
B$_{12}$	2	mcg
Niacin mg equivalents	9.5	
Pantothenic acid	3	mg
Folic acid	50	mcg
Choline	85	mg
Inositol	26	mg
Biotin	35	mcg
Calcium	600	mg
Phosphorus	420	mg
Sodium	190	mg

Continued on next page

Wyeth-Ayerst—Cont.

Potassium	700	mg
Chloride	355	mg
Magnesium	65	mg
Manganese	0.2	mg
Iron	12	mg
Copper	0.45	mg
Zinc	3.5	mg
Iodine	65	mcg

Preparation: *Ready-to-Feed* (32 fl. oz. cans of 20 calories per fluidounce formula)—shake can, open and pour into previously sterilized nursing bottle; attach nipple and feed. Cover opened can and immediately store in refrigerator. Use contents of can within 48 hours of opening.
Concentrated Liquid—For normal dilution supplying 20 calories per fluidounce, use equal amounts of NURSOY® liquid and cooled, previously boiled water. *Note: Prepared formula should be used within 24 hours.*
Powder—For normal dilution, add 1 scoop (8.9 grams or 1 standard tablespoonful) of NURSOY POWDER, packed and leveled, to 2 fluidounces of water. For larger amounts of formula add ¼ standard measuring cup of powder (35.5 grams), packed and leveled, to 8 fluidounces (1 standard measuring cup) of water.
Note: Prepared formula should be used within 24 hours.

How Supplied: *Ready-to-Feed*—presterilized and premixed, 32 fluidounce (1 quart) cans, cases of 6; *Concentrated Liquid*—13 fluidounce cans, cases of 24; *Powder*—1 pound cans, cases of 6.
Shown in Product Identification Section, page 437

RESOL®
[ree'sol]
Oral Electrolyte Rehydration and Maintenance Solution

RESOL® is intended for replacement and maintenance of water and electrolytes in diarrhea with mild to moderate dehydration. RESOL is ready to feed and presterilized, and water should not be added. Sterilized nipples should be used.

Ingredients: Water, glucose, sodium chloride, potassium citrate, citric acid, disodium phosphate, magnesium chloride, calcium chloride, and sodium citrate.
Proximate Analysis:
One fluidounce supplies about 2.5 Calories.

	mEq/liter	Approximate mEq/8 fl. oz. (237 mL)
Sodium	50	12
Potassium	20	4.7
Calcium	4	0.95
Magnesium	4	0.95
Chloride	50	12
Citrate	34	8.0
Phosphate (HPO_4^{-2})	5	1.2

	gram/liter
Glucose	20

How Supplied: Ready-to-feed—presterilized, 8 fluidounce bottles, cartons of 6 bottles (Hospital Package only); ready-to-feed—presterilized, 32 fluidounce cartons, cases of 6 cartons.
Shown in Product Identification Section, page 437

SMA®
Iron fortified
Infant formula
READY–TO–FEED
CONCENTRATED LIQUID
POWDER

Breast milk is the preferred feeding for newborns. Infant formula is intended to replace or supplement breast milk when breast feeding is not possible or is insufficient, or when mothers elect not to breast feed.
Good maternal nutrition is important for the preparation and maintenance of breast feeding. Extensive or prolonged use of partial bottle feeding, before breast feeding has been well established, could make breast feeding difficult to maintain. A decision not to breast feed could be difficult to reverse.
Professional advice should be followed on all matters of infant feeding. Infant formula should always be prepared and used as directed. Unnecessary or improper use of infant formula could present a health hazard. Social and financial implications should be considered when selecting the method of infant feeding.
SMA® is unique among prepared formulas for its fat blend, whey-dominated protein composition, amino acid pattern and mineral content. SMA, utilizing a hybridized safflower (oleic) oil, became the first infant formula offering fat and calcium absorption equal to that of human milk, with a physiologic level of linoleic acid. Thus, the fat blend in SMA provides a ready source of energy, helps protect infants against neonatal tetany and produces a ratio of vitamin E to polyunsaturated fatty acids (linoleic acid) more than adequate to prevent hemolytic anemia.
By combining reduced minerals whey with skimmed cow's milk, SMA adjusts the protein content to within the range of human milk, reverses the whey-protein to casein ratio of cow's milk so that it is like that of human milk, and reduces the mineral content to a physiologic level.
The resultant 60:40 whey-protein to casein ratio provides protein nutrition superior to a casein-dominated formula. In addition, the essential amino acids, including cystine, are present in amounts close to those of human milk. So the protein in SMA is of high biologic value.
The physiologic mineral content makes possible a low renal solute load which helps protect the functionally immature infant kidney, increases expendable water reserves and helps protect against dehydration.

Use of lactose as the carbohydrate results in a physiologic stool flora and a low stool pH, decreasing the incidence of perianal dermatitis.

Ingredients: SMA® Concentrated Liquid or Ready-to-Feed. Water; nonfat milk; reduced minerals whey; lactose; oleo, coconut, oleic (safflower), and soybean oils; soy lecithin; calcium carrageenan. *Minerals:* Potassium bicarbonate; calcium chloride and citrate; potassium chloride; sodium citrate; ferrous sulfate, sodium bicarbonate; zinc, cupric, and manganese sulfates. *Vitamins:* Ascorbic acid, alpha tocopheryl acetate, niacinamide, vitamin A palmitate, calcium pantothenate, thiamine hydrochloride, riboflavin, pyridoxine hydrochloride, beta-carotene, folic acid, phytonadione, activated 7-dehydrocholesterol, biotin, cyanocobalamin.
SMA® Powder. Nonfat milk; reduced minerals whey; lactose; oleo, coconut, oleic (safflower), and soybean oils; soy lecithin.
Minerals: Calcium chloride; sodium bicarbonate; calcium hydroxide; ferrous sulfate; potassium hydroxide and bicarbonate; potassium chloride; zinc, cupric, and manganese sulfates.
Vitamins: Ascorbic acid, alpha tocopheryl acetate, niacinamide, vitamin A palmitate, calcium pantothenate, thiamine hydrochloride, riboflavin, pyridoxine hydrochloride, beta-carotene, folic acid, phytonadione, activated 7-dehydrocholesterol, biotin, cyanocobalamin.

PROXIMATE ANALYSIS
at 20 calories per fluidounce
READY-TO-FEED, POWDER, and CONCENTRATED LIQUID:

	(w/v)
Fat	3.6%
Carbohydrate	7.2%
Protein	1.5%
60% Lactalbumin (whey protein)	0.9%
40% Casein	0.6%
Ash	0.25%
Crude Fiber	None
Total Solids	12.6%
Calories/fl. oz.	20

Vitamins, Minerals: In normal dilution each quart contains 2500 IU vitamin A, 400 IU vitamin D_3, 9 IU vitamin E, 55 mcg vitamin K_1, 0.67 mg vitamin B_1(thiamine), 1 mg vitamin B_2(riboflavin), 55 mg vitamin C (ascorbic acid), 0.4 mg vitamin B_6(pyridoxine hydrochloride), 1 mcg vitamin B_{12}, 9.5 mg equivalents niacin, 2 mg pantothenic acid, 50 mcg folic acid, 14 mcg biotin, 100 mg choline, 420 mg calcium, 312 mg phosphorus, 50 mg magnesium, 142 mg sodium, 530 mg potassium, 355 mg chloride, 12 mg iron, 0.45 mg copper, 3.5 mg zinc, 150 mcg manganese, 65 mcg iodine.

Preparation: *Ready-to-Feed* (8 and 32 fl. oz. cans of 20 calories per fluidounce formula)—shake can, open and pour into previously sterilized nursing bottle; attach nipple and feed. Cover opened can and immediately store in refrigerator. Use contents of can within 48 hours of opening.

Powder —(1 pound can)—For normal dilution supplying 20 calories per fluidounce, use 1 scoop (or 1 standard tablespoonful) of powder, packed and leveled, to 2 fluidounces of cooled, previously boiled water. For larger amount of formula, use ¼ standard measuring cup of powder, packed and leveled, to 8 fluidounces (1 cup) of water. Three of these portions make 26 fluidounces of formula. *Concentrated Liquid* —For normal dilution supplying 20 calories per fluidounce, use equal amounts of SMA® liquid and cooled, previously boiled water.
Note: Prepared formula should be used within 24 hours.

How Supplied: *Ready-to-Feed* —presterilized and premixed, 32 fluidounce (1 quart) cans, cases of 6; 8 fluidounce cans, cases of 24 (4 carriers of 6 cans). *Powder* —1 pound can with measuring scoop, cases of 6. *Concentrated Liquid* —13 fluidounce cans, cases of 24.
Also Available: SMA® lo-iron. For those who appreciate the particular advantages of SMA®, the infant formula closest in composition nutritionally to mother's milk, but who sometimes need or wish to recommend a formula that does not contain a high level of iron, there is SMA® lo-iron with all the benefits of regular SMA® but with a reduced level of iron of 1.4 mg per quart. Infants should receive supplemental dietary iron from an outside source to meet daily requirements.
Concentrated Liquid —13 fl. oz. cans, cases of 24. *Powder* —1 pound cans with measuring scoop, cases of 6. *Ready-to-feed* —32 fl. oz. cans, cases of 6.
Preparation of the standard 20 calories per fluidounce formula of SMA® lo-iron is the same as SMA® iron fortified given above.
Shown in Product Identification Section, page 437

WYANOIDS® Relief Factor
[wi 'a-noids]
Hemorrhoidal Suppositories

Description: Active ingredients: Live Yeast Cell Derivative, Supplying 2,000 units Skin Respiratory Factor Per Ounce of Cocoa Butter Suppository Base and Shark Liver Oil 3%. Inactive Ingredients: Beeswax, Glycerin, Phenylmercuric Nitrate 1:10,000 (as a preservative), Polyethylene Glycol 600 Dilaurate.

Indications: To help shrink swelling of hemorrhoidal tissues and provide prompt, temporary relief from pain and itching.

Usual Dosage: Use one suppository up to five times daily, especially in the morning, at night, and after bowel movements, or as directed by a physician.

Directions: Remove wrapper and insert one suppository rectally using gentle pressure. Frequent application and lubrication with Wyanoids® Relief Factor provide continual therapy which will lead to more rapid improvement of rectal conditions.

Caution: In case of bleeding or if the condition persists, the patient should consult a physician. Keep this and all medicines out of the reach of children. Do not store above 80°F.

How Supplied: Boxes of 12 and 24.
Shown in Product Identification Section, page 437

Zila Pharmaceuticals, Inc.
777 EAST THOMAS ROAD
PHOENIX, AZ 85014

ZILACTIN® Medicated Gel
[zī-lăc-tĭn]

Description: ZILACTIN® is a patent protected,* film forming, Medicated Gel for topical administration. Its active ingredient is tannic acid (7%) suspended in SD alcohol 37 (80.8% by volume).

Indications and Usage: ZILACTIN® Medicated Gel is for use in the fast relief of the pain, itching or burning of inside the mouth ulcers (canker sores) as well as fever blisters and cold sores on or around the lips. Clinical studies have demonstrated that when properly applied, ZILACTIN forms a smooth, comfortable and very tenacious film. Even inside the mouth on canker sores, mucosal abrasions from dental procedures, braces, dentures and other appliances, etc., a single application can last up to six or more hours. During this time, ZILACTIN gives lasting protection and pain relief as it holds the medication in place to speed healing. Inside the mouth, the film is opaque white; outside the mouth on fever blisters and cold sores, it is transparent. At first symptoms, ZILACTIN should be applied four (4) times a day for the first two (2) days. The affected area should be dried with a clean tissue, cotton swab or gauze pad and a thin layer of ZILACTIN applied. The gel should be allowed to air dry as the film forms within sixty (60) seconds. When applied inside the mouth, the film will normally withstand eating and drinking as it prevents saliva, food particles and drink from coming in contact with the sore. Even citrus beverages may be consumed without difficulty.

Precautions: A slight, but temporary, burning sensation may be experienced when applying ZILACTIN® to an open sore or blister.
If infection persists beyond ten days, discontinue use and consult your physician. Keep all medications out of children's reach.

DO NOT USE IN OR AROUND EYES
In the event of accidental contact with eye tissues, flush immediately and continuously with clear water for 10 minutes. Seek immediate medical attention if pain or irritation persists.

Professional Labeling: Same.

How Supplied: ZILACTIN® Medicated Gel is available in .25 oz. (7.1 grams) tube (NDC #51284-468-02) and in 1.0 gram foil "Medipack", for professional use (NDC #51284-468-04).
*U.S. patent numbers 4,285,934 and 4,381,296

Distributed by:
ZILA Pharmaceuticals, Inc.
Phoenix, AZ 85014
Shown in Product Identification Section, page 437

Diagnostics Devices and Medical Aids

This section is intended to present product information on Diagnostics, Devices and Medical Aids designed for home use by patients. The information concerning each product has been prepared, edited and approved by the manufacturer.

The Publisher has emphasized to manufacturers the necessity of describing products comprehensively so that all information essential for intelligent and informed use is available. In organizing and presenting the material in this edition the Publisher is providing all the information made available by manufacturers.

In presenting the following material to the medical profession, the Publisher is not necessarily advocating the use of any product.

Boehringer Mannheim Diagnostics
Division of Boehringer Mannheim Corp.
**9115 HAGUE ROAD
INDIANAPOLIS, IN 46250**

ACCU–CHEK® II
BLOOD GLUCOSE MONITOR

The Accu-Chek® II Blood Glucose Monitor, Cat.No.792, is the one recommended by 8 out of 10 doctors who specialize in treating people with diabetes.[1] It uses dual optics and specific programming for fine tuned accuracy: the only system that is F.D.A. cleared for use in the neonatal clinical setting.[2]
This monitor uses the #1 selling Chemstrip bG® Test Strips[3], which can also be read visually.
[See table below].

1. Reference on file: Boehringer Mannheim Diagnostics.
2. As of March, 1987.
3. Open-Call Survey, *Am Druggist*, Sept. 1987, p. 146.

ACCU–CHEK® II
DIABETES CARE KIT

Accu-Chek II Diabetes Care Kit, Cat. No.794, is the easy, economical way to be outfitted for self blood glucose testing. This complete kit contains: monitor, Chemstrip bG® Test Strips, Soft Touch™ Lancet Device, Glucose Control Solutions, Supply Case, Training Tape, Lancets, and cotton balls.

TRACER™ II
BLOOD GLUCOSE MONITOR

Tracer™ II Blood Glucose Monitor, Cat.No.780, is the latest addition to the B.M.D. family of monitors. Accurate, reliable, and affordable, this monitor uses Tracer bG™ Test Strips, Cat.No.00535. These smaller strips utilize the superior chemistry of Chemstrip bG Strips, but need even less blood.

EDUCATIONAL MATERIAL

Meal Planner
A simple dietary planner which uses exchange lists and selects portion sizes based upon the caloric allowance of one's diet.

Talking About Diabetes
A general discussion of diabetes, including current management techniques of the 1980's.

Lavoptik Company, Inc.
**661 WESTERN AVENUE N.
ST. PAUL, MN 55103**

LAVOPTIK® Eye Cups

Description: Device—Sterile disposable eyecups.

How Supplied: Individually bagged eyecups are packed 12 per box, NDC 10651-01004.

Ortho Pharmaceutical Corporation
**Advanced Care Products Division
RARITAN, NJ 08869**

ADVANCE®
Pregnancy Test

Active Ingredients: Human Chorionic Gonadotropin (HCG) alpha chain specific monoclonal antibody HCG, beta-chain specific antibody/enzyme conjugate, chromogenic substrate solution, and buffer solution.
Indications: An in-vitro pregnancy test for use in the home that can detect the presence of HCG in the urine as early as one (1) day past last missed period.
Actions: ADVANCE will accurately detect the presence or absence of HCG in urine in just thirty minutes. It is as accurate as pregnancy test methods used in many hospitals.
Dosage and Administration: Perform the test according to instructions. If, after thirty minutes, a blue color appears on the rounded end of the COLORSTICK, the patient can assume she is pregnant. If the rounded end of the COLORSTICK remains white, and no blue color can be seen, no pregnancy hormone has been detected and the patient is probably not pregnant. The test results may be affected by certain health conditions such as an ovarian cyst or ectopic pregnancy and by certain medications such as thiazide diuretics, plurothiazine, hormones, steroids, chemotherapeutics, and thyroid drugs. For additional reassurance, a toll-free telephone number is included in each package insert. This service is staffed by Registered Nurses who can answer any questions the patient may have about her results, or how she performed the test.
How Supplied: Each ADVANCE test contains a plastic COLORSTICK, a plastic vial containing buffer solution, a glass tube containing dried test chemicals, a glass tube containing color developing

solution, a test stand with urine collection and instructions for use.

Storage: Store at room temperature (59°–86°F). Do not freeze.
Shown in Product Identification Section, page 417

DAISY 2®
Pregnancy Test

Active Ingredients: Human Chorionic Gonadotropin (HCG) alpha chain specific monoclonal antibody HCG, beta chain specific antibody/enzyme conjugate, chromogenic substrate solution, and buffer solution.

Indications: An in-vitro pregnancy test for use in the home that can detect the presence of HCG in the urine as early as one (1) day after a missed period.

Actions: DAISY 2 will accurately check the presence or absence of HCG in urine in just thirty minutes. It is as accurate as pregnancy testing methods used in many hospitals.

Dosage and Administration: Perform the test according to instructions. If, after thity minutes, a blue color appears on the rounded end of the COLORSTICK, the patient can assume she is pregnant. If the rounded end of the COLORSTICK remains white, and no blue color can be seen, no pregnancy hormone has been detected and the patient is probably not pregnant. All home pregnancy test kits recommend a second test if the first test indicates that the patient is not pregnant and her period does not begin within a week. This second test may be needed because the patient may have miscalculated her period, or her body may not have accumulated enough hormone for a true reading. Many women like the reassurance that comes from double-checking the results. DAISY 2 makes this double checking easy and convenient by providing two complete and identical tests in each kit. For additional reassurance a toll-free telephone number is included in each package insert. This service is staffed by Registered Nurses who can answer any questions the patient may have about her results, or how she performed the test. The test results may be affected by certain health conditions such as a ovarian cyst or ectopic pregnancy and certain medications such as thiazide diuretics, plurothiazine, hormones, steroids, chemotherapeutics, and thyroid drugs.

How Supplied: Each DAISY 2 kit contains everything needed to perform two tests, two plastic COLORSTICKS, two plastic vials containing buffer solution, two glass tubes containing dried test chemicals, two glass tubes containing color developing solution, a test stand, two urine collection cups and instructions for use.

Storage: Store at room temperature (59–86°F). Do not Freeze.
Shown in Product Identification Section, page 417

Test Strip Size/ Cat.No.	Visual	Accu- Chek bG®	Accu- Chek® II
Chemstrip bG® 25 00501	•		
Chemstrip bG® 50 00502	•		•
Chemstrip bG® 50 00503	•	•	
Chemstrip bG® 100 00508	•		

FACT PLUS™
Pregnancy Test

Active Ingredients: Human Chorionic Gonadotropin (HCG) antibody, HCG antibody/enzyme conjugate, and chromogenic substrate solution.

Indications: An in-vitro pregnancy test for use in the home that can detect the presence of HCG in the urine as early as the first day of a missed period.

Actions: FACT PLUS will accurately detect the presence or absence of HCG in urine in just 5–8 minutes. It is the same pregnancy test method used in many hospitals.

Dosage and Administration: Perform the test according to instructions. If, after 5–8 minutes, a plus (+) sign has formed in the center of the test cube, the patient is probably pregnant. If a minus (−) sign appears, no pregnancy hormone has been detected and the patient is probably not pregnant. In the unlikely event that neither sign appears the test system has not worked properly and the patient should call the toll free number included in each package insert. This toll free number is staffed by Registered Nurses who can answer any questions the patient may have about her results, or how she performed the test. The test results may be affected by various other factors and medications such as thiazide diuretics, plurothiazine, hormones, steroids, chemotherapeutics, and thyroid drugs.

How Supplied: Each FACT PLUS kit contains a plastic test cube, a glass tube containing dried test chemicals, a plastic vial containing color developing solution, a test stand with a urine collection cup and urine dropper, a test stand with urine collector and complete instructions for use.

Storage: Store at room temperature (59–86°F). Do not freeze.

Shown in Product Identification Section, page 417

Parke-Davis
Consumer Health Products Group
Division of Warner-Lambert Company
201 TABOR ROAD
MORRIS PLAINS, NJ 07950

e·p·t® plus™
Early Pregnancy Test

- Results as early as one day after missed period.
- Simple color change test.
- Easy to perform—just one chemical step.
- Proven 99% accurate in laboratory tests.

How EPT PLUS works

When you're pregnant, you produce a hormone called HCG—(Human Chorionic Gonadotropin), which is found in your urine. EPT PLUS detects the presence of this pregnancy hormone in your urine. When you perform the test, a color change in the test tube shows you whether the hormone is there. **Any color change** from the initial purplish red color means you are pregnant and should therefore see your doctor. No color change means you are not pregnant.

When to use EPT PLUS

When a woman becomes pregnant a special hormone begins to be produced and will appear in her urine. EPT PLUS measures whether this hormone is present or not. If you **are** pregnant, this hormone usually reaches a level which EPT PLUS can detect one day after a missed period. In some cases, however, detectable levels may not be reached until several days later. EPT PLUS can be used one day after a missed period as well as any day thereafter.

EPT PLUS can tell you if you are pregnant in as fast as 10 minutes. To verify negative results the test should be rechecked at 30 minutes. During this time, you can carry the test tube with you since EPT PLUS is completely portable, and movement will not affect the test. Any color change during this 30 minute period indicates a positive result.

Use only the first morning urine

Use only your first urine of the morning. This is because the pregnancy hormone is most concentrated in the first urine specimen of the day. You should collect it in the clear plastic lid that covers the test kit. Be sure to rinse the lid thoroughly in clear tap water before you deposit the urine in it.

You will need only a few minutes to set up the test. If you do not have time to do the test the first thing in the morning, you can cover and store your first morning urine specimen in the refrigerator. However, be sure to do the test the same day the urine was collected. Let the urine warm to room temperature before testing.

(**Note:** After your urine has been stored for several hours a sediment may form at the bottom of the container. DO NOT mix or shake the urine. Use only the urine at the top of the container.)

The EPT PLUS Test Kit

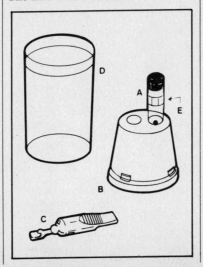

A. **Glass test tube** with rubber stopper,* which contains the special test chemicals. Leave stopper in place until you perform the test.
B. **Test holder.**
C. **Plastic vial,*** which contains the proper amount of buffer solution.
D. **Plastic lid.** Use this to collect and hold the urine for the test.
E. **Test result illustrations,** for easy reading of test results.
*Double Kit contains two.

EPT PLUS is simple to perform

Before you start, read all the directions and recommendations carefully. Remove the rubber stopper from the glass test tube (A) and save it for later. Hold up the plastic vial (C) to be sure that no liquid is in the neck of the vial. Twist the top off and squeeze out entire contents into the glass test tube (A).

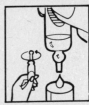

Now fill the empty plastic vial (C) with urine as you would with a medicine dropper.

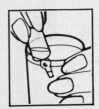

Carefully squeeze 3 drops of urine into the test tube (A).

Put the rubber stopper back on the test tube (A) and shake the tube gently to mix the contents. **Please note the color of the liquid in the tube.** In most cases, the liquid will be a deep purplish red color, however the exact shade will vary among women.

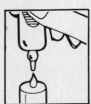

If the result is positive, the color change can begin to show as early as 10 minutes. If there is **any** change from the original purplish red color this indicates a positive result. If the solution has not changed within that time, check the solution again at 30 minutes. (If necessary, you may carry the test tube with you.) If there is still no color change the test result is negative. Any color change during

Continued on next page

Parke-Davis—Cont.

this 30 minute period indicates a positive result.

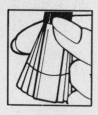

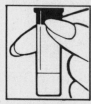

NEGATIVE (−)

If there is no color change, this means that no pregnancy hormone has been detected in your urine and you are probably not pregnant. In the unlikely event that a week passes and you still have not menstruated, you may have miscalculated your period, or the test might have been performed incorrectly. In this case, you should perform another test using a new EPT PLUS kit. If the second test still gives you a negative result—and you still have not menstruated—there could be other important reasons why your period has not begun and you should see your physician. Among other conditions, this could be a sign of ectopic pregnancy, which, unlike a usual pregnancy, is one in which the fertilized egg is implanted in a position other than the uterus (such as in the Fallopian tube). This requires immediate medical supervision.

POSITIVE (+)

If the liquid **clearly does** change color (as indicated in the color swatch shown below on right), your urine does contain the pregnancy hormone, and you can assume you are pregnant.

You should now plan to consult your physician, who is best able to advise you. (In certain rare cases HCG levels may be elevated even though you are not pregnant. Your physician can determine this. Also, use of oral contraceptives should not affect test results.)

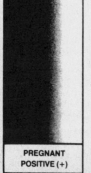

NOT PREGNANT NEGATIVE (−)	PREGNANT POSITIVE (+)

EPT PLUS accuracy

EPT PLUS is 99% accurate in laboratory tests.

EPT PLUS is as accurate as leading hospital and lab urine tests, so you can trust the result.

INGREDIENTS*

Each test kit contains:
1. Gold sol particles coated with monoclonal HCG antibodies.
2. A special aqueous buffer solution.

*Not to be taken internally.
For in-vitro diagnostic use.
Store at 59°–86°F

Questions about EPT PLUS?

CALL US TOLL FREE. . . 8 AM TO 5 PM EST
WEEKDAYS AT 1-800-562-0266.
IN NEW JERSEY, CALL COLLECT AT (201) 540-2458.
Registered Nurses are available to answer your calls.

Shown in Product Identification Section, page 419

e·p·t® STICK TEST
Early Pregnancy Test

- **Results as early as one day after missed period.**
- **Easy to perform—one chemical step.**
- **Easy to read—a pink color at the end of the test stick signals a positive result.**
- **Proven 99% accurate in laboratory tests.**

EPT STICK PREGNANCY TEST

The ept stick test uses advanced technology to make home pregnancy testing simple and gives a clear and highly accurate result. The key element of this test is a stick which changes color to indicate pregnancy. Any shade of pink that appears on the tip of the stick and remains after rinsing, indicates that you are pregnant.

HOW EPT STICK WORKS

When a woman becomes pregnant, her body produces a special hormone known as HCG (Human Chorionic Gonadotropin), which appears in the urine. The ept stick test can detect this hormone as early as the first day after a missed period.

If you obtain a positive result, you can assume you are pregnant and should see your doctor. A negative result means that no HCG has been detected and you can assume you are not pregnant.

WHEN TO USE THE EPT STICK TEST

The ept stick test can detect HCG hormone levels in your urine as early as one day after a missed period. In some cases, however, detectable levels may not be reached until several days later. The ept stick test can be used one day after a missed period as well as any date thereafter.

BEFORE YOU BEGIN:

- Read through this entire pamphlet carefully.

- If you have any questions, call the toll free number provided on the back page of this pamphlet. Registered Nurses are available to answer your questions.

THE EPT STICK PREGNANCY TEST KIT

A. **Glass test tube** with rubber stopper, which contains the special test chemicals. Leave stopper in place until you perform the test.
B. **Test holder.**
C. **Plastic vial,** which contains the proper amount of buffer solution.
D. **Plastic lid.** Use this to collect and hold the urine for the test.
E. **White pouch** containing the test stick with one end coated with test chemicals.

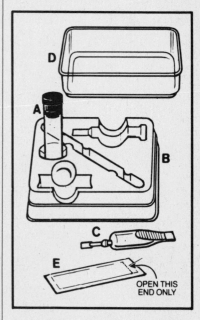

The ept stick test is easy to perform, simply follow the pictures as indicated. (Starting below)

Urine collection

Use only first morning urine to conduct this test. Why? Because if you are pregnant, the pregnancy hormone is most concentrated in the first urine specimen of the day. You should collect it in the clear plastic lid that covers the test kit (D). Be sure to rinse the lid thoroughly in clear tap water before you deposit the urine in it. If you do not have enough time to do the test the first thing in the morning, you can cover and store your first morning urine specimen in the refrigerator. However, be sure to do the test the same day the urine was collected. Let the urine warm to room temperature before testing.

(**NOTE:** *After your urine has been stored for several hours, a sediment may form at the bottom of the container. DO NOT mix or shake the urine. Use only the urine at the top of the container.*)

Remove the rubber stopper from the glass test tube (A) and save it for later.

Hold up the plastic vial (C) to be sure that no liquid is in the neck of the vial. Twist the top off and squeeze out entire contents into the glass test tube (A).

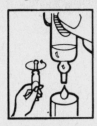

Now fill the empty plastic vial (C) with urine as you would with a medicine dropper.

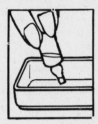

Carefully squeeze 5 drops of urine into the test tube (A).

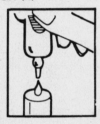

Put the rubber stopper back on the test tube (A) and shake the tube gently to mix the contents. Put the test tube back in the stand and remove the stopper.

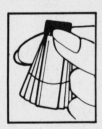

Remove the test stick from the white pouch (E) by tearing along **the line indicated**. Take out the stick handling it **only** by the thicker end. **DO NOT TOUCH THE OTHER THINNER END OF THE STICK AS THIS MAY VOID THE TEST.**

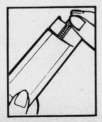

Put the test stick in the test tube (A) with the coated thinner end in the liquid. Leave the test stick in the test tube for 10 minutes.

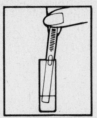

Turn on the **cold water** faucet and allow water to run gently until water is cool. Holding the thick end of the test stick, remove it from glass tube (A). Rinse both sides of the stick under **cool, gently flowing** tap water for a slow count of 3.

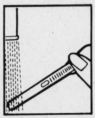

Reading your test results

If the tip of the test stick has turned any shade of *pink*, this is a positive result. You can assume you are pregnant and should consult your doctor.

If the tip of the stick is still white, and no pink color can be seen, this signals a negative result. To verify negative results, replace the test stick into the test tube and wait another 20 minutes. Remove and rinse again with tap water. If it is still white, you are probably not pregnant. If there is any shade of pink on the tip of the stick at this point it is a positive result.

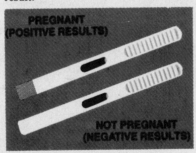

PREGNANT (POSITIVE RESULTS)

NOT PREGNANT (NEGATIVE RESULTS)

EPT STICK ACCURACY

Although the ept stick test is proven 99% accurate in laboratory tests, a low incidence of false results (positive when no pregnancy exists or negative when pregnancy is present) can occur. Check with your doctor if you get unexpected or inconsistent test results. Certain health conditions such an ovarian cyst or an ectopic pregnancy (a pregnancy outside the uterus) can cause a false or irregular result with your test.

INGREDIENTS*

Each test kit contains:

1. Gold sol particles coated with monoclonal HCG antibodies.
2. A special aqueous buffer solution.
3. Test stick coated with monoclonal antibodies.

*Not to be taken internally. For in-vitro diagnostic use.

Store at 59°–86°F.

Marketed by
PARKE-DAVIS Consumer Health Products Division
Warner-Lambert Co., Morris Plains, NJ 07950 USA

Shown in Product Identification Section, page 419

Tambrands Inc.
LAKE SUCCESS, NY 11042

FIRST RESPONSE®
Home Diagnostic Test Kits
Ovulation Predictor Test
(New 10 Minute Test Available Early 1989)

Description: This accurate, easy-to-perform and easy-to-read home ovulation predictor test gives a "Yes" or "No" result in just 10 minutes. It will help a woman find the time in her monthly cycle that she is most able to become pregnant, and it can also help her plan the timing of her pregnancy. She can do the test at home and get her results in just 10 minutes. The Test is easy to read since she simply compares her result to a furnished reference color—no need for day-to-day color comparisons.

How the test works: The test measures luteinizing hormone (LH), which is always present in urine, but increases on the most fertile day of a woman's cycle. This increase or "surge" in LH triggers ovulation. FIRST RESPONSE® detects this LH surge via a simple-to-read color change. Unlike other home ovulation tests, FIRST RESPONSE® does not require day-to-day color comparisons since the FIRST RESPONSE® result is simply compared to a furnished reference color. If the test result is equal to or darker than the reference color, a woman knows she is about to ovulate. Most women will ovulate within 12 to 24 hours after the surge. Predicting ovulation in advance is important because the egg can only be fertilized for up to 24 hours after ovulation. Therefore, a woman is most likely to become pregnant if she has intercourse within 24 hours of her surge.

How Supplied: The new FIRST RESPONSE® Ovulation Predictor Test contains all the materials needed for 5 days of testing, which is enough to detect

Continued on next page

Tambrands—Cont.

the hormone surge for about two-thirds of ovulating women. However, since menstrual cycles can be irregular, approximately one-third of the women may need to continue testing with a 3-day refill kit. When a woman detects her surge, she may stop testing and save any unused tests to use the following month, if she does not become pregnant.

Instructions for use: The package contains simple, easy-to-follow, illustrated directions on how to perform the test. If there are any questions, a member of the FIRST RESPONSE® medical information staff is available to answer them at 1-800-523-0014, Monday through Friday, from 7 AM to 5 PM Eastern Time.

Shown in Product Identification Section, page 432

Professional Labeling
FIRST RESPONSE®
Home Diagnostic Test Kits
Pregnancy Test

Description: FIRST RESPONSE® Pregnancy Test gives a "yes" or "no" result in only 5 minutes. FIRST RESPONSE® is easy to use and takes only a few simple steps. In just 5 minutes it turns pink for pregnant; it stays white if not pregnant. FIRST RESPONSE® is so sensitive it can be used the first day a woman misses her period. No other home pregnancy test can be used earlier. And a woman can test any time of day.

FIRST RESPONSE® Pregnancy Test is available in both single and double test kits.

How the test works: If conception occurs, a woman's body begins to produce the pregnancy hormone hCG (human chorionic gonadotropin). The FIRST RESPONSE® Pregnancy Test detects this hormone in a woman's urine. The test gives a pink color result if hCG is present in the urine. If no hCG has been detected, FIRST RESPONSE® gives a white color result, indicating that the woman is not pregnant. However, if a woman does not have her period within a few days, the test should be repeated. This is because she may have ovulated and conceived late in her cycle, resulting in a slower buildup of hCG. Also, it is possible that she may have miscalculated the day her period was due. If the result is negative in the second test and her period does not start within a week, she should consult a doctor.

Instructions for use: The package insert contains simple easy-to-follow, illustrated directions on how to perform the test. If there are any questions or additional information is needed, please call 1-800-523-0014.
FIRST RESPONSE® Pregnancy Test and Ovulation Predictor Test are manufactured exclusively for and distributed by Tambrands Inc., Lake Success, NY 11042. FIRST RESPONSE is a registered trademark of Tambrands® Inc. © 1989 Tambrands, Inc.

Shown in Product Identification Section, page 432

EDUCATIONAL MATERIAL

Health Information Series #2
Patient/Consumer Pamphlets:
Ovulation Prediction
Detecting Pregnancy
Free to Pharmacists, Physicians and Consumers (patients).

Warner-Lambert Company
Consumer Health Products Group
201 TABOR ROAD
MORRIS PLAINS, NJ 07950

EARLY DETECTOR™
In-Home Test for the Detection of Hidden Blood in the Stool

Description: Early Detector is an *in-vitro* diagnostic test to detect hidden blood in the stool.

Indications: There is uniform medical agreement that the earlier colorectal cancer is diagnosed and appropriate treatment instituted, the more favorable the disease prognosis. Among the early warning signs, rectal bleeding is considered the most significant symptom. The primary at-risk groups include people over the age of 40, plus those with a family history of colorectal cancer, or the presence, or family history of familial polyposis of the colon.
In-home tests such as Early Detector are considered one of the most effective methods for large-scale screening.

Actions: Early Detector is a gum guaiac based, *in-vitro* diagnostic kit that tests for occult blood in three successive bowel movements. The procedure is simple, more acceptable to patients, and easy to perform in the privacy of the home.

Directions for Use: Complete, illustrated, easy-to-follow directions are included with each test. People who are actively bleeding from other conditions such as hemorrhoids or menstruation should not take the test. Some medications such as aspirin, iron supplements, vitamin C (over 250 mg. per day), rectal ointments, and anti-inflammatory drugs can cause an error in results. For two days before and throughout the test period, patients should avoid red or rare meat, turnips, horseradish and vitamin C supplements in their diets.

How Supplied: The Early Detector In-Home Test contains 3 specimen pads with Activity Indicator® test verification spots, developer solution, a packet containing a developer tablet and an instruction booklet.

Early Detector
The Early Detector in-home test finds hidden blood in the stool. The test is fast, painless, and simple. Blood in the stool can be a sign of a number of conditions. Some of these are ulcers, diverticulosis, hemorrhoids and cancer of the colon and rectum. Early Detector can alert you and your doctor to conditions which may require medical help. Read all the instructions before you perform the test. Follow the step-by-step guide with care to get accurate results.

Why should I use Early Detector?
Blood in the stool can be a sign of various conditions, including ulcers, diverticulosis, hemorrhoids and cancer of the colon and rectum. But you may not be aware of this blood. Therefore, you may not seek

Warner-Lambert

Familiarize yourself with the Early Detector test kit

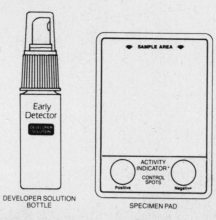

DEVELOPER SOLUTION BOTTLE　　　　SPECIMEN PAD

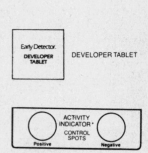

Positive Activity Indicator ® will turn blue after you spray with developer solution.
Negative Activity Indicator will not change color.

the medical treatment you may need. Now there's Early Detector. The Early Detector Test is a fast, painless, and simple method of finding hidden blood in the stool. The Early Detector Test can be done in the privacy of your own home. There is nothing to mail in. You perform the test. You read the results.

How does Early Detector work?

Early Detector is a simple version of a standard laboratory test for hidden blood in the stool. The test is easy to do. After a bowel movement, you use a specimen pad to pat the anal area to get a stool specimen. The Early Detector Developer Solution is applied to the stool specimen. A chemical reaction will take place between the solution and stool specimen. If there is hidden blood in the stool, the area around the specimen will turn blue.

How often should I use Early Detector?

After age 40, when colorectal disease is most prevalent, annual screening for hidden blood in the stool with Early Detector is advisable. However, people who have a medical history of hidden blood in the stool or have a family history of gastrointestinal medical disorders should perform the test more often. The ease and convenience of Early Detector allows for more frequent and convenient screening.

What chemicals are found in Early Detector?

The final prepared Developer Solution has a stable mixture of hydrogen peroxide, gum guaiac, and denatured ethyl alcohol in water.

Each specimen pad has a positive Activity Indicator® which contains hematin, a chemical which when sprayed with Developer Solution will turn blue.

What are the precautions I should take?

The chemicals in Early Detector are not for internal use. Early Detector is made for outside the body use (**FOR IN VITRO DIAGNOSTIC USE**). Do not eat or drink this test.

Use the developer solution within two months after adding the tablet. (Record Date on Page 13).

EARLY DETECTOR DEVELOPER SOLUTION MAY BE IRRITATING. DO NOT GET IN EYES. IF CONTACT OCCURS, FLUSH PROMPTLY WITH WATER.

Keep the Early Detector Developer Solution away from heat and light. Keep the bottle tightly capped when not in use. CAUTION: FLAMMABLE. DO NOT USE NEAR OPEN FLAME. KEEP OUT OF REACH OF CHILDREN.

How should Early Detector be stored?

Store at room temperature (59°F–86°F)—do not refrigerate. Keep away from light and heat. Protect from direct sunlight. Keep developer solution tightly capped when not in use. Your Early Detector Test has:

3 Individually wrapped Specimen Pads with Activity Indicator®
1 Bottle Developer Solution
1 Packet Containing Developer Tablet
1 Instruction Booklet With Photographs.

How do I prepare myself to use the Early Detector Test Kit?

● Do not perform the test if you are actively bleeding from other conditions that may show up in the stool specimen. Some conditions are hemorrhoids or menstrual bleeding.

● **INTERFERING SUBSTANCES**

Some medicines such as aspirin, iron supplements and anti-inflammatory drugs for arthritis may cause the test to turn blue, even when blood due to a medical problem is not present in the stool (false positive result). Vitamin C (over 250 mg. daily) may prevent blood which may be present in the stool from turning the paper blue (false negative result). Such medicines should not be taken two (2) days prior to or during the test period. If your doctor has prescribed any of these medicines for you, check with him/her to see if it is permissible for you to stop taking your drugs for a few days. The use of rectal ointments should also be avoided while taking the test.

● Instructions for Special Diet. **FOR TWO DAYS BEFORE AND THROUGHOUT THE TEST PERIOD, FOLLOW THE SPECIAL DIET GUIDELINES BELOW.**

Do not eat:	Do eat foods such as:
Red or Rare Meat	Poultry
Turnips	Fish
Horseradish	Vegetables
Vitamin C Supplements	Fruit
(over 250 mg daily)	Peanuts
	Popcorn
	Bran Cereal

If you know that any of the above cause you discomfort, or if you are on a special diet or taking prescription medications check with your doctor before performing the test.

Instructions

Follow these with care to insure accurate results. Read all instructions before starting test.

NOTE: DEVELOPER SOLUTION SHOULD HAVE BEEN PREPARED AT LEAST 60 MINUTES PRIOR TO USE. To properly perform the test you will need to sample and test three successive bowel movements. It is important to do this test on all three bowel movements in a row. (If you miss one, continue test until three samples have been tested.) Gastrointestinal problems often bleed off and on. If you test three stool specimens in a row, you will have a better chance of finding hidden blood in the stool. You should do all three tests even if the first and second tests do not show hidden blood.

USE THESE INSTRUCTIONS FOR EACH TEST

STEP 1.

Wash hands thoroughly before using this test. Have a specimen pad and developer solution bottle close to the toilet or sink.

STEP 2.

After a bowel movement, take a specimen pad and **fold the Activity Indicator spots under to keep them free of stool.**

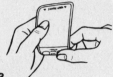

STEP 3.

Gently pat (*do not wipe*) the anal area to get a smear of stool.

STEP 4.

Shake bottle well. Remove the clear plastic overcap from developer solution bottle. Hold bottle upright and specimen pad 1–3 inches away. Press firmly on the bottle top and spray repeatedly to wet the entire stool specimen. Be sure to spray the two Activity Indicator spots on bottom of pad. Five sprays should fully soak the pad.

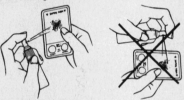

Caution: Do not spray on clothing or furniture.

STEP 5.

READ THE RESULTS IN 30–60 SECONDS. COLOR MAY FADE AFTER 60 SECONDS.

The Activity Indicator spots on the bottom of the specimen pad will show that the test is working. **The spots do not show whether there is blood in the stool.** When you spray the spots, the positive spot will turn blue and the negative spot will not change color.

NOTE: If the positive spot is blue before you spray the pad the specimen pad should not be used. If the spot does not turn blue after you have sprayed it with developer solution, do not continue test. Call toll free number (Page 11) for assistance.

Now look at the area on and around the stool specimen **Any trace of blue color of any shade or intensity is a positive result** (except in the Activity Indicator positive spot). No trace of blue color on or around the stool specimen is a negative result. See color photo for examples of positive/negative test results (Page 12 of booklet). After reading results, flush the specimen pad in the toilet.

NOTE: If you are color blind, have someone help you read the test.

STEP 6.

Record each test result in the space provided in the Record of Early Detector Test Results (last page).

Continued on next page

Warner-Lambert—Cont.

IMPORTANT: If any of the three tests show a trace of blue color, you should consult with your doctor as soon as you can. Discontinue testing and consult with your doctor if your first or second test is positive.

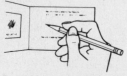

STEP 7. Wash hands thoroughly after using each test.

What do the results mean?

If a blue color (positive reading) is anywhere on the specimen pad (except in the positive circle of the Activity Indicator) this shows that there may be blood in the stool. Be sure to check edges of the smear area. If you see **ANY** blue anywhere on the specimen pad area (except in the positive circle of the Activity Indicator) within 30–60 seconds after you have sprayed the developer solution on the stool sample, the test is positive. This does not always mean that you have a serious medical problem. The blue color may be caused by the food you have eaten or the medicines you are taking or other conditions such as ulcers or hemorrhoids. As with all tests for hidden blood, the results do not give conclusive evidence of any specific disease. Early Detector is a screening tool, a diagnostic aid. It is **not** made to take the place of routine physical examinations or other tests your doctor may wish to perform. If you have a positive result from your test, you should consult with your doctor as soon as you can. Remember **only one** specimen pad of the three tests you have done has to show a blue color for you to consult with your doctor.

If your tests showed no trace of blue color this means that at the time of taking the test there was no detectable blood in the stool. However, this does not mean you are free of disease. Not all gastrointestinal disorders bleed. You may have other symptoms which led you to use this test, such as bowel habit changes (e.g. diarrhea or constipation lasting longer than 2 weeks), unexplained weight loss lasting 2 or more weeks or visually evident blood in the stool (red or black). If so, even if your tests are negative, you should consult with your doctor.

What are the limitations of the test?

As with all tests for hidden blood, results with Early Detector cannot prove the presence or absence of bleeding or illness. Early Detector is not made to replace tests that your doctor may wish to perform.

Tests to find hidden blood are being used and evaluated both in clinical practices and at leading medical centers.

Past results show that:

● In health screening surveys, the positive rate has been about 2% to 5%. Positive means any trace of blue color. However, this does not always mean

that you have a serious medical problem. The blue color may be caused by the food you have eaten or the medicines you are taking.

Tests have shown that consumers can perform this test and read the results as well as a testing laboratory.

FOR ANY INFORMATION OR ASSISTANCE YOU MAY NEED CONCERNING EARLY DETECTOR YOU MAY CALL TOLL FREE 1-800-E.D. HELPS

Shown in Product Identification Section, page 433

Whitehall Laboratories Inc.

**Division of American Home Products Corporation
685 THIRD AVENUE
NEW YORK, NY 10017**

CLEARBLUE EASY™
Pregnancy Test Kit

Clearblue Easy is a rapid, one-step pregnancy test for home use which detects tiny amounts of the pregnancy hormone HCG (Human Chorionic Gonadotropin) in the urine. This hormone is produced in increasing amounts during the first part of pregnancy. Clearblue Easy uses sensitive monoclonal antibodies to detect the presence of the hormone from the first day of a missed period.

Clearblue Easy is the easiest and fastest pregnancy test available because all you have to do is hold the absorbent tip in your urine stream, replace the cap, and in 3 minutes you'll know the test is complete when a blue line appears in the small window. The large window shows the test result. If there is a blue line in the large window, you are pregnant. If there is no line, you are not pregnant. The pregnancy hormone HCG is most concentrated in the first urine specimen of the day, so you must use this urine to conduct the test.

A negative result means that no pregnancy hormone was detected and you are probably not pregnant. If your period does not start within a week, you may have miscalculated the day your period was due. Repeat the test using another Clearblue Easy test. If the second test still gives a negative result and you still have not menstruated, you should see your doctor.

Clearblue Easy is specially designed for easy use at home. However, if you do have questions about the test or results, give the Clearblue Easy TalkLine a call at 1-800-223-2329. A specially trained staff of advisors is available 24 hours a day to answer your questions.

Produced by Unipath Ltd., Bedford, U.K. Unipath, Clearblue Easy and the fan device are trademarks

Distributed by Whitehall Laboratories, New York, NY 10017

Shown in Product Identification Section, page 435

CLEARPLAN™
Ovulation Predictor

CLERAPLAN Ovulation Predictor is an easy-to-use in-home test which employs highly sensitive monoclonal antibody technology to accurately predict the onset of ovulation, and consequently, the best time each month for a woman to try to become pregnant. The test monitors the changing level of Luteinizing Hormone (LH) in a woman's urine. Small amounts of LH are present during most of the menstrual cycle, but the level normally rises sharply up to 36 hours before ovulation (which is when an egg is released from the ovary). CLEARPLAN detects this LH surge which precedes ovulation so that a woman knows 24–36 hours beforehand the time she is most able to become pregnant.

CLEARPLAN is the easiest ovulation predictor to use because of its unique technological design, which consists of only two components— a sampler stick and a base unit. To use CLEARPLAN, a woman simply urinates on the test stick (a woman can use either morning or evening urine) and places it in each of the three wells of the base unit for ten minutes each. The procedure is completed in 30 minutes and results are easily obtained by reading the end of the test stick. An increase in blue color indicates that there is an LH surge and ovulation will occur in the next 24–36 hours, while a white color indicates that little or no LH is present.

A woman will be most fertile during the 2 to 3 days after the first rise in blue color. Sperm can fertilize an egg for many hours after sexual intercourse. So, if sexual intercourse occurs during the 2–3 days after a significant increase in blue color is observed, the chances of getting pregnant are maximized.

Laboratory studies confirm that CLEARPLAN is over 98% accurate as shown by radioimmunoassay (RIA) and ultrasound in predicting ovulation.

CLEARPLAN contains 10 days of tests so that it can predict ovulation in more women. This is because women can have both regular and irregular menstrual cycles, and CLEARPLAN's 10 days of tests will better cover this variation. In fact, CLEARPLAN can detect the LH surge in over 90% of women. If the LH surge occurs before 10 tests are used, the unused tests can be used in future cycles, if needed.

CLEARPLAN offers users the support of a 24-hour TalkLine (1-800-223-2329).

This service is operated by trained advisors who are available to answer any questions about using the test or reading the results.

Produced by Unipath Ltd., Bedford, U.K. Unipath, Clearplan and the fan device are trademarks

Distributed by Whitehall Laboratories, New York, NY 10017

Shown in Product Identification Section, page 435

Certified regional poison control centers

The regional poison control centers in the following list are certified by the American Association of Poison Control Centers. To receive certification, each center must meet certain criteria. It must, for example, serve a large geographic area; it must be open 24 hours a day and provide direct dialing or toll-free access; it must be supervised by a medical director; and it must have registered pharmacists or nurses available to answer questions from the public.

Staff members of these regional centers are trained to resolve toxicity situations in the home of the caller, but, in some instances, hospital referrals are given.

The regional centers have a wide variety of toxicology resources, including a computer capability covering some 350,000 substances that are updated quarterly. They also offer a range of educational services to the public as well as to the health-care professional. In some states, these large centers exist side by side with smaller poison control centers that provide more limited information.

AMERICAN ASSOCIATION OF POISON CONTROL CENTERS

Centers are listed by region, alphabetically.

FAR WEST

Los Angeles County Medical Association Regional Poison Control Center
1925 Wilshire Blvd.
Los Angeles, CA 90057
(213) 664-2121 (Administration)
(213) 484-5151
1-(800) 777-6476 (California only)
1-(800) 825-2722

Medical Director:
Marc Bayer, M.D.
(213) 484-5151

Supervisor:
Corrine Ray, R.N., B.S.
(213) 484-5151

Oregon Poison Center
The Oregon Health Sciences University
3181 SW Sam Jackson Park Road
Portland, OR 97201
(503) 279-7799 (Administration)
(503) 279-8968 (Local)
(800) 452-7165 (OR only)

Medical Director:
Brent T. Burton, M.D.
(503) 279-7799

Associate Director for Poison Control:
Terryll S. Putnam, R.N.
(503) 279-7799

San Diego Regional Poison Center
U.C.S.D. Medical Center
225 Dickinson St.
San Diego, CA 92103-1990
(619) 543-3666 (Administration)
(619) 543-6000

Medical Director:
George M. Shumaik, M.D., F.A.C.E.P.
(619) 543-3666

Director:
Anthony S. Manoguerra, Pharm.D.
(619) 543-3666

San Francisco Bay Area Regional Poison Control Center
San Francisco General Hospital

Room 1E86
1001 Potrero Ave.
San Francisco, CA 94110
(415) 821-8324 (Administration)
(415) 476-6600
(800) 523-2222 (Bay area only)

Medical Director:
Charles Becker, M.D.
(415) 821-5200

Toxic Information Center
(415) 821-5338
(800) 233-3360

Medical Director:
Kent R. Olson, M.D.
(415) 821-8324

Regional Poison Center
UC Davis Medical Center
2315 Stockton Blvd.
Sacramento, CA 95817
(916) 453-3414 (Administration)
(916) 453-3692
(800) 342-9293 (northern California)

Medical Director:
Timothy Albertson, M.D., Ph.D.
Coordinator:
Judith Alsop, Pharm.D.

GREAT LAKES

Blodgett Regional Poison Center
1840 Wealthy, S.E.
Grand Rapids, MI 49506
(616) 774-7854 (Administration)
(800) 632-2727
Medical Director:
John R. Maurer, M.D.
(616) 774-7854
Director:
Daniel J. McCoy, Ph.D.
(616) 774-7854
Associate Director:
John H. Trestrail III, R.Ph.

Central Ohio Poison Center
Columbus Children's Hospital
700 Children's Dr.
Columbus, OH 43205
(614) 461-2012 (Administration)
(614) 228-1323
(800) 682-7625
Medical Director:
Mary Mortensen, M.D.
Administrative Director:
Judith G. D'Orsi
(614) 461-2717

Children's Hospital of Alabama Poison Control Center
1600 7th Avenue South
Birmingham, AL 35233
(205) 933-4050
(800) 292-6678
Medical Director:
Edward Kohaut, M.D.
(205) 933-4050
Director:
William King, Ph.D
(205) 933-4050

Kentucky Regional Poison Center of Kosair Children's Hospital
P.O. Box 35070
Louisville, KY 40232-5070
(502) 562-7264 (Administration)
(502) 589-8222
(800) 722-5725 (KY only)
Medical Director:
George C. Rodgers Jr., M.D., Ph.D.
(502) 562-8837
Director:
Nancy J. Matyunas, Pharm.D.
(502) 562-7264

NEW ENGLAND
Massachusetts Poison Control System
300 Longwood Ave.
Boston, MA 02115
(617) 735-6609 (Administration)
(617) 232-2120, (800) 682-9211
Medical Director:
Allen Woolf, M.D.. M.Ph
Assistant Director:
Patricia Grbcich, Pharm.D., J.D.

Rhode Island Poison Center
Rhode Island Hospital
593 Eddy St.
Providence, RI 02902
(401) 277-5906 (Administration)
(401) 277-5727
(401) 277-8062 (TTD)
Medical Director:
William J. Lewander, M.D.
(401) 277-5906
Associate Director:
Philip N. Johnson, Ph.D.
(401) 277-5906

ROCKY MOUNTAINS
Arizona Poison Control System
Arizona Health Sciences Center,
Room 3204K, University of Arizona
Tucson, AZ 85724
(602) 626-7899 (Administration)
(602) 626-6016 (Tucson)
(602) 253-3334 (Phoenix)
(800) 362-0101 (AZ only)
Medical Directors:
John Sullivan, M.D.
(602) 626-7899
Donald Kunkel, M.D., J.D.
(602) 239-6690
Director:
Theodore G. Tong, Pharm.D.
(Tucson)
(602) 626-7899
Joyce M. Bradley, R.N., M.S.
(Phoenix)
(602) 253-0813

Component Centers:
Arizona Poison and Drug Information Center
Arizona Health Sciences Center
Rm. 3204K
University of Arizona
Tucson, AZ 85724

Samaritan Regional Poison Center
Good Samaritan Medical Center
1111 E. McDowell
Phoenix, AZ 85062

Intermountain Regional Poison Control Center
50 N. Medical Dr., Building 528
Salt Lake City, UT 84132
(801) 581-7504 (Administration)
(801) 581-2151
(800) 456-7707 (UT only)
Medical Director:
Douglas Rollins, M.D., Ph.D.
(801) 581-5117
Director:
Joseph C. Veltri, Pharm.D.
(801) 581-7504

New Mexico Poison and Drug Information Center
University of New Mexico Room 125
Albuquerque, NM 87131
(505) 277-4261 (Administration)
(505) 843-2551
(800) 432-6866 (NM only)
Medical Director:
Dan Tandberg, M.D.
(505) 277-5062
Director:
William G. Troutman, Pharm.D.
(505) 277-4261

Rocky Mountain Poison Center
645 Bannock St.
Denver, CO 80204-4507
(303) 893-7774 (Administration)
(303) 629-1123
(800) 332-3073 (CO only)
(800) 525-5042 (MT only)
(800) 442-2702 (WY only)
Medical Director:
Barry H. Rumack, M.D.
(303) 893-7774
Associate Director:
Kathleen M. Wruk, R.N., B.S.N.
(303) 893-7774

SOUTH ATLANTIC

Duke University Poison Control Center
Box 3007
Duke University Medical Center
Durham, NC 27710
(919) 684-4438 (Administration)
(919) 684-8111
(800) 672-1697 (NC only)
Medical Director:
Shirley K. Osterhout, M.D.
(919) 684-4438
Director for Administration:
Christine Rudd, Pharm.D.

Triad Poison Center
Cove Memorial Hospital
1300 N. Elm St.
Greensboro, N.C. 27401-1020
(919) 379-4105
Medical Director
John Lelonde, M.D.
Director
David Wheeler
(919) 379-4105

Georgia Poison Control Center
Box 26066
80 Butler St., S.E.
Atlanta, GA 30335
(404) 589-4400
(800) 282-5846
(404) 525-3323 (TTY)
Medical Director:
Robert Geller, M.D.
(404) 589-3545
Managing Director:
Gaylord Lopez, Pharm D.
(404) 827-7043

Maryland Poison Center
20 N. Pine St.
Baltimore, MD 21201
(301) 328-7604 (Administration)
(301) 528-7701
(800) 492-2414 (MD only)
Medical Director:
Richard L. Gorman, M.D.
(301) 328-7604
Director:
Gary M. Oderda, Pharm.D., M.P.H.
(301) 328-7604

National Capital Poison Center
Georgetown University Hospital
3800 Reservoir Rd., N.W.
Washington, DC 20007
(202) 784-2087 (Administration)
(202) 625-3333
Medical Director/Director:
Toby L. Litovitz, M.D.
(202) 784-2088

Florida Poison Information Center
at the Tampa General Hospital
P.O. Box 1289
Tampa, FL 33601
(813) 251-7044 (Administration)
(813) 253-4444, (800) 282-3171
Medical Director:
James V. Hillman, M.D.
(813) 251-6911
Director:
Sven Normann, Pharm.D.
(813) 251-7044

Indiana Poison Center
Methodist Hospital of Indiana
1701 N. Senate Blvd. P.O. Box
1367
Indianapolis, IN 46206
(317) 929-2331 (Administration)
(317) 929-2323
(800) 382-9097
(317) 924-6411

Medical Director:
Brent Furbee, M.D.
(317) 924-8035

Director:
James B. Mowry, Pharm.D.
(317) 924-2329

Poison Control Center
Children's Hospital of Michigan
3901 Beaubien Blvd.
Detroit, MI 48201
(313) 745-5329 (Administration)
(313) 745-5711
(800) 462-6642 (Michigan)

Medical Director:
Regine Aronow, M.D.
(313) 745-5335

Administrative Affairs:
Richard E. Dorsch Jr., M.D.

**Regional Poison Control Center
and Cincinnati Drug and Poison
Information Center**
231 Bethesda Ave., M.L. #144
Cincinnati, OH 45267-0144
(513) 558-5111
(800) 872-5111

Medical Director:
Clifford G. Grulee Jr., M.D.

Director:
Leonard T. Sigell, Ph.D.
(513) 558-9182

GREAT PLAINS
**Cardinal Glennon Children's
Hospital Regional Poison Center**

1465 S. Grand Blvd.
St. Louis, MO 63104
(314) 772-8300 (Administration)
(314) 772-5200
(800) 392-9111 (MO only)
(800) 366-8888 (U.S.)

Medical Director:
Anthony J. Scalzo, M.D.
(314) 772-8300

Managing Director:
Michael W. Thompson, B.S. Pharm
(314) 772-8300

Program Director:
Robert W. Jaeger, B.S. Pharm.
314) 772-8300

**Hennepin Regional Poison
Center**
Hennepin County Medical Center
701 Park Ave.
Minneapolis, MN 55415
(612) 347-3144 (Administration)
(612) 347-3141
(612) 347-6219 (TTY)
Medical Director:
Louis Ling, M.D.
(612) 347-3174
Supervisor:
Michael J. Wieland, R.Ph.
(612) 347-3144

Mid-Plains Poison Center
8301 Dodge St.
Omaha, NE 68114
(402) 390-5434 (Administration)
(402) 390-5400
(800) 642-9999 (NE only)
(800) 228-9515 (surrounding
states)
Medical Director:
David Tolo, M.D.
Director: James O'Donnell, R.Ph.
Manager: Jeff Benson, R.Ph.

**Minnesota Regional Poison
Center**
St. Paul-Ramsey Medical Center
640 Jackson St.
St. Paul, MN 55101
(612) 221-3096 (Administration)
(612) 221-2113
(800) 222-1222

Medical Director:
Samuel Hall Jr., M.D.
(612) 221-3470
Managing Director:
Leo Sioris, Pharm.D.
(612) 221-3192

MIDDLE ATLANTIC

**Long Island Regional Poison
Control Center**
Nassau County Medical Center
2201 Hempstead Tpk.
East Meadow, NY 11554
(516) 542-3707 (Administration)
(516) 542-2323
Medical Director:
Howard C. Mofenson, M.D.
(516) 542-3707
Clinical Coordinator:
Thomas R. Caraccio, Pharm.D.
(516) 542-3707

**Hudson Valley Poison Control
Center**
Nyack Hospital, N. Midland Ave.,
Nyack, N.Y. 10960
(914) 353-1000
Medical Director:
Stanley H. Oransky
Director:
Patricia Urello, M.S., M.P.
(914) 353-1000

**New Jersey Poison Information
and Education System**
201 Lyons Ave.
Newark, NJ 07112
(201) 926-7443 (Administration)
(800) 962-1253 (NJ only)

Medical Director:
Steven M. Marcus, M.D.
(201) 926-7443

**New York City Poison Control
Center**
455 First Ave., Room 123
New York, NY 10016
(212) 340-4497 (Administration)
(212) 340-4494
(212) POISONS

Medical Director:
Lewis Goldfrank, M.D.
(212) 561-3346

Director:
Richard Weisman, Pharm.D.
(212) 340-4494

Pittsburgh Poison Center
One Children's Place
3705 Fifth Ave. at DeSoto St.
Pittsburgh, PA 15213
(412) 647-5600 (Administration)
(412) 681-6669

Medical Director:
Robert McDonald, M.D.
(412) 624-2591

Director:
Edward P. Krenzelok, Pharm.D.
(412) 647-5600

**Delaware Valley Regional Poison
Control Program**
One Children's Center
Philadelphia, PA, 19104
(215) 386-2066 (Administration)
(215) 386-2100

Medical Director:
Dr. Fred Henretig, M.D.
(215) 386-2066

Director:
Thomas Kearney, Pharm D.
(215) 386-2066

MID-SOUTH

Alabama Poison Center
809 University Blvd. E.
Tuscaloosa, AL 35401
(205) 345-0600 (Administration)

(800) 462-0800 (AL only)

Medical Director:
Perry Lovely, M.D.
Co-Medical Directors:
Phillip K. Bobo, M.D.
John G. Fisher III, Pharm.D.
(205) 345-0600

Nursing Director:
Lois Dorough, R.N.
Executive Director:
Richard Looser

West Virginia Poison Center
West Virginia University
School of Pharmacy
3110 MacCorkle Ave., S.E.
Charleston, WV 25304
(304) 347-1212 (Administration)
(304) 348-4211
(800) 642-3625 (WV only)

Medical Director:
David E. Seidler, M.D.
(304) 347-1212
Director:
Gregory P. Wedin, Pharm.D.
(304) 347-1212

SOUTH

North Texas Poison Center
P.O. Box 35926
Dallas, TX 75235
(214) 590-5000 (Administration)
(800) 441-0040 (TX only)

Medical Director:
Gary Reed, M.D.
(214) 590-5000
Head Nurse:
Teri Gale, R.N.
(214) 590-5000

Texas State Poison Center
University of Texas Medical Branch
Galveston, TX 77550-2780
(409) 761-3332 (Administration)
(409) 765-1420
(713) 654-1701 (Houston)
(516) 478-4490 (Austin)
(800) 392-8548 (TX only)

Medical Director:
Wayne R. Snodgrass, M.D., Ph.D.
(409) 761-1677
Director:
Michael Ellis, M.S.
(409) 761-3332